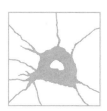

Encyclopedia of the

Neurological
Sciences

M–Ph
VOLUME 3

Associate Editors

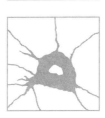

Encyclopedia of the
Neurological
Sciences

Editors

Michael J. Aminoff
School of Medicine, University of California
San Francisco, California

Robert B. Daroff
University Hospitals of Cleveland
Cleveland, Ohio

M–Ph

VOLUME 3

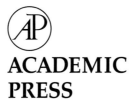

ACADEMIC
PRESS
An imprint of Elsevier Science

Amsterdam Boston Heidelberg London New York Oxford Paris San Diego San Francisco Singapore Sydney Tokyo

Academic Press
An imprint of Elsevier Inc.
525 B Street, Suite 1900, San Diego, California 92101-4495, USA
http://www.academicpress.com

Elsevier Science Ltd.
The Boulevard, Langford Lane, Kidlington, Oxford OX5 1GB, UK
http://www.elsevier.com

Library of Congress Catalog Card Number: 2003104629

International Standard Book Number: 0-12-226870-9 (set)
International Standard Book Number: 0-12-226871-7 (Volume 1)
International Standard Book Number: 0-12-226872-5 (Volume 2)
International Standard Book Number: 0-12-226873-3 (Volume 3)
International Standard Book Number: 0-12-226874-1 (Volume 4)

Printed in the United States of America
03   04   05   06   08   MM   9   8   7   6   5   4   3   2   1

Subject Areas

AUTONOMIC NERVOUS SYSTEM
Sudhansu Chokroverty, Editor

BACTERIAL AND FUNGAL INFECTIONS
Karen L. Roos, Editor

CLINICAL NEUROPHYSIOLOGY
Sudhansu Chokroverty, Editor

EPILEPSY
Jerome Engel, Jr., Editor

HISTORY (BIOGRAPHIES)
Kenneth L. Tyler, Editor

IMPAIRED CONSCIOUSNESS
G. Bryan Young, Editor

INTENSIVE CARE UNIT
Daryl Gress, Editor

METABOLIC DISEASES
Bruce O. Berg, Editor

MOVEMENT DISORDERS
Christopher G. Goetz, Editor

NEUROANATOMY AND CLINICAL LOCALIZATION
Joseph C. Masdeu, Editor

NEUROBIOLOGY AND PHYSIO-LOGICAL BASIS OF SYMPTOMS
Michael J. Aminoff and Robert B. Daroff, Editors

NEUROENDOCRINOLOGY
James L. Roberts, Editor

NEUROEPIDEMIOLOGY
John F. Kurtzke, Editor

NEUROGENETICS
Stefan M. Pulst, Editor

NEUROIMMUNOLOGY
Richard Ransohoff, Editor

NEUROMUSCULAR DISORDERS
Hiroshi Mitsumoto, Editor

NEUROONCOLOGY
Lisa M. DeAngelis, Editor

NEUROOPHTHALMOLOGY AND NEUROTOLOGY
Mark J. Morrow, Editor

NEUROPATHOLOGY
Michael J. Aminoff and Robert B. Daroff, Editors

NEUROPHARMACOLOGY
David A. Greenberg, Editor

NEUROPSYCHOLOGY AND BEHAVIORAL NEUROLOGY
Bruce L. Miller, Editor

NEURORADIOLOGY AND IMAGING
William J. Powers and Colin P. Derdeyn, Editors

NEUROSURGERY
Robert F. Spetzler, Editor

NEUROTOXICOLOGY
Christopher G. Goetz, Editor

NEUROVIROLOGY AND PRION DISEASES
Kenneth L. Tyler, Editor

PAIN
Nathaniel Katz, Editor

PARASITIC INFECTIONS
Marylou V. Solbrig, Editor

PEDIATRIC AND DEVELOPMENTAL NEUROLOGY
Bruce O. Berg, Editor

PERIPHERAL NEUROLOGY
Hiroshi Mitsumoto, Editor

PSYCHIATRY AND PSYCHOPHARMACOLOGY
Lowell Tong, Editor

SLEEP AND SLEEP DISORDERS
Sudhansu Chokroverty, Editor

STROKE, ISCHEMIA, AND HEADACHE
K. Michael Welch, Editor

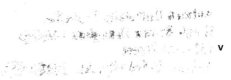

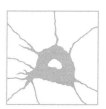

Preface

DURING the past 25 years, remarkable advances have occurred in the clinical sciences of neurology, neurosurgery, and psychiatry, as well as the many different branches of the clinical and basic neurosciences that impact on these fields. Because of the pace of these advances, those not engaged in a particular discipline have difficulty keeping abreast with the field, and those who are not involved in the neurosciences are faced with a daunting task when attempting to seek information on a particular topic. These difficulties created the need that prompted us to develop this four-volume *Encyclopedia of the Neurological Sciences*.

The encyclopedia is an alphabetically organized compendium of more than 1,000 entries that relate to different aspects of the neurosciences. It is comprehensive in scope, with entries related to clinical neurology, neurosurgery, neuroanatomy, neurobiology, neuroepidemiology, neuroendocrinology, neurogenetics, neuroimaging, neurotoxicology, neuroimmunology, neuropharmacology, pediatric neurology, neurooncology, neuropathology, developmental neurology, behavioral neurology, neurophysiology, applied electrophysiology, neuroophthalmology, neurotology, pain, psychiatry, psychopharmacology, rehabilitation, critical care medicine, and the history of the neurosciences. We designed most entries to be understandable without

detailed background knowledge in the subject matter. The entries are not intended for those working directly in the field under consideration, but rather for individuals from other disciplines who wish to gain an understanding of the subjects. Students and the lay public should benefit most from entries providing general overviews of particular topics, and might skip the more technical entries. Cross references assist the reader to follow a theme from a simple to a more advanced level, and from a general to a focused outlook, or the reverse.

The entries are intended to provide relatively succinct accounts. We have not included exhaustive referencing but, rather, have placed suggestions for further reading at the end of each entry. There is some inevitable overlap between entries and, in some instances, the same topic is discussed in several. This overlap was deliberate, as we intended to provide coherent accounts of topics without forcing the reader to go from one entry to another, as if traversing an obstacle course, to obtain the desired information. In some instances, particularly with areas of controversy, we included two entries on the same topic, reflecting conflicting viewpoints, and hope that this will stimulate readers to pursue the topic further.

We are indebted to the many people who helped in the creation of this encyclopedia. The associate editors (listed on page ii) guided the selection of contributors and reviewed the individual entries in their subject area. The contributors, all acknowledged experts in their fields, prepared the entries. We reviewed all of these entries, making suggestions for improvement in content, style, and clarity, and are grateful to the contributors and associate editors for working with us in achieving the final product that we intended. Dr. Graham Lees conceived this project while he was at Academic Press, and his joyous encouragement and support allowed the concept to evolve. Thereafter, Dr. Jasna Markovac assumed oversight at Academic Press (now part of Elsevier Science), providing excellent advice and unfailing assistance at all stages of the endeavor. Karen Dempsey of Academic Press displayed great patience, good humor, and efficiency in bringing the encyclopedia to fruition. She attended painstakingly to a seemingly endless number of administrative details, and coordinated all communications between us, the contributors, associate editors, and publisher. She not only ensured that necessary deadlines were met, but did so with grace and charm. The production of this encyclopedia involved many other people at Academic Press, including Christopher Morris, with his particular expertise in the production of major reference works. Our secretaries provided invaluable assistance. In San Francisco, the arrival electronically of each new batch of entries brought the office staff a certain respite as MJA disappeared behind his computer screen. In Cleveland, the computer literacy of Vicki Fields, RBD's secretary, compensated for his Luddite predisposition. Finally, we must record our indebtedness to our wives and families, whose patience, forbearance, and support enabled us to complete this undertaking.

Michael J. Aminoff
San Francisco, California

Robert B. Daroff
Cleveland, Ohio

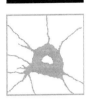

Contributors

GARY M. ABRAMS
University of California, San Francisco

LAUREN E. ABREY
Memorial Sloan-Kettering Cancer Center

JOHN ADAIR
University of New Mexico School of Medicine

BASSAM MOHAMED J. ADDAS
Dalhousie University, Halifax, Nova Scotia

LAMIA AFIFI
Stanford University

BERNARD W. AGRANOFF
University of Michigan

TABASSUM AHMED
University of Pennsylvania School of Medicine

FELIPE ALBUQUERQUE
Barrow Neurological Institute

RICHARD P. ALLEN
Johns Hopkins University

ANTHONY AMATO
Brigham and Women's Hospital, Harvard Medical School

CHRISTOPHER AMES
Barrow Neurosurgical Associates

JONATHAN C. AMINOFF
University of California, Berkeley

MICHAEL J. AMINOFF
University of California, San Francisco

AMIT ANAND
Indiana University School of Medicine

JAMBUR ANANTH
University of California, Los Angeles

SONIA ANCOLI-ISRAEL
Veterans Affairs Healthcare System, San Diego

V. ELVING ANDERSON
University of Minnesota

JOHN C. ANDREFSKY
Wadsworth-Rittman Hospital, Wadsworth, Ohio

CARL F. ANSEVIN
Northeastern Ohio Universities College of Medicine

PATRICIA A. AREÁN
University of California, San Francisco

RONALD L. ARIAGNO
Stanford University

KARA L. ARVIN
Washington University, St. Louis School of Medicine

STEPHEN ASHWAL
Loma Linda University School of Medicine

GENEVIÈVE AUBERT
Université Catholique de Louvain

RICHARD J. AUCHUS
University of Texas Southwestern Medical Center, Dallas

GIULIANO AVANZINI
Instituto Neurologico Nazionale "C. Besta," Milan

ISSAM A. AWAD
Yale University School of Medicine

FELICIA B. AXELROD
New York University Medical Center

MISHA-MIROSLAV BACKONJA
University of Wisconsin Medical School

ALISON E. BAIRD
National Institutes of Health

J. KEVIN BAIRD
U.S. Naval Medical Research Unit, Jakarta, Indonesia

JESSE BALLENGER
Case Western Reserve University

ROBERT W. BALOH
University of California, Los Angeles

PETER BANYS
Veterans Affairs Medical Center, San Francisco

RICHARD J. BAROHN
University of Kansas Medical Center

MICHELE BARRY
Yale University School of Medicine

JUAN BARTOLOMEI
Yale University School of Medicine

JASON J. BARTON
Beth Israel Deaconess Medical Center

JONATHAN J. BASKIN
Neurosurgery Group of Chatham, New Jersey

NANCY BASS
Rainbow Babies and Children's Hospital, Cleveland

H. HUNT BATJER
Northwestern University Medical School

RANJAN BATRA
University of Mississippi Medical Center

STEPHEN BEALS
Southwest Craniofacial Center, Phoenix

KIRSTEN BECHTEL
Yale University School of Medicine

ANTHONY BÉHIN
Groupe Hospitalier Pitié-Salpêtrière

JERRY M. BELSH
University of Medicine and Dentistry of New Jersey

EDUARDO E. BENARROCH
Mayo Clinic

BERNARD R. BENDOK
Northwestern University Medical School

SUSAN BENLOUCIF
Northwestern University Medical School

JEFFREY L. BENNETT
University of Colorado Health Sciences Center

M. BENOIT
Hospital Pasteur, Nice

MARINA BENTIVOGLIO
University of Verona

ETTY BENVENISTE
University of Alabama, Birmingham

BRUCE O. BERG
University of California, San Francisco

JOSEPH R. BERGER
University of Kentucky

MITCHEL S. BERGER
University of California, San Francisco

MEETA BHATT
St. Vincent's Catholic Medical Center, New York

ANITA BHATTACHARYYA
University of Wisconsin

ITALO BIAGGIONI
Vanderbilt University Medical Center

MATT T. BIANCHI
University of Michigan

PAOLO BIGLIOLI
University of Milan

PIERRE LOUIS ALFRED BILL
Wentworth Hospital, Durban, South Africa

JOSE BILLER
Indiana University

VALÉRIE BIOUSSE
Emory University School of Medicine

SHAWN J. BIRD
University of Pennsylvania Hospital

THOMAS D. BIRD
Veterans Affairs Medical Center, Seattle

PETER M. BLACK
Children's Hospital, Boston

MICHAEL BLAW
University of Texas Southwestern Medical Center

BRUNO BLONDEL
Institut Pasteur, Paris

SERGIU C. BLUMEN
Hillel Yaffe Medical Center, Hadera, Israel

JOHN B. BODENSTEINER
Barrow Neurological Institute

NICHOLAS BOGDUK
University of Newcastle, Royal Newcastle Hospital

THOMAS W. BOHR
Loma Linda University School of Medicine

DIANE B. BOIVIN
Douglas Hospital, Verdun, Quebec

MICHEL BONDUELLE
Université de Paris VI

ANU BONGU
Northwestern University Medical School

EDUARDO BONILLA
Columbia University College of Physicians and Surgeons

DAVID BONOVICH
University of California, San Francisco

ISTVAN BONYHAY
Beth Israel Deaconess Hospital

JOHN BOOSS
Department of Veterans Affairs, West Haven, Connecticut

PERSEPHONE BORROW
Edward Jenner Institute for Vaccine Research, Compton, Berkshire, UK

DAVID BORSOOK
Massachusetts General Hospital

BERNARD BOUTEILLE
University of Limoges, France

ADAM BOXER
University of California, San Francisco

RAYMOND BRADLEY
Veterinary Laboratories Agency, Addlestone, UK

JAN LEWIS BRANDES
Vanderbilt University Medical Center

THOMAS BRANDT
Neurologische Klinik, Universität München

PAUL W. BRAZIS
Mayo Clinic

CATHERINE S. BRENNAN
University of California, Davis

HANNAH R. BRIEMBERG
Brigham and Women's Hospital, Harvard Medical School

THOMAS BRIESE
University of California, Irvine

GAVIN W. BRITZ
Harborview Medical Center, University of Washington

LOUANN BRIZENDINE
University of California, San Francisco

PER BRODAL
University of Oslo

MARK B. BROMBERG
University of Utah School of Medicine

STEVEN M. BROMLEY
Neurological Institute of New York

KENNETH H. BROOKLER
Neurotologic Associates, New York

STEPHEN N. BROOKS
Stanford University

PAUL W. BROWN
National Institute of Neurological Disorders and Stroke

STEPHEN P. BRUEHL
Vanderbilt University Pain Control Center

ALAIN F. BRUNET
McGill University and Douglas Hospital Research Centre

J. EDWARD BRUNI
University of Manitoba

RICHARD C. BURGESS
Cleveland Clinic Foundation

ROBERT E. BURKE
National Institute of Neurological Disorders and Stroke

JORGE G. BURNEO
University of Alabama

DANIEL J. BUYSSE
University of Pittsburgh School of Medicine

DAVID B. BYLUND
University of Nebraska Medical Center

LEONARD H. CALABRESE
Cleveland Clinic Foundation

CAROL CAMFIELD
IWK Grace Health Center, Halifax, Nova Scotia

PETER CAMFIELD
IWK Grace Health Center, Halifax, Nova Scotia

MICHAEL CAMILLERI
Mayo Clinic and Mayo Foundation

IAIN L. CAMPBELL
Scripps Research Institute

ALDO CANNATA
University of Milan

STEPHEN CALDWELL CANNON
University of Texas Southwestern Medical Center, Dallas

LOUIS R. CAPLAN
Beth Israel Deaconess Medical Center

THOMAS J. CARLOW
University of New Mexico Health Science Center

PETER CARMEL
New Jersey Medical School

STIRLING CARPENTER
University of Porto, Portugal

FRANCISCO JAVIER CARRILLO-PADILLA
Universidad de La Laguna, Tenerife, Canary Islands

ROSALIND D. CARTWRIGHT
Rush-Presbyterian-St. Luke's Medical Center

SUSAN CASTRO-OBREGÓN
Buck Institute for Age Research, Novato, California

GASTONE G. CELESIA
Loyola University, Stritch School of Medicine, Maywood, Illinois

FERNANDO CERVERO
McGill University

DAVID A. CHAD
University of Massachusetts

DAVID CHADWICK
Walton Centre for Neurology and Neurosurgery, Liverpool

R. ANDREW CHAMBERS
Yale University School of Medicine

CHIH-JU CHANG
Cathay General Hospital, Taipei, Taiwan

DAE-IL CHANG
Kyung Hee University, Seoul

SANDRA BOND CHAPMAN
University of Texas

FADY T. CHARBEL
University of Illinois

ZAHID F. CHEEMA
University of Oklahoma Health Sciences Center

THOMAS C. CHELIMSKY
Case Western Reserve University School of Medicine

MING CHENG
Barrow Neurological Institute

MICHAEL CHERINGTON
St. Anthony Hospital, Denver

NATHAN I. CHERNY
Shaare Zedek Medical Center, Jerusalem

BARBARA JEAN CHERRY
University of Southern California

DAVID A. CHESNUTT
Duke University Eye Center

ANDREW L. CHESSON
Louisiana State University Medical Center

VERONICA CHIANG-MOY
Yale University School of Medicine

WINSTON CHIONG
University of California, San Francisco

HYUNMI CHOI
Columbia-Presbyterian Medical Center

CHADWICK W. CHRISTINE
University of California, San Francisco

OK YUNG CHUNG
Vanderbilt University Medical Center

KENNETH J. CIUFFREDA
State University of New York/State College of Optometry

DAVID B. CLARKE
Dalhousie University

RICHARD E. CLATTERBUCK
Barrow Neurological Institute

MAIRAV COHEN-ZION
San Diego State University

BRADLEY A. COLE
Beaver Medical Group, Highland, California

MONROE COLE
University Hospitals of Cleveland

JAMES F. COLLAWN
University of Alabama

JAMES E. CONWAY
Johns Hopkins Hospital

MICHAEL C. CORBALLIS
University of Auckland

JAMES J. CORBETT
University of Mississippi Medical Center

JOHN R. CORBOY
University of Colorado Health Sciences Center

JODY COREY-BLOOM
University of California, San Diego

H. BRANCH COSLETT
University of Pennsylvania School of Medicine

JAMES R. COUCH
University of Oklahoma College of Medicine

THERESE COUDERC
Institut Pasteur, Paris

DAVID L. COULTER
Harvard Medical School

PAUL DAMIAN COX
University of California, Davis

TERRY A. COX
National Eye Institute

ELIZABETH C. CRABTREE
Tulane University

BRUCE A. CREE
University of California, San Francisco

DIDIER CROS
Massachusetts General Hospital

DEWITTE T. CROSS
Washington University School of Medicine, St. Louis

ESTHER CUBO
Hospital de la Zarzuela, Madrid

ANTONIO CULEBRAS
Veterans Affairs Medical Center, Syracuse

JEFFREY L. CUMMINGS
University of California, Los Angeles

VALERIE A. CWIK
Arizona Health Science Center, Tucson

MARINOS DALAKAS
National Institute of Neurological Disorders and Stroke

JOSEP O. DALMAU
University of Arkansas for Medical Sciences

FERNANDO DANGOND
Brigham and Women's Hospital, Harvard Institutes of Medicine

DEAN DANNER
Emory University

ROBERT B. DAROFF
University Hospitals of Cleveland

ROBERT B. DAROFF, JR.
San Francisco Veteran's Adminstration Medical Center

KAUSHIK DAS
St. Vincent's Hospital and Medical Center, New York

WILLIAM DAVID
Hennepin County Medical Center, Minneapolis

ROBERT A. DAVIDOFF
University of Miami School of Medicine

LARRY DAVIDSON
Yale University School of Medicine

LARRY E. DAVIS
Albuquerque Veterans Affairs Hospital

TED M. DAWSON
Johns Hopkins University School of Medicine

VALINA L. DAWSON
Johns Hopkins University School of Medicine

HANNEKE DE BOER
International Bureau for Epilepsy, Heemstede, The Netherlands

LAURA DE GREGORIO
University of California, San Diego

JACQUES L. DE REUCK
University of Ghent

RONALD K. DE VENECIA
Massachusetts Eye and Ear Infirmary

LISA M. DEANGELIS
Memorial Sloan-Kettering Cancer Center

GREGORY DEL ZOPPO
Scripps Research Institute

GAYLE M. V. DELANEY
Association for the Study of Dreams

JEAN-YVES DELATTRE
Groupe Hospitalier Pitié-Salpêtrière

LOUIS F. DELL'OSSO
Veterans Affairs Medical Center, Cleveland

COLIN P. DERDEYN
Washington University School of Medicine, St. Louis

ROLF DERMIETZEL
University of Bochum, Germany

VIVEK DESHMUKH
Barrow Neurological Institute

PAUL W. DETWILER
Tyler Neurosurgical Associates, Tyler, Texas

MICHELLE DEVERELL
University of California, San Francisco

L. DANA DeWITT
Newton-Wellesley Hospital

UPINDER K. DHAND
University of Missouri Health Sciences Center

SUHAYL DHIB-JALBUT
University of Maryland School of Medicine

ANDRÉ DIEDRICH
Vanderbilt University

SALVATORE DiMAURO
Columbia University

ROBERT L. DODD
Stanford University

MICHAEL DONAGHY
Radcliffe Infirmary, University of Oxford

RICHARD L. DOTY
University of Pennsylvania Hospital

JACK DRESCHER
New York, New York

ANTOINE DRIZENKO
Hôpital Roger Salengro, Lille, France

NINA F. DRONKERS
Veterans Affairs Northern California Health Care System

DEEPAK CYRIL D'SOUZA
West Haven Veterans Affairs Medical Center

GEORGE H. DU BOULAY
National Hospital, London

GARY DUCKWILER
University of California, Los Angeles

JOHN DUDA
University of Pennsylvania

MICHEL DUMAS
University of Limoges, France

ROBERT H. DWORKIN
University of Rochester School of Medicine and Dentistry

PAUL R. DYKEN
Mobile, Alabama

NANCY PIPPEN ECKERMAN
Indiana University School of Medicine

ERIC EGGENBERGER
Michigan State University Clinical Center

DAVID EIDELBERG
North Shore University Hospital, Manhasset, New York

ANDREW A. EISEN
Vancouver General Hospital

STUART J. EISENDRATH
University of California, San Francisco

WENDY ELDER
Barrow Neurological Institute

ANDREW G. ENGEL
Mayo Clinic

JEROME ENGEL
University of California, Los Angeles

GREGORY M. ENNS
Stanford University

ERIK R. ENSRUD
Brigham and Women's Hospital, Harvard Medical School

FRED J. EPSTEIN
Beth Israel Medical Center, New York

ROBERT J. ERNST
University of Cincinnati

OWEN B. EVANS
University of Mississippi Medical Center

CRAIG EVINGER
State University of New York, Stony Brook

JIN FAN
Weill Medical College of Cornell University

MARTHA J. FARAH
University of Pennsylvania

MICHEL FARDEAU
Institut de Myologie, Paris

MARTIN R. FARLOW
Indiana University School of Medicine

JOHN T. FARRAR
University of Pennsylvania

WILLIAM O. FAUSTMAN
Palo Alto Veterans Affairs Health Care System

ROBERT D. FEALEY
Mayo Clinic

ADRIANA FEDER
Columbia-Presbyterian Medical Center

TODD E. FEINBERG
Beth Israel Medical Center, New York

WILLIAM H. FEINDEL
Montreal Neurological Institute

H. K. P. FEIRABEND
University of Leiden

IMAN FEIZ-ERFAN
Barrow Neurological Institute

NATALIO FEJERMAN
Hospital de Pediatria, Buenos Aires

JOSEPH D. FENSTERMACHER
Henry Ford Hospital, Detroit

DONNA M. FERRIERO
University of California, San Francisco

ROBERT D. FIELD
Parkinsons Institute, Sunnyvale, California

R. DOUGLAS FIELDS
National Institute of Child Health and Human Development

TERRY D. FIFE
Barrow Neurological Institute

OMAR FIGUEROA
George Washington University School of Medicine

CHRISTOPHER MARK FILLEY
University of Colorado Health Sciences Center

EDWARD J. FINE
State University of New York, Buffalo

STANLEY FINGER
Washington University, St. Louis

JOHN K. FINK
University of Michigan

MORRIS A. FISHER
Hines Veteran's Affairs Hospital, Chicago

EDMOND J. FITZGIBBON
National Eye Institute

ANNE FLEMING
University of California, San Francisco

LOMA K. FLOWERS
University of California, San Francisco

ROD FOROOZAN
Willis Eye Hospital, Philadelphia

FRANCIS M. FORSTER
Cincinnati, Ohio

ANNE L. FOUNDAS
Tulane University School of Medicine

GLENN W. FOWLER
University of California, Irvine

MARK STEVEN FREEDMAN
University of Ottawa

MARSHALL FREEMAN
Columbia University College of Physicians and Surgeons

ROY FREEMAN
Beth Israel Deaconess Hospital

J. K. FRENKEL
Santa Fe, New Mexico

ROBERT P. FRIEDLAND
Case Western Reserve University School of Medicine

NEIL FRIEDMAN
Cleveland Clinic Foundation

GEORG FRIES
Klinikum Johannes-Gutenberg, Mainz, Germany

JOSEPH M. FURMAN
University of Pittsburgh School of Medicine

PIERLUIGI GAMBETTI
Case Western Reserve University

PAUL D. GAMLIN
University of Alabama

ROSALIE GEARHART
University of California, San Francisco

PHILIP R. GEHRMAN
San Diego State University

DOUGLAS J. GELB
University of Michigan Medical School

DOUGLAS L. GELOWITZ
Yale University School of Medicine

MARK S. GEORGE
Medical University of South Carolina

MARK S. GERBER
Barrow Neurological Institute

DANIEL H. GESCHWIND
University of California, Los Angeles

MICHAEL GESCHWIND
University of California, San Francisco

CHRISTOPHER C. GETCH
Northwestern University Medical School

STEFAN GEYER
Heinrich Heine University, Düsseldorf, Germany

GHANASHYAM D. GHADGE
University of Chicago Medical Center

JORGE M. GHISO
New York University School of Medicine

SASHA E. B. GIBBS
University of California, Berkeley

RICHARD F. GILLUM
National Center for Health Statistics, Centers for Disease Control and Prevention

JOSÉ M. GIMÉNEZ-AMAYA
Universidad Autónoma de Madrid

CHRISTOPHER G. GOETZ
Rush-Presbyterian-St. Luke's Medical Center

EDWARD J. GOETZL
University of California, San Francisco

ANDREW C. GOLDMAN
State University of New York, Brooklyn Health Science Center

FERNANDO GONZALEZ
Barrow Neurological Institute

CLIFTON L. GOOCH
Columbia University

DOUGLAS S. GOODIN
University of California, San Francisco

MARIANNE S. GOODMAN
Mount Sinai School of Medicine and Bronx Veterans Affairs Medical Center

ROBERT R. GOODMAN
Neurological Institute of New York

JAMES TAIT GOODRICH
Montefiore Medical Center, Albert Einstein College of Medicine

ANDREA C. GORE
Mount Sinai School of Medicine, New York

PHILIP B. GORELICK
Rush Medical College

GLENN R. GOURLEY
Oregon Health Sciences University

MANUEL B. GRAEBER
Imperial College School of Medicine, London

NEILL R. GRAFF-RADFORD
Mayo Clinic

STEVEN B. GRAFF-RADFORD
Cedars-Sinai Medical Center, Los Angeles

SCOTT T. GRAFTON
Dartmouth Brain Imaging Center

DAVID I. GRAHAM
University of Glasgow

KIM S. GRAHAM
MRC Cognition and Brain Sciences Unit, Cambridge

ALAN C. GREEN
University of California, Los Angeles

BARTH A. GREEN
University of Miami

DAVID A. GREENBERG
Buck Institute for Age Research, Novato, California

STEPHANIE GREENE
Children's Hospital, Boston

JOHN E. GREENLEE
Veterans Affairs Medical Center, Salt Lake City

MICHAEL D. GREICIUS
Stanford University School of Medicine

CARLA DELASSUS GRESS
University of California, San Francisco Voice Center

FRANCESCO GRILLO
University of Milan

KALANIT GRILL-SPECTOR
Stanford University

CHARLES GROB
University of California, Los Angeles

CHARLES GROSE
University of Iowa Hospital

MURRAY GROSSMAN
University of Pennsylvania

BLAIR P. GRUBB
Medical College of Ohio

JAMES D. GUEST
University of Miami School of Medicine

ROBERTO GUGIG
University of California, San Francisco

CHRISTIAN GUILLEMINAULT
Stanford University

MICHAEL Z. GUO
Columbia University College of Physicians and Surgeons

KERN H. GUPPY
University of Illinois

DAVID A. HAFLER
Brigham and Women's Hospital

TIMOTHY C. HAIN
Northwestern University Medical School

DUANE E. HAINES
University of Mississippi Medical Center

ELLEN HALLER
University of California, San Francisco

MICHAEL HALMAGYI
Royal Prince Alfred Hospital, Sydney

PATRICK P. HAN
Barrow Neurological Institute

IFTIKHARUL HAQ
University of Miami School of Medicine

YADOLLAH HARATI
Baylor College of Medicine

GADY HAR-EL
State University of New York Health Science Center at Brooklyn

SHAILAJA HARI
Henry Ford Hospital, Detroit

TIMOTHY R. HARRINGTON
Barrow Neurological Institute

GREGORY S. HARRISON
Cleveland Clinic Foundation

ERNEST L. HARTMANN
Sleep Disorders Center, Newton, Massachusetts

HANS-PETER HARTUNG
Heinrich Heine University, Düsseldorf, Germany

W. ALLEN HAUSER
Columbia University College of Physicians and Surgeons

ARTHUR P. HAYS
Columbia University

E. TESSA HEDLEY-WHYTE
Massachusetts General Hospital, Harvard Medical School

KENNETH M. HEILMAN
University of Florida College of Medicine

CATHY M. HELGASON
University of Illinois

JANET ODRY HELMINSKI
Midwestern University, Downers Grove, Illinois

J. CLAUDE HEMPHILL
San Francisco General Hospital

MATTHEW T. HENDELL
Children's Hospital of Philadelphia

VICTOR W. HENDERSON
University of Arkansas for Medical Sciences

WAYNE A. HENING
New York, New York

DEANA M. HENN
Barrow Neurological Institute

JEFFREY S. HENN
Barrow Neurological Institute

PETER HERSCOVITCH
National Institutes of Health

SCOTT HERSHBERGER
California State University, Long Beach

MAX J. HILZ
New York University Medical Center

STEPHEN P. HINSHAW
University of California, Berkeley

MICHIO HIRANO
Columbia University

MAX HIRSHKOWITZ
Houston Veterans Affairs Medical Center

TONY HO
Neuronyx, Inc., Malvern, Pennsylvania

JOHN ALLAN HOBSON
Massachusetts Mental Health Center

GEORG F. HOFFMAN
Universität Heidelberg, Germany

RALPH EDWARD HOFFMAN
Yale University School of Medicine

ERIC HOLLAND
Memorial Sloan-Kettering Cancer Center

DAVID HOLTZMAN
Washington University School of Medicine, St. Louis

KEITH J. HOLYOAK
University of California, Los Angeles

CHANG-ZERN HONG
University of California, Irvine

L. NELSON HOPKINS
State University of New York, Buffalo

MADY HORNIG
University of California, Irvine

JONATHAN HOTT
Barrow Neurological Institute

CRAIG E. HOU
University of California, San Francisco

ERIC A HOUPT
University of Virginia School of Medicine

FRED M. HOWARD
University of Rochester School of Medicine and Dentistry

RONA JANE HU
Stanford University

ROBERT W. HURST
University of Pennsylvania Medical Center

JOSHUA ISRAEL
San Francisco Veteran's Administration Medical Center

BRIAN J. IVINS
Walter Reed Army Medical Center

ROBERT K. JACKLER
University of California, San Francisco

ALAN C. JACKSON
Queen's University, Kingston, Ontario

CARLAYNE E. JACKSON
University of Texas Health Science Center, San Antonio

LUCIA F. JACOBS
University of California, Berkeley

MARC JACOBS
University of California, San Francisco

DANIEL M. JACOBSON
Marshfield Clinic, Wisconsin

GEORGE I. JALLO
Beth Israel Medical Center, New York

ROBERT NEWLIN JAMISON
Brigham and Women's Hospital

SAM P. JAVEDAN
Barrow Neurological Institute

ERIC JAVEL
University of Minnesota Medical School

DAVID T. JECK
Washington University, St. Louis School of Medicine

JOANNA C. JEN
University of California, Los Angeles

J. DAVID JENTSCH
University of California, Los Angeles

ANNE B. JOHNSON
Albert Einstein College of Medicine

J. PATRICK JOHNSON
Cedars-Sinai Medical Center, Los Angeles

RICHARD T. JOHNSON
Johns Hopkins Hospital

ROBERT W. JOHNSON
University of Bristol and Bristol Royal Infirmary

STEVEN JOHNSON
University of Colorado Health Sciences Center

INGRID S. JOHNSRUDE
MRC Cognition and Brain Sciences Unit, Cambridge

S. CLAIBORNE JOHNSTON
University of California, San Francisco

BARRY D. JORDAN
Burke Rehabilitation Hospital, White Plains, New York

RYUI KAJI
Tokushima University Hospital, Japan

YOUSUF KANJWAL
Medical College of Ohio

RAJU KAPOOR
National Hospital for Neurology and Neurosurgery, London

HANS KARBE
Neurological Rehabilitation Center, Bonn, Germany

EDWARD J. KASARSKIS
University of Kentucky Medical Center

BASHAR KATIRJI
Case Western Reserve University

JOEL KATZ
York University, Toronto

NATHANIEL KATZ
Brigham and Women's Hospital

DANIEL IAN KAUFER
University of Pittsburgh Medical Center

DAVID I. KAUFMAN
Michigan State University Clinical Center

HORACIO C. KAUFMANN
Mount Sinai School of Medicine, New York

PETRA KAUFMANN
Neurological Institute of New York

WALTER E. KAUFMANN
Johns Hopkins University School of Medicine

SHARON KEENAN
School of Sleep Medicine, Inc., Palo Alto, California

DAVID ALEXANDER KEITH
Massachusetts General Hospital

G. EVREN KELES
University of California, San Francisco

RHONA S. KELLEY
Southern Illinois University School of Medicine

JOHN J. KELLY
George Washington University School of Medicine

WILLIAM R. KENNEDY
University of Minnesota Hospital

MICHAEL KERN
Humboldt University, Berlin

ANDREW KERTESZ
St. Joseph's Health Center, London, Ontario

JOHN A. KESSLER
Northwestern University Medical School

SHAUKAT A. KHAN
Yale University School of Medicine

RAMESH KHURANA
Johns Hopkins University School of Medicine

MATTHEW C. KIERNAN
Prince of Wales Hospital, Randwick, Australia

BERND C. KIESEIER
Heinrich Heine University, Düsseldorf, Germany

JAWAD F. KIRMANI
State University of New York, Buffalo

BETTE K. KLEINSCHMIDT-DEMASTERS
University of Colorado Health Sciences Center

AMI KLIN
Yale University School of Medicine

RICHARD J. KNAPP
Aventis Pharmaceuticals, Inc.

NERISSA U. KO
University of California, San Francisco

THOMAS K. KOCH
Doernbecher Children's Hospital, Portland, Oregon

PETER J. KOEHLER
Atrium Medical Centre, Heerlen, The Netherlands

NOBUO KOHARA
Kobe City General Hospital, Japan

MAX K. KOLE
Henry Ford Hospital, Detroit

STEFAN KÖLKER
Universität Heidelberg, Germany

WILLIAM C. KOLLER
University of Miami School of Medicine

SPYROS S. KOLLIAS
University Hospital of Zurich

EDWIN H. KOLODNY
New York University School of Medicine

KATIE KOMPOLITI
Rush-Presbyterian-St. Luke's Medical Center

DOUGLAS KONDZIOLKA
University of Pittsburgh Medical Center

AMOS D. KORCZYN
Tel Aviv University Medical Center

JULIE P. KORENBERG
Cedars-Sinai Medical Center, Los Angeles

DANIEL J. KOSINSKI
Medical College of Ohio

ROLF KÖTTER
Heinrich Heine University, Düsseldorf, Germany

JOEL H. KRAMER
University of California, San Francisco

GERALD KREFT
Johann Wolfgang Goethe-Universität, Frankfurt

MARTINA L. KREUTZER
Stanford University

LUDMILA A. KRYZHANOVSKAYA
University of Virginia

PETRI KURSULA
University of Oulu

JOHN F. KURTZKE
Georgetown University (emeritus)

CLETE A. KUSHIDA
Stanford Sleep Disorders Clinic

JUTTA KÜST
Neurological Rehabilitation Center, Bonn, Germany

ALBERT R. LA SPADA
University of Washington Medical Center

ENRIQUE LABADIE
Veterans Affairs Medical Center, Tucson

DAVID LACOMIS
University of Pittsburgh School of Medicine

JENNIFER M. A. LAIRD
AstraZeneca R&D, Montreal

MICHELLE V. LAMBERT
Institute of Psychiatry, London

ELIZABETH L. LANE
North Shore University Hospital, Manhasset, New York

HANS LASSMANN
University of Vienna

PATRICK J. LAVIN
Vanderbilt University Medical Center

MICHAEL H. LAVYNE
Weill Medical College of Cornell University

MICHAEL T. LAWTON
University of California, San Francisco

PETER D. LE ROUX
University of Pennsylvania

JOHN PAUL LEACH
Walton Centre for Neurology and Neurosurgery, Liverpool

MARTIN H. LEAMON
University of California, Davis

XAVIER LECLERC
Hôpital Roger Salengro, Lille, France

RICHARD J. LEDERMAN
Cleveland Clinic Foundation

ANDREW G. LEE
University of Iowa Hospitals and Clinics

KAREN LEE
University of California, San Francisco

KEWCHANG LEE
San Francisco Veteran's Administration Medical Center

VIRGINIA M. Y. LEE
University of Pennsylvania

ALAN D. LEGATT
Montefiore Medical Center, Albert Einstein College of Medicine

R. JOHN LEIGH
University Hospitals of Cleveland

A. ARTURO LEIS
Mississippi Methodist Rehabilitation Center

G. MICHAEL LEMOLE
Barrow Neurological Institute

RUTH LEMOLE
Barrow Neurological Institute

GREGORY A. LESKIN
Stanford University and Veterans Affairs Palo Alto Healthcare System

CATHERINE A. LESLIE
University of Virginia

DORA LEUNG
Neurological Institute of New York

JOHN M. LEVENTHAL
Yale University School of Medicine

KERRY H. LEVIN
Cleveland Clinic Foundation

BRIAN LEVINE
Baycrest Centre for Geriatric Care, Toronto

RUTH E. LEVINE
University of Texas Medical Branch, Galveston

RICHARD A. LEWIS
Wayne State University School of Medicine

PETER A. LEWITT
Clinical Neuroscience Center, Southfield, Minnesota

DESCARTES LI
University of California, San Francisco

JUN LI
Wayne State University School of Medicine

YANSHENG LI
Baylor College of Medicine

JONATHAN LICHTMACHER
University of California, San Francisco

YELENA LINDENBAUM
Neurological Institute of New York

MICHAEL LINK
Mayo Clinc

W. IAN LIPKIN
University of California, Irvine

JAMES K. LIU
University of Utah Health Sciences Center

CHRISTOPHER M. LOFTUS
University of Oklahoma College of Medicine

LINDA LOHR
State University of New York, Buffalo

ELAN D. LOUIS
Neurological Institute of New York

PHILLIP A. LOW
Mayo Clinic

SAMUEL K. LUDWIN
Queen's University, Kingston, Ontario

ELIO LUGARESI
Universita di Bologna

W. DAVID LUST
Case Western Reserve University School of Medicine

LINDA M. LUXON
Great Ormond Street Hospital for Sick Children

PATRICK D. LYDEN
University of California, San Diego

JAMES LYNCH
Sierra Neurosurgery Group, Reno, Nevada

TIMOTHY LYNCH
Mater Misericordiae Hospital, Dublin

WILLIAM LYTTON
State University of New York Downstate Medical Center

MIA M. MacCOLLIN
Massachusetts General Hospital

R. LOCH MACDONALD
Pritzker School of Medicine, University of Chicago

ROBERT L. MACDONALD
Vanderbilt University

STEVEN H. MADONICK
Yale University School of Medicine

JOSEPH R. MADSEN
Children's Hospital, Boston

GARY MAGRAM
New Jersey Neuroscience Institute

JASON D. MAGUIRE
U.S. Naval Medical Research Unit, Jakarta, Indonesia

MARK W. MAHOWALD
Hennepin County Medical Center, Minneapolis

MICHAEL J. MAJSAK
New York Medical College

EWA MALATYNSKA
Indiana University of School of Medicine

ROLF MALESSA
Klinik für Neurologie, Weimar, Germany

GHAUS M. MALIK
Henry Ford Hospital, Detroit

TIMOTHY W. MALISCH
Northwestern University Medical School

BETH A. MALOW
University of Michigan Medical Center

BALA V. MANYAM
Texas A&M University College of Medicine

E. MARANI
University of Leiden

OMKAR N. MARKAND
Indiana University School of Medicine

A. JULIO MARTINEZ[†]
University of Pittsburgh Medical Center

VICENTE MARTINEZ
Novartis Pharma AG, Basel, Switzerland

CAROLINA MARTINS
University of Florida

JOSEPH C. MASDEU
University of Navarre Medical School, Spain

ROBERTO MASFERRER
Masferrer Neurosurgical Professional, Colorado Springs

KIMBERLEE MICHALS MATALON
University of Houston

RUEBEN MATALON
University of Texas Medical Branch, Galveston

CATHERINE A. MATEER
University of Victoria, British Columbia

NINAN T. MATHEW
Houston Headache Clinic

RICHARD H. MATTSON
Yale Medical Center

DARIUS MATUSEVICIUS
University of Ottawa

WILLIAM L. MAXWELL
University of Glasgow

PAUL J. MAY
University of Mississippi Medical Center

RICHARD MAYEUX
Columbia University

JUSTIN C. McARTHUR
Johns Hopkins Hospital

W. VAUGHN McCALL
Wake Forest University Baptist Medical Center

ROBERT W. McCARLEY
Harvard Medical School, Veterans Affairs Medical Center

ALEXANDER J. McDONALD
University of South Carolina School of Medicine

MATTHEW J. McDONALD
University of Miami School of Medicine

CAMERON G. McDOUGALL
Barrow Neurological Institute

ROBERT C. McKINSTRY
Washington University School of Medicine, St. Louis

KIMFORD J. MEADOR
Georgetown University Hospital

MARK F. MEHLER
Albert Einstein College of Medicine

SYNTHIA H. MELLON
University of California, San Francisco

RONALD MELZACK
McGill University

MARIO MENDEZ
University of California, Los Angeles

MICHELLE MENDOZA
California Pacific Medical Center, San Francisco

DANIEL L. MENKES
University of Tennessee

GUNDELA MEYER
Universidad de La Laguna, Tenerife, Canary Islands

JOHN STERLING MEYER
Veterans Affairs Medical Center, Houston

R. CHRISTOPHER MIALL
University of Oxford

GABRIELE MICELI
Catholic University of Rome

EDWARD MICHNA
Brigham and Women's Hospital

DRAGUS MIHAILA
Clinical Neuroscience Center, Southfield, Minnesota

BRUCE L. MILLER
University of California, San Francisco

DAVID H. MILLER
North Shore University Hospital, Manhasset, New York

[†]Deceased

HANNAH A. MILLER
University of California, San Francisco

ROBERT G. MILLER
California Pacific Medical Center, San Francisco

ROBERT H. MILLER
Case Western Reserve University

J. GORDON MILLICHAP
Northwestern University Medical School

ALIREZA MINAGAR
University of Miami School of Medicine

MAJID MIRMIRAN
Stanford University Medical Center

SOHAIL K. MIRZA
Harborview Medical Center, University of Washington

PANAYIOTIS MITSIAS
Henry Ford Hospital, Detroit

HIROSHI MITSUMOTO
Columbia-Presbyterian Medical Center

EDSON MIYAWAKI
Brigham and Women's Hospital

ELI M. MIZRAHI
Baylor College of Medicine

CHARLES V. MOBBS
Mount Sinai School of Medicine, New York

GÉRARD MOHR
Hôpital Général Juif, McGill University

BAHRAM MOKRI
Mayo Clinic

NISHA N. MONEY
University of California, San Diego

SAKTI MOOKHERJEE
Veterans Affairs Medical Center, Syracuse

PHILIP G. MORGAN
University Hospitals Health System, Cleveland

CHARLES M. MORIN
Université Laval, Quebec

MARTHA J. MORRELL
Columbia-Presbyterian Comprehensive Epilepsy Center

ROBERT G. MORRISON
University of California, Los Angeles

MARK J. MORROW
Hattiesburg Clinic, Mississippi

HUGO W. MOSER
Kennedy Krieger Institute, Baltimore

SHIMON MOSES
Soroka Medical Centre, Beer Sheva, Israel

MARK L. MOSTER
Albert Einstein Medical Center

GRAHAM MOUW
University Hospitals of Cleveland

MICHAEL JON MUFSON
Brigham and Women's Hospital

TODD MULDERINK
Northwestern University Medical School

TURHON A. MURAD
Chico State University

JENNIFER MURPHY
University of California, San Francisco

BRIAN EAMON MURRAY
Mater Misericordiae Hospital, Dublin

MALINA NARAYANAN NADIG
Children's Hospital, Boston

ARIF NAJIB
Medical University of South Carolina

JEFFREY J. NEIL
St. Louis Children's Hospital

CLAIRE NEILAN
Memorial Sloan-Kettering Cancer Center

EDWARD GEORGE NEILAN
Harvard Medical School

GINA M. NELSON
University of Alabama

ROBERT NEUMAR
University of Pennsylvania

DAVID W. NEWELL
Harborview Medical Center, University of Washington

KATHY NEWELL
University of Kansas Medical Center

NANCY J. NEWMAN
Emory University School of Medicine

PETER K. NEWMAN
Middlesbrough General Hospital, UK

CHARLES D. NICHOLS
Vanderbilt University

CHARLES E. NIESEN
Cedars-Sinai Medical Center, Los Angeles

ERIC W. NOTTMEIER
Barrow Neurological Institute

TATJANA NOVAKOVIC-AGOPIAN
California Pacific Medical Center, San Francisco

MARC R. NUWER
University of California, Los Angeles

LARS NYBERG
Umeå University, Sweden

WILLIAM L. NYHAN
University of California, San Diego

ANNE LOUISE OAKLANDER
Massachusetts General Hospital

JOSE A. OBESO
University of Navarre Medical School, Spain

HERBERT N. OCHITILL
San Francisco General Hospital

JENNIFER OGAR
Veterans Affairs Northern California Health Care System

SHIN J. OH
University of Alabama

RICHARD K. OLNEY
University of California, San Francisco

ROGER J. PACKER
Children's National Medical Center, Washington, D.C.

SEYMOUR PACKMAN
University of California, San Francisco

DEEPAK N. PANDYA
Boston University School of Medicine

ANDRE PARENT
Université Laval, Robert-Giffard, Quebec

JACK M. PARENT
University of Michigan Medical Center

SHAHRAM PARTOVI
Barrow Neurological Institute

RUTI PARVARI
Ben Gurion University, Beer Sheva, Israel

ALVARO PASCUAL-LEONE
Beth Israel Deaconess Medical Center

GAVRIL W. PASTERNAK
Memorial Sloan-Kettering Cancer Center

GREGORY M. PASTORES
New York University School of Medicine

ROY A. PATCHELL
University of Kentucky Medical Center

NARESH P. PATEL
Mayo Clinic, Scottsdale

MARC C. PATTERSON
Columbia University

DONALD W. PATY
University of British Columbia

NEAL S. PEACHEY
Cleveland Clinic Foundation

WARWICK J. PEACOCK
University of California, San Francisco

RAFAEL PELAYO
Stanford University Medical Center

JOHN M. PELLOCK
Virginia Commonwealth University School of Medicine

ALAN PERCY
University of Alabama

PERLA I. PERIUT
Neurological Center of South Florida

AXEL PERNECZKY
Klinikum Johannes-Gutenberg, Mainz, Germany

RICHARD J. PERRY
National Hospital for Neurology and Neurosurgery

CAROL K. PETITO
University of Miami

MICHELLE PETRI
Johns Hopkins University School of Medicine

WILLIAM A. PETRI
University of Virginia Health Sciences Center

LA PHENGRASAMY
University of California, San Francisco

MICHEL PHILIPPART
University of California, Los Angeles

LAWRENCE H. PITTS
University of California, San Francisco

MICHAEL A. POLLACK
Nemours Children's Clinic, Orlando, Florida

FRANCISCO A. PONCE
Barrow Neurological Institute

RANDALL W. PORTER
Barrow Neurological Institute

MICHAEL I. POSNER
Sackler Institute, Weill Medical College

MARC N. POTENZA
Yale University

ARTISS L. POWELL
Robert Wood Johnson Medical School

JAMES H. POWERS
University of California, San Francisco

PAULINE POWERS
University of South Florida

WILLIAM J. POWERS
Washington University School of Medicine, St. Louis

VIRGINIA PRENDERGAST
Masferrer Neurosurgical Professional, Colorado Springs

DAVID C. PRESTON
Case Western Reserve University

SUSAN PRESTON-MARTIN
Keck School of Medicine, University of Southern California

MARK C. PREUL
Barrow Neurological Institute

JEAN-PIERRE PRUVO
Hôpital Roger Salengro, Lille, France

ADAM PUCHE
University of Maryland School of Medicine

WILLIAM A. PULSINELLI
University of Tennessee, Memphis

STEFAN M. PULST
Cedars-Sinai Medical Center, Los Angeles

ADNAN I. QURESHI
State University of New York, Buffalo

TONSE N. K. RAJU
National Institutes of Health

ANIL NATESAN RAMA
Stanford University Medical Center

KATHERINE P. RANKIN
University of California, San Francisco

ALAN M. RAPOPORT
New England Center for Headache

STANLEY I. RAPOPORT
National Institute on Aging

DISYA RATANAKORN
Ramathibodi Hospital, Mahidol University, Thailand

ROBERT A. RATCHESON
Case Western Reserve University School of Medicine

STEVEN D. RAUCH
Massachusetts Eye and Ear Infirmary

LEE RAWITSCHER
San Francisco General Hospital

AMIR RAZ
Weill Medical College of Cornell University

JEREMY H. REES
Institute of Neurology, London

HAROLD L. REKATE
Barrow Neurological Institute

ALBERT L. RHOTON
University of Florida College of Medicine

DANIELE RIGAMONTI
Johns Hopkins Hospital

HOWARD RIINA
Weill Medical College of Cornell University

ANDREW J. RINGER
University of Cincinnati

MICHAEL W. RISINGER
Stanford University Medical Center

VICTOR M. RIVERA
Baylor College of Medicine

MATTHEW RIZZO
University of Iowa

E. STEVE ROACH
Wake Forest University School of Medicine

AHMAD ROBBIE
Neurological Associates of the Ozarks, Springfield, Missouri

PHILIPPE ROBERT
Hospital Pasteur, Nice

MAURIZIO ROBERTO
University of Milan

DAVID ROBERTSON
Vanderbilt University

JULIUS ROCCA
Karolinska Institute

M. RODRIGUEZ
Universidad de La Laguna, Tenerife, Canary Islands

M. C. RODRIGUEZ-OROZ
University of Navarre Medical School, Spain

NICHOLETTE ROEMER
University of California, San Francisco, Veteran's Administration Medical Center

WILLIAM R. ROESKE
University of Arizona College of Medicine

C. LELAND ROGERS
St. Joseph's Hospital, Phoenix

WILLIAM E. ROLAND
Harry S. Truman Memorial Veterans' Hospital

GABRIELE V. RONNETT
Johns Hopkins University School of Medicine

KAREN L. ROOS
Indiana University School of Medicine

RAYMOND P. ROOS
University of Chicago Medical Center

F. CLIFFORD ROSE
London Neurological Centre

HOWARD J. ROSEN
University of California, San Francisco

MICHAEL ROSENBERG
New Jersey Neuroscience Institute

JEFFREY ROSENFELD
Carolinas Medical Center, Charlotte, North Carolina

NICHOLAS Z. ROSENLICHT
San Francisco Veteran's Administration Medical Center

PETER B. ROSENQUIST
Wake Forest University School of Medicine

PHILIP ROSENTHAL
University of California, San Francisco

EDGAR L. ROSS
Brigham and Women's Hospital

JUDITH LEVINE ROSS
Thomas Jefferson University

MARK A. ROSS
University of Kentucky Medical Center

AGUEDA ROSTAGNO
New York University School of Medicine

JOHN F. ROTHROCK
USA Medical Center, Mobile, Alabama

JOHN C. ROTHWELL
Institute of Neurology, London

DONALD ROYALL
University of Texas Health Science Center, San Antonio

MARC RUBENZIK
University of Arizona College of Medicine

ROBERT L. RUFF
Louis Stokes Cleveland Veterans Affairs Medical Center

SEAN D. RULAND
Rush Medical College

BARRY S. RUSSMAN
Shriners Hospital For Children, Portland, Oregon

ROBERT S. RUST
University of Virginia Health Systems

THOMAS SABIN
New England Medical Center

ALFREDO A. SADUN
Keck School of Medicine, University of Southern California

SAM SAFAVI-ABBASI
Barrow Neurological Institute

LORA S. SALANDANAN
Cedars-Sinai Medical Center, Los Angeles

VIRGILIO D. SALANGA
Cleveland Clinic of Florida

ANDRES M. SALAZAR
Walter Reed Army Medical Center

HOWARD W. SANDER
Weill Medical College of Cornell University

DONALD B. SANDERS
Duke University Medical Center

ELAINE SANDERS-BUSH
Vanderbilt University

CARLOS S. SANTANA
University of South Florida

JOEL R. SAPER
Michigan Head Pain and Neurological Institute

RAMA SAPIR
Shaare Zedek Medical Center, Jerusalem

HARVEY B. SARNAT
Cedars-Sinai Medical Center, Los Angeles

SUSUMU SATO
National Institute of Neurological Disorders and Stroke

RICHARD SATRAN
University of Rochester

ELIANA SCEMES
Albert Einstein College of Medicine

HERBERT H. SCHAUMBURG
Albert Einstein College of Medicine

ARNOLD B. SCHEIBEL
University of California, Los Angeles

CARLOS H. SCHENCK
Hennepin County Medical Center, Minneapolis

KENNETH E. SCHMADER
Duke University Medical Center

HELMUT S. SCHMIDT
Ohio Sleep Medicine and Neuroscience Institute

MARKUS H. SCHMIDT
Ohio Sleep Medicine and Neuroscience Institute

THOMAS J. SCHNITZER
Northwestern University Medical School

HERBERT A. SCHREIER
Children's Hospital, Oakland, California

KAREN SCHWAB
Walter Reed Army Medical Center

PHILIP A. SCHWARTZKROIN
University of California, Davis

DANIEL R. SCOLES
Cedars-Sinai Medical Center, Los Angeles

ALVIN B. H. SEAH
Emory University School of Medicine

JONATHAN V. SEHY
Washington University, St. Louis

WARREN R. SELMAN
Case Western Reserve University School of Medicine

SHARON J. SHA
University of California, San Francisco

JEFFRY ROWLAND SHAEFER
Harvard School of Dental Medicine

BHAGWAN T. SHAHANI
University of Illinois

ABU S. M. SHAMSUZZAMAN
Mayo Clinic

BARBARA E. SHAPIRO
Case Western Reserve University School of Medicine

KHEMA RAM SHARMA
University of Miami School of Medicine

SANSAR C. SHARMA
New York Medical College

JAMES A. SHARPE
Toronto Hospital

JEREMY M. SHEFNER
State University of New York, Syracuse Health Science Center

JAVAID I. SHEIKH
Stanford University

RAVINDER SHERGILL
Stanford Sleep Disorders Clinic

DAVID G. SHERMAN
University of Texas Health Science Center, San Antonio

ELLIOTT H. SHERR
University of California, San Francisco

ANDREW G. SHETTER
Barrow Neurological Institute

ROBERT W. SHIELDS
Cleveland Clinic Foundation

TINA T. SHIH
Columbia-Presbyterian Medical Center

VIVIAN E-AN SHIH
Massachusetts General Hospital

KYUNG SHIK-SUH
Ajou University School of Medicine, Suwon, Korea

MICHAEL T. SHIPLEY
University of Maryland School of Medicine

RODNEY A. SHORT
Neurology Consultants, Davenport, Iowa

MICHAEL W. SHY
Wayne State University School of Medicine

PETER SIAO
Massachusetts General Hospital

MAMADOU SIDIBE
Emory University

BO K. SIESJÖ
Lund University, Sweden

MICHAEL H. SILBER
Mayo Clinic

STEPHEN D. SILBERSTEIN
Jefferson Headache Center, Philadelphia

ROSALIA SILVESTRI
Brigham and Women's Hospital

DAVID SIMON
Beth Israel Deaconess Medical Center

JON S. SIMONS
University College, London

P. JEANETTE SIMPSON
Johns Hopkins University School of Medicine

RAYMOND S. SINATRA
Yale University School of Medicine

DAVID SINCLAIR
Montreal Neurological Hospital, McGill University

CHRISTOPHER M. SINTON
Harvard Medical School, Veterans Affairs Medical Center

CLAIRE SIRA
University of Victoria

JOSEPH SIRVEN
Mayo Clinic

CATINA Y. SLOAN
Mayo Clinic and Mayo Foundation

JONATHAN R. SLOTKIN
Children's Hospital, Boston

KRIS A. SMITH
Barrow Neurological Institute

VIRGINIA E. SMITH
University of California, Berkeley

WADE S. SMITH
University of California, San Francisco

YOLAND SMITH
Emory University

MATTHEW D. SMYTH
University of California, San Francisco

JULIE S. SNOWDEN
Manchester Royal Infirmary

LOUIS SOKOLOFF
National Institute of Mental Health

MARYLOU V. SOLBRIG
University of California, Irvine

SEYMOUR SOLOMON
Montefiore Medical Center, Bronx, New York

VIREND K. SOMERS
Mayo Clinic

VOLKER K. H. SONNTAG
Barrow Neurological Institute

JULIO SOTELO
National Autonomous University of Mexico

NORBERTO E. SOTO
National Center for Complementary and Alternative Medicine

GAREN SPARKS
University of Texas, Dallas

ROBERT F. SPETZLER
Barrow Neurosurgical Associates

ARTHUR J. SPIELMAN
City University of New York

ANTONIO SPINA-FRANCA
University of Sao Paulo, Brazil

RITA SPIRITO
University of Milan

ALLA SPIVAK
University of California, San Francisco

STEPHEN R. SPRANG
University of Texas Southwestern Medical Center, Dallas

DAVID C. SPRAY
Albert Einstein College of Medicine

JAYASHREE SRINIVASAN
Seattle Neurosurgery Clinic, University of Washington

JOHN S. STAHL
University Hospitals of Cleveland

JEFFREY ROBERT STARKE
Texas Children's Hospital

SERGIO STARKSTEIN
Buenos Aires Neuropsychiatric Center

JEFFREY M. STATLAND
University of Kansas School of Medicine

GARY K. STEINBERG
Stanford University

JEANNE L. STEINER
Yale University School of Medicine

MIRCEA STERIADE
Université Laval School of Medicine, Quebec

BARNEY J. STERN
Emory Clinic

JOHN M. STERN
University of California, Los Angeles

MARCUS A. STOODLEY
Prince of Wales Medical Research Institute, Randwick, Australia

STEPHEN E. STRAUS
National Center for Complementary and Alternative Medicine

DAVID A. STUMPF
Northwestern University

DONALD T. STUSS
Baycrest Centre for Geriatric Care, Toronto

AUSTIN J. SUMNER
Louisiana State University Medical Center

CLIVE SVENDSEN
University of Wisconsin

EVA SVOBODA
Baycrest Centre for Geriatric Care, Toronto

RAYMOND A. SWANSON
San Francisco Veteran's Administration Medical Center

THOMAS R. SWIFT
Medical College of Georgia

YVETTE TACHE
University of California, Los Angeles

TZE-CHING TAN
Queen Elizabeth Hospital, Hong Kong

CAROLINE M. TANNER
Parkinsons Institute, Sunnyvale, California

JINNY TAVEE
Cleveland Clinic Foundation

CHRISTOPHER L. TAYLOR
University Hospitals of Cleveland

CHARLES H. TEGELER
Wake Forest University Baptist Medical Center

SIBEL TEKIN
University of California, Los Angeles

STEWART J. TEPPER
New England Center for Headache

JOHN B. TERRY
Via Christi Regional Medical Center, Wichita, Kansas

WENDY TODARO THANASSI
Yale University School of Medicine

NICHOLAS THEODORE
Barrow Neurological Institute

PHILIP V. THEODOSOPOULOS
University of California, San Francisco

TODD P. THOMPSON
Straub Clinic and Hospital, Honolulu

GRETCHEN E. TIETJEN
Medical College of Ohio

THOMAS A. TOMSICK
University of Cincinnati

GANG A. TONG
University of California, San Diego

JEANNETTE J. TOWNSEND
University of Utah School of Medicine

MARK H. TOWNSEND
Louisiana State University School of Medicine

DORIS A. TRAUNER
University of California, San Diego

ADAM TRAVIS
University of California, San Francisco

DAVID M. TREIMAN
Barrow Neurological Institute

ROSARIO R. TRIFILETTI
New York Cornell Medical Center

MICHAEL TRIMBLE
National Hospital for Neurology and Neurosurgery, London

JONATHAN D. TROBE
Kellogg Eye Center, Ann Arbor, Michigan

JOHN Q. TROJANOWSKI
University of Pennsylvania

B. TODD TROOST
Wake Forest University School of Medicine

ALEX TSELIS
Wayne State University

ROGER E. TURBIN
University of Medicine and Dentistry of New Jersey

DENNIS C. TURK
University of Washington

RONALD J. TUSA
Emory University

ATUL TYAGI
General Infirmary, Leeds

H. RICHARD TYLER
Boston, Massachusetts

KENNETH L. TYLER
University of Colorado Health Sciences Center

BETTY ANN TZENG
University of California, San Francisco

JOSÉ ULLÁN
Universidad Panamericana, Zaropan, Mexico

DAVID R. VAGO
University of Utah

EDWARD VALENSTEIN
University of Florida

CRAIG VAN DYKE
University of California, San Francisco

J. VAN GIJN
University of Utrecht Medical Centre

DOUGLAS VANDERBURG
New York University School of Medicine

EVA V. VARGA
Sarver Heart Center, Tucson

LEONARDO VECCHIET
"G. d'Annunzio" University, Chieti, Italy

V. V. VEDANARAYANAN
University of Mississippi Medical Center

JOSÉ LUÌS VELAYOS
University of Navarre, Spain

ANTONIUS JOHANNES VERBERNE
University of Melbourne

MICHAEL VERTINO
Upstate Medical University, Syracuse

GILBERT VEZINA
Childrens National Medical Center, Washington, D.C.

BELINDA A. VICIOSO
University of Texas Southwestern Medical Center

SOPHIA VINOGRADOV
University of California, San Francisco

GOVINDA S. VISVESVARA
National Center for Infectious Diseases

FRED VOLKMAR
Yale University School of Medicine

JEAN PAUL G. VONSATTEL
Massachusetts General Hospital

TUAN VU
Columbia University

ANNE M. WALBERER
University of Utah

MATTHEW T. WALKER
Northwestern University Medical School

MICHAEL WALL
University of Iowa

GENE V. WALLENSTEIN
University of Utah

MITCHELL T. WALLIN
Veterans Affairs Medical Center, Washington, D.C.

JAMES ANDREW WALTZ
Max Planck Institute for Brain Research, Frankfurt

DAJIE WANG
University of Pennsylvania

NANPING WANG
University of California, Riverside

STEVEN WARACH
National Institutes of Health

KEVIN R. WARD
Virginia Commonwealth University

ELIZABETH WARRINGTON
National Hospital for Neurology and Neurosurgery, London

ROBERT T. WATSON
University of Florida College of Medicine

MARKUS WEBER
Kantonsspital St. Gallen, Switzerland

LOUIS H. WEIMER
Columbia University

BRYCE WEIR
Pritzker School of Medicine, University of Chicago

DANIEL S. WEISS
University of California, San Francisco

K. MICHAEL WELCH
Finch University/Chicago Medical School

ROY O. WELLER
Southampton General Hospital

GWEN WENDELSCHAFER-CRABB
University of Minnesota

MICHAEL WEST
University of Manitoba

MARY ANNE WHELAN
Bassett Hospital, Utica, New York

PETER J. WHITEHOUSE
Case Western Reserve University

RICHARD J. WHITLEY
University of Alabama

ROBERT J. WIENECKE
University of Oklahoma Health Science Center

HEINZ-GREGOR WIESER
Neurologische Klinik, Universität Zurich

ASA J. WILBOURN
Cleveland Clinic Foundation

OLAJIDE A. WILLIAMS
Columbia-Presbyterian Medical Center

H. RICHARD WINN
Harborview Medical Center, University of Washington

FRANZ J. WIPPOLD
Washington University School of Medicine, St. Louis

JONATHAN D. WIRTSCHAFTER
University of Minnesota

KRYSTYNA WISNIEWSKI
New York State Institute for Basic Research

TIMOTHY F. WITHAM
University of Pittsburgh School of Medicine

DAVID R. WITT
Kaiser Permanente Medical Center, San Jose, California

RONA F. WOLDENBERG
North Shore University Hospital, New York University School of Medicine

GIL I. WOLFE
University of Texas Southwestern Medical Center

SHIRLEY H. WRAY
Massachusetts General Hospital

CHEN-SEN WU
National Institutes of Health

NANCY SHENG-SHIH WU
University of California, San Francisco

KRISTINE YAFFE
San Francisco Veteran's Administration Medical Center

ABUTAHER M. YAHIA
State University of New York, Buffalo

THORU YAMADA
University of Iowa College of Medicine

HENRY I. YAMAMURA
University of Arizona College of Medicine

CHIEN-MING YANG
Fu Jen Catholic University, Hsinchuang, Taiwan

CLAIRE C. YANG
University of Washington School of Medicine

KEITH O. YEATES
Children's Hospital, Columbus, Ohio

GORSEV YENER
Dokuz Eylul University Medical School, Izmir, Turkey

EDWARD N. YETERIAN
Colby College

GEORGE K. YORK
Kaiser Permanente Stockton Medical Center and The Sôa Institute

G. BRYAN YOUNG
Victoria Hospital, London, Ontario

WILLIAM L. YOUNG
University of California, San Francisco

DONALD YOUNKIN
Children's Hospital of Philadelphia

KIN YUEN
Stanford Sleep Disorders Clinic

W. K. ALFRED YUNG
University of Texas M. D. Anderson Cancer Center

JOSEPH M. ZABRAMSKI
Barrow Neurological Institute

LOLITA ZALIAUSKIENE
University of Alabama, Birmingham

PHYLLIS C. ZEE
Northwestern University Medical School

LEONARD S. ZEGANS
University of California, San Francisco

DENNIS ZGALJARDIC
North Shore University Hospital, Manhasset, New York

IRINA V. ZHDANOVA
Boston University

BRIAN M. ZIMNITZKY
Clifton T. Perkins Hospital Center, Jessup, Maryland

DOUGLAS W. ZOCHODNE
Heritage Medical Research, Calgary, Alberta

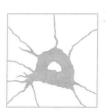

Guide to Using The Encyclopedia

THE *Encyclopedia of the Neurological Sciences* is a comprehensive study of the nervous system and of the various conditions and disorders that affect or involve the nervous system. This major reference work consists of four separate volumes and about 3,500 pages, and it includes more than 1,000 different entries covering all aspects of neurology. The following Guide will explain how the work is organized and how the information within it can be located.

ORGANIZATION

For the purpose of this Encyclopedia, chief editors Dr. Michael Aminoff and Dr. Robert Daroff, in consultation with the various associate editors, have defined the field of neurological science as consisting of 32 distinct subject areas. (Please see page v of this section for a complete listing of these areas.)

This organization by subject area served not only to establish a thematic overview of the entire discipline, but also to provide a practical means of approaching the task of developing the Encyclopedia. By means of the subject-area scheme, the massive entry list of more than 1,000 topics was divided into manageable sections averaging about 30 entries per section. Each of these subject areas was then assigned by the chief editors to an associate editor with particular expertise in that discipline. The editor in question was primarily responsible for the selection of topics and authors in this area, and for the review and approval of manuscripts.

ENTRY FORMAT

The *Encyclopedia of the Neurological Sciences* is arranged in a single alphabetical sequence according to title. Entries whose titles begin with the letters A to De are in Volume 1, entries with titles from Di- to L are in Volume 2, entries from M to Ph- are in Volume 3, and Pi- to Z in Volume 4, along with the Subject Index. In addition to this alphabetical sequence, the entries are also grouped according to their specific discipline within the overall field of neurological science. (Please see the subsequent section "Contents by Subject Area" for information on this grouping.)

The editors have made every effort to provide each entry with a succinct, precise title so that the reader will know immediately what is covered in this entry. In addition, each entry begins with a short introductory statement defining the issue to be discussed.

So that they can be easily located, entry titles generally begin with the key word or phrase indicating the topic, with any generic terms following. For example, "Myopathy, Congenital" is the entry title rather than "Congenital Myopathy," and similarly "Acoustic Neuroma, Treatment" is the title rather than "Treatment of Acoustic Neuroma."

CROSS REFERENCES

Virtually all the entries in the Encyclopedia have cross references to other entries. These appear at the end of the entry text. The cross references indicate related entries that can be consulted for further information on the same topic, or for other information on a related topic. The Encyclopedia contains nearly 6,000 cross references in all. For example, the entry "Schizophrenia, Treatment" provides the following cross references:

See also–Antipsychotic Pharmacology; Dopamine; Electroconvulsive Therapy (ECT); Hallucinations, Visual and Auditory; Lobotomy; Neuropsychiatry, Overview; Schizophrenia, Biology

FURTHER READING

The Further Reading section appears as the last element in an entry. It lists recent secondary sources to aid the reader in locating more detailed or technical information. Review articles and research papers that are important to an understanding of the topic are also listed. For example, the entry "Phantom Limb and Stump Pain" has the following references:

Fields, H. L. (1987). *Pain.* McGraw-Hill, New York.
Jensen, T. S., and Nikolajsen, L. (1999). Phantom pain and other phenomena after amputation. In *Textbook of Pain* (P. D. Wall and R. Melzack, Eds.), 4th ed., pp. 799–814. Churchill-Livingstone, Edinburgh, UK.
Katz, J., (1997). Phantom limb pain. *Lancet* **350**, 1338–1339.
Katz, J., and Gangliese, L. (1999). Phantom limb pain: A continuing puzzle. In *Psychosocial Factors in Pain: Critical Perspectives* (R. J. Gatchel and D. C. Turk, Eds.), pp. 284–300. Guilford, New York.
Katz, J., and Melzack, R. (1990). Pain "memories" in phantom limbs: Review and clinical observations. *Pain* **43**, 319–336.
Nikolajsen, L., Ilkjaer, S., Kroner, K., *et al.* (1997). Randomised trial of epidural bupivacaine and morphine in prevention of stump and phantom pain in lower-limb amputation. *Lancet* **350**, 1353–1357.
Sherman, R. A. (1989). Stump and phantom limb pain. *Neurol. Clin.* **7**, 249–264.

The Further Reading references are for the benefit of the reader; they provide the author's recommendations for more information on the given topic. Thus they consist of a limited number of entries. They do not represent a complete listing of all the sources consulted by the author in preparing the paper.

INDEX

A Subject Index is located at the end of Volume 4. This index is the most convenient way to locate a desired topic within the Encyclopedia and thus it should be the starting point for any reader seeking to find a topic. The subjects in the index are listed alphabetically and indicate the volume and page number where information on this topic can be found.

CONTENTS BY SUBJECT AREA

Preceding the Index in Volume 4 is a Table of Contents by Subject Area. This listing provides a breakdown of the entries in the Encyclopedia according to the topical area to which they were assigned. For example, the first subject area is **Autonomic Nervous System**, and it begins with the entry "Autonomic Dysreflexia."

The purpose of this listing is to display to the reader the nature and scope of all 32 subject areas, so that a person who is interested in (for example) the area of **Neurosurgery** as a whole can see which topics throughout the work fall into this category. Or, a person who wishes to read a series of the biographical entries for famous scientists can do so by consulting the section called **History (Biographies)**.

In the interests of conserving space and maintaining consistency, each topic in the Encyclopedia is listed only under one area heading. However, this does not imply that the entry has relevance only in this field; many entries could be classified in two or more areas. For example the topic "Epilepsy, Epidemiology" appears in the **Epilepsy** subject area but also applies to the **Neuroepidemiology** area. The entry "Melatonin" is listed under **Sleep and Sleep and Disorders** because of its role in the sleep process, but could also have been placed in **Neuroendocrinology** because of its classification as a hormone.

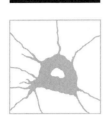

COLOR PLATE SECTION
FOR VOLUME 3

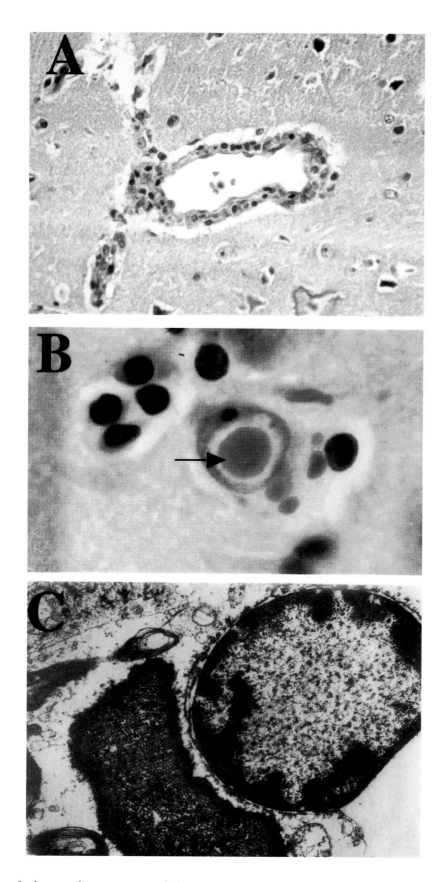

Pathological features of subacute sclerosing panencephalitis (SSPE). (A) Perivascular inflammatory cells and neuronal loss in brain tissue from an SSPE patient (H & E stain). (B) An eosinophilic intranuclear inclusion body. (C) Electron microscopy of intracytoplasmic (crescent-shape) inclusion bodies and intranuclear filamentous course inclusions (magnification, ×19,000). See entry MEASLES VIRUS, CENTRAL NERVOUS SYSTEM COMPLICATIONS OF.

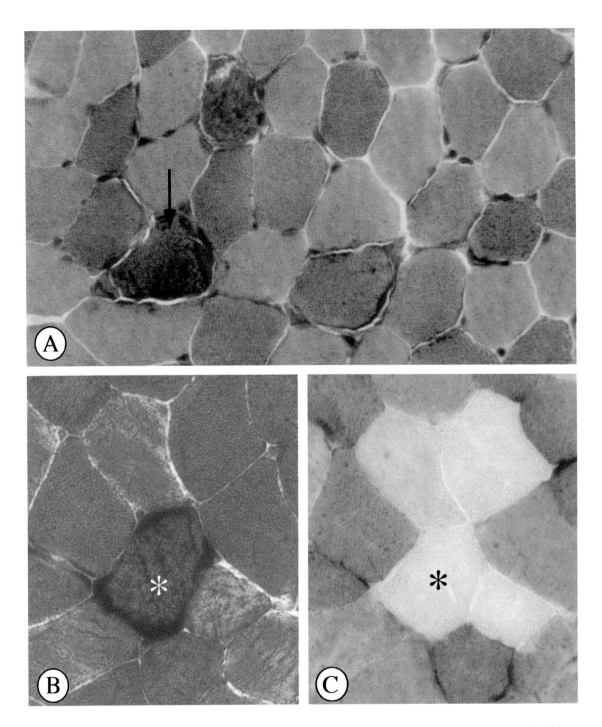

(A) Ragged-red fibers (RRFs) revealed by the modified Gomori trichrome stain. Abnormal accumulations of mitochondria appear as reddish blotches, mostly at the periphery of muscle fibers. (B and C) Serial cross sections from the muscle biopsy of a patient with Kearns–Sayre syndrome. In B, an RRF (asterisk) is highlighted by the histochemical stain for succinate dehydrogenase, which is entirely encoded by nuclear DNA. In C, the same RRF (asterisk) shows no activity for cytochrome c oxidase, an enzyme that contains three subunits encoded by mtDNA. See entry MITOCHONDRIAL ENCEPHALOMYOPATHIES, OVERVIEW.

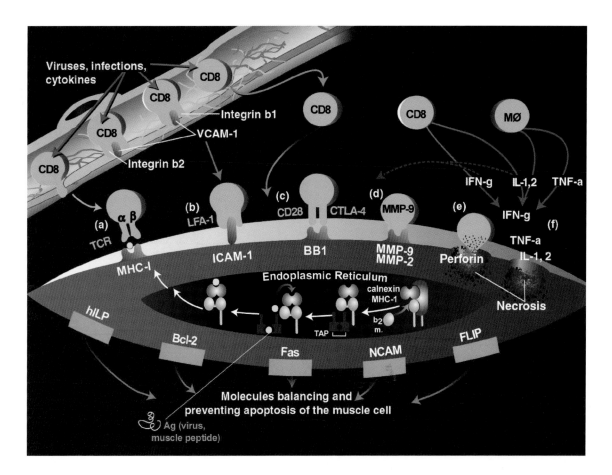

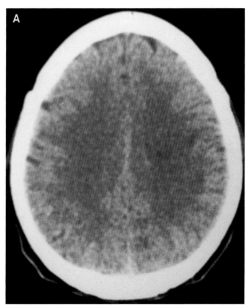

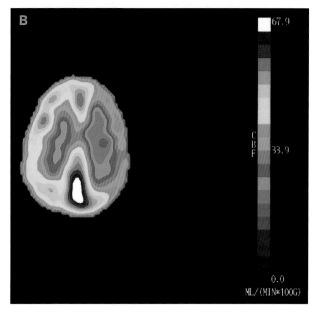

Top: Molecules, receptors, and their ligands involved in exiting of T cells through the endothelial cell wall and recognizing muscle antigens on the surface of muscle fibers. Sequentially, the LFA-I/ICAM-I binding anchors cytoskeletal molecules in the nascent immunological synapse. This allows interaction of TCR/MHC with the sampling of MHC–peptides complex and engagement of BB1 and CD40 costimulatory molecules with their ligands CD28, CTLA, and CD40L—prerequisites for antigen recognition. Metalloproteinases facilitate attachment of T cells to the muscle surface. Muscle fiber necrosis occurs via perforin granules released by the autoinvasive T cells. A direct myocytotoxic effect exerted by released IFN-γ, IL-1, or TNF-α may also occur. See entry MYOSITIS, INFLAMMATORY. Bottom: Structural and functional neuroimages from a man with right carotid occlusion and transient ischemic attacks manifested by left arm and leg weakness. (A) The structural x-ray CT image shows normal gray and white matter in both hemispheres with no evidence of any structural abnormality. (B) The physiological PET cerebral blood flow image shows reduced cerebral blood flow in the part of the brain supplied by the occluded carotid artery. See entry NEUROIMAGING, OVERVIEW.

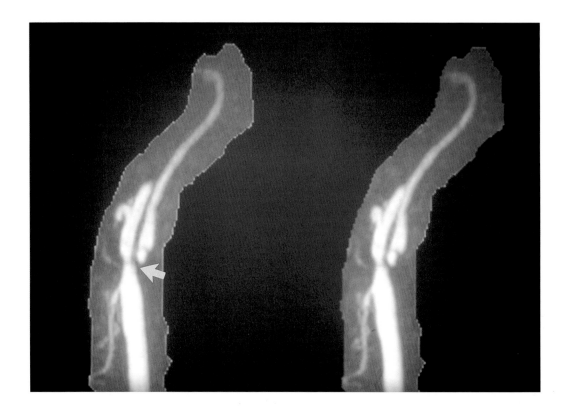

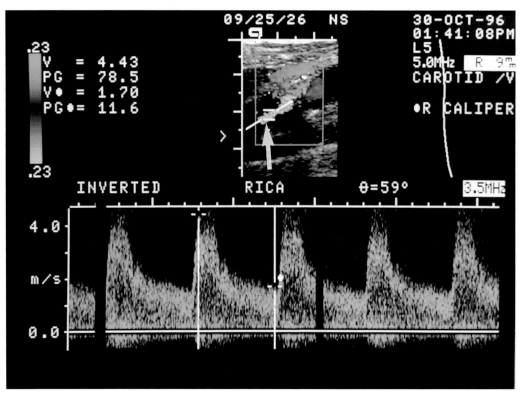

Top: Magnetic resonance angiogram of a high-grade stenosis (arrow) of the origin of the internal carotid artery. Bottom: Color Doppler ultrasound of a high-grade stenosis of the right internal carotid artery. The Doppler cursor (arrow) is placed at the site of the highest velocity. The waveform on the lower aspect of the figure shows high peak systolic velocities, consistent with a high-grade stenosis, and high diastolic flow rates, characteristic of the low-resistance cerebral circulation. See entry NEURORADIOLOGY, DIAGNOSTIC.

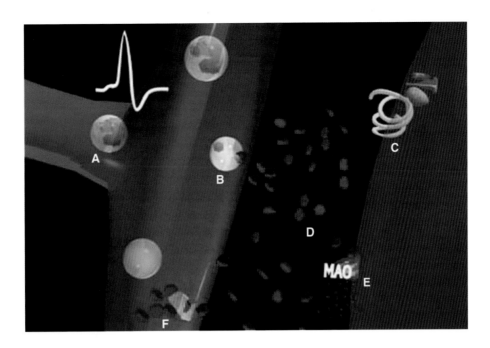

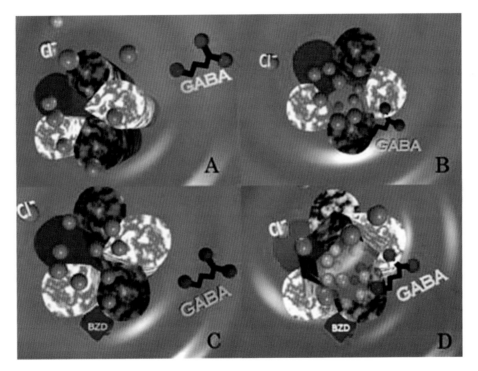

Top: The synthesis, storage, action, and termination of norepinephrine, a representative brain neurotransmitter. (A) Norepinephrine is synthesized in the nerve cell and packaged into vesicles. In preparation for release, these vesicles are transported to the nerve terminal. (B) Upon arrival of an action potential at the axon terminal and the resultant calcium entry, vesicles fuse with the nerve terminal membrane, thereby releasing their contents into the synapse. (C) Released neurotransmitter diffuses across the synaptic cleft and can interact with postsynaptic receptor targets to cause excitatory or inhibitory postsynaptic potentials and/or stimulate second messenger systems. Termination of the response is accomplished by removing free neurotransmitter from the synapse. (D) Simple diffusion can carry the neurotransmitter out of the synapse, or (E) enzymes [e.g., monoamineoxidase (MAO)] can degrade or chemically modify the neurotransmitter, rendering it incapable of further action. (F) Finally, reuptake of neurotransmitter back into the presynaptic neuron or into surrounding cells can terminate the signal as well as recycle some of the neurotransmitter. Bottom: Ionotropic receptors (ligand-gated ion channels) are pore-forming proteins that can be activated and opened by neurotransmitter binding. (A) The γ-aminobenzoic acid (GABA) chloride channel is also the site of action of a group of drugs called benzodiazepines (BZDs) (e.g., alprazolam). (B) The receptor is composed of five subunits and allows influx of chloride into the cell when the neurotransmitter GABA binds to it. (C) BZD binding alone is not sufficient to open the channel. (D) The binding of both GABA and BZDs allows greater chloride influx than GABA binding alone. See entry NEUROTRANSMITTER RECEPTORS.

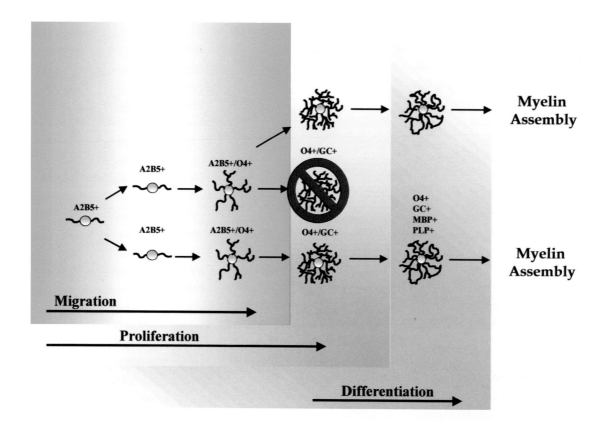

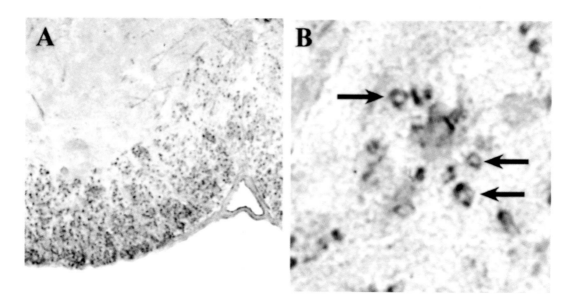

Top: Overview of the development of oligodendrocytes. Immature bipolar oligodendrocyte precursors recognized by labeling with the mAb A2B5 proliferate extensively in response to PDGF, are highly migratory, and mature into multiprocessed pro-oligodendroblasts. Oligodendroblasts proliferate primarily in response to bFGF and can be recognized by labeling with mAb O4. Expression of the major glycolipid of myelin galactocerebroside (GC) and cessation of proliferation accompany differentiation of the precursors into oligodendrocytes. This is a particularly susceptible stage in the lineage, and in the absence of survival signals many of the cells die by apoptosis. Maturation of oligodendrocyte is accompanied by increased expression of myelin components (MBP and PLP) and assembly of the myelin sheath. Bottom: Developing myelin in the mouse spinal cord detected by antibodies to myelin basic protein (MBP). (A) Transverse section through the ventral region of the P7 mouse spinal cord. The myelin develops in a patchy manner, reflecting the differentiation and maturation of individual oligodendrocytes. (B) Higher power micrograph of an individual MBP-labeled oligodendrocyte in the developing spinal cord that is myelinating several adjacent axons (arrows). The MBP myelin sheaths cut in transverse section appear as dark circles with an unlabeled axon in the center. See entry OLIGODENDROCYTES.

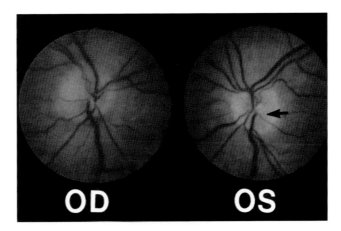

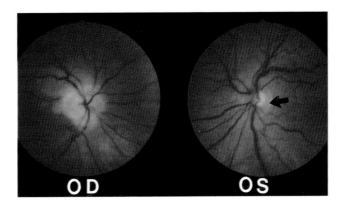

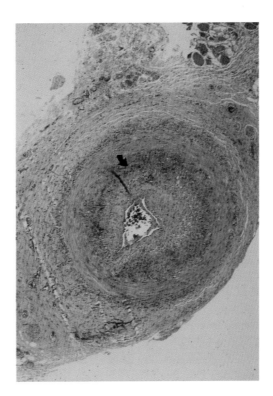

Top: A 68-year-old man had sudden onset of painless visual loss in the right eye. The right optic nerve is edematous. The left optic nerve has a cup to disk ratio of less than 0.1 (arrow). These are typical features of nonarteritic anterior ischemic optic neuropathy. Middle: Milky swelling of the right optic nerve in an 80-year-old patient with giant cell arteritis. The normal left eye has a cup to disk ratio of 0.4 (arrow). Bottom: Positive temporal artery biopsy performed 3 weeks after starting steroids. There are numerous lymphocytes present in the internal elastic lamina (arrow), a pathognomoic sign of arteritis. See entry OPTIC NERVE DISORDERS.

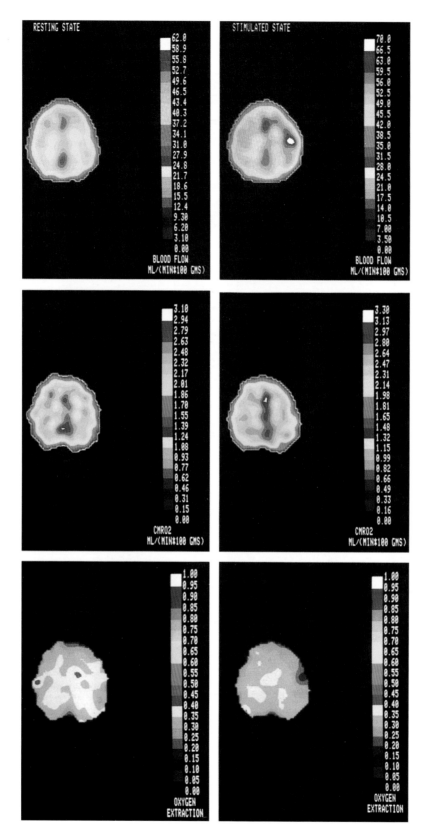

Effect of physiological brain stimulation on regional cerebral blood flow (CBF) and oxygen metabolism. All images are from the same subject. The left-hand column shows images of cerebral blood blow, cerebral oxygen metabolism (CMRO$_2$), and oxygen extraction fraction (OEF) obtained with the eyes closed. OEF is normally uniform throughout the resting brain, reflecting the close coupling of CBF and CMRO$_2$. Corresponding images in the right-hand column were obtained during vibrotactile stimulation of the left fingers. During stimulation, there is increased CBF in the contralateral sensorimotor cortex (top right) but no increase in CMRO$_2$ (middle right). OEF is decreased (lower right), reflecting the fact that CBF has increased more than CMRO$_2$. This decrease in OEF results in increased oxygen content of venous blood which can be detected by BOLD MRI. See entry PHYSIOLOGICAL BRAIN IMAGING.

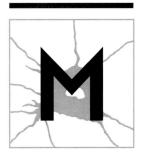

MacEwen, William

Encyclopedia of the Neurological Sciences
Copyright 2003, Elsevier Science (USA). All rights reserved.

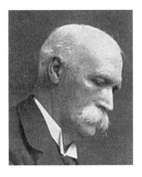

WILLIAM MACEWEN (1848–1924) was born in Scotland. After completing his primary education he attended the University of Glasgow, from which he graduated in 1869. He then became house surgeon at the Royal Infirmary to Sir George MacLeod (1828–1892), the recently appointed successor to Joseph Lister (1827–1912). Later, he accepted an appointment at the Glasgow Fever Hospital at Belvidere to earn extra income. During his tenure here, he started his classic work on laryngeal intubation, which was a revolutionary concept because airway intubation typically required a tracheotomy or laryngotomy.

During this same period, MacEwen continued his education, receiving a medical degree in 1872 from the University of Glasgow—a degree his American colleagues much appreciated because they could address him as "doctor" rather than as "mister." In November 1874, he was elected to the dispensary staff of the Royal Infirmary and began the most productive and illustrious segment of his career. From this point on, MacEwen devoted himself totally to a surgical practice. In 1876, he was appointed surgeon-in-charge of the wards and lecturer in clinical medicine at the School of Medicine at the young age of 28.

MacEwen fully adopted and refined Joseph Lister's principles of antisepsis principles, a key factor in his later success in cerebral surgery. Lister's aseptic principles were based on the use of a carbolic spray misting the operating room during surgery; the surgical instruments and dressings were sterilized with the same solution. MacEwen's operating room was meticulously clean and he required the surgeons to dress in sterilized operating gowns, a dress policy that made him the object of much derision by his colleagues. MacEwen's attention to aseptic details was so great that he would not allow the use of wood or bone-handled surgical instruments and even went so far as to not allow the use of instruments with proprietary engravings out of concern that their crevices could harbor organisms. As reported by many of his students, MacEwen was a tough taskmaster who worked extraordinarily long hours with meticulous attention to detail. When he spoke, his words were considered both instructive and as commands not to be questioned.

In the 1880s, MacEwen flowered to his full potential, becoming one of the leading surgeons in the world. It was a time of incredible productivity, with the earliest period of neurosurgery only just beginning. Having firmly adopted the antiseptic principles of Lister, a surgeon could now operate on the brain with a markedly reduced risk of infection. The recently introduced concepts of cerebral localization gave the surgeon reasonable guidelines of where to look for an intracerebral lesion. MacEwen had avidly followed and put into practice the techniques of Pierre Paul Broca (1824–1881), David Ferrier (1843–1928), and Jean-Martin Charcot (1825–1893) of Paris. He was also concurrently doing experimental work on bone transplants and was advancing important concepts on bone growth. His brilliant presentation at the British Medical Association meeting in Glasgow in 1888 opened to the world the feasibility of safe surgical operations on the brain.

As often happens, certain precipitous events occur that spark the prepared mind to investigate further. In MacEwen's case, this involved an 11-year-old boy who presented with a left frontal skull injury, focal seizures, and aphasia. MacEwen believed that the child had a pyogenic intracerebral abscess located in Broca's area. He requested permission to operate but this request was refused by the family. The family did allow an autopsy, from which MacEwen's hunch of an abscess in Broca's area proved to be correct. From this original case, MacEwen went on to eventually operate on a number of brain lesions and in 1893 published a seminal work in neurosurgery, *Pyogenic Infective Diseases of the Brain and Spinal Cord*. For the first time, a textbook had been produced that was based on antiseptic principles, cerebral localization, and neurological diagnosis and with results that were shockingly good for the time; in fact, the results were so good that no surgeon was able to exceed MacEwen's surgical outcomes until the introduction of antibiotics in the 1930s.

MacEwen's seminal work on pyogenic abscesses influenced a generation of future neurosurgeons, including Hermann Oppenheim (1858–1919), Harvey Cushing (1869–1939), Victor Horsley (1857–1916), Walter Dandy (1886–1946), and Fedor V. Krause (1857–1937).

In 1892, at the age of 44, MacEwen was appointed regius professor of surgery at Glasgow. MacEwen replaced Sir George MacLeod, who had in turn replaced Lord Lister. MacEwen had now come full circle in the academic world: Lister's most illustrious student was now to occupy the regius chair. In writing a testimonial for MacEwen, Lord

Lister made the following observation:

> Dr. MacEwen has acquired more than European fame by the originality and brilliancy of his contributions to surgery. His reputation is eminently calculated to excite the enthusiasm of his students, and to enhance the renown of any school with which he may be connected. He thus possesses claims of the highest order to the vacant chair in the University of Glasgow.

MacEwen received many honors during his lifetime. He was knighted in 1902 and was honored with a number of prestigious corresponding memberships in scientific and surgical societies throughout the world.

Sir William MacEwen, Regius Professor of Surgery at the University of Glasgow and pioneer in the field of cerebral surgery, died on the evening of Saturday, March 22, 1924.

—*James Tait Goodrich*

See also–Broca, Pierre-Paul; Charcot, Jean-Martin; Ferrier, David (see Index entry Biography for complete list of biographical entries)

Further Reading

Bowman, A. K. (1942). *The Life and Teaching of Sir William MacEwen. A Chapter in the History of Surgery*. Hodge, London.

Canale, D. J. (1996). William MacEwen and the treatment of brain abscesses: Revisited after one hundred years. *J. Neurosurg.* 84, 133–142.

Lyons, A. E. (1997). The crucible years 1880–1900: MacEwen to Cushing. In *A History of Neurosurgery in Its Scientific and Professional Contexts* (S. H. Greenblatt, Ed.), pp. 153–166. American Association of Neurological Surgeons, Park Ridge, IL.

MacEwen, W. (1880). Tracheal tubes introduced through the mouth for administration of chloroform during an operation for the removal of an epithelioma from the tongue and pharynx. *Lancet* 2, 906.

MacEwen, W. (1881). Intra-cranial lesions illustrating some points in connexion with the localisation of cerebral affections and the advantages of antiseptic trephining. *Lancet* 2, 541–543, 581–583.

MacEwen, W. (1888). An address on the surgery of the brain and spinal cord delivered at the annual meeting of the British Medical Association held in Glasgow, August 9, 1888. *Br. Med. J.* 2, 302–309, 322–324.

MacEwen, W. (1912). *The Growth of Bone: Observations on Osteogenesis. An Experimental Inquiry into the Development and Reproduction of Diaphyseal Bone*. MacLehose, Glasgow.

Mad Cow Disease

see Bovine Spongiform Encephalopathy

Magendie, François

Encyclopedia of the Neurological Sciences
Copyright 2003, Elsevier Science (USA). All rights reserved.

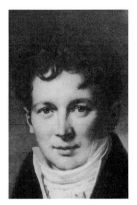

François Magendie (courtesy of the Collège de France, Paris)

FRANÇOIS MAGENDIE (1783–1855) was born the son of a surgeon in Bordeaux, France. The family moved to Paris in 1791, one year before the revolution. At age 16, he became apprenticed to Alexis Boyer (1757–1833), surgeon at the Hôtel Dieu, and Magendie was soon appointed his prosector of anatomy, teaching other students. He became doctor of medicine in 1808 and started experimental research on vegetable poisons. This is often considered the start of experimental pharmacology as a research field. He became prosector of anatomy at the Faculty of Medicine in 1811 but resigned two years later, starting a medical practice and private courses in experimental physiology. According to Claude Bernard (1813–1878), Magendie's successor at the Collège de France, this was the start of a new physiology based on experiments on living animals. The reason for the resignation is an issue of debate. Possibly a conflict with professors at the faculty, including the professor of surgery Guillaume Dupuytren (1777–1835), played a role.

Magendie studied the action of the stomach and, applying emetics, the mechanism of vomiting. In 1816, he published *Précis Élémentaire de Physiologie*, a textbook that would go through four French editions until 1836 and was translated into several languages (American edition in 1845). The physiological experiments covered various aspects, including swallowing, digestion, heart action, blood temperature, and blood sugar. Starting in the 1820s, the nervous system became the major field of his interest. In the second edition of *Précis* (1825) are the experiments on the nervous system that have been referred to often. Despite his dedication to experimental physiology, he did not neglect medical teaching and practice and made his rounds at the Hôtel Dieu hospital. His students considered him impulsive and brusque of manner.

In 1821, he founded *Journal de Physiologie Expérimentale*, to which he added *et Pathologie* one year later. In the second volume are the descriptions of experiments on the spinal roots. He had tried to perform these experiments in the past, but they were difficult to carry out. Finally, he succeeded to cut some lumbar and sacral dorsal roots of eight young puppies without damaging the spinal cord: "I saw it [the hind leg] move in a very obvious manner, although sensibility was still quite extinct in it." He supposed the posterior roots were destined for sensibility and had a different function from that of the anterior roots. The cutting of the anterior roots was more difficult, but Magendie succeeded and observed that "the limb was completely motionless and flaccid, whilst it preserved an unequivocal sensibility." He was able to confirm the results in other animals and by stimulation experiments with galvanic currents. However, he did not state that the respective roots served only sensory or motor functions since he observed some motor function on stimulation of the dorsal roots (which in retrospect must be attributed to reflex phenomena).

Some believed Charles Bell (1774–1842) had priority of the discovery of the function of the posterior and anterior roots. In fact, he only demonstrated that cutting the posterior roots did not influence motion, whereas touching the anterior roots with the point of the knife resulted in convulsion of the back muscles. The results had been printed on a pamphlet that was circulated among acquaintances (1811). Bell interpreted his results supposing that the anterior roots were connected with the cerebrum, conveying motor as well as sensory impressions, whereas the dorsal roots were supposed to be connected with the cerebellum, conveying involuntary impressions (probably autonomic pathways). Thus, he did not indicate the functions of the posterior and anterior roots as clearly as did Magendie. Nevertheless, the law resulting from the experiments by Bell and Magendie (i.e., that the anterior roots convey motor functions and the posterior roots convey sensory functions) is still known as the Bell–Magendie law.

Another phenomenon associated with Magendie's name is the syndrome of Hertwig–Magendie, which is now known as skew deviation, a vertical divergent deviation of the eyes. First described by Karl Heinrich Hertwig (1798–1881), Magendie observed it after dissection of the medial cerebellar peduncle in a rabbit (1825).

In 1828, he described the connection between the subarachnoid space and the fourth ventricle, which is now known as Magendie's foramen. However, he erroneously supposed the cerebrospinal fluid to be produced in the arachnoid membrane and enter the fourth ventricle, pass through the aqueduct, and flow into the lateral ventricles. The paper evoked much criticism abroad.

Throughout his career, Magendie vascillated in his beliefs between 18th century vitalism and the new scientific determinism, and in this respect he stood between François-Xavier Bichat (1771–1802), whose vitalistic ideas he contested, and Claude Bernard.

In 1830, Magendie married the wealthy widow Henriette Bastienne de Puisaye, and 1 year later he was appointed to the chair of medicine at the Collège de France, where he continued the lectures that previously had been given privately. In 1837, he was chosen president of the authoritative Académie des Sciences. In 1841, Claude Bernard became his *préparateur* and in 1847 his *suppléant* (deputy) at the Collège de France. After Magendie died at age 72 in 1855, Bernard succeeded him on the chair at the Collège de France in 1856.

—*Peter Koehler*

See also–Bell, Charles (see Index entry Biography for complete list of biographical entries)

Further Reading

Cranefield, P. F. (1974). *The Way in and the Way out. François Magendie, Charles Bell and the Roots of the Spinal Nerves.* Futura, New York.
Magendie, F. (1822). Expériences sur les fonctions des racines des nerfs rachidiens. *J. Physiol. Exp. Pathol.* **2**, 276–279.
Olmsted, J. M. D. (1944). *François Magendie. Pioneer in Experimental Physiology and Scientific Medicine in the 19th Century France.* Schuman, New York.

Magnetic Resonance Angiography (MRA)

Encyclopedia of the Neurological Sciences
Copyright 2003, Elsevier Science (USA). All rights reserved.

MAGNETIC resonance angiography (MRA) in neurovascular imaging noninvasively images flowing blood in the large blood vessels of the intracranial and extracranial circulations. Clinical MRA techniques include time of flight (TOF), phase contrast (PC), and gadolinium enhancement. The technique chosen depends on the region of interest being imaged, the clinical question being asked, and the capabilities of the available equipment. MRA complements catheter angiography in the diagnostic algorithm for many vascular problems and may replace catheter angiography in certain situations.

Each MRA technique employs a different strategy to distinguish the MR signal coming from the water in blood versus water in surrounding tissues. (The signal measured in MRA comes from the ^{1}H nuclei, or "protons," in water molecules. For simplicity, we use "protons" or "water" to mean water ^{1}H nuclei unless otherwise indicated.) In the TOF technique, multiple radio frequency (RF) pulses are rapidly applied to a selected slice of tissue during image acquisition. Following the series of "saturating" RF pulses, MR signal from water within the slice is suppressed, meaning the tissue appears dark on an MR image. This tissue signal will recover, and the time constant describing the recovery is the T1 relaxation time constant. Tissues with lesser values for T1 recover magnetization or signal more quickly. For brain water at typical magnetic field strength, this recovery takes approximately 1 sec after the last RF pulse. The saturating RF pulses reduce signal from both tissue and blood within the slice, but blood present in the selected slice when the saturating pulses were applied is replaced by incoming, flowing blood that has not been subjected to any saturating RF pulses. The incoming unsaturated blood has greater magnetization or signal compared to the saturated background. When the MR image is obtained, the unsaturated blood will contribute much stronger MR signal to the final image than the saturated tissue. This phenomenon, called flow-related enhancement, is the basis of TOF imaging (Fig. 1).

Two variations of the TOF technique, two-dimensional (2D) and three-dimensional (3D), are widely used in clinical practice. In 2D TOF, MR signal is acquired one slice at a time until a region of interest is covered. For example, more than 50 separate acquisitions are normally used to image the extracranial carotid arteries. A mathematical technique, called a 2D Fourier transform, is used to create a source image of each slice (Fig. 2A). The source images are then analyzed using a maximum intensity projection (MIP) algorithm to form the final MRA. The images are displayed in multiple obliquities to

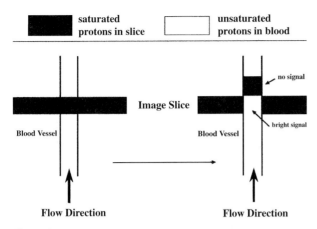

Figure 1
Flow-related enhancement. Unsaturated blood replaces the blood that was present in the slice when the saturation pulse was applied (adapted with permission from Paul Hsieh).

resemble a conventional angiogram (Fig. 2B). The MIP algorithm extracts the brightest pixels in each source image from multiple different projections and then stacks the information to form the final image. One potential source of artifact in this method is related to tissues with protons that recover quickly from the saturating pulse (i.e., have a short T1 relaxation time constant). Examples include protons in fat and water protons in areas of hemorrhage. The MIP algorithm does not discriminate between bright pixels from flow and bright pixels from these other causes. The source images must be carefully reviewed when these factors are present. In 3D TOF, the MR signal is generated from blood flowing through a larger tissue volume or slab. The entire slab is saturated with rapid RF pulses. Phase encoding gradients in two directions and a readout gradient in the third dimension and are used to partition the MR signal collected from the slab. These data are decoded into source images using a 3D Fourier transform (Fig. 3A). Source images are then transformed into the final MRA using a MIP algorithm similar to 2D MRA (Fig. 3B).

In both 2D and 3D TOF, flowing blood is evaluated predominately in one chosen direction. Blood flowing in the opposite direction may cause unwanted signal. In the evaluation of the extracranial carotid arteries, for instance, only signal from arterial flow is desired. Signal from the jugular veins flowing in the opposite direction may interfere with interpretation of the MR angiogram. Saturation bands are used to eliminate this type of signal. Applying RF pulses to a band of tissue distal to the selected slice or slab saturates the blood flowing into the region of interest from the opposite direction and prevents this blood from contributing any signal to the final image. While imaging the cervical extracranial carotid arteries, a superior saturation band is positioned over the intracranial dural sinuses to eliminate interference from the jugular veins.

Two phenomena may cause areas of signal loss in both 2D and 3D TOF techniques. Blood that travels within rather than through an imaged slice or slab remains in the imaged volume for a longer period of time. This blood is subjected to a number of RF pulses and thereby becomes partially saturated. This phenomenon, called in-plane saturation, decreases contrast between flowing blood and stationary tissue. For this reason, normal flow in a section of a tortuous vessel that travels within a slice of tissue may be misinterpreted as an area of absent blood flow.

Intravoxel dephasing also may cause signal loss in TOF images. A voxel represents the smallest unit of volume from which an MR signal is obtained. Magnetic field gradients are applied during RF pulses in order to provide spatial localization. Protons in blood moving through the magnetic gradient obtain phase shifts proportional to their velocity. A voxel must contain protons with similar or coherent phase to contribute adequate signal. If all the protons in blood are traveling at the same velocity, they will acquire the same net phase shift and signal will be recovered. If blood is traveling at different velocities, protons will acquire different phase shifts. Voxels

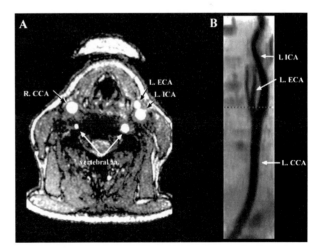

Figure 2
(A) 2D TOF source image of the neck. (B) 2D TOF MIP image of the left carotid artery. Dotted line represents the level of the source image. Only the left carotid is shown. CCA, common carotid artery; ECA, external carotid artery; ICA, internal carotid artery.

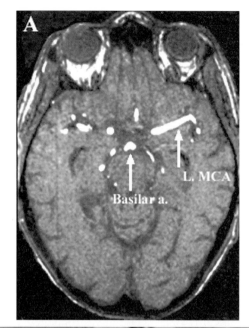

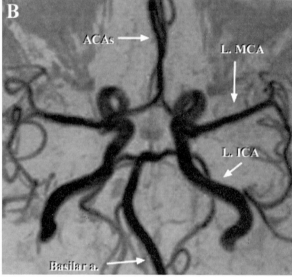

Figure 3
(A) 3D TOF source image of the circle of Willis. (B) 3D MIP image of the circle of Willis. L. MCA, left middle cerebral artery; ACAs, anterior cerebral arteries; L. ICA, left internal carotid artery.

vessels. Intravoxel dephasing also may cause signal loss in stenotic vessels. Areas of stenosis, commonly found in patients with atherosclerotic disease, may cause turbulent blood flow, which is characterized by an increased range of velocities. This may lead to an area of signal loss even when flow is present. Overestimating the degree of stenosis or misinterpreting a high-grade stenosis as an occlusion may result. Adjusting imaging parameters can help offset the signal loss from intravoxel dephasing.

In 3D TOF, signal from incoming unsaturated blood must traverse a thicker slab during the image acquisition than in 2D TOF. The number of saturating RF pulses affecting the blood increases with the slab thickness. Near the distal end of the slab the blood becomes partially saturated and loses contrast with the background tissue. This limits the slab thickness in 3D TOF. Acquiring the imaged volume in multiple overlapping thin section acquisitions (MOTSA) may diminish the loss of signal resulting from a thicker slab. The circle of Willis, for example, is often acquired as two separate slabs. 3D TOF is also less sensitive in detecting slow flow compared to 2D TOF. With slower flow, blood is also affected by more saturating RF pulses as it crosses the slab and consequently loses signal. Advanced techniques have been developed to compensate for the previously mentioned effects and maintain adequate contrast between blood and stationary tissue.

The fundamental difference between 2D and 3D TOF is the way in which the source images are acquired. 2D TOF collects data for source images one slice at a time. The data collected from each slice are directly transformed into one source image. 3D TOF collects data from an entire region of interest. Data are then mathematically decoded into separate source images. 3D TOF achieves greater spatial resolution and signal to noise ratios than 2D TOF but is limited by the slab thickness and longer imaging times. 3D TOF MRA is commonly used for the intracranial arterial vasculature. A typical study requires between 12 and 15 min. 2D and 3D TOF MRA are often used together to image the extracranial carotid arteries. Because it is faster, 2D TOF is used to image the entire course of the extracranial carotid artery from the aortic arch to the skull base. 3D TOF limited to the carotid bifurcation region may then be performed in a reasonable amount of time. This provides higher resolution of this area, where most clinically significant stenoses occur. These sequences require approximately 5 and

that contain protons with different or incoherent phases will contribute less or no signal. This phenomenon is referred to as intravoxel dephasing. Intravoxel dephasing commonly results in normal vessels due to laminar flow. Laminar flow causes the velocity of blood to vary between the periphery and center of a blood vessel. The widest range of velocities occurs near the edge of the vessel. This causes artifactual signal loss near the edges of normal

7 min, respectively. The quality of the study in both techniques may be compromised by patient motion. In 2D TOF, patient motion and pulsatile fluctuations in the size of blood vessels may result in a staircase artifact due to slight misalignment between slices.

Recent work with gadolinium-enhanced 3D MRA in neurovascular imaging is very promising and this technique is replacing TOF techniques at many centers. Gadolinium is an intravascular contrast agent used in MRI that shortens the T1 relaxation time constant of nearby water protons. Gadolinium-enhanced MRA is based on the marked shortening effect of gadolinium on the T1 relaxation time constant of water protons in blood compared to stationary tissue. Because of the shortened T1 relaxation time constant, the magnetization of blood recovers more quickly than the stationary tissue and contributes more signal. Excellent contrast between flowing blood and stationary background tissue results because most image acquisition is performed during the first pass of gadolinium, when it is confined to the intravascular space. Rapid imaging time is possible since magnetization in blood recovers quickly. The reduced imaged time helps decrease the number of problems related to patient motion. Using this method, the aortic arch to the base of the skull may be imaged in less than 30 sec. A thicker slab than 3D TOF may be imaged because the quick recovery of magnetization from blood eliminates the saturation effects related to traveling through a thick slab of tissue. In-plane saturation and intravoxel dephasing effects that complicate TOF are also reduced. Appropriately timing the onset of imaging following gadolinium injection, interference from venous signal, and rapid digital collection strategies are the main challenges of gadolinium-enhanced MRA. More powerful and faster magnetic field gradients and novel methods of collecting and organizing the MR signal continue to improve gadolinium-enhanced MRA.

Phase contrast (PC) is another useful MRA technique for selected applications. This method is based on the phase shift that moving protons acquire when they pass through a magnetic field gradient as described previously. Stationary protons do not develop a phase shift. PC requires acquisition of two data sets for each area that is imaged. A bipolar motion-sensitive gradient is used to induce a phase shift in moving protons. The only difference between the two acquisitions is the reversal of this gradient. Moving protons will develop opposite phase shifts during the two acquisitions. Signal from stationary tissue in the two data sets will be identical since no phase shift occurs during either acquisition. Subtraction of the two data sets thus eliminates signal from stationary tissue, leaving signal only from flowing blood. This eliminates the artifacts caused by tissues with short T1 relaxation time on TOF images discussed earlier.

The PC technique may be adjusted to target flow of certain velocities. This is particularly useful in areas of slow flow and may be useful in distinguishing slow flow from occlusions. The PC technique is very useful, for instance, in MR venography for discriminating normal slow venous flow from venous sinus thrombosis. PC MRA also allows imaging of thicker slabs than does 3D TOF. PC MRA is hampered by longer acquisition times since multiple data sets must be obtained for a given region of interest. This technique is very sensitive to motion artifact.

MRA complements conventional angiography in many clinical situations, and in certain situations it is the study of choice. The most common indication for MRA is evaluating the degree of stenosis of the extracranial carotid arteries. Multiple large studies have defined the role of carotid endarterectomy versus medical therapy in the treatment of patients with carotid atherosclerotic disease depending on the severity of stenosis and the presence or absence of symptoms. In these trials, the degree of carotid stenosis was determined by catheter angiography. Numerous studies have attempted to define the accuracy of MRA in measuring the severity of stenosis compared with catheter angiography. Various clinical strategies now incorporate screening MRA into the decision of whether a patient should have surgery or be treated with medical therapy. If the MRA is normal or demonstrates mild stenosis, one may avoid the possible complications and cost of catheter angiography. If moderate to severe stenosis is present and surgery is being considered, catheter angiography is usually needed for further evaluation. Some surgeons, however, will operate based on MRA and Doppler ultrasound results without catheter angiography.

MRA may incidentally detect intracranial aneurysms and be used to screen for intracranial aneurysms in carefully selected situations. Small aneurysms (<5 mm), aneurysms located in tortuous sections of vessels or near the petrous bone, and aneurysms with slow flow or thrombus all pose challenges to detection with MRA. Correlation with standard MRI of the brain should always be performed to evaluate for a potentially thrombosed aneurysm or aneurysm with slow flow that is not visualized with MRA. Some investigators advocate MRA screening in certain high-risk patients, such as those with adult polycystic kidney disease or a family history of aneurysms, but the benefit is controversial. It must be remembered that the sensitivity for detecting aneurysms is lower than that of catheter angiography and the consequences of a missed aneurysm are potentially devastating. MRA does not have any routine role in aneurysm detection or evaluation in the acute setting of subarachnoid hemorrhage or symptoms.

MRA can also add valuable information by identifying occluded or diseased vessels in stroke patients. MRA may be the initial study of choice for suspected carotid or vertebral artery dissections, an important cause of stroke in young and middle-aged patients. (Dissections are caused by hemorrhage into the wall of a blood vessel. This results in narrowing of the lumen of the vessel that may be detected with MRA.) Correlation with the source images and standard MRI sequences for areas of hemorrhage within the vessel wall increases the sensitivity for detecting dissections. Rarer causes of vascular disease, such as Takayasu's arteritis, fibromuscular dysplasia, and moyamoya, may also be detected with MRA.

MRA is a very useful method to noninvasively image intracranial and extracranial circulations. MRA provides an important complementary role to catheter angiography in many cases. In certain situations, the cost and potential risks of catheter angiography may be avoided. MR angiograms can be generated using a variety of techniques. Each exam should be tailored to best address the clinical question at hand. As equipment and sequences improve, MRA will play an even larger role in neurovascular imaging.

—Dave Jeck, Jeff Neil, and Robert McKinstry

See also–Angiography; Cerebral Angiography; Computerized Axial Tomography (CAT); Magnetic Resonance Imaging (MRI); Neuroimaging, Overview; Neuroradiology, Diagnostic; Physiological Brain Imaging; Positron Emission Tomography (PET); Single-Photon Emission Computed Tomography (SPECT)

Further Reading

Amoli, S. R., and Turski, P. A. (1999). The role of MR angiography in the evaluation of acute stroke. *Neuroimaging Clin. North Am.* **9**, 423–438.

Atlas, S. W. (1994). MR angiography in neurologic disease. *Radiology* **193**, 1–16.

Executive Committee for the Asymptomatic Carotid Atherosclerosis Study (1995). Endarterectomy for asymptomatic carotid artery stenosis. *J. Am. Med. Assoc.* **273**, 1421–1428.

Leclerc, X., Gauvrit, J. Y., Nicol, L., *et al.* (1999). Contrast-enhanced MR angiography of the craniocervical vessels: A review. *Neuroradiology* **41**, 867–874.

North American Symptomatic Carotid Endarterectomy Trial Collaborators (1991). Beneficial effect of carotid endarterectomy in symptomatic patients with high-grade carotid stenosis. *N. Engl. J. Med.* **325**, 445–453.

Mitchell, D. G. (1999). Vascular techniques. *MRI Principles*, pp. 237–255. Saunders, Philadelphia.

Rosovsky, M. A., Litt, A. W., and Krinsky, G. (1996). Magnetic resonance carotid angiography of the neck. Clinical implications. *Neuroimaging Clin. North Am.* **6**, 863–874.

Wardlaw, J. M., and White, P. M. (2000). The detection and management of unruptured intracranial aneurysms. *Brain* **123**, 205–221.

Magnetic Resonance Imaging (MRI)

Encyclopedia of the Neurological Sciences

IN STANDARD magnetic resonance imaging (MRI), an image is constructed using signal from the ^{1}H nuclei in tissues. One reason for choosing this particular nucleus is that a substantial fraction of the human body is made up of water, which contains ^{1}H. Furthermore, the concentration equivalent of ^{1}H nuclei in water is on the order of 110 M. For comparison, the concentration of sodium in the body, which is also MR detectable, is approximately 1000 times smaller (approximately 40 mM). Thus, the water ^{1}Hx signal offers an unparalleled signal-to-noise ratio for imaging.

A major step in obtaining an MR image is to distinguish radio frequency (RF) signal coming from ^{1}H atoms in various parts of the body—that is, to spatially localize them. In general, all water ^{1}H atoms have the same resonance frequency and phase unless steps are taken to cause them to vary from location to location. As described previously, the resonance frequency for a particular MR-detectable nucleus is directly related to the magnetic field (B_{eff}) surrounding the nucleus. Most imaging methods exploit this relationship to cause the resonance frequency and/or phase of water ^{1}H to vary with position in such a way as to make MRI possible.

Historically, a number of approaches have been used to ensure that the water hydrogen nuclei at different locations in the body have different signal characteristics. One of the first was to create a magnet in which the main magnetic field is saddle shaped. The saddle-shaped field is very inhomogeneous except at a single point in the center of the magnet. Since resonance frequency is proportional to B_{eff}, the ^{1}H atoms at the center of the inhomogeneous magnetic field have a characteristic and unique resonance frequency when compared with ^{1}H nuclei in other locations. Using this method, an RF pulse can be applied at the resonance frequency corresponding to ^{1}H nuclei at the center of the magnetic field, exciting only nuclei at that location. The RF signal received following the excitation can be filtered in such a way as to measure only that resonance frequency corresponding to the single point in the magnet. For this method, the magnet contains a motorized bed that moves the patient through the magnetic field in a stepwise fashion. The MR experiment is repeated point by point until a sufficient number of points have been obtained to produce an image. This method was referred to as field-focused nuclear magnetic resonance (FONAR) and developed by Raymond Damadian at the Down State Medical Center of the University of New York. Although this method created some of the first MR images, it is far too slow to be practical.

More practical approaches to MRI involve the application of magnetic field gradients. In contrast to the scanner described previously, modern MR scanners are designed so that the main magnetic field is very uniform. To alter the shape of the main magnetic field, special coils of wire are included in the bore of the magnet. When current is passed through these coils of wire, they cause a carefully controlled distortion of the main magnetic field. The resulting magnetic field gradient causes the magnetic field (B_{eff}) to vary in a linear fashion through space. The gradient coils can be switched on and off at will during imaging and magnetic field gradients can be applied in any orientation desired (e.g., from the front to back of the magnet, side to side, and up and down). If a magnetic field gradient is applied to a sample, the water molecules at different locations have different resonance frequencies because B_{eff} varies with position. The spectrum (i.e., the plot of signal amplitude vs frequency) of the signal obtained while the gradients are turned on represents a profile of the sample as shown in Fig. 1. If the strength of the magnetic field gradient is known, then the resonance frequency (in units of hertz) on the abscissa can be replaced with location in the magnet (in units of

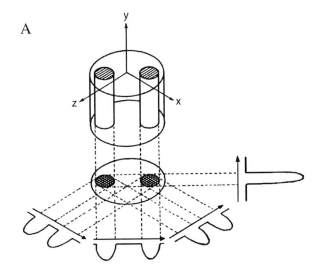

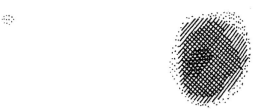

Figure 1
(A) The relationship between a three-dimensional object, its two-dimensional projection along the y axis, and four one-dimensional projections at 45° intervals in the xz plane. The arrows indicate the applied gradient direction corresponding to each projection. (B) An MR image made of two glass capillary tubes filled with water and oriented as indicated in A (adapted with permission from Lauterbur, 1973).

centimeters). Several different profiles of the sample can be combined to reconstruct an image using a method known as filtered back projection. The concept of associating frequency and location was originally described by one of the pioneers of MRI methods, Paul Lauterbur, at State University of New York, Stony Brook. He applied the term "zeugmatography" to this idea. Although the term never caught on, the method of employing linear magnetic field gradients remains the cornerstone of modern MRI.

In a further key advance, Richard Ernst at the Swiss Federal Institute of Technology in Zurich (and a winner of the 1991 Nobel Prize in chemistry) demonstrated how to manipulate the magnetic field gradients so that a two-dimensional Fourier transform could be employed to reconstruct MR images efficiently. Present-day MRI is most commonly done using variations on this Fourier refinement of the filtered back projection method. In a typical imaging sequence (Fig. 2), a gradient is turned on during application of the RF pulse. As described previously, this causes the resonance frequency of water ^{1}H in the sample being imaged to vary linearly with position. A frequency-selective RF pulse is then applied so that nuclei within only a slice of the sample are excited. Once this is accomplished, the "slice-select" magnetic field gradient pulse is turned off. A second magnetic field gradient pulse is then applied perpendicular to the slice-select gradient. This phase encode magnetic field gradient pulse has the effect of causing the resonance phase to vary linearly along one direction of the face of the excited slice. Finally, a readout gradient is applied during signal acquisition, orthogonal to the first two, so that frequency varies linearly across the second direction within the slab during acquisition. The differences in phase and frequency can be used to assign signal amplitudes to the points (known as voxels) within the slice. Numerous adaptations of this basic sequence have been developed, each optimized for a particular body system, use, or situation. For example, fast imaging sequences, in which an image

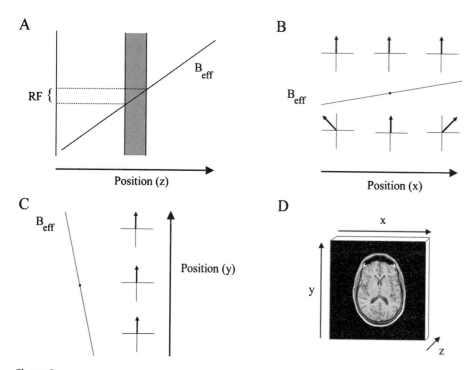

Figure 2

Methods of spatial encoding for MRI. (A) A slice-selective RF pulse. When a slice-select magnetic field gradient is applied, B_{eff} varies linearly along the z axis of the magnet as shown. Since the resonance frequency of ^{1}H atoms is proportional to B_{eff}, it is possible to apply an RF pulse with a carefully chosen frequency bandwidth such that it excites ^{1}H atoms within only a "slice" of the sample as represented by the shaded area. (B) A phase encoding magnetic field gradient pulse, which is applied next. The three arrows in the top row represent three ^{1}H atoms at different positions along the x axis of the excited slice. Prior to the application of the phase encoding magnetic field gradient pulse, all three atoms have the same resonance frequency and phase so the arrows can be viewed as turning clockwise in synchrony. While the gradient pulse is applied, the atom in the left is in a lower B_{eff} and has a lower resonance frequency. It can thus be thought of as slowing down its rotation and falling behind the other atoms. Likewise, the atom on the right is in a higher B_{eff} and rotates faster, moving ahead of the other atoms. When the gradient pulse is turned off, the three atoms once again rotate at the same frequency, although now they are out of phase with one another. As shown in the bottom row, the phase difference is a function of position. (C) Application of the readout gradient. Again, three ^{1}H atoms are shown, although they are not the same three shown in B. These three atoms are all at the same position along the x axis of the sample and hence all have the same phase. A magnetic field gradient pulse is applied during signal acquisition as shown. This has the effect of causing signal frequency to vary with position while the signal is detected. By assigning signal intensities to locations within the selected slice based on phase and frequency, an image can be reconstructed as shown in D.

of a slice is obtained in a few tens of milliseconds, are used to image the beating heart. Advances in MR pulse sequence design, magnet system hardware design, and image analysis methods continue to occur at a rapid pace.

In the images shown in Fig. 3, there is contrast (difference in signal intensity) between various brain regions, such as gray matter and white matter. If all the signal arises from ^{1}H atoms in water molecules, what distinguishes water in gray matter from water in white matter? The answer lies in the fact that gray and white matter provide different microenvironments for water molecules and this affects some of their MR properties. Two such properties are the T1 and T2 relaxation time constants. Although a detailed description of these relaxation mechanisms is beyond the scope of this entry, it is possible to obtain the image in such a way that the intensity of the signal from a given region depends on the T1 or T2 relaxation time constant of the water in that region. Such images are referred to as T1-weighted and T2-weighted images, respectively. Other common forms of contrast include contrast based on the translational motion of water (diffusion imaging) and contrast based on the level of blood oxygenation (functional MRI). It is also possible to alter pulse sequences so that signal arises only from moving blood within blood vessels, making MR angiography possible. MRI methods have likewise been developed for assessing tissue perfusion

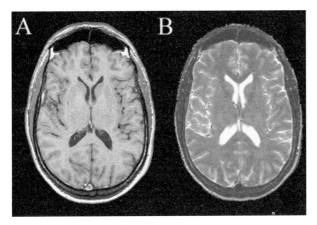

Figure 3
Two axial images from the level of the basal ganglia in a human. (A) Image is T1 weighted. Note that white matter is brightest, gray matter is less bright, and CSF spaces are darkest. (B) Image is a T2-weighted image of the same slice. Note that white matter is darkest, gray matter is somewhat brighter, and CSF is brightest. The differences in signal intensity in the images are due to the relative water T1 (A) and T2 (B) relaxation time constants.

either with or without the addition of exogenous contrast agents.

Another means by which to obtain more information from MR images is the use of contrast agents. A common approach is to make an intravenous injection of a compound that decreases the T1 relaxation time constant of water that comes into contact with it (e.g., a gadolinium-containing compound). Such agents typically are confined to the intravascular space except where the blood–brain barrier (BBB) is disrupted. As a result, they cause signal on T1-weighted images to be bright in areas of high vascularity or BBB disruption. These compounds are analogous to the contrast agents used for computed tomography (CT) scanning. A more sophisticated approach is to administer contrast agents that are relatively concentrated in brain areas dependent on factors other than vascularity or BBB integrity. One contrast agent, which has been used in animals but is thus far impractical for human use, is manganese. Being a calcium analog, manganese is taken up and trapped preferentially in electrically active presynaptic terminals, where it decreases water T1 relaxation time constant. Thus, manganese infused into the brain (because it does not cross the BBB well) will highlight areas of activation. Furthermore, this contrast enhancement persists for hours following infusion. Similar contrast agents are currently under development for human use and for detection of a wide variety of compounds or physiological states.

MRI is the central nervous system (CNS) imaging modality of choice for many clinical situations, including the detection of CNS tumors, infection, stroke, and malformations. MRI offers unparalleled clarity for images of the brainstem and spinal cord—regions in which CT images suffer from beam-hardening artifact caused by the surrounding bony structures. MRI also offers better contrast between white and gray matter than does CT. On the other hand, CT offers advantages for evaluation of acute intracranial hemorrhage, intracranial calcification, bony lesions, and emergency scanning following trauma. With regard to evaluation of bone, MRI does not typically provide detailed bony anatomy because bone has relatively less water than soft tissues and hence provides less signal from which to construct an image. It is interesting to note, however, that MR of bone can be used to detect the bone edema that accompanies fracture. In certain circumstances, MR has been used to detect nondisplaced fractures of the wrist and knee before they become detectable by conventional CT or x-ray.

When considering an MR scan for a patient, two other factors should be taken into account. The first is risk to the patient. MR scanner magnets tend to be large, with the patient placed into a cylindrical space approximately 3 ft in diameter and 10 ft deep. This may present a problem for markedly obese patients, who do not fit in the scanner, or patients with claustrophobia, who may not tolerate the enclosed space. In addition, quick access to the patient in the event of an emergency is somewhat hindered. Of note, MR magnets of newer design tend to be more open and are comparable to CT scanners for patient access. Another factor is the presence of the strong magnetic field required for MR scanning. This field affects nearby equipment, particularly electric motors and metal components such as syringe pumps or gas cylinders. For example, patients requiring assisted ventilation must be maintained with a specially designed, MR-compatible mechanical ventilator or be ventilated by hand. Furthermore, the field may affect cardiac pacemakers or implanted metal hardware from orthopedic procedures. The second consideration is cost. The cost of MR scans is two or three times that of CT scans and much more than that of conventional x-ray studies. As with all medical diagnostic studies, the relative risks and benefits should be weighed carefully.

—*Jeff Neil*

See also–Computerized Axial Tomography; Magnetic Resonance Angiography; Magnetic Resonance, Overview; Magnetic Resonance Spectroscopy; Neuroimaging, Overview; Neuroradiology, Diagnostic; Physiological Brain Imaging; Positron Emission Tomography

Further Reading

Damadian, R. (1980). Field focusing NMR (FONAR) and the formation of chemical images in man. *Philos. Trans. R. Soc. London B* **289**, 503–510.

Kumar, A., Welti, D., and Ernst, R. R. (1975). NMR Fourier zeugmatography. *J. Magn. Reson.* **18**, 69–83.

Lauterbur, P. (1973). Image formation by induced local interactions: Examples employing nuclear magnetic resonance. *Nature* **242**, 190–191.

Lin, Y.-J., and Koretsky, A. P. (1997). Manganese enhances T1-weighted MRI during brain activation: An approach to direct imaging of brain function. *Magn. Reson. Med.* **38**, 378–388.

Vaughan, B. (1989). A short illustrated history of magnetic resonance imaging. *Austr. Radiol.* **33**, 390–398.

Magnetic Resonance (MR), Overview

Encyclopedia of the Neurological Sciences

THE PHENOMENON of nuclear magnetic resonance (NMR) in bulk materials was discovered independently and virtually simultaneously in 1946 by two research groups—Bloch, Hansen, and Packard at Stanford University and Purcell, Torrey, and Pound at Harvard University. Bloch and Purcell shared the Nobel Prize for physics in 1952 for their discovery. A relatively simple description of this phenomenon is that it represents the net absorption of electromagnetic energy by nuclei of a naturally occurring, nonradioactive isotope referred to as a nuclear spin system. In more concrete terms, if a nuclear spin system (e.g., a glass of water) is placed in a magnetic field, it is possible to excite the nuclei (hydrogen atoms in the water) using a radio frequency (RF) pulse. This excitation causes the hydrogen atomic nuclei to make the transition between ground and excited spin states and vice versa—stimulated absorption and emission—as predicted by quantum mechanics. In the original experiments by Bloch and Purcell, RF energy was applied to the sample at a series of RF frequencies. A very slight excess absorption of RF energy was measured at the frequency corresponding to the energy difference between the ground and excited states of the spin system. In addition to detection of magnetic resonance by RF absorption, excitation of a nuclear spin system creates a nonequilibrium spin state that can be detected using an RF antenna or receiver. The frequencies and intensities at which the electromagnetic field interacts with the spin system contain considerable information about the physical environment of the nuclei being studied. In modern pulsed Fourier transform NMR experiments, it is the nonequilibrium response of the sample's spin system that is measured as an RF signal composed of signal frequencies and intensities.

One characteristic of magnetic resonance (MR) is that the energies involved are very small—many orders of magnitude smaller than the typical energy of a chemical bond. As a result, the method is nondestructive. It has been safely and routinely applied to human subjects in the form of magnetic resonance imaging (MRI).

A second characteristic is that not all atomic nuclei are MR detectable; only those that possess nonzero nuclear angular momentum or "spin" are detectable. Typically, these are nuclei that are nonradioactive, although there are exceptions. For example, all three isotopes of hydrogen, ^{1}H ("protons"), ^{2}H (deuterium), and ^{3}H (tritium), are MR detectable. ^{1}H is the naturally abundant isotope, meaning that 99.98% of hydrogen atoms in a glass of ordinary water are ^{1}H. ^{2}H is a rare, nonradioactive isotope of hydrogen and comprises only 0.015% of the hydrogen atoms in an ordinary glass of water. Finally, ^{3}H, which is present at even lower concentrations than ^{2}H, is both radioactive and MR detectable. Each of these isotopes of hydrogen has its own characteristic radiofrequency, or resonance frequency, when placed in a magnetic field. This difference in resonance frequencies makes it possible to distinguish the various isotopes from one another in NMR experiments. In contrast to hydrogen, the naturally most abundant isotope of oxygen, ^{18}O, is not MR detectable, whereas the ^{17}O isotope is (0.04% natural abundance). Other nuclei that are MR detectable include phosphorus (^{31}P, ~100% natural abundance), carbon (^{13}C, 0.01%), sodium (^{23}Na, ~100%), fluorine (^{19}F, ~100%), and many others. It is worth noting that electrons, which have spin magnetic moments, are detectable through electron spin resonance.

Since its discovery, MR has found a myriad of uses. In medicine, it provides static anatomic images as well as maps of tissue activation and blood flow. It has been used to determine the structure of complex biomolecules such as proteins. Furthermore, MR spectra can be obtained from solid samples and MR has made contributions to material science. MR has been used by the food industry to determine moisture content of food during processing. MRI of seeds provides information regarding their composition prior to planting. MR has even been used by oil explorers in well logging (a small MR probe is lowered into the sample, which in this case is the ground).

—*Jeff Neil*

See also—Computerized Axial Tomography; Magnetic Resonance Angiography; Magnetic Resonance Imaging; Magnetic Resonance Spectroscopy; Neuroimaging, Overview; Neuroradiology, Diagnostic; Physiological Brain Imaging

Further Reading

Bloch, F. (1946). Nuclear induction. *Phys. Rev.* **70**, 460–474.
Purcell, E. M., Torrey, H. C., and Pound, R. V. (1946). Resonance absorption by nuclear magnetic moments in a solid. *Phys. Rev.* **69**, 37–38.

Magnetic Resonance Spectroscopy (MRS)

Encyclopedia of the Neurological Sciences

ANALYSIS of the levels (or frequencies) at which energy is absorbed (or emitted) by a nuclear spin system may provide considerable information about the system. The precise resonance frequency of a given nucleus is determined by two factors: the magnetogyric ratio of the particular nucleus being studied (γ, a physical constant that is unique for a particular nucleus) and the magnetic field (B_{eff}) in which it resides at the time of the magnetic resonance (MR) experiment. This relationship can be written as

$$\omega = \gamma \times B_{eff}$$

where ω is the resonance frequency. In a magnetic field (B_{eff}) of 11.8 T, for example, the resonance frequency of ^{1}H atoms is 500 MHz. Thus, an MR study of ^{1}H in an 11.8-T magnet would be done using radio frequency (RF) excitation and detection at a frequency of 500 MHz (about five times that of a typical FM radio station). On the other hand, if one wished to study deuterium (^{2}H) in the same magnetic field, one would use a frequency of 76.8 MHz because ^{2}H has its own characteristic value for γ. A magnetic field of 11.8 T is considered quite strong by today's standards and is nearly 250,000 times that of the earth's magnetic field.

The RF signal obtained from an MR sample contains fine gradations in the resonance frequencies for particular atoms in a molecule. This is due to the fact that some atoms are relatively more shielded from the applied magnetic field than others. This frequency shift, referred to as the chemical shift, is caused by shielding of nuclei by nearby electrons. This shielding causes the B_{eff} for a particular ^{1}H atom in an 11.8-T magnetic field to be slightly less than 11.8 T. The resultant chemical shifts are quite small relative to the overall resonance frequency. For example, the spectrum of ethanol (HO–CH$_2$–CH$_3$) shown in Fig. 1 was obtained at 500 MHz. In this example, the abscissa of the spectrum is the resonance (RF signal) frequency and the ordinate is the resonance (RF signal) amplitude. The resonance frequency is typically expressed as parts per million (ppm). In Fig. 1, 1 ppm corresponds to one-millionth of 500 MHz, or 500 Hz. As shown in the spectrum,

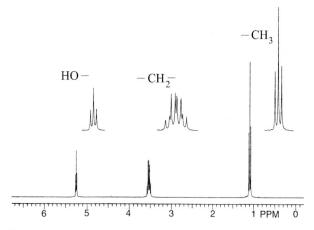

Figure 1
A ^{1}H MR spectrum of dry ethanol. The abscissa is the chemical shift in parts per million (ppm). The ordinate represents the relative resonance amplitude. Each resonance line contains a multiplet structure that is expanded as an inset. The multiplet at 5.2 ppm corresponds to the OH group, the one at 3.5 ppm to the CH$_2$ group, and the one at 1.1 ppm to the CH$_3$ group (spectrum provided by Andre D'Avignon and Joseph J. H. Ackerman).

^{1}H atoms at different positions in ethanol have resonance frequencies spread over approximately 2500 Hz or 5 ppm.

In addition to chemical shift, the RF signals from each ^{1}H group are split into closely spaced resonance frequencies known as multiplets. The splitting is a consequence of magnetic interactions between adjacent ^{1}H nuclei in the molecule. One way of explaining this phenomenon is to regard each ^{1}H nucleus as a small magnetic dipole that generates its own extremely small magnetic field. This small field alters the B_{eff} of nearby ^{1}H atoms. The magnetic dipole of a given ^{1}H atom can be thought of as oriented either parallel or antiparallel to the applied magnetic field (the field generated by the large magnet into which the sample was placed). This orientation determines whether the B_{eff} for neighboring ^{1}H nuclei is increased or decreased by a tiny amount, thus either slightly increasing or decreasing the resonance frequency of those nuclei. This phenomenon is known as through-bond or scalar coupling. For example, the two ^{1}H atoms of the CH$_2$ group in a particular ethanol molecule may be oriented in three possible configurations: both parallel to the field, both antiparallel, or one parallel and one antiparallel. As a result, there are three possible states to affect the ^{1}H atoms of the neighboring OH and CH$_3$ groups. In the first case, the resonance of adjacent nuclei is shifted to a

slightly higher resonance frequency, in the second to a lower frequency, and in the third it is unchanged because the small fields generated by the two dipoles cancel. When the spectrum from all the ethanol molecules in the sample together is measured, the resulting OH and CH$_3$ resonances are triplets representing the signal from molecules with ^{1}H atoms of the CH$_2$ groups in each of the three configurations. These triplets are enlarged and shown as insets in Fig. 1. The presence of multiplets can be useful for inferring molecular structure by providing information about how the ^{1}H nuclei in the spectrum are positioned relative to one another. Note that it is possible to have multiplets of multiplets as a result of scalar coupling. The CH$_2$ resonance of ethanol is split into a quartet through scalar coupling with ^{1}H atoms of the CH$_3$ group and simultaneously split into a doublet through scalar coupling with the ^{1}H atom of the OH group. This results in a multiplet with 2×4 or eight peaks as shown in Fig. 1.

MR spectra also contain information about the relative number of nuclei contributing to each resonance. The amplitude of a resonance multiplet is proportional to the relative number of equivalent nuclei in the molecule that contribute to it. In the example given, the OH, CH$_2$, and CH$_3$ resonances (the peaks of each multiplet added together) have relative amplitudes of 1:2:3 because there one, two, and three atoms at each position. Thus, it is possible to use MR spectroscopy of brain metabolites to estimate their concentration in the brain.

Although MR spectroscopy can be used to elegantly evaluate the chemical structure of a sample contained in a test tube, its application to intact human brain introduces a number of complexities and challenges. First, the many molecules of the human brain are detected simultaneously, with their resonance peaks overlapping throughout the spectrum. Second, many of the molecules are considerably larger than ethanol, and their spectra are correspondingly more intricate. Third, the metabolites detected from human brain are typically present in low concentrations (on the order of millimoles per liter) and provide correspondingly lower signal. Finally, there are technical limitations to the quality of spectra that can be obtained from the human brain. One technical limitation is related to the magnetic field strength at which the spectra are obtained. It is desirable to obtain MR spectra at high magnetic field strength for two reasons. First, spectral dispersion increases as field strength increases, so the resonance peaks are spread out over a wider range of frequencies. Thus, signals that tend to overlap at lower magnetic field strengths may not overlap at higher field strengths. This improvement in spectral dispersion simplifies spectral analysis. Another desirable attribute of higher magnetic field strength is that MR signals are stronger at higher magnetic field, providing a better signal-to-noise ratio in the spectra. Currently, high-resolution MR spectroscopy of small samples (those that can be contained in a small glass tube) is typically done at magnetic fields >7 T. Because of difficulties in constructing a high-field magnet large enough to fit a whole human inside, as well as other technical difficulties, studies of humans are generally done at fields <7 T. Thus, spectra obtained from live humans suffer from poorer signal-to-noise ratio and spectral dispersion than spectra obtained at high field.

A wide variety of methods are available for obtaining MR spectra from the human brain. The primary task is to obtain RF signal from the brain region of interest while discarding that arising from other parts of the "sample" (i.e., other brain areas, scalp, bone, etc.). The methods in use today can be classified into two major categories: single voxel methods and chemical shift imaging (CSI). In single voxel methods, a single region of interest is chosen (e.g., the occipital lobe) and a spectrum is obtained from it only. Examples of single voxel methods are point-resolved spectroscopy and stimulated echo acquisition mode. One advantage of single voxel methods is that signal may be acquired relatively quickly but only from a single region of interest. For CSI, signal is obtained from a "slab" of tissue. This slab is typically more than 1 cm thick (as compared with typical imaging "slices," which are generally less than 5 mm thick). Once the data have been obtained, the slab can be analyzed as a two-dimensional grid and spectra can be displayed from individual regions of interest from the slab. CSI offers greater coverage of the brain than single voxel methods but can be more time-consuming. The method used depends on the information desired in a given situation and differences in signal-to-noise ratio between the methods as a function of acquisition time and region of interest size.

Detection of ^{1}H metabolite signals from the brain provides a unique hurdle compared with detection of others, such as ^{31}P or ^{23}Na. When ^{1}H spectra are obtained there is an enormous signal from ^{1}H in brain water with which to contend. The concentra-

tion of equivalent ^{1}H nuclei in water is on the order of 110 M. This is an extraordinary advantage in standard MR imaging, which is based on detection of signal from water ^{1}H. For spectroscopy, however, the ^{1}H signal from water interferes with detection of signal from metabolites of interest, which are present in concentrations of tens of millimolar or less (approximately 10,000 times less than the water ^{1}H concentration). The problem arises because the massive signal from water ^{1}H overwhelms the smaller signal from metabolites. The RF signal detected is generally digitized by an analog-to-digital converter (ADC). If a full water signal is present, most of the range of the ADC is applied to digitizing the water signal, leaving a much smaller dynamic range over which to digitize the metabolite signal. As a result, most ^{1}H spectroscopy of human brain employs some sort of water signal suppression. This commonly involves excitation of the ^{1}H resonance of water alone and then suppressing the signal by dephasing the water magnetization.

With current technology, ^{1}H spectra from human brain typically show three or four readily detected resonances. As shown in Fig. 2, they are choline, creatine (both creatine and phosphocreatine as a single resonance), N-acetyl-containing compounds (NAA), and lactate. The reason that these resonances are more easily detected than others is related to the

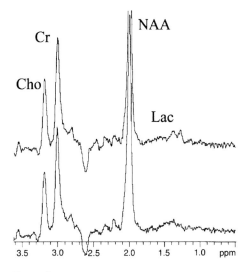

Figure 2
^{1}H MR spectra obtained from a human brain at 1.5 T. Two spectra are shown, one above the other. The top spectrum was obtained after intravenous infusion of lactate. Note that the lactate resonance is visible in this spectrum but not in the lower one. Cho, choline; Cr, creatine; NAA, N-acetyl-containing compounds; Lac, lactate.

fact that the particular resonances have relatively less splitting due to scalar coupling than others and that these metabolites are present in relatively higher concentrations. Choline serves as a component of membranes and is also a constituent of the neurotransmitter acetylcholine. Creatine, when phosphorylated, stores energy in the form of phosphate bonds. Phosphocreatine levels reflect the cellular energy state, but its detection requires ^{31}P nuclear magnetic resonance (NMR) because creatine and phosphocreatine are indistinguishable using ^1H NMR. The precise role of NAA in brain metabolism is unclear, although it is widely believed that NAA is found primarily in neurons and not glia. As a result, changes in NAA level may reflect changes in the number of neurons present in a given region of interest. Lactate is an intermediary of energy metabolism. Its levels may be increased under a variety of conditions. For example, if brain tissue is alive but receiving inadequate oxygen for aerobic glycolysis, lactate levels may increase due to anaerobic glycolysis. Lactate levels may also be increased by the presence of inflammatory cells, which often utilize anaerobic glycolysis. Note that the ^1H signal from the methyl group of lactate is a doublet due to scalar coupling with the ^1H atom on the α carbon of lactate.

As mentioned previously, the amplitude of an MR resonance can be used to measure metabolite concentration. However, the absolute amplitude of a resonance signal depends on many factors, including the particular RF coil used, its tuning, coil loading by the sample, and the gain of the receiver amplifiers. Because absolute resonance amplitudes are difficult to relate directly to concentrations, resonance amplitudes are typically presented as ratios, with the understanding that most of the factors affecting resonance amplitude are the same for all resonances in the spectrum. For example, ratios of various resonance amplitudes to creatine are often used (e.g., NAA:creatine), assuming that creatine levels are relatively constant in the brain. A more sophisticated approach is to use an external standard. This is a small amount of a compound that is not found in the brain but has an easily detectable resonance. The standard, containing a known concentration of the reference compound, is placed within the sensitive volume of the RF coil during data acquisition. The resultant spectrum contains the resonances of interest and the reference resonance. The absolute concentration of brain metabolites can be calculated by taking the ratio of the metabolite resonance amplitude to that of the standard, the concentration of which is known. A third approach is to obtain a nonwater-suppressed spectrum from the same region of interest as the water-suppressed ^1H spectrum. The ratio of metabolite resonance amplitude detected on the water-suppressed spectrum to water resonance amplitude detected on the nonsuppressed spectrum can be used to calculate metabolite concentration as the ratio of metabolite to water, giving concentration in millimoles per liter.

Overall, MRS has the potential to provide a wealth of information regarding metabolite levels in living human brain. Currently, human spectroscopy experiments have just begun to scratch the surface and MRS has not yet found a place in everyday patient care. With time, it is likely that improvements in magnetic field strength and MR equipment, coupled with advances in pulse sequence design (spectral editing), will enable routine detection of lower amplitude resonances in spectra from human brain.

—*Jeff Neil and Jonathan Sehy*

See also—Computerized Axial Tomography; Magnetic Resonance Angiography; Magnetic Resonance Imaging; Magnetic Resonance, Overview; Neuroimaging, Overview; Neuroradiology, Diagnostic; Physiological Brain Imaging

Further Reading

Becker, E. D. (1993). A brief history of nuclear magnetic resonance. *Anal. Chem.* **65**, 295A–302A.

Magnetic Stimulation

Encyclopedia of the Neurological Sciences
Copyright 2003, Elsevier Science (USA). All rights reserved.

EARLY experiments in humans using high-voltage, short-duration electrical stimulation applied to the scalp overlying the motor cortex were quite uncomfortable and inappropriate for routine clinical use. In 1985, Barker and colleagues introduced the technique of transcranial magnetic stimulation (TMS), which led to a new era of research in motor control and cortical function with a rapidly growing number of publications on healthy and diseased subjects. The technique and its modifications, such as double-stimulus paradigms, repetitive transcranial magnetic stimulation (rTMS), and peristimulus time histograms (PSTH), proved to be powerful investigational methods. rTMS is also used as a therapeutic tool in central nervous system disorders such as depression and movement disorders and will likely have other therapeutic applications in the future.

MAGNETIC STIMULATOR AND COILS

The components of a magnetic stimulator consist of a capacitor and an inductor (the stimulating coil). The energy for stimulation is derived from charging a bank of capacitors to approximately 4 kV that when discharged induces a current of up to 5000 A that passes through the copper coil creating a brief but intense magnetic field. Tissues, skull, and scalp present little or no impedance to a magnetic field of rapidly changing intensity. The current direction in the coil is opposite the direction of the induced currents in the nervous tissue.

The intensity of the magnetic field is represented by flux lines around the coil and is measured in tesla. The stimulating current, which is maximal in an annulus underneath the coil, may be either biphasic or monophasic. Since the direction of current flow determines which neuronal elements are activated within the cortex, a biphasic impulse may stimulate different populations of cells than a monophasic impulse. Large round coils penetrate deepest and the magnetic fields are distributed through a larger volume of tissue that results in nonfocal stimulation. Smaller coils, especially butterfly or figure-eight-shaped coils, are much more focal, with activation occurring beneath the intersection site, but they produce a relatively weak magnetic field.

WHICH ELEMENTS OF THE MOTOR CORTEX ARE STIMULATED?

Since the introduction of TMS there has been a debate over which structures are activated by the magnetic stimulus. A single low-intensity anodal electrical stimulus delivered to the exposed surface of the cortex in monkeys preferentially activates pyramidal tract neurons directly in the region of the axon hillock (Fig. 1, left). This results in a single descending volley recordable from the pyramidal tract that has been termed D wave or direct wave. Increasing the stimulus intensity activates input cells, causing trans-synaptic activation of pyramidal tract neurons. A series of recordable volleys termed I waves to indicate their indirect origin follow the initial D wave. The I waves are separated by intervals

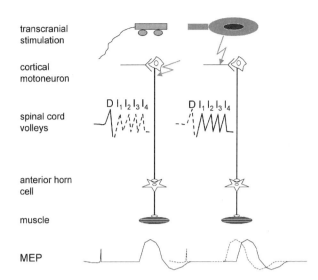

Figure 1

Preferential excitation of pyramidal cells at the axon hillock by electrical stimulation (left) versus trans-synaptical activation by magnetic stimulation (right). Higher stimulus intensities result in a shorted latency (dashed line) of the magnetically evoked MEP. For D and I wave activity, see text.

of approximately 1.5–2 msec. Epidural recordings of multiple descending volleys from the spinal cord of conscious human patients have provided evidence that transcranial electrical stimulation activates the motor cortex in humans and animals in the same way. The same experiments have also confirmed that subthreshold transcranial magnetic stimuli at least over the hand area of the motor cortex preferentially activate the pyramidal cells trans-synaptically (Fig. 1, right). The onset latency of the motor evoked potential (MEP) from small hand muscles occurs approximately 2 msec later than the electrically induced response (Fig. 1, right, bottom). However, with higher stimulus intensities and/or certain lateral coil positions, the latency may shorten consistent with D wave activation. Response of lower limb muscles has a similar latency with electric and magnetic stimulation, which indicates that both techniques have the same activation site and readily produce D wave activity.

TMS also activates the local circuit inhibitory interneurons. Several ipsi- and contralateral inhibitory phenomena have been revealed with double (conditioning)-stimulus paradigms and rTMS.

METHODS AND MEASUREMENTS

For routine studies, the magnetic stimulator is connected with a standard electromyograph (EMG) machine (Fig. 2). The discharge of the stimulator triggers a sweep that will display the recorded motor response (MEP) of a target muscle. Measurements include the cortical threshold, latency and central motor conduction time (CMCT), amplitude, and MEP:CMAP (compound muscle action potential after peripheral electrical nerve stimulation) ratio.

Cortical Threshold

In a relaxed target muscle, the threshold reflects the global excitability of the motor pathway, including large pyramidal cells, cortical excitatory and inhibitory interneurons, and spinal motoneurons. Even slight voluntary contraction of the target muscle reduces the cortical threshold (facilitation). The position of a circular coil centered over the vertex is less critical than the positioning of the figure-eight coil. Threshold is independent of age, gender, and hemisphere but varies with different target muscles. It is lowest for hand muscles and highest for proximal arm muscles, leg muscles, and axial muscles. This is in keeping with the more extensive cortical representation of hand versus more proximal muscles.

Latency and Central Conduction Time

Latency of the cortical response and subsequently CMCT depends on whether the MEP was recorded at rest or with activation, which shortens the latency by several milliseconds. The onset of the MEP is usually readily identifiable. The shortest of four or five responses is measured. In some diseases, the MEP may be markedly reduced in amplitude and, when facilitation is used, partially buried in the

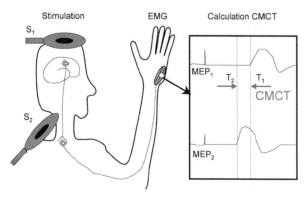

Figure 2
Principle of TMS and calculation of CMCT. MEP_1 is recorded after transcranial magnetic stimulation (S_1), and MEP_2 is recorded after cervical stimulation (S_2). CMCT is estimated by onset latency (T_1) minus onset latency (T_2).

background EMG. To calculate the CMCT, the peripheral segment of the motor pathway (anterior horn cell muscle) is estimated and then subtracted from the onset latency of the MEP (Fig. 2).

For cervical root stimulation, the most active part of the coil is positioned just rostral to the spinous process of C7, midline, or within 2 cm lateral to this position. Since a peripheral nerve is being stimulated, it is of no consequence which way the coil faces. Positioning the coil with the midpoint of its leading inner edge midline over the particular vertebral body of interest can stimulate the lumbosacral roots. The main aim is to elicit several responses from which an accurate onset latency can be measured. Stimulating the nerve roots either magnetically or electrically excites the nerve roots in the region of the intervertebral foramen. Therefore, the onset latency does not include the conduction time from the anterior horn cell (AHC) to the intervertebral foramen and the CMCT will be estimated slightly too long. This is not the case when using the F wave method. The CMCT is given by the formula $(F + M - 1)/2$, where F is the shortest F wave latency, M is the onset of the direct muscle response, and 1 msec is allowed for the turnaround time at the anterior horn cell. Latency varies with height and arm length; thus, central motor conduction is slightly faster in women than in men. With age, latency and central conduction increase in a linear fashion.

Amplitude and MEP:CMAP Ratio

The absolute amplitude of the MEP is dependent on complex interactions between the cortico-motoneuron and the anterior horn cell at the moment of stimulation. There can be considerable intertrial as well as intra-individual variation, especially when stimulating with threshold or slightly suprathreshold intensities. With increasing stimulus intensity, the response becomes more stable. Many factors account for this variability, most of which are difficult or impossible to control in the clinical setting. Coil position is critical and minimal angulation of the coil even at the same site may drastically change the amplitude of subsequent responses. Even modest muscle contraction greatly facilitates the response. The amplitude is usually measured peak to peak.

Because of its variability, the absolute amplitude is of limited clinical value, but in patients without lower motor neuron disease a side-to-side difference of 50% or more can be regarded as abnormal. The MEP:CMAP ratio takes account of the lower motor neuron contribution and is a more useful indicator of disease originating in the cortex. A ratio of <20% can be considered abnormal.

Cortical Mapping

The motor cortex is organized in terms of movements rather than muscles. Individual muscles have multiple representations (convergence) and a given cortical motoneuron may give input to several spinal motoneurons of different muscles (divergence). Since TMS preferentially activates fast-conducting, monosynaptic (cortico-motoneuronal) connections, maps reflect only the output function and distribution of this subpopulation of cortical motoneurons. For motor mapping, usually a butterfly (figure-eight) coil is used because the more focused field gives more accurate maps. Using the magnetic coil, motor mapping experiments in conscious humans have clearly documented plasticity of the motor cortex and its ability to reorganize in certain circumstances.

Reorganization of the motor cortex output map has been shown with piano practice, congenital atresia of the forearm, altered sensory input associated with immobilization, ischemic nerve block, dystonia, stroke, facial palsy, and in blind Braille readers.

TMS of the occipital cortex can evoke phosphenes in different areas of the visual field, and TMS of the sensorimotor cortex can occasionally trigger somatotopically organized paresthesias.

The Cortical Silent Period

As mentioned earlier, TMS also produces inhibitory phenomena, the most consistent being the presence of a long period of EMG silence during a sustained voluntary contraction (Fig. 3). This is akin to the silent period obtained by stimulating a peripheral motor nerve during contraction of a muscle. The duration of the silent period, usually defined as the time from the beginning of the MEP to the return of voluntary EMG activity, is linearly related to stimulus intensity but independent of the level of background contraction. For clinical consistency, measurements are made with defined stimulus intensities in relation to individual motor thresholds. Silent periods are longest in small hand muscles (200–300 msec) and less prominent in proximal arm muscles and leg muscles. Weak stimuli can depress EMG activity while not eliciting motor response; this indicates that the threshold for this inhibitory effect is less than that for the excitatory effect. Spinal inhibitory mechanisms such as the Renshaw inhibition are considered to contribute only to the first

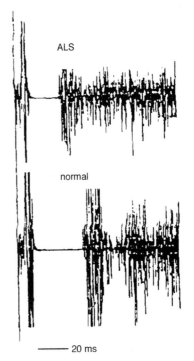

ALS

normal

——— 20 ms

Figure 3
Silent period in a normal subject and an ALS patient.

50–60 msec of the silent period, whereas most of the suppression is due to different cortical inhibitory mechanisms.

Paired Cortical Stimulation

Two transcranial magnetic stimuli delivered in a conditioning test paradigm can be used to assess intracortical inhibitory and excitatory mechanisms. The effects depend on the type of stimulus (electric or magnetic), the scalp site, the intensity of both the conditioning and test stimulus, the muscle activity, and the interstimulus interval (ISI). With the muscle at rest, the response of a suprathreshold stimulus is inhibited by a subthreshold conditioning stimulus at intervals of 1–5 msec and facilitated from approximately 10 to 20 msec. The inhibitory effect is reduced with voluntary contraction. The inhibition is due to the effects of local circuit inhibitory interneurons and also the result of inhibitory collaterals from excited corticospinal fibers. Subthreshold pairs of stimuli of equal strength result in inhibition of the test response at ISI 5–30 msec and facilitation at ISI 40–90 msec. A different pattern occurs with higher stimulus intensities: ISI of 25–50 msec cause facilitation and ISI of 60–200 msec inhibition. Paired cortical stimulation paradigms can be used to assess drug effects and pathological conditions.

Repetitive Transcranial Magnetic Stimulation

rTMS is only possible with special stimulators that have technical features allowing the fast rates. The technique is able to modulate corticospinal excitability. The effects, ranging from inhibition to facilitation, depend on the stimulation parameters (stimulus intensity, interstimulus interval, number of stimuli, and interval between successive trains) and may last beyond the duration of the rTMS. Lasting effects of high-frequency rTMS (>1 Hz) on clinical symptoms have been seen in Parkinson disease and depressed patients, whereas low-frequency rTMS can transiently improve symptoms in patients with task-specific dystonia. Further clinical applications are treatment of focal epilepsy, cortical myoclonus, spasticity, and obsessive–compulsive disorders. Other effects outside the motor areas include interference with language, cognitive processes, and memory. rTMS at high frequency and intensity may cause epileptic seizures.

Peristimulus Time Histograms

The cortico-motoneuronal system can be investigated using PSTHs. The firing probability of a voluntarily activated motor unit is modulated when it is subjected to a series of transcranial magnetic stimuli. The PSTH recorded from forearm and hand muscles typically shows a marked increase in the firing probability occurring approximately 20–25 msec after the stimulus referred to as the primary peak. The onset latency of the primary peak is in keeping with a volley descending through the fast-conducting monosynaptic (corticospinal) pathway. The configuration of the primary peak (amplitude, duration, and dispersion) reflects the rising phase of the composite excitatory postsynaptic potential at the anterior horn cell induced by the descending cortical volley. This technique has been applied to several diseases but has been of particular value in amyotrophic lateral sclerosis (ALS).

USE OF THE MAGNETIC COIL FOR PERIPHERAL NERVE STIMULATION

Use of the magnetic coil for study of the peripheral nervous system has been limited by its inability to deliver a focal, supramaximal stimulus. However, advances in coil design promise improvement in the precision of the stimulus and thus the utility of magnetic peripheral nerve stimulation.

Peripheral nerves are most readily stimulated by the magnetic coil at sites where there is an abrupt change in the volume conductor or at sites of nerve bending. This may explain the paradoxical ease with which proximal versus distal nerves are stimulated. The direction of current flow is critical in cortex stimulation but not in peripheral nerve stimulation. However, the CMAP latency may change by a fraction of a millisecond when the current direction is reversed, possibly as a result of cathodal–anodal reversal effect and/or shallower rise time in the strength of the magnetic field with reversed flow.

STIMULATION OF CRANIAL NERVES

The intracranial portions of the motor cranial nerves V, VII, XI, and XII are readily stimulated through the magnetic coil. For eliciting responses from muscles innervated through the cranial nerves at their intracranial–extramedullary portion, the magnetic coil is positioned approximately 6 or 7 cm lateral to the vertex on the bimastoid line ipsilateral to the recording site. Evidence indicates that the nerves are excited close or just distal to their exit foramina. Since proximity of the stimulus to the surface recording electrodes can be a problem, a concentric needle electrode often provides better results. An enoral "permucosal" recording device is also helpful to reduce artifact. The central, crossed, corticopontine portion of the motor cranial nerve conduction is more difficult to assess. The coil is optimally placed 4 cm lateral to the vertex on a line joining the vertex (Cz) and the external auditory meatus. Activation of the target muscle is usually required to obtain a response.

SAFETY CONSIDERATIONS AND SIDE EFFECTS

Adverse effects of single pulse magnetic stimulation of the motor cortex are extremely rare. Induction of epileptic seizures and kindling has caused most concern, but there have only been a few anecdotal reports of seizures occurring at or shortly after the time of magnetic stimulation. Formal studies on known epileptics have failed to induce either clinical seizures or electroencephalographic epileptic activity. However, it has become clear that rTMS, depending on the stimulation parameters, can evoke seizures in normal subjects and patients with neurological disease. As a general guide, previous cranial neuro-surgery with insertion of metal clips, the wearing of a biomedical devices such as a cardiac pacemaker, and a history of seizures are relative contraindications.

MAGNETIC STIMULATION IN DISEASE

Many abnormalities revealed by magnetic stimulation are not disease specific and, as for other neurophysiological tests, the results must be considered in light of clinical data. The major abnormalities of the cortical response are delayed onset, small amplitude, and dispersed morphology (Fig. 4). Frequently, the correlation between clinical deficit and degree of MEP abnormalities is poor. In general, demyelination of central motor pathways is associated with more marked conduction slowing, whereas in neuronal disease the MEP, if recordable, is of small amplitude but usually only modestly prolonged in latency.

Amyotrophic Lateral Sclerosis

Earlier studies in ALS using electrical stimulation of the cortex showed modest prolongation of central motor conduction time, frequently marked attenuation, and, in some cases, the absence of the MEP. TMS reveals similar abnormalities. The prominent abnormality is an absent or small MEP that is frequently dispersed. In general, the correlation of central motor conduction prolongation with other MEP abnormalities and with clinical upper motor neuron signs (hyper-reflexia, finger flexion, and impaired fine finger movement) is poor.

Various neurophysiological methods employing TMS have indicated hyperexcitability of the motor cortex in ALS. The threshold required to stimulate

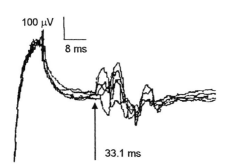

Figure 4
Small, dispersed MEP of late onset (upper limit 19.3 msec) recorded from the ADM in an MS patient at 85% stimulator output. Threshold is 75%.

the motor cortex with a magnetic coil is reduced early in the disease, and the cortical silent period, a measure of corticospinal inhibition, is shortened compared to that of normal subjects (Fig. 3). PSTHs in patients with ALS show a diversity of abnormalities ranging from the primary peak being small (or absent) to being large and increased in temporal dispersion. Indirect evidence suggests that these abnormalities are supraspinal in origin and are not the result of anterior horn cell disease. Patients with primary lateral sclerosis show significantly elevated thresholds to TMS and longer CMCT to both upper and lower limbs.

Multiple Sclerosis

Demyelination induces conduction block, slowed conduction, and inability to faithfully sustain rapid trains of impulses. These characteristic physiological disturbances in multiple sclerosis (MS) individually or in combination account for prolongation of CMCT, reduced MEP:CMAP ratio, increased variability of onset latency of the MEP (latency jitter), and dispersed morphology. Slowing of central motor conduction, the most commonly seen abnormality, can be very marked and correlates to some degree with the presence of upper motor neuron signs and clinical deficit. A common site of demyelination in MS is the corpus callosum and interhemispheric conduction through the corpus callosum is significantly slowed in this disease. A significantly increased threshold in resting or preactivated muscles is frequent. This is usually associated with prolonged central conduction but may also occur as an isolated abnormality. MEP studies may detect subclinical involvement of motor pathways and the overall sensitivity is comparable to that of visual evoked potentials.

Studies with PSTHs in MS have shown delayed and dispersed primary peaks consisting of multiple subpeaks. A similar abnormality is seen in ALS, but the underlying mechanism is likely different.

Movement Disorders

Conduction time through the descending motor pathways is normal in Parkinson's disease (PD), Huntington's disease, primary dystonia, essential tremor, and myoclonus. Determining the cortical threshold in PD has produced inconsistent results; decreased, normal, or elevated thresholds have been reported. The cortical silent period is shortened or normal and, when short, the abnormality can be reversed after L-DOPA therapy. Corticocortical inhibition tested at short conditioning test intervals, and with the muscle at rest, is reduced in PD. On the other hand, interstimulus intervals between 40 and 75 msec show greater than normal inhibition of the test response. The physiological abnormalities in PD revealed by TMS probably result from a combination of increased inhibition and reduced excitation occurring at both cortical and subcortical levels. In dystonia and Huntington's disease, double-stimulation paradigms have produced conflicting findings, most likely due to different stimulation parameters. Nevertheless, it is likely that future studies will provide useful insight into the pathophysiological mechanisms and mode of drug action.

Stroke

TMS is of value for the examination of motor deficits in stroke and appears to be a good predictor of stroke outcome. A recordable MEP in early stages correlates with a favorable outcome, whereas an absent response predicts poor recovery. Patients with delayed but present MEP recover more slowly than those with normal MEPs, but recovery is similar at 12 months. The CMCT correlates well with the grade of weakness; an increased threshold correlates with the presence of brisk tendon jerks. Using mapping studies, cortical reorganization after stroke can be demonstrated.

Hereditary Spastic Paraplegia and Spinocerebellar Ataxias

In patients with hereditary spastic paraplegia, lower limb responses are almost always abnormal: absent, small, or delayed. Upper limb responses, however, may be normal even in the presence of clinical upper motor neuron signs. A similar pattern can be seen in patients with hereditary motor and sensory neuropathy with pyramidal signs (HMSN type V). The CMCT to small hand muscles in Friedreich's ataxia is most often prolonged and the MEP is frequently of small amplitude and dispersed. The sensitivity is greater when recording from lower limb muscles. Prolongation of central motor conduction is also a common finding in patients with HTLV-I-associated tropical spastic paraparesis. Responses of lower limbs typically show marked prolongation. Upper limb responses may be normal or show slowing of central conduction that is less prominent than from recordings from leg muscles.

Epilepsy and Drugs

Attempts have been made to use TMS for localizing epileptic foci, but it appears that the epileptic focus cannot be localized with sufficient resolution. One would expect that cortical excitability might be increased in patients with epilepsy, but threshold measurements have revealed conflicting results. Intracortical inhibition in epilepsy is reduced, but this is a nonspecific finding that can be seen in many other disorders. It is unclear whether changes in cortical excitability are due to medication or to epilepsy. Antiepileptic drugs (AEDs) that act on sodium channels (carbamazepine, phenytoin, and lamotrigin) increase motor threshold but do not have a significant effect on intracortical inhibition. In contrast, AEDs or medication modulating activity of GABA receptors (e.g., lorazepam and diazepam) have no significant effect on motor threshold but enhance intracortical inhibition and suppress intracortical facilitation. In patients evaluated for epilepsy surgery, rTMS applied to the dominant hemisphere reliably arrests speech, which corresponds to Wada test results.

Radiculopathy and Spondylotic Myelopathy

Magnetic stimulation over the spinal enlargements excites the nerve roots a few centimeters distal to the anterior horn cell in the vicinity of the intervertebral foramen. The response latency is reproducible but the stimulus is usually submaximal. This precludes commentary about the amplitude of the response and detection of a more distal conduction block and limits the value of magnetic root stimulation to evaluate radiculopathies. As with other conduction techniques used to evaluate radiculopathies (F waves, sensory evoked potentials [SEPs], H reflexes, and magnetic stimulation), conduction block is difficult to interpret given the variability of MEP amplitude and uncertainty in obtaining a maximum amplitude potential. However, a side-to-side amplitude difference >50%, in the absence of EMG evidence of denervation (fibrillation and positive sharp waves), is suggestive of conduction block.

A high percentage of abnormalities in the MEP has been described in spondylotic myelopathy. The CMCT is frequently prolonged, the threshold raised, and the response dispersed and of small amplitude. Abnormalities of central conduction may precede clinical evidence of myelopathy. Slowed central conduction may be an early manifestation of cord compression before this is evident on magnetic resonance imaging.

Plexopathy

The coil can be used to a greater advantage in plexopathies. For example, a neuropraxic lesion of the upper trunk of the brachial plexus cannot be detected by stimulation of Erb's point, which is usually below the lesion. Accurate localization would require direct electrical stimulation of the spinal roots through a monopolar needle. This can be achieved noninvasively by magnetic stimulation. Eliciting a response from the deltoid or biceps is clear evidence of nerve muscle continuity and significant slowing of onset latencies would indicate demyelination. MEP amplitudes after magnetic plexus stimulation are quite variable and one cannot comment as to the presence or otherwise of conduction block. Once there has been significant axon loss, needle EMG is the best method of determining axonal continuity. Reinnervation, subsequent to an axonopathy, can be documented by the ability to recruit motor units, which occurs some time before nerves can be either electrically or magnetically stimulated.

Peripheral Neuropathies

As previously mentioned, magnetic stimulation has some limitations with regard to the peripheral nervous system because of lack of focallity and the inability to elicit a potential of consistent maximum amplitude. This precludes accurate detection of conduction block. However, there are at least two situations in which use of the coil is advantageous. In children who do not tolerate electrical stimulation, magnetic stimulation often allows measurement of conduction velocities sufficient to differentiate between a demyelinating versus an axonal neuropathy. Second, in demyelinating neuropathies, cortical stimulation can reveal marked conduction slowing in the most proximal nerve segments. The F wave can often do the same, but when the neuropathy is severe, it may be absent.

Respiratory Dysfunction

Diaphragmatic recording is used routinely to diagnose and monitor patients with impaired respiratory function. Although electrical stimulation of the phrenic nerve is well established, cervical magnetic stimulation of the phrenic nerves is less painful and achieves a more constant degree of diaphragmatic recruitment. The diagnosis of impaired central respiratory drive can often be accomplished by transcortical magnetic stimulation of the motor cortex with recording from the diaphragm and phrenic nerve conduction studies. These studies are of particular value in critically ill patients in whom both the central and peripheral lesions may impair respiration. Phrenic nerve pacing is becoming a more frequent substitute to positive pressure ventilation via tracheotomy in patients with high cervical cord lesions or central hypoventilation. TMS may help identify patients who may benefit from this treatment.

Intraoperative Monitoring of MEPs

The ability to evoke MEPs during surgery has been a useful addition to the battery of neurophysiological tests that can be used to monitor and prevent the development of clinical deficits during surgery. Motor evoked potential monitoring is particularly relevant in surgery that may damage the motor pathways independently of the sensory pathways. Examples of this include resection of spinal cord tumors, cross-clamping of cerebral blood vessels, and resection of tumors and AVMs involving the motor cortex and subcortical motor pathways.

—*Markus Weber and Andrew Eisen*

See also–Brain Mapping and Quantitative EEG; Deep Brain Stimulation; Electrostimulation; Magnetic Resonance Imaging; Magnetic Resonance, Overview; Magnetoencephalography; Silent Period

Further Reading

Berardelli, A., Rona, S., Inghilleri, M., *et al.* (1996). Cortical inhibition in Parkinson's disease. A study with paired magnetic stimulation. *Brain* **119**, 71–77.

Boniface, S. J., Mills, K. R., and Schubert, M. (1991). Responses of single spinal motoneurons to magnetic brain stimulation in healthy subjects and patients with multiple sclerosis. *Brain* **114**, 643–662.

Chen, R., Classen, J., Gerloff, C., *et al.* (1997). Depression of motor cortex excitability by low-frequency transcranial magnetic stimulation. *Neurology* **48**, 1398–1403.

Chokroverty, S., Picone, M. A., and Chokroverty, M. (1991). Percutaneous magnetic coil stimulation of human cervical vertebral column: Site of stimulation and clinical application. *Electroencephalogr. Clin. Neurophysiol.* **81**, 359–365.

de Noordhout, A. M., Myressiotis, S., Delvaux, V., *et al.* (1998). Motor and somatosensory evoked potentials in cervical spondylotic myelopathy. *Electroencephalogr. Clin. Neurophysiol.* **108**, 24–31.

Di Lazzaro, V., Oliviero, A., Profice, P., *et al.* (1999). Direct recordings of descending volleys after transcranial magnetic and electric motor cortex stimulation in conscious humans. *Electroencephalogr. Clin. Neurophysiol. Suppl.* **51**, 120–126.

Heald, A., Bates, D., Cartlidge, N. E., *et al.* (1993). Longitudinal study of central motor conduction time following stroke. 1. Natural history of central motor conduction. *Brain* **116**, 1355–1370.

Weber, M., and Eisen, A. (1999). Assessment of upper and lower motor neurons in Kennedy's disease: Implications for corticomotoneuronal PSTH studies. *Muscle Nerve* **22**, 299–306.

Ziemann, U., Steinhoff, B. J., Tergau, F., *et al.* 1998 Transcranial magnetic stimulation: Its current role in epilepsy research. *Epilepsy Res.* **30**, 11–30.

Zifko, U., Remtulla, H., Power, K., *et al.* (1996). Transcortical and cervical magnetic stimulation with recording of the diaphragm. *Muscle Nerve* **19**, 614–620.

Magnetoencephalography

Encyclopedia of the Neurological Sciences
Copyright 2003, Elsevier Science (USA). All rights reserved.

MAGNETOENCEPHALOGRAPHY (MEG) is a measurement of the magnetic field generated by a current source that has a tangential (parallel) orientation to the brain surface (skull). In principle, it is similar to electroencephalography (EEG), but EEG measures radial sources as well. The latter, however, is a measurement of field potential that is smeared by tissue conductivity, whereas the magnetic field is only minimally affected, resulting in better spatial resolution. The strength of the magnetic field, however, falls off rapidly, making measurement of distant sources from deep within the brain difficult. This is one reason why combined EEG and MEG may yield more information than either one alone. One method for combining the two, thought to improve the localization of active sources, is to first decide whether EEG or MEG most appropriately determines signal amplitude and then selectively attenuate the least appropriate signal components from both methods. The consensus is that EEG and MEG both measure the same current sources, although each may be looking at the sources from a different angle. The right-hand rule of physics illustrates this, namely that the magnetic signal (fingers) encircles the source current (the thumb). Furthermore, EEG and MEG waveforms often differ, suggesting a different source configuration between them. There is an apparent signal–phase difference between interictal electric and magnetic spikes.

When MEG is used to evaluate brain function and to correlate with brain anatomy, analysis of the measured magnetic field distribution outside the brain will only give a most likely location of signal origin. This is an inverse solution performed by modeling the current source as a single dipolar point, which may also represent a center of gravity when it represents a wide region of magnetic activity. A model with multiple dipoles is also used, but it is difficult to model an extended (widely distributed) source. The head is simply modeled as a sphere, but it has become common practice to use the actual head as a realistic model, both to improve localization accuracy and to make a better anatomical correlation.

The brain's magnetic field is very small, approximately one-billionth of the earth's magnetic field, ranging from 10^{-15} to 10^{-12} T (1 femto-T to 1 pico-T). It is essential to have a device that can record such a minute signal. The device used is the superconducting quantum interference device (SQUID). The superconducting condition is a state in which no resistance to the flow of electrical current exists and can be attained by cooling the metal niobium to a temperature of 23 K and by using liquid helium (4.2 K).

The elimination of signal contamination is essential. One way to achieve this is to use a magnetically shielded room, although some machines have been developed to work in an electromagnetically hostile environment.

Each sensor is a round coil 15–20 mm in diameter. Two coil designs of axial or planar gradiometer types are used and are strategically stacked to make various kinds of gradiometers (first, second, and so on). Recent MEG machines, however, predominantly use a magnetometer with a single coil configuration to increase sensitivity.

The pioneering MEG work was performed by David Cohen, a physicist at Massachusetts Institute of Technology, in 1968. In 1982, the first MEG measurement in epileptic patients using a single-channel system led to an explosion of research in the field. A few years later, 7- to 9-channel systems were developed, and toward the end of the 1980s 24- to 37-channel systems became available that also incorporated a magnetometer design of sensor coils instead of gradiometers. Within the past several years, a helmet-shaped whole head system has been developed with 122 and up to more than 300 channels.

In contrast to EEG recording, MEG does not require the application of electrodes, but it does require immobility, which makes its use in long-term epilepsy monitoring problematic. Any magnetic objects, such as hair pins or surgical clips, will interfere with the MEG recording. Various stimulators for evoked magnetic field measurement can be devised and are usually positioned outside the shielded room.

The application of MEG has expanding throughout the years. In fact, it is sometimes chosen over EEG for selected research questions, but the cost has made its use almost prohibitive, being nearly 100 times more expensive than EEG. Although proving an excellent research tool, the real value of MEG has yet to be firmly established.

The most notable application is in the field of epilepsy research (Fig. 1). Wheless *et al.* studied 58 patients with refractory partial epilepsy and found MEG to be a promising presurgical diagnostic method. Combined positron emission tomography and MEG provide supportive information relative to the location of epileptogenic zones. MEG can guide the placement of subdural electrodes and can differentiate between patients with mesial and lateral temporal seizure onsets. Ictal MEG, being a non-invasive procedure, despite its long recording time, may be useful when invasive studies are contemplated.

MEG 40-Hz activity has been recorded in wakefulness and rapid eye movement sleep and has been linked to cognition. Mental calculation and intensive thinking have been associated with 5- to 7-Hz MEG activity in the frontal regions. Evoked responses are easily obtained with MEG and are often used not only to identify functional anatomy but also to locate important landmarks in cases of anticipated brain surgery. Following stimulation of the median nerve, for example, somatosensory evoked fields are elicited. MEG has been extensively

used to study the readiness potential of self-paced movement.

MEG has recently been applied to studying hemisphere dominance for language and has reportedly shown almost 100% accuracy using clusters of dipole analysis. Combined MEG and EEG studies have suggested that the fusiform gyrus might play an important role in face perception.

MEG localization of the sensorimotor cortex, together with magnetic resonance images, has been incorporated into an intraoperative neuronavigation system that provides neurosurgeons with the best surgical strategy when treating cerebral lesions. MEG has also been used to study pain perception and migraine, where a slowly shifting magnetic field of large amplitude was noted to coincide with migraine attacks. MEG can be used to monitor brain and heart activity of a fetus in utero.

—*Susumu Sato*

See also–Electroencephalogram (EEG); Epilepsy, Diagnosis of; Magnetic Stimulation

Further Reading

Baillet, S., Garnero, L., Marin, G., *et al.* (1999). Combined MEG and EEG source imaging by minimization of mutual information. *IEEE Trans. Biomed. Eng.* **46**, 522–534.

Eliashiv, D., Squires, K., Fried, I., *et al.* (1999). Ictal magnetic source imaging (MSI) in focal epilepsy. *Epilepsia* **40**, 222.

Ganslandt, O., Fahlbusch, R., Nimsky, C., *et al.* (1999). Functional neuronavigation with magnetoencephalography: Outcome in 50 patients with lesions around the motor cortex. *J. Neurosurg.* **91**, 73–79.

Lamusuo, S., Forss, N., Ruottinen, H. M., *et al.* (1999). [18F]FDG–PET and whole scalp MEG localization of epileptogenic cortex. *Epilepsia* **40**, 921–930.

Llinas, R., and Ribary, U. (1993). Coherent 40-Hz oscillation characterizes dream state in humans. *Proc. Natl. Acad. Sci. USA* **90**, 2078–2081.

Merlet, I., Paetau, R., Garcia-Larrea, L., *et al.* (1997). Apparent asynchrony between interictal electric and magnetic spikes. *NeuroReport* **8**, 1071–1076.

Okada, Y., Lahteenmaki, A., and Xu, C. (1999). Comparison of MEG and EEG on the basis of somatic evoked responses elicited by stimulation of the snout in the juvenile swine. *Clin. Neurophysiol.* **110**, 214–229.

Rose, D. F., Smith, P. D., and Sato, S. (1987). Magnetoencephalography and epilepsy research. *Science* **238**, 329–335.

Watanabe, S., Kakigi, R., Koyama, S., *et al.* (1999). Human face perception traced by magneto- and electro-encephalography. *Brain Res. Cogn. Res.* **8**, 125–142.

Wheless, J. W., Willmore, L. J., Breier, J. I., *et al.* (1999). A comparison of magnetoencephalography, MRI, and V-EEG in patients evaluated for epilepsy. *Epilepsia* **40**, 931–941.

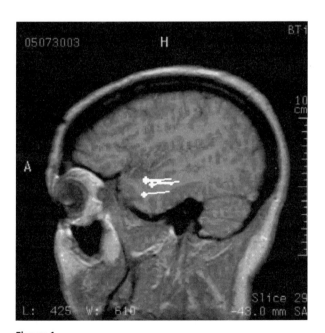

Figure 1
An example of epilepsy localization showing a cluster of dipoles in the temporal lobe (courtesy of Biomagnetic Technologies, Inc., San Diego).

Malaria

Encyclopedia of the Neurological Sciences

FOUR species in the protozoan coccidian genus *Plasmodium* cause malaria, a disease typically marked by episodic fevers and chills. These parasites depend on human beings as intermediate hosts. The definitive hosts, mosquitoes of the genus *Anopheles*, transmit the infection among people.

EPIDEMIOLOGY AND TRANSMISSION

Among the plasmodia that routinely infect human beings—*P. falciparum*, *P. vivax*, *P. malariae*, and *P. ovale*—only infection by *P. falciparum* carries significant risk of death. Clinical malaria occurs in approximately 300–500 million people each year, killing between 1.5 and 2.7 million. Endemic malaria occurs throughout most of the tropical latitudes, but seasonal transmission may occur anywhere between the polar circles where infectious human beings mix with locally abundant and receptive anopheline mosquito populations.

Endemic malaria disappeared from North America, Japan, Australia, Korea, Taiwan, and most of Europe during the 1950s when DDT and effective new antimalarial drugs were aggressively applied. Nonetheless, during the past 20 years sporadic outbreaks of *P. falciparum* and *P. vivax* have occurred in New York City and many other areas in North America and Europe. These rare outbreaks in developed temperate regions reflect a much broader and serious global resurgence of malaria that has occurred since approximately 1970 in the wake of the emergence of resistance to antimalarial drugs and the social reluctance to apply residual insecticides such as DDT.

PATHOGENESIS

Sporozoites from the salivary glands of infected anophelines feeding on humans rapidly transit through the bloodstream to invade hepatocytes, where they transform to schizonts. Each invading sporozoite becomes a schizont that matures to yield up to 40,000 merozoites over a period of one to several weeks (long-term latent forms of *P. vivax* and *P. ovale* called hypnozoites may remain quiescent for many months or years). The mature schizont bursts, releasing merozoites into the bloodstream. Sporozoite inoculation, schizont development, and rupture do not cause disease. Liberated merozoites invade red blood cells, becoming trophozoites that develop to schizonts containing 6 to 12 merozoites. Some merozoites instead develop to sexual forms called gametocytes (distinctive male and female forms appear separately) that fuse and undergo meiosis in the gut of anopheline mosquitoes to produce sporozoites in the salivary glands.

The rupture of schizont-infected red blood cells marks the onset of clinical malaria. The parasite amplifies its numbers and provokes disease through cycles of schizogony and reinvasion of red blood cells. Spiking fever, episodic chills, headache, nausea, vomiting, and muscle pain typically occur with acute malaria in people who lack the naturally acquired immunity to disease that comes with chronic exposure to infection.

DIAGNOSIS

Diagnosis in endemic areas, where malaria causes most febrile disease, is often made based on the presentation of this clinical spectrum. Standard light microscopic demonstration of the specific morphological features of plasmodia within red blood cells in films stained by Giemsa reagents provides a definitive diagnosis (Fig. 1).

CLINICAL FEATURES

Malaria may be broadly classified as either uncomplicated or severe/complicated. Symptoms of

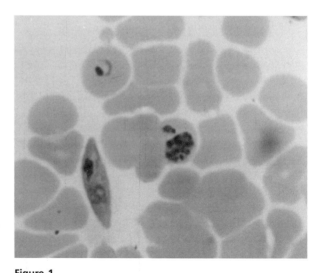

Figure 1
High-powered oil immersion light microscopy (40×) of Giemsa-stained thin blood smear. Center, gametocyte; top, ring stage infected red blood cell; right, schizont.

uncomplicated malaria range from none (as in most semi-immune adults in holoendemic areas) to debilitating (e.g., confinement to the home or even bed usually occurs in travelers stricken by malaria). These patients almost always fully recover with appropriate outpatient management.

In children, febrile seizures may occur with uncomplicated malaria of *P. vivax* or *P. falciparum* species and alone do not constitute cerebral malaria. Demonstration of plasmodia in the blood of patients with central nervous system dysfunction who lack evidence of other contributing causes constitutes the basis of the diagnosis of cerebral malaria. Cerebral malaria represents the greatest threat to travelers and young children living where moderate transmission occurs. Severe anemia is the greater risk to infants and young children where malaria is holoendemic.

The precise case definition of cerebral malaria is a syndrome characterized by signs of cerebral dysfunction unexplained by hyperpyrexia or detectable metabolic abnormalities. In practice, however, severe disease may manifest with both cerebral and systemic symptoms. Severe and complicated malaria includes those infections marked by hyperparasitemia (>100,000 parasites/μl of blood), cerebral involvement, severe anemia, hypoglycemia, or evidence of organ dysfunction, renal failure, lactic acidosis, Gram-negative sepsis, and hemorrhage (Table 1). These cases typically require management in the intensive care setting. The cerebrospinal fluid is usually normal but may have elevated protein levels (up to 200 mg/dl) or mild lymphocytic pleocytosis.

In most clinical or epidemiological studies, cerebral malaria carries a poor prognosis, with approximately one in five patients admitted to hospital with a diagnosis of cerebral malaria dying, regardless of the level of care available. In contrast, there is one Vietnam War-era case series in which all patients with significant neurological dysfunction received steroids and recovered. Unfortunately, the general lack of specific effective interventions beyond intravenous quinine therapy remains a major obstacle to care.

Table 1   NON-NEUROLOGICAL SEVERE/COMPLICATED MALARIA SIGNS

Severe anemia	Hypoglycemia
Kidney failure	Liver dysfunction
Blood acidosis	Lung edema
Shock	Spontaneous bleeding
Spleen rupture	Massive hemolysis

The pathogenesis of cerebral malaria probably lies in the process of sequestration of late blood stage forms in the vasculature of deep organs, including capillary beds in the brain. *Plasmodium falciparum* expresses proteins on the surface of infected red blood cells that bind to thrombospondin receptors on the surface of endothelial cells. Occlusion of narrow venules by the so-called sludging of adherent infected red blood cells probably contributes to anoxia, but ischemic necrosis is not a prominent pathological feature of cerebral malaria. Risk of cerebral malaria and a fatal outcome has been correlated to parameters reflecting a vigorous cellular immune response, especially cytokines such as tumor necrosis factor, nitric oxide synthase, and interleukins-4, -6, and -10. Pathological findings with cerebral malaria include ring hemorrhage, demyelination, microglial accumulation, prominent neutrophilic and lymphocytic infiltrates, and histiocytes laden with parasitized red blood cells and malaria pigment.

Recovery from cerebral malaria may be complete or carry permanent neurological sequelae. The prognosis correlates directly with duration of unconsciousness, worsening as coma lengthens. Although rare in adults who survive cerebral malaria, neurological sequelae are common in children, occurring in more than 10% of cases. These may include chronic learning disability, hemiplegia, psychosis, tremors, cortical blindness, epilepsy marked by generalized or focal seizures, cranial nerve abnormalities (particularly oculovestibular), cerebellar ataxia, Guillain–Barré syndrome, polyneuropathies, muscular spasticity or hypotonia, and dysarthria.

Delayed or late neurological complications, designated the postmalaria neurological syndromes, also occur. These occur in patients who recover from cerebral malaria and then relapse 1 or 2 days later into coma. Inflammatory spinal fluids with elevated protein with or without a lymphocytic pelocytosis occur.

Paradoxically, another important neurological aspect of malaria is the side effects associated with quinine therapy. Quinine often provokes a syndrome called cinchonism that may include one or more of the following symptoms: ringing in the ears, high tone deafness, nausea, vomiting, headache, dizziness, amblyopia, photophobia, diplopia, diarrhea, urticarial rash, and dysphoria. Overdose may be associated with permanent damage to retinal and auditory ganglion cells and severe neurological complications, such as blindness, deafness, seizures, and coma.

Quinine should also be used cautiously in patients with myasthenia gravis because of its curare-like effect on motor end plates, lengthening the refractory period of the skeletal muscle membrane.

TREATMENT AND PREVENTION

Uncomplicated malaria is treated by oral administration of a blood schizonticide, such as chloroquine, mefloquine, or halofantrine; a combination of blood schizonticides, such as pyrimethamine/sulfadoxine (Fansidar), quinine/doxycycline, and atovaquone/proguanil (Malarone); or any number of standard drugs combined with one of the artemisinin derivatives. Among these therapies, neuropsychological effects have been most frequently observed with mefloquine, occurring in 10–12% of individuals taking prophylactic doses and in a higher percentage of individuals taking treatment doses. Most of these minor effects are transient and include headache, fatigue, insomnia, vivid dreams, short-term memory disturbance, blurred vision, dizziness, fine tremor, unsteady gait, depressed mood, and anxiety. Mefloquine can exacerbate underlying Axis I psychiatric conditions, such as mood disorders or psychoses, and reduce seizure threshold in people with underlying seizure disorders, particularly those who are taking valproic acid. In both cases, mefloquine is generally contraindicated.

Widespread resistance to antimalarial drugs, especially but not exclusively by *P. falciparum*, complicates the clinical management of patients with malaria. Apart from the obvious clinical factors, therapeutic decisions must be based on the species involved as well as the geographic origin of the infection and the corresponding risk of therapeutic failure due to drug resistance. The World Health Organization (http://www.who.int/) and the U.S. Centers for Disease Control and Prevention (http://www.cdc.gov/) offer specific guidance. These organizations also offer specific guidance on the prevention of malaria in locations with drug-resistant parasites. Personal protective measures, including use of bed nets, repellants, and protective clothing and avoidance of contact with anopheline mosquitoes, diminish but do not eliminate risk of infection.

—*Jason D. Maguire and J. Kevin Baird*

See also—Parasites and Neurological Diseases, Overview; Tropical Neurology

Further Reading

Daroff, R. B. (1999). Neurology in a combat zone: Vietnam 1966. *J. Neurol. Sci.* **170**, 131–137.

Daroff, R. B., Deller, J. J., Jr., Kastl, A. J., Jr., *et al.* (1967). Cerebral malaria. *J. Am. Med. Assoc.* **202**, 679–682.

Deloran, P., Dumont, N., Nyongabo, T., *et al.* (1994). Immunologic and biochemical alterations in severe falciparum malaria: Relation to neurologic symptoms and outcome. *Clin. Infect. Dis.* **19**, 480–485.

Gilles, H. M., and Warrell, D. A. (1993). *Bruce–Chwattis Essential Malariology*, 3rd ed. Oxford Univ. Press, New York.

Urquhart, A. D. (1994). Putative pathophysiological interactions of cytokines and phagocytic cells in severe human falciparum malaria. *Clin. Infect. Dis.* **19**, 117–131.

World Health Organization (1995, November). Fact sheet No., 94 World Health Organization, Geneva.

Malignant Hyperthermia

Encyclopedia of the Neurological Sciences

MALIGNANT HYPERTHERMIA (MH) is a hypermetabolic state that can be induced by exposure of susceptible patients to any of the volatile anesthetics (with the notable exception of nitrous oxide). In addition, the muscle relaxant succinylcholine is a potent triggering agent for MH. Clinical onset is often sudden and dramatic, although it may be delayed; however, once the onset is initiated, the progression is usually extremely rapid. The signs of malignant hyperthermia include muscular contractions, increased oxygen uptake and carbon dioxide production, increased heart rate, and profound hyperthermia with recorded temperatures as high as 108°F (42.2°C). Development of muscle rigidity, particularly of the masseter muscle, is commonly seen after intravenous injection of succinylcholine and is often considered a hallmark of the disease. As a result of the increased metabolic rate, both respiratory and metabolic acidosis are associated features. These findings are the sequelae of massively increased metabolism in skeletal muscle caused by abnormal calcium metabolism.

In 1960, Denborough and Lovell reported a case of MH in a 21-year-old male who underwent general anesthesia during treatment of a broken leg. The patient reported anesthetic deaths in his family, 10 members of which had died under ether anesthesia. Investigation of this and other families suggested that MH was inherited as an autosomal dominant trait with so-called incomplete penetrance (carriers of the mutant gene vary in the severity with which it is expressed). Given the fact that MH is characterized by a triggered dramatic increase in calcium ion flux into striated muscle cells, the most probable explanation seemed to be an altered gene product.

However, caveats were acknowledged early in the search for the responsible gene. Autosomal dominance with variable penetrance may not describe the inheritance in all MH families. Moreover, testing for MH depended on nonstandardized batteries of pharmacological indices, such as testing muscle biopsies for contractures induced by halothane or caffeine, or measuring increases in concentrations of the muscle enzyme creatine kinase in the plasma of patients exposed to volatile anesthetics. These secondary indices of MH were not ideal in either specificity or sensitivity in identifying susceptible families.

Britt screened 56 families with MH and found that approximately 30 families did not fit a pattern of dominant inheritance. McPherson and Taylor reviewed the literature in 1981 and found that only 49 of 93 families showed a clear or possible autosomal dominant mode of inheritance. In 20 families, a recessive pattern could not be excluded, and in the remaining families the patterns were unclear but multifactorial inheritance or environmental influences were possible. It was believed that most of the nondominant pedigrees indicated a polygenic mode of inheritance, although recessive inheritance could not be excluded in some cases.

The search for a gene causing MH has been helped by the identification of a porcine model of the disease. In pigs the halothane-responsive MH phenotype cosegregates with mutation (*RYR1*) in the gene for the ryanodine receptor, a calcium-release channel that links the sarcoplasmic reticulum to the T tubule. The mutation is a change from C to T at position 1843 in the cDNA of this gene, which substitutes an arginine for cystine at position 614 of the receptor protein. When MH-susceptible pigs with the *RYR1* marker were crossed with normal pigs, the marker segregated with the MH phenotype in all 376 of the descendants. These observations were taken as overwhelming evidence that they *RYR1* mutation causes MH in the porcine model.

McCarthy mapped MH susceptibility in a human family with autosomal dominant inheritance and localized it to a region on the long arm of the chromosome 19—q12–13.2 (the prefix q designates the long arm). MacLennan mapped the ryanodine receptor in some families with autosomal dominant

inheritance and localized it to the region q13.1. The results of these and related studies clearly showed that mutations in the ryanodine receptor were causative for many cases of MH. However, the same group analyzed the molecular change in the ryanodine receptor in 35 other families predisposed to MH. In only 1 family did the change correspond exactly with the arginine-to-cystine substitution found in pigs. It should be noted that the myopathy, central core disease, also results from mutations in the ryanodine receptor. Patients with this rare myopathy are at significantly increased risk for developing MH.

Levitt and coworkers have shown that in three families with MH-susceptible members, the MH phenotype does not cosegregate with markers for chromosome 19, a finding confirmed by other authors studying other families. Recent studies have shown that mutations in a related calcium channel, the dihydropyridine receptor, can also be causative for MH susceptibility. In addition, in some families at least two other genetic loci seem to be associated with MH, although the precise genes involved are not known. Therefore, MH susceptibility is clearly a complex disease, with obvious genetic and molecular variability even among families with unequivocal autosomal dominant inheritance. If changes in calcium fluxes are the cause, there are several ways in which it might be altered.

The previously mentioned studies indicate that some families with MH susceptibility have a defect in the ryanodine receptor similar to that seen in pigs; however, other types of MH also exist, indicating that if Ca^{2+} flux is the cause of MH, there is more than one way to adversely alter it. Currently, the only other syndromes known to be associated with MH are central core disease and King Denborough syndrome. Increased susceptibility to MH has been suggested for a variety of other myopathies, such as Duchenne's muscular dystrophy, but evidence has not supported such associations.

TREATMENT

Since MH results from abnormal calcium flux, it is perhaps not surprising that a calcium channel blocker is used as the main treatment. The calcium channel blocker dantrolene has reduced the mortality of MH from >90% to <10%. Recent work has confirmed that dantrolene interacts directly with the ryanodine receptor. In addition to treatment with dantrolene, exposure to volatile anesthetics must be discontinued immediately and cooling techniques started. If surgery must continue, nitrous oxide, narcotics nondepolarizing muscle relaxants, and the intravenous agent propofol are believed to be safe alternatives. In patients known to be susceptible to MH, these drugs may be safely given as an anesthetic combination.

NEUROLEPTIC MALIGNANT SYNDROME

Neuroleptic malignant syndrome has a presentation similar to that of MH. The syndrome is triggered by chronic administration of psychoactive drugs, primarily phenothiazines, monoamine oxidase inhibitors, or butyrophenones. The onset of symptoms and signs, however, is slower than that seen with MH, and recovery usually occurs with discontinuation of the triggering drugs. Dantrolene is not indicated for treatment.

—*Philip G. Morgan*

See also–Calcium; Hyperthermia; Hypothermia

Further Reading

Britt, B. A., Endrenyi, L., Peters, P. L., *et al.* (1976). Screening of malignant hyperthermia susceptible families by creatine phosphokinase measurement and other clinical investigations. *Can. Anaesth. Soc. J.* **23**, 263–284.

Denborough, M. A., and Lovell, R. R. H. (1960). Anaesthetic deaths in a family. *Lancet* **2**, 45.

Healy, J. M., Lehane, M., Heffron, J. J., *et al.* (1990). Localization of the malignant hyperthermia susceptibility locus to human chromosome 19q12–q13.2. *Biochem. Soc. Trans.* **18**, 326.

Jurkat-Rott, K., McCarthy, T., and Lehmann-Horn, F. (2000). Genetics and pathogenesis of malignant hyperthermia. *Muscle Nerve* **23**, 4–17.

Levitt, R. C., Nouri, N., Jedlicka, A. E., *et al.* (1991). Evidence for genetic heterogeneity in malignant hyperthermia susceptibility. *Genomics* **11**, 543–547.

MacLennan, D. H., and Phillips, M. S. (1992). Malignant hyperthermia. *Science* **256**, 789–794.

McPherson, E., and Taylor, C. A., Jr. (1982). The genetics of malignant hyperthermia: Evidence for heterogeneity. *Am. J. Med. Genet.* **11**, 273–285.

Malingering

Encyclopedia of the Neurological Sciences
Copyright 2003, Elsevier Science (USA). All rights reserved.

MALINGERING is the intentional production of false or exaggerated symptoms. These symptoms may appear to be physical or psychological. Patients who malinger are motivated by a conscious desire to obtain secondary gain, which is a tangible external benefit. This is distinguished from primary gain, which is an internal psychological desire to be taken care of by others. Examples of secondary gain include the following: financial reward, admission to the hospital to obtain shelter and food, drug-seeking behavior to obtain narcotics, and avoidance of noxious situation (e.g., military duty, criminal responsibility, jail, and work responsibilities).

Patients who are malingering differ from patients with somatoform and factitious disorders in a number of ways. In somatoform disorder, the symptoms are not intentionally produced and the patients do not seek obvious secondary gain. Patients with factitious disorder intentionally produce symptoms, but they do this mainly for primary gain. They may also get disability or financial benefits from their symptoms, but this is not their main goal. Malingering patients, on the other hand, are not focused on obtaining sympathy or attention from others. Their symptoms will cease as soon as there is no longer potential secondary gain. It is actually rare for patients to be "pure" malingerers. It is more common to see patients with evidence of both primary and secondary gain interests at some point in their history. Often, these patients will appear to have varying degrees of awareness about the validity of their condition. It is usually difficult to make a definitive diagnosis in patients who fall between the ranges of somatoform disorder versus factitious disorder versus malingering.

DIAGNOSIS

Medical providers should consider malingering in the differential diagnosis if the objective clinical evaluation of a patient differs greatly from the patient's complaints. The clinicians should investigate whether there is an obvious secondary gain and the context of the situation. For example, in a clinical setting, the patient might be suspected of exaggerating symptoms if they ask for a letter to get a medical leave of absence from work while showing little interest in treatment or follow-up. In a legal setting, a clinician might give more attention to the possibility of malingering if the patient presents for an evaluation that will be used in a civil or criminal court case.

Psychological testing such as the Minnesota Multiphasic Personality Inventory and neuropsychological testing contain scales to detect if patients are exaggerating symptoms. There are also symptom validity tests in which the patient is given a set of questions to answer. Patients who are malingering will do much worse than random chance, indicating they may be consciously choosing the wrong answers. There are standard assessment tests to detect a patient exaggerating the cognitive symptoms, such as the Rey 15 Item Test or the Test of Memory Malingering.

Malingering may also be suspected if there is evidence from outside observers that contradicts the patient's claims. For example, a patient might claim they have a work-related back injury. They would be discovered to be malingering if covert videotaping showed them lifting heavy loads at home.

EVALUATION AND MANAGEMENT

There are a number of ways that a malingering patient might enter the clinical setting. The appropriate response to a malingering patient varies depending on the context in which the patient is seen. If the patient presents in a clinical setting such as a clinic or emergency room, the clinician should evaluate the patient and make a careful differential diagnosis. Patients who are malingering often have histories of true illness overlapping their exaggerated complaints and there may be a genuine comorbid medical or psychiatric condition. A patient with genuine depression related to work stress might be motivated to elaborate on the symptoms to get disability compensation so that they do not have to return to work. If the patient is suspected of malingering, the clinician might simply tell the patient that the clinical findings do not match the patient's report of symptoms and that treatment is not indicated. The clinician may also offer to help the patient think of alternative ways the patient can achieve their goals besides getting medical care. For example, if a patient wants admission to the hospital because they are homeless, they may be given other suggestions for housing, such as shelters. If there is a comorbid illness, the clinician should offer treatment or referral as indicated.

If the patient is being evaluated as evidence for a claim such as a lawsuit or for a workman's compensation case, the clinician usually reports the diagnosis to the court and not to the patient. Since the physician is not in a treatment relationship with the patient, confronting the patient that they are malingering is usually not necessary or helpful. The symptoms may stop when the patient's goal is achieved or hope of gain is futile.

—Betty Ann Tzeng and Stuart Eisendrath

See also–Delusions; Factitious Disorder; Malingering; Münchausen Syndrome; Somatoform Disorders

Further Reading

Gorman, W. F. (1982). Defining malingering. *J. Forensic Sci.* **27**, 401–407.
Rundell, J., and Wise, M. (Eds.) (1996). *Textbook of Consultation–Liaison Psychiatry*, pp. 368–401. American Psychiatric Press, Washington, DC.

Manganese

Encyclopedia of the Neurological Sciences
Copyright 2003, Elsevier Science (USA). All rights reserved.

MANGANESE poisoning results primarily from inhalation of manganese dust in industry, mining, and agriculture. Exposure in the United States occurs in industrial mills separating manganese from other ores and through its use as an antiknock additive in gasoline. Clinical signs of manganese poisoning have been reported in agricultural workers exposed to the fungicide Maneb (manganese–ethylene-bis-diothiocarbamate). In Chile and India, intoxication occurs mainly among manganese miners. Manganese is widely used in industry in the manufacture of chlorine gas, storage batteries, paints, and linoleum. It is also used for cleaning and coloring molten glass and in the production of soap products. Workers exposed to manganese dust inhale and swallow particles, which are then absorbed from the lungs and the gastrointestinal tract. In patients with chronic liver failure who cannot eliminate manganese well, accumulation is especially hazardous.

Several lines of evidence demonstrate that the brain regions known as the striatum and globus pallidum are particularly vulnerable to manganese intoxication. These areas are involved in the circuitry that is abnormal in Parkinson's disease, which is characterized by tremor, rigidity, slowness of movement, and balance problems. Likewise, one of the hallmarks of manganese intoxication is a parkinsonian syndrome. Toxic symptoms occur in approximately 15% of exposed miners and include dystonia or cramping spasms, bradykinesia or slowness, tremor, and gait dysfunction These signs may appear as early as $1\frac{1}{2}$ months after exposure to manganese dust, although there is usually a delay of 6–9 months. The onset is usually gradual, with increasing weakness and fatigability progressing to the point that the subject is unable to work. The gait becomes awkward and is particular in that the subjects fall backwards or find themselves propelled forward when walking. The upper limbs, trunk, and head develop a coarse, rhythmic tremor that is debilitating. Although it may be difficult to differentiate manganese toxicity from idiopathic Parkinson's disease, the tremor in manganese intoxication is typically larger in amplitude with a flapping quality. Although frank weakness is unusual, patients complain of slowness, weakness and fatigue, and difficulty performing tasks that require fine motor control, such as writing and buttoning. Involvement of the autonomic nervous system can cause heart rate irregularities, blood pressure alterations, and impotency.

Because of these clinical similarities to Parkinson's disease, occupational physicians and epidemiologists have questioned whether manganese exposure may play a role in the pathogensisis of Parkinson's disease. Statistical analytical techniques (meta-analyses) have been applied to case reports and worker cohort studies in order to clarify toxic ranges for extrapyramidal signs in different occupational settings. Data from 18 references on 60 individual case reports and population studies in 325 workers and control subjects formed the basis of one analysis. Of 117 workers, 6% with an exposure >5 mg/m^3 had acute extrapyramidal features, and in follow-up studies 14% exposed to manganese dust had parkinsonism 11–20 years after cessation of exposure. The median latency period between exposure and development of parkinsonism ranged from 6 months to 2 years. This important issue of the role of low-dose, chronic exposure to manganese in terms of a cause of parkinsonism and possibly Parkinson's disease remains an intense area of research.

Outside of the occupational setting, hospitalized patients who cannot eat and receive their entire nutrition through intravenous therapy [total parenteral nutrition (TPN)] can develop toxic signs from high levels of infused manganese. Subjects develop distinctive abnormalities on magnetic resonance (MR) scanning that involve a hyperintense pattern in the region of the globus pallidus. These lesions disappear after cessation of the TPN, and in some patients the MR abnormalities correlate with the development of clinical parkinsonism and high manganese blood levels.

Other signs of manganese intoxication include personality change consisting of irritability, lack of sociability, uncontrollable laughter, tearfulness, mild euphoria, and suspiciousness. Patients become abusive or even assaultive during brief emotional explosions. If the exposure to manganese continues, mental languor and extreme lack of energy and muscular weakness may occur; patients frequently fall asleep immediately after sitting down, even while at work. Tingling sensations or paresthesias have been reported, but no other sensory disturbances occur. Other symptoms and signs include sialorrhea, profuse sweating, impotence, insomnia, hallucinations, terrifying dreams, and muscle cramps.

Diagnosis of manganese intoxication requires a strong exposure history and documentation of high levels of urinary manganese. Approximately 43% of the body burden of manganese is in the bone. Excretion is biphasic with a rapid phase having a half-life of 4 days and a second slower phase having a half-life of 39 days. Methods of biological monitoring are poor and individual manganese levels in blood and urine do not correlate with either present or past exposure.

Management involves removal from the exposure source, and no specific treatment is available. Both 2,3-dimercapto-1-propanol and CaNa$_2$EDTA have been used without success. Based on the clinical similarities to Parkinson's disease, manganese intoxication has been treated with levodopa and dopaminergic drugs with symptomic success. Once parkinsonism develops, however, full recovery is rare, even with prolonged removal from the toxic source. Signs and symptoms remain prominent for many months after cessation of exposure and then slowly begin to wane. However, clinical improvement does not correlate well with reductions in the body concentrations of manganese.

—*Christopher G. Goetz*

See also–Corpus Striatum; Environmental Toxins; Globus Pallidus; Intoxication; Lead; Mercury; Methyl Alcohol; Neuropathy, Toxic; Neurotoxicology, Overview; Tropical Neurology

Further Reading

Calne, D. B., Chu, N.-S., Huang, C.-C., *et al.* (1994). Manganism and idiopathic parkinsonism: Similarities and differences. *Neurology* 44, 1583–1586.

Feldman, R. G. (1992). Manganese as a possible eco-etiologic factor in Parkinson's disease. *Ann. N. Y. Acad. Sci.* **648**, 266–267.

Goetz, C. G., Kompoliti, K., and Washburn, K. (1996). Neurotoxic agents. In *Clinical Neurology*. (R. J. Joynt and R. C. Griggs, Eds.), Vol. 2, pp. 1–112. Lippincott–Raven, Philadelphia.

Meco, G., Bonifati, V., Vanacore, N., *et al.* (1994). Parkinsonism after chronic exposure to the fungicide Maneb (manganese-bis-dithiocarbamate). *Scand. J. Work Environ. Health* **20**, 301–305.

Mirowitz, S. A., and Westrich, T. J. (1992). Basal ganglial signal intensity alterations: Reversal after discontinuation of parenteral manganese administration. *Radiology* **185**, 535–536.

Wolters, E. Ch., Huang, C.-C., Clark, C., *et al.* (1989). Positron emission tomography in manganese intoxication. *Ann. Neurol.* **26**, 647–651.

Mania

Encyclopedia of the Neurological Sciences
Copyright 2003, Elsevier Science (USA). All rights reserved.

MANIA is a disturbance of mood characterized by euphoria and associated physical and psychosomatic symptoms. Mania is not merely the opposite of depression. Patients suffering from mania may also experience irritability or a mixture of irritability and euphoria. A common idea among clinicians is that mania is so pleasant as to be intoxicating. Although for many patients this is no doubt sometimes the case, holding this as a clinical ideal may, in fact, lead to mania's misdiagnosis as agitated depression or disorganized schizophrenia.

The key feature of mania is that the affected person's rate of speech, thought processes, and goal-directed behavior are increased compared to the usual level for that particular person rather than a universal norm. Because mania can begin gradually, and because the state may cause little distress on the part of the patient, finding friends and family to verify the patient's condition can be essential to the diagnosis. Like all psychiatric conditions, mania causes functional impairment; unfortunately, those who experience it often minimize its consequences.

For diagnostic purposes, a manic episode requires that symptoms of disturbed mood last for at least 1 week. The mood is elevated, expansive, or irritable, and it is associated with a number of related features, including grandiosity, decreased need for sleep, excessive or pressured talking, racing thoughts, distractibility, and excessive and/or potentially dangerous activity. It is important to keep in mind that manic behavior is not disorganized but represents a goal-directed increase such that the person's functioning is impaired. In addition, the diagnosis of mania requires that these symptoms are not the result of another medical condition (e.g., a generalized sepsis) or alcohol and substance abuse.

The presence of mania is sufficient for the diagnosis of bipolar disorder: Individuals need not experience distinct periods of depression alternating with periods of mania in order to qualify for the condition. Most patients with bipolar disorder usually experience some depression, but those who experience mania as their first episode are thought to have a better prognosis. Mania that alternates with periods of normal mood, or euthymia, often goes undiagnosed if the increase in activity is helpful in some way (e.g., to an employer). Unfortunately, over time, people with mania may experience shorter, more intense manic episodes that alternate with periods of severe depression. The diagnostic criteria for hypomania are similar to those for mania, except that the episodes need only last 4 days, do not cause marked impairment, necessitate hospitalization, or co-occur with psychosis.

Patients who have had mania in the past will present to their mental health professionals with major depression; they may be unable or unwilling to accurately describe past mania episodes. Antidepressants may precipitate a manic episode in a patient who may be unable to recollect that they had one. In addition, antidepressants may cause patients with depression to experience a manic or a hypomanic episode. Physicians must be familiar with signs of past manic episodes in order to avoid causing iatrogenic mania. Signs include frequent moves, multiple jobs and career changes, and disordered relationships.

The brain pathways and structures involved with the phenomenon of mania are unknown; however, several theories have been put forth. Damage to the orbitofrontal region can cause euphoria and disinhibition, and orbitofrontal leukotomies have been used as a treatment for severe depression. Another theory is that mania results from lack of orbitofrontal control by a deeper structure, the amygdala, through dysregulation of the connecting neural pathways.

Other conditions besides schizophrenia can mimic mania. For example, patients with severe generalized anxiety disorder may report sleeplessness, poor concentration, irritability, and racing thoughts. In addition, patients may demonstrate restlessness during the examination. A key feature distinguishing generalized anxiety from mania is the absence of a decreased need for sleep, and the primary cognition is worry, not grandiosity. Patients with attention-deficit hyperactivity disorder (ADHD) may also display symptoms suggestive of mania, especially children and adolescents. When attempting to differentiate ADHD from mania, whether in children or adults, the clinician must keep in mind that mania is a disorder of mood, not of behavior or concentration, and they must search for a predominance of euphoria or irritability. Finally, a high comorbidity exists between mania and alcohol and stimulant abuse (such as cocaine and methamphetamines), which makes mania all the more difficult to diagnose. In genuine "dual-diagnosis" cases, however, alcohol and substance intoxication usually remits prior to the mania, allowing for the clinician to distinguish between them.

—*Mark H. Townsend*

See also–Amygdala; Anxiety Disorders; Attention-Deficit/Hyperactivity Disorder (ADHD); Bipolar Disorder; Borderline Personality Disorder; Depression; Hysteria; Mood Disorders, Biology; Mood Disorders, Treatment; Mood Stabilizer Pharmacology; Schizophrenia, Biology

Further Reading

Akiskal, H. S. (1999). Bipolarity: Beyond classic mania. *Psychiatr. Clin. North Am.* **22**, 512–703.
George, M. S., Ketter, T. A., Kimbrell, T. A., *et al.* (1997). Brain imaging in mania. In *Mania* (P. J. Goodnick, Ed.). American Psychiatric Press, Washington DC.
Ghaemi, S. N., Boiman, E. E., and Godwin, F. K. (2000). Diagnosing bipolar disorder and the effect of antidepressants: A naturalistic study. *J. Clin. Psychiatry* **61**, 804–808.
Jamison, K. R. (1995). *An Unquiet Mind.* Knopf, New York.
Solomon, D. A., Keitner, G. I., Miller, I. W., *et al.* (1995). Course of illness and maintenance treatments for patients with bipolar disorder. *J. Clin. Psychiatry* **56**, 5–13.

Maple Syrup Urine Disease

Encyclopedia of the Neurological Sciences

INBORN errors of metabolism most often result from rare single-gene defects that follow Mendelian patterns for an autosomal recessive trait. This implies that both alleles at a single gene locus harbor a mutation. By definition, parents of the affected individual are obligate carriers for a single mutant allele but they express no phenotype of the disease. Left untreated, many of these disorders present with neurological complications resulting in impaired function of the brain and central nervous system that can proceed to death. By understanding the affected metabolic pathway, treatments have been designed that correct or greatly minimize the neurological pathologies for many of these disorders. Maple syrup urine disease (MSUD) serves as an example of such a single gene trait in which the use of protein-modified diets (PMDs) has allowed most of the affected individuals to become productive members of society. However, severe neurological crisis remains a constant threat to even the most well-managed MSUD patient. Therefore, individuals with MSUD require greater clinical vigilance than do patients with phenylketonuria, the better known inborn error of amino acid metabolism. Thus, management of the MSUD patient presents a constant challenge to the dietitian and physician.

HISTORY OF MAPLE SYRUP URINE DISEASE

In the mid-1950s, as a physician in resident training, John Menkes was intrigued by a family whose child he saw had severe physical and mental complications and died in infancy. The family history revealed that previous sibs had died in infancy of unknown cause but all emitted a sweet odor from their body fluids. These findings brought Menkes to the realization that he was observing the consequences of an inborn error of metabolism. He went on to identify the source of the odor, which he likened to maple syrup, as resulting from the accumulation of the branched-chain amino acids (BCAAs) (leucine, isoleucine, and valine) and their transaminated ketoacid derivatives (BCKAs) in body tissues and fluids. Hence the name coined for this inborn error of branched-chain amino acid metabolism was maple syrup urine disease. Further studies confirmed the inherited nature of MSUD with transmission following Mendelian patterns for an autosomal recessive trait placing each pregnancy within a family at risk for MSUD with a 25% chance of producing an affected child. Heterozygote parents tolerate high-protein diets without clinical consequences. MSUD is known to exist in all races, with an overall incidence of approximately 1/150,000 live births. Within certain ethnic groups, for example the Mennonites in the United States, the incidence has reached 1/176 and has been attributed to a founder effect. The founder effect is based on families in a defined popular tracing their origin to a common ancestor, thereby increasing the probability for inheriting the mutant allele.

By the early 1960s, the metabolic block was found to be due to defective function of the mitochondrial branched-chain α-ketoacid dehydrogenase [BCKD] complex. This enzyme catalyzes the irreversible oxidative decarboxylation of the BCKAs, the second step in BCAA catabolism, and commits them to their degradation (Fig. 1). Since BCAAs are essential amino acids, they must be supplied by dietary protein or through autophagy of cellular protein. The ability of cells to sense the concentrations of the BCAAs plays important roles in maintaining normal cellular homeostasis. This may be why all cells with mitochondria have the ability to catabolize the BCAAs. This is quite different from most other amino acids, whose metabolism is mainly confined to hepatocytes. When cellular leucine concentration is maintained within normal limits by dietary intake, autophagy of cellular protein turnover is low. A reduction in cellular leucine concentration prompts endogenous protein degradation to reestablish the norm. The importance of maintaining BCAA concentration is further evidenced in conditions in which their oxidation is increased. Cachexia associated with many chronic diseases, such as cancer and AIDS, and the normal process of aging is associated with increased BCAA oxidation rates. Since BCKD is the only pathway for BCAA oxidation, increased BCKD activity must be occurring in this condition. When cellular isoleucine concentration is low, the cell cycle is arrested at the G_1 stage and results in disorders of the hair, skin, and eyes. In brain, BCAAs are the major source of nitrogen for formation of glutamate as a neural transmitter. The reason relates to the

rapid access BCAAs have in crossing the blood–brain barrier. Likewise, the transaminated BCKA in turn serves as the nitrogen acceptor in glutamate conversion back to α-ketoglutarate. The rapid formation and breakdown of glutamate is critical for proper synaptic function. Severe neurological consequences occur with increased BCAA as found in untreated MSUD, that can result in death. Thus, the importance of maintaining a cellular balance of BCAA appears to be the main reason for all cells retaining the capacity to metabolize the BCAAs.

Since irreversible loss of the BCAAs can only occur by the action of BCKD, the activity state of BCKD serves to control the cellular concentration of these amino acids. However, BCKD is not functioning in individuals with MSUD; therefore, control of BCAA concentration must rely on dietary intake of protein. Enough BCAAs must be supplied so that synthesis of new protein can occur in the rapidly developing newborn. BCAAs must also be supplied to the brain for normal synaptic activity. The fact that PMDs are successful in treating MSUD provided the emphasis to include measurements of plasma leucine in newborn screening programs used in many areas throughout the world. These programs have proved beneficial in providing early identification and intervention to minimize complications of physical and mental development for a number of inborn errors of metabolism in addition to MSUD. Commercially available BCAA-free infant formulas are supplemented with appropriate amounts of BCAAs unique to each individual's need. In older children and adults with MSUD, natural foods low in BCAAs are included in the diet and the MSUD formula is used only to balance the nutritional requirements not met by natural foods. Plasma BCAA is monitored on a regular basis to obtain optimal growth based on height and weight charts. Some physicians choose to supplement the PMDs with pharmacological amounts of vitamin B_1 since some forms of MSUD are reported to be helped by this supplement. Diet therapy remains the primary treatment and must be continued throughout life. Only a few clinics include computed tomography, magnetic resonance imaging, and/or electroencephalography in the monitoring of the MSUD patient.

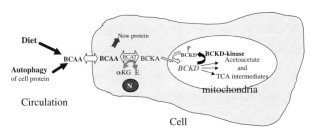

Figure 1

Schematic representation of branched-chain amino acid (BCAA) metabolism. BCAT, branched-chain amino transferase; BCKA, branched-chain ketoacids; BCKD, branched-chain ketoacid dehydrogenase; α-KG, α-ketoglutarate; E, glutamate; N, nucleus; TCA, tricarboxylic acid cycle.

THE BCKD COMPLEX

It was not until the late 1970s that the BCKD complex was isolated, purified, and shown to oxidatively decarboxylate all three BCKAs. Four proteins are used for the catalytic function. These reactions are diagrammed in Fig. 2. Decarboxylation activity resides in an $\alpha_2\beta_2$ tetramer that requires thiamin pyrophosphate (vitamin B_1 derivative) as a cofactor. The α and β subunits are products of two separate genes located on human chromosome 19 and 6, respectively. Transfer of the resulting branched-chain acyl group to coenzyme A (CoA) occurs by the action of a lipoate containing acyltransferase (E2) that forms the scaffold core of the complex. The two sulfur residues in lipoate are reduced during the process and must be reoxidized by the flavoprotein dihydrolipoamide dehydrogenase (E3). NAD serves as the ultimate acceptor of the hydrogen molecules. The gene for E2 is found on chromosome 1 and that for E3 on chromosome 7. BCKD activity commits the BCKAs to their catabolic fate, with each CoA ester now following a separate substrate-specific pathway to acetoacetate from leucine, acetoacetate and succinyl CoA from isoleucine, or succinyl CoA from valine.

The fact that all mammalian cells with mitochondria have the BCKD complex means that in order to prevent uncontrolled catabolism of the BCAAs, the activity of BCKDs must be regulated. Regulation is accomplished by expression of a gene on chromosome 16 that encodes a complex-specific kinase (BCKD-kinase). Activity of BCKD-kinase phosphorylates two serine residues in the E1α protein blocking the substrate binding site, thus effectively stopping the overall function of BCKDs. Tissue-specific control of BCKD activity by the kinase is best illustrated by comparing kinase expression in skeletal muscle and liver. The high-protein content of skeletal muscle must be maintained to prevent wasting as found in cachexia. Therefore, BCKD activity must remain low, a feat accomplished by a high expression of the BCKD-kinase. In contrast, hepatocytes express low amounts of BCKD-kinase, rendering most of the BCKD active for ready catabolism of BCKAs brought to the liver from peripheral tissues such as muscle. Tissues such as brain and kidney have intermediate levels of kinase expression, but very little is known about the importance of BCKD activity in brain and the subregions of this organ. Hormones and nutritional state will increase or decrease the expression of BCKD-kinase with the appropriate concomitant changes in the activity of BCKD. Our current understanding is that regulation of BCKD activity in the various tissues is controlled by BCKD-kinase expression. A countering BCKD-phosphatase that dephosphorylates E1α with apparent reactivation of the complex has been reported, but no studies have implicated the activity or expression of this component in regulating the BCKD activity state. The genes responsible for this phosphatase activity are not known.

MUTATIONS CAUSING MSUD

In 1985, the first cDNA clone for E2 of the BCKD was isolated and characterized. Genomic and cDNA clones have been prepared and studied for all components of the BCKD complex except for the putative BCKD-phosphatase. DNA mutations in the genes for E1α, E1β, and E2 have been shown as causative of MSUD. The E3 flavoprotein also functions in other mitochondrial multienzyme complexes; therefore, mutations in this gene present with a phenotype distinct from MSUD and lethality in the neonate period. Attempted treatments for individuals with mutations in the E3 gene have met with failure. All types of DNA alterations have been reported, including genomic deletions, base insertions and deletions, and base substitutions that change the codons or splice site junctions. More than 50 different mutant alleles have been described among the three genes. Amino acid substitutions over the entire coding regions of each gene product have been demonstrated as disruptive of enzyme function. Since MSUD is expressed as an autosomal recessive trait, mutations in one allele for two different genes of the BCKD complex do not result in disease. Both alleles at a single locus must be mutated to present the

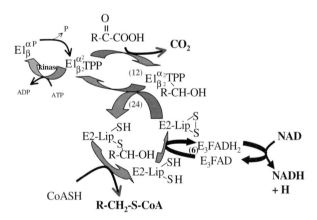

Figure 2
Reactions of BCKD. E1 decarboxylase is an $\alpha_2\beta_2$ tetramer using thiamin PP (TPP) as a cofactor. E2 acyltransferase forms the core and E3 dihydrolipoamide dehydrogenase is a homodimer. The numbers of subunits in the complex are shown in parentheses.

clinical phenotype. No dominant negative alleles have been identified. Only the 1325T>A transition in the cDNA for E1α that results in a Y438N substitution in the protein is found with any frequency in the general population. This mutation accounts for approximately 100% of the MSUD found in the Mennonite population. However, in most families without consanguinity, each parent holds a different mutant allele. Progeny of these matings expressing MSUD are therefore compound heterozygotes having two different mutant alleles at the single gene locus. In several ethnic groups, consanguineous matings are encouraged and thus increase the probability for expression of rare disorders such as MSUD. Recent data indicate that mutation frequency for causing MSUD is approximately the same for each of the three genes.

The identification of mutations within the three genes has allowed a new classification for MSUD as Ia, Ib, and II for mutations in E1α, E1β, and E2, respectively. However, the significance for clinical outcome with regard to the gene that harbors the mutation has not been defined. A clinical definition of varying phenotypes for MSUD is still found in the literature. The "classic" form presents in the newborn period with apnea, poor sucking, ketosis, seizures, coma, and possible death. Plasma leucine levels range from 1000 to >5000 μM (normal, 140 μM) and BCKD activity is <2% of control values. "Intermediate" or "severe variant" presents from infancy to young adulthood with plasma leucine between 400 and 2000 μM and BCKD activity <10% of control. The "intermittent" form becomes evident in childhood to young adulthood usually after a high-protein insult. Plasma leucine concentrations are between 150 and 1000 μM with <20% of control BCKD activity. A thiamine-responsive form has been described, but the mechanism for this effect is not defined. To date, the well-characterized thiamine-responsive patients have mutations in the gene for E2. As more nucleotide changes are defined, it will be possible to develop a clearer relationship of genotype to clinical phenotype. A genetic basis for each clinical descriptor will then be possible. The phenotype should include BCAA tolerance, susceptibility to crisis and development of brain edema, ease of correction of the crisis, and any other clinically relevant signposts.

Several factors contribute to the lack of a clear relationship between genotype and phenotype. First, BCKD is a multiprotein complex and most individuals with MSUD are compound heterozygotes. This condition allows for extensive variation among the components forming the complex that can result in functional variation. Both catalytic and protein interaction can be altered. Second, the use of PMDs minimizes or eliminates the full clinical phenotype. Third, some MSUD patients will tolerate a higher protein diet when provided with pharmacological doses of thiamine. Lastly, the genetic background of all humans, except identical twins, is unique to the individuals and therefore will influence the expression of a single gene trait. Together, these factors, and possibly others, make it necessary to tailor the treatment and management to each patient, even for affected siblings within a single family.

PATHOPHYSIOLOGY

Newborn infants with MSUD are full-term products of an uncomplicated pregnancy. Screening programs that test for elevated plasma leucine concentrations should detect infants at risk for MSUD. If newborn screening is not available or fails for any reason, infants with classic MSUD present in the newborn period with irritability, hypertonicity, a poor sucking response, and can progress rapidly into seizures, coma, and death. The clinical key to the attending physician is the sweet odor easily detected in the ear wax, and that to the parent is the same odor in the urine noticed most when changing the diaper. Whether identified by newborn screen or an alert pediatrician, the infant should be tested with a complete plasma amino acid profile. An alternative is to test the urine for ketoacids using 2,4-dinitrophenylhydrazine, which forms yellow crystals when BCKAs are present. The presence of allo-isoleucine in plasma is the hallmark of MSUD. Confirming diagnosis is made by an enzyme assay for BCKD activity using isolated peripheral white cells or cultured fibroblasts or lymphoblasts prepared from the patient. BCKD activity in the suspected patient cells should be compared to that found in a known MSUD cell line and a normal control cell line. All cells should be treated to induce dephosphorylation of the BCKD complex so that total BCKD activity is compared among the cell types.

Leucine is the most detrimental among the three BCAAs and can reach concentrations in excess of 5000 μM. Normal plasma concentrations are 100–140 μM and clinical signs can appear with concentrations higher than 400 μM. It is critical that leucine concentrations be reduced as rapidly as possible, which has been accomplished through the use of hemodialysis or peritoneal dialysis or administration of total parenteral nutrition without the BCAAs. The choice depends mainly on the stage of decompensation and the age of the child. Care must be taken to monitor the isoleucine and valine levels because additional complications can result if these are not present in adequate amounts for growth. These two BCAAs do not usually reach the concentrations observed for leucine and therefore can rapidly decrease to zero by this treatment. As a consequence of low valine and/or isoleucine, there have been reported ophthalmic, hair, and dermal lesions. These management problems are now well recognized and physicians familiar with treatment of metabolic disorders are alert to early signs of distress.

With the advent of newborn screening, early recognition with elevated plasma leucine has enabled treatment of the MSUD infant within the first 3–10 days after birth. The use of tandem mass spectrometry in newborn screening methods, with its speed and accuracy, should greatly enhance the early diagnosis.

In the early years after discovery of MSUD, autopsies were done to seek the pathophysiological basis of the disease and identify markers unique to the phenotype. Brain tissue showed status spongiosis, reduced myelination, decreased lipid content, and increased cerebral water content. The naturally occurring animal model, the Poll Hereford cow, has authentically replicated these findings in cow brain. Both white and gray matter are affected, but none of these findings are different from those seen in many other conditions that result in brain edema. These findings do explain the vomiting, lethargy, seizures, coma, and death for the clinical progression of the untreated newborn.

Identification and treatment with PMDs in the newborn period has resulted in near normal development of the MSUD patient according to some parameters. However, there remain a few individuals whose mental development is compromised. The IQ values in the MSUD population range from <75 to >130. It is not clear whether this relates to the specific gene that is mutated, is the result of other genes in this family, or relates to the environmental factors surrounding the individual.

Another dilemma remains because even patients in excellent metabolic control can experience decompensation and a rapid progression to a life-threatening condition. This occurs most often with viral or bacterial infections that trigger cellular breakdown of endogenous protein. Immunizations have also been reported to initiate a crisis, but any insult that causes a deviation to a high protein load can induce this scenario. Several reports in the literature document this situation and many others cases go unreported. The initial signs are often vomiting, ataxia, and dehydration that bring about the need for hospitalization. After the initial presentation, the condition parallels the untreated newborn. Unfortunately, even the best treatment in hospital with a rapid decrease in plasma BCAAs can still not be enough and death will result. In all cases that have been examined, the brain shows extensive edema. A positron emission tomography scan of the brain in one patient revealed decreased glucose utilization. In cases in which patients survive the insult and plasma BCAA concentrations are normalized, the edema usually resolves by 14 days. Despite efforts to identify some unique feature for the MSUD phenotype, the underlying cause for the pathophysiology remains unknown. It is suggested that repeated insults have a cumulative effect, resulting in compromised brain function. Only one longitudinal study covering 20 years and 26 patients followed by electroencephalograph (EEG) monitoring has been reported. The results showed no direct correlation between BCAA plasma concentrations and the EEG pattern. A general conclusion was that EEG data are like those seen for a number of conditions presenting with brain edema. Support for the cumulative effects of repeated episodes of edema comes from the observed residual atrophy in brain tissue after each incidence.

One possible explanation for the pathophysiology that is actively being investigated is the glutamate, GABA, neurotransmitter cycle in neuron function. BCAAs serve as the major contributor of nitrogen for the formation of glutamate from α-ketoglutarate. In turn, the BCKAs will accept the amino group from glutamate to reduce its presence. The rapid formation and loss of glutamate plays an important role in synaptic reactions. Thus, excess BCAAs can interfere with this process, and this disturbance may be responsible for the observed MSUD phenotype.

FUTURE CONCERNS

Despite the success of newborn screening programs in identification and the use of PMDs in managing the MSUD individual, many challenges remain. Protein insults still hold the threat of coma and death within 24 hr of the insult. Constant vigilance is needed and the health care provider must be aware of the special needs of these patients. Another challenge is maternal MSUD, in which the mother has MSUD and therefore cannot tolerate a high-protein diet that is needed for optimal fetal development. In most cases, the fetus will be heterozygous and therefore can catabolize BCAAs. Whether fetal metabolism will adequately handle any excess BCAAs to spare the mother, this insult requires additional testing. Three such pregnancies have been reported, with all infants presenting as small for gestational age and having the consequences of this condition. Another concern is whether new problems will emerge as these PMD-treated patients age. It remains to be resolved whether newly emerging complications are the result of the single gene defect or the treatment rendered.

—*Dean J. Danner*

See also–Menkes' Disease; Micturition; Organic Acid Disorders

Further Reading

Chuang, D. T., and Shih, V. E. (1995). Disorders of branched chain amino acid and keto acid metabolism. In *The Metabolic Basis of Inherited Disease*. (C. R. Scriver, A. L. Beaudet, W. S. Sly, and D. Valle, Eds.), Vol. 1, pp. 1239–1277. McGraw-Hill, New York.

Danner, D. J., and Doering, C. B. (1998). Human mutations affecting branched chain α-ketoacid dehydrogenase. *Front. Biosci.* **3**, 517–524.

Ellerine, N. P., Herring, W. J., Elsas, L. J., *et al.* (1993). Thiamine-responsive maple syrup urine disease in a patient antigenically missing dihydrolipoamide acyltransferase. *Biochem. Med. Metab. Biol.* **49**, 363–374.

Fisher, C. R., Chuang, J. L., Cox, R. P., *et al.* (1991). Maple syrup urine disease in Mennonites: Evidence that the Y393N mutation in E1alpha impedes asssembly of the E1 component of branched-chain α-ketoacid dehydrogenase complex. *J. Clin. Invest.* **88**, 1034–1037.

Grunewald, S., Hinrichs, F., and Wendel, U. (1998). Pregnancy in a woman with maple syrup urine disease. *J. Inherit. Metab. Dis.* **21**, 89–94.

Heindel, W., Kugel, H., Wendel, W., *et al.* (1995). Proton magnetic resonance spectroscopy reflects metabolic decompensation in maple syrup urine disease. *Pediatr. Radiol.* **25**, 296–299.

Korein, J., Sansaricq, C., Kalmijn, M., *et al.* (1994). Maple syrup urine disease: Clinical, EEG, and plasma amino acid correlations with a theoretical mechanism of acute neurotoxicity. *Int. J. Neurosci.* **79**, 21–45.

Nellis, M. M., and Danner, D. J. (2001). Gene preference in maple syrup urine disease. *Am. J. Hum. Genet.* **68**, 232–237.

Peinemann, F., and Danner, D. J. (1994). Maple syrup urine disease, 1954 to 1993. *J. Inherit. Metab. Dis.* **17**, 3–15.

Marie, Pierre

Encyclopedia of the Neurological Sciences
Copyright 2003, Elsevier Science (USA). All rights reserved.

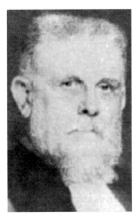

Pierre Marie (reproduced with permission from the Louis D. Boshes archives at the University of Illinois at Chicago).

PIERRE MARIE (1842–1940) was born in Paris and died in Normandy 1 year after the onset of World War II. He came from a wealthy family and remained financially secure. His private undergraduate education was rich in classic studies. He had a strong interest in medicine but acquiesced to the desire of his father, who preferred law as the profession for his son. Marie secured his law degree in Paris and immediately enrolled in medical school to follow his choice of profession. His mentors during his training years were Charcot and Bouchard. He was successful in the very competitive public examination for internship in the Hospitals of Paris and was regarded as one of the most able students of Charcot. Charcot was supportive of Marie's career and appointed him as chief of his clinic as well as chief of his laboratory. At the Salpetriere, the neurological institute established by Charcot, Marie's contemporaries included Brissaud, Babinski, and Gilles de la Tourette. During the brief time that Sigmund Freud spent in Paris (1885 and 1886), he became acquainted with Marie. Both were interested in cerebral palsy. Marie proposed a study concerned with hysteria but later withdrew from the project. Freud later singly published his observations concerning hysterical paralysis. In 1893, Brissaud and Marie established the *Revue Neurologique*, which became the journal of the French Society of Neurology. In 1899, he successfully competed for the position of agrege. This nontenured associate professor appointment placed him in a position for a possible later professorial chair.

In common with his mentor, Charcot, Marie was not concerned with experimental medicine or laboratory research. Early in his career he sought to correlate gross and microscopic pathology with his clinical observations. In 1886, he made fundamental observations regarding pituitary tumors and acromegaly. Some cite Marie as the father of modern endocrinology. In the same year, Charcot and Marie described a familial progressive muscle atrophy (Charcot–Marie–Tooth disease). His other clinical discoveries included hereditary disease of the cerebellum and the bone and joint changes seen in chronic pulmonary disease. The latter was designated as hypertrophic pulmonary osteoarthropathy. He also authored a text on diseases of the spinal cord and was most interested in the localization of brain function and language.

Beginning in 1882, he wrote frequently on aphasia and its varieties. His style was incisive, critical, and uncompromising. For some years, Marie had expressed concerns about the existing concepts of aphasia. He raised these to a new height in 1906 with his polemical paper, "The Third Left Frontal Convolution Plays No Special Role in the Function of Language." The controversies associated with speech disorders were considered at length at aphasia meetings in Paris in 1908 by prominent neurologists. Heated discussions followed by Marie and the Dejerines and those supporting their respective positions. The formulations and conclusions of Marie regarding language disturbances tended to be based on his clinical impressions rather than the correlation of clinical and neuropathological findings of the Dejerines. At the final meeting of the conference, they stressed that their anatomic data supported the classic traditional concept of motor aphasia. Marie held that his observations, conclusions, and position were completely contrary to those of the Dejerines. Klippel, the chairman of the conference, concluded that it remained necessary to revise certain questions regarding aphasia.

In 1909, in an attempt to reduce lingering tensions and enmity arising from the heated 1908 conference, Achard, the president of the French Society of Neurology, suggested,

> Everyone has his own way of interpreting what he has seen, and perhaps it's not bad that all firm beliefs continue to be presented. We should take care not to forget that our revisions of yesterday may be revised tomorrow.

After Dejerine's death in 1917, Marie finally succeeded to Charcot's chair in neurology, but by this time he was past the prime of his academic career. During World War I, along with his neurological contemporaries, his efforts were dedicated to the care of war casualties. The most notable of his students during these later years were Guillain, Foix, Lhermitte, and Percival Bailey. Bailey, later a prominent figure in neurology and neurosurgery in the United States, worked as an assistant in the laboratory of Marie. Bailey observed,

> Pierre Marie's influence in the Parisian medical world was immense. His great wealth made him independent; his honesty made him respected; his innate courtesy and dignity made him friends and disarmed his opponents; and his creative intelligence spread his reputation throughout the world. He is a good example of the best in French medicine.

In the mid-1920s, following the successive deaths of his daughter, wife, and son, Marie resigned from the faculty of medicine and gradually withdrew from the medical community. However, he did maintain contact with the *Revue Neurologique*. His mood at that time was best indicated by his comment, "You see it is better to love nature and the arts, since contact with mankind is very often disillusioning; Nature never deceives us."

The remarkable clinical observations and discoveries made by Marie early in his brilliant career have stood the test of time. As he aged, his perspectives and conclusions notably in the area of aphasia were less secure. His unique style, however, resulted in a broader perspective and significant review of brain function and language, a subject that continues to hold the interest of many neuroscientists.

—Richard Satran

See also–Aphasia; Charcot, Jean-Martin; Charcot–Marie–Tooth Disease; Freud, Sigmund (see Index entry Biography for complete list of biographical entries)

Further Reading

Achard, M. (1909). Allocution. *Rev. Neurol.* 17, 93–94.
Bailey, P. (1970). Pierre Marie. In *Founders of Neurology* (W. Haymaker and F. Schiller, Eds.), 2nd ed. Thomas, Springfield, IL.
Cole, M. F., and Cole, M. (1971). *Pierre Marie's Papers on Speech Disorders.* Hafner, New York.
Lhermitte, J. (1941). Pierre Marie 1853–1940. *Paris Med.* 119, Annexe XI–XII.
Meyer, A. (1940). Dr. Pierre Marie. *J. Nerv. Mental Dis.* 92, 416–418.
Satran, R. (1990). Pierre Marie. In *The Founders of Child Neurology* (S. Ashwall and M. Steele, Eds.), pp. 313–318. Norman, San Francisco.

Marijuana

Encyclopedia of the Neurological Sciences
Copyright 2003, Elsevier Science (USA). All rights reserved.

CANNABINOL (marijuana) is one of the most commonly abused drugs. It has been used since 3000 B.C. in cultures as diverse as those found in the Middle East and Asia. The drug has a number of names, including hashish, ganja, and bhang. The active product in marijuana is derived primarily from the flowering of hemp plants, although all parts of both the male and female plant contain psychoactive compounds. Among the cannabinoids are cannabinol, cannabidiol, cannabiolic acid, and several other congeners.

The most active compound responsible for most of the psychological and physiological symptoms is δ-tetrahydrocannabinol (THC). Low to moderate doses of the drug cause very few psychological and physiological symptoms. The pharmacological actions and the long-term effects of chronic use are unclear. The drug can be smoked, eaten, or taken intravenously. In man, THC exerts its most prominent effects on the central nervous and the cardiovascular systems. The nervous system effects differ depending on the dose, route of administration, and the experience and expectation of the subject. When smoked, the psychological effects do not develop for 20–30 min. The effects can last up to 3 hr. However, THC is absorbed and accumulates in tissues such as the testes and the brain.

THC causes euphoria, alterations in memory and motor coordination, feelings of relaxation, and heightened sexual arousal. Some individuals experience increased hunger; others have reported increased suspiciousness, paranoia, and aggressiveness, whereas some become withdrawn socially. In an isolated environment, sleepiness may be a prominent feature. Abnormal eye movements (nystagmus), wide-based gait (ataxia), and tremors have also been reported. The drug can precipitate seizures in patients with known seizure disorders. In addition, balance and stability of stance may be affected, and driving and tasks requiring complex integration of perception and attention are impaired with as little as one or two cigarettes. Behavioral effects of alcohol are additive to those of marijuana. Cardiac effects include increased heart frequency rate and increased blood pressure.

Treatment of patients with acute toxic reactions involves reassurance that the problems will resolve within a few hours. Because of the possible high concentration of the drug in various tissues, the neurological effects of the drug may take up to 8 hr to resolve. No antidote is available, although a mild sedative might be useful. In cases of acute psychotic states, haloperidol in divided doses of 5–20 mg/day has been used successfully.

—*Esther Cubo and Christopher G. Goetz*

See also–Alcohol-Related Neurotoxicity; Amphetamine Toxicity; Cocaine; Endocannabinoids; Heroin; LSD (Lysergic Acid Diethylamide); PCP (Phencyclidine Hydrochloride); Smoking and Nicotine; Substance Abuse

Further Reading

Chang, L. W., and Dyer, R. S. (Eds.) (1995). *Handbook of Neurotoxicology*. Dekker, New York.
Jaffe, J. H. (1980). Drug addiction and drug abuse. In *Pharmacologic Basis of Therapeutics* (A. G. Goodman, L. S. Gilman, and A. Gilman, Eds.), pp. 535–584. Macmillan, New York.

Mass Effect

Encyclopedia of the Neurological Sciences
Copyright 2003, Elsevier Science (USA). All rights reserved.

MASS EFFECT is the pathological situation in which a component of the central nervous system (CNS) is compressed by intrinsic or extrinsic pathology. It is often a compelling indication for urgent neurosurgical intervention.

HISTORY

The consequences of intracranial mass lesions from trauma were recognized as far back in antiquity as the Edwin Smith surgical papyrus, the first written record about the nervous system dating back to 1700 B.C. In the 1870s, cerebral localization of function allowed rational neurosurgical therapy to be developed for mass lesions. Pioneer neurosurgeons have since popularized surgical techniques for removing mass lesions. At that time, however, mass lesions were diagnosed very late in their course, and neurological morbidity and mortality were high. Until the 1970s, other than nucleotide brain scanning, the only radiographic tools available were plain radiography, cerebral angiography, pneumoencephalography, and myelography. These invasive methods were not easily repeatable, did not image the tissues directly, and were associated with significant risks. In 1973, computed tomography (CT) became available commercially and facilitated our current understanding of mass effect and timely intervention.

ETIOLOGY AND PATHOPHYSIOLOGY

The potential causes of mass effect can be broadly classified as those associated with an early or a late increase in intracranial pressure (ICP). The slower the growth of the mass, the more likely the intracranial contents will accommodate the mass as extracellular fluid spaces shrink, cerebrospinal fluid (CSF) production decreases, cerebral atrophy occurs, and cerebral plasticity allows cortical functions to relocate to unaffected areas over time. As a result, ICP tends to remain normal until the late stages of compression by CNS tumors, other mass lesions of the CNS (e.g., giant aneurysms), and tumors of surrounding bone and soft tissues. In contrast, traumatic lesions and primary intracerebral hematomas manifest acutely or subacutely with a sudden increase in ICP. Thus, a 5-cm slow-growing meningioma may be asymptomatic, whereas a similarly sized hemorrhage is likely to cause hemiplegia and alter the patient's level of consciousness.

Regardless of the origin of a mass lesion, the mechanisms by which they cause detrimental effects include focal distortion of neuronal tissue directly inhibiting cellular function, compression of vessels causing ischemia in local areas or in the area supplied by the vessels, and increased ICP with or without obstruction of CSF flow with resultant secondary hydrocephalus.

SYMPTOMS AND SIGNS

Headaches are a universal warning sign of expanding mass lesions and often precede more specific and localizing symptomatology. Headaches can be accompanied by visual obscurations (if there is papilledema), vomiting, or disturbances of consciousness when ICP is elevated acutely. More specific clinical manifestations of space-occupying lesions depend on their location and etiology. Lesions in frontal, occipital, and intraventricular locations are less likely to manifest with overt focal symptomatology than those in the temporal and parietal lobes, diencephalon, brainstem, or spinal cord. Pressure gradients across intracranial compartments caused by the nonuniform distribution of pressures can cause the intracranial contents to shift and ultimately herniate. This process occurs in the classic uncal, tentorial, tonsillar, and subfalcine clinical herniation syndromes. The associated cerebral injury can be compounded by compression of adjacent major vasculature and secondary infarction.

DIAGNOSIS

Space-occupying lesions that cause mass effect are usually diagnosed either incidentally in the course of evaluation of nonspecific symptoms such as headache or in the setting of localizing neurological symptoms. CT and magnetic resonance imaging used with intravenous contrast agents allow precise anatomical localization and often provide clues about differential diagnoses.

TREATMENT

The ideal treatment of mass effect is surgical removal of the mass without inflicting further neurological injury. Other options include decompressive craniectomy or lobectomy to alleviate compromise of residual neural structures. If surgical options are not feasible, therapy should be aimed at normalizing ICP, relieving herniation, minimizing the effects of cerebral edema, and decreasing the likelihood of secondary infarcts by maximizing perfusion and the delivery of essential nutrients to sustain normal neural metabolism.

Head Position

Traditionally, neurosurgical patients have been nursed with a minimum of 30° of head elevation to try to maximize venous drainage from the cerebral circulation. Recent literature suggests that this practice is neither detrimental nor essential. More important, neck kinking should be avoided to prevent obstruction of jugular venous outflow.

Ventilation

Hyperventilation effectively decreases ICP acutely by causing CSF alkalosis and secondary cerebrovasoconstriction, thus decreasing intracranial blood volume. Its chronic use, however, is problematic due to cerebral ischemia in areas of already compromised blood flow and the risks of rebound intracranial hypertension when the P_aCO_2 is corrected. Normocapnia should therefore be maintained when possible (normocapnia is defined as a P_aCO_2 of 35–45 mmHg), and a P_aCO_2 of approximately

35 mmHg is advocated when ICP is elevated (usually higher than 30 mmHg). Positive end-expiratory pressure has variable effects on ICP. A minimal level should be used to maintain the arterial oxygen level between 80 and 100 mmHg and optimal P_aCO_2.

Osmotic and Diuretic Agents

Mannitol is the agent of choice. Bolus doses (0.25–1 g/kg) every 6 hr offer the greatest benefit and the least side effects when treating ICP. Although its mechanism of action is unknown, mannitol decreases the cerebral content of H_2O, decreases the viscosity of blood, and shrinks endothelial cells, thereby improving blood flow through compressed vessels, transiently increasing plasma volume and therefore cerebral perfusion, and decreasing CSF production. It also possesses antioxidant properties. Its side effects are the development of hyperosmolar states (serum osmolarity > 320 mOsm/liter), renal failure, and electrolyte imbalance. Furosemide has been used primarily or to enhance the effect of mannitol in reducing ICP.

CSF Drainage

In the presence of hydrocephalus, ventricular catheterization is a rapid and simple method of relieving ICP. The risks of its use include cerebral tissue injury, hemorrhage, and infection of violated tissues. However, not all cases of elevated ICP can be treated by CSF drainage because compressed or displaced ventricular spaces can be difficult to cannulate. Lumbar drainage of CSF also incurs the risk of precipitating tonsillar herniation.

Corticosteroids

The indications for the use of steroids are limited to peritumoral edema and spinal cord injury. Corticosteroids offer no benefit in the treatment of cerebral infarct or trauma and may increase the incidence of nosocomial infections and other metabolic complications.

Adjuvant Cerebroprotectants

Sedatives such as short-acting benzodiazepines, propofol, barbiturates, and paralytics can be used judiciously to help control ICP. However, barbiturates have many side effects, including depression of the cardiorespiratory and immune system. Consequently, they are only used for the acute situation of intractably elevated ICP when mass effect is likely to resolve relatively quickly. Additional brain protection from hypothermia is promising and under investigation. Anticonvulsants have no direct effect on ICP but are recommended in selected patients with mass lesions when a seizure could suddenly increase ICP and cause clinical deterioration.

CONCLUSION

The early recognition and accurate identification of mass effect are essential to minimize neurological injury. Tailored therapy, including the resection of the lesion, decompressive surgery, and adjuvant treatments, can help minimize secondary damage and hasten recovery of neurological function.

—*Veronica Chiang and Issam Awad*

See also–Craniectomy; Hydrocephalus; Intracranial Pressure; Intracranial Pressure Monitoring; Lobectomy

Further Reading

Artru, A. A. (1987). Reduction of cerebrospinal fluid pressure by hypocapnia: Changes in cerebral blood volume, cerebrospinal fluid volume, and brain tissue water and electrolytes. *J. Cereb. Blood Flow Metab.* **7**, 471–479.

Bittar, R. G., Olivier, A., Sadikot, A. F., *et al.* (2000). Cortical motor and somatosensory representation: Effect of cerebral lesions. *J. Neurosurg.* **92**, 242–248.

Cottrell, J. E., Robustelli, A., Post, K., *et al.* (1977). Furosemide- and mannitol-induced changes in intracranial pressure and serum osmolality and electrolytes. *Anesthesiology* **47**, 28–30.

Feldman, Z., Kanter, M. J., Robertson, C. S., *et al.* (1992). Effect of head elevation on intracranial pressure, cerebral perfusion pressure, and cerebral blood flow in head-injured patients. *J. Neurosurg.* **76**, 207–211.

Fortune, J. B., Feustel, P. J., Graca, L., *et al.* (1995). Effect of hyperventilation, mannitol, and ventriculostomy drainage on cerebral blood flow after head injury. *J. Trauma* **39**, 1091–1099.

Lundberg, N., Kjallquist, A., and Bien, C. (1959). Reduction of increased intracranial pressure by hyperventilation. A therapeutic aid in neurological surgery. *Acta Psychiatr. Scand.* **34**, 1–64.

Marion, D. W., Obrist, W. D., Carlier, P. M., *et al.* (1993). The use of moderate therapeutic hypothermia for patients with severe head injuries: A preliminary report. *J. Neurosurg.* **79**, 354–362.

Oldendorf, W. H. (1980). *The Quest for an Image of the Brain.* Raven Press, New York.

Rossini, P. M., Caltagirone, C., Castriota-Scanderbeg, A., *et al.* (1998). Hand motor cortical area reorganization in stroke: A study with fMRI, MEG and TCS maps. *NeuroReport* **9**, 2141–2146.

Signorini, D. F., and Alderson, P. (2000). Therapeutic hypothermia for head injury. *Cochrane Database Syst. Rev.* **2**, CD001048.

McArdle's Disease
see Glycogen Storage Diseases

Measles Virus, Central Nervous System Complications of

Encyclopedia of the Neurological Sciences

MEASLES (or rubeola) was recognized as early as the 10th century by a Persian physician, Al-Rhazes. In 1911, Goldberger and Anderson showed that measles was caused by a virus, and in 1954 Enders and Peebles isolated the virus and were able to propagate it in cell culture. This led to the preparation of the attenuated live virus vaccines in the early 1960s and the subsequent near eradication of measles in the developed world. However, measles remains a worldwide health care problem, particularly in Third World countries in which mass vaccination programs are lacking. Approximately 30–40 million cases of measles are reported annually, and at least 1 million people die from complications of the acute infection. Even in industrialized countries, measles epidemics occur in young adults despite childhood vaccination, suggesting that unlike natural infection, the vaccine may not endow lifelong immunity. Central nervous system (CNS) complications of measles are rare but serious. These include postinfectious measles encephalitis (PME), subacute sclerosing panencephalitis (SSPE), and subacute measles encephalitis with immunosuppression (SME), also known as measles inclusion body encephalitis. Although recent epidemiological studies suggest an association between measles and autism, this association is controversial. This entry highlights the clinical, pathological, and pathogenic aspects of measles CNS complications. Currently, there is no effective treatment for these complications, and patients either die or are left with considerable disability.

THE VIRUS

Measles virus (MV) is a negative-stranded RNA virus that belongs to the paramyxovirus family (Fig. 1).

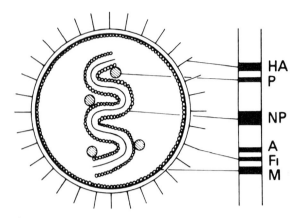

Figure 1
A schematic representation of the measles virus and its major structural proteins (courtesy of Dr. Peggy Swoveland, Department of Veteran's Affairs).

The virus consists of a lipid envelope that anchors the hemagglutinin (HA) and fusion (F) proteins, which are responsible for the attachment of the virus on the cell surface and fusion of the infected cells, respectively. Both HA and F are also critical for induction of neutralizing antibodies. The virus core contains the RNP complex, which consists of the nucleocapsid (N) protein and the polymerase complex (L and P units). A matrix (M) protein links the envelope proteins (HA and F) with the RNP complex and is critical for the assembly and budding of new virions from infected cells. In addition, the MV genome encodes for three nonstructural proteins (C, R, and V), some of which may serve virulence function. MV infects cells through the attachment of the HA protein to cell surface receptors including CD46, a complement regulatory protein also known as membrane cofactor protein (MCP). An additional receptor for MV, CDw150 or SLAM (signaling lymphocyte activation molecule), was recently identified. It is not clear whether the SSPE virus uses the CD46 receptor to infect neurons. The paucity of CD46 expression in the CNS and the inability of wild-type MV to bind CD46 suggest an alternative receptor. However, studies in CD46 transgenic mice indicate that although CD46 is required for the initial infection, neuronal spread can occur independently.

THE ACUTE INFECTION

Humans are the natural host and reservoir for the virus. Measles is transmitted by aerosol and replicates initially in the upper respiratory tract epithelium followed by lymphatic spread and viremia within 3 days of exposure. The viremia leads to a transient suppression of cell-mediated immune responses that lasts 1–4 weeks. Immunosuppression is believed to be due to virus interception of cytokine synthesis pathways, including interleukin-12 and interferon-γ, induction of T cell apoptosis, and T cell anergy. After 7–10 days of infection, the virus spreads to epithelial tissues, and clinical symptoms of fever, cough, coryza, conjunctivitis, and oral mucosal lesions (Koplik spots) appear. This is followed a few days later by the appearance of a maculopapular skin rash that begins on the head and neck and then spreads to the entire body. By the time the rash appears, the clinical symptoms begin to improve. IgM antibodies to MV can be detected during the first week and IgG antibodies begin to increase 2 weeks after infection. Determination of MV antibody titers confirms the diagnosis when in doubt. In some cases, pneumonia and otitis media complicate the acute illness and bacterial superinfection can occur. In immunocompromised patients, lethal giant cell pneumonia can develop. Protein-losing enteropathy secondary to viremic spread to the intestine can be a fatal complication in children residing in developing countries. An atypical form of measles has been described in individuals who received the killed measles vaccine and were later exposed to the virus. The symptoms of atypical measles are similar to those of measles except that they can be more severe.

POSTINFECTIOUS MEASLES ENCEPHALITIS

PME strikes 1 in 1000 measles cases and accounts for 95% of the neurological complications associated with measles. Much less frequently, PME may complicate measles vaccination (1 in 1 million vaccinations). The onset is abrupt, usually occurring 4 or 5 days after onset of the rash, but can predate the rash by a few days or occur up to 3 weeks later. Headache, fever, seizures, and multifocal neurological deficits evolve quickly and the patient may become obtunded. Magnetic resonance imaging (MRI) may show demyelinating lesions (Fig. 2). Cerebrospinal fluid (CSF) examination may be normal, but in some patients there is mononuclear pleocytosis and elevated protein levels, including those for myelin basic protein. The electroencephalograph (EEG) may show diffuse slowing. The disease is invariably monophasic, but mortality is high, ranging from 10 to 40%. Survivors are usually left with variable degrees of disability, including mental retardation, motor deficits, and ataxia.

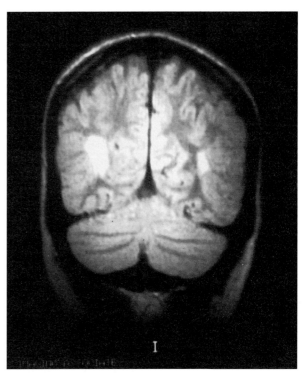

Figure 2
MRI from a 10-year-old boy who had onset of motor weakness and seizures 10 days following live measles vaccination. The T2 MRI shows diffuse white and gray matter disease (courtesy of Dr. Ajay S. Gupta, Caylor-Nickel Clinic, Bluffton, IN).

Pathologically, there is perivenular inflammation and demyelination with striking similarities to experimental autoimmune encephalomyelitis. MV cannot be recovered from the CNS, but in very few cases it has been cocultivated from the CSF. *In situ* hybridization studies failed to detect MV RNA in brain, but reverse transcriptate polymerase chain reaction- based *in situ* hybridization detected an infection of endothelial cells in some cases. Approximately half of patients with PME demonstrate a lymphoproliferative response against myelin basic protein. The pathogenesis of PME is not known, but it is widely believed to be due to immune dysregulation triggered by MV, resulting in molecular mimicry and in a misguided attack on myelin antigens. Additional mechanisms may include an attack on the myelin-producing cell (the oligodendrocyte) with rapid clearance of the virus (hit-and-run mechanism) or an attack by MV-specific cytotoxic T cells on infected endothelial cells. Although no specific HLA haplotype correlates with PME, other genetic elements involving the T cell receptor makeup could influence susceptibility to disease. Treatment is generally supportive, and there is anecdotal experience in favor of intravenous steroid use.

SUBACUTE SCLEROSING PANENCEPHALITIS

Described by Dawson in 1933 (Dawson's encephalitis) and subsequently by Van Bogaert in 1945 (Van Bogaert's encephalitis), the causation of SSPE by MV was not established until 1967 when Connolly and colleagues demonstrated elevated anti-MV antibodies in SSPE serum and CSF and MV antigen in SSPE brain. In 1969, MV was rescued from SSPE brain tissue by cocultivation techniques.

SSPE is a rare complication of measles currently affecting less than 1 in 1 million measles cases in the developed world. The incidence of the disease declined markedly following the introduction of the measles vaccine. The typical age of onset is between 5 and 10 years but can be as early as 2 years and as late as 30 years following measles. The most common clinical presentation is mood and intellectual dysfunction and declining school performance (stage 1) (Fig. 3A). This is followed months to years later by the onset of motor dysfunction, myoclonic jerks, ataxia, and seizures (stage 2) (Fig. 3A). Ocular signs consisting of retinal pigmentation, optic atrophy, chorioretinitis, optic neuritis, and papilledema occur

in two-thirds of patients. After a period of a few months to a year, the patient enters stage 3, which is characterized by decorticate or decerebrate posturing, loss of brainstem function, and coma. Approximately two-thirds of patients die during this stage. Those who survive enter stage 4, in which the patient appears awake but is in fact mute and has lost cortical function. Pathological crying and laughter and startle responses to auditory stimuli are common. The patient usually succumbs to an infection or vasomotor collapse after an average duration of illness of 3 or 4 years. Some patients die rapidly within a few weeks and some can survive as long as 12 years. Substantial improvement has been observed in 10% of patients usually during stage 2 and some of the remissions were sustained for several years.

The diagnosis of SSPE is confirmed by the demonstration of elevated anti-measles virus antibodies in serum and CSF. CSF IgG index is elevated, indicating intrathecal IgG synthesis, and CSF oligoclonal IgG bands react specifically with measles antigens. The EEG shows a characteristic pattern of periodic slow wave complexes with some associated sharp transients (Fig. 3B) with a repetition rate of once every 5–15 sec; the complexes are time locked to the myoclonic jerks. Brain MRI demonstrates both gray and white matter disease with cortical atrophy and ventricular dilatation (Figs. 3C and 3D).

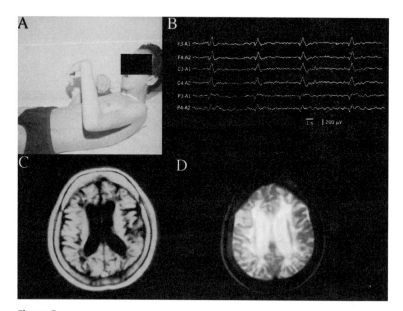

Figure 3
Clinical and laboratory features of SSPE. (A) An SSPE patient during a myoclonic jerk. (B) An EEG tracing in clinical stage II showing bilaterally synchronous periodic spike and wave complexes occurring at regular intervals. (C) MRI showing ventricular dilatation and cortical atrophy and (D) the corresponding T2-weighted image showing diffuse white matter disease.

SSPE affects the cerebral cortex and brainstem, with less involvement of the cerebellum and spinal cord. Perivascular infiltration with lymphocytes and macrophages is found in the gray and white matter, with widespread neuronal loss, variable degrees of demyelination, and gliosis. Eosinophilic, intranuclear, and cytoplasmic viral particles are seen in neurons and oligodendroglia and react with measles antibodies. Electron microscopy shows viral nucleocapsids with a fuzzy appearance in the cytoplasm and a smooth appearance in the nucleus (Fig. 4).

Although rare, SSPE continues to fascinate scientists interested in mechanisms of virus persistence in

Table 1 POTENTIAL PATHOGENIC MECHANISMS IN SSPE

Proposed factors leading to MV persistence in SSPE
  Abnormal host response
  Defective virus
  A second agent
Factors contributing to maintenance of virus persistence
  Defective cytotoxic T lymphocyte (CTL) response
  Lack of HLA expression in the CNS
  Lack of viral epitopes critical for CTL recognition
  Failure of infected neurons to produce interferon-β
  Interferon-resistant strains of measles virus

the CNS. Although the etiological agent in SSPE has been identified as measles or a measles-like virus, the pathogenetic events that initiate and maintain persistence remain unclear. There are two central questions regarding the pathogenesis of SSPE: (i) Why does measles virus in rare cases enter and persist in the CNS and (ii) why does the immune system fail to eliminate the infection? A number of mechanisms have been proposed and are summarized in Table 1.

There is indirect evidence that MV invades the brain during acute infection since EEG abnormalities and CSF pleocytosis have been observed in approximately 30% of uncomplicated measles cases. Although SSPE patients do not have history of acute encephalitis, it is possible that virus invasion of the CNS occurs during acute measles followed by a latent period of months or years. Measles at an early age appears to increase the risk of SSPE, perhaps related to the maturation stage of the immune response and CNS cells as suggested by animal models of persistent measles encephalitis. The presence of maternal antibodies to MV may result in the conversion of an acute to a subacute infection as indicated by animal models of SSPE.

Mutations affecting the expression of the measles envelope proteins (HA and F) and matrix (M) protein have been described. Perhaps the most relevant mutation is that of the M protein, which disables the packaging and maturation of newly formed virions, resulting in a nonproductive infection. However, it is unlikely that SSPE is due to a defective virus since outbreaks of SSPE have not been observed in families or communities. It is more likely that mutations occur after MV has infected the CNS perhaps due to host cell factors that restrict viral gene expression, hyperactive antibody response, or the presence of maternal antibodies. The presence of an overactive anti-measles antibody response in the CNS contributes to restriction of viral gene

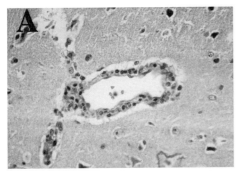
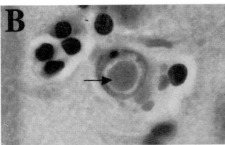
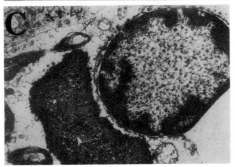

Figure 4
Pathological features of SSPE. (A) Perivascular inflammatory cells and neuronal loss in brain tissue from an SSPE patient (H & E stain). (B) An eosinophilic intranuclear inclusion body (courtesy of Dr. Robert Herndon), and (C) electron microscopy of intracytoplasmic (crescent-shape) inclusion bodies and intranuclear filamentous course inclusions (magnification, ×19,000). (See color plate section.)

expression, a phenomenon referred to as antibody-induced antigenic modulation. Although infected cells fail to produce mature virus, they are able to spread the infection to adjacent cells, perhaps explaining the slowly progressive disease course.

Epidemiological studies indicate a higher incidence of SSPE in rural areas, suggesting exposure to a second, perhaps zoonotic, agent. However, no such agent has been found in SSPE tissue. It is also possible that MV persists outside the CNS following acute infection but is then triggered by a second agent later in life, leading to CNS invasion and SSPE.

Failure of the immune system to clear MV-infected neurons contributes to the maintenance of virus persistence. During the past decade, a number of mechanisms have been identified that could impair the elimination of MV from the CNS in SSPE, including a defect in the generation of MV-specific cytotoxic T lymphocytes (CTLs); failure of infected neurons to express HLA class I molecules necessary for recognition of infected cells by the cellular immune response; and an inability of infected neurons to produce interferon-β, a cytokine critical for the host innate antiviral defense mechanisms. Additionally, in humans the MV CTL response is higher for the HA and F proteins than for the core proteins. Thus, mutations affecting HA and F genes could result in deletions of viral epitopes that are critical for CTL recognition and consequently lysis of infected cells. Furthermore, interferon-resistant strains of MV have been identified in SSPE and acute measles. Such strains are more likely to persist and could play a role in the pathogenesis of SSPE. Antibodies could also contribute to persistence by stripping viral antigen from the surface of infected cells, thus reducing their susceptibility to lysis by complement. Although the previously mentioned mechanisms impair the ability of the immune system to rid neurons of the infection, they can also be viewed as beneficial responses that have evolved to protect a postmitotic cell population (neurons) from cell death. As such, persistently infected neurons can survive but at the expense of compromised function.

SSPE is a lethal disease and treatment with antiviral and immunomodulating agents has been disappointing. Isoprinosine, a drug with antiviral and immunopotentiation effects, has been reported to stabilize or significantly improve the clinical condition in some patients, whereas other studies concluded that the drug is ineffective. Clinical improvement with intrathecal or intraventricular injection of α-interferon has been reported in some patients, but this treatment is costly, requires hospitalization, and has not been shown to cure the disease. A multinational study with combined Isoprinosine and intraventricular interferon-α-2b in SSPE is currently under way. Fortunately, measles vaccination has virtually eliminated the disease in many countries.

SUBACUTE MEASLES ENCEPHALITIS WITH IMMUNOSUPPRESSION

SME is a rare complication of immunosuppression and is distinct from SSPE. SME occurs in patients with defects in cell-mediated immunity, those receiving immunosuppressive drugs for the treatment of lymphoproliferative disorders, and in patients with acquired immunodeficiency syndrome (AIDS). Rarely, the condition can result from vaccinating an immunosuppressed patient. A history of measles or measles exposure precedes the onset of neurological deficit by 1–6 months. The disease is characterized by the onset of seizures, motor deficits, coma, and death within days to a few weeks. The CSF shows no abnormalities

Table 2   COMPARATIVE FEATURES OF THE CNS COMPLICATIONS CAUSED BY MEASLES VIRUS

	Postmeasles encephalomyelitis	Subacute sclerosing panencephalitis	Subacute measles encephalitis
Measles age	>2 years	<2 years	Any age
Onset after measles	Within 3 weeks	Months to years	Weeks to months
Course and outcome	Improvement (80%)	Fatal in years	Fatal in months
Antibody to MV	Normal	Elevated	Deficient
Cellular immunity	Normal	Defective MV CTL	Suppressed
CSF	Pleocytosis, elevated protein	Ab to MV in oligoclonal IgG bands	Normal
EEG	Slowing	Periodic complexes	Slowing
Pathology	White matter periventricular inflammation	Panencephalitis, inclusions, inflammation	Inclusions, no inflammation
Measles in CNS	Absent	Present	Present

and, in contrast to SSPE, antibodies to MV are not found. Pathologically, there is neuronal loss with eosinophilic inclusion bodies in neurons and glia but no inflammation. Virus can be recovered from the brain and measles proteins are detectable in infected cells. Treatment with the antiviral drug Ribavarin has produced encouraging results in some patients. Despite the occurrence of SME following measles vaccination, it is recommended that patients with AIDS be vaccinated because the benefits outweigh the risks.

CONCLUSION

In summary, measles virus can produce serious complications in the CNS that can be distinguished clinically and pathologically. Table 2 summarizes the characteristic features of each of these complications. The underlying pathogenic mechanisms are not totally understood and continue to be investigated. Although treatment is largely symptomatic, prevention with mass vaccination, combined with the development of a better vaccine, could potentially eliminate measles and its complications in the future.

—*Suhayl Dhib-Jalbut*

See also–Central Nervous System Infections, Overview; Demyelinating Disease, Pathology of; Encephalitis, Viral; HIV Infection, Neurological Complications of; Meningitis, Viral; Rubella Virus; Varicella-Zoster Virus

Acknowledgments

This work was supported by grants from the Departments of Veterans Affairs (Merit Review) and Health and Human Services (NIH/NINDS K-24 award).

Further Reading

Dhib-Jalbut, S., and Johnson, K. P. (1994). Measles virus diseases. In *Handbook of Neurovirology* (R. R. McKendall and W. G. Stroop, Eds.), pp. 539–554. Dekker, New York.
Dhib-Jalbut, S., Xia, Q., Drew, P., *et al.* (1995). Differential up-regulation of HLA class I molecules on neuronal and glial cell lines by virus infection correlates with differential induction of IFN-β. *J. Immunol.* **155**, 2096–2108.
Gogate, N., Swoveland, P., Yamabe, T., *et al.* (1996). Major histocompatibility complex class I expression on neurons in subacute sclerosing panencephalitis and experimental subacute measles encephalitis. *J. Neuropathol. Exp. Neurol.* **55**, 435–443.
Johnson, R. T. (1998). *Viral Infections of the Nervous System*, pp. 227–239. Lippincott–Raven, Philadelphia.
Liebert, U. G. (1997). Measles virus infections of the central nervous system. *Intervirology* **40**, 176–184.
Norrby, E., and Kristensson, K. (1997). Measles virus in the brain. *Brain Res. Bull.* **44**, 213–220.
Patterson, J. B., Manchester, M., and Oldstone, M. B. A. (2001). Disease model: Dissecting the pathogenesis of the measles virus. *Trends Mol. Med.* **7**, 85–88.
Schneider-Schaulies, J., Niewiesk, S., Schneider-Schaulies, S., *et al.* (1999). Measles virus in the CNS: The role of viral and host factors for the establishment and maintenance of a persistent infection. *J. Neurovirol.* **5**, 613–622.

Median Nerves and Neuropathy

Encyclopedia of the Neurological Sciences
Copyright 2003, Elsevier Science (USA). All rights reserved.

ENTRAPMENT of the median nerve proximal to the carpal tunnel can occur at different sites. These conditions are rare when compared with carpal tunnel syndrome (CTS), estimated at a frequency of 2 in 1000. However, these two conditions can be confused because they can cause similar symptoms of arm and hand pain, sensory disturbances, and motor weakness.

ANATOMY

The median nerve receives contributions from the C5–T1 nerve roots. The nerve fibers are organized in clusters within the nerve according to how they branch off the main nerve trunk. This anatomical characteristic can explain why in a compressive injury, certain branches of the nerve can be affected while others are spared.

The median nerve is formed from the medial (C5–C7) and lateral (C8–T1) cords of the brachial plexus. It passes through the axilla and descends along the medial arm in close proximity to the brachial artery. In the antecubital fossa, the median nerve is posterior to the bicipital aponeurosis and median vein and anterior to the brachialis muscle and the elbow joint. The only branches of the median nerve above the elbow are articular branches to the elbow joint. The first motor branches arise near the elbow crease. In the forearm, the median nerve passes between the two heads of the pronator teres (PT) muscle in 80–95% of the population.

MOTOR INNERVATION

The median nerve commonly innervates 12 muscles in the arm: the pronator teres (PT), flexor carpi radialis (FCR), palmaris longus (PL), flexor digitor-um sublimis (FDS), lateral portion of the flexor digitorum profundus (FDP), pronator quadratus (PQ), flexor pollicis longus (FPL), abductor pollicis brevis (APB), superficial head of flexor pollicis brevis (FPB), the first and second lumbricals, and opponens pollicis (OP) (Fig. 1). The first motor branch of the median nerve supplies the PT muscle as it courses between the two heads of the muscle in the proximal forearm. The median nerve then gives off multiple branches to supply the FDS muscle below the medial epicondyle. The FCR is usually the next muscle innervated by the median nerve. The anterior interosseous nerve (AION) then

branches off the main nerve distal to FDS, and courses with the anterior interosseous artery deep in the forearm along the interosseous membrane and between the FPL and lateral FDP muscles. The AION supplies three muscles—FPL, lateral FDP and lastly the PQ but carries no cutaneous sensory fibers. The main trunk of the median nerve continues to the forearm and enters the carpal tunnel after it supplies the FDS and FCR. Once past the carpal tunnel and into the hand, it supplies the APB, OP, superficial head of the FPB and lumbricals I and II.

SENSORY INNERVATION

The median nerve carries cutaneous sensation from the wrist and hand. It also supplies sensation from the brachial artery, the elbow joint, and the radio-ulnar, radiocarpal, and carpal joints. The first cutaneous sensory branch is the palmar cutaneous nerve, which branches proximal to the flexor retinaculum and thus is not affected in CTS. It supplies sensation to the skin over the thenar eminence. The remaining fibers of the median nerve travel under the flexor retinaculum, through the carpal tunnel, and end in the hand. The median nerve supplies the sensation to the lateral aspects of the palm, thumb, and index, middle, and lateral half of the ring finger as well as the dorsal aspects of the distal phalanges of these fingers. The median nerve also supplies sensation to the blood vessels and bony structures of the lateral hand and $3\frac{1}{2}$ fingers. This sensory territory is present in approximately 72% of the population, with the most common variation being the extent of median innervation to the ring finger.

ENTRAPMENT SITES

High median nerve entrapment is usually located in the regions around the shoulder or the elbow. The syndrome of high median nerve entrapment around the shoulder is usually due to trauma, such as humeral fracture, anterior shoulder dislocation, or crutch palsy. The median nerve can also be injured with a tourniquet around the mid-arm. In this situation, the ulnar and radial nerves are also usually affected, resulting in a "trinerve" palsy. If the cause of the high median palsy is trauma such as compression from crutches, the treatment is con-servative and prognosis is good, especially if there is only partial functional loss or if recovery begins

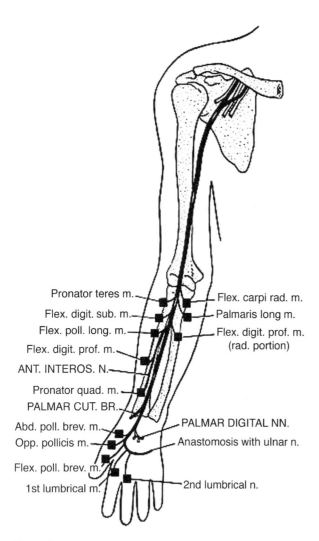

Figure 1
Muscles in the arm commonly innervated by the median nerve (copyright Joe F. Jabre. Reprinted with permission from TeleEMG.com).

early. The time of recovery depends on the severity of the initial injury.

More commonly, median nerve entrapment occurs near the elbow. The sites are at the Ligament of Struthers (LS) above the elbow and below the elbow at the lacertus fibrosis, the head of the PT muscle, and the sublimis bridge of the FDS muscle. Isolated entrapment of the AION also occurs.

Ligament of Struthers (LS Compression)

The LS is a fibrous band that can run from a supracondylar process (aberrant bony spur) to the medial epicondyle. When present, the median nerve and brachial artery and vein pass under this band, which is present in 1 or 2% of the population, although only a small percentage of this group develops this syndrome. Clinically, patients complain of pain around the elbow and possibly sensory changes and paresthesia in the lateral palm, thenar eminence, and median nerve innervated digits. When present, motor weakness can involve all median innervated muscles, including the pronator teres. The symptoms may worsen with forceful extension of the wrist and elbow with the forearm supinated. Since the brachial artery also runs under the ligament with the median nerve, the blood vessel can be compressed during elbow extension and can cause a diminished radial pulse at the wrist. Plain x-ray of the elbow can help diagnose this syndrome if it shows the supracondylar process; however, the ligament can be present even without the aberrant bony spur.

Pronator Teres Syndrome

In the region of proximal forearm where the PT muscle originates, there are several sites at which median nerve compression can occur. As the median nerve crosses the elbow to enter the forearm, it passes underneath the lacertus fibrosis, which is a fascial band extending from the biceps tendon to forearm fascia. The nerve then passes between the superficial and deep heads of the PT muscle and then beneath the flexor digitorum superficialis arch. In this region, the median nerve can be compressed by a thickened lacertus fibrosus, a hypertrophied pronator teres muscle, or a tight flexor digitorum superficialis arch.

The most common cause of entrapment in this region is probably a hypertrophied PT muscle. Clinically, patients complain of aching pain in the proximal forearm. Pain and paresthesia can be present in the median nerve distribution and tend to be intermittent and activity dependent. Most symptoms can be exacerbated by extension and pronation of the forearm. Weakness in the median nerve distribution can be variable and depends on the severity of compression. The PT muscle can be weak in this syndrome because this muscle can receive median nerve supply via multiple branches, some of which may leave the nerve trunk prior to the site of compression.

On exam, the pronator compression test can be performed to help evaluate proximal median nerve entrapments. This is accomplished by applying pressure at the lateral and proximal edge of the PT muscle for approximately 30 sec. A positive test is pain and paresthesia in the median distribution. The Tinel sign can also be elicited in the forearm, and when present it is helpful in the diagnosis. Other tests to evaluate the syndrome include resistance to pronation with elbow flexion in PT syndrome and resisted flexion of the proximal interphalangeal joint of the middle digit when caused by a tight FDS arch. These tests are positive if they increase the pain and paresthesia in the median distribution.

AION Syndrome

The AION branches off from the median nerve approximately 5–8 cm distal to the lateral epicondyle, and it is the last major branch of the median nerve. It innervates three muscles in the forearm: FPL, FDP to the index and middle fingers, and the PQ. The common locations for AION entrapment are at the tendinous origin of the FDS muscle to the middle finger, at an accessory head of the FPL muscle, and at the tendinous origin of the deep head of the PT muscle. AION paralysis has also been reported as a result of trauma and injuries, such as fractures, lacerations, and penetrating wounds.

AION dysfunction can also be caused by inflammation, focal neuritis, or vasculitis and may represent an incomplete variant of brachial neuritis. In cases of AION palsy unrelated to trauma, patients commonly complain of constant or intermittent pain in the proximal volar forearm. Patients may report that as pain began to improve, they noticed weakness and loss of motor dexterity.

Unlike the previously described syndromes of proximal median neuropathy, the AION syndrome does not cause sensory loss or paresthesia. Weakness also does not involve the muscles affected in CTS. On physical examination, when weakness is present there is decrease or loss of ability to flex the interphalangeal joint of the thumb and the distal interphalangeal joint of the index finger. Due to anatomical variations with possible innervation contributed by the ulnar nerve, the distal interphalangeal joint of the middle finger may or may not be affected. Weakness of the FPL and FDP muscles is manifested by an inability to oppose the tips of the thumb and index finger (as in making an OK sign) but may be seen only if compression is severe. Additionally, there is weakness of the PQ muscle. To examine the PQ muscle, pronation of the forearm is tested with the elbow flexed to minimize contribution from PT. In cases of Martin–Gruber anastomosis between the median and ulnar nerves, which occurs in approximately 15% of limbs, half have ulnar nerve arising from the AION. Thus, in the AION syndrome, the ulnar innervated intrinsic hand muscles may also become affected and weak.

ETIOLOGY

The causes of proximal median nerve compression are usually trauma (especially acute cases) and repetitive use associated with anatomic anomalies in the forearm, such as hypertrophied PT muscle, a tight lacertus fibrosis, or a tight FDS arch. Hobbies and occupations (e.g., butcher, carpenter, or leather cutter) that require repetitive elbow flexion and pronation have been associated with proximal median nerve entrapments. Other causes of proximal median neuropathy include persistent median artery, a thrombosed artery of an epineural vessel, and pseudoaneurysms of the axillary or brachial artery. Compression can also be caused by forearm fractures, elbow dislocations, injection injuries, compartmental syndrome, or hemorrhage into nerve sheath. Plain x-ray or magnetic resonance imaging (MRI) can be useful in the diagnosis of compression injuries caused by structural abnormality, such as mass lesions or LS.

Trauma caused by bone fractures that leads to median nerve injury can do so from the direct force that caused the fracture, from nerve stretch or laceration from displaced bone fragment, or from injury to blood vessels that supply the nerve. The most common fracture associated with median nerve injury is at the elbow, with a frequency of 0.5–16%. The median nerve is also susceptible to injury with a wrist fracture or dislocation, and in this situation the ulnar nerve can also be compromised.

DIFFERENTIAL DIAGNOSIS

Proximal median neuropathy can be difficult to diagnose because it rarely presents with all the expected features. Often, it presents as a partial syndrome because nerve fibers travel in fascicles and the compression or injury affects different fibers unevenly or selectively. Thus, if only fibers designated to become the AION are entrapped in a proximal lesion, the clinical picture is that of an AION syndrome suggestive of more distal involvement.

CARPAL TUNNEL SYNDROME

If the carpal tunnel syndrome (CTS) is advanced, it is not difficult to differentiate from proximal median neuropathy. However, in early cases the symptoms may be more nonspecific with sensory changes in the hand. The sensory exam should be helpful because the region over the thenar eminence should be normal in CTS. Weakness of median innervated forearm muscles on exam also indicates a more proximal lesion. It is important to establish the correct diagnosis because CTS is common in the population and frequently treated with surgical release, which is of no benefit for proximal median neuropathy.

CERVICAL RADICULOPATHY

Patients with C6 or C7 radiculopathy may present with symptoms similar to proximal median nerve compression. Both conditions can have prominent forearm pain, sensory loss/changes in the hand, and arm weakness if severe. However, cervical radiculopathy usually also presents with neck or shoulder pain that radiates down the arm and can be aggravated by neck movement. When weakness is present, muscles not innervated by the median nerve are affected in cervical radiculopathy, such as the biceps and triceps muscles. Also, tendon reflexes can be diminished or absent in cervical radiculopathy, with biceps tendon reflex affected in C6 lesion and triceps reflex in C7 lesion. Clinicoradiographic correlation with cervical spine MRI can confirm the diagnosis.

BRACHIAL PLEXOPATHY

Brachial plexopathy may present as proximal median neuropathy if only the median nerve fibers are involved. However, in many instances other nerves are also affected, and a careful sensory and motor examination will reveal weakness and sensory loss outside of median nerve distribution. Additional sensory and/or motor involvement suggests a more diffuse process rather than a focal compressive lesion of the median nerve.

ELECTROPHYSIOLOGICAL DIAGNOSIS

Electrophysiological testing in proximal median neuropathy is useful for localizing the lesion as well as for evaluating the severity of the neuropathy. The electrodiagnostic results may be normal when complaints are mainly of pain and dysesthesias without sensory loss or weakness. In this situation, nerve conduction studies and electromyography may be most useful in eliminating other causes, such as cervical radiculopathy or brachial plexopathy.

In proximal median nerve entrapment at the PT, nerve conduction studies may show slowing across the elbow as well as a decreased median sensory nerve action potential (SNAP) amplitude. The decrease in velocity and amplitude is seen because demyelination usually occurs before axonal loss in compressive lesions, and sensory fibers are more susceptible to injury than motor fibers. Distal latencies and F wave latency studies are usually normal and do not aid in the diagnosis of proximal median nerve compression. As the lesion progresses, there may be secondary axonal loss, resulting in decreased compound muscle action potential and SNAP amplitudes.

In AION syndrome, there are no abnormalities in routine conduction studies of the median nerve, and the diagnosis is more dependent on an abnormal needle electromyography of innervated muscles. Conduction studies using needle electrodes to measure distal latencies to PQ muscle when stimulating median nerve at the elbow may show abnormal distal latencies. Rosenberg described a technique that involves simultaneous recording over PQ and APB muscles while stimulating the elbow, with AION syndrome diagnosed if distal latency to PQ is prolonged and that to APB is normal.

Needle electromyography (NEMG) is more useful for diagnosis of proximal median neuropathy by examining the median innervated muscles. The muscles proximal to the lesion should be normal, whereas those distal to the lesion may show abnormal neurogenic changes, including signs of denervation (fibrillations, positive sharp waves, reduced recruitment patterns, and increased motor unit amplitude and duration).

If the compression is at the LS, then on NEMG all the muscles innervated by the median nerve may show abnormalities. In the pronator syndrome, the PT muscle may or may not be spared because its innervation may branch off from the median nerve distal to the site of compression.

Of the three muscles supplied by the AION—PQ, FDP and FPL—only the pronator quadratus has sole innervation by AION. The FDP has dual innervation from median and ulnar nerves, and the FPL can have innervation from both the AION and the main branch of the median nerve (31). Because the FCR muscle is usually innervated by the median nerve before the AION branches off, the muscle should be normal on electrophysiological testing in the AION syndrome. Therefore, the FCR is an important muscle for EMG examination to aid in localization of the median nerve lesion.

It is also important to examine other nerves in the arm for comparison to determine whether the cause of the patient's symptoms is a mononeuropathy versus a diffuse polyneuropathy or plexopathy. The most common nerves used for comparison are the ulnar and radial nerves. It is also prudent to study the contralateral median nerve because bilateral median neuropathies have been reported.

TREATMENT

Treatment depends on the severity of symptoms caused by the compression, as determined by clinical examination and electrodiagnostic testing. In patients whose symptoms are mild, intermittent, and use dependent, avoiding the provoking movement, such as elbow flexion and pronation, may be sufficient.

If symptoms persist despite conservative treatment, then surgery is needed to relieve the site of compression. Surgical exploration for pronator syndrome usually begins with an incision above the flexor crease of the elbow, which enables visualization of the LS if present. Surgery necessitates removal of the suprachondylar process and resecting the ligament. Periosteum is also removed due to the chance that the spur can regenerate, causing a recurrence of symptoms. If LS is not the cause of compression, then surgical incision is extended into the forearm following the course of the median nerve. At the pronator teres muscle, a major site of compression, care is taken to manipulate the nerve only from the radial aspect because branches to the flexor and pronator muscles usually branch off from the ulnar side. If the entrapment is a tendinous band within the pronator teres muscle, then dissection of the band or a portion of the muscle can relieve the constriction.

Treatment of the AION syndrome depends on the etiology. Compressions caused by traumatic penetrating lesions need timely surgical exploration and repair; compartmental syndrome or hematomas also require immediate surgical intervention. However, in spontaneous nontraumatic AION syndrome, some have recommended conservative treatment and observation for at least 1 year because many patients have spontaneous recovery up to 12 or more months after onset. This is especially the case when the AION syndrome is a manifestation of brachial neuritis, which may be diagnosed by additional involvement of other nerves by clinical exam or electrophysiological testing. In situations in which symptoms are exacerbated by specific movements, resting or immobilizing the arm in supination and a trial of antiinflammatory medication are indicated as part of conservative management. If surgical exploration is indicated, the incision is similar to that for pronator syndrome, and the superficial head of the pronator teres muscle is separated from the deep head to trace the AION as it goes under the sublimis arch of the flexor digitorum superficialis, which is released to decompress the nerve. Occasionally, the fascial plane between the PT and FCR muscles has to be separated to improve visualization of the nerve as it goes under the sublimis arch.

PROGNOSIS

Prognosis for mild proximal median neuropathy is good. Fifty percent of patients with pronator syndrome usually recover in 4 months with conservative management. Surgical results depend on the cause and severity of the median nerve lesion as well as the duration of symptoms. In acute nerve compression associated with blunt trauma or hematoma, immediate decompression should have favorable prognosis. Of patients who have received surgery for proximal median neuropathy syndromes, approximately half had partial recovery, approximately 25% had complete improvement, and approximately 25% showed no change in their deficits. In a long-term follow-up, patients with only sensory symptoms appeared to have complete

recovery after surgery. The best results are reported in patients with definite anatomical constriction seen during surgery.

—*Dora Leung*

See also–Brachial Plexopathies; Carpal Tunnel Syndrome; Neuropathies, Entrapment; Radiculopathy

Further Reading

Dawson, D. M., Hallett, M., and Wilbourn, A. J. (Eds.) (1999). Median nerve entrapment. In *Entrapment Neuropathies*, 3rd ed., pp. 95–122. Lippincott–Raven, Philadelphia.
De Araujo, M. P. (1996). Electrodiagnosis in compression neuropathies of the upper extremities. *Orthop. Clin. North Am.* **27**, 237–244.
Gross, P. T., and Tolomeo, E. A. (1999). Proximal median neuropathies. *Neurol. Clin.* **17**, 425–445.
Mody, B. S. (1992). A simple clinical test. *Br. J. Hand Surg.* **17**, 513–514.
Rennels, G. D., and Ochoa, J. (1980). Neuralgic amyotrophy manifesting as anterior interosseous nerve palsy. *Muscle Nerve* **3**, 160–164.
Rosenberg, J. N. (1990). Anterior interosseous/median nerve latency ratio. *Arch. Phys. Med. Rehab.* **71**, 228–230.
Seror, P. (1996). Anterior interosseous nerve lesion: Clinical and electrophysiological features. *J. Bone Jt. Surg.* **78**, 238–241.
Stewart, J. D. (2000). *Focal Peripheral Neuropathies*, 3rd ed. Lippincott Williams & Wilkins, Philadelphia.
Sunderland, S. (1978). The median nerve. Anatomical and physiological features. In *Nerves and Nerve Injury*, 2nd ed.; pp. 672–677, 691–727. Churchill Livingstone, London.
Wilborn, A. J. (1996). Nerve injuries caused by injections and tourniquets. *Syllabus: 1996 AAEM Plenary Session. Physical Trauma of Peripheral Nerves*, p. 15. American Association of Electrodiagnostic Medicine, Rochester, MN.

Medulla Oblongata

Encyclopedia of the Neurological Sciences
Copyright 2003, Elsevier Science (USA). All rights reserved.

THE MEDULLA OBLONGATA, the lowermost portion of the brainstem, is composed of ascending and descending fiber pathways, which control motor (voluntary) functions of the body, and neuronal cell groups, which are major sites of visceral sensory processing and the control of cardiovascular, respiratory, gastrointestinal, and other physiological functions. Many of the homeostatic functions of the nervous system are dependent on groups of medullary neurons, which are integral components of the central neuronal circuits controlling autonomic function.

The medulla oblongata (Fig. 1) is also known as the myelencephalon and forms the caudal half of the rhombencephalon, so named because of its shape. A comparison of the structure of the human medulla oblongata with that of the rat reveals a remarkable level of consistency, indicating that the medulla is one of the earlier evolved components of the central nervous system.

In the embryo, neurons of the medulla arise from the lower part of the cranial portion of the neural tube. The primitive central canal widens to form a four-sided pyramid shape with a rhomboid floor that becomes the fourth ventricle extending over the medulla and pons.

ANATOMICAL FEATURES

Descending Pathways

A number of major axonal bundles traverse the rostrocaudal axis of the medulla. Although these pathways may not synapse within the confines of the medulla, their disruption by traumatic lesions may seriously impair the functions they subserve.

Corticospinal Tract: The precentral motor cortex and the premotor area contain the neuronal cell bodies of a major fiber bundle that descends through the medulla oblongata in the medullary pyramids or pyramidal tract (Figs. 1 and 2). These major conduits of the corticospinal tract convey motor impulses to the spinal cord and control voluntary movement. An important feature of the pyramidal tract is the decussation or crossing-over point of the majority

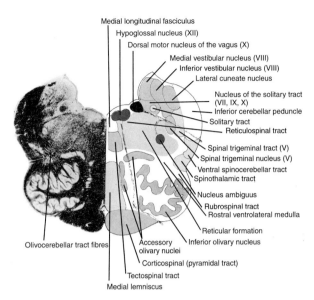

Figure 2
The medulla at the level of the olive. Motor neuronal cell groups and fiber tracts are dark red and pale red, respectively. Sensory neuronal cell groups and fiber tracts are dark blue and pale blue, respectively [reproduced with permission from Heimer, L. (1983). *The Human Brain and Spinal Cord.* Springer-Verlag, New York].

of corticospinal tract fibers that, in addition to demarcating the boundary between the medulla oblongata and the spinal cord, allows the right side of the brain to send signals to the left side of the body, whereas the left cerebral hemisphere communicates with the right side. Whereas the caudal boundary of the medulla oblongata is delineated by the pyramidal decussation (Fig. 1), its junction with the pons, the pontomedullary groove, defines its rostral extent.

Corticobulbar Tract: Corticobulbar pathway axons travel into the brainstem with those of the corticospinal tract. These axons project to cranial nerve motor neurons of the trigeminal nucleus, the facial nucleus, the nucleus ambiguus, and the hypoglossal nucleus (Fig. 2) and are involved in the control of the muscles of the head and face, including the tongue. Corticobulbar projections to the cranial nerve motor neurons are crossed. Motor neurons of the trigeminal nucleus, nucleus ambiguus, and facial nucleus, but not the hypoglossal nucleus, also receive input from the ipsilateral cerebral cortex.

Medial Forebrain Bundle: The medial forebrain bundle contains axons from neurons projecting from the hypothalamus as well as axons projecting to the

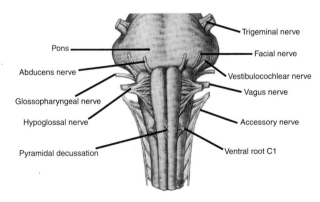

Figure 1
Ventral aspect of the brainstem [reproduced with permission from Carpenter, M. B., and Sutin, J. (1983). *Human Neuroanatomy.* Williams & Wilkins, Baltimore].

hypothalamus from other structures. An important descending projection in the medial forebrain bundle is that which arises from neurons of the paraventricular hypothalamic nucleus that project to dorsal medullary structures, such as the nucleus of the solitary tract and the dorsal motor nucleus of the vagus (Fig. 2) and via a diffuse projection through the medullary reticular formation to sympathetic preganglionic neurons in the thoracic spinal cord.

Vestibulospinal Tract: Axons of the lateral vestibulospinal tract, emanating from the lateral vestibular nucleus, descend uncrossed through the medulla into the ventral white matter of the spinal cord. Similarly, axons of the medial vestibulospinal tract arising from the medial vestibular nucleus (Fig. 2) descend to the cervical cord as both crossed and uncrossed components. These vestibulospinal pathways facilitate rapid movement in response to changes in body position and provide control of antigravity muscles.

Rubrospinal Tract: Arising from the contralateral red nucleus of the midbrain, this fiber system descends through the lateral medulla (Fig. 2) to the spinal cord and is involved in somatic motor function.

Reticulospinal Tract: This system arises from the midbrain, pontine, and medullary reticular formation (Fig. 2) and descends to the cord as both crossed and uncrossed pathways. Axons terminating in the spinal dorsal gray matter modulate somatic sensory transmission (e.g., pain) and originate, in part, from the ventral midline medullary raphé neurons, some of which produce the monoamine neurotransmitter serotonin. Neurons in the midline medullary raphé region also project to sympathetic preganglionic neurons of the thoracic spinal cord.

A region of the rostral ventrolateral medulla contains presympathetic vasomotor neurons (or premotor sympathoexcitatory vasomotor neurons) that send axons to the sympathetic preganglionic neurons. Located ventral to the motor neurons of the compact formation of the nucleus ambiguus and dorsal to the presympathetic vasomotor neurons of the rostral ventrolateral medulla are groups of respiratory premotor neurons that send axons to phrenic nerve motor neurons and thoracic inspiratory motor neurons. These respiratory neurons of the Bötzinger complex, pre-Bötzinger complex, and rostral and caudal ventral respiratory groups form a more or less continuous column in the ventrolateral medulla.

Tectospinal Tract: The tectum or roof of the midbrain, the superior colliculus, contains neuronal cell bodies whose axons descend through the medulla close to the midline (Fig. 2) to the contralateral ventral spinal cord. These neurons are involved in head movements (turning) in response to visual and auditory stimuli.

Medial Longitudinal Fasciculus: The axons of neurons found in the vestibular nuclei form an additional fiber tract that descends close to the tectospinal tract and is involved in coordinating eye and head movements (Fig. 2).

Ascending Pathways

Dorsal column tracts: The dorsal column tracts, or medial lemniscal system (Fig. 2), convey sensory information pertinent to fine touch, vibration, point discrimination, and positioning (proprioception) associated with the skin and joints. Ascending axons in the gracile and cuneate fasciculi convey information from the upper and lower halves of the body, respectively, to terminate in the gracile and cuneate nuclei of the dorsal medulla oblongata. In turn, the axons of neurons of the gracile and cuneate nuclei ascend, crossing in the midline at the lemniscal decussation of the medial lemniscus, relaying in the thalamus en route to the somatosensory cortex.

Spinothalamic Tracts: The lateral spinothalamic tract (Fig. 2) conveys pain and temperature information, whereas the anterior spinothalamic tract carries information about light touch. These tracts arise from spinal dorsal column neurons that receive input from afferent fibers entering the dorsolateral fasciculus or Lissauer's tract of the spinal cord.

Spinoreticular Tract: This less clearly defined tract consists of axons carrying information about deep pain. It originates from ventrolateral spinal cord neurons and terminates onto neurons of the midline medullary raphé and rostral ventrolateral medulla.

Spinocerebellar Tracts: Dorsal and ventral spinocerebellar pathways (Fig. 2) ascend through the lateral medulla oblongata to the cerebellum via the cerebellar peduncle. Both pathways are involved in movement control conveying sensory information from muscle spindles, tendon organs, and touch and pressure receptors.

Cranial Nerves and Cranial Nerve Nuclei

In addition to the major ascending and descending pathways traversing its length, somatic motor, somatic sensory, visceral motor, and visceral sensory neurons are major features of the medulla oblongata. Cranial nerves that contain fibers arising from or projecting to medullary structures include the facial nerve (cranial nerve VII), the glossopharyngeal nerve (cranial nerve IX), the vagus nerve (cranial nerve X), the accessory nerve (cranial nerve XI), and the hypoglossal nerve (cranial nerve XII) (Fig. 3).

Facial Nerve (Cranial Nerve VII): The facial nerve arises from neurons in the facial motor nucleus in the rostral medulla/caudal pons (Fig. 3). It contains predominantly somatic motor axons supplying muscles of the face and scalp, ear, the posterior belly of the digastric muscle, and the stylohyoid muscle. In particular, motoneurons of the facial nucleus control the muscles of the forehead, lips, and cheeks, which together are called the muscles of facial expression. Neurons of the superior salivatory nucleus give rise to parasympathetic preganglionic neurons that project in the facial nerve via the submandibular and sphenopalatine ganglia to the submandibular and sublingual glands.

Glossopharyngeal Nerve (Cranial Nerve IX): The glossopharyngeal nerve contains somatic and visceral sensory as well as somatic and visceral motor components (Fig. 3). Somatic motor fibers originate from neurons of the nucleus ambiguus to innervate the stylopharyngeus muscle. Parasympathetic neurons of the inferior salivatory nucleus exit the medulla in the glossopharyngeal nerve and, via the

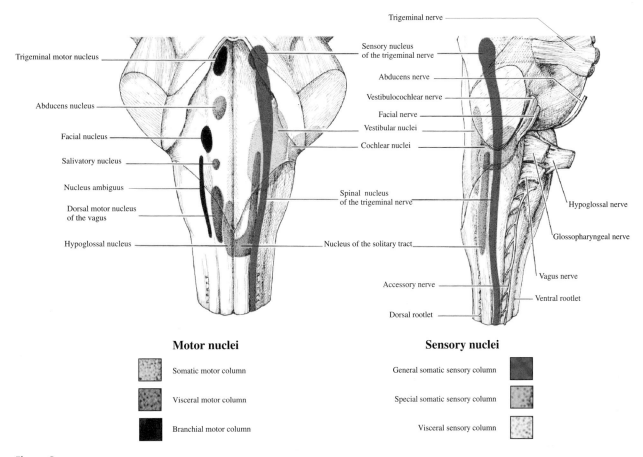

Figure 3

Motor and sensory neuronal cell groups of the medulla oblongata and caudal pons. The somatic motor (hypoglossal nucleus and the abducens nucleus), visceral motor (dorsal motor nucleus of the vagus and the salivatory nucleus), and branchial motor (nucleus ambiguus, facial nucleus, and trigeminal motor nucleus) columns are depicted on the left. The somatic sensory (trigeminal sensory nucleus), special somatic sensory (vestibular nucleus and cochlear nucleus), and visceral sensory (nucleus of the solitary tract) columns are depicted on the right [reproduced with permission from Nauta, W., and Feirtag, M. (1986). *Fundamental Neuroanatomy.* Freeman, New York].

tympanic nerve, project to the otic ganglion to innervate the parotid gland. Visceral sensory afferent fibers arising from the carotid sinus baroreceptors and chemoreceptors travel in the glossopharyngeal nerve. The cell bodies of these afferents are found in the jugular and petrosal ganglia, and they terminate in the nucleus of the solitary tract onto second-order neurons of the baroreflex and chemoreflex.

Vagus Nerve (Cranial Nerve X): Three visceral motor cell groups consisting of parasympathetic preganglionic neurons are found in the medulla oblongata: the dorsal motor nucleus of the vagus, the nucleus ambiguus, and the rostral medullary salivatory nuclei (Fig. 3). The vagus or "wanderer," so named because of its diverse array of peripheral projection targets, contains afferent fibers that arise from abdominal visceral and thoracic structures as well as parasympathetic preganglionic motor nerve fibers. Parasympathetic motor neurons coursing in the vagus nerve innervate parasympathetic ganglia located close to or within a diverse range of cervical, thoracic, and abdominal visceral structures. The most caudal group of parasympathetic neurons that contributes efferent fibers to the vagus, the dorsal motor nucleus of the vagus, lies ventral to and at approximately the same level as the hypoglossal nucleus. It supplies preganglionic parasympathetic vagal outflow to the smooth muscle and glands of the gastrointestinal tract as well as to the heart and respiratory tract via the vagus and glossopharyngeal nerves. Vagal stimulation activates gastrointestinal peristalsis and gastric, hepatic, and pancreatic secretory activity and reduces heart rate. An additional group of neurons contributing preganglionic parasympathetic to the vagus nerve are found in the vicinity of the nucleus ambiguus. The nucleus ambiguus has two major components: the compact formation, which consists of motoneurons projecting to the esophagus and upper airways, and the external formation, which contains a loose collection of parasympathetic preganglionic neurons that project to the heart, lungs, and airways.

Vagal preganglionic neurons of the dorsal motor nucleus of the vagus receive input from a broad range of medullary and supramedullary sources, including cerebral cortical regions, the amygdala, the lateral hypothalamic area, the paraventricular hypothalamic nucleus, the midbrain central gray area, the pontine A5 and parabrachial nuclei, as well as intramedullary neuronal groups. Similarly, neurons within the nucleus ambiguus and its surroundings receive input from hypothalamic, midbrain, and pontine structures.

Vagal afferent fibers arise from a diverse array of structures of the abdominal viscera and the cardiopulmonary region. These convey information from chemoreceptors and mechanoreceptors of the gastrointestinal tract, heart and lungs, and hepatic glucoreceptors to neurons of the nucleus of the solitary tract. Vagal afferent projections to the nucleus of the solitary tract are regarded as pseudobipolar, and their cell bodies are clustered within the nodose ganglion. Destruction of the nucleus of the solitary tract in anesthetized experimental animals interrupts a number of reflexes, including the baroreceptor reflex and the chemoreflex. In animals that are allowed to recover, this treatment produces fulminating hypertension and pulmonary edema reminiscent of neurogenic pulmonary edema that may occur secondary to head trauma in humans. Neurogenic pulmonary edema caused by trauma to intramedullary structures may involve interruption of pathways involved in cardiovascular and respiratory control.

Accessory Nerve (Cranial Nerve XI): The accessory nerve includes medullary and spinal branches. The former contains axons arising from motor neurons of the nucleus ambiguus that project to the larynx, whereas the latter contains motor fibers arising from the anterior horns of the first five or six cervical spinal cord segments. These supply the trapezius and sternocleidomastoid muscles.

Hypoglossal Nerve (Cranial Nerve XII): The caudally located hypoglossal nucleus lies bilaterally on either side of the dorsal medulla and innervates the striated muscles of the tongue via the hypoglossal nerve (Fig. 3). Motor fibers emerge from the medulla between the inferior olive and the pyramids. Neurons in the hypoglossal nucleus receive input from the cerebral cortex and other supramedullary sources as well as sensory input from the trigeminal nerve and the nucleus of the solitary tract, an elongated structure located bilaterally in the dorsal medulla oblongata.

Spinal Trigeminal Tract

Sensory information from the face, mouth, and nose is conveyed to the nervous system by the trigeminal nerve. Many trigeminal (cranial nerve V) primary afferent cell bodies are found within the trigeminal ganglion (also known as the Gasserian or semilunar ganglion), although a small number are also found in the trigeminal mesencephalic nucleus. The latter group are the only primary afferent neuronal cell bodies located within the central nervous system.

Trigeminal ganglion neurons enter the brainstem at the level of the pons and synapse within the trigeminal nuclear complex, which consists of the principal sensory nucleus and the spinal trigeminal nucleus located in the lateral medulla oblongata (Fig. 3). The caudal one-third of the spinal trigeminal nucleus is found within the medulla oblongata in the subnucleus caudalis. Primary afferent fibers conveying pain and temperature signals project caudally in the spinal trigeminal tract to the subnucleus caudalis. These neurons, in turn, send crossed projections to the thalamus via the ventral trigeminothalamic tract.

PHYSIOLOGICAL FUNCTIONS

Arousal and Nociception

Despite the long-standing concept of the reticular activating system, first proposed by Moruzzi and Magoun as an explanation of brainstem control of cortical arousal, it has failed to stand up to close inspection. The reticular activating system concept developed in conjunction with descriptions of brainstem neuroanatomy that focused on nonspecificity of neuronal function and projection patterns. This may have arisen from observations that arousal could be produced by a wide variety of stimuli, including pain, sounds, odors, or sudden movements. Modern views of the mechanisms associated with arousal have largely abandoned this nonspecific approach to understanding mechanisms of arousal, although the concept survives in most textbooks of neurology. In fact, although the mechanisms of arousal are still under investigation, it is apparent that specific groups of neurons in the medulla oblongata and other supramedullary structures process sensory information that has an impact on the level of arousal. At the level of the medulla oblongata, neurons of the nucleus of the solitary tract that respond to specific sensory stimuli are roughly topographically organized such that the rostral nucleus of the solitary tract receives largely gustatory input while caudal and intermediate zones receive respiratory and general visceral inputs. These neurons synapse with intramedullary relay neurons but also contribute to a major ascending projection.

The medulla is also a major site of nociceptive (pain) processing. In particular, neurons of the raphé magnus have long been associated with nociceptive

function. It is unlikely that these spinally projecting neurons function specifically to modulate nociceptive processing. A modern view suggests that medullary raphé neurons modulate a range of sensory and motor functions, including nociception, thermoregulation, sympathetic vasomotor control, and some aspects of sexual organ function.

Nociceptive signals from peripheral pain receptors are relayed in the substantia gelatinosa of the spinal dorsal horn to medullary and supramedullary neurons via a number of ascending pathways, including the spinothalamic tract, the spinoreticular tract, and the spinomesencephalic tract. Neurons within the ventral medullary midline (raphé magnus nucleus) play an important role in nociceptive processing by modulating the activity of the ascending nociceptive pathways. These, in turn, are influenced by neurons in the midbrain periaqueductal gray area.

Eating and Digestion

Food consumption is influenced by a wide variety of factors, such as food odors, taste, appearance, and hunger. Anticipation of food consumption, as well as the act of food consumption, promotes salivation, gastric acid secretion, and changes in gastrointestinal motility and blood flow. Although a number of mechanisms regulate satiety, release of the neuropeptide cholecystokinin from enteroendocrine cells of the gastrointestinal mucosa in response to the presence of nutrients in the intestinal lumen signals the nervous system via vagal afferents terminating in the nucleus of the solitary tract. These signals are relayed to the hypothalamus by ascending pathways to modulate the function of other groups of neurons that control food consumption.

The gastrointestinal tract is largely under the control of the complex network of intrinsic sensory and motor neurons known as the enteric nervous system. Gastrointestinal propulsion, absorption, blood flow, and gastric secretion are under the influence of local reflexes controlled by this system. However, elements of gastrointestinal function are modulated by sensory and motor pathways that relay and are integrated in the medulla oblongata. Therefore, digestion is also influenced by extrinsic neurons that originate within the medulla oblongata. The presence of nutrients within the gastrointestinal tract is sensed by specialized vagal afferents that terminate in the nucleus of the solitary tract. Sugars, lipids, peptides, and other substances are detected and subtly alter gastrointestinal function. Mechanical distension of the stomach and intestinal walls is detected by stretch receptors whose afferent fibers travel in the vagus. Gastrointestinal motility, gastric emptying, gastric acid secretion, pancreatic secretion, and other gastrointestinal functions are under vagal parasympathetic control arising principally from the dorsal motor nucleus of the vagus. Gastrointestinal blood flow is modulated throughout the digestive process and, apart from local mechanisms, is influenced by the splanchnic sympathetic vasomotor outflow.

Taste

Gustatory (taste) signals arising from taste buds of the tongue, palate, pharynx, epiglottis, and upper esophagus are communicated to the gustatory region (rostral third) of the nucleus of the solitary tract by primary afferent fibers in cranial nerves VII (facial nerve), IX (glossopharyngeal nerve), and X (vagus nerve). The ganglion cells associated with these primary afferents are located in the geniculate ganglion (nerve VII), petrosal ganglion (nerve IX), and nodose ganglion (nerve X). Taste receptors in the tongue and oropharyngeal mucosa give rise to primary afferent fibers in the chorda tympani, a branch of the facial nerve, the lingual branch of the glossopharyngeal nerve, and the superior laryngeal branch of the vagus. The second-order neurons of the gustatory region of the nucleus of the solitary tract (the gustatory nucleus of Nageotte) then relay gustatory signals to the parabrachial nucleus and the somatosensory thalamus (ventral posteromedial thalamic nucleus), which in turn projects to the insular cortex and gustatory region of the postcentral gyrus of the cortex. Disorders of taste sensation are usually associated with defective olfaction (ability to smell odors).

Salivation

Salivation or saliva production by the submandibular, sublingual, and parotid glands is controlled by the activity of neurons of the salivatory nuclei located near the dorsal pontomedullary junction. Preganglionic parasympathetic axons arising from cells in the superior salivatory nucleus travel in the chorda tympani branch of the facial nerve to terminate within the submandibular ganglion. Postganglionic cholinergic fibers then pass to the sublingual and submandibular glands, where they stimulate salivary secretion. Neurons in the superior salivatory nucleus also control secretion from the lacrimal, nasal, and palatine glands. Their axons travel in the facial nerve to the sphenopalatine ganglion, whose postganglionic fibers innervate the lacrimal gland and glands of the nasal epithelium.

Neurons in the inferior salivatory nucleus innervate the parotid gland via the glossopharyngeal nerve and the otic ganglion. These preganglionic parasympathetic neurons respond to taste, smell, and mechanical stimulation of other structures of the mouth. They also receive inputs from higher centers of the neuraxis.

Vestibular Function

The vestibular system helps maintain body stance and posture, and it coordinates body, head, and eye movements and visual fixation. Peripheral vestibular transducers of the vestibular labyrinth, the vestibular ganglion cells of the vestibulocochlear nerve (cranial nerve VIII), the vestibular nuclei, and other supramedullary structures are the major components of this system.

Although most of the components of the vestibular system lie rostral to the medulla and are found in the caudal half of the dorsal pons, the inferior olivary nucleus is a prominent feature of the ventral medulla oblongata that provides a source of climbing fiber input via the olivocerebellar tract to the Purkinje cells of the cerebellum. These interconnections are important for regulating the movements that help to maintain body equilibrium and eye movements that occur in response to vestibular signals.

Autonomic Function and the Medulla Oblongata

Despite the implication that some physiological functions are self-governing or autonomic, most of these functions are closely integrated with motor activity, affective states, and behavior. Thus, changes in behavioral state that involve activation of motor functions are accompanied by changes in the function of the body's internal organs. The physiological changes that accompany exercise, such as redistribution of cardiac output and augmentation of the rate and depth of respiration, are an example of this phenomenon. The autonomic nervous system is the motor system controlling the viscera, and in large part but not exclusively, its activity occurs below our level of awareness. Thus, we are usually unaware of the minor changes in the beating of our hearts or the normal processes of digestion, but when we are faced with a stressful situation (e.g., public speaking), we are all too aware of signs such as tachycardia and increased gastrointestinal activity. Most aspects of autonomic function are inextricably linked to the maintenance of homeostasis and are modulated by sensory input arising from the organs they control.

Thus, mechanoreceptors in the heart, lungs, gut, and major thoracic arteries, as well as specialized sensors that detect circulatory oxygen levels or gut and hepatic concentrations of lipids or glucose, play a vital role in the maintenance of bodily homeostasis.

Cardiovascular Regulation—Sympathetic Vasomotor and Cardiovagal Control: The cardiovascular system, operating in concert with the respiratory system, transports oxygenated blood to the tissues of

the body. A major controller of the caliber of the resistance vessels of the arterial system is the sympathetic vasomotor neural outflow (Fig. 4). The sympathetic vasomotor outflow arises from preganglionic nerves in the intermediolateral cell column of the thoracic spinal cord. These cholinergic fibers synapse with noradrenergic postganglionic neurons in the sympathetic ganglia and innervate vascular smooth muscle and the heart. Although local chemical factors can modulate and fine-tune regional

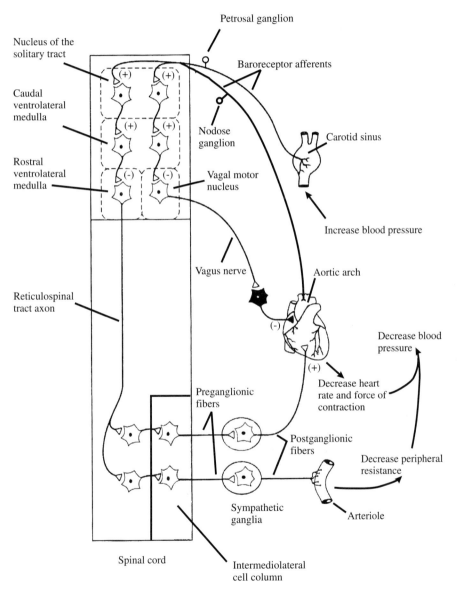

Figure 4
Neuronal circuits that control the cardiovascular system. Sympathetic vasomotor outflow is driven by premotor sympathoexcitatory (presympathetic) neurons of the rostral ventrolateral medulla whose axons travel in the reticulospinal tract. Negative feedback control is provided by baroreceptor input to the nucleus of the solitary tract [reproduced with permission from Kandel, E. R., Schwartz, J. H., and Jessel, T. M. (1991). *Principles of Neural Science*, 3rd ed. Elsevier, New York].

blood flow, sympathetic vasomotor neural outflow is a major determinant of vascular resistance and therefore arterial blood pressure.

A recurring feature of the homeostatic bodily functions under the control of neuronal networks located within the medulla oblongata is the importance of negative feedback provided by afferent information relayed to the brain via the cranial nerves. A well-characterized example of this phenomenon is arterial baroreceptor reflex regulation of sympathetic vasomotor discharge and heart rate. A trisynaptic model of the intramedullary circuitry has been developed and involves arterial baroreceptor afferent (mechanosensitive) fibers that travel in the aortic depressor and carotid sinus nerves to synapse within the nucleus of the solitary tract (Fig. 4). Inhibition of sympathetic vasomotor neurons of the rostral ventrolateral medulla occurs via an inhibitory pathway in the caudal ventrolateral medulla. The caudal ventrolateral medulla is an additional neuronally heterogeneous region that, if damaged by trauma, can lead to neurogenic pulmonary edema.

Although frequently viewed as separate physiological systems, the functioning of the respiratory system and that of the cardiovascular system are strongly interdependent. This is clearly evident within the neural networks of the medulla oblongata, in which neurons that control respiratory function and sympathetic vasomotor function are closely situated and interconnected.

Sympathetic vasomotor outflow to the heart and blood vessels is critically dependent on neurons located in the rostral ventrolateral medulla, whose axons synapse directly with sympathetic preganglionic neurons of the thoracic spinal cord. Early views of central sympathetic vasomotor control processes were based on the concept of a vasomotor center. It is now recognized that such a view is an oversimplification and that multiple groups of premotor neurons, interneurons, sensory neurons, and supramedullary neurons all have important functions.

The activity of the presympathetic neurons may be an important determinant of elevated sympathetic vasomotor outflow observed in congestive cardiac failure and essential hypertension. Compression of the ventrolateral medulla by components of the cerebral vasculature lying adjacent to the ventrolateral medullary surface has also been associated with some cases of essential hypertension. In patients with multiple-system atrophy, in which symptoms of autonomic failure including orthostatic hypotension are accompanied by parkinsonian symptoms, cate-

cholamine-containing neurons of the rostral ventrolateral medulla are depleted along with the loss of neurons from other brain regions.

Centrally acting antihypertensive drugs (clonidine, rilmenidine, and moxonidine) likely exert their effects, at least in part, through inhibition of rostral ventrolateral medulla presympathetic neurons via actions at pre- and postsynaptic α_2-adrenoceptors. The importance of rostral ventrolateral medulla presympathetic neurons is further indicated by their pivotal position in the circuitry that mediates a number of cardiovascular reflexes and their role as a relay for descending pathways emanating from the cerebral cortex, hypothalamus, and midbrain periaqueductal gray.

Respiration: Rhythmic, coordinated movements of the diaphragm, intercostal muscles of the chest, and the muscles of the upper airways, including the pharynx, larynx, tongue, lips, and nostrils, control respiration. Respiration has both voluntary and involuntary components. Expiration and inspiration may be modified by voluntary actions (e.g., whistling, blowing up a balloon, inhalation, and speech) but usually occur unnoticed by the individual and do not require conscious thought to occur.

The neural network responsible for the generation of rhythmic respiratory activity is the central respiratory generator and includes neurons of the Bötzinger and pre-Bötzinger complex and the rostral and caudal ventral respiratory groups of neurons. Although its precise functions are not well understood, it is apparent that the central respiratory generator is influenced by peripheral signals transmitted via the vagus nerve (mechanoreceptors in the lungs) and from specialized nerve endings (chemoreceptors) that signal the level of oxygenation of the arterial blood in the carotid sinus. Afferent fibers arising from chemoreceptors travel in the carotid sinus nerve and terminate within the nucleus of the solitary tract.

The central respiratory generator network determines the timing (breath length and interbreath interval) as well as the depth of respiration. Many of the features of the timing, depth, and shaping of the neural output to respiratory motoneurons are retained when the medulla is isolated at the medullary pontine junction. The function of the central respiratory generator remains intact under anesthesia, although very deep anesthesia produces respiratory arrest. Natural and synthetic opioid drugs, such as morphine, meperidine, and heroin, have a profound influence on respiration, and respiratory arrest is most frequently the cause of death in cases of overdose with these drugs.

Although normal respiration continues largely unnoticed, it is also subject to limited voluntary control. A signal from the cerebral cortex can initiate breath-holding or rapid breathing to produce hyperventilation. Ultimately, voluntary inhibition of respiratory activity succumbs to the increasingly overwhelming urge to breathe as the arterial oxygen tension plummets and intramedullary sensors are driven by elevated extracellular concentrations of carbon dioxide.

CLINICAL SIGNIFICANCE OF LESIONS OF THE MEDULLA OBLONGATA

Lesions of the medulla oblongata produce symptoms that are related to the involvement of sensory and motor pathways traversing its length as well as the involvement of the cranial nerve neurons. Thus, lesions producing syndromes involving the hypoglossal nerve may involve the hypoglossal nerve rootlets close to the medullary pyramids or the dorsal medullary hypoglossal motoneurons. Lesions influencing the rootlets of one or more of the medullary cranial nerves may be produced by trauma, tumors, or inflammatory disease. Lesions of the basal medulla may damage the medullary pyramids and the nerve roots of the cranial nerves. These lesions may occur as a result of an infarct involving blood vessels supplying the basal medulla. If the lesion does not involve the medial brainstem pathways, a syndrome similar to corticospinal tract (or pyramidal tract) syndrome results. Lesions of the dorsal medulla frequently result in coma, and the associated damage to neuronal cell groups in the reticular formation is often life threatening. Lesions of the lateral medulla can damage the fibers of the spinal trigeminal tract, causing a loss of pain and temperature sensation in the ipsilateral face and contralateral medulla.

CONCLUSION

The medulla oblongata may be regarded as the "spinal cord of the head" when viewed from the perspective of its importance in the control of head and facial musculature. The medulla oblongata is not an independent entity in the central nervous system. It does not participate in a single function that is not, at some level, dependent on input from and modulation by other regions of the nervous system. The medulla oblongata acts as a pipeline for ascending and descending pathways involved in a wide variety of nervous system functions and also as a processor of input from a diverse array of sources located within the periphery as well as from all levels of the nervous system. Many of the homeostatic functions of the nervous system are regulated by neurons confined to the medulla oblongata, although these processes are fine-tuned through a host of interactions with most levels of the neuraxis.

—*Anthony J. M. Verberne*

See also–Accessory Nerve (Cranial Nerve XI); Brain Anatomy; Central Nervous System, Overview; Facial Nerve (Cranial Nerve VII); Glossopharyngeal Nerve (Cranial Nerve IX); Hypoglossal Nerve (Cranial Nerve XII); Vagus Nerve (Cranial Nerve X)

Further Reading
Loewy, A. D., and Spyer, K. M. (1990). *Central Regulation of Autonomic Functions.* Oxford Univ. Press, Oxford.
Niewenhuys, R., Voogd, J., and van Huijzen, C. (1988). *The Human Central Nervous System*, 3rd ed. Springer-Verlag, New York.
Paxinos, G. (Ed.) (1990). *The Human Nervous System.* Academic Press, San Diego.
Steward, O. (2000). *Functional Neuroscience.* Springer-Verlag, New York.

Medulloblastoma
see Childhood Brain Tumors

Megalencephaly

Encyclopedia of the Neurological Sciences
Copyright 2003, Elsevier Science (USA). All rights reserved.

MEGALENCEPHALY is a condition in which the occipitofrontal head circumference exceeds the mean by at least two standard deviations adjusted for age, sex, and race. It is a descriptive term referring to an abnormally large head rather than indicating any specific diagnosis. However, it is an important physical sign suggesting a variety of disease states,

Table 1 DISEASE STATES OF MEGALENCEPHALY

Familial
Hydrocephalus
  Noncommunicating
  Communicating
Subdural fluid collections
Cerebral edema
Bony abnormalities
  Familial
  Myotonic dystrophy
  Anemia
  Cranioskeletal dysplasias

each of which must be excluded in the neurological evaluation of the patient (Table 1). The head circumference may be abnormally large at birth, although in some cases it is within normal limits only to later increase at a rate greater than normal for head circumference growth. Some megalencephalic persons are otherwise quite normal and have other normal family members with megalencephaly. There is no known genetic basis for this familial megalencephaly.

One syndrome of benign extracerebral fluid collections (idiopathic external hydrocephalus or benign enlargement of extracerebral spaces) has been associated with megalencephaly. There is a notable enlargement of the extracerebral spaces during the first year of life that levels off during the second year. In this group of patients, the extracerebral spaces are decreased during the next several years without treatment, and the development of the patient is generally within normal limits. The cause of this condition is unknown.

—*Bruce Berg*

***See also**–Alexander's Disease; Brain Development, Normal Postnatal; Dysmorphology; Hydrocephalus; Microcephaly*

Further Reading

Alvaarez, L. A., Maytel, J., and Shinnar, S. (1986). Idiopathic external hydrocephalus: Natural history and relationship to benign familial macrocrania. *Pediatrics* 77, 901–907.
Bodensteiner, J. B., and Chung, C. O. (1993). Macrocrania and megalencephaly in the neonate. *Semin. Neurol.* 13, 84.
DeMyer, W. (1994). *Technique of Neurologic Examination: A Programmed Text*, 4th ed. McGraw-Hill, New York.
Hamza, M., Bodensteiner, J. B., Noorani, P. A., *et al.* (1987). Benign extracerebral fluid collection: A source of macrocrania in infancy. *Pediatr. Neurol.* 3, 218–221.

Melatonin

Encyclopedia of the Neurological Sciences
Copyright 2003, Elsevier Science (USA). All rights reserved.

MELATONIN (*N*-acetyl-5-methoxytryptamine) is the major hormone of the pineal gland. It was isolated and identified in 1958 by Professor Aaron Lerner at Yale University. Although Our knowledge of melatonin physiology is far from complete, there are several well-established facts about this hormone that should be considered while discussing its role in sleep.

MELATONIN AS PART OF "BIOLOGICAL CLOCK" SYSTEM

The pineal gland (epiphysis cerebri), the eyes, and the suprachiasmatic nuclei (SCN) of the hypothalamus develop from the roof of the diencephalon. These are the major structures of the biological clock system. They are involved in the perception and/or translation of photic information and thereby facilitate an organism's adaptive adjustment to rhythmic changes in environmental illumination due to the earth's daily rotation under the sun. In phylogenetically primitive vertebrates, whose pineal glands have direct access to light, a light stimulus elicits an acute physiological response via photoreceptor cells in the pineal and can inhibit melatonin production or entrain a circadian rhythm of intrinsic pineal oscillator. However, in mammals, including humans, the pineal gland is shielded from direct light input and lacks photoreceptors or an active endogenous oscillator. A near-24-hr (circadian) rhythm of activity in the human pineal gland depends on the periodic signal from SCN. The neurons of this small hypothalamic structure are capable of sustaining a circadian pattern of activity even in the absence of a rhythmic environmental input and are normally active during the day and slow down at night. The activation of SCN neurons has an inhibitory effect on the pineal, defining a nocturnal pattern of melatonin secretion. However, the amplitude and the phase of the periodic signal from SCN can be modified by endogenous and exogenous factors. If SCN neurons are activated at night (e.g., by environmental light perceived by the retina), melatonin production declines. Melatonin, in turn, can attenuate the activity of SCN. This melatonin action supports a normal decline in the activity of the major circadian pacemaker at night, further promotes melatonin secretion, and contributes to an overall increase in the amplitude of circadian body rhythms. Melatonin can also produce a shift in the circadian phase of SCN activity, advancing or delaying it. The magnitude and the direction of the phase-shifting effect largely depend on the time of melatonin administration.

CIRCULATING MELATONIN LEVELS IN HUMANS

Temporal changes in the activity of SCN are promptly reflected in the pattern of melatonin production. The lipid-soluble melatonin does not accumulate in a small pea-size gland, but it is secreted directly into the cerebrospinal fluid and general circulation. Therefore, rhythmic changes in circulating melatonin levels follow the temporal pattern of melatonin secretion and, if measured, can provide the most reliable information on an individual's circadian phase. Under the same light–dark cycle, the timing of the onset and offset of melatonin secretion tends to remain constant for a given individual. When the light–dark cycle is altered, for example, following a jet flight across several time zones, SCN gradually readjusts its phase of activity, bringing the individual in tune with the new environment. The pattern of melatonin secretion closely follows the dynamics of this process. Thus, by repeatedly measuring melatonin in saliva or blood samples, it is possible to track an individual's pace of circadian entrainment. The sample collection procedure, however, requires strict control of the environmental lighting conditions to avoid an acute suppression of melatonin secretion by light.

Daytime blood levels of melatonin in young adults do not normally exceed 2 or 3 pg/ml, whereas at night they increase to approximately 100 pg/ml, peaking in the early morning hours (1–5 AM) (Fig. 1). Marked interindividual variations in nocturnal melatonin levels are observed in all age groups. The human fetus and newborn infant do not produce their own melatonin but rely instead on hormone supplied via the placental blood and, postnatally, via the mother's milk. At 9–12 weeks of age, infants' rhythmic melatonin production increases rapidly, with the highest nocturnal melatonin levels observed in children younger than 5 years of age. Although no adequate longitudinal studies of human melatonin production have been conducted, it is suggested from cross-sectional studies that melatonin levels decrease with physiological aging (Fig. 1). To what extent such a decline is the result of normal physiological

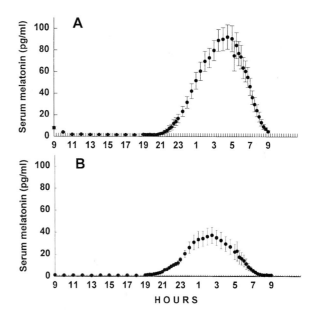

Figure 1
Profile of endogenous serum melatonin levels in (A) young and (B) aged adults (mean ± SEM, $n = 18$ for each group). Serum samples were taken at 15- to 60-min intervals during a 25-hr period.

aging, pineal calcification, comorbidity, or effects of pharmacological or nutritional factors is not clear.

ENDOGENOUS MELATONIN AND SLEEP PHYSIOLOGY

The earliest observations on melatonin levels in humans by Harry J. Lynch documented the concurrence of melatonin release from the pineal gland and the habitual hours of sleep at night. Recent reports correlate the daily onset of melatonin secretion with the onset of nocturnal sleepiness. Observations in human infants also reveal a correlation between the time of consolidation of nocturnal sleep and the normal onset of rhythmic melatonin secretion, both of which occur when infants are approximately 3 months old. The declines of both melatonin secretion and sleep efficiency with age are thought to be related phenomena. Studies of circadian phase shifts in humans also show that a change in the timing of the onset of melatonin secretion correlates with a change in the timing of evening sleepiness, a phenomenon widely observed in shift workers and in transmeridian jet travelers. Acute changes in circulating melatonin levels after pinealectomy or from the suppression of melatonin production by, for example, treatment with adrenergic β-blockers are reported to cause insomnia. In contrast, an increase in circulating melatonin induced by suppression of melatonin-metabolizing liver enzymes results in sleepiness. Although these correlational observations do not prove a causal relationship between melatonin secretion and sleep, they tend to substantiate direct experimental results.

EFFECTS OF MELATONIN TREATMENT ON SLEEP

There are two major effects of melatonin treatment on sleep, which can manifest jointly or separately. One is a phase-shifting effect of melatonin, which helps to resynchronize the sleep phase with the dark phase of the environmental light–dark cycle. By inducing a circadian phase advance, melatonin shifts the onset of evening sleepiness to an earlier hour, promoting easier sleep initiation and earlier morning awakening. In contrast, by causing a phase delay, melatonin postpones both the onset of evening sleepiness and morning awakening. This effect can be beneficial to those experiencing a transmeridian flight, those who do shift work, or patients with phase delay or phase advance syndromes. Such melatonin action can also help to entrain circadian rhythms in blind people, whose intrinsic circadian oscillator "free-runs" (i.e., has a period of more or less than 24 hr) in the absence of the synchronizing effect of environmental light. To produce a circadian phase shift, melatonin must be administered at particular circadian hours of the day, according to its phase–response curve. Late afternoon melatonin treatment, approximately 4–6 hr prior to the individual onset of melatonin secretion, would promote a phase advance. The administration of melatonin early in the morning, at the time of the individual offset of melatonin production by the pineal gland, would cause a circadian phase delay. This effect of melatonin can be achieved by increasing circulating melatonin levels to within physiological or pharmacological concentrations. Employing high pharmacological doses or slow-release formulation, however, might cause some reduction in melatonin efficacy if the long duration of melatonin signal causes it to affect opposite portions of the melatonin phase–response curve (i.e., phase advance in the evening and phase delay in the morning).

Melatonin also has an acute sleep-promoting effect that does not seem to critically depend on the time of administration. Both physiological (3–5 μg/kg) and pharmacological melatonin doses promote sleep onset or sleep maintenance (Fig. 2), supporting the

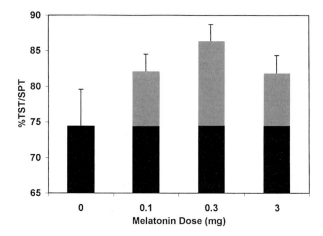

Figure 2
Increase in sleep efficiency in elderly insomniacs (TST/SPT <85%) after treatment with different oral doses of melatonin (mean ± SEM, $n = 12$).

notion that normal nocturnal surge in melatonin production might be an important factor in human sleep regulation. Lack of clear dose dependency of this effect with doses in excess of those that result in normal nocturnal melatonin levels (i.e., approximately 100 pg/ml) might be explained on the basis of the saturation levels of melatonin receptors, which are reported to be less than 100 pg/ml. Thus, if the hypnotic effect of melatonin is indeed receptor mediated, a dose increase may not only fail to elicit an improved response but also even promote a downregulation of receptors and a partial loss or modification of effect.

The effect of melatonin on sleep initiation is typically manifest within 30–60 min after the treatment is administered orally. Observations also suggest that an increase in serum melatonin levels within the physiological range, occurring either during the daytime or late in the evening, is not an imperative signal for sleep. It is rather a gentle promoter of general relaxation and sedation, elements of sleepiness that in favorable conditions might significantly facilitate sleep onset and are typical of a period immediately prior to sleep initiation conventionally called quiet wakefulness. Such a melatonin quality might also be related to its reported anxiolytic effects.

Melatonin's effect on sleep initiation is not accompanied by any dramatic changes in electrophysiological sleep architecture, a common complication encountered with many existing hypnotics. However, the tendencies observed include a modest decrease in the duration of stage 4 and an increase in the duration of stage 2 sleep in some of the people studied. Unlike some popular hypnotics, melatonin does not inhibit rapid eye movement sleep. In contrast, melatonin treatment can reportedly facilitate subjects' dreaming. It is not clear whether these subjective reports reflect an increase in dreaming per se or a better recall of dreams.

MECHANISMS OF MELATONIN EFFECTS ON SLEEP

Acute effects of melatonin on sleep and its ability to shift a circadian phase of sleep–wake cycle suggest that it might play the role of a physiological link between circadian and homeostatic mechanisms of sleep regulation. The nature of phase-shifting and hypnotic effects of melatonin is not clear, but current research on the underlying mechanisms is vigorous. Melatonin has specific binding sites, some of which are identified as G protein-coupled melatonin receptors, in various central and peripheral tissues. The effects of melatonin on circadian phase shift are likely linked to its action on the level of SCN activity. The acute suppression of SCN activity by melatonin might also help to attenuate the activating pressure of the circadian pacemaker and underlie its acute sleep-promoting effect. However, melatonin might also facilitate sleep initiation or maintenance by affecting other sleep-related structures. Functional melatonin receptors or binding sites have been identified in thalamic nuclei or preoptic areas of the hypothalamus—brain regions critical for sleep regulation. The peripheral effects of melatonin (e.g., those promoting a decrease in core body temperature or peripheral vasodilation) might also be cofactors of the hypnotic properties of the pineal hormone. Although it is likely that the physiological effects of melatonin are mediated via its G protein-bound receptors, a high lipid solubility of the hormone, which enables it to easily cross cell membranes, does not exclude the possibility of direct intracellular effects.

One of the well-tested ways of exploring the mechanism of a physiological or pathophysiological process is through the development of an adequate animal model. Although circadian effects of the pineal hormone have been found in many species, there are only a few animal studies of its acute effects, which has led to contradictory interpretations. These inconsistencies may be explained, in part, by the choice of experimental animals—nocturnally active rodents whose melatonin is high at night when they are at the peak of their active phase. Thus, melatonin might have a quite different biological meaning in nocturnal compared to diurnal animals. Our recent observations in several diurnal species of nonhuman primates and in diurnal zebrafish indicate their high sensitivity to melatonin's sleep-promoting effects and provide hope that such animal models will help in deciphering the mechanisms of hypnotic effects of melatonin.

MELATONIN THERAPY

Melatonin's ability to promote sleep and help shift the phase of the circadian rhythms makes this pineal hormone a potentially useful therapeutic agent. Lack of significant changes in sleep architecture or memory function after melatonin treatment and its low toxicity are additional advantages of such medication compared to some other hypnotics. However, all available information from animal and human studies suggests that melatonin may participate in diverse physiological processes that include circadian rhythms, sleep, reproduction, temperature regulation, and immune responses. In dealing with something so multipurpose, one must be very careful, especially if long-term administration of the hormone is considered, avoiding the hazards of either deficiency or excess. Adjusting individual melatonin dose and time of treatment would help to avoid possible side effects of melatonin therapy, including daytime grogginess, headaches, or excessively vivid dreaming.

Melatonin treatment might be beneficial to those with stress-related, shift work-related, or jet lag-related insomnia or for people suffering from circadian sleep disorders or blindness. When the goal of melatonin treatment is to resynchronize the circadian body rhythms, melatonin should be administered either at subjective afternoon (3 or 4 hr before habitual bedtime) to advance sleep propensity or in the morning (immediately after awakening) to delay the onset of sleepiness. If an acute sleep-promoting effect of melatonin is desired or melatonin is used to maintain the entrainment of the circadian body rhythms in a free-running blind patient, treatment should be administered approximately 30 min prior to one's habitual bedtime. In this way, the time of melatonin administration is coordinated with the time of its normal increase in secretion, thus minimizing the possibility of an undesired phase-shifting effect of melatonin treatment.

Using physiological or pharmacological doses of the hormone, melatonin treatment was also successfully applied in children with neurological disorders (e.g., children affected by Angelman syndrome, who suffer from severe insomnia). In such children, an increase in sleep quantity and quality after melatonin (0.3 mg) administration was not accompanied by significant changes in their daytime behavior. However, in some patients, parents and teachers noticed a decrease in hyperactivity, and this effect correlated with an increase in the children's attention. Since children with neurological disorders are often prone to seizures, the reported antiseizure properties of melatonin might provide an additional benefit for such patients. If long-term melatonin treatment in such children is initiated, it is important to use physiological rather than pharmacological doses of the hormone, since excess melatonin might affect the development of the reproductive system.

Many people older than 50 years of age have relatively low blood melatonin levels and complain of an age-related decline in sleep quantity and quality. Melatonin treatment was repeatedly shown to promote sleep initiation or to help maintain overnight sleep in elderly insomniacs. However, older individuals exhibit a substantially higher variability in the sleep-promoting effect of melatonin and often much higher circulating melatonin levels after treatment. This might be related to age-related changes in the absorption or metabolism of ingested melatonin. Changes in receptor sensitivity with age might also contribute to less predictable results of melatonin treatment in the elderly. This notion emphasizes an important issue—the need to individually adjust a melatonin dose used for therapeutic purposes and to keep circulating melatonin concentration within the physiological levels (i.e., <200 pg/ml in blood or <50 pg/ml in saliva). There are several obvious benefits to such a strategy. It allows maintaining nighttime circulating melatonin levels within the normal physiological range, which might be important since it is not known what kind of long-term effects pharmacological levels of melatonin might cause. It also prevents a significant daytime increase in circulating melatonin concentrations. The latter is vital since melatonin's daily rhythm is an important periodic neuroendocrine signal for the rest of the body, including the circadian clock SCN, helping to promote a temporal synchronization of other circadian rhythms. Thus, it is imperative to avoid blunting the amplitude of SCN's signal by elevating melatonin levels during the day.

Modern assay techniques allow accurate monitoring of endogenous melatonin levels, or those caused by melatonin treatment, by sampling saliva or blood. To estimate the circadian phase based on the onset of melatonin secretion, such samples should be collected repeatedly (at 30-min intervals or more frequently) for 5 or 6 hr, starting approximately 4 hr before an individual's habitual bedtime. To estimate peak endogenous melatonin levels, samples should be collected overnight, at least once an hour. Sampling should be conducted under a low environmental light intensity (<10 lx) since melatonin production is easily suppressed by light. A maximum increase in the circulating level of the hormone after its oral administration can be estimated by collecting blood or saliva 1 hr after daytime treatment. Since individuals have different sensitivities to the phase-shifting effects of melatonin or light exposure, such measurements might also help in choosing an appropriate timing and dose regime for phase-adjusting therapy.

Available data on the effects of melatonin on sleep suggest that the hormone may have a normal role in human sleep initiation and maintenance, perhaps serving as a humoral link between circadian and homeostatic sleep mechanisms. They further suggest that melatonin deficiency might be expected to impair the integrity, quantity, and quality of nocturnal sleep, and that melatonin replacement therapy might offer an effective and innocuous approach to the treatment of such insomnia without disturbing normal sleep architecture. Perhaps melatonin therapy would also play a beneficial role supporting other physiological functions that involve melatonin, including the entrainment and coordination of various biological rhythms. However, the benefits of melatonin treatment and the suppression of unwanted effects can be fully realized only if the pineal hormone is administered at an appropriate dose and at an appropriate circadian time.

—*Irina V. Zhdanova*

See also–Drowsiness; Excessive Daytime Sleepiness; Fatigue; Insomnia; Jet Lag; Light Therapy; Serotonin; Sleep Disorders; Sleep–Wake Cycle; Suprachiasmatic Nucleus (SCN)

Further Reading

Dollins, A. B., Zhdanova, I. V., Wurtman, R. J., *et al.* (1994). Effect of inducing nocturnal serum melatonin concentrations in daytime on sleep, mood, body temperature and performance. *Proc. Natl. Acad. Sci. USA* **91**, 1824–1828.

Kräuchi, K., Cajochen, C., Werth, E., *et al.* (2000). Functional link between distal vasodilation and sleep-onset latency? *Am. J. Physiol.* **278**, R741–R748.

Lewy, A. J., Bauer, V. K., Ahmed, S., *et al.* (1998). The human phase response curve (PRC) to melatonin is about 12 hours out of phase with the PRC to light. *Chronobiol. Int.* **15**, 71–83.

Lockley, S. W., Skene, D. J., Arendt, J., *et al.* (1997). Relationship between melatonin rhythms and visual loss in the blind. *J. Clin. Endocrinol. Metab.* **81**, 2980–2985.

Shochat, T., Luboshitzky, R., and Lavie, P. (1997). Nocturnal melatonin onset is phase locked to the primary sleep gate. *Am. J. Physiol.* **273**, R364–R370.

Tzischinsky, O., and Lavie, P. (1994). Melatonin possesses time-dependent hypnotic effects. *Sleep* **17**, 638–645.

Zhdanova, I. V., Lynch, H. J., and Wurtman, R. J. (1997). Melatonin: A sleep promoting hormone. *Sleep* **20**, 899–907.

Zhdanova, I. V., Wurtman, R. J., Balcioglu, A., *et al.* (1998). Endogenous melatonin levels and the fate of exogenous melatonin: Age effects. *J. Gerontol. Biol. Sci.* **53A4**, B293–B298.

Zhdanova, I. V., Wurtman, R. J., and Wagstaff, J. (1999). Effects of low dose of melatonin on sleep in children with Angelman syndrome. *J. Pediatr. Endocrinol. Metab.* **12**, 57–67.

Membrane Potential

Encyclopedia of the Neurological Sciences

AN EXCITABLE MEMBRANE will have a stable potential when there is no net ion current flowing across the membrane. Two factors determine the net flow of ions across an open ionic channel: the membrane potential and the differences in ion concentrations between the intracellular and extracellular spaces. Since cells have negative intracellular potentials, the electrical force will tend to direct positively charged ions (cations such as sodium, potassium, and calcium) to flow into a cell. Hence, electrical forces will direct an inward flow of sodium, potassium, and calcium ions and an outward flow of chloride ions. The direction of ion movement produced by the "concentration force" depends on the concentration differences for the ion between the intracellular and extracellular compartments. Sodium, calcium, and chloride ions have higher extracellular concentrations compared with intracellular concentrations. The intracellular concentration of potassium is greater than the extracellular concentration. Concentration forces direct an inward flow of sodium, calcium, and chloride ions and an outward flow of potassium ions. The membrane potential at which the electrical and concentration forces are balanced for a given ion is called the equilibrium or Nernst potential for a given ion. At the equilibrium potential, inward and outward current movements are balanced for a specific ion due to balancing of the electrical and concentration forces. For a given cation, at membrane potentials that are negative compared with the equilibrium potential, ions flow into the cell, and at membrane potentials that are more positive than the equilibrium potential, current carried by the specific ion will flow out of the cell. The direction of current movement for a specific ion always tends to bring the membrane potential back to the equilibrium potential for that specific ion. Examples of approximate equilibrium potentials for ions in skeletal muscle are shown in Table 1.

The membrane potential represents a balance among the equilibrium potentials of the ions to which the membrane is permeable. The greater the conductance of an ion, the more that ion will influence the membrane potential of the cell. The principal conductances responsible for establishing the resting membrane potential are chloride conductance, potassium conductance, and sodium conductance. Chloride conductance is large in skeletal muscle fibers, in which it is mediated by skeletal muscle chloride channels. Peripheral nerve fibers have smaller chloride conductances. In skeletal muscle, chloride is the dominant membrane conductance, accounting for approximately 80% of the resting membrane conductance. Chloride channels in skeletal muscle are unusual in that they are gated by the presence of ions at the intracellular and extracellular orifices rather than by the membrane potential. The channel is likely to open when a chloride ion presents itself. The unique gating properties of chloride channels result in the chloride ions being distributed across the membrane in accord with the membrane potential. Consequently, chloride conductance does not set the membrane potential.

Table 1 EQUILIBRIUM POTENTIALS

Ion	Equilibrium potential (mV)
Sodium	65
Potassium	−105
Calcium	>100
Chloride	−95 (resting potential)
Resting potential	−95

Table 2 MEMBRANE POTENTIAL UNDER DIFFERENT CONDITIONS

Membrane state	Dominant membrane conductance	Membrane potential
Resting	K^+	Close to K^+ equilibrium potential, approximately -95 mV
Peak of action potential	Na^+	Close to Na^+ equilibrium potential, approximately 40 mV

Instead, chloride conductance acts as a brake to make it more difficult for the membrane to depolarize. Therefore, chloride conductance provides an important stabilizing influence on the membrane potential.

The dominant ion in setting the resting membrane potential is potassium. Potassium conductance accounts for approximately 20% of the resting membrane conductance in skeletal muscle and accounts for most of the resting conductance in neurons and nerve fibers. The small amount of sodium conductance in the resting skeletal muscle, or nerve membrane, results in the resting membrane potential being slightly positive or depolarized compared to the equilibrium potential for potassium (Table 2). The specific class of potassium channels that determines the resting membrane potential is the inward or anomalous rectifier potassium channel. Resting calcium conductance is exceeding small. Therefore, calcium does not contribute to the resting membrane potential.

During an action potential, Na^+ channels open and the dominant membrane conductance is that of Na^+. Consequently, the membrane potential is approximately the same as the Na^+ equilibrium potential (Table 2).

—*Robert L. Ruff*

See also–Action Potential, Generation of; Action Potential, Regeneration of; Impulse Conduction; Ion Channels, Overview; Motor Unit Potential; Muscle Contraction, Overview

Acknowledgment

This work was supported by the Office of Research and Development, Medical Research Service of the Department of Veterans Affairs.

Further Reading

Ruff, R. L. (1986). Ionic channels: I. The biophysical basis for ion passage and channel gating. *Muscle Nerve* **9**, 675–699.

Shapiro, B. E., and Ruff, R. L. (2002). Disorders of skeletal muscle membrane excitability: Myotonia congenita, paramyotonia congenita, periodic paralysis and related syndromes. In *Neuromuscular Disorders in Clinical Practice* (B. Katirji, H. J. Kaminski, B. E. Shapiro, D. Preston, and R. L. Ruff, Eds.), pp. 987–1021. Butterworth–Heinemann, Boston.

Memory, Autobiographical

Encyclopedia of the Neurological Sciences
Copyright 2003, Elsevier Science (USA). All rights reserved.

FACETS OF MEMORY have been subjected to scientific scrutiny for well over a century, but a surprisingly small proportion of this research has directly examined the most human of all memory processes—memory for information and experiences pertaining to one's own life, or autobiographical memory. Although the encoding, retention, and retrieval processes discovered in laboratory studies are relevant to our everyday autobiographical memory experiences, autobiographical memory has an added layer of complexity. Unlike the word lists or pictures studied in the laboratory, it is implicated in one's protracted self-awareness across time and self-identity. Indeed, it is this close connection to the self that makes autobiographical memory an unpopular topic among experimentalists, who prefer a greater degree of control over the encoding process than can be achieved in an autobiographical memory study.

Like other memory domains, autobiographical memory is not unitary. Contrasting autobiographical systems and processes can be identified in healthy people and can be affected differentially by brain disease. Storage and retrieval of autobiographical information depends on complex and widely distributed mechanisms. Generation of autobiographical information is a reconstructive, strategic, and often fallible cognitive operation that is affected by both the characteristics of the subject and the nature of the information being retrieved.

THE COGNITIVE NEUROSCIENCE OF AUTOBIOGRAPHICAL MEMORY

Recollection of perceptual, cognitive, and emotional details allows one to reexperience a prior event that is specific in time and place. Knowledge of facts and themes from one's autobiography, on the other hand, relates to self-identity but is not time locked to any single prior episode. These reexperiencing and self-knowledge components overlap with the domains of episodic and semantic memory that have influenced experimental memory research.

The Episodic/Semantic Distinction within Autobiographical Memory

Episodic memory was defined by Tulving as the retrieval of an event specific in time and place and has been traditionally assessed through tests of word lists, text, or pictures. Semantic memory was defined as the retrieval of undated, generic knowledge about the world and oneself, for which standard assessment includes tests of vocabulary, object naming, and recognition of famous faces and news events. Within the framework of autobiographical memory, episodic autobiographical memory refers to the reexperiencing of specific past episodes and their details, and semantic autobiographical memory refers to factual information about oneself (e.g., schools attended, previous jobs, skills, and personality traits). In comparison to semantic autobiographical memory, episodic autobiographical reexperiencing probably evolved relatively late, is unique to humans, and stabilizes late in development (at approximately age 4). Episodic and semantic memory can be dissociated in patients with brain disease and in healthy adults with functional neuroimaging.

Conway and colleagues have also proposed a model of autobiographical memory that overlaps with the episodic/semantic distinction. In the Self Memory Model, autobiographical memory is organized into levels of knowledge specificity: life time periods, general events, and event-specific knowledge. Life time periods (knowledge about primary school, university, and working for company X) and general events (themes of repeated events, single extended events, or a clustering of activities thematically related by a goal) broadly overlap with semantic autobiographical memory, whereas event-specific knowledge (episodic fragments such as sensory and perceptual details) is analogous to episodic autobiographical memory.

Strategic Retrieval Processes in Autobiographical Remembering

Recollection of autobiographical episodes is a complex multistage cyclic retrieval process that does not necessarily result in a high-fidelity representation of the original experience. The frontal lobes serve a controlling and monitoring function in this process.

In the first step, a memory template is developed in response to internal or external cues and demands. Following search initiation, sensory and phenomenal properties are brought to consciousness through patterns of transregional neocortical activation. The medial temporal lobes (including the hippocampus) probably contain the indices or "combinatory codes" to these regions. The resulting pattern is verified against the original template until a satisfactory outcome occurs, which may require numerous cycles of template elaboration and verification of activation patterns. Reexperiencing may also occur more spontaneously through associative or direct activations in response to highly specific or elaborate cues (e.g., odor). Autobiographical memories are thus not stored as distinct units but are rather diffusely represented and reactivated through hippocampal–neocortical interaction. Access to semantic knowledge, either personal or public, which is by definition free of temporal and contextual components, is thought to be less dependent on hippocampal–neocortical interactions.

Since autobiographical memory is reconstructive in nature, faulty retrieval attempts may occur, specific details may be lost or inconsistently retrieved, and the description may change with changes in personal goals and self-schemas. In cases of frontal brain damage, this distortion can reach pathological levels in the form of confabulation. More subtle forms of memory distortion can be observed in healthy people. Researchers have manipulated false memory by exploiting the tendency of individuals to create a coherent and internally consistent representation of experience.

Autobiographical Retrieval across the Life Span

The pattern of autobiographical memory retrieval varies across the life span. What is referred to as the life span retrieval curve is most evident when subjects are asked to recall freely and date memories that come to mind in response to a list of cue words. The number of memories recalled across the life span is represented by a retrieval curve with three components. First, there is an overall decrease in memories recalled over time, with superior autobiographical recall for memories occurring in recent years. Second, there is a reduction of memories during early childhood years referred to as childhood amnesia. The third component, observed in middle-aged and older adults, is an increase in recall of memories from adolescence and young adult years, known as the reminiscence bump. The latter component may be related to memory enhancement of events that are both novel and important in the formulation and stabilization of one's self-identity and personal goals.

AUTOBIOGRAPHICAL MEMORY IN PATIENTS WITH NEUROPSYCHOLOGICAL DISORDERS

Contributions of the Medial Temporal, Diencephalic, and Basal Forebrain Regions

Selective impairment of specific memory systems or processes in patients with amnesia provides useful information about the organization of memory in the brain. One clear finding from such studies is that episodic memory is more sensitive to brain damage than is semantic memory. This finding is consistent with the previously described conceptualization of autobiographical episodic and semantic retrieval processes. That is, retrieval of personal semantic information derives from stable memory traces that are more redundantly represented than those traces mediating episodic reexperiencing.

Patients with classic forms of anterograde amnesia due to medial temporal, diencephalic, or basal forebrain damage are severely impaired in the acquisition, retention, and retrieval of novel experiences. These structures act as bottleneck regions during the encoding and retrieval of episodes. The hippocampus and related medial temporal lobe structures play an important role in the binding of spatial and other contextual event details that are represented throughout the neocortex. Damage to the medial temporal region results in the loss of contextual specificity that contributes to the recollection of unique episodes. Retrieval of general or semantic information that is independent of contextual specificity is less prone to disruption. Medial temporal lobe damage is associated with a temporal gradient of retrograde amnesia (originally described by Ribot) by which information acquired relatively recently is more vulnerable to damage than remotely acquired information. The precise nature and determinants of this gradient are currently under debate. The temporal extent of retrograde amnesia is related to the amount of medial temporal damage. Recent evidence suggests that the gradient most aptly describes the pattern of remote semantic memory loss and that remote episodic memory follows a more temporally extensive gradient.

Damage to the diencephalic structures, either by focal lesions or more commonly by Wernicke–Korsakoff syndrome due to chronic alcoholism, causes a temporally extensive retrograde amnesia. The basal forebrain, the final bottleneck structure, has projections to other systems important to memory, namely the hippocampal and amygdalar systems. Numerous pathways that have been linked to memory pass through or nearby this region. Due to its anatomical complexity, its contributions to memory are not well understood.

Although a semantic deficit can be demonstrated in amnesic patients, it is almost invariably less severe than the episodic deficit. New knowledge and skills (e.g., motor tasks and computer knowledge) can be acquired with repeated trials under conditions of minimal interference, even in severe amnesics who cannot form new episodic memories. Such patients can therefore show remarkable demonstrations of learning in the absence of recollection of any learning episode.

Retrograde amnesia is nearly always accompanied by anterograde amnesia that is greater in degree, although an increasing number of cases of disproportionate (also called isolated or focal) retrograde amnesia are being reported. An exception to this pattern can be found in patients with bilateral inferolateral temporal cortical damage (e.g., semantic dementia), in which semantic memory is more impaired.

Prefrontal Contributions to Autobiographical Amnesia

The prefrontal cortex is involved in the organization, storage, search, retrieval, and reconstruction of autobiographical memories. Patients with prefrontal damage often show autobiographical memory deficits due to impairments in one or more of these processes. These patients, however, derive more benefit from retrieval support than do patients with medial temporal lobe damage.

Frontal lesions also appear to be requisite to amnesic syndromes in which self-awareness is clearly disrupted, most notably in confabulation. Confabulation is the unintentional recollection of erroneous information that can be either plausible or completely bizarre. In either case, the patient is unaware or unconcerned about his or her memory deficits and will hold his or her views with absolute conviction. Confabulation is most frequently reported for autobiographical information, although it has also been reported for semantic information. In amnesics, confabulation is typically associated with damage to the ventromedial frontal region, prefrontal cortex, and basal forebrain, although damage to these regions does not necessarily imply the presence of confabulation. Confabulation occurs with greater frequency in conjunction with Wernicke–Korsakoff syndrome and hemorrhage after a ruptured communicating artery aneurysm, but it may also accompany trauma to the frontal lobes, herpes simplex encephalitis, frontal lobe dementia, and cerebral infarction. Confabulations differ from delusions in that they occur in the context of amnesia or a transient confusional state rather than in the context of psychosis.

The predominant explanation of confabulation is that it is a symptom of impaired search and monitoring processes during memory retrieval. These processes are also of particular importance in successful autobiographical remembering. Without the proper functioning of these mechanisms, memories and their fragments may be retrieved out of context, out of order, or be overly influenced by the immediate social or physical environment. The ability to differentiate real events from thought content or imagined events may also be impaired.

Psychogenic Retrograde Amnesia in Autobiographical Memory

Psychogenic or functional amnesia is the sudden loss of autobiographical memory and personal identity, and it is commonly precipitated by a traumatic event, severe stress, or depression. Individuals are often unaware of their previous lives and unconcerned about their amnesic condition. In the fugue state, a person may wander for days in pursuit of a particular destination or goal, usually related to precipitating circumstances, unaware and oblivious to his or her lack of identity or personal history. Although episodic autobiographical memory is predominantly affected in psychogenic amnesia, recollection of semantic or general information (e.g., famous faces and news events) may or may not be impaired. The extent of autobiographical memory loss may encompass an entire lifetime or a specific stressful event or time period. Autobiographical memory loss in these cases is usually temporary. Memory for ongoing events during the amnesic state is temporarily intact, but this information may be lost upon recovery. Psychogenic symptoms vary from case to case because they are idiosyncratic in nature. Many cases of psychogenic amnesia have a history of brain disease, giving rise to speculation that retrograde amnesia is neither purely organic nor psychogenic but a mixture of the two.

FUNCTIONAL IMAGING OF AUTOBIOGRAPHICAL REMEMBERING

With the recent development of functional imaging techniques, a handful of studies have investigated the neuroanatomical correlates of autobiographical remembering in healthy adults. Brain activity studied *in vivo* during autobiographical remembering has begun to extend the knowledge from neuropsychological research to normal autobiographical memory. Consistent with the roles of prefrontal and hippocampal structures in patients with brain disease, imaging studies have demonstrated the activation of these areas in healthy adults during autobiographical recollection. Further investigation is required to clarify the differential contributions of the right and left hemispheres as well as possibly distinct dorsal/ventral and medial/lateral contributions from the frontal lobes.

ASSESSMENT OF AUTOBIOGRAPHICAL MEMORY

Although autobiographical memory impairment can have significant implications for patients' quality of life, it is typically not assessed or is informally assessed using one or two questions. Detailed neuropsychological test batteries often leave autobiographical memory unexamined. Although it is obviously difficult to assess such inherently subjective information, impoverished autobiographical recollection can be reliably detected. In cases of suspected confabulation, verification against significant others' reports is required.

Two widely used tools for the assessment of autobiographical memory are the Crovitz technique and the Autobiographical Memory Interview (AMI). The Crovitz technique is used extensively in the experimental study of autobiographical memory. The basic testing procedure comprises giving subjects a list of words and asking them to recall an event related to each word. The administration and scoring of this instrument, however, vary from laboratory to laboratory. The AMI is the only commercially available clinical measure. It is a semistructured interview that separately assesses episodic and personal semantic autobiographical memory across three broad lifetime periods. Each episode or component is given a qualitative 0–3 rating reflecting the degree of reexperiencing conveyed by the patient's recollection.

—E. Svoboda and B. Levine

See also–Memory, Episodic; Memory, Explicit/
Implicit; Memory, Overview; Memory, Semantic;
Memory, Spatial; Memory, Working; Transient
Global Amnesia

Further Reading

Conway, M. A., and Pleydell-Pearce, C. W. (2000). The construc-
    tion of autobiographical memories in the self-memory system.
    Psychol. Rev. 107, 261–288.
Kapur, N. (1999). Syndromes of retrograde amnesia: A conceptual
    and empirical synthesis. *Psychol. Bull.* 125, 800–825.
Kopelman, M. D., Wilson, B. A., and Baddeley, A. D. (1989). The
    Autobiographical Memory Interview: A new assessment of
    autobiographical and personal semantic memory in amnesic
    patients. *J. Clin. Exp. Neuropsychol.* 11, 724–744.
Rubin, D. C., Rahhal, T. A., and Poon, L. W. (1998). Things
    learned in early adulthood are remembered best. *Mem. Cognit.*
    26, 3–19.
Tulving, E. (1989). Remembering and knowing the past. *Am. Sci.*
    77, 361–367.

Memory, Episodic

Encyclopedia of the Neurological Sciences
Copyright 2003, Elsevier Science (USA). All rights reserved.

ALTHOUGH human memory systems encompass several different types of learning phenomena, episodic memory is what most people are referring to when they discuss memory. Episodic memory is our ability to learn, store, and later retrieve new information, and it is often referred to as recent memory or anterograde memory. Recent models of memory place episodic memory within the declarative memory system, which refers to memories that are directly accessible to conscious recollection. Retrieval of information from declarative memory is usually intentional and done with the awareness of the individual. Episodic memory specifically refers to memory for events or episodes in one's life that are associated with a particular time and place. Episodic memory can be contrasted with semantic memory, which is another component of the declarative memory system and refers to a person's fund of general information. Unlike episodic memory, semantic memory holds information that does not depend on a particular time or place. Thus, knowing that Cleopatra was a queen of Egypt is part of semantic memory; remembering a time when one

saw Shakespeare's *Anthony and Cleopatra* is part of episodic memory. Similarly, learning a list of words is a function of episodic memory; knowing what the words mean depends on semantic memory.

Episodic memory is a complex set of cognitive operations and is mediated by multiple neurological pathways and systems. To illustrate some of these components, consider a friend's account of a recent trip to Europe. She describes how the trip began in Paris and then continued to Nice, Monaco, Venice, Vienna, and finally Frankfurt. She also recounts a boat trip on the Seine during which a tour guide informed her that the Eiffel Tower was completed in 1889 and is 300 m high. She exclaims that Venice was one of the trip's highlights and describes in detail the view of St. Mark's Basilica from her hotel window.

Extensive research with primate and neurological patients has demonstrated that your friend's ability to store information about events that occurred several months previously depends on the integrity of structures in the medial temporal lobes. One of the first structures linked to new learning was the hippocampus, a small structure shaped like a seahorse tucked deep in the medial portion of each temporal lobe. Patients with bilateral lesions in the hippocampus typically present with dense amnesia or an inability to learn new information. Old information and basic perceptual and intellectual functioning can be entirely unaffected. Controlled lesion studies with primates also revealed that even incomplete damage to the hippocampus can produce significant memory impairment. More extensive experiments have shown that the hippocampus is just one part of an extensive information processing network that contributes to memory performance. Information being processed in all parts of the neocortex projects to parahippocampal gyrus, perirhinal cortex, and entorhinal cortex prior to being sent to the hippocampus. The hippocampus has been subdivided into key components: Information projects first to the dentate gyrus and then to the C3 and C1 regions. Information leaving the hippocampus enters the subiculum and entorhinal cortex prior to being projected back to the cortex. Projections to the cortex are widely distributed, with multiple cortical regions contributing to a memory trace. Because memories are stored in multiple cortical regions, memories can be triggered by initial access to only a limited portion of the memory; this explains why memories for specific events are preserved following focal cortical lesions. Although the hippocampus appears critical for normal memory function, damage to other parts of the medial temporal system can also impair memory. Similarly, damage to the hippocampus alone does not seem to impair memory as much as when there is concurrent damage to entorhinal and perirhinal cortex.

Your friend recalled several facts that were verbal in nature and some images of St. Mark's Basilica that were visual in nature. Hemispheric specialization of memory largely parallels that of cognitive operations in general, with verbal memory predominately mediated by the left hippocampus and visual memory predominately mediated by the right hippocampus. Memories are typically multimodal, however, and both hemispheres generally contribute to the formation of new memory traces.

One of the mechanisms by which learning occurs in this information-processing system may be long-term potentiation, which is a long-term increase in synaptic sensitivity and postsynaptic output that occurs when a neural loop has been activated. This change in synaptic activity can last for hours or days after the original stimulus has disappeared, thereby leading many neuroscientists to suggest that long-term potentiation may be the basis for more permanent synaptic changes and the formation of a durable memory trace. Ironically, the role of the medial temporal system in long-term storage of information may be time limited. Several studies have shown that damage to the hippocampus may not affect retrieval of information that was learned months or years prior to the lesion. Patients with focal amnesia typically present with intact memory for old semantic and autobiographical facts. This implies that the medial temporal system may serve to link together previously unconnected cortical sites; once these neural loops are established, however, the hippocampus is no longer necessary for activation of that memory.

Your friend's account of her European trip also illustrates other features of episodic memory. She not only recalled several facts about the Eiffel Tower but also could specify where and when she learned them. This is an example of source memory. Source memory is memory for the source of a fact or message (e.g., who said something rather than what was said). The frontal lobes appear to be the critical structure for this kind of learning. In one study, patients with frontal lobe lesions recalled as many facts as their age-matched controls and younger subjects, but they frequently attributed facts to incorrect sources. A study of Huntington's disease patients, who have subcortical and frontal dysfunc-

tion, also demonstrated impaired memory for the source of learned information, even though fact recall did not differ significantly between early stage Huntington's patients and an age- and education-equated group of healthy control subjects. In contrast, although Alzheimer's disease patients recall fewer facts than healthy controls, when they remember information, they attribute their learning to the correct source.

The frontal lobes are also important for other aspects of episodic memory. In recounting her travels, your friend was able to report on where her trip began, where she went next, and so on. This depends on the ability to store and retrieve not only the events but also when they occurred in relationship to other events. Patients with frontal lobe lesions are impaired at placing items in the correct temporal order, even when memory for the items is intact, and may have difficulty giving biographical details or stating recent U.S. presidents in the correct chronological order. Temporal ordering and source memory are examples of contextual memory—that is, encoding not just the events but also the context within which they occur—and it appears that frontal structures provide the foundation for this cognitive skill. The frontal lobes also play a key role in how information to be learned is organized during encoding and retrieval. For example, in one study using positron emission tomography in normals, activation in left prefrontal cortex was linked to semantic clustering, which is a measure of active regrouping of words into semantic categories during free recall.

Episodic memory is a complex cognitive ability subserved by multiple brain systems, and it can therefore be disrupted by several different types of neurological disorders. The hippocampus and surrounding structures play a central role in new learning, so disorders causing hippocampal pathology are almost always associated with significant deficits in new learning. Perhaps the most common disorder producing extensive hippocampal damage is Alzheimer's disease. The neuropathological changes of Alzheimer's disease—neuritic plaques, neurofibrillary tangles, and neuronal cell loss—typically begin in the medial temporal lobe (entorhinal cortex and hippocampus), which explains why episodic memory is so impaired in Alzheimer's disease patients. Herpes encephalitis also differentially affects the temporal lobes and can produce severe amnesia. The hippocampus is also very sensitive to oxygen and glucose deprivation. Consequently, events that produce acute anoxia, such as cardiac arrest, drowning, and asphyxiation, commonly result in damage to the hippocampus and deficits in episodic memory. Another type of memory disorder thought to be linked to the medial temporal lobe system is transient global amnesia, which is a syndrome in which a previously well person suddenly becomes confused and amnesic for a period of usually less than 24 hr. Language, attention, visuospatial skills, and semantic memory are well preserved. Blood flow studies have shown changes in the medial temporal lobes, presumably due to ischemia in the vertebrobasilar system.

Structural damage in other areas of the brain can also produce episodic memory impairment. Studies of patients with Korsakoff's disease and patients with focal injury have shown that lesions in the dorsal–medial nucleus of the thalamus can produce an amnesia as severe as that following hippocampal damage. Neurological disorders such as multiple sclerosis, Huntington's disease, Parkinson's disease, progressive supranuclear palsy, and subcortical ischemic vascular disease can also compromise normal memory functions. In these disorders, the neurological damage is in subcortical structures such as the basal ganglia, midbrain, and white matter, and the rich interconnections between subcortical structures and the frontal lobes are disrupted. The nature of the episodic memory impairment in these subcortical syndromes tends to be different than the amnesia following medial temporal injury. Medial temporal injury interferes with the consolidation of new information; consequently, new information is rapidly forgotten after relatively short delay periods. In subcortical syndromes, patients may have difficulty learning new material because of slowed information processing and inefficient encoding. They are better able to retain what they have learned, however, and their recognition memory is often better than their spontaneous recall.

Individual differences in episodic memory abilities have also been a subject of considerable research. Age is a very strong predictor of how well information is stored and retrieved. Significant improvement in recall levels, recognition, and application of learning strategies (e.g., organization and rehearsal) occurs during childhood and into early adolescence. Large cross-sectional and longitudinal studies have further suggested that age-related declines in memory performance begin in the fourth and fifth decades of life and continue throughout the life span. Although atrophic changes in the hippocampus may explain some of the age-related changes in episodic memory, cognitive psychologists have also found that older normals are less likely to spontaneously organize information to be learned than are younger normals. For example, younger subjects cluster together list items that share semantic properties to a much greater degree than do older subjects. Several researchers have also found that source and temporal order memory are more affected by normal aging than is fact memory, further suggesting that changes in the frontal lobes may also contribute to age-related episodic memory decline.

Gender differences in episodic memory have also been studied. Females tend to outperform males on a host of verbal memory tasks, whereas studies examining visuospatial memory have yielded less consistent results. These frequently reported sex differences in verbal episodic memory have generated considerable debate regarding their underlying mechanisms. Estrogen has been considered as one possible contributing factor. Experimental studies in postmenopausal women have generally found a protective effect of estrogen on verbal memory, and longitudinal studies found that women who were estrogen users performed better on verbal memory tasks than nonusers of similar age.

Advances in our understanding of the cognitive and neuroanatomical bases of episodic memory have made important contributions to clinical practice and the differentiation of learning and memory disorders, and they offer a framework for future research aimed at improving episodic memory functions.

—*Joel H. Kramer*

***See also*–Hippocampus; Memory, Autobiographical; Memory, Explicit/Implicit; Memory, Overview; Memory, Semantic; Memory, Spatial; Memory, Working**

Further Reading

Brandt, J., Bylsma, F. W., Aylward, E. H., et al. (1995). Impaired source memory in Huntington's disease and its relation to basal ganglia atrophy. *J. Clin. Exp. Neuropsychol.* **17**, 868–877.

Caine, D., and Watson, J. D. (2000). Neuropsychological and neuropathological sequelae of cerebral anoxia: A critical review. *J. Int. Neuropsychol. Soc.* **6**, 86–99.

Goldman, W. P., Winograd, E., Goldstein, F. C., et al. (1994). Source memory in mild to moderate Alzheimer's disease. *J. Clin. Exp. Neuropsychol.* **16**, 105–116.

Janowsky, J. S., Shimamura, A. P., and Squire, L. R. (1989). Source memory impairment in patients with frontal lobe lesions. *Neuropsychologia* **27**, 1043–1056.

Savage, C. R., Deckersbach, T., Heckers, S., *et al.* (2001). Prefrontal regions supporting spontaneous and directed application of verbal learning strategies: Evidence from PET. *Brain* **124**, 219–231.

Sherwin, B. B. (2000). Oestrogen and cognitive function throughout the female lifespan. *Novartis Found. Symp.* **230**, 188–196.

Shimamura, A. P., Janowsky, J. S., and Squire, L. R. (1990). Memory for the temporal order of events in patients with frontal lobe lesions and amnesic patients. *Neuropsychologia* **28**, 803–813.

Squire, L. R., and Kandel, E. (2000). *Memory: From Mind to Molecules.* Scientific American Library, New York.

Strupp, M., Bruning, R., Wu, R. H., *et al.* (1998). Diffusion-weighted MRI in transient global amnesia: Elevated signal intensity in the left mesial temporal lobe in 7 of 10 patients. *Ann Neurol.* **43**, 164–170.

Memory, Explicit/Implicit

Encyclopedia of the Neurological Sciences
Copyright 2003, Elsevier Science (USA). All rights reserved.

MEMORY is the capacity to utilize facts, events, and skills previously experienced or learned. This mental process can be performed either consciously or unconsciously in humans. Explicit memory is remembering that is conscious and effortful, such as in trying to recall someone's name. Implicit memory, on the other hand, refers to remembering that is outside of an individual's awareness and is considered automatic. Knowing how to deal a deck of cards or ride a bike exemplifies this type of memory. Individuals with certain neurological conditions have demonstrated dissociations between the two types of memory, suggesting multiple mechanisms and/or locations for these memory processes.

EXPLICIT MEMORY

Tasks

Memory for words, paragraphs, digits, and/or objects has been used to study episodic memory or memory for facts and events within a temporal context (Table 1). For example, individuals are asked to recall, recognize, and/or draw stimuli previously seen or heard. Individuals may be asked to read a series of words then report them back. Recall may be immediate or after some delay (minutes or days). Subjects may also be asked to identify among a series of words, digits, or objects those that they have seen before—a process called recognition memory.

Table 1 EXAMPLES OF EXPLICIT AND IMPLICIT MEMORY

Explicit memory: conscious, effortful
Episodic: knowledge, facts, events within a temporal context
Semantic: knowledge, facts
Working: manipulation of information held in temporary storage
Source: knowledge of when, where, or from whom information is acquired
Metamemory: awareness of one's memory capabilities and strategies; monitoring, control

Implicit memory: unconscious, automatic
Procedural: skill learning, habits, with and without a motor component
Associative (classic conditioning, learned conditioned response probabilistic associations, artificial grammar, category learning): knowledge of associations or categories over multiple trials without explicit awareness of rules or learning
Priming: change in reaction time or accuracy in response to prior exposure to a stimulus

Recognition is less effortful than recall, as reflected in better memory performance for recognition than recall tasks. Individuals may also view or copy line drawings and then be asked to reconstruct them from memory.

To assess semantic memory or memory for knowledge and facts, individuals may be asked to name common objects. Alternatively, they may be asked to perform a fluency task; that is, to name as quickly as possible either items from a particular category or any objects that begin with a particular letter. The number of items generated in a short period of time (usually 1 or 2 min) is a measure of this type of memory function.

Working memory refers to the manipulation of information held in temporary store, such as adding 317 and 286 without the aid of paper and pencil. Tasks typically used to assess this type of memory are two-component or dual tasks, such as reading a series of sentences and then attempting to recall the last word from each sentence. Source memory (knowing the context in which information was acquired) and metamemory (the awareness of one's memory capabilities and strategies) are assessed with direct questions to individuals regarding where and when they learned a particular fact or by having them rate their confidence in regard to knowing certain information or not.

Biological Bases of Explicit Memory

Neuroanatomical loci for explicit episodic and semantic memory are the medial temporal area and diencephalic midline structures. This includes the hippocampal formation, entorhinal cortex, parahippocampal cortex, and perirhinal cortex. In addition, "word-finding" difficulties on fluency tasks used to assess semantic memory are often found in patients with left hemisphere frontal lesions.

Working memory is associated with prefrontal cortex. There is also frontal cortex involvement for recall of source and temporal order information (e.g., when information is on the "tip of the tongue").

IMPLICIT MEMORY

Procedural and associative learning and memory are acquired over multiple trials (with the possible exception of taste aversion), whereas priming can occur after a single trial. Different implicit memory tasks may also be dissociable within certain populations or within subgroups of populations (e.g., Alzheimer's or Parkinson's disease), suggesting that independent processes and/or different anatomical substrates are required to perform these processes.

Implicit Memory Tasks

Procedural learning tasks reflect motor skills learning and include such tasks as pursuit rotor and mirror drawing. Associative learning refers to classic conditioning in which individuals learn an association between an unconditioned and conditioned stimulus to produce a conditioned response. Pavlov's dogs are a classic example. In humans (as well as in rabbits), individuals can learn to blink to a tone alone after a series of trials in which a tone is paired with an air puff to the eye. Associative learning can also include cognitive associations such as probabilistic associations, artificial grammar learning, and category level learning. Subjects learn a set of associations over a series of trials—for example, forecasting the weather based on cues, learning an artificial grammar system by being shown a series of letter strings adhering to a novel grammar system, or classifying novel stimuli after exposure to a series of training stimuli. Patients with amnesia and other individuals with explicit memory impairment can perform these tasks without specific knowledge of training sessions or recognition of stimuli used in individual trials.

Priming is an unconscious change in performance due to prior exposure to a stimulus. This change most typically facilitates memory but can also be inhibitory. Tasks commonly used to assess priming include fragment-stem completion and repetition priming. Fragment-stem completion involves expo-sure to a list of words and then completion of a list of fragment stems (e.g., someone may respond "street" to the stimulus "str___"). Individuals are more likely to complete stems with words from a prior list rather than generate new words. Stimuli used in repetition priming can be either words or pictures, with prior exposure typically eliciting either faster or more accurate responses over a series of trials.

Biological Bases of Implicit Memory

Motor skills learning and memory, including procedural memory and sequence learning, occur primarily in motor cortex, basal ganglia, and the supplementary motor area. Classic condition associative learning and memory, perhaps the best studied pathways in mammals, involve regions of the cerebellum. In addition, the hippocampus has a modulating effect on some conditioned responses. For example, ablation of the hippocampus does not affect the learned response, whereas electrical or chemical modification of the hippocampus does. Probabilistic classification is most likely related to functioning of the caudate nucleus. For example, both Huntington's and Parkinson's disease patients are impaired on this task and have known caudate nucleus pathology. Artificial grammar and category learning may depend on neocortical functioning. Loci for category learning may also include the striatum.

There may be two types of priming: perceptual and conceptual priming. Perceptual priming refers to the presemantic form and structure of the stimulus and is considered modality specific. It is associated with right extrastriate occipital cortex for visual presentation and the sensory cortex relevant for the task plus the striatum for stimuli presented in other modalities. Conceptual priming refers to activation of the semantic store or stimulus meaning, with locations most likely involving left temporal cortex and/or polymodal association cortices.

MEMORY IMPAIRMENT IN CLINICAL POPULATIONS

A loss of memory is the inability to remember past events, facts, or knowledge. Clinical conditions for which memory losses are common are organic amnesia, traumatic brain injury, Alzheimer's disease, stroke, mental retardation, Down's syndrome, Korsakoff's syndrome (memory loss due to alcoholism), Huntington's disease, and Parkinson's disease. Various clinical conditions demonstrate dissociations between explicit and implicit memory systems. Moreover, dissociations have been demonstrated within these classification systems as well. For example, loss of explicit memory and relative sparing of implicit memory are well documented in patients with amnesia, traumatic brain injury, and Korsakoff's and Down's syndrome. A loss of implicit memory has been evidenced in patients with Huntington's and Parkinson's disease. A hallmark clinical feature of Alzheimer's disease is explicit memory loss. This may be episodic or semantic or both. Certain implicit memory processes may be impaired as well, such as classic conditioning, whereas other implicit memory tasks may remain intact.

Noted brain injury cases also demonstrate dissociations between different aspects of memory. For example, patient HM underwent surgery in 1953 for intractable epilepsy. Surgeons removed parts of his temporal lobes, including the hippocampus. The seizures stopped, but HM no longer had the ability to transfer information from short- to long-term memory. Thus, he could meet and carry on a conversation with someone, but if the person left and returned a few minutes later, he had no memory of meeting that person. He could, however, perform certain implicit memory tasks, such as mirror tracing.

LIFE SPAN AND RISK OF MEMORY IMPAIRMENT

Memory problems are different during different stages of the life span. There is evidence that both children and older adults demonstrate age-related increases and decreases in explicit memory, respectively, whereas implicit memory is relatively intact in both age groups. Even children with mental retardation and those with Down's syndrome show impaired explicit but spared implicit memory.

Age-related declines in explicit memory begin to occur in approximately the fourth decade. Classic conditioning (associative learning) also shows decline beginning at approximately this time. In addition, the risk of diseases associated with memory loss increases with age. For example, there is increased risk of stroke-related dementia and memory impairment as well as dementia due to Parkinson's disease. Also, Alzheimer's disease increases exponentially with age. The prevalence of Alzheimer's disease is approximately 6–8% at age 65, whereas estimates of prevalence range from 20 to

50% after age 85. Finally, Down's syndrome patients who survive to the age of 35 begin to exhibit both the behavioral and neuropathological features typical of Alzheimer's disease.

—*Barbara J. Cherry*

See also–Alzheimer's Disease; Down's Syndrome; Memory, Autobiographical; Memory, Episodic; Memory, Overview; Memory, Semantic; Memory, Spatial; Memory, Working

Further Reading

Anooshian, L. J. (1998). Implicit and explicit memory in childhood: A review of relevant theory and research. *Child Study J.* **28**, 17–52.

Cabeza, R., Kapur, S., Craik, F. I. M., *et al.* (1997). Function neuroanatomy of recall and recognition: A PET study of episodic memory. *J. Cogn. Neurosci.* **9**, 254–265.

Fleischman, D. A., and Gabrieli, J. D. E. (1998). Repetition priming in normal aging and Alzheimer's disease: A review of findings and theories. *Psychol. Aging* **13**, 88–119.

Reder, L. M. (Ed.) (1996). *Implicit Memory and Metacognition.* Erlbaum, Mahwah, NJ.

Schacter, D. L., Chie, C.-Y. P., and Ochsner, K. N. (1993). Implicit memory: A selective review. *Annu. Rev. Neurosci.* **16**, 159–182.

Shimamura, A. P. (1995). Memory and frontal lobe function. In *The Cognitive Neurosciences* (M. S. Gazzaniga, Ed.). MIT Press, Cambridge, MA.

Squire, L. R., and Zola, S. M. (1996). Structure and function of declarative and nondeclarative memory systems. *Proc. Natl. Acad. Sci. USA* **93**, 13515–13522.

Vicari, S., Bellucci, S., and Carlesimo, G. A. (2000). Implicit and explicit memory: A function dissociation in persons with Down syndrome. *Neuropsychologia* **38**, 240–251.

Memory, Overview

Encyclopedia of the Neurological Sciences
Copyright 2003, Elsevier Science (USA). All rights reserved.

THE HUMAN brain has the remarkable capacity to continually assimilate new information and form new associations. Our memories include factual information and personal events, and they represent verbal, auditory, spatial, tactile, olfactory, and even emotional experiences. Importantly, this new information can be stored for extended periods of time and retrieved when needed. This ability to encode, store, and later retrieve information is a multifactorial and complex biological function requiring numerous mental operations and brain regions. It stands to reason, then, that these abilities can be easily disrupted by a host of neurological and psychiatric disorders. Memory deficits are often the first symptom in progressive dementing disorders and can be the only cognitive deficit in disorders such as mild head trauma and multiple sclerosis. In addition, memory problems are among the most frequent complaints of normal elderly and patients with major psychiatric disorders, such as depression and schizophrenia. The frequency of memory problems underscores the importance of understanding the different ways in which learning and memory occur and the different ways in which they can break down.

Our knowledge of human memory is derived from studies of both normal individuals and patients with specific neurological disorders. The study of memory has inspired several different theories, many of which divide memory into various subsystems. These divisions are not mutually exclusive, of course, and often the differences between them reflect differing areas of emphasis rather than opposing views about the underlying nature of memory. The most widely used memory constructs have been developed by cognitive psychologists and neuroscientists and help show how different neurological syndromes produce dramatically different types of memory disorders.

One of the most important advances in memory research in recent years has been the distinction between declarative and nondeclarative memory systems. Declarative memory refers to memories that are directly accessible to conscious recollection. It deals with facts, data, and experiences that are acquired through learning; the retrieval of this information is usually intentional and within the awareness of the individual. Because the act of remembering within the declarative system is typically explicit, the term explicit memory is often used.

The neuroanatomical structures mediating the declarative memory system have been extensively studied during the past several decades. The association between amnesia and medial temporal lobe structures became firmly established in the 1950s when patients with extensive, bilateral temporal lobe resections were found to have severe impairments in new learning. It is now understood that declarative memory is the product of several interacting subsystems that rely on multiple brain regions. Perhaps most critical for the storage of new information is the hippocampal region (hippocampus proper, dentate gyrus, and subiculum) and its adjacent cortical regions, the parahippocampal, perirhinal, and entorhinal cortices. Because the hippocampus has extensive neural connections with the dorsomedial nucleus of the thalamus and mamillary bodies,

diencephalic lesions have also been found to produce amnesic syndromes.

Awareness of nondeclarative memory systems evolved when it became clear that amnesic patients were still able to demonstrate intact learning and memory under certain conditions. Nondeclarative memory refers to several different memory systems that are behaviorally and neuroanatomically distinct from the declarative memory system. The most studied types of nondeclarative memory are priming and skills learning. Priming is the phenomenon by which prior exposure of material facilitates an individual's later performance with that same material. For example, subjects may be shown a list of words and later be given a word fragment and asked to identify what the word might be. Even amnesic patients who display no conscious recollection of the previous list of words (i.e., no declarative memory) complete the word fragment faster when the word was presented previously. The fact that prior exposure to a word can influence subsequent behavior clearly reflects some type of memory for the information. Skills learning or procedural memory is another type of nondeclarative memory. Procedural memory is demonstrated when patients exhibit learning of a skill. For example, patients with amnesia and dementia are often capable of learning new perceptual and motor skills (e.g., mirror-reading) and can even become more proficient at complex problem solving. Importantly, this increased proficiency can take place in the absence of the patient's conscious recollection of any prior learning trials. Priming and procedural learning are sometimes referred to as implicit memory because memory for the to-be-learned material is implicit in the patient's normal performance. Classic conditioning, in which learning takes the form of establishing new stimulus–response associations, is another form of nondeclarative memory. The presence of classic conditioning in primitive organisms offers fairly convincing evidence that learning can take place in the absence of a medial temporal memory system.

The distinction between declarative and nondeclarative memory is most dramatic in patients with amnesic disorders. Amnesic patients have declarative memory impairment, whereas nondeclarative memory systems are often intact. Numerous studies of amnesic patients with focal damage to medial temporal structures have demonstrated preservation of priming, habit formation, skills learning, and conditioning. Studies of the memory impairment associated with primary degenerative dementias, however, have revealed a more complex picture. Although all dementia patients have declarative memory deficits, they may differ in nondeclarative memory function. For example, Alzheimer's patients show impaired word-completion priming but have preserved procedural learning. Huntington's and Parkinson's disease patients, on the other hand, typically perform normally on priming tasks but exhibit impairments on measures of procedural memory. These different patterns of declarative and nondeclarative memory loss, in conjunction with functional imaging studies with healthy controls, suggest a particular neuroanatomy for nondeclarative memory. Association cortex appears to be a critical substrate for priming, whereas the basal ganglia, particularly the caudate, appears critical for procedural learning. Studies with nonhuman mammals have further linked the cerebellum with classic conditioning of musculoskeletal responses, and the amygdala with conditioned associations that have an emotional response.

Some investigators have further subdivided declarative memory into episodic and semantic memory. Episodic memory refers to memory for specific events, that is, episodes in one's life that can be assigned to a particular point in time. Semantic memory, on the other hand, refers to our storehouse of general information. Unlike episodic memory, semantic memory is not temporally coded; it holds information that does not depend on a particular time or place. Semantic memory also holds information such as words, symbols, and grammatical rules that are necessary in the use of language. Thus, our concept of what a sandwich is forms part of semantic memory; our recollection of the sandwich we ate for lunch yesterday is stored within episodic memory. When clinicians evaluate memory in their patients, they typically assess episodic memory. Even when the to-be-remembered information is a word list, the meaning of the words (i.e., semantic memory) is presumed to be intact; what is intended to be measured is the patient's memory for the contents of that particular list (i.e., episodic memory). When neurological syndromes impair memory, it is typically episodic memory that is affected. Most amnesic patients are very impaired in their ability to learn new information but have normal access to general facts and information that was acquired prior to their illness. There have even been reports of patients with hippocampal damage and impaired episodic memory that could still acquire factual (i.e., semantic) knowledge. Conversely, patients with semantic

dementia, caused by left anterior temporal neocortical atrophy, have relatively spared episodic memory and severely impaired semantic memory. Alzheimer's disease patients, who have both medial temporal and cortical temporal neuronal loss, suffer impairments in episodic and semantic memory.

Another important division of memory, first proposed in 1890 by William James, makes the distinction between short-term and long-term memory. Short-term memory (STM) generally refers to recall of material immediately after it is presented or during uninterrupted rehearsal of the material; it is thought to be limited in its capacity, and in the absence of rehearsal, it undergoes rapid decay, probably lasting less than 30 sec. Long-term memory (LTM) refers to recall of information after a delay interval during which the examinee's attention is focused away from the target items. It is thought to have an extraordinarily large capacity and to be fairly durable over time. The clinical significance of this distinction is exemplified in patients with amnesic syndromes. These patients tend to perform within the normal range on immediate recall of limited amounts of new material; their ability to repeat digit and letter sequences, for example, is intact. The locus of their deficit is in encoding and storing new information into LTM and thus they are unable to remember any information once a delay interval is imposed between presentation and recall.

Although the distinction between STM and LTM is well established in the experimental psychology and behavioral neurology literature, the terms STM and LTM are often used differently by other disciplines and the lay public. Typically, when patients refer to problems with their short-term memory, they are describing difficulties remembering recently acquired information after delays (i.e., LTM). Patients often label their memory for events from a long time ago as long-term memory. Consequently, caution must be exercised in clinical practice when using the terms STM and LTM. Clinicians should also be cognizant of how well a particular clinical procedure permits a clear differentiation between the various theoretical constructs. For example, during most immediate recall tasks, examinees are typically relying on a combination of STM and LTM, particularly when the amount of information to be learned exceeds the individual's immediate memory span. Therefore, inferences about the integrity of a patient's LTM cannot be based solely on the results of an immediate memory task.

The concept of STM has been extended in recent years to incorporate the idea that it is more than just a temporary and passive storage system. It is now understood that a considerable degree of information processing can occur with memories that are being held "on-line." This capacity to hold information in STM storage while at the same time carrying out other mental operations is referred to as working memory. Working memory is a complex system, hypothesized to have multiple on-line storage components (e.g., one for auditory information and one for visual information) and a central executive component that allocates processing resources between the various subsystems. The working memory system enables us to multitask–that is, perform such tasks as mental arithmetic or organizing information as it is presented. Unlike STM, which can be well preserved in many neurological disorders, working memory tends to be very vulnerable to cerebral insult. Functional imaging has begun to shed light on the neuroanatomy of working memory. Parietal structures play a major role in mediating the more passive, STM component of working memory. The multitasking component primarily involves frontal structures, particularly dorsolateral prefrontal cortex.

Another important distinction often made in clinical studies of memory is retrograde vs anterograde amnesia. Acute insult to neural systems responsible for memory can disrupt recall of information acquired prior to the injury (retrograde amnesia) as well as information presented for learning after the insult (anterograde amnesia). Retrograde memory can be assessed by asking the patient to recall autobiographical information. Assessing retrograde memory overlaps with "remote memory" because both are concerned with information that has been encoded and stored in LTM prior to central nervous system injury or disease. Both of these constructs further overlap with semantic memory to the extent that semantic memory is composed largely of information stored prior to the onset of most memory disorders. Anterograde memory is evaluated whenever a patient is asked to learn new material and thus overlaps significantly with the constructs of LTM and episodic, declarative memory.

Studies of retrograde amnesia in patients have helped refine our understanding of episodic memory. It is apparent that initial acquisition of information does not guarantee permanent storage. Rather, a process must take place during which the neural circuitry underlying a particular memory undergoes consolidation. The precise parameters and biological mechanisms of consolidation are poorly understood, but it is clear that consolidation can take place over a period of years. Studies of patients with focal medial temporal lesions have found temporally limited retrograde amnesias extending for a year or more prior to their insult. Consolidation can be similarly disrupted in patients receiving electroconvulsive shock therapy and in patients suffering traumatic brain injury. In fact, it is not uncommon for head-injured patients to have no recall of events 24–48 hr prior to their accident. Consolidation is also an active process that involves an ongoing interaction between how often the memory is retrieved, which details are forgotten, and the influence of new information on the to-be-remembered event. Consequently, the mental and neural representations of an event may go through a process of reorganization over time. The hippocampal memory system appears to be the critical structure for this process of consolidation, although the conscious availability of old memories following medial temporal damage offers strong evidence that the permanent storage site for episodic memory is outside the hippocampus.

Advances in cognitive neuroscience have begun to delineate key memory constructs and have identified several neuroanatomical structures that are integral to the process of learning. Importantly, when applied to clinical practice, these constructs assist in the differentiation of learning and memory disorders.

—*Joel H. Kramer*

***See also*–Intelligence; Language, Overview; Learning, Overview**

Further Reading

Baddeley, A. (1998). Working memory. *C. R. Acad. Sci. III* **321**, 2167–2173.

Schacter, D. L. (1992). Understanding implicit memory: A cognitive neuroscience approach. *Am. Psychol.* **47**, 559–569.

Squire, L. R. (1991). The medial temporal lobe memory system. *Science* **253**, 1380–1386.

Squire, L. R., and Zola, S. M. (1996). Structure and function of declarative and nondeclarative memory systems. *Proc. Natl. Acad. Sci. USA* **93**, 13515–13522.

Tulving, E. (1972). Episodic and semantic memory. In *Organization and Memory* (E. Tulving and W. Donaldson, Eds.). Academic Press, New York.

Vargha-Khadem, F., Gadian, D. G., Watkins, K. E., *et al.* (1998). Differential effects of early hippocampal pathology on episodic and semantic memory. *Science* **277**, 376–380.

Memory, Semantic

Encyclopedia of the Neurological Sciences

SEMANTIC MEMORY encompasses that body of knowledge held in common by members of a cultural or linguistic group. It is a mental thesaurus of the organized knowledge an individual possesses about the meaning of objects, words, symbols, and all manner of facts. During the course of development, the normal individual acquires a vast storehouse of knowledge. which is relatively stable with use and disuse. Our verbal vocabulary is one example of semantic memory: The average adult comprehends and is able to retrieve many thousands of word meanings. Our visual vocabulary is at least as important as our verbal vocabulary. Objects, quite apart from having verbal labels, have clearly defined attributes and functions. Semantic memory of our visual environment is in fact even more basic and is acquired earlier in life than verbal semantics. Consider the implications of not knowing which objects are edible or which objects are dangerous.

Historically, semantic memory is a recent concept that evolved from the debate in the early 1970s regarding the organization and properties of long-term memory. The realization that an individual's long-term memory for autobiographical events unique to the individual and memory for semantic knowledge must be differentiated was strengthened by studies of patients with brain damage. At that time, it was known that amnesic patients with circumscribed bilateral lesions of the medial temporal lobe have a grave loss of autobiographical memory but have no impairment of their semantic memory. Knowledge of word meanings is intact; visual object knowledge is normal; and reading, writing, and arithmetic—all classes of semantic memory—are unimpaired. On the other hand, selective impairments of word knowledge, an individual's verbal semantics, have been observed in certain rare aphasic syndromes, and selective impairments of visual object knowledge have been investigated in the context of perceptual disorders. In neither case was autobiographical memory necessarily compromised. This evidence of a double dissociation of word and object knowledge from autobiographical memory aided in the emergence of the concept of semantic memory.

The concept of a selective impairment of semantic memory derived from the investigation of patients with cortical degenerative conditions, such as Alzheimer's disease and frontotemporal dementia, that affect both structures subserving word comprehension and visual object knowledge. Thus, it became possible to yoke deficits from two distinct domains of inquiry that hitherto had been considered from two entirely different frameworks of enquiry. In the original study that proposed a selective impairment of semantic memory, three patients were studied in-depth and their preserved and impaired cognitive skills were documented. They were all university graduates, still able to complete abstract reasoning tests at a good level, and their autobiographical memory was relatively detailed. They were able to read, write, and express themselves fluently within the limitations imposed by the loss of individual word meanings. Their ability to repeat words and sentences was average or above average. However, they were unable to recall many word meanings that were obviously once within their vocabulary. A comparable impairment in the visual domain was documented: Although their perceptual skills were intact, they had difficulty in identifying common objects. In both the verbal and the visual domain, very clear-cut frequency effects were observed. Uncommon words and objects appeared to be lost entirely, whereas very common words and objects appeared to be retained. However, there appeared to be impoverished or partial knowledge of an item. For example, when asked to define a word such as "hammer," they might know it was a tool but not which tool. Shown a picture of a pear, they might know it was a fruit but not which fruit. These observations provided evidence of a hierarchical organization with the cortical semantic representations of both words and visual objects.

Two other points of interest emerged from this original investigation. First, there was no one-to-one relationship between knowledge of a stimulus item in the verbal and the visual domain. Both preservation of knowledge in the visual domain and loss of knowledge of the same item in the verbal domain and the converse, preservation of item knowledge in the verbal domain and loss in the visual domain, were documented. This led to the speculation that our knowledge base is organized in multiple modality-specific meaning systems. Second, tentative evidence for category-specific semantic deficits was observed. One patient had much less difficulty in defining words with an abstract referent than words with a concrete referent. For example, he was able to define "supplication" as "making a serious request for help" and "arbiter" as "a man who arbitrates to produce a peaceful solution." By comparison, the best he could do for "needle" was "I've forgotten," and his response for "geese" was "an animal but I've forgotten precisely." This early observation anticipated the demonstration of many more semantic category dissociations: Many unexpected selective category impairments and selective category preservations are now on record.

CATEGORY SPECIFICITY

Neuropsychological disorders of semantic memory are frequently selective to particular categories of semantic information. During the past two decades, an increasingly fine-grain categorical organization of semantic memory has emerged. The most widely documented of the various category-specific phenomena is the selective impairment of knowledge of animate objects with sparing of knowledge of man-made objects. This dissociation was first observed in a small group of patients recovering from herpes simplex encephalitis. They were tested in both the verbal domain by asking them to define names of man-made objects and living things (animals and plants) and in the visual domain by asking them to identify pictorial representations of the same items. Dramatic differences in their knowledge of these two categories in both modalities were observed; indeed, their knowledge of living things was all but obliterated. In this group, knowledge of foods was also impaired. The converse dissociation has also been documented; in other words, in some patients there is a relative sparing of animate items and a loss of knowledge of inanimate objects. This classic example of a double dissociation effectively rules out the possibility that such category effects are merely a product of the inherent difficulty in assigning meaning to either the animate or inanimate semantic category.

The animate/inanimate distinction, though given most prominence in many accounts of category effects in the organization of semantic memory, by no means exhausts the range of category-specific disorders that have been documented. There are many categories of knowledge not encompassed by the abstract/concrete or the animate-inanimate distinctions. An early recognized category effect was the selective loss or selective preservation of proper nouns compared with common nouns. There are patients whose language is entirely fluent and who are able to use a wide vocabulary with the exception of names of people. It is common for the recall of proper names to be more elusive than that of object names; consequently, selective difficulty with peoples' names has been considered the more difficult task. However, the selective sparing of proper names can be quite remarkable. The first account of a patient with grave word comprehension difficulties documented a selective preservation of country names (not peoples' names), a pattern that has since been observed in other patients. A patient with a global dysphasia who had no viable speech production and appeared to have little or no comprehension of spoken language was assessed using picture arrays and printed word arrays from which she had to choose the spoken target. She was either at chance or significantly impaired on all categories of common nouns. However, her performance was virtually flawless with countries, famous people (e.g., Churchill and Picasso), and famous buildings (e.g., the Parthenon and the Kremlin).

Orthogonal to these category dissociations within the noun vocabulary, there are equally unexpected dissociations between parts of speech. This has been documented most frequently for nouns compared with verbs. There are studies showing impaired verb use and comprehension in patients with excellent ability to comprehend and retrieve both proper and common nouns. For example, one remarkable patient was unable to demonstrate the actions "push" and "pull" or to point to pictures representing these actions. Nevertheless, he obtained high scores on stringent naming tests that included items such as sextant, trampoline, Lenin, and Virginia Woolf. There is also evidence of many more fine-grain categorical deficits. Selective difficulty in comprehending names of colors, parts of the body, fruits, small manipulable objects, and buildings have all been recorded and attributed to loss of categorical knowledge.

Is there a principled account of these category-specific semantic memory phenomena? It has been suggested that the origin of these effects can be traced to the acquisition of these concepts in childhood. There are intrinsic differences between semantic categories, which in turn dictate different weightings of sensory and motor information during the learning process. The weightings from various sensory and motor channels are very different for animate and inanimate objects and differ for subcategories within each of these broad categories. For example, the distinction between animals often relies on shape (giraffe and camel), size (bee and bird), and movement (pigeon and duck). Flowers are distinguished mainly by shape differences (tulip and daffodil), fruits by taste and texture (plum and peach), small manipulable tools by proprioception (pencil and crayon), and action verbs by kinesthesis (jump and hop). These sensory and motor channels of information each have distinctive topographically organized input channels. It seems likely that the observed patterns of category specificity reflect the topographical organization of the neural systems that are involved in semantic processing. Some evidence for this theory is provided by imaging studies, which have demonstrated different areas of activation for different semantic categories.

MODALITY SPECIFICITY

The categorical organization of the semantic knowledge base is firmly established. However, it is not known whether this level of representation is stored in a unitary all-purpose amodal system or whether there are multiple meaning systems. Is information from the verbal and visual domain integrated within a unified core semantic representation? Alternatively, do verbal semantics and visual semantics operate in parallel and have a degree of autonomy? Much neuropsychological data favor the multiple meaning systems theory for the following reasons. First, some patients have highly selective verbal semantic deficits that spare entirely the visual knowledge base. Equally important is evidence of comparable patients with selective visual semantic loss that spares verbal knowledge. This double dissociation of verbal and visual knowledge impairments effectively rules out a cerebral organization in which either verbal or visual knowledge is more or less vulnerable to the effects of brain damage. Second, patients with category-specific deficits confined to one modality provide further and even more powerful evidence. A patient was described who, within the verbal domain, had lost knowledge of animals but not of objects. Because there was a clear-cut categorical deficit, this pattern of impairment was believed to arise at the level of semantic and not to be due to a disconnection from the auditory input processes. However, this pattern was not observed within the visual domain because his knowledge of both animals and objects was intact. He was asked to define the word "dolphin" and he replied "a fish or a bird." Shown a picture of a dolphin, he stated "lives in water ... they are trained to jump up and come out. ... In America during the war years they started to get this particular animal to

go through to look into ships." A recurrent theme throughout investigations of semantic memory deficits is the lack of concordance between verbal knowledge and visual knowledge. This modality-specific organization of meaning can perhaps also be traced to the development of knowledge systems in childhood. Visual semantics are well established prior to verbal semantics. Perhaps the basic categorical organization of visual knowledge provides a blueprint for acquisition of verbal knowledge that with use and the passage of time acquires a degree of autonomy.

ANATOMICAL CONSIDERATIONS

The localization of function is a central issue for understanding the functional architecture of the brain. Rare individual case studies of focal brain lesions can help to identify critical brain areas that may subserve particular cognitive skills. The territory of the left middle cerebral artery is invariably implicated in stroke cases that have impairments of verbal semantic knowledge with sparing of visual semantics. In contrast, damage to the posterior cerebral artery may selectively impair visual object knowledge. However, the co-occurrence of damage to verbal and visual semantic knowledge systems can be observed in patients with focal cortical atrophy. Indeed, semantic dementia is now recognized as a specific syndromic variant of frontotemporal degeneration associated with asymmetrical atrophy primarily of the anterior left temporal lobe. It is characterized by a fluent dysphasia with loss of comprehension in the context of intact syntax and speech production and loss of visual object knowledge in the context of intact visual perceptual skills. Semantic dementia provides good evidence of a modular organization, not only for input and output systems but also for the core cognitive system—an individual's knowledge base.

—*Elizabeth K. Warrington*

See also–Agnosia; Language and Discourse; Language, Overview; Memory, Autobiographical; Memory, Episodic; Memory, Explicit/Implicit; Memory, Overview; Memory, Spatial; Memory, Working

Further Reading

Hodges, J. R., Patterson, K., Oxbury, S., *et al.* (1992). Semantic dementia: Progressive fluent aphasia with temporal lobe atrophy. *Brain* **115**, 1783–1806.

McCarthy, R. A., and Warrington, E. K. (1990). *Cognitive Neuropsychology*. Academic Press, London.

Snowden, J. S., Goulding, P. J., and Neary, D. (1989). Semantic dementia: A form of circumscribed cerebral atrophy. *Behav. Neurol.* **2**, 167–182.

Snowden, J. S., Neary, D., and Mann, D. M. (1996). *Fronto-Temporal Lobar Degeneration*. Churchill Livingstone, New York.

Warrington, E. K. (1975). The selective impairment of semantic memory. *Q. J. Exp. Psychol.* **27**, 187–199.

Warrington, E. K., and McCarthy, R. A. (1987). Categories of knowledge: Further fractionations and an attempted integration. *Brain* **110**, 1273–1296.

Warrington, E. K., and Shallice, T. (1984). Category specific semantic impairments. *Brain* **107**, 829–853.

Memory, Spatial

Encyclopedia of the Neurological Sciences
Copyright 2003, Elsevier Science (USA). All rights reserved.

SPATIAL MEMORY, the memory for the spatial location and organization of objects in our environment, plays a critical role in daily life. Even the momentary loss of memory for the location one's keys, glasses, or daily parking place can be unsettling. The dramatic degeneration of spatial memory in neurological disorders such as Alzheimer's disease greatly disrupts a person's ability to function and control his or her life.

SPATIAL MEMORY AND SPATIAL COGNITION

Spatial memory is one component of spatial cognition (Fig. 1). Spatial cognition embraces a range of mental representations of spatial relations in the external world. It includes the manipulation and orientation of single objects (e.g., mental rotation and knowing the location of an object relative to a reference point such as the body) and spatial orientation, which is orienting in large-scale space (e.g., spatial navigation and way finding). Together,

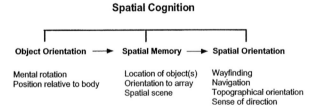

Figure 1
The relationship of spatial memory to other forms of spatial cognition.

these cognitive abilities are used to manipulate, recall, and navigate through space, whether in the real world or in mental imagery. The different abilities are also dependent on each other. Remembering the location of an object may require that one remember its orientation in space, and being able to remember the location of objects is necessary for large-scale spatial navigation. Thus, these three subcategories of spatial cognition are related in a hierarchical fashion. They are also mediated by different neural structures, as discussed later. Hence, spatial cognition is not a unitary trait that can be assessed with a single test; it is a complex of cognitive abilities that can function in concert or independently. Therefore, different neurological insults can produce a wide variety of changes in spatial cognition. To determine which subsystem has been affected, one must identify the kind of spatial cognition that has been damaged.

The location of an object can be remembered in reference to different kinds of spatial information (Fig. 2). First, the object can be coincident with a conspicuous landmark or beacon. Second, the object's location can be remembered as a triangulation from an array of objects. Here, the subject has to remember not only what objects are where but also how they are oriented (e.g., vertical or horizontal). If they are being viewed from a novel vantage point, the subject may have to mentally rotate them to determine the triangulation. Finally, the object's location may be encoded as in the direction of a distant landmark or compass mark; this is a landmark that is so far away that the navigator cannot use it to determine distance accurately—only direction.

Space can also be encoded using different reference frames according to the situation. For example, one can encode a location relative to one's own body, such as to one's left or right. This egocentric encoding, mediated largely by the parietal cortex, is different from that of structures, such as hippocampus, that mediate orientation in a global sense, independent from one's body. An example of such allocentric encoding is a mental image of the layout of a city. A spatial memory encoding of an object's position can be either egocentric or allocentric, depending on the frame of reference.

LOCALIZATION AND FUNCTION OF SPATIAL MEMORY

Just as spatial cognition is not a single phenomenon but a complex of cognitive abilities, so too is memory

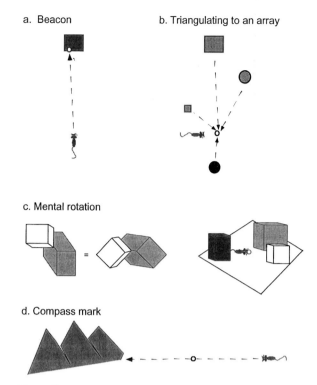

a. Beacon

b. Triangulating to an array

c. Mental rotation

d. Compass mark

Figure 2
Mechanisms underlying spatial memory. (a) Orienting toward a beacon, an object whose location is coincident with that of the goal's. (b) Triangulating toward an array, where the location of a goal is defined relative to nearby landmarks. (c) Mental rotation of landmarks in an array. (d) Orienting toward a compass mark, a landmark that supplies directional information, like a compass.

composed of several systems organized in hierarchical levels, all mediated by different brain structures. As with other types of memory, spatial memory can be classified as short (i.e., minutes or hours) or long term (i.e., weeks to months). An important component of working or short-term memory, as proposed by Baddeley, is a visuospatial scratch pad. This "structure" encodes the memory of object locations, a memory that may last only a few seconds before it is forgotten or rehearsed and consolidated into long-term memory. Like short-term verbal memory, short-term memory for object locations is subject to interference, giving credence to the notion of a short-term spatial memory system. In humans, there is additional lateralization of spatial memory, given the specialization of the right cerebral hemisphere for spatial processing.

Neural Encoding of Spatial Memory

Neuroimaging studies in humans suggest that both the right posterior parietal cortex and the right

lateral prefrontal cortex are important in the processing of spatial working memory. However, the right medial temporal lobe, including the hippocampus, has been implicated in long-term spatial memory.

Behavioral studies of memory for object locations typically require subjects to study groups of stimulus items located on an array and then to recall and replace those objects after a delay interval (Fig. 3). This technique was developed by Brenda Milner in the 1980s while studying patients who underwent unilateral temporal lobectomies for the treatment of epilepsy. Patients were asked to view 16 toy objects laid out on an array and to estimate a price for each object. After a delay, the subjects were then asked to recall each object from memory and then to place each object in its original location. After a long delay, both the right and the left lobectomy patients were impaired on the object recall task, with the left patients performing worse than the right patients. In the object location task, however, the right lobectomy patients were severely impaired, whereas the left lobectomy patients performed at normal levels.

Although spatial memory impairment only occurs with right medial temporal lobe damage, deficits in visual memory and object recall have also been demonstrated, making it difficult to completely

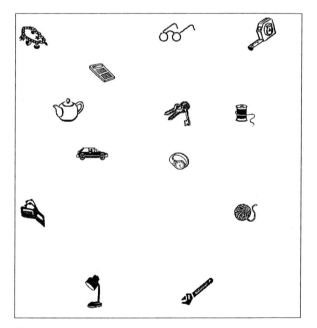

Figure 3
Spatial memory recall task developed by Brenda Milner. In this task, subjects are asked to recall the location of household objects that they have seen previously arrayed on an open surface.

dissociate spatial memory from other types of memory. Long-term spatial memory appears to be dissociable among cerebral hemispheres, even within the same temporal lobe. Nunn and colleagues replicated the Milner study but included a temporal titration procedure. Here, the delay between viewing the array and recall was varied for the right and left lobectomy groups. In this way, they could match performance on the object location (spatial) memory function with the object recall (nonspatial) memory function. Only the right temporal lobectomy patients were impaired on the spatial version of the task.

Also at issue are the exact medial temporal structures involved in spatial memory and their relative roles. Although focal lesion studies have laid the groundwork for models of hippocampal involvement in human spatial memory, they are flawed because control of lesion size is almost impossible, leading to variability within studies of the structures involved. This is alleviated somewhat by lesion analysis, a procedure measuring the size of the lesions, and only subjects with specific lesion measurements are included in the study. Nunn *et al.* included only those patients with specific hippocampal lesions that did not encroach upon surrounding structures to demonstrate the importance of right hippocampus in spatial memory. Functional neuroimaging studies have also been utilized to study spatial memory, but different results have been obtained from different laboratories and/or different techniques (positron emission tomography and functional magnetic resonance imaging). The cognitive/behavioral research is generally consistent, however, with the view that the right hippocampus is specialized in some way for spatial memory, although it does not have an exclusive role in this capacity.

This raises the issue of the independence of spatial memory from other types of memory. Even if spatial memory can be dissociated in this way, this does not mean that spatial memory is a separate memory system. Its status, however, is currently a matter of debate. For example, some argue that spatial memory may serve as the foundation for broad concepts such as episodic memory, whereas others argue that it is simply a subcomponent of the broader declarative memory system. These questions are at the forefront of an active area of research and are being pursued employing many techniques, including electrophysiological recordings in laboratory rodents and humans, genetic and pharmacological lesions in rodents, and neuroimaging studies in humans.

Evidence from Animal Models of Spatial Memory

Data from nonhuman animals offer an important perspective on the nature of spatial memory. There are two complementary lines of evidence, one from patterns of space use in wild animals and the other from neurophysiological recordings from laboratory rodents orienting in space.

Studies of the natural patterns of space use in wild rodents and wild birds have found a remarkable pattern: The larger the territory or the greater the need for spatial memory, the larger the hippocampus is relative to the whole brain in that species. Thus, small rodents and birds that store food like squirrels (e.g., kangaroo rats and chickadees), putting a single seed in a cache and returning weeks later to retrieve it, have relatively larger hippocampi than closely related species that do not store food in this way. Within species, individuals of the sex that must search widely for mates or nest sites during the breeding season (e.g., voles and cowbirds) also have a relatively larger hippocampus. Thus, data from the naturally occurring patterns of hippocampal size in both birds and mammals indicate the role of the hippocampus in spatial cognition.

More direct evidence comes from neurophysiological studies of spatial memory in the laboratory rodent. Recordings from single hippocampal neurons during exploration of a novel place have led to a sophisticated understanding of the role of the hippocampus in this process. Much of this work began with the theory of the hippocampus as a cognitive map, first proposed by John O'Keefe and Lynn Nadel in 1978. This theory developed from O'Keefe's finding that pyramidal neurons in the rat hippocampus are active only in a particular point in space, such as only at the end of one arm of a radial arm maze (Fig. 4a). These "place cells" have receptive fields that can be altered by changing the environment. As shown in Fig. 4b, if the landmarks around the outside of the radial arm maze are rotated, the place fields also rotate, firing only when the rat is in the same spatial position relative to those landmarks. Thus, neural activity in hippocampal place cells closely parallels the spatial behavior of the rodent.

Experimental lesions of the hippocampus also confirm its role in spatial memory. After a lesion, the rodent will make repeated revisits in the radial arm maze. In the water maze, although the rodent can learn a path to the platform after many trials, it cannot quickly adapt its behavior if released from a

a. Radial arm maze

b. Using landmarks to encode a position

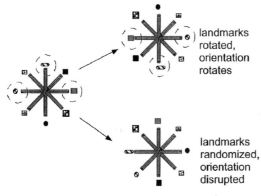

landmarks
rotated,
orientation
rotates

landmarks
randomized,
orientation
disrupted

c. Water maze

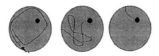

Figure 4
Methods used to study spatial memory in laboratory animals. (a) Radial arm maze developed by David S. Olton. The goal of this task is to retrieve eight rewards, each placed on the end of a maze arm (●). Over several days, the rodent naturally learns to avoid revisiting an arm that has recently been explored (○). Performance is quantified as the number of revisits per trial. The same maze can also be used to study long-term memory by training the rodent that only a certain subset of arms are ever rewarded. Performance on this task is quantified as the number of incorrect visits, either to never-baited arms or arms already visited in that trial. (b) The use of landmarks by laboratory rodents to encode a position in space on the radial arm maze. The unique shapes represent unique local landmarks. The dashed line encircles three of the landmarks available during training to facilitate the visualization of the manipulations. After rats learn the landmarks, they are either rotated or randomized. After rotation (top), the rats simply rotate their orientation and continue to orient accurately. After randomization (bottom), the rats must completely relearn the maze. Note that the circles with dashed lines could also represent the shape and location of three place fields encoded by three hippocampal neurons; place fields would rotate with the landmarks. (c) Water maze developed by Richard G. M. Morris. The goal of this task is to find a hidden platform whose surface is several centimeters beneath the water's surface. Until the platform is found, the rodent must keep swimming. Over the course of several trials in a few days, the rodent learns to take increasingly shorter paths to the platform, even when it is released from a different location on each trial. Representative swim paths from three points during the learning of the task are shown, arranged chronologically from left to right. ●, hidden platform location.

novel start point, but must painstakingly memorize a new route.

HORMONAL INFLUENCES

Male and female humans and laboratory rats show a remarkable difference in the visual cues that they use to orient. In rats, Williams has shown that male performance on the radial arm maze is severely disrupted if the maze is curtained, even if positional landmarks are still visible. Female performance is only slightly impaired under this condition. In contrast, if the positional landmarks are removed or randomized female performance is severely impaired, whereas this manipulation has less effect on male performance. For example, if male and female rats were trained on a radial arm maze (Fig. 4b), female performance would be completely disrupted if the landmarks were randomized. In contrast, males would continue to orient to other cues, such as the geometrical shape of the room.

Similar patterns are seen in humans: There are female or male advantages on different spatial tasks. The largest sex difference, and one that has been documented in different cultures and age groups, is mental rotation. However, in the recall of the relative position of objects, women are more accurate than men. This is seen for the recall of a large number of objects (>20), whether drawn on a sheet of paper or actual objects in a small room such as an office. In contrast, Postma demonstrated a male advantage when the absolute location of fewer objects (<10) must be recalled.

The explanation for this difference may lie in the preference of males to encode in terms of direction and distance and females to encode in terms of relative position. The same effect is seen in map recall studies. When given fictitious maps to remember, women remember more distinctive landmarks, whereas men are more accurate at reproducing accurate Euclidean directions and distances. Men and women also differ in their response to virtual mazes, with men navigating more accurately by direction of movement, whereas women are more accurate regarding the identity and location of landmarks. Recent neuroimaging studies of this phenomenon suggest that both men and women employ right hippocampal activation during virtual maze navigation. However, there are subtle sex differences in the parallel involvement of the prefrontal and parietal cortices during navigation. Unfortunately, results from imaging are contradictory, and further research is needed before any strong conclusions can be drawn regarding the neural basis of such sex differences in spatial navigation.

EFFECTS OF AGING

As with other types of memory, the accuracy of spatial memory recall declines with age. The parameters surrounding the objects to be remembered, however, have a major effect on this age difference in recall.

A common technique to study changes with aging is the recall of distinctive objects or patterns on a small matrix (e.g., 5×5) on a display board or computer screen. Performance is measured as the number of objects recalled after a delay. Older subjects show reduced accuracy on this task compared to young adults, particularly when the task is set up as incidental learning. In this case, subjects are not instructed to remember but simply do so incidentally while paying attention to another instruction (e.g., estimate the cost of the object). However, even when instructed to remember (intentional learning), a deficit is seen in older subjects. Older subjects do particularly poorly when the objects to be remembered are similar to each other (e.g., all poker chips compared to different household objects). A similar age difference in spatial memory recall is seen on more naturalistic tasks, such as placing objects on maps. Again, there is an added effect if the learning is incidental, not intentional, and an effect of type of object: Real objects are recalled more readily than paper-and-pencil versions of the same task. Evidence suggests that objects are also confused if they are too similar to each other in type (e.g., tool vs furniture), suggesting that the semantic encoding of an object contributes to age-related declines in recall.

—*Lucia F. Jacobs*

See also–Aging, Overview; Alzheimer's Disease; Memory, Autobiographical; Memory, Episodic; Memory, Explicit/Implicit; Memory, Overview; Memory, Working; Motion and Spatial Perception

Further Reading
Baddeley, A. (1993). *Your Memory: A User's Guide*, 2nd ed. Penguin, London.
de Haan, E. H. F., Kappelle, L. J., and Postma, A. (2001). Varieties of human spatial memory: A meta-analysis on the effects of hippocampal lesions. *Brain Res. Rev.* 35, 295–303.
Jacobs, L. F. (1996). Sexual differentiation and cognitive function. In *Gender and Society* (C. Blakemore and S. Iversen, Eds.). Oxford Univ. Press, Oxford.
Kausler, D. H. (1994). *Learning and Memory in Normal Aging.* Academic Press, San Diego.
Kimura, D. (1999). *Sex and Cognition.* MIT Press, Cambridge, MA.
Kolb, B., and Whishaw, I. Q. (1996). Spatial behavior. In *Human Neuropsychology*, 4th ed. Freeman, New York.
Isgor, C., and Sengelaub, D. R. (1998). Prenatal gonadal steroids affect adult spatial behavior, CA1 and CA3 pyramidal cell morphology in rats. *Horm. Behav.* 34, 183–198.
Nunn, J. A., Graydon, F. J. X., Polkey, C. E., *et al.* (1999). Differential spatial memory impairment after right temporal lobectomy demonstrated using temporal titration. *Brain* 122, 47–59.
O'Keefe, J., and Nadel, L. (1978). *The Hippocampus as a Cognitive Map.* Oxford Univ. Press, Oxford.
O'Keefe, J., Burgess, N., Donnett, J. G., *et al.* (1998). Place cells, navigational accuracy, and the human hippocampus. *Philos. Trans. R. Soc. London B* 353, 1333–1340.
Sherry, D. F., and Hampson, E. (1997). Evolution and the hormonal control of sexually dimorphic spatial abilities in humans. *Trends Cogn. Sci.* 1, 50–56.
Sherry, D. F., Jacobs, L. F., and Gaulin, S. J. C. (1992). Adaptive specialization of the hippocampus. *Trends Neurosci.* 15, 298–303.
Squire, L. R. (1987). *Memory and Brain.* Oxford Univ. Press, Oxford.
Williams, C. L., and Meck, W. H. (1993). Organizational effects of gonadal hormones induce qualitative differences in visuospatial navigation. In *The Development of Sex Differences and Similarities in Behavior* (M. Haug, R. E. Whalen, C. Aron, and K. L. Olsen, Eds.). Kluwer, Dordrecht.

Memory, Working

Encyclopedia of the Neurological Sciences
Copyright 2003, Elsevier Science (USA). All rights reserved.

THE CONCEPT of working memory, which has also been described by the terms active memory and on-line memory, emerged in the field of cognitive psychology and describes a particular kind of short-term memory (STM) function in which information is kept active for the purpose of performing cognitive operations on it. Because it involves executive processes as well as those related to the maintenance of information, working memory differs from others kinds of STM, such as the simple rehearsal of new information en route to long-term memory (LTM). Working memory capacities are essential for cognitive processes described as controlled, attentive, and non-routine, and are involved, for example, in the ability to repeat a set of digits in the reverse order in which they were presented, because cognitive operations must be performed on the incoming information in order to re-represent it. The ability to repeat a set of digits in the order in which they were presented, on the other hand, depends only on STM for a string of phonological information. Rather than serving only as an intermediate step between perception and LTM, working memory serves as a kind of mental scratchpad, fundamental to higher level cognitive processes such as reasoning and abstract problem solving.

WORKING MEMORY AND HIGHER LEVEL COGNITION

The observations of Baddeley and colleagues first indicated that rather than consisting of a single buffer for the temporary storage of information to be encoded in LTM, the human working memory is a multicomponent system. These researchers used a dual-task paradigm in which subjects were required to perform cognitive tasks concurrent with various distractor tasks designed to occupy specific working memory buffers. In such experiments, a spatial tracking or tapping task is often used to probe the dependence of a cognitive task on spatial working memory. The dependence of a cognitive task on phonological STM is typically assessed through the use of tasks that interfere with the subvocal rehearsal of phonological information, such as a digit retention task or a task in which the subject is required to continuously repeat the word "the." By showing that the disabling of hypothesized working memory buffers specific for a particular information domain (e.g., phonological information) impairs the solution of problems dependent on the processing of information in that domain, the results of these studies provide evidence for the existence of domain-specific working memory buffers. Additional experimental results point to the existence of other domain-specific working memory buffers, such as a purely visual buffer and a conceptual buffer. Together, these studies have established a role for working memory in the performance of higher level cognitive tasks, such as mental arithmetic and other forms of abstract problem solving. In addition, the investigations of the human working memory system performed by Baddeley and associates accomplished much in establishing that various domain-specific STM processes can operate largely independently.

Evidence indicating that a strong relationship exists between abstract problem solving and demands placed on working memory also comes from correlational analyses. These studies have attempted to quantify the working memory demands of problems a priori in terms of the number of cognitive representations or "chunks" that an individual must keep concurrently active in the course of solving problems. These methods have been used to establish that a strong correlation exists between working memory span and cognitive processes such as sentence comprehension and reasoning.

Based on the results of psychological investigations, Baddeley proposed what is now the most prevalent model of working memory, consisting of a set of domain-specific STM buffers that interface with a common executive control module (Fig. 1). In comparison to domain-specific working memory buffers, executive processes of working memory have proved particularly difficult to study; as a consequence, existing models of working memory are vague regarding the nature of functions of the central executive module of the working memory system, and no unified concept of executive functions exists. Evidence that an executive control mechanism is critical to the function of a multimodal working memory system comes from dual-task studies using a random number-generation task or a simple decision-making task in which the subject must make a specific response to each of a set of stimuli (such as tones) in order to occupy the hypothesized executive module of working memory. However, there is no agreement regarding which aspects of these tasks characterize the essence of executive function.

More detailed formulations of executive processes in working memory are available from computational models of complex cognition, which formalize cognitive processes such as working memory in the

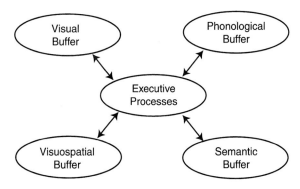

Figure 1
Multicomponent model of the human working memory system, developed by Baddeley (1986). Visual and semantic buffers have been added to those included in the original model, and other functionally independent buffers may exist as well.

context of a system. One example is Anderson's ACT model, in which mental representations take the forms of systems of rules consisting of actions that are selected based on the satisfaction of sets of conditions. Working memory in this system comprises the presently active subset of conditions and actions and thus involves the retention of conceptual information, as well as possible action plans, in the form of goal hierarchies. This idea of executive processes suggests that action plans for working with memory may be limited in terms of the number of representations of subgoals that can be concurrently active. Experimental support for this formulation of executive processes, and their relation to higher level cognition, is provided by Carpenter, Just, and Shell, who found that subjects' success rates in solving abstract problems correlated highly with both the number and types of rules that a problem required the test-taker to induce.

A more general hypothesis regarding the unifying characteristic of higher level cognitive tasks dependent on executive processes of working memory proposes that such tasks require the ability to provide different responses to the same stimuli in different contexts. In turn, this ability requires the capacity to actively represent relations, or bindings, between stimuli and between stimuli and concepts, such as roles that stimuli could possibly play in the context of a past event or plan for future action. This idea is instantiated in another set of computational models and is supported by the results of recent studies showing that the need to actively represent bindings is a source of working memory capacity limitations. These studies indicate, for example, that limitations on STM for objects arise from limitations on the number of object–location bindings that must be retained simultaneously.

NEURAL SUBSTRATES UNDERLYING WORKING MEMORY BUFFERS

Studies of STM using both lesion and electrophysiological techniques, with both human and infrahuman subjects, have helped to determine the cortical networks underlying working memory processes. These studies have revealed that working memory function depends on complex interactions between prefrontal cortical areas and posterior cortical areas subserving domain-specific processing.

In studies with nonhuman primates, working memory function has typically been assessed using a delayed-response paradigm, one example of which

is the delayed matching-to-sample (DMS) task. In this task, the subject is presented with a stimulus, called a sample, and after a delay of several seconds during which the screen is blank, the subject is shown one or more test stimuli and is prompted to indicate whether the stimulus it just saw (or heard or felt) was the same as or different from the sample. Researchers have long observed that monkeys with lesions of prefrontal cortex show impaired performance on delayed-response tasks. Such studies have often implicated an area of monkey dorsolateral prefrontal cortex (DLPFC) surrounding the principal sulcus (Brodmann area 46), as well as areas of posterior parietal cortex, in the performance of delayed-response tasks dependent on spatial working memory. In contrast, the results of lesion studies have typically found that the performance of nonspatial DMS tasks depends on intact ventrolateral prefrontal cortex as well as areas of inferior temporal cortex.

Electrophysiological studies indicate that rather than just playing a role in the encoding of new information or in the retrieval of stored information, neurons in prefrontal cortex are involved in keeping memory representations active in preparation for behavioral responses. Specifically, it has been found that when monkeys are made to perform delayed response, certain cells in prefrontal cortex increase their firing rates at the start of the delay in which the monkey is required to retain a stimulus in memory, maintain high rates of firing during the delay, and decrease firing rates immediately following the delay. The idea that principal sulcus neurons are involved in working memory is supported by findings that individual cell clusters show delay activity that is specific to particular objects, as well as locations in space, and that performance on delayed response tasks is impaired when the activity of cells during the memory delay is attenuated.

A role for prefrontal cortex in the function of short-term working memory has been demonstrated by numerous studies with human subjects as well. The deficits exhibited by rhesus monkeys with prefrontal lesions in performance of delayed response tasks, for example, are also observed in human subjects with prefrontal lesions. In the past decade, neuroimaging investigations have provided additional evidence that prefrontal cortex in humans is essential for the performance of tasks dependent on working memory. Brain imaging studies using both positron emission tomography and functional magnetic resonance imaging techniques indicate that increased activation in prefrontal cortex is associated with the performance of tasks dependent on working memory for objects, spatial locations, and verbal stimuli. In addition, brain imaging data indicate that the performance of spatial and verbal working memory tasks by humans produces increased activation in distinct cortical networks, analogous to those identified in the macaque, and that prefrontal cortical activation increases correspondent with the working memory load of the task.

NEURAL SUBSTRATES UNDERLYING EXECUTIVE FUNCTIONS OF WORKING MEMORY

A long history of clinical and experimental observations involving patients with brain lesions indicates that intact prefrontal cortex is critical to the executive control of thought, especially in terms of the structuring of flexible, goal-directed behavior. Clinically, lesions of prefrontal cortex are associated with deficits in the performance of psychological tasks dependent on executive control, especially tasks such as the Wisconsin Card Sort Task, the Stroop Task, and the antisaccade task, which require the inhibition of an overlearned response. A role for prefrontal cortex in executive control is also supported by a host of experimental studies involving humans and nonhumans with prefrontal cortical lesions. Work by Petrides and associates, for example, indicates that dorsolateral prefrontal areas play an essential role in the performance of sequencing tasks, and that DLPFC lesions impair memory for behavioral sequences that are both self-generated and external.

The idea that dorsolateral prefrontal cortex provides the essential substrate for executive processes of working memory is also supported by results of electrophysiological studies in primates using variations of traditional "working memory" tasks. These studies identified sets of neurons in monkey prefrontal cortex whose activity, rather than reflecting the retention of a particular stimulus, predicted the response of the animal. This function has been termed prospective memory, the activation of a memory for a stimulus or event in anticipation of its reoccurrence.

Findings linking prefrontal cortical function to the executive control of cognition have been interpreted in several different ways, corresponding to different psychological theories. One view is that lesions of dorsolateral prefrontal cortex disrupt executive processes related to the execution of action plans, which involves the scheduling of goals, and can be seen as fitting well with the formulations of Anderson and Carpenter, Just, and Shell. Petrides and colleagues, however, suggested that impairment shown by both human and nonhuman primates with lesions of dorsolateral prefrontal cortex on sequencing tasks may be attributed to a more general impairment in working memory for events. A third view proposes that a role for prefrontal cortex in the ability to actively represent relationships might explain a role for it in the structuring of responses, the retention of past event sequences, and other cognitive capacities associated with executive function. This hypothesis is supported by recent evidence indicating that the ability to actively represent relationships depends on intact prefrontal cortex. The results of recent electrophysiological experiments in primates, for example, indicate that neurons in prefrontal cortex show activity corresponding to the retention of specific relationships between stimulus dimensions. Additionally, studies with brain-lesioned patients indicate that damage to prefrontal cortex results in a reduced capacity to represent conceptual relations.

PARCELLATION OF PREFRONTAL CORTEX IN TERMS OF WORKING MEMORY FUNCTIONS

A number of recent experimental studies have sought to answer the question of whether working memory capacities are anatomically segregated in the manner formulated in existing psychological models. The results of these studies suggest that some modularity may exist in the anatomical organization of executive and domain-specific working memory functions.

Several recent experimental studies using functional brain imaging techniques provide support for the idea that dorsolateral areas of prefrontal cortex play an essential role in executive aspects of working memory but not in the rehearsal of domain-specific information. These studies found that requiring subjects to perform multiple tasks simultaneously led to increases in activation in DLPFC compared to conditions in which subjects performed the tasks separately. Based on these observations, Petrides and colleagues proposed a two-stage concept of prefrontal cortical function that dissociates higher level working memory functions related to event memory and planning, attributed to mid-dorsolateral regions (Brodmann areas 9 and 46), and domain-specific working memory functions, thought to be carried out in more ventral areas of lateral prefrontal cortex (Brodmann area 47; Fig. 2).

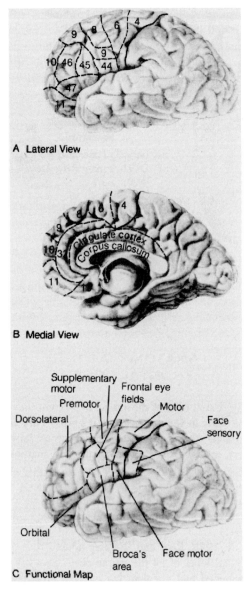

A Lateral View

B Medial View

C Functional Map

Figure 2
(A) Lateral and (B) medial views of Brodmann's cytoarchitectonic map of the frontal lobe of the human. (C) Approximate boundaries of functionally distinct areas of human prefrontal cortex [reproduced with permission from Kolb, B., and Whishaw, I. Q. (1990). *Fundamentals of Human Neuropsychology*. Freeman, New York].

Based on the framework of Baddeley, it has been proposed that each domain-specific STM buffer may be subserved not only by a unique ensemble of areas in posterior cortex but also by a distinct area of prefrontal cortex. The idea that the subregions of prefrontal cortex are devoted to domain-specific processing has received support from a number of primate studies, suggesting that dorsolateral areas

of prefrontal cortex are preferentially involved in the performance of tasks dependent on spatial working memory as opposed to working memory for object identity.

This issue is complicated by the results of a number of recent studies that suggest that many neurons in DLPFC respond to multiple modalities rather than being specific for a certain domain. These experiments reveal the existence of cells in DLPFC whose firing rates correspond to the retention of cross-modal information in cases in which visual information is used to discriminate between test stimuli distinguished by texture and vice versa. In addition, experiments involving the cooling of tissue in the principle sulcus area indicate that delayed-response deficits result from inactivation of DLPFC regardless of whether memoranda are spatial or not, and that this finding applies in the case of visual, tactile, and auditory stimuli. The issue is further complicated by knowledge that many areas of prefrontal cortex receive projections from multiple regions in posterior cortex responsible for domain-specific processing and that prefrontal cortical areas are interconnected in complex ways. Currently, no consensus exists as to what level of anatomical segregation characterizes working memory functions. The different views are not necessarily contradictory; the DLPFC might be subdivided into areas involved in domain-specific processing and areas involved in supramodal executive functions. Further study is required to resolve this issue.

NEUROMODULATORY INFLUENCES ON WORKING MEMORY

Characterizing the psychological nature of working memory processes and their neurophysiological basis is an enterprise of particular clinical importance based on the considerable evidence indicating a role for working memory dysfunction in cognitive impairments present not just in patients with focal brain lesions but also in those with particular neuropsychiatric disorders. A large body of research implicates impairments in working memory in neuropsychiatric disorders of cognition such as schizophrenia and in neurological disorders, such as Alzheimer's disease and Parkinson's disease. Together with a considerable body of evidence indicating that neuropsychiatric conditions often involve disturbances in the function of diffuse modulatory systems such as those involving the neurochemicals dopamine and acetylcholine, these findings suggest that working memory is subject to neuromodulatory influences. These results fit well with results of a growing number of experimental studies providing direct evidence for neuromodulatory influences on working memory function in both human and nonhuman primates.

CONCLUSIONS

The term working memory refers to active manipulation of information in the service of goal-directed behavior. Although questions remain regarding the issues of what exactly constitutes an executive process, what the cognitive representations are on which executive processes operate, and the precise sources of working memory capacity limitations, clear evidence points to a role for working memory in higher level cognition, for prefrontal cortical function in domain-specific and executive aspects of working memory function, and for neuromodulatory influences on neural mechanisms of working memory. Integrating psychological conceptions of the role of working memory in higher level cognition with knowledge of the neural basis of and neuromodulatory influences on working memory function is critical to understanding the link between dysfunctional neural processing and disordered cognition. An increased understanding of the role of working memory in higher level cognition is of clinical interest in that it should help researchers to better characterize the cognitive deficits precipitated by neuropsychiatric disorders. Due to the dependence of higher level cognitive processes on working memory function, a better knowledge of neural mechanisms of working memory has potentially important clinical implications in that therapies that are developed for disorders of cognition are likely to exert their effect by influencing neural mechanisms of working memory function.

—*James A. Waltz*

See also–Executive Function; Memory, Autobiographical; Memory, Episodic; Memory, Explicit/Implicit; Memory, Overview; Memory, Semantic; Memory, Spatial; Motion and Spatial Perception; Problem Solving

Further Reading

Anderson, J. R. (1983). *The Architecture of Cognition*. Harvard Univ. Press, Cambridge, MA.
Baddeley, A. D. (1986). *Working Memory*. Oxford Univ. Press, Oxford.
Carpenter, P. A., Just, M. A., and Shell, P. (1990). What one intelligence test measures: A theoretical account of the processing in the Raven Progressive Matrices Test. *Psychol. Rev.* **97**, 404–431.
Fuster, J. M. (1995). *Memory in the Cerebral Cortex: An Empirical Approach to Neural Networks in the Human and Nonhuman Primate*. MIT Press, Cambridge, MA.
Jonides, J., (1995). Working memory and thinking. In *Thinking: An Invitation to Cognitive Science* (E. E. Smith and D. N. Osherson, Eds.), 2nd ed., Vol. 3, pp. 215–265. MIT Press, Cambridge, MA.
Kopelman, M. D. (1994). Working memory in the amnesic syndrome and degenerative dementia. *Neuropsychology* **8**, 555–562.
Luck, S. J., and Vogel, E. K. (1997). The capacity of visual working memory for features and conjunctions. *Nature* **390**, 279–281.
Miller, E. K. (2000). The prefrontal cortex and cognitive control. *Nat. Rev. Neurosci.* **1**, 59–65.
Roberts, A. C., Robbins, T. W., and Weiskrantz, L. (1998). *The Prefrontal Cortex: Executive and Cognitive Functions*. Oxford Univ. Press, Oxford.
Smith, E. E., and Jonides, J. (1997). Working memory: A view from neuroimaging. *Cogn. Psychol.* **33**, 5–42.
Waltz, J. A., Knowlton, B. J., Holyoak, K. J., *et al.* (1999). A system for relational reasoning in human prefrontal cortex. *Psychol. Sci.* **10**, 119–125.

Ménière's Disease

Encyclopedia of the Neurological Sciences

PROSPER MÉNIÈRE first described the symptom complex known as Ménière's disease in 1861. In 1938, Hallpike and Cairns first proposed fluid dilation of the endolymphatic space (endolymphatic hydrops) as the underlying mechanism of hearing loss and vertigo in the disorder. Although this mechanism has been widely accepted to explain Ménière's syndrome, its precise cause is unclear.

The term Ménière's disease refers to idiopathic endolymphatic hydrops. The terms secondary Ménière's syndrome and delayed or secondary endolymphatic hydrops are sometimes used to distinguish from idiopathic Ménière's when there appears to be an underlying mechanism, such as autoimmune inner ear disease, previous viral infection, or syphilis.

CLINICAL FEATURES

The symptoms of Ménière's disease include the classic triad of unilateral hearing loss, tinnitus, and attacks of vertigo. Table 1 outlines criteria for making the diagnosis. Hearing may become noticeably diminished or muffled just prior to and during attacks of severe

Table 1 CRITERIA FOR DIAGNOSING MÉNIÈRE'S DISEASE[a]

Vertigo
    Recurrent, well-defined episodes of spinning or rotation
    Duration ranging from 20 min to 24 hr
    Nystagmus associated with attacks
    Nausea and vomiting during vertigo spells
    No focal neurological symptoms during attacks
Deafness
    Fluctuating hearing
    Sensorineural hearing loss, unilateral
    Progressive hearing loss, typically unilateral
Tinnitus
    Variable low-pitched, intensifies during attacks
    Present on the affected side
    Subjective

[a] Modified from American Academy of Otolaryngology, Head and Neck Surgery definitions. Adapted from Pearson and Brachmann (1985) and Alford (1972).

spinning vertigo. Vertigo typically lasts 1–6 hr and is commonly associated with roaring tinnitus. Reduced hearing and tinnitus occur in association with vertigo in the vast majority of cases and always localize to the same ear, except in bilateral active Ménière's disease. During the vertigo episodes, patients are generally incapacitated and, as for vertigo in general, head motion or movement intensify the discomfort.

In the initial stages of Ménière's disease, attacks of vertigo are commonly very severe and hearing is affected only briefly. As Ménière's disease progresses, the duration of vertigo attacks may diminish, but the hearing loss usually progresses and begins to persist even between attacks.

Some patients experience "drop attacks," which are sudden perceptions of violent tilting or flipping of the environment that cause them to fall without loss of consciousness. Drop attacks have been referred to as otolithic crises of Tumarkin and may be caused by sudden deformation of the utricle, the gravity-sensing organ of the inner ear. This causes the sudden feeling of falling and a reflexive loss of muscular tone that precipitates the fall.

The diagnosis of Ménière's disease should be made with caution unless there is characteristically low-frequency hearing loss or fluctuating unilateral hearing loss associated with prolonged attacks of spinning vertigo. The term vestibular Ménière's disease is somewhat outdated and refers to a condition with attacks of vertigo with no hearing loss or tinnitus. Although early Ménière's disease can occasionally present this way, unrelated conditions can cause prolonged attacks of vertigo including vestibular migraine. Since the treatment for vestibu-

lar migraine is quite different from that of Ménière's disease, distinguishing these conditions is important.

MECHANISM

The pathophysiology of Ménière's disease has been a subject of much study. The endolymphatic duct and sac drain endolymph from the auditory and vestibular apparatus. Endolymph is produced continuously. It is drained and its fluid secretion is regulated via the endolymphatic sac. The sac has fenestrated blood vessels that are leaky and can allow fluid to pass between their membranes. In this sense, the sac acts like a sponge or sieve to clean and drain debris from the inner ear and to regulate its fluid production. If the endolymphatic duct narrows and the flow of endolymph to the sac is decreased, the sac responds by secreting glycoproteins that increase endolymph production. In Ménière's disease, recurrent attacks could be caused by congenital narrowing, acquired scarring, or fibrosis of the duct or by blockage of the sac by cellular debris or immune complexes as depicted in Fig. 1. The possible causes of Ménière's disease include postviral infection, allergy mediated, and autoimmune. The main site of immune activity in the inner ear is the sac. Approximately one-third of patients with Ménière's disease have specific anti-cochlear antibodies by Western blot assay.

Delayed effects of viral labyrinthitis probably account for some cases of Ménière's syndrome. Viruses may gain access to the labyrinth either via

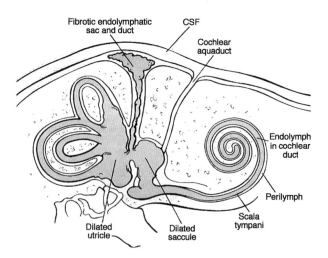

Figure 1
Schematic of endolymphatic duct scarring as a possible cause of endolymphatic hydrops (Ménière's syndrome). CSF, cerebrospinal fluid.

the bloodstream or from the upper pharynx and then through the middle ear and round window membrane. The latency between viral exposure and viral symptoms such as vestibular neuritis is thought to be on the order of days to weeks. Despite the significant circumstantial evidence of a viral mechanism in some cases of Ménière's disease, viral genetic material has not been consistently identified in patients with the condition.

TREATMENT

The goals of treatment in Ménière's disease are to control attacks of vertigo and, it is hoped, to limit progression of hearing loss. Currently, there is no treatment proven to arrest progression. Sodium restriction sufficient to stop attacks of vertigo may reduce permanent hearing loss.

Diet and Medication

Initial treatment usually consists of a severe sodium-restricted diet, sometimes with the addition of a diuretic agent, such as hydrochlorothiazide or acetazolamide. Betahistine can be used as an adjunct, and some clinicians recommend adding niacin and avoiding caffeine. If disabling attacks of vertigo continue despite these medical measures, surgical intervention is usually necessary.

Surgical Intervention

Surgical treatments include endolymphatic shunting, vestibular nerve sectioning, labyrinthectomy, and gentamicin chemodenervation. Although one study of endolymphatic shunting suggested that it is no more effective than sham surgery, many otologists believe that this procedure has a role in the treatment of Ménière's syndrome. It has the advantage of being a relatively minor procedure with a reasonably low risk of significant hearing loss. Vestibular nerve sectioning entails destruction of the vestibular portion of the eighth cranial nerve. This disconnects the affected inner ear from the rest of the body and can thus stop attacks of vertigo. The hearing portion of the nerve is left intact so that tinnitus and hearing loss are likely to continue even after surgery. Labyrinthectomy is a simpler destructive procedure reserved for patients with no useful hearing in the affected ear. Both vestibular nerve sectioning and labyrinthectomy result in unilateral peripheral vestibular loss; consequently those patients are at higher risk of ending up with bilateral vestibular loss if Ménière's disease later affects the other side. Gentamicin

chemodenervation (or streptomycin) is a procedure by which the antibiotic gentamicin, a toxin to vestibular hair cells (and, to a lesser extent, the auditory hair cells), is administered to the inner ear. The drug is injected directly through the eardrum into the middle ear or, occasionally, via a round window catheter. Once the gentamicin-induced damage to the balance system is sufficient, endolymphatic swelling no longer produces vertigo. Although gentamicin injections are much less invasive and potentially less expensive, they are also less reliable and may place the patient at greater risk of hearing loss.

—*Terry D. Fife*

See also–Hearing Loss; Tinnitus; Vertigo and Dizziness

Further Reading

Alford, B. R., for the Committee on Hearing and Equilibrium (1972). Ménière's disease: Criteria for diagnosis and evaluation of therapy for reporting. *Trans. Am. Acad. Opthalmol. Otolaryngol.* **67**, 1462–1464.

Andrews, J. C. (1997). Laboratory experience with experimental endolymphatic hydrops. *Otolaryngol. Clin. North Am.* **30**, 969–976.

Arnold, W., and Altermatt, H. J. (1995). The significance of the human endolymphatic sac and its possible role in Ménière's disease. *Acta Oto-Laryngol. Suppl.* **519**, 36–42.

Brookes, G. B. (1997). Medical management of Ménière's disease. *Ear Nose Throat J.* **76**, 634–640.

Fife, T. D. (1999). Ménière's syndrome. *Curr. Treat. Options Neurol.* **1**, 57–67.

LaRouere, M. J. (1996). Surgical treatment of Ménière's disease. *Otolaryngol. Clin. North Am.* **29**, 311–322.

Pearson, B. W., and Brachmann, D. E., for the Committee on Hearing and Equilibrium (1985). Guidelines for reporting treatment results in Ménière's disease. *Otolaryngol. Head Neck. Surg.* **93**, 579–581.

Ruckenstein, M. J. (1999). Immunologic aspects of Ménière's disease. *Am. J. Otolaryngol.* **20**, 161–165.

Meningiomas

Encyclopedia of the Neurological Sciences

THE CURRENT World Health Organization classification of meningiomas is shown in Table 1. These tumors are defined as typical, atypical, or malignant. Typical meningiomas are subclassified into several histological subtypes that are descriptive only and have no prognostic significance; these include meningothelial, fibroblastic, transitional, psammomatous, angiomatous, microcystic, secretory, clear cell,

Table 1   WORLD HEALTH ORGANIZATION CLASSIFICATION OF TUMORS OF THE MENINGES[a]

Tumors of meningothelial cells
  Meningiomas
    Meningothelial
    Fibrous (fibroblastic)
    Transitional (mixed)
    Psammomatous
    Angiomatous
    Microcystic
    Secretory
    Clear cell
    Chordoid
    Lymphoplasmacyte-rich
    Metaplastic
  Atypical meningioma
  Papillary meningioma
  Anaplastic (malignant) meningioma
Mesenchymal nonmeningothelial tumors
  Benign neoplasms
    Osteocartilaginous tumors
    Lipoma
    Fibrous histiocytoma
    Others
  Malignant neoplasms
    Hemangiopericytoma
    Chondrosarcoma
      Variant: mesenchymal chondrosarcoma
    Malignant fibrous histiocytoma
    Rhabdomyosarcoma
    Meningeal sarcomatosis
    Others
  Primary melanocytic lesions
    Diffuse melanosis
    Melanocytoma
    Malignant melanoma
      Variant: meningeal melanomatosis
  Tumors of uncertain histogenesis
    Hemangioblastoma (capillary hemangioblastoma)

[a] Based on Kleihues and Cavanee (1997).

choroidal, lymphoplasmacyte-rich, and metaplastic tumors. Papillary meningiomas tend to be more aggressive than other types, with a high rate of extraneural metastases and recurrence. Atypical meningiomas have frequent mitoses, increased cellularity, prominent nucleoli, a high nuclear/cytoplasmic ratio, sheet-like growth, and necrosis. Malignant meningiomas have "histological features of frank malignancy far in excess of the abnormalities noted in atypical meningiomas," including nuclear atypia, a high mitotic index, and conspicuous necrosis. Malignant meningiomas are known as particularly aggressive tumors that invade adjacent brain and blood vessels.

Jaskalainen *et al.* applied a point system to assess clinicopathological behavior in meningiomas. This system assigned points for loss of architecture, increased cellularity, nuclear pleomorphism, mitotic figures, focal necrosis, and the presence or absence of brain infiltration. Grade I (benign tumors) had 0–2 points, grade II ("atypical" tumors) had 3–6 points, grade III ("anaplastic" tumors) had 7–11 points, and grade IV (sarcomatous) had 12–18 points. By these criteria, 94.3% of 657 meningiomas were benign, 4.7% were atypical, and 1.0% were anaplastic. Twenty-six percent of atypical and anaplastic tumors had the same computed tomography (CT) appearance as benign tumors, suggesting that imaging does not by itself predict malignancy. The recurrence rate at 5 years for benign tumors was 3%, for atypical tumors 38%, and for anaplastic tumors 78%. Benign tumors recurred at 7.5 years as the median interval, atypical tumors at 2.4 years, and anaplastic tumors at 3.5 years. For benign tumors, the recurrence rate was 21% at 25 years.

Features having biological significance in meningiomas include their clonality, their tendency to occur twice as often in women as in men, their association with previous radiation exposure and increasing age, their expression of growth factors including those stimulating angiogenesis, and their involvement in the syndrome of neurofibromatosis (NF) type 2. The clonal derivation of a tumor can be delineated with the knowledge that in women, one X chromosome is inactivated by methylation in each cell. Analysis of which of these X chromosomes is inactivated in tumor cells determines whether the tumor cells are derived from the same maternal cell. The analysis can be done through loss of heterozygosity (LOH) analysis for a specific gene sequence, differential expression of genes, or differential methylation. Using LOH analysis in nine patients, Jacoby *et al.* showed that meningiomas appeared to be monoclonal; however, in four of the tumors, the clonality ratios were less than 3.0, leaving the interpretation ambiguous. The conclusion is that most meningiomas are monoclonal, but there is definite evidence for polyclonality in a minority. This may mean that some tumors can "recruit" other cells that were not initially neoplastic to become neoplastic via paracrine or other transformation process, a heretical concept in oncology.

Most meningiomas display deletions of the long arm of chromosome 22, primarily at the site for the NF 2 gene. This is likely one of the "meningioma" genes, and it is responsible for the high rate of occurrence of meningiomas in NF type 2 patients. The mechanism by which chromosome 22 loss leads to tumor formation in meningiomas is unknown. The product of the NF 2 gene is involved in cytoskeletal stability; one hypothesis is that if it is abnormal or deleted, contact inhibition is impaired and there is gradual uncontrolled growth because the cell does not recognize its neighbors.

Long-term studies on children radiated for tinea capitis showed that their chance of developing a meningioma as adults was 10 times greater than normal. Meningiomas can also occur after cranial radiation for other childhood tumors. The propensity for meningiomas to develop following radiation therapy may indicate that chromosomal mutations underlie the majority of spontaneous meningioma formation.

Meningiomas are found twice as often in women as in men, are prone to increase in size during pregnancy, and are found with increased frequency in patients with breast carcinoma. One possible explanation of these data is that sex hormone receptors are important in their pathogenesis. A number of receptor studies strongly suggest that these are tumors responsive to sex hormones, much like breast and prostate cancer. Our laboratory group has shown that the progesterone receptor is the major sex hormone receptor expressed in meningiomas. Its presence can be demonstrated by Northern blot analysis, competitive binding assays, and immunocytochemistry. In our series, meningiomas from 81% of women and 19% of men had expression of functional progesterone receptors. The role of the estrogen receptor is more complex. There are several types of estrogen receptors, the strongest and most common type of which is found in meningiomas. However, the current consensus is that estrogen receptor activity is not an important element in meningioma growth control. Androgen receptor mRNA is also expressed in meningiomas, more often in women than in men; the role of the androgen receptor in meningioma pathogenesis is unknown.

Meningiomas express growth factor receptors more robustly than do more malignant tumors. They express receptors for platelet-derived growth factor (PDGF), vascular endothelial growth factor (VEGF), and epidermal growth factor (EGF); in some cases, there is expression of both receptor and ligand, setting the stage for an autocrine loop stimulatory pathway. While analyzing meningiomas for the presence of PDGF, we performed Northern blot analysis to demonstrate that meningiomas express transcripts for three members of the PDGF family, including PDGF-A and -B, and the beta form of the

PDGF receptor. The *ras* oncogene is activated as an intermediate messenger when PDGF-B is added to short-term meningioma cultures. The PDGF-β receptor is present in activated form in meningiomas, again supporting its potential importance for these tumors. The EGF receptor, activated by transforming growth factor-α in most instances, is expressed in meningiomas. It has been well characterized in these tumors and can be demonstrated in its activated form by anti-phosphotyrosine antibody techniques. VEGF is an important agent in stimulating blood vessel formation and is expressed in meningiomas. KDR and Flt-1, the receptors for VEGF, are expressed in vascular endothelial cells within these tumors.

Meningioma biology is reflected in important ways in imaging. Meningiomas arise from the arachnoid layer of the coverings of the brain, but may infiltrate the dura and bone, and a dural "tail" or bony hyperostosis adjacent to the tumor reflect this growth feature (Figs. 1 and 2). On unenhanced CT or magnetic resonance imaging (MRI), they are isointense with brain and may be partially calcified.

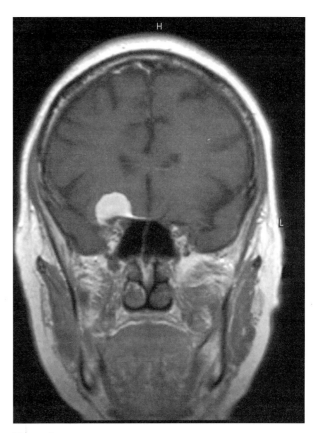

Figure 1
Note the dural thickening adjacent to this optic nerve sheath meningioma, the classic "dural tail."

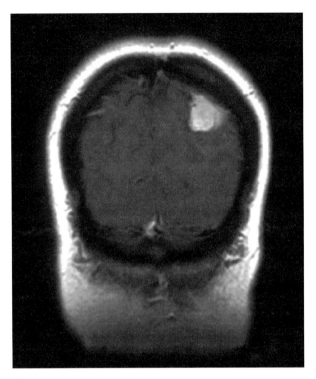

Figure 2
Hyperostosis of the skull commonly occurs adjacent to meningiomas.

When contrast material is given, they enhance homogeneously and brightly, demonstrating the absence of a blood–brain barrier in the extracranial circulation that supplies meningiomas (see Figs. 3 and 4). Their extraaxial location, enhancement pattern, and relationship to the dura usually allow the diagnosis to be made readily.

Special features may change the imaging characteristics in individual meningiomas; in approximately 15%, necrosis, cyst formation, or hemorrhage may be seen. Indistinct margins, marked peritumoral edema, mushroom-like projections from the tumor, invasion deep into the brain, and heterogeneous enhancement suggest aggressive behavior radiographically. However, malignant meningiomas cannot be distinguished absolutely from more benign forms by either CT or MRI. Edema, demonstrated by low signal intensity surrounding meningiomas, is a particularly interesting example of the relationship between molecular biology and clinical behavior. Kalkanis *et al.* demonstrated that the production of VEGF by a tumor correlates with the amount of surrounding edema. Provias *et al.* showed that VEGF production was related to new blood vessel formation. Thus, the edema occurs because of newly

formed "leaky" blood vessels, which are more prominent in some meningiomas than in others.

Because meningiomas are slow growing (Fig. 5) and occur in elderly patients, the decision about whether they should be treated is not always easy (Figs. 4 and 5). It is our belief that tumors that are symptomatic, demonstrably changing, have significant edema peritumoral edema, or are likely to become symptomatic during the next few years, deserve consideration of surgical resection. The decision must be made in conjunction with the patient's age, general medical condition, and personal preference. In general, it is often easier to remove a tumor when it is smaller and less symptomatic than when it is large and producing critical symptoms.

The interpretation of survival data following meningioma surgery is difficult because many meningioma patients are elderly. At 15 years, the survival rate is 63% for patients with meningiomas compared to 78% for patients of the same age without meningiomas; thus, a meningioma can shorten one's life expectancy. Surgical mortality in published series varies from 1 to 14%. Poor preoperative clinical condition, compressive symptoms from the tumor,

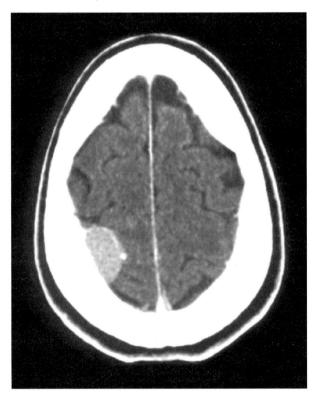

Figure 3
Meningiomas enhance brightly with contrast administration on CT and MRI scans, because of their vascularity.

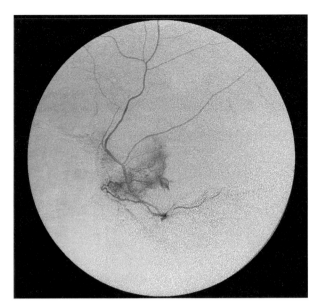

Figure 4
Meningiomas have a characteristic "blush" on angiogram due to their highly vascular nature; they most commonly fill from the middle meningeal artery, as does this one.

incomplete tumor removal, pulmonary embolism, and intracranial hematoma all increase mortality. Some studies have shown that surgery in patients older than age 70 has the same risk as surgery in patients younger than age 70.

Radiation therapy can be useful both as initial adjunctive treatment and as a treatment option for recurrent disease. For benign tumors, radiation appears to put cells into an apoptotic state; thus, the goal is not shrinkage of the tumor but cessation of growth. Conventional radiotherapy after subtotal resection may have a role in preventing or retarding tumor progression. External beam radiation therapy may offer substantial benefit in diminishing recurrence but may have unacceptable neurological side effects. The major problem with external beam radiation for meningiomas is the effect of radiation on the surrounding brain. To avoid this, there has been the increasing use of radiosurgery for treatment of recurrent or residual meningiomas. Newly developed conformal techniques, such as radiosurgery and stereotactic radiotherapy, greatly lessen the likelihood of injury to brain surrounding the tumor.

Because of the complications associated with single-dose radiosurgery, Brigham and Women's Hospital and the Joint Center for Radiation Therapy have developed a form of repeated stereotactic radiation using a relocatable frame. Designated stereotactic radiotherapy allows treatment of tumors adjacent to the optic nerves and brainstem, which is not feasible with single-dose radiosurgery. This procedure has now been used in more than 100 patients with meningiomas, using a 6-week course of daily therapy and avoiding the acute complications of radiosurgery. This may allow for the advantages of external beam radiation therapy without its risks.

Medical adjunctive therapy is still being investigated. Antiestrogen therapy is not effective for meningiomas, although antiprogesterone therapy may have a role. Grunberg *et al.* used RU486, a progesterone receptor antagonist, and found that one-third of recurrent meningiomas that were enlarging at the time of initial treatment diminished in size during treatment. This drug is currently being investigated in a cooperative multi-institutional study in the United States and Europe. Several studies have suggested that there may be a benefit to treatment with α-interferon or hydroxyurea.

Meningiomas are fascinating and important tumors whose understanding and management are changing significantly. New knowledge of their biology helps to explain the role of sex hormones, growth factors,

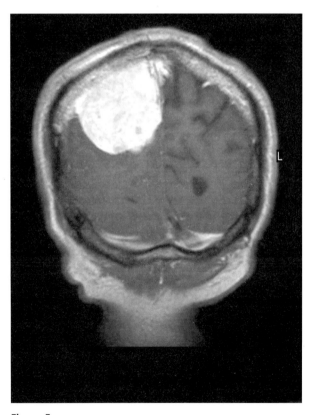

Figure 5
Meningiomas can grow to be quite large before becoming symptomatic, because of their slow rate of growth.

radiation, and chromosomal alterations in their pathogenesis. They express progesterone receptors and lose part of the long arm of chromosome 22; they also express PDGF, EGF, and VEGF and their receptors. The roles of both surgery and radiation have recently been clarified. It has been shown that surgery can be performed safely in the elderly patients in whom these tumors typically occur. Skull base surgery has become increasingly effective. Image-guided surgery may increase the likelihood of safe and complete resection, and the new intraoperative MRI scanners provide real-time assessment of the degree of resection. Radiation has been recognized as an important adjunct to surgery, especially as focal radiation in the form of stereotactic radiosurgery or stereotactic radiotherapy. Ongoing research ensures that our understanding of this tumor and its treatment will continue to increase exponentially.

—Stephanie Greene and Peter Black

See also–Acoustic Neuroma; Brain Tumors, Biology; Brain Tumors, Genetics; Central Nervous System Tumors; Childhood Brain Tumors; Glial Tumors; Nerve Sheath Tumors; Pituitary Tumors; Primary Central Nervous System Lymphoma and Germ Cell Tumors; Spinal Cord Tumors, Biology of

Further Reading

Black, P. M., Carroll, R., Glowacka, D., et al. (1994). Platelet-derived growth factor expression and stimulation in human meningiomas. J. Neurosurg. 81, 388–393.

Carroll, R. S., Glowacka, D., Dashner, K., et al. (1993). Progesterone receptor expression in meningiomas. Cancer Res. 53, 1312–1316.

Carroll, R. S., Black, P. M., Zhang, J. P., et al. (1997). Expression and activation of epidermal growth factor receptors in meningiomas. J. Neurosurg. 87, 315–323.

Grunberg, S. M., Weiss, M. H., Spitz, I. M., et al. (1991). Treatment of unresectable meningiomas with the antiprogesterone agent mifepristone. J. Neurosurg. 74, 861–866.

Hakim, R., Alexander, E., III, Loeffler, J. S., et al. (1998). Results of linear accelerator-based radiosurgery for intracranial meningiomas. Neurosurgery 42, 446–453.

Jaaskelainen, J., Haltia, M., and Servo, A. (1986). Atypical and anaplastic meningiomas: Radiology, surgery, radiotherapy and outcome. Surg. Neurol. 25, 233–244.

Jacoby, L. B., Pulaski, K., Rouleau, G., et al. (1990). Clonal analysis of human meningiomas: Radiology, surgery, radiotherapy, and outcome. Surg. Neurol. 25, 233–242.

Kalkanis, S. N., Carroll, R. S., Zhang, J. P., et al. (1996). Correlation of vascular endothelial growth factor messenger RNA expression with peritumoral vasogenic cerebral edema in meningiomas. J. Neurosurg. 85, 1095–1101.

Kleihues, P., and Cavenee, W. K. (Eds.) (1997). Pathology and Genetics of Tumours of the Nervous System. International Agency for Research on Cancer, Lyon, France.

Provias, I., Claffey, K., del Aguila, L., et al. (1997). Meningiomas: Role of vascular endothelial growth factor/vascular permeability factor in angiogenesis and peritumoral edema. Neurosurgery 40, 1016–1026.

Meningitis, Eosinophilic

Encyclopedia of the Neurological Sciences

PATIENTS with eosinophilic meningitis generally present with clinical signs indistinguishable from those of viral meningitis; 50% of patients will have headache, neck stiffness, nausea, and paresthesias. Eosinophilic meningitis is defined as clinical signs of meningitis associated with the presence of >10 eosinophils/μl cerebrospinal fluid (CSF) and/or ≥10% eosinophilia among CSF leukocytes.

ETIOLOGY AND EPIDEMIOLOGY

Although eosinophilic meningitis can occur under a variety of conditions, including parasitic and fungal infections, myeloproliferative diseases, and foreign bodies (Table 1), the most common cause is invasion of the central nervous system (CNS) by the rat lungworm, Angiostrongylus (Parastrongylus) cantonensis (Fig. 1). Discovered in rat lungs by Chen in Canton, China, in 1935, human infection has been reported from islands of the South Pacific, Hawaii, Australia, Malaysia, India, Indonesia, Papua New Guinea, Thailand, Guam, Vietnam, Madagascar, Reunion, Ivory Coast, Egypt, Puerto Rico, and Cuba. The April 2000 outbreak of eosinophilic meningitis among eight Chicago medical students on spring break in Jamaica has been demonstrated to be due to A. cantonensis.

Angiostrongylus cantonensis-infected rats have been identified in nonendemic locations from Southeast Asia to the Americas, apparently transported aboard intercontinental ships.

PARASITIC CAUSES OF EOSINOPHILIC MENINGITIS

The three most common parasitic causes of eosinophilic meningitis are A. cantonensis, Gnathostoma sphingerum, and Baylisascaris procyonis. Less common parasitic diseases described in case reports to cause CSF eosinophilia and occasional clinical signs of meningitis include cerebral and spinal schistosomiasis,

Table 1   CAUSES OF EOSINOPHILIC MENINGITIS

Parasitic etiologies
  Common
    Angiostrongylus cantonensis
    Gnathostoma spingerum
    Baylisascaris procyonis
  Less common
    Taenia solium (neurocysticercosis)
    Schistosomiasis (ectopic CNS/spinal)
    Paragonimiasis (ectopic CNS/spinal)
    Toxocariasis (migrating larvae)
    Strongyloidiasis (migrating larvae)
    Onchocerciasis
    Ascariasis (migrating larvae)
    Echinococcosis (ectopic CNS cysts)
    Trichinosis
    Fascioliasis
    Coenurosis (ectopic CNS cysts)
Nonparasitic infectious etiologies
  Coccidiomycosis
  Cryptococcosis (rare)
  Myiasis (ectopic CNS penetration)
  Rarely bacterial, rickettsial, or viral meningitis (usually low-
    level CSF eosinophilia)
  Meningeal tuberculosis (rare)
Drugs
  Antimicrobials—ciprofloxacin, cotrimoxazole, intraventricular
    gentamicin/vancomycin
  NSAIDS (ibuprofen)
  Contrast myelography
Myeloproliferative diseases
  Hypereosinophilic syndrome
  Hodgkin's disease
  Leukemia
  Lymphoma
  Disseminated glioblastoma
  Paraneoplastic syndrome associated with lung cancer
Foreign bodies
  Ventriculoperitoneal shunts
Miscellaneous conditions
  Sarcoidosis
  Eosinophilic granuloma
  Multiple sclerosis

neurocysticercosis, cerebral or spinal paragonimiasis, fascioliasis with ectopic CNS localization, migrating CNS ascaris, CNS strongyloidiasis, CNS echinococcus, migrating larvae of toxocara and trichinella, and onchocercus volvulus. CSF eosinophilic counts in these less common parasitic causes are usually lower than those seen in cases caused by the three most common parasites.

Angiostrongylus Eosinophilic Meningitis

There are 20 species of the nematode Angiostrongylus that infect animals, but only 3 species are believed to cause eosinophilic meningitis in humans: *A. cantonensis* (the most common cause), *A. malaysiensis*, and *A. mackerrasae*. Based on its morphology, *A. cantonensis* has recently been transferred to the genus *Parastrongylus*.

Pathogenesis: Adults of the rat lungworm *A. cantonensis* reside and lay their eggs in the pulmonary arteries of rats. After hatching, larvae migrate out of the respiratory tract and are swallowed to later pass out with feces. They develop into second- and third-stage larvae within their natural intermediate hosts, slugs and snails. Freshwater prawns, land crabs, and frogs have been found to harbor third-stage larvae as well, presumably as a result of eating the intermediate hosts. Sexually mature worms measure 20–35 mm.

Humans become infected by ingesting infected mollusks, including freshwater crabs and shrimp, and unwashed ground produce such as watercress or lettuces, where infected small slugs can be inadvertently eaten or contaminate produce with infected slime. Infection may be acquired by tourists or residents in endemic areas who consume snails as a delicacy.

Clinical Presentation: Larvae of *A. cantonensis* are neurotropic and clinical manifestations occur 2–35 days after ingestion. The disease usually presents as a transient meningitis with excruciating headache, neck stiffness, nausea, and vomiting. Severe peripheral parasthesias are frequent and may persist for

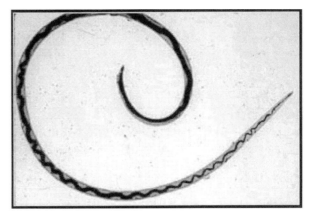

Figure 1
Angiostrongylus cantonesis adult female. Note the "barber pole" appearance of the dark red intestinal tract filled with blood and intertwined with the white genital tract (from http://www.medicine.cmu.ac.th/dept/parasite/official/nematode/AcAd1.htm).

weeks after other symptoms resolve. Cranial nerve involvement and visual disturbances also occur, whereas urinary retention, ataxia, and spinal cord lesions are very rare. Fever exceeds 38°C in 30% of patients. Other clinical findings are generalized weakness, optic neuropathy, periorbital edema, and unilateral facial paralysis.

Laboratory Diagnosis: Diagnosis is predominately based on the clinical presentation of CSF eosinophilia, exposure history, and the lack of focal lesions on computed tomography (CT) or magnetic resonance imaging (MRI). CSF examination reveals leukocyte counts that range from 20 to 5000 cells (usually 150–2000). CSF eosinophilia is usually in the range of 20–70%, with normal or minimally low glucose and slightly elevated CSF protein. Although the eosinophil's bilobed nucleus and prominent cytoplasmic granules may be distinguished from other leukocytes in an unstained CSF sample, a more reliable approach is examination of a centrifuged CSF preparation stained with Wright's solution or Giemsa stain to enumerate the number of eosinophils within the CSF. Larvae are rarely recovered from the CSF antemortem.

Serum and CSF immunodiagnosis (enzyme-linked immunosorbent assay) for Angiostrongylus has the greatest accuracy, and recent assays with monoclonal antibodies against CSF antigens appear even more promising. Large-scale sensitivity and specificity data have yet to be collated. Peripheral blood eosinophilia does not correlate with CSF eosinophilia and is usually slightly abnormal. Other parasitic eosinophilic meningitides, such as gnathostomiasis, neurocysticercosis, and baylisascaris, or other migrating larvae would cause an abnormal CT or MRI scan.

Management and Treatment: Because *A. cantonensis* cannot complete its life cycle in humans, larvae usually die within 1 or 2 weeks and most patients recover without sequelae. Nonsteroidal anti-inflammatory agents and occasionally narcotics are used for headache. Although steroids and repeated lumbar punctures have been used with some success in cases with increased intracranial pressure, no controlled studies have been performed. Thiabendazole, mebendazole, and ivermectin have been reported to kill migrating *A. cantonensis* larvae in infected rodents, but only rare, nonenthusiastic case reports of use in humans have been described. The *Medical Letter* cautions that using antiparasitic drugs can provoke neurological symptoms. One report described two patients in New Hebrides treated with thiabendazole; both patients became markedly more symptomatic with treatment. Several other studies have shown no appreciable clinical improvement with its use. Surgical removal of larvae is recommended for patients with ocular involvement.

Gnathostomiasis

Gnathostomiasis is caused by the migration of larvae of *Gnathostoma spinigerum*. The disease is endemic in Southeast Asia, parts of China, and Japan, and it occurs sporadically in Europe, Africa, the Middle East, and the Americas. *Gnathostoma spinigerum* larvae are not neurotropic and clinical symptoms are caused by the migration of larvae into cutaneous, visceral, ocular, and neural tissue. Adult *G. spinerum* worms are gastrointestinal parasites of domestic wild dogs and cats. Eggs passed in canine or feline feces hatch in water to release first-stage larvae, which are then ingested by the Cyclops water flea. The infected Cyclops flea is in turn ingested by fish, frogs, eels, snakes, chickens, and ducks. Humans acquire infection by eating raw or undercooked fish, poultry, frogs, or reptiles.

Clinical Symptoms: Larvae penetration into the CNS is usually through migration along neural roots. Thus, radicular pain and paresthesias occur prior to headache. Paralysis of extremities and cranial nerves is common, along with an acute meningoencephalitis. Severe tissue destruction can result in acute cerebral hemorrhages.

Diagnosis: CSF examination usually reveals an eosinophilic pleocytosis with elevated protein and normal glucose levels. CT examinations reveal areas of hemorrhage. Peripheral blood eosinophilia is more striking than that which occurs with angiostrongyliasis. Serological tests have been developed but are difficult to obtain outside of endemic areas.

Management: Supportive care and corticosteroids are the mainstay of treatment. Adequate preparation (cooking) of fish and poultry prevents primary disease.

Baylisacariasis

Baylisacaris procyonis has rarely been a cause of meningoencephalitis in the United States, although the high prevalence of infected raccoons and their ever-increasing proximity to people in many suburban areas may provide increased opportunity for human infection to occur. *Baylisacaris procyonis* is an ascaris of raccoons and is shed in their feces.

The larvae are neurotropic and rare cases of eosinophilic meningoencephalitis have been described in the United States. Definitive diagnosis requires morphologic examination of larvae, but clinical features of an eosinophilic meningoencephalitis in a child with pica and exposure to raccoon-contaminated soil are highly suggestive of the diagnosis.

RARE PARASITIC CAUSES OF EOSINOPHILIC MENINGITIS

Occasionally, ectopic eggs or larvae of other parasites can cause an eosinophilic pleocytosis, although usually without a frank clinical meningitis. These include schistosomiasis, toxocariasis, trichinosis, neurocysticercosis, cerebral paragonimiasis, ascariasis, echinococcosis, strongyloidiasis, onchocerciasis, and fascioliasis. Either spinal or cerebral migration of larvae can cause the eosinophilic pleocytosis.

NONPARASITIC INFECTIOUS ETIOLOGIES OF EOSINOPHILIC MENINGITIS

The one fungal infection associated with striking CSF eosinophilia when it disseminates to the CNS is coccidiomycosis. CSF eosinophilia has been described for CNS and, rarely, viral, bacterial, and rickettsial diseases, but not to the levels seen with angiostrongyliasis or gnathostomiasis.

MYELOPROLIFERATIVE AND NEOPLASTIC ETIOLOGIES OF EOSINOPHILIC MENINGITIS

Eosinophilic meningitis has been described with such myeloproliferative diseases as Hodgkin's disease, leukemia, carcinomatous meningitis, and non-Hodgkin's lymphoma. Case reports of disseminated glioblastoma and paraneoplastic syndromes secondary to bronchogenic carcinoma have been associated with a CSF eosinophilic pleocytosis. Idiopathic hypereosinophilic syndrome may have CNS infiltration with eosinophils. Patients always have a striking peripheral eosinophilia, often higher than 1500/μl, concomitant with the meningitis.

OTHER NONINFECTIOUS CAUSES OF EOSINOPHILIC MENINGITIS

A variety of other noninfectious causes have been known to trigger eosinophilic meningitis. Foreign bodies in the CSF, particularly ventriculoperitoneal (VP) shunts, have caused eosinophilic meningitis. In one study of children with VP shunts, 30% had ≥8% CSF eosinophilia. Case reports of eosinophilic meningitis have been described with nonsteroidal agents such as ibuprofen, antibiotics (especially intraventricular antibiotics), and myelography contrast agents. Miscellaneous conditions, such as CNS sarcoidosis, multiple sclerosis, and eosinophilic granuloma, have also been described to present with CSF eosinophilia.

SUMMARY

Although a variety of parasitic, fungal, neoplastic, and noninfectious conditions can cause eosinophilic meningitis, the predominant infectious agents are three parasites that have migrating CNS invasive larvae: *A. cantonensis*, *G. spiningerum*, and *B. procyonis*. When CSF eosinophilia is discovered, a thorough epidemiological history is the physician's best tool for etiological diagnosis because the collection and identification of live larvae from CSF is unusual.

—*Michele Barry and Wendy Thanassi*

See also–Bacterial Meningitis; Fungal Meningitis; Meningitis, Viral; Parasites and Neurological Diseases, Overview; Tropical Neurology

Further Reading

Bia, F., and Barry, M. (1986). Parasitic infections of the central nervous system. *Neurol. Clin.* **4**, 171–206.
Epi Update (2000, May 10). Eosinophilic meningitis, CDC confirmed—USA (Chicago). http://www.doh.state.fl.us.
Fuller, A., Munckhoff, W., Kiers, L., *et al.* (1993). Eosinophilic meningitis due to *Angiostrongylus cantonensis*. *West. J. Med.* **159**, 78–80.
Klikas, M., Kroenke, K., and Hardman, J. (1982). Eosinophilic radiculomyeloencephalitis: An angiostrongyliasis outbreak in American Samoa related to the ingestion of *Achatina fulica* snails. *Am. J. Trop. Med. Hyg.* **31**, 1114–1122.
Koo, J., Pien, F., and Kliks, M. (1988). *Angiostrongylus* (*Parastrongylus*) eosinophilic meningitis. *Rev. Infect. Dis.* **10**, 1155–1162.
Medical Letter (2000, March). Drugs for parasitic infections. Medical Letter, New Rochelle, NY.
Weller, P. (1993). Eosinophilic meningitis. *Am. J. Med.* **95**, 250–253.
Wilson, M., and Weller, P. (1999). Eosinophilia. In *Tropical Infectious Diseases Principles, Pathogens and Practice* (R. Guerrant and P. Weller, Eds.), pp. 1400–1419. Churchill Livingstone, London.

Meningitis, Viral

Encyclopedia of the Neurological Sciences

THE CONCEPT that agents other than bacteria can invade the central nervous system began with the emergence of poliomyelitis as an epidemic infection and, subsequently, the realization that similar meningeal inflammation and cerebrospinal fluid (CSF) pleocytosis occurred in some patients during mumps parotitis. That meningitis could be caused by other "filterable agents" (i.e., viruses) was demonstrated by Rivers and Scot, who in 1935 recovered lymphocytic choriomeningitis virus from the CSF of an affected patient. It is now known that a wide variety of viral agents may invade the central nervous system to produce meningitis or encephalitis.

Viral meningitis is important in three regards. First, viral meningitis must be differentiated from the much more dangerous condition, bacterial meningitis: Until this is accomplished, patients presenting with signs and symptoms of meningitis must be considered medical emergencies, and antibiotic treatment for presumptive meningitis must be instituted if there is serious question of bacterial rather than viral infection. Second, viral meningitis, although rarely fatal, may produce clinical impairment that may persist from weeks to months. Finally, "lymphocytic" or "aseptic" meningitis may be caused by agents other than viruses, and the possibility of other, more readily treated (and sometimes more dangerous) conditions must be kept in mind when diagnosing a patient with presumed viral meningitis.

PATHOGENESIS

Before meningitis can occur, the causative agent must first penetrate the body from the external environment and then gain entry to the nervous system across the blood–brain barrier. Initial entry of the virus into the host may occur by gastrointestinal inoculation (as is the case with the enteroviruses), cutaneous inoculation (as occurs with the arthropod-borne agents), the respiratory route (as is the case with mumps), or transmucosal penetration or intravenous inoculation (as occurs with HIV). Early workers in the field of viral central nervous system (CNS) infections believed that invasion of the nervous system occurred by spread of viruses within neurons. Currently, however, it is known that the majority of viral meningitides result from hematogenous dissemination of virus following symptomatic or clinically inapparent systemic infection. Penetration across the blood–brain barrier may occur at the choroid plexus or through meningeal capillaries. Exceptions to this are unusual but include meningitis following genital herpes simplex infection, meningitis associated with herpes zoster, and Mollaret's meningitis, in which reactivated infection of herpes simplex virus type 2 within dorsal root ganglia leads to repeated episodes of meningitis. Replication of viruses in cells of the meninges, superficial brain or spinal cord parenchyma, and the ventricular system elicits an inflammatory response, which is predominantly lymphocytic, and results in alteration of the blood–brain barrier so that protein levels increase within CSF. Unlike bacteria or fungi, however, replication of viruses does not consume glucose within CSF, nor does it usually result in altered transport of glucose across the blood–brain barrier. Thus, in contrast to bacterial, mycobacterial, or fungal infections, CSF glucose concentrations in viral meningitis are usually normal.

EPIDEMIOLOGY

Meningitis is the most common CNS infection caused by viruses, and viral meningitis is a far more common condition than bacterial or fungal meningitis. Approximately 10,000–15,000 cases of lymphocytic or presumed viral meningitis are reported each year, with an incidence of 5–10 cases per 100,000 individuals. Unreported cases, however, may be as much as 10-fold higher. CSF pleocytosis has also been reported in random individuals infected with measles, mumps, and HIV, and similar asymptomatic CNS involvement probably occurs with other viral agents as well. Although viral meningitis may affect all age groups, it is predominantly a disease of childhood.

The agents causing viral meningitis can be divided into three broad groups: common agents of viral meningitis, including the enteroviruses, arthropod-borne agents, and herpesvirus type 2; less common agents, including HIV, mumps, lymphocytic choriomeningitis virus, and human herpesvirus 6 and parvovirus B19; and agents known to cause lymphocytic meningitis only in rare cases. In addition, a number of nonviral, and occasionally noninfectious, conditions may present with CSF findings indistinguishable from those of viral meningitis.

Major Agents Causing Viral Meningitis

Enteroviruses: Enteroviruses account for approximately 90% of cases in which the causative virus is

Table 1   VIRUSES CAUSING MENINGITIS

Major causes of viral meningitis
   Enteroviruses (coxsackie and echoviruses)
   Arboviruses
   Herpes simplex virus type 2
   Human immunodeficiency virus
Less common causes of viral meningitis
   Herpes simplex virus type 1
   Epstein–Barr virus
   Mumps virus (rare in Western countries; common in
   underdeveloped countries)
   Lymphocytic choriomeningitis virus
   Parvovirus B19
Rare causes of viral meningitis
   Varicella-zoster virus (usually in the setting of cutaneous zoster)
   Influenza A and B viruses
   Parainfluenza viruses
   Rotaviruses
   Cat scratch fever virus
   Measles virus
   Coronaviruses
   Adenoviruses

identified (Table 1). Enteroviruses are small, unenveloped single-stranded RNA viruses within the family Picornaviridae. Although more than 70 serotypes of enteroviruses have been identified, coxsackievirus A9 and echoviruses E7, E9, E11, E19, and E30 account for 70% of all cultured isolates of CSF. Polioviruses, although not associated with viral meningitis in developed countries, still cause aseptic meningitis in underdeveloped countries as well as paralytic disease. Enteroviruses are disseminated by fecal–oral spread, and cases in developed countries tend to cluster during summer months when conditions of sanitation tend to be most relaxed. Recent studies employing polymerase chain reaction methods, however, confirm older observations that enteroviral CNS infections occur throughout the year, and many previously undiagnosed cases of viral meningitis

occurring during winter months are also caused by these agents. Coxsackieviruses and echoviruses may cause encephalitis and, rarely, paralytic disease.

Arthropod-Borne Agents: Arthropod-borne viruses, or arboviruses, include agents from several different families that are not human viruses but rather agents of small mammals or birds and are spread to human hosts through the bite of an arthropod vector (Table 2). Although these agents are most commonly considered to cause encephalitis, all of them, with the exception of Eastern equine encephalitis, more frequently cause an illness in which meningitis symptoms predominate. The most common arthropod-borne agents associated with viral meningitis include St. Louis encephalitis virus, the California/LaCrosse group of viruses, Colorado tick fever, and, as an emerging pathogen, West Nile virus. These agents, like enteroviruses, have a peak incidence in summer and early fall. The exception to this rule is Colorado tick fever, which is more frequently transmitted in the spring and early summer.

Herpesviruses: Herpesviridae are enveloped, double-stranded DNA viruses. Herpes simplex virus types 1 and 2, varicella-zoster virus, Epstein–Barr virus, cytomegalovirus, and human herpesvirus 6 have all been recovered from cases of viral meningitis. Of these, however, only herpes simplex virus has been associated with significant numbers of cases. Older data suggest that herpes simplex virus type 2 accounts for 2 or 3% of cases of viral meningitis. Recent work employing polymerase chain reaction methods suggests that it may be the most common cause of viral meningitis in adult women. Herpes simplex type 2 most often causes meningitis following primary genital infection. Occasional cases may also follow primary genital infection with herpes simplex virus type 1; nonprimary genital infection with either serotype only rarely causes disease. CSF

Table 2   ARBOVIRAL AGENTS ASSOCIATED WITH MENINGITIS IN THE UNITED STATES

Family	Genus	Virology	Agents	Vector	Seasonal incidence
Togaviridae	Alphaviruses	Single-stranded positive sense RNA	Western equine encephalitis	Mosquito	Summer, early autumn
	Flaviviruses	Single-stranded positive sense RNA	St. Louis encephalitis	Mosquito	Summer, early autumn
			West Nile virus	Mosquito	
Bunyaviridae	Bunyavirus	Single-stranded negative sense RNA	California/LaCrosse encephalitis virus	Mosquito	Summer, early autumn
Reoviridae	Orbivirus	Double-stranded RNA	Colorado tick fever	Tick	Spring, early summer

pleocytosis occurs during both chicken pox and herpes zoster with or without skin lesions; this pleocytosis is usually asymptomatic but may occasionally be associated with meningitic symptoms.

HIV: HIV has been associated with both acute and persistent lymphocytic meningitis. Onset is most commonly at the time of seroconversion. The course may be uniphasic, chronic, or, occasionally, recurrent. HIV RNA can be identified in CSF using reverse transcriptase-polymerase chain reaction (RT-PCR) methods, which also allow assessment of viral burden. It must be kept in mind, however, that most patients with HIV will experience viral invasion of the CNS, and meningitis, even in the presence of known HIV infection, may be due to other bacterial, viral, or fungal agents.

Less Frequent Causes of Viral Meningitis

Other Herpesviruses: As discussed previously, herpes simplex virus type 1, human herpesvirus 6, varicella-zoster virus, cytomegalovirus, and Epstein–Barr virus may occasionally cause meningitis.

Mumps Virus: Mumps virus, like measles virus, is a paramyxovirus, containing a single-stranded RNA genome. Prior to the advent of mumps vaccine, mumps was the second most common cause of viral meningoencephalitis, accounting for more than 15% of isolates. Currently, mumps virus meningitis is rare in developed countries, as is mumps encephalitis due to vaccinations. The virus is still a common cause of CNS infection in underdeveloped countries, where it also is an important cause of virus-induced deafness. In experimental animals infected *in utero*, mumps can cause aqueductal stenosis. Infected ependymal cells can be detected in human CSF during mumps encephalitis, and rare cases of mumps encephalitis have been complicated by aqueductal stenosis.

Lymphocytic Choriomeningitis Virus: Lymphocytic choriomeningitis virus (LCMV) is an arenavirus containing single-stranded RNA. Like arthropod-borne agents, LCMV is not a human virus but is a virus of wild and laboratory mice. LCMV is associated with human cases of meningoencephalitis as a consequence of exposure to laboratory or wild mice and in rare epidemics it is associated with pet hamsters. Cases tend to be more common under conditions of impoverished living and poor hygiene. Only approximately 15% of infected individuals develop meningitis. LCMV meningitis typically occurs during autumn and early winter, and it has been suggested that this reflects more extensive mouse–human contact as mice move inside to escape winter weather. In studies prior to 1960, the virus was thought to account for 9–11% of cases of viral meningitis. In recent years, reports of meningitis due to LCMV have been rare. However, congenital LCMV infection is a significant, often unrecognized cause of chorioretinitis, hydrocephalus, microcephaly or macrocephaly, and mental retardation. Acquired LCMV infection likewise may be an underappreciated illness. The meningitis caused by LCMV may be extremely persistent and has been associated with symptoms and CSF abnormalities lasting months. Acquired LCMV infection may also be associated with encephalitis, transverse myelitis, a Guillain–Barré-type syndrome, and both transient and permanent acquired hydrocephalus.

Parvovirus B19: Parvovirus B19 most commonly causes an acute febrile illness, accompanied by erythema infectiosum. The virus can also produce meningitis and meningoencephalitis in both immunocompetent and immunocompromised patients. The combination of rash and signs of meningeal irritation may mimic acute meningococcal infection. CSF findings, however, are typical of viral infection. Occasionally, CSF may be normal.

Rare Causes of Viral Meningitis

Rare causes of viral meningitis include influenza A and B viruses, parainfluenza viruses, rotaviruses, cat scratch fever virus, coronaviruses, measles virus, and adenoviruses, although this last group of agents more commonly cause encephalitis.

CLINICAL SYMPTOMS AND SIGNS

Onset of viral meningitis may occur following a symptomatic, systemic illness or as an isolated event following inapparent systemic infection. Patients present with headache, photophobia, and, in many instances, symptomatic neck stiffness or back pain. Significant alteration of consciousness is far less common than in bacterial meningitis but does occasionally occur. Seizures or focal neurological signs are unusual and raise concerns about concomitant viral encephalitis or infection due to some other process, such as brain abscess. Patients are usually uncomfortable but do not appear severely ill. Physical examination may reveal evidence of systemic illness, including rash, lymphadenopathy, pharyngitis, or splenomegaly, depending on the infectious agent. Neurological examination will reveal nuchal rigidity. The patient may be unable to touch chin to chest. Resistance to passive neck flexion and Kernig's and/or Brudzinski's signs may be present but are inconsistent, and both signs may be absent in milder cases. A useful test of nuchal rigidity is to ask the patient to touch forehead to knee; this will often be positive when all other tests of meningeal irritation are questionable or absent. Papilledema is rare. Focal neurological signs are unusual and raise concerns about more serious infections, including viral encephalitis and brain abscess. Routine blood studies may reveal a lymphocytic pleocytosis. Liver function tests may be elevated if there is hepatic involvement.

LABORATORY DIAGNOSIS OF VIRAL MENINGITIS

The most important diagnostic test in viral meningitis is lumbar puncture. This should be preceded by head magnetic resonance imaging or, less optimally, computed tomography if focal signs are present or if there is any suspicion of increased intracranial pressure. Spinal fluid will usually show mildly elevated opening pressure, lymphocytic pleocytosis, elevated protein, and normal glucose (Table 3). A mononuclear pleocytosis is seen in the majority of cases, and the cell count is usually less than 300 cells/ mm^3. Protein is usually in the range of 50–100 mg/dl. Exceptions exist to this CSF formula, however. Cell count may be as high as 1000 cells/mm^3. During the first 24–48 hr of infection, CSF may contain a mixture of polymorphonuclear leukocytes and lymphocytes. Recent studies suggest that the persistence of neutrophils in CSF during viral meningitis may be more prolonged than previous appreciated. Glucose concentrations, although usually >50% of blood values, may be significantly depressed: This has been reported with meningitis due to herpes zoster, mumps, and lymphocytic choriomeningitis virus. Return of CSF to normal may be extremely prolonged following viral meningitis, and isolated reports have described persistent CSF pleocytosis and elevated protein over periods of weeks to months.

Prior to the advent of PCR, diagnosis of viral meningitis was difficult and often an exercise in futility: viruses may take considerable time to grow in culture, and many viral agents cannot be readily grown from CSF. Viral serologies comparing acute and convalescent sera have been used for retrospective diagnosis, and serological diagnosis can be accelerated by comparing serum and CSF antibody titers to identify synthesis of specific antiviral antibody within the nervous system; however, serological tests only rarely allow rapid enough diagnosis to direct therapy.

The advent of PCR methods has revolutionized the diagnosis of both meningitis and encephalitis. PCR diagnostic methods for enteroviruses and HIV are readily available in many laboratories, and PCR diagnosis of other agents is often available through larger commercial laboratories or the Centers for Disease Control. In the case of HIV, RT-PCR methods are available not only for diagnosis infection but also for determining viral load. Additional PCR tests for viral agents continue to be described. Even with the use of PCR, the causative agents in many cases of viral meningitis remain undiagnosed.

Table 3 CSF FINDINGS IN BACTERIAL, VIRAL, TUBERCULOUS, AND FUNGAL MENINGITIS

	Bacterial meningitis	Viral meningitis	Tuberculous meningitis	Fungal meningitis
Protein	Elevated	Mildly elevated	Elevated	Elevated
Glucose	<50% blood glucose	Normal[a]	<50% blood glucose	<50% blood glucose
Cells	Polys	Lymphs or lymphs + polys[b]	Lymphs + polys	Lymphs
Other	Gram stain, culture[c]	PCR (viral culture)	AFB stain culture (20 ml CSF) PCR	India ink prep cryptococcal Ag culture (20 ml CSF) PCR

[a] CSF glucose may occasionally be depressed in meningitis due to mumps, lymphocytic choriomeningitis virus, or herpes zoster.

[b] CSF during the first 24 hr of viral meningitis may contain a mixture of lymphocytes and polymorphonuclear leukocytes. In these cases, in contrast to bacterial meningitis, CSF glucose is usually normal and follow-up lumbar puncture 24 hr later will often but not always show lymphocytes only.

[c] Positive Gram's stain requires approximately 10^5 colony-forming untis (CFU)/ml of CSF. Approximately 25% of Gram's stains will be positive if CSF contains 10^3 CFU/m. Prior antibiotic treatment will reduce this amount by 20%.

OTHER CAUSES OF LYMPHOCYTIC MENINGITIS

Viral meningitis should be considered in the differential diagnosis of any patient presenting with headache, photophobia, and neck stiffness. However, the presence of these findings also makes it mandatory to exclude bacterial infection. Although patients with viral meningitis are less severely ill than those with bacterial meningitis, bacterial meningitis may also appear mild in its early stages. Furthermore, antibiotic therapy in bacterial meningitis may sometimes cause a shift in CSF cells from polymorphonuclear leukocytes to lymphocytes.

Many other conditions may also cause a lymphocyte meningitis, in which CSF findings may be similar to those seen in viral infections. These include *Mycobacterium tuberculosis*, Lyme disease, infections due to Ehrlichiae or, rarely, other Rickettsial agents, *Mycoplasma pneumoniae*, and fungi (particularly *Cryptococcus neoformans* and, rarely, *Toxoplasma gondii*). Tuberculous and fungal meningitis are often, but not always, accompanied by a significant decrease in CSF glucose. Lyme meningitis may produce CSF findings identical to those seen in viral meningitis. However, papilledema, erythema migrans, and cranial neuropathies are common features of Lyme meningitis, whereas they are distinctly unusual in viral meningitis. Similarly, patients with Lyme meningitis tend to have fewer white blood cells (mean, 80 vs 301/mm^3) and a significantly greater percentage of mononuclear cells than patients with viral meningitis. Both *M. tuberculosis* and *Mycoplasma pneumoniae* are difficult to culture but are readily detectable by PCR; PCR tests for Ehrlichiae are in limited use but may not be available in all hospital laboratories. Aseptic meningitis may also occur as a complication of therapy with a number of agents, including nonsteroidal antiinflammatory drugs, carbamazepine, and trimethoprim sulfamethoxazole. Patients with recurrent (Mollaret's) meningitis often have recurrent infection due to herpes simplex type 2. However, a very similar picture can be seen in patients in whom there is period leakage from dermoid or epidermoid cysts abutting the meninges. In such patients, the diagnosis may be made by careful MRI examination of brain and spinal cord. In cases of suspected viral meningitis, CSF should always be sent for bacterial culture, with inclusion of tests for other agents if clinically indicated.

TREATMENT

Most cases of viral meningitis are self-limited, and antiviral chemotherapy is usually not indicated. Controlled studies of antiviral agents in viral meningitis have not been reported in detail. Recent data from controlled studies presented in abstract form, however, suggest that virological and clinical improvement are better in patients with severe enteroviral meningoencephalitis treated with the antiviral agent pleconaril than with placebo. Similarly, depending on the severity of illness, consideration should be given to therapy of herpes simplex meningitis with acyclovir or similar agents. Use of antiviral agents in viral meningitis is still essentially experimental and must be balanced against the severity of disease and complications of the therapy. An exception to this is HIV meningitis, in which diagnosis of HIV infection is in itself an indication for highly active antiretroviral therapy.

PROGNOSIS

Viral meningitis is almost always a self-limited disease. Recovery may occur within days. However, symptomatic illness is not infrequently prolonged, and patients may require weeks or months to return to full health. Permanent neurological deficits or intellectual impairment are rare.

—*John E. Greenlee*

***See also*—Bacterial Meningitis; Central Nervous System Infections, Overview; Encephalitis, Viral; Enteroviruses; Fungal Meningitis; Human Herpes Viruses; Lymphocytic Choriomeningitis Virus (LCMV); Measles Virus, Central Nervous System Complications of; Meningitis, Eosinophilic**

Further Reading

Adair, C. V., Gauld, R. L., and Smadel, J. E. (1953). Aseptic meningitis, a disease of diverse etiology: Clinical and etiologic studies on 854 cases. *Ann. Intern. Med.* **39,** 675–704.
Barton, L. L., and Hyndman, N. J. (2001). Lymphocytic choriomeningitis virus: Reemerging central nervous system pathogen. *Pediatrics* **105,** E35.
Greenlee, J. E., and Carroll, K. (1997). Cerebrospinal fluid in central nervous system infections. In *Infections of the Central Nervous System* (W. M. Scheld, R. J. Whitley, and D. T. Durack, Eds.), 2nd ed., pp. 899–922. Raven Press, New York.
Henquell, C., Chambon, M., Bailly, J. L., *et al.* (2001). Prospective analysis of 61 cases of enteroviral meningitis: Interest of systematic genome detection in cerebrospinal fluid irrespective of cytologic examination results. *J. Clin. Virol.* **21,** 29–35.

Jahrlin, P. B., and Peters, C. J. (1992). Lymphocytic choriomeningitis virus: A neglected pathogen of man. *Arch. Pathol. Lab. Med.* **116**, 486–488.

Johnson, R. T. (1998). *Viral Infections of the Nervous System*, 2nd ed. Lippincott–Raven, Philadelphia.

Najioullah, F., Bosshard, S., Thouvenot, D., *et al.* (2001). Diagnosis and surveillance of herpes simplex virus infection of the central nervous system. *J. Med. Virol.* **61**, 468–473.

Nash, D., Mostashari, F., Fine, A., *et al.* (2001). The outbreak of West Nile virus infection in the New York City area in 1999. *N. Engl. J. Med.* **334**, 1807–1814.

Negrini, B., Kelleher, K. J., and Wald, E. R. (2001). Cerebrospinal fluid findings in aseptic versus bacterial meningitis. *Pediatrics* **105**, 316–319.

Read, S. J., and Kurtz, J. B. (1999). Laboratory diagnosis of common viral infections of the central nervous system by using a single multiplex PCR screening assay. *J. Clin. Microbiol.* **37**, 1352–1355.

Rotbart, H. A. (2000). Viral meningitis. *Semin. Neurol.* **20**, 277–292.

Rotbart, H. A., and Webster, A. D. (2001). Treatment of potentially life-threatening enterovirus infections with pleconaril. *Clin. Infect. Dis.* **32**, 228–235.

Rotbart, H. A., McCracken, G. H., Jr., Whitley, R. J., *et al.* (1999). Clinical significance of enteroviruses in serious summer febrile illnesses of children. *Pediatr. Infect. Dis. J.* **18**, 869–874.

Tabak, F., Mert, A., Ozturk, R., *et al.* (1999). Prolonged fever caused by parvovirus B19-induced meningitis: Case report and review. *Clin. Infect. Dis.* **29**, 446–447.

Menkes' Disease

Encyclopedia of the Neurological Sciences

MENKES' DISEASE is a neurodegenerative and connective tissue disorder, inherited as an X-linked recessive trait, that was first described by Menkes in 1962. In the subsequent decade, the disorder was shown by Danks and colleagues to involve defective copper homeostasis with a copper-deficiency phenotype due to failure of copper absorption from the small intestine. At the cellular level, defective cellular copper export causes trapping of copper in some cell types (e.g., intestinal mucosa and kidney tubule), leading to systemic copper insufficiency and failure of copper delivery to tissues such as the central nervous system. The disorder was recently shown to be due to mutations in a gene encoding a copper-transporting P-type ATPase, ATP7A or MNK. The MNK transporter appears to function ubiquitously in the mediation of intracellular translocation and cellular efflux of copper in multiple cell types.

CLINICAL FEATURES

Classic and lethal Menkes' disease (estimated incidence 1/90,000 to 1/254,000 live births) presents in the immediate newborn period or in early infancy with nonspecific neurological manifestations, such as lethargy, poor feeding, failure to thrive, and twitching. Myoclonic seizures and hypothermia are frequent. There are various degrees of spasticity, with limited spontaneous movement. At least two severe cases have been described with neonatal cutis laxa. Growth may be retarded and development is generally severely delayed; death occurs in early childhood.

There is a facial resemblance (described as "pudgy" or "cherubic") among patients due in part to the distinct craniofacial configuration, decreased facial movements, and abnormalities of the hair (steely depigmented hair) that may be observed in the newborn period. The disorder was formerly known as kinky hair disease or steely hair disease. The hair is fragile and frequently broken; pili torti is seen on microscopic examination. Seborrheic dermatitis can be a persistent skin manifestation.

Central nervous system features include demyelination, reactive gliosis, and neuron loss in the cerebral hemispheres, the cerebellum, and the spinocerebellar tracts. Magnetic resonance angiography (MRA) brain scan shows intracranial vascular tortuosity as well as decreased cortical mass, white matter atrophy, and ventricular dilatation. Central nervous system manifestations in Menkes' disease include not only neurodegenerative changes of a diffuse and unspecified nature but also selective defects that may be of developmental origin. These include abnormal dendritic arborization of pyramidal neurons, primary cellular degeneration in the thalamus, and reduced number and abnormal dendritic arborization of Purkinje cells. The developmental nature of these defects, the early onset of central nervous system disease, and the distinct craniofacial configuration of severely affected hemizygotes suggest that Menkes' disease must be considered in part a malformation syndrome of prenatal onset.

Skeletal and connective tissue changes include wormian bones in the lambdoid and sagittal sutures (present in the newborn period), flaring or cupping of the anterior ribs, and lateral or medial spur formation of the proximal and distal femoral and humeral metaphyses (present by age 2 months). Osteoporosis can be seen after age 6 months. There is tortuosity, narrowing, and dilatation of cerebral, visceral, and limb arteries related to intimal hyperplasia, fragmentation, and beading of elastic tissue. Lobular bladder diverticuli are found in some patients.

Patients with less severe or atypical manifestations have shown a milder phenotype in general, with later onset of symptoms and a less severe clinical course. As such, Menkes' disease must be considered a disorder of varied severity, with implications for clinical evaluation of children with psychomotor retardation of unknown etiology.

A specific variant of mild Menkes' disease is the occipital horn syndrome, previously called X-linked cutis laxa. Documentation of abnormal copper metabolism and definitive molecular genetic analyses have confirmed that the occipital horn syndrome is a distinct allelic variant of Menkes' disease and presents as a connective tissue disorder caused by a secondary deficiency of the cuproenzyme, lysyl oxidase. The syndrome is characterized by hyperelastic and bruisable skin, bladder diverticulae, varicosities, hypermobile joints, and multiple skeletal abnormalities (short and broad clavicles, fused carpal bones, thoracic malformations, and bony exostoses of the occiput). The occipital horn syndrome is sometimes accompanies by mild neurological impairment, in contrast to the severe neurological degeneration of Menkes' disease.

As with other X-linked recessive disorders, genetic counseling and medical practice are often experientially based on a presumption of the benign nature of heterozygosity. However, it is reasonable to consider that a fraction of heterozygotes may exhibit connective tissue or central nervous system manifestations in varying degrees, dependent on the severity of mutation, skewing of lyonization, or other disease mechanisms. Such patients may undergo diverse medical interventions without a diagnosis or with an incorrect diagnosis. In particular, female heterozygotes may show some measure of mild impairment on cognitive testing or neurological examination or both. Subtle and patchy skin or skeletal abnormalities may be present, and in a recent study heterozygotes showed vessel tortuosity or premature volume loss or both on MRA brain scans. Therefore, it appears that there is a finite risk of clinically significant manifestations in carriers of severe Menkes' disease mutations. Such possibilities should be considered in diagnostic protocols, genetic counseling, and in making decisions on whether treatment may be indicated for some heterozygotes.

BASIC DEFECT

In patients with Menkes' disease, oral copper is poorly absorbed and there is abnormal distribution of body copper. For example, low levels are found in plasma, liver, and brain, whereas excessive accumulation has been documented in other tissues, such as intestinal mucosa, kidney, and placenta. Measurements of cuproenzyme activities in tissues of patients with Menkes' disease have confirmed reduced specific activities, and it is therefore reasonable to ascribe many of the clinical manifestations to deficiencies of cuproenzymes in multiple tissues. Deficiencies in the function of cuproenzymes such as cytochrome c oxidase (mitochondrial respiratory chain), superoxide dismutase (free radical eradication), and dopamine-β-hydroxylase (synthesis of catecholamines and neurological development) may be implicated in the pathogenesis of neurological manifestations.

Based on studies in cell culture, defective copper efflux from cells, with cellular copper accumulation, is the basic cellular phenotype. Under this construction, copper would be taken up by intestinal mucosal (or renal tubular) cells but not released across the serosal membrane, thereby causing systemic copper insufficiency, reduced cuproenzyme activities, and Menkes' disease.

The Menkes' gene, designated as MNK or ATP7A, is expressed in all tissues except liver, a pattern consistent with a housekeeping role for this P-type ATPase in cell copper homeostasis and with the Menkes' disease phenotype. The MNK protein is localized in the membrane of the trans-Golgi network and cycles between the trans-Golgi and plasma membrane localizations in response to basal conditions or conditions of copper excess, respectively. The MNK protein contains specific motifs that govern trafficking of the protein to the trans-Golgi network and retrieval from the plasma membrane. Therefore, copper dyshomeostasis and disease can result not only from mutations that abolish the transport function of MNK but also from mutations leading to incorrect intracellular localization.

Diverse mutations of the MNK gene have been described in severe Menkes' disease, and all are predicted to result in severe impairment of the expression, structure, or function of the protein. Approximately 20–40% of patients with severe Menkes' disease have partial nonoverlapping deletions or deletion/insertions. Additional mutations are unique for each family and include nonsense, missense, and splice-site mutations and small deletions or insertions. Analyses in patients with milder disease, especially those with the occipital horn syndrome, have revealed splice-site mutations in splice donor or acceptor sites that are not in the invariant dinucleotide sequences at the intron boundaries. In such instances, expression of some fraction of correctly spliced, full-sequence mRNA would presumably result in the synthesis of a small amount of normal MNK protein and in the milder occipital horn cell phenotype.

DIAGNOSIS

Menkes' disease should be considered in any male infant with unexplained seizures, mental retardation, and hypothermia. The hair changes and radiological findings are helpful differential features and might be used in initial clinical evaluations for possible heterozygosity in female patients with unexplained neurodevelopmental presentations.

Serum copper and ceruloplasmin concentrations are decreased when measured after the first 2 weeks of life, but these may be indistinguishable from normal when measured in cord blood or during the first or second week of life. The hepatic copper content is markedly decreased, even in the immediate perinatal period. Daily urine copper excretion may be increased during the first year of life. Finally, the measurement of plasma and cerebrospinal fluid catecholamine levels is increasingly being used in the diagnosis of Menkes' disease (and in the monitoring of treatment). In particular, elevations of dihydroxyphenylalanine (DOPA) and dihydroxyphenylacetic acid (DOPAC) can be found, with decreased levels of specific norepinephrine metabolites or of norepinephrine or epinephrine. Elevations in the ratios of DOPA or DOPAC to norepinephrine or derivatives thereof likely reflect dopamine-β-hydroxylase deficiency due to the reduced availability of copper to the central nervous system.

Menkes' disease and occipital horn syndrome are expressed in cultured skin fibroblasts, and an elevated copper content can be detected by atomic absorption spectrophotometry or as the accumulation of radioactive copper. Characteristically, kinetic studies reveal a markedly reduced efflux of copper in mutant fibroblasts. Such studies should be performed by laboratories experienced in these analyses. Although the analyses may be employed in the initial assessment of heterozygosity in the presence of a positive family history, there may be as high as a 50% rate of false negativity, and the results must be interpreted with caution.

Once the diagnosis is confirmed in a proband by biochemical or molecular studies, genetic counseling proceeds as with other X-linked disorders. In the instance of a singleton case of severe Menkes' disease, and absent definitive data on maternal heterozygosity, conventional Bayesian calculations may be employed as for other X-linked recessive disorders with male lethality. Diagnosis in a proband can be confirmed biochemically, whereas mutation identification is usually required for definitive categorization of a potential heterozygote.

Second-trimester prenatal diagnosis of male fetuses at risk has been performed by copper accumulation and kinetic studies in cultured amniotic fluid cells. First-trimester prenatal diagnosis has been accomplished by measurement of copper content in chorionic villus samples. Because of specific sources of ambiguity in both kinds of prenatal measurements, biochemical prenatal diagnosis must be performed by a laboratory with extensive experience in tissue copper biochemistry.

Prenatal diagnosis and heterozygote detection have also been accomplished by mutation detection in instances in which the mutation in a given family was already known or identified as part of the clinical diagnostic sequence. With respect to the genetic counseling of heterozygotes, it should be noted that there have been instances of recurrence in women who are not carriers of mutations, suggesting that germline mosaicism cannot be excluded as a mechanism in the transmission of the Menkes' disease mutations.

In practice, clinical molecular diagnosis and the availability of mutation identification may be problematic since, with one exception, all mutations appear to be unique to each family. If, in a given family, the mutation is not already known, the identification of a mutation may take some time, and treating physicians should be prepared to avail themselves of accurate biochemical testing protocols for diagnosis and management.

TREATMENT

Postnatal, postsymptomatic treatment is predicated on the bypassing of the intestinal absorptive block; copper is administered parenterally, usually as copper histidine, as early in the course of the disease as possible. Results of earlier treatment attempts were not encouraging; however, there have been recent reports of therapeutic amelioration of symptoms in milder or atypical patients or when treatment is begun very early in life. In some instances, significant improvements in neurological status have occurred, but patients have developed some of the severe connective tissue manifestations of the occipital horn syndrome. It has been hypothesized that treatment outcome is primarily predicated on the existence of residual functioning MNK protein. A different hypothesis emphasizes that positive effects can be achieved, even in the face of severe mutations, if treatment is begun very early, perhaps in a baby intentionally delivered prematurely. This last hypothesis is consonant with the notion that some of the pathology begins *in utero*, and that parenteral copper is more likely to enter the brain prior to the maturation of exclusionary brain transport mechanisms. Given all these uncertainties, both empirical and theoretical, it must be emphasized that the treatment of Menkes' disease is investigational, and patients should be referred for treatment to centers with ongoing systematic treatment protocols. Except for such an investigational endeavor, a patient with Menkes' disease should be managed by an experienced multidisciplinary medical team, including neurologists, nutritionists, gastroenterologists, pulmonologists, urologists, and social service personnel.

—*Seymour Packman*

See also–Maple Syrup Urine Disease

Further Reading

Cox, D. (1999). Disorders of copper transport. *Br. Med. Bull.* 55, 544–555.

Danks, D. (1975). Steely hair, mottled mice and copper metabolism. *N. Engl. J. Med.* 293, 1147–1149.

Ferenci, P., Gilliam, T., Gitlin, J., *et al.* (1996). An international symposium on Wilson's and Menkes' disease. *Hepatology* 4, 952–958.

Harris, E. (2000). Cellular copper transport and metabolism. *Annu. Rev. Nutr.* 20, 291–310.

Horn, N., Tonnesen, T., and Tumer, Z. (1995). Variability in clinical expression of an X-linked copper disturbance, Menkes' disease. In *Genetic Response to Metals* (B. Sarkar, Ed.), pp. 285–303. Dekker, New York.

Kaler, S. (1998). Metabolic and molecular bases of Menkes' disease and occipital horn syndrome. *Pediatr. Dev. Pathol.* 1, 85–98.

Menkes, J. (1997). Disorders of copper metabolism. In *The Molecular and Genetic Basis of Neurological Disease* (R. Rosenberg, S. Prusiner, S. DiMauro, and R. Barchi, Eds.), pp. 1273–1290. Butterworth-Heinemann, Boston.

Menkes, J., Alter, M., Steigleder, G., *et al.* (1962). A sex-linked recessive disorder with retardation of growth, peculiar hair, and focal cerebral and cerebellar degeneration. *Pediatrics* 26, 764–779.

Packman, S., Vulpe, C., Levinson, B., *et al.* (1995). Menkes' disease: From patients to gene. In *Genetic Response to Metals* (B. Sarkar, Ed.), pp. 275–284. Dekker, New York.

Vulpe, C., and Packman, S. (1995). Cellular copper transport. *Annu. Rev. Nutr.* 15, 293–322.

Mental Retardation

Encyclopedia of the Neurological Sciences

ALMOST NO DISEASE CATEGORY arouses more controversy within the medical field than mental retardation because it raises issues such as eugenics and the balance between nature (genetics) and nurture in influencing a behavioral phenotype. Even the term is subject to critique. Major issues that impact these affected individuals are highlighted along with recent advances in the genetics and pathophysiology of mental retardation.

In 1992, the American Association on Mental Retardation stated that "mental retardation ... is characterized by significantly subaverage intellectual functioning, existing concurrently with related limitations in ... adaptive skill areas." This definition recognizes that it is possible and meaningful to measure an individual's cognitive abilities and that mental retardation is a composite of a deficiency in these abilities and in the practical application of adaptive skills that are essential for participating in society. Any definition of a deficiency in cognitive skills must be normative. Thus, an IQ of 70 merely reflects the percentile within the total population who scored at that level. For most standardized tests this corresponds to two standard deviations below the mean. This has served as a practical cutoff for mental retardation, with mild mental retardation equal to an IQ between 50 and 70, moderate to severe <50, and borderline mental retardation between 71 and 80. Therefore, these terms reflect society's threshold for a minimal level of intelligence and daily functioning. If this threshold is utilized as a "litmus test" to instigate a search for causes and to initiate a network of educational and support services, then we have begun to address the needs of these vulnerable members of our society. However, the treatment of the mentally retarded throughout history, even in the past century in the United States, has frequently reflected less well-intentioned motivations.

HISTORY

The plight of individuals with mental retardation has been dependent on the customs and beliefs of the era and the locale. In ancient Greece and Rome, infanticide was common and children with disabilities were sold for entertainment or amusement (the circus of P. T. Barnum offered similar fates for the physically unusual). The Middle Ages provided only minimal relief for the mentally retarded because they were frequently sold into slavery or abandoned. However, with the Age of Enlightenment there was a shift in the attitude and treatment of the mentally retarded. In 1690, John Locke published *Essay Concerning Human Understanding*, in which he put forth his theory that the mind was a *tabla rasa*; this theory would have a significant impact on the care and training of individuals with mental retardation. He was also the first to draw a distinction between mental retardation and mental illness: "Herein seems to lie the difference between idiots and madmen, that madmen put wrong ideas together and reason from them, but idiots make very few or no propositions and reason scarce at all."

The modern era in the education and care of individuals with mental retardation began with the work of French physician Jean Marc Itard (1774–1838). He was famous for his attempts to educate a child found in the mountains outside Aveyron whom he named Victor. The systematic training program that he developed for Victor, although it achieved minimal success, inspired the work of Edouard Seguin. Seguin also undertook the training of a cognitively impaired child and in 1837 established a program for "educating" these children at the Salpetriere in Paris. Seguin immigrated to the United States in 1848 and founded an organization that became the American Association on Mental Retardation.

In 1905, Alfred Binet and Theodore Simon created the first intelligence test. This was used as a screen for students in French schools. In 1911, Henry Goddard translated the test into English, and in 1916 Lewis Terman of Stanford University refined the test into what became known as the Stanford–Binet. Intimately connected with these advances, however, was the rise of the eugenics movement in the United States. Goddard published *The Kallikak Family: A Study in the Heredity of Feeble-Mindedness* (1913), which promulgated views about the coheritability of criminality and mental retardation. The eugenics movement reached its zenith in the United States at this time. As many as 27 states had involuntary sterilization laws, and immigration was markedly curtailed by the Immigration Restriction Act of 1924 primarily to prevent the entry of potential "dysgenics" from southern and eastern Europe. It is in this light that we must interpret the current advances in genetic technology. As we are reminded by George Santayana, "those who forget the past are condemned to repeat it."

Positive change occurred for individuals with mental retardation after World War II. The National Association for Retarded Children was founded in 1950 and has been a strong advocate for support services, research, and enhanced rights for retarded individuals. Between 1950 and 1975, enrollment of mentally retarded children in special education programs in the United States increased from less than 50,000 to more than 1.3 million. This movement culminated in the passing of the Education for All Handicapped Children Act, now titled the Individuals with Disabilities Education Act. This act guarantees appropriate education and intervention for all children with disabilities from birth to age 21. Recent U.S. Census Bureau data show that 5,339,400 children are receiving services through this act. Despite these impressive recent gains, there remains much to be done. For instance, testing for certain metabolic disorders is inconsistent from state to state, thus resulting in missed opportunities to prevent new cases of mental retardation. These missed opportunities are even more prevalent in countries less prosperous than the United States.

EPIDEMIOLOGY

As stated previously, mental retardation is functionally defined as the combination of intelligence two standard deviations below the mean and poor adaptive skills. The Wechsler Intelligence Scale for Children III and most other standardized intelligence tests utilize similar scales, thus allowing for quantitative classification of mild, moderate to severe, and borderline mental retardation. Numerous population-based studies have estimated the prevalence of mental retardation. The majority of these studies have found that mild mental retardation affects 15 per 1000 individuals and that moderate to severe mental retardation affects approximately one-third of these individuals or 5 per 1000. There is variability between populations that reflects neonatal and prenatal genetic and metabolic screening programs. Some variability exists as a result of higher consanguinity and levels of nutrition and poverty, and other differences reflect cultural biases toward testing and labeling intellectually challenged children. Most of these individuals come to medical attention because of delays in developmental milestones, particularly speech; however, some continue to be detected as late as 10 years of age.

Many mildly retarded or borderline individuals are able to function independently and are active members of the workforce. However, some require full-time assistance and the care of multidisciplinary medical teams (the cardiac, neurological, and endocrine issues of Down's patients provide a compelling example). The care of the mentally retarded represents a significant percentage of overall health care expenditures. A recent Dutch study determined that the economic costs to society for mental retardation were nearly equal to those for heart disease, stroke, and cancer combined, thus highlighting the need for prevention, early detection, and treatment.

ETIOLOGY

The known causes of mental retardation are too numerous to be delineated here; Table 1 is a list of the more common etiologies. Generally, etiologies are classified into the following categories: prenatal, perinatal, and postnatal. The prenatal group includes known genetic syndromes, central nervous system malformations (which overlap with many other causes), and toxic (e.g., fetal alcohol syndrome) and infectious causes. Perinatal conditions include birth asphyxia, stroke, and meningitis. Using this classification, a recent study of mental retardation in school-age children in metropolitan Atlanta found that 87% of children with mild mental retardation and 57% of moderate to severely affected children did not have identified causes. A similar skew was reported in a landmark Swedish study of all children born in Göteborg between 1966 and 1970, although the percentages of known diagnoses were higher. In many studies, a significant percentage of children with no identifiable diagnosis have a strong family history. Recent discoveries highlight the continued importance that careful genetic analysis will have on the diagnosis and treatment of the mentally retarded.

GENETICS

Since the description of "mongolism" by J. Langdon Down in 1866 and the discovery of trisomy 21 by

Table 1 CATEGORIES AND CAUSES OF MENTAL RETARDATION

Category	Causes
Prenatal	Genetic
	Chromosomal (e.g., trisomy 21, mosaics, translocations)
	Mutant gene (e.g., fragile X, Rubinstein–Taybi, Coffin–Lowry)
	Metabolic (e.g., phenylketonuria, galactosemia, Smith–Lemli–Opitz)
	Acquired
	Fetal alcohol syndrome
	Other maternal subtance abuse
	Nutritional (e.g., rubella, toxoplasmosis, CMV)
	Unknown
	Syndrome (e.g., Schinzel–Giedeon, FG and KBG syndromes)[a]
	Multiple congenital anomaly and mental retardation
Perinatal	Birth asphyxia
	Infection (HSV encephalitics or group B Strep meningitis)
	Stroke (embolic or hemorrhagic)
	Very low birth weight, extreme prematurity
	Metabolic (e.g., hypoglycemia, hyperbilirubinemia)
Postnatal environmental	Toxins (e.g., lead)
	Infection (H. influenza b meningitis, arbovirus encephalitis)
	Trauma (consider nonaccidental)
Undetermined	Familial
	Nonfamilial

[a] These are labeled as unknown; they are mostly likely genetic but can be acquired.

Lejeune in 1960, considerable progress has been made in uncovering genetic causes of mental retardation. Currently, there are 948 separate entries for mental retardation in the *Online Mendelian Inheritance of Man*. Many of these are rare single gene disorders resulting in mental retardation through a metabolic defect or through aberrations early in embryology. Examples of these disorders include tyrosinemia and holoprosencephaly, respectively. The majority of syndromes do not have an identified causative gene. Most individuals with mental retardation cannot be given a syndromic diagnosis, despite a family history. Recent work, however, has identified a previously unrecognized chromosomal mutation that may be second only to

Down's syndrome as a common genetic cause of mental retardation.

In 1995, Jonathan Flint and colleagues reported the development of a system by Southern blot analysis (and now refined to a fluorescence *in situ* hybridization approach) that could detect submicroscopic deletions or rearrangements at the ends of chromosomes. It had been known for some time that these telomeric regions are more susceptible to translocations and deletions. These investigators showed that these "subtelomeric" rearrangements could be detected sensitively by their methods and that a not insignificant percentage of patients with mental retardation were found to have these chromosomal changes. A recent study by this group systematically addressed this association and reported that 7% of patients with mental retardation and some dysmorphic features and 0.5% of patients with isolated mental retardation have these deletions or translocations, which were not detected by traditional 600-band karyotyping. Moreover, they discovered that in approximately 50% of these cases, one parent had a previously undetected balanced translocation. This generation transfer has important genetic counseling implications. This approach should provide an important clinical tool for diagnosing mental retardation and also will provide more general information on gene alleles that can cause mental retardation. Indeed, a recent paper by Higgins *et al.* that reported a family with nonsyndromic mental retardation localized to the telomeric region of chromosome 3q is a confirmation of this potential.

Another area in which there has been considerable progress in the identification of disease-causing mutations is X-linked mental retardation (Fig. 1). This reflects years of work that began with the recognition that familial mental retardation is more common in males, with an average reported ratio of 1.2:1. Fragile X is the most common X-linked disorder of mental retardation. Identified by the susceptibility of metaphase chromosomes to breakage in the presence of folate, this disorder (and its *in vitro* "fragility") is caused by methylation of an expanded CCG repeat and subsequent inactivation of the *fmr1* gene. This encodes a protein (fmrp) thought to be involved in mRNA transport and regulation of protein translation. Interestingly, the triplet repeat region can be demethylated *in vitro* with 5-azadeoxycytidine, leading to normal transcription of the gene. This might pave the way for the development of pharmacological therapy for these patients. Another "fragile" site, FRAXE, has also

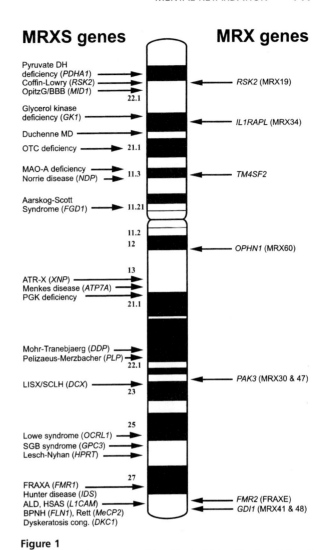

Figure 1

Map of the X chromosome (G banding) with localization of cloned genes responsible for syndromic (MRXS) and nonsyndromic (MRX) mental retardation transmitted in an X-linked fashion. The syndrome name is followed by the name of the gene in brackets for MRXS, whereas for MRX genes the name is followed by the number of the MRX family in brackets in which mutations of that gene were found. OTC, ornithine transcarbamylase; MAO-A, monoamino oxidase A; PGK, phosphoglycerol kinase; LISX/SCLH, lissencephaly X/subcortical laminar heterotopia; SGB, Simpson–Golabi–Behmel; ALD, adrenoleukodystrophy; HSAS, hydrocephalus with stenosis of the aqueduct of Silvius; BPNH, bilateral periventricular nodular heterotopia (reprinted with permission of Dr. Ben Oostra).

been linked to mental retardation; the gene *fmr2* encodes a putative transcription factor. Although mental retardation is rarely associated with methylation-based inactivation of this gene, there are reports linking microdeletions of *fmr2* with mental retardation and premature ovarian failure.

Many families have been reported in which individuals affected by mental retardation span multiple generations. Multiplex families that have an autosomal mode of inheritance are usually not large enough to permit localization of the causative mutation by classic genetic analysis. This analysis is simplified when the inheritance pattern implicates the X chromosome, and numerous families have been documented with an X-linked form of mental retardation. Many of these families do not have detectable physical or medical features to accompany the cognitive impairment. Therefore, the terms nonsyndromic or isolated mental retardation apply. As a first approximation, the genes causing mental retardation may be directly involved in synaptic plasticity. To date, six genes (including *fmr2*) have been implicated in the pathogenesis of mental retardation: *OPHN1*, *GDI1*, *PAK3*, *IL1RAPL*, and *TM4SF2*. The first three have been indirectly implicated in neurite outgrowth and synaptic vesicle recycling. The last two are cell surface molecules; *TM4SF2* is part of a class of proteins called tetraspanins, which have been shown to play a role in cell–cell signaling. It will be interesting to determine if any of these mutations shed light on general mechanisms of synaptic plasticity and if the pathways identified by this research will inform studies on the more common polygenic forms of mental retardation.

CONCLUSION

During the past 50 years, there has been considerable progress in the services and rights accorded to individuals with mental retardation. Also, much information has been learned regarding the genetic causes of mental retardation. We hope that the rapid advances in biotechnology will lead to meaningful treatments for these individuals.

—*Elliott H. Sherr and Donna M. Ferriero*

See also–Autism; Brain Development, Normal Postnatal; Child Neurology, History of; Cognitive Impairment; Developmental Neuropsychology; Down's Syndrome; Genetic Testing, Molecular; Intelligence; Learning Disabilities; Learning, Overview; Mental Status Testing

Further Reading

Cabezas, D. A., Arena, J. F., Stevenson, R. E., *et al.* (1999). XLMR database. *Am. J. Med. Genet.* **85**, 202–205.

Higgins, J. J., Rosen, D. R., Loveless, J. M., *et al.* (2000). A gene for nonsyndromic mental retardation maps to chromosome 3p25-pter. *Neurology* **55**, 335–340.

Knight, S. J., Regan, R., Nicod, A., *et al.* (1999). Subtle chromosomal rearrangements in children with unexplained mental retardation. *Lancet* **354**, 1676–1681.

McKusick, V. A. (2000). *Online Mendelian Inheritance in Man, OMIM*. McKusick–Nathans Institute for Genetic Medicine, Johns Hopkins University/National Center for Biotechnology Information, National Library of Medicine, Baltimore, MD/Bethesda, MD. http://www.ncbi.nlm.nih.gov/omim.

Micklos, D., Witkowski, J. (2000). *Image Archive on the American Eugenics Movement*. Cold Spring Harbor Laboratory, Cold Spring Harbor, NY. http://vector.cshl.org/eugenics.

Mental Status Testing

Encyclopedia of the Neurological Sciences
Copyright 2003, Elsevier Science (USA). All rights reserved.

THE MENTAL status examination (MSE) is a standard component of health care practice for general medical practitioners, neurologists, and mental health professionals. It should be used to evaluate the cognitive and psychiatric status of any patient who is known or suspected to have neurological or psychiatric symptoms. Because it functions largely as a screening tool, the MSE not only can help identify aspects of the patient's mental health that are in need of more detailed investigation but also can elicit information that alerts practitioners to the need for referral to a specialist. Although a variety of structured MSE instruments exist and can be quite useful for aspects of the assessment, unstructured or semistructured forms of the MSE are best able to provide a comprehensive picture of an individual patient's functioning. Clinicians can expand or contract the unstructured MSE to provide information that is more applicable to their specialty, and they may tailor it to focus in on particular areas of suspicion for a single patient. The three main components of the MSE—history, psychiatric status, and cognitive status—are described here.

HISTORY

Whenever possible, a comprehensive MSE should involve taking a history before the formal mental status testing begins. The primary goal of this history should be to obtain current and past information pertaining to the patient's behavioral, neurological, and psychiatric status. An attempt should always be made to elicit a clear timeline from the patient for any problem because diagnostic accuracy in mental disorders often relies on factors such as age of onset, rate of progression, episodicity, duration, and frequency.

The history should begin with a complete description of the patient's current complaints and symptoms, and the interviewer should be sure to fully investigate changes or problems in the areas of behavior, cognition, and psychological status, including current stressors. Next, a medical history should be taken, again with a particular focus on medical issues that pertain to cognitive and psychiatric functioning. Questions should be asked regarding general medical disease or injury, neurological disease or injury, medications, seizures, head injury, toxic exposure, and substance use (including alcohol, tobacco, caffeine, and drug use). Third, the interviewer should obtain a psychiatric history from the patient, including any past or present diagnoses, assessment, and treatment. Fourth, any relevant social history should be noted. This should include educational attainment, vocational history (including military service), and a criminal history to provide information about any significant behavioral problems. Lastly, the patient's family history should be obtained. This will focus on any significant history of neurological or psychiatric problems in family members, but it should also obtain information about general medical conditions that could impact neurological status (e.g., hypertension and stroke). It may also be helpful to ask the patient about family members with behavioral oddities because the proverbial "funny uncle" may have had an undiagnosed neurological or psychiatric disease.

PSYCHIATRIC STATUS

Making an assessment of the patient's psychiatric status is the first phase of the formal mental status examination. It relies heavily on behavioral observation on the part of the interviewer, and much of the information will have already been gathered as an implicit part of the history-taking process. Psychiatric status is the foundation for the rest of the MSE because a patient who is seriously disordered in this domain may not be able to perform well on the cognitive portion of the examination. Interpretation of patients' higher level functioning must be guided by an awareness of the psychiatric factors that may be limiting them.

Appearance

Although this has been a standard component of mental status examination in the past, it has recently become a controversial category due to accusations of clinician insensitivity and bias. Thus, evaluation in this area should be done cautiously, avoiding statements that could be interpreted as solely the opinion of the examiner (e.g., "attractive") and focusing on aspects of appearance that have direct relevance to the issue of the patient's mental status. Common inclusions in this category are statements about the patient's apparent level of consciousness (alert, drowsy, stuporous, etc.), apparent age (differentiated from actual age), eye contact, clothing, hygiene and grooming, position (sitting or lying down), as well as indication of any physical abnormalities, disabilities, or relevant features not included elsewhere.

Attitude

This is an assessment of the patient's degree of cooperation with the assessment process as well as their attitude toward the clinician. Any positive or negative deviation from the norm should be noted, including hostility, guardedness, apathy, eagerness, or jocularity; otherwise, the patient is usually described as cooperative. A statement is often made in this section noting whether or not the clinician was able to establish rapport with the patient, with an indication if the patient was particularly engaging or inappropriate (e.g., seductive, disinhibited, or abusive).

Motor Activity/Behavior

Most items in this category correspond with observations of gross neurological function. Statements should be made about the patient's general level of activity (from restless hyperactivity to bradykinesia, or abnormally slow movement), coordination, gait, and posture (e.g., spasticity or rigidity). Any unusual motor behavior should also be included, such as tremor, rhythmic movements, tics, or abnormal facial expression. This may also include odd mannerisms or behaviors such as frequent grimacing or a tendency to place objects from throughout the room in their mouth (hyperorality).

Mood

There are many different definitions of mood; however, one analogy used in the psychotherapy-oriented disciplines is that mood is distinguished from affect as climate is distinguished from weather. It is less variable and superficial than affect and represents the deeper, more typical emotional tone experienced by the patient over a longer period of time (days to weeks). Thus, mood is best derived primarily from history and patient self-report, unless the clinician has opportunity to observe the patient over the course of multiple visits.

Affect

This is the visible, expressed emotional state of the patient during the evaluation. Facial expression, tone of voice, content of speech, physical tension, and posture may all be used to form a statement about the patient's affect. Extreme fluctuations in affect (labile affect), as well as the absence of normal variation (flattened affect), are important and should be noted. It is standard practice to include a statement comparing affect to mood, and any disjunction among modalities should be noted (e.g., smiling broadly while discussing an emotionally upsetting event, or tearfulness in the context of reportedly positive mood).

Thought Process

This is an assessment of the quality of the patient's thought, particularly with regard to its degree of connection and organization. Common observations include whether the patient's thought process is linear and understandable or whether the patient evidences significant tangentiality (getting off topic), flight of ideas, perseveration (repeatedly returning to the same topic or word), loose associations, or circumstantiality (excessive attention to detail, usually at the expense of the main topic of conversation). Echolalia, neologisms, and clang associations (connecting words because of their sound rather than their meaning; e.g., "cuff tough rebuff") are examples of disordered thought processes occurring at the level of words or short phrases.

Thought Content

This category includes observations about the nature of the patient's thoughts as well as perceptions. Delusions, hallucinations, homicidal or suicidal ideation, obsessions, and compulsive thoughts are commonly described in this section. Any significant preoccupation, paranoia, or phobia should be noted here, along with any dissociative phenomena, such as derealization or depersonalization.

COGNITIVE STATUS

As with the psychiatric portion of the MSE, each component of the cognitive status evaluation builds upon what has preceded it. Impairment in language, for instance, must be considered in the evaluation of abstract reasoning because the patient may be able to clearly conceptualize their response but cannot communicate it. The cognitive component of the MSE is more scripted than the history or psychiatric status examination, and it relies heavily on the patient's performance of various tasks. A number of structured cognitive examinations have been created to provide comprehensive screening; however, flexibility in response to an individual patient's pattern of cognition will always provide a more complete, accurate assessment. Some of the most widely used structured MSEs include versions of the Folstein Mini-Mental State Exam (Table 1), although it has an updated version, the 3MS. The American Neuropsychiatric Association also recommends the use of the Neurobehavioral Cognitive Status Examination, updated under the name COGNISTAT. For dementia screening in older patients, the Mattis Dementia Rating Scale is quite thorough.

Attention

If the patient is having difficulty maintaining attention and concentration, this will be observable by the clinician. The patient may miss questions or instructions, or they may become easily distracted. Simple attention can best be quantified using a digit repetition task, in which the patient is asked to repeat back increasingly longer sequences of digits. Adult patients should be able to repeat back five to seven digits; if they are unable to repeat a span of five digits after two trials, their attention is probably impaired.

Orientation

The three major domains to which the patient should be oriented are person (who they are), place (location and how they got there), and time (date and time of day). Orientation is actually a measure of recent memory functioning because it is dependent on attending to and learning the continually changing facts about one's environment. It may be assessed by asking the patient questions about the city, state, name of the hospital, and floor of the building on which the interview is taking place as well as the full date, day of the week, season, and time of day.

Language

A number of aspects of both expressive and receptive language can be assessed fairly easily during the course of the MSE. First, the patient's spontaneous speech should be rated for fluency (i.e., are their words unusually slow or halting), prosody (rising and falling voice inflection),

Table 1   MINI-MENTAL STATE[a]

Maximum points	Question
5	What is the: Year? Season? Date? Day? Month?
5	Where are we: State (Country)? County (Province)? City? Hospital (Place)? Floor (Street)?
3	Name three objects (Apple, Penny, Table) using 1 second to say each. Then ask the patient to repeat all three after you have said them. 1 point for each correct. Then repeat them until the patient learns them. Count the number of trials and record ——.
5	Serial 7's: Subtract 7 from 100 and stop at 5 answers. 1 point for each correct. OR, Spell "WORLD" backwards. Number correct is the number of letters in correct order (e.g., "dlorw" = 3 points).
3	Ask for the names of the three objects (Apple, Penny, Table). 1 point for each correct.
2	Point to a pencil and a watch. Ask the patient to name them as you point.
1	Have the patient repeat the phrase, "No ifs, and, or buts."
3	Have the patient follow a three-stage command, only after all three steps have been given: "Take the paper in your right hand, fold it in half, and put it on the floor."
1	Write "CLOSE YOUR EYES" in large letters. Show this to the patient and ask them to do what it says.
1	Have the patient write a sentence spontaneously.
1	Have the patient copy the intersecting pentagons below.

Total: 30

[a] From Folstein *et al.* (1975).

appropriate grammatical structure, articulation, and gross comprehension. Then, more structured assessments are usually done. Repetition is assessed by having the patient repeat simple and then more complex words and phrases after the examiner (e.g., "No ifs, ands, or buts"). Verbal fluency can be assessed by having the patient name as many animals as they can in 1 min. Normal adults should name approximately 18–22 animals, decreasing slightly in the elderly. An assessment of confrontation naming can be done by simply pointing at various objects around the office and asking the patient to name them. However, structured stimulus booklets (such as Kaplan's *Boston Naming Test*) are available that contain pictures of objects that are increasingly difficult to name. Utilizing such structured assessments is preferable due to their sensitivity as well as the availability of extensive normative data. The patient's comprehension can be assessed by asking them to follow grammatically complex commands (e.g., "Before touching your chin, point to your eye") and answer complex statements (e.g., "If a lion was killed by a tiger, which animal is dead?"). Finally, an assessment for alexia and agraphia can be done by asking the patient to read and write various words or sentences. Spontaneous writing as well as writing to dictation should be assessed.

Construction

Assessment of visuospatial skills in the MSE is usually limited to construction tasks, in which the patient is asked to either copy drawings or draw objects from memory. Mental status examinations often include only one complex two-dimensional drawing, a pair of interlocking pentagons. This is usually scored on a pass–fail basis, allowing the patient to "pass" if both of the pentagons have five angles of any shape and they intersect. Ideally, however, the patient should be asked to copy multiple stimuli that begin simply (e.g., a diamond or a circle) and become more complex (e.g., a cube), moving from two to three dimensions. Common errors include rotation, perseveration (drawing the same component repeatedly), and stimulus-bound behavior, in which the patient attempts to draw their copy immediately next to or even on top of the stimulus picture. For drawing on command, patients are often asked to draw the face of a clock that indicates the time 11:10. This measure is particularly sensitive to visuospatial neglect, micrographia, and spatial disorganization. Errors in correctly reproducing the time may suggest attentional problems, memory deficits, or executive dysfunction.

Memory

Both verbal and nonverbal memory should be assessed in a thorough MSE. Remote verbal memory for autobiographical information can be obtained by asking the patient for information about their childhood. Both recent and remote semantic memory can be assessed by asking the patient questions about important world events or famous people from successive decades of their life, including the current year. When a patient has recent memory loss, it is helpful diagnostically to ascertain the time period in the patient's life in which their memories become fragmented (e.g., the patient can tell detailed stories about the Vietnam war but cannot identify any U.S. presidents after Ford).

There are a number of ways to assess patients' ability to learn new information during the course of an MSE, all of which include a learning trial followed by memory assessment after a delay. Clinicians often name three or four words, ask the patient to repeat the words back, then ask the patient to remember them for later. After performing a different task for 30 sec to 10 min, the examiner asks the patient to recall the objects. Another way to assess new learning that is particularly useful when the patient has a language deficit is to show the patient five small objects (such as a coin, pen, or comb) and then hide the objects around the office, showing the patient each hiding place. Then, after a delay of 5 min, the clinician asks the patient where the objects are located. Patients younger than age 60 should be able to find four or all five of the objects. This test can also be done with stimuli that are more salient to the patient, such as money. Visuospatial memory can be assessed by asking the patient to draw one or more of the visuoconstruction stimuli from memory 5–10 min after they copied them. Assessment with more complex stimuli provides greater sensitivity to mild memory impairment.

Higher Cognitive Functioning

There are a variety of tasks that can be done during a MSE that elicit information regarding the patient's higher level functions. For instance, abstract reasoning can be assessed by asking the patient to explain similarities (e.g., "How are an eye and an ear alike?") or by asking the patient to interpret proverbs. These are scored according to both the degree of concrete-

ness and the accuracy of the patient's answers. Another aspect of higher function, calculation, can easily be assessed by asking the patient to perform a series of math problems either on paper or mentally (although the latter relies on complex attention and working memory in addition to calculation skills). The patient's judgment can also be assessed by both listening carefully during the history and asking the patient questions about how they would behave in situations requiring good judgment and reasoning (e.g., "If you were stranded in the Denver airport with only one dollar, what would you do?"). The patient's level of insight can also be described in this section, although it is most often assessed during the history by asking questions about the nature of the patient's symptoms in order to determine the patient's level of awareness of their problems.

CONCLUSION

There are as many ways to conduct an MSE as there are individual patients, but an assessment containing the previously discussed components will be both thorough and edifying. A good MSE can render a valuable snapshot of the patient that guides the clinician toward providing the best assessment, diagnosis, and treatment.

—*Katherine P. Rankin*

See also–Cognitive Impairment; Diagnostic and Statistical Manual of Mental Disorders (DSM-IV); Neuropsychiatry, Overview; Neuropsychology, Overview

Further Reading

Folstein, M. F., Folstein, S. E., and McHugh, P. R. (1975). "Mini-Mental State": A practical method for grading the cognitive state of patients for the clinician. *J. Psychiatr. Res.* **12**, 189–198.

Kaplan, E. F., Goodglass, H., and Weintraub, A. (1983). *The Boston Naming Test*, 2nd ed. Lea & Febiger, Philadelphia.

Kiernan, R. J., Mueller, J., and Langston, J. W. (1987). The Neurobehavioral Cognitive Status Examination: A brief but quantitative approach to cognitive assessment. *Ann. Intern. Med.* **107**, 481–485.

Malloy, P. F., Cummings, J. L., Coffey, C. E., *et al.* (1997). Cognitive screening instruments in neuropsychiatry: A report of the committee on research of the American Neuropsychiatric Association. *J. Neuropsychiatr. Clin. Neurosci.* **9**, 189–197.

Mattis, S. (1988). *Dementia Rating Scale: Professional Manual*. Psychological Assessment Resources, Odessa, FL.

Strub, R. L, and Black, F. W. (2000). *The Mental Status Examination in Neurology*. Davis, Philadelphia.

Teng, E. L., and Chui, H. C. (1987). The Modified Mini-Mental State (3MS) Examination. *J. Clin. Psychiatry* **48**, 314–318.

Meralgia Paresthetica

Encyclopedia of the Neurological Sciences
Copyright 2003, Elsevier Science (USA). All rights reserved.

MERALGIA PARESTHETICA refers to the clinical condition resulting from entrapment of the lateral femoral cutaneous nerve (LFCN) in the thigh. The nerve branches off the lumbar plexus and conveys fibers from the L2 and L3 nerve roots. The nerve courses through the pelvis, running adjacent to the lateral edge of the psoas muscle. It enters the leg underneath or through the inguinal ligament, just medial to the anterior superior iliac spine; it is in this location that entrapment can occur. The nerve is purely sensory, relaying sensory information from the anterolateral and lateral thigh.

CLINICAL SYNDROME

Meralgia paresthetica (from *meros*, meaning thigh, and *algo*, meaning pain) is characterized by abnormal sensations or paresthesias from the upper lateral thigh. Patients typically describe their symptoms as a burning, tingling, or pins and needles–type sensation, superficially in the skin. Individuals may complain of hyperpathia, in which light touch to the skin (from clothing or a hand) results in unpleasant sensations. Symptoms may be reproduced by tapping over the lateral aspect of the inguinal ligament (Tinel's sign). Symptoms are usually unilateral and are often exacerbated by prolonged walking, standing, or thigh extension, and they are improved by sitting. Clinical signs include a loss of light touch or pinprick sensations in the upper lateral thigh, often in a more restricted area than the zone of paresthesias. Over time, the paresthesias may slowly resolve, although mild sensory loss may persist.

ETIOLOGY

Meralgia paresthetica is most commonly caused by mechanical entrapment of the LFCN as it runs underneath or through the inguinal ligament. Reported causes include blunt or penetrating trauma, tight-fitting pants/corsets/belts, compression from a wallet, carrying heavy objects supported on the thigh or groin, or prolonged leaning of a thigh against a bench or table. Nerve injury has also been associated with surgical procedures, such as harvesting the iliac bone for grafting, external compression from

prolonged lithotomy position, direct injury from laparoscopic inguinal herniorrhaphy, and compression from a retractor during gastroplasty for morbid obesity. Meralgia has also been associated with retroperitoneal masses such as tumors and bleeds. Meralgia may be seen in pregnant or obese individuals or in patients with ascites, with symptoms resolving following weight loss or delivery; presumably, abdominal distension and increased lumbar lordosis in these conditions eventuates in stretch and/or angulation of the nerve.

DIFFERENTIAL DIAGNOSIS

Other conditions that may mimic meralgia paresthetica include lumbar radiculopathies (e.g., from disk disease), lumbar plexopathies (e.g., from retroperitoneal masses), or femoral neuropathies. These conditions usually involve weakness of hip flexion and knee extension, atrophy of thigh muscles, and loss of the knee reflex (if the L4 nerve root is involved). Radiculopathies secondary to nerve root compression typically involve radiating pains to the thigh.

ELECTRODIAGNOSIS

Meralgia paresthetica is principally a clinical diagnosis. Electrophysiological examinations [nerve conduction studies and needle electromyography (EMG)] can assist in defining the diagnosis and in excluding radiculopathies, femoral neuropathies, and plexopathies. Sensory nerve conduction studies of the LFCN are technically difficult to perform, particularly in obese individuals. The LFCN sensory nerve action potential in the affected leg may be absent or reduced in size compared with the response obtained in the asymptomatic, contralateral leg. A slowed LFCN sensory conduction velocity may be seen across the compression site. The needle EMG study is normal in meralgia parasthetica but abnormal in characteristic patterns in radiculopathies, femoral neuropathies, and plexopathies.

TREATMENT

Treatment is usually conservative, with oral analgesics. Precipitating factors (e.g., tight belts, corsets, and weight gain), if identified, should be eliminated. Weight loss and abdominal exercises may be helpful. Nerve blocks and steroid injections at the lateral end of the inguinal ligament have been attempted with variable results. Surgery has been recommended in refractory cases, although this should be reserved for patients with disabling pain because symptoms typically remit spontaneously with time. Surgical release of the entrapped nerve under the inguinal ligament as well as transection and neurolysis have all been employed.

—*William S. David*

See also–Neuropathies, Entrapment

Further Reading

Aldrich, E. F., and Van den Heeven, C. M. (1989). Suprainguinal ligament approach for surgical treatment of meralgia paresthetica. *J. Neurosurg.* **70**, 492.
Keegan, J. J., and Holyoke, E. A. (1962). Meralgia paresthetica: An anatomical and surgical study. *J. Neurosurg.* **19**, 341.
Sarala, P. K., Nisihara, T., and Oh, S. J. (1979). Meralgia paresthetica: Electrophysiologic study. *Arch. Phys. Med. Rehab.* **60**, 30.
Stevens, A., and Rosselle, N. (1970). Sensory nerve conduction velocity of N. cutaneous femoris lateralis. *Electromyogr. Clin. Neurophysiol.* **10**, 397.

Mercury

Encyclopedia of the Neurological Sciences
Copyright 2003, Elsevier Science (USA). All rights reserved.

HUMAN mercurial intoxication results from exposure to the metal, to its inorganic salts, and to organic mercury-containing compounds that are degraded to the inorganic metal. Another form of mercurialism, with different chemical and clinical manifestations, results from intoxication with alkyl compounds, particularly methyl and ethyl mercury.

Inorganic mercury poisoning occurs as an industrial disease during paper manufacture, in the preparation of chlorine, and as a result of exposure to certain other chemical processes. Historically, mercurialism was associated with the hat manufacturing industry because mercuric nitrate was used for processing felt. Acute poisoning has also occurred followed the use of mercuric chloride as a local antiseptic, following the excessive use of calomel as a diuretic, and following merthiolate ear irrigations. Although dental amalgams release small amounts of mercury, available data do not indicate that this exposure represents a significant clinical risk of intoxication.

The main atmospheric source of mercury pollution is through the burning of coal and other fossil fuels.

Metallic mercury volatilizes at room temperature and condenses on skin and respiratory membranes. It is absorbed from the skin and the gastrointestinal and respiratory tracts. Elemental, nonionized mercury is transported in the blood, bound to plasma proteins and hemoglobin. Inorganic mercury has remarkable affinity for the kidney; as a result, symptoms of intoxication relate predominantely to that organ. Brain uptake varies, depending on chemical form, but under appropriate conditions the brain incorporates mercury rapidly. Once incorporated into the nervous system, mercury is very slowly eliminated.

Serum concentrations are unreliable indicators of inorganic mercury toxicity, but toxic symptoms are usually present when concentrations exceed 500 mg/liter. Blood concentrations less than 100 mg/liter are considered safe. Urinary excretion is similarly an untrustworthy measure of toxicity. Inorganic mercury produces its toxic effects by altering membranes, particularly through combination with sulfur-containing bonds. Mercury inhibits energy metabolism by interacting with several enzyme systems that contain sulfur and by effects on chemicals including lipoic acid, coenzyme A, and pantetheine. Unlike lead, however, mercury forms complexes with amino groups of proteins.

Acute poisoning is usually manifest by an inflammation of the mouth, marked salivation, and severe gastrointestinal disturbances, such as colic and diarrhea. The breath has a fetid odor, often described as "metallic." A brownish mercurial line may be visible along the margin of the teeth. In many cases, there is a marked emotional irritability and a rapid onset of weakness in the lower limbs. Acute psychotic episodes with delirium, hallucinations, and marked motor activity may occur.

The chronic form of mercurialism is more common and occurs in industries that use mercury in low doses. The onset of illness may be subtle, with mild tremor and weakness of the limbs, or involve a progressive personality change. Other involuntary movements, muscle cramps, clonic spasms, or even convulsions may develop. Occasionally, a clinical picture resembling Parkinson's disease, with slowness, gait difficulty, rigidity, and tremor, develops. Personality changes generally accompany or precede the motor phenomena. Marked fatigability, irritability, insomnia, and an extreme muscular weakness appear early. This picture may persist for weeks or months and is referred to as mercurial neurasthenia. These symptoms may be interrupted or accompanied by periods of excitability and irritability, as typified in Lewis Carroll's Mad Hatter. The hyperirritability becomes extremely violent, with the patient being assaultive or even homicidal. Some of these cases terminate in a severe psychosis. In the more severe cases, there is predominant apathy that progresses to lethargy and may become so severe that patients fall asleep as soon as they sit down.

Neurologically, there is often a wide variety of findings, such as vertigo, nystagmus, blurred vision, narrowing of the visual fields, optic neuritis and atrophy of the optic nerve, instability or ataxia, and convulsive seizures. There may be tingling sensations (dysesthesias) and extreme pains in the extremities (peripheral neuritis) with muscle wasting.

Measurement of nerve conduction velocity has been suggested as a means of determining safety of mercury levels in the workplace. Slowing of median motor nerve conduction was found to correlate with increased levels of mercury in the blood and urine as well as with increased numbers of neurological symptoms.

The major form of chronic inorganic mercurialism in children is called acrodynia, a syndrome that has also been observed in adults. The principal manifestations include personality changes varying from extreme irritability (particularly in infants) to general bad temper. There is tachycardia and hypertension. The hands are pink or red and swollen. The feet are usually cold and moist and may become swollen and desquamated. Profuse sweating on the trunk may give rise to a miliary rash. Insomnia, anorexia, weight loss, and constipation are often present. The condition can be reversed with therapy, but recovery is slow.

Organic mercury readily enters the brain from the blood, and brain turnover is slow. In chronic exposure, approximately 10% of the body burden localizes in the brain. With acute intoxication, less than 3% is degraded into inorganic brain mercury, but this rate may change with time. Specifically, inorganic mercury levels may account for 82–100% of brain mercury after organic mercury exposure if the autopsy is done several years after exposure. Once biotransformation to inorganic mercury occurs, excretion rates are extremely low since inorganic mercury cannot leave the brain easily. Anatomical changes in the brain involve especially the primary visual cortex and cerebellum followed by the frontal and parietal lobes of the brain and the deep brain area called the putamen. Peripheral nerves are also damaged. Because organic mercury is converted to inorganic metal, the intoxication syndrome seen after organic mercury exposure largely mimics the signs seen with inorganic exposure.

Alkyl mercury poisoning has followed ingestion of contaminated seafood or exposure to alkyl mercury used in seed grain as an antifungal additive. Massive intoxication occurred in individuals living in the vicinity of Minamata Bay, Japan, as a result of ingestion of fish and shellfish containing methyl mercury. Similar problems occurred, to a lesser degree, in Scandinavia. The Minamata Bay area incident resulted in at least 111 cases of mercurialism, with 42 known deaths. Because mercury crossed the placental barrier, fetal injury was particularly severe. During the involvement, 42 of 400 live births exhibited evidence of brain damage despite lack of clinical symptoms in all but one mother. In reconstructing the history of this form of mercury intoxication, researchers discovered that the original contamination resulted from discharge of an effluent containing inorganic mercury from an adjacent chemical plant. The mercury was then methylated by microorganisms in the sediment of the bay. The methyl mercury so formed was incorporated into the protein of fish and shellfish, and the alkyl mercury remained bound to protein for long periods because the half-life is several years. The intoxication occurred after humans consumed the contaminated seafood. In 1972, another catastrophic epidemic of methyl mercury poisoning occurred in Iraq. A total of 6530 patients were hospitalized for treatment, and 459 known fatalities occurred, principally as a result of eating homemade bread prepared from seed treated with a methyl mercury fungicide.

Alkyl mercury compounds share many of the biochemical effects of their inorganic counterparts because they also complex with sulfhydryl radicals. The blood–brain barrier provides little impediment to the crossing of alkyl mercurials. When they reach the brain, turnover is slower than in other organs. After chronic exposure, approximately 10% of the total body burden of alkyl phosphates localizes in the brain. Strong affinity for the sulfhydryl group of amino acids exists so that the alkyl mercury is quickly bound to protein or polypeptides and tends to remain in bound organic form. Less than 3% of the total mercury is degraded to inorganic mercury.

No warning symptoms occur in individuals exposed to alkyl mercurials until toxic or even fatal amounts have been incorporated. The most frequent initial manifestations are dysesthesias of the extremities, beginning in the fingers and toes and extending to a glove-stocking distribution. The visual fields may be concentrically constricted, and this alteration appears as the initial symptom in approximately half the cases. The visual impairment may proceed to include optic atrophy and, ultimately, blindness. As the condition progresses, almost all patients demonstrate evidence of cerebellar involvement, with unsteady gait, slurred speech, and poor coordination. Neurogenic deafness is another commonly observed finding. Less common manifestations include resting or postural tremor, chorea, athetosis, myoclonus, rigidity, decerebrate posturing, lability of affect, mental deterioration, comatose states, akinetic mutism, contractions, and excessive sweating.

A family that ingested mercury-contaminated pork during a 3-month period in 1969 was examined at the time of intoxication and followed for 22 years. Four children developed severe methyl mercury poisoning acutely, and the most profound signs occurred in the youngest, a neonate exposed *in utero*. Signs included balance and coordination problems, weakness, and cortical blindness. The adults, although exposed, had no symptoms of intoxication acutely. At 22-year follow-up, the two oldest children had cortical blindness. The two youngest ones had died during early adulthood, each demented, mute, diffusely weak with involuntary movements in the extremities, and with seizures. One adult had developed poor tandem gait. In the autopsy specimen, regional mercury levels correlated with the extend of brain damage, which was most marked in the paracentral and parietal–occipital cortex. Since most mercury was inorganic, the authors suggested that methyl mercury had entered the brain but was endogenously biotransformed over many years and thereafter remained in high concentrations in the inorganic form because this chemical does not easily cross the blood–brain barrier.

It is difficult to diagnose mercury toxicity from laboratory data because of variability of blood and urine measurements. Although measurements in blood and hair are less variable than those in urine, these do not accurately reflect the degree of mercury toxicity. In urine, levels higher than 35 μg/g creatinine are considered elevated. Hair samples must be collected according to specific protocols. For example, head samples must be taken close to the scalp and then washed to remove contaminants, such as hair dyes or hair treatments. The advantage of hair samples is that they provide exposure information for the past year. Pubic hair has the advantage of being more likely free of mercury-containing surface contaminants.

For treatment, mercury-binding compounds augment excretion of the metal in intoxicated patients regardless of the type of mercury exposure. The agents employed include D-penicillamine, n-acetyl-DL-penicillamine, and thiol resins. Dimer-caprol is no longer utilized because it increased cerebral mercury concentrations in animals experimentally receiving the methyl form. Administration of chelating agents results in only irregular removal of mercury from the body. When chelating agents are administered, mercury concentrations of blood increase for 1–3 days, presumably as a result of rapid mobilization from the tissues and a slower rate of urinary and fecal excretion. After this period, blood concentrations decline. Thiol resins are not absorbed from the gastrointestinal tract so they can be administered orally to bind mercury in bile and other fluids within the intestine. Fecal excretion is then enhanced by preventing reabsorption of methyl mercury so that redistribution of mercury in the body will not occur. Because thiol resins cannot reenter the body, they have no potentially adverse systemic effects. Spironolactone has also been employed in the experimental treatment of inorganic mercury poisoning. The protective effect appears to be related to increasing stool excretion through an unknown mechanism.

Most patients with severe mercury poisoning die within a few weeks of symptom onset, and those who survive have major neurological disability. In those with mild or moderate neurological symptoms, especially children and young adults, improvement may occur within the first 6 months. Cases have also been reported of ataxic, bedridden individuals who regained the ability to walk and of children who were totally blind but regained vision.

—*Christopher G. Goetz*

See also—Dioxin; Environmental Toxins; Lead; Manganese; Neuropathy, Toxic; Neurotoxicology, Overview

Further Reading

Davis, L. E., Kornfeld, M., Mooney, H. S., *et al.* (1994). Methyl mercury poisoning: Long-term clinical, radiological, toxicologic, and pathologic studies of an affected family. *Ann. Neurol.* 35, 680–688.

Franchi, E., Loprieno, G., Ballardin, M., *et al.* (1994). Cytogenetic monitoring of fishermen with environmental mercury exposure. *Mutat. Res.* 320, 23–29.

Goetz, C. G., and Washburn, K. R. (1999). Metals and neurotoxicology. In *Medical Neurotoxicology* (P. G. Blain and J. B. Harris, Eds.), pp. 181–200. Arnold, London.

Grandjean, P., Weihe, P., and White, R. F. (1995). Milestone development in infants exposed to methylmercury from human milk. *Neurotoxicology* **16**, 27–33.

Levy, M. (1995). Dental amalgam: Toxicological evaluation and health risk assessment. *J. Can. Dent. Assoc.* **61**, 667–668, 671–674.

Sharma, D. C. (1987). Biochemical basis of the toxicity of mercury. *Med. Hypotheses* **23**, 259–263.

Singer, R., Valciukas, J. A., and Rosenman, K. D. (1987). Peripheral neurotoxicity in workers exposed to inorganic mercury compounds. *Arch. Environ. Health* **42**, 181–184.

Merritt, H. Houston

Encyclopedia of the Neurological Sciences
Copyright 2003, Elsevier Science (USA). All rights reserved.

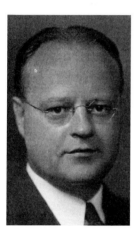

H. HOUSTON MERRITT (1902–1979), the outstanding clinical neurologist of his time in the United States, was a superb teacher, gifted researcher in the neurological field, author, and an excellent medical administrator from the departmental level to the vice presidency of a great university.

Merritt was born in Wilmington, North Carolina. He attended the Universities of North Carolina and Vanderbilt. In 1926, he received his M.D. degree from Johns Hopkins University. His postgraduate training included a year at Yale in internal medicine, two years at the Boston City Hospital in neurology, and a year in Berlin in neuropathology.

He began his academic career as an assistant professor of neurology (later associate professor) at the Harvard Neurological Unit of the Boston City Hospital (BCH). This neurological training program was supported by the Rockefeller Foundation, staffed by Harvard, and the BCH supplied the space and the numerous patients. Tracy J. Putnam chaired the unit. Merritt, as second in command, was the

mainstay. His brilliant diagnostic ability became legendary. Often, as a case was being presented to him, he would interrupt with the diagnosis before the history had begun. The diagnosis often was quite esoteric, such as an ependymoma of the filum terminale in a young man, but it proved correct. House officers highly respected him and were at ease with him, as he was with them. He was remarkable in his ability to avoid the use of rank, to lead rather than to drive. Therefore, an unusual camaraderie developed between Merritt and his residents.

Merritt's research required diligent, time-consuming effort. All the spinal fluids from the entire BCH were sent to his laboratory for chemical analysis. The results were reviewed daily. Patients not known to the department but with cerebrospinal fluid (CSF) abnormalities had their diagnoses verified by consultation. His landmark book, *The Cerebrospinal Fluid*, coauthored with Fremont-Smith, was based on approximately 21,000 spinal fluid examinations. In retrospect, this CSF monitoring was, as a by-product, a novel approach to improving the treatment of the neurological patients in a large hospital.

In the 1930s, phenobarbital was the mainstay of anticonvulsant therapy. The search for new medications was often empiric, based on some similarity in structure origin. The time was ripe for a scientific approach. Working with Tracy Putnam, the seizure threshold was established for the untreated, individual animal and again after phenobarbital and other barbiturates had been administered. Thus, the relative value of other barbiturates to phenobarbital was established. Moreover, new medications could be synthesized using molecules shown to have anticonvulsant possibilities. Thus, phenytoin (Dilantin) was discovered and its clinical efficacy determined. The floodgates were opened for new and better medications, thus improving the care of patients with epilepsy.

Early in academic life, one often has a delightful period when every day is a pleasure to live. Clinical achievements are satisfying. The challenges of research are being met. Teaching is thrilling. The relationships with patients, students, residents, and colleagues are ideal. This is often followed by a period of disillusionment. Most of Merritt's 13 years on the Harvard faculty were such a period. The unpleasant period followed when Putnam, the director, resigned. It was almost universally expected that Merritt would succeed. Instead, the Harvard trustees appointed Dr. Derek Denny-Brown. A few weeks later, England and Germany went to war with each other. This delayed, for more than a year, Denny-Brown's arrival. This interim was exceedingly difficult for Merritt. He met the challenge with extraordinary efforts, never complaining, holding the unit together for an indefinite period and for someone else.

In 1944, Merritt moved to New York to be professor of clinical neurology at Columbia University and chief of the Division of Neuropsychiatry at Montefiore Hospital. In 1948, he became professor and chairman of the Department of Neurology at Columbia University and director of the neurological services at the New York Neurological Institute (NYNI). He proved so effective in upgrading the NYNI that he is generally regarded as its first director.

His uncanny abilities for development and improvement led to his being appointed dean of the College of Physicians and Surgeons of Columbia University and vice president of the University for Health Affairs. These were not easy times in university administration because the anti-Vietnam War movements were in full force among students, including those of Columbia University.

With all these administrative duties, he maintained his clinical and teaching efforts. In 1955, the first edition of *A Textbook of Neurology* was published. This he kept current for six editions. The sixth edition was published just 2 weeks after his death.

Merritt's clinical acumen was widely sought after. His famous patients included President Eisenhower, Premier António de Oliviera Salazar of Portugal, and composer Dimitri Shostakovich. Approximately 38 of his former residents became department chairs, and he was frequently asked to be the visiting professor at their institutions. Thus, he shared his tremendous knowledge of clinical neurology with another generation.

His many achievements were recognized by awards. At Columbia the chair of neurology is endowed in his name, a conference room is named for him, and he was given the Distinguished Service Award of the Columbia University College of Medicine and Surgery. Both Harvard and Columbia awarded him honorary degrees.

He served as president of the American Neurological Association, the Association for Research in Nervous and Mental Diseases, the American Board of Psychiatry and Neurology, and the Ninth International Congress of Neurology. Voluntary health organizations—the Multiple Sclerosis, Muscular Dystrophy, Cerebral Palsy, and Epilepsy Societies—recognized his efforts with awards.

Merritt and his wife, Mabel Carmichael Merritt, although childless, enjoyed their nieces, nephews, and the children of their young associates. At their home, be it in Cambridge, Bronxville, or, in the summer, New Bedford, they graciously welcomed their many colleagues.

Merritt served as the role model for a generation of neurologists, not only as the brilliant clinician but also in his perseverance in clinical research and administrative fields. With a ready wit, he never complained but, despite difficulties, kept steadfastly proceeding on course. Thus, he achieved so much.

—*Francis M. Forster*

***See also*—Antiepileptic Drugs (see Index entry Biography for complete list of biographical entries)**

Further Reading

Merritt, H. H. (1955). *A Textbook of Neurology.* Lea & Febiger, Philadelphia.

Merritt, H. H., and Fremont-Smith, F. (1938). *The Cerebrospinal Fluid.* Saunders, Philadelphia.

Merritt, H. H., Putnam, T. J., and Schwab, D. H. (1938). A new series of anticonvulsant-drugs tested by experiments in animals. *Arch. Neurol. Psychiatry* 39, 1003.

Merritt, H. H., and Putnam, T. J. (1938). Sodium diphenyl hydantoinate in the treatment of convulsive disorders. *J. Am. Med. Assoc.* 111, 1068.

Metastases, Brain

Encyclopedia of the Neurological Sciences
Copyright 2003, Elsevier Science (USA). All rights reserved.

THERE ARE TWO main types of brain tumors. Primary brain tumors arise from cells native to the central nervous system (CNS) and originate in the brain. Metastatic brain tumors begin growth in tissues outside the CNS and then spread secondarily to involve the brain.

Of the two types, metastases to the brain are much more common and outnumber primary brain tumors by at least 10 to 1. The exact frequency of brain metastases is difficulty to determine with precision, but they are estimated to affect 20–40% of cancer patients. These percentages may increase in the future as the ability to detect small tumors with magnetic resonance imaging (MRI) improves. The frequency of brain metastases may also increase due to the longer survival of cancer patients in general.

Not all cancers in the body produce brain metastases at the same rate. In adults, the most common sources of brain metastases are the lung, breast, gastrointestinal tract, genitourinary tract, and skin (malignant melanoma), in that order. In patients younger than 21 years of age, brain metastases arise most often from sarcomas (osteogenic sarcoma, rhabdomyosarcoma, and Ewing's sarcoma) and germ cell tumors. Cerebral metastatic disease in children is less frequent than in adults and affects approximately 6–10% of children with cancer. The clinical presentation and neurological manifestations of cerebral metastases in children are similar to those seen in adults, and the approach to diagnosis and treatment is the same.

Most tumor cells are carried to the brain by the blood, almost always through the arterial circulation. Most commonly, the metastasis originates in the lung from either a primary lung cancer or a metastasis to the lung. Metastases do not appear randomly in the brain, and most are found in the area of the gray/white junction. This is due to a change in the size of blood vessels at that point; the narrowed vessels act as a trap for emboli. Brain metastases tend to be more common at the terminal watershed areas of arterial circulation (the zones on the border of or between the territories of the major cerebral vessels). The distribution of metastases among the large vascular subdivisions of the CNS follows approximately the relative weight and blood flow to each area. Accordingly, approximately 80% of brain metastases are located in the cerebral hemispheres, 15% in the cerebellum, and 5% in the brainstem.

Brain metastases may be single or multiple. The proportion of multiple metastases is high, and two-thirds to three-fourths of patients have multiple brain metastases at diagnosis. It is probable that with the widespread use of MRI and improvements in MRI contrast agents and resolution, the proportion of multiple metastases will be even higher in the future. Metastases from colon, breast, and renal cell carcinoma are often single, whereas malignant melanoma and lung cancer have a greater tendency to produce multiple cerebral lesions.

Metastases to the brain usually produce symptoms, and more than two-thirds of patients with brain metastases have some neurological symptoms during the course of their illness. More than 80% of brain metastases are discovered after the diagnosis of systemic cancer has been made. The clinical presentation of brain metastases is similar to that of other mass lesions in the brain. Headache is a common presenting symptom, and this may be followed after an interval of days or weeks by other focal symptoms or signs. However, the headache may be mild and is rarely of localizing value. Early morning headache (usually thought to be associated with raised intracranial pressure) is a presenting symptom in only 40% of patients with brain metastases. Headaches are more common with multiple metastases or posterior fossa lesions. Focal weakness is the second most common presenting symptom of metastases to the brain. Seizures, either focal or generalized, occur in approximately 10% of patients at diagnosis. They are more common in patients with multiple metastases. Abnormalities of higher mental function may take the form of a nonfocal encephalopathy (1 or 2% of patients with brain metastases exhibit this symptom complex), but more commonly neurological symptoms are due to localized dysfunction (e.g., aphasia caused by a metastasis in the speech area). Five to 10% of patients may present with acute neurological symptoms caused by hemorrhage into the tumor or cerebral infarction from embolic or compressive occlusion of a blood vessel. Hemorrhage into a metastasis is particularly common with choriocarcinoma and melanoma, although it can occur in a metastasis from any primary brain tumor. Indeed, the signs and symptoms related to cerebral metastatic lesions are extremely varied, and the suspicion of brain metastases should be raised in all patients with known systemic cancer in whom new neurological findings develop.

The best diagnostic test for brain metastases is contrast-enhanced MRI. If the clinical history is typical and lesions are multiple, usually there is little doubt about the diagnosis. However, it is important that metastases be distinguished carefully from primary brain tumors (benign or malignant), abscesses, cerebral infarction, and hemorrhages. One study showed that the false-positive rate, even when using contrast MRI for the diagnosis of single brain metastases, is approximately 11%. Other diagnostic tests, such as arteriography or biopsy, may be needed to firmly establish the diagnosis.

The optimum therapy of brain metastases (single or multiple) is still evolving. Several methods of treatment are available for patients with intracranial metastases. Corticosteroids, radiotherapy, and surgical therapy all have an established place in management, and as a result of recent randomized trials the role of radiosurgery is also becoming clearer. In addition, chemotherapy is useful in some patients with chemosensitive tumors. When determining the best treatment for each patient, the following must be considered: the extent of systemic disease, neurological status at diagnosis, and the number and site of metastases. Regardless of treatment, brain metastases are associated with a poor prognosis. Untreated patients have a median survival of only approximately 4 weeks. Nearly all untreated patients die as a direct result of the brain tumor, with increasing intracranial pressure leading to obtundation and terminal cerebral herniation.

ANTICONVULSANTS

Seizures occur in approximately 25% of patients with brain metastases and are the presenting complaint in 10–15% of patients. Randomized studies have shown that prophylactic anticonvulsants do not reduce the frequency of first seizures in patients with newly diagnosed brain metastases. Therefore, anticonvulsants should only be given to patients who have actually had seizures and should not be given routinely to all patients when brain metastasis is diagnosed.

CORTICOSTEROIDS

Almost all patients with brain metastases should be started on corticosteroid (steroid) therapy. Patients with small, completely asymptomatic lesions may not need steroids; however, steroids may reduce the side effects of cranial radiotherapy and are rarely harmful for short periods of time. The mechanism of action of corticosteroids is not completely understood, although a reduction in the edema surrounding the metastatic tumors is a frequent finding. The beneficial effects of steroids are noticeable within 6–24 hr after the first dose and reach maximum effect in 3–7 days. The median survival time of patients treated with steroids alone is approximately 2 months.

RADIOTHERAPY

Radiotherapy is the treatment of choice for most patients with brain metastases. Unfortunately, there is no consensus on the optimum radiation dose and schedule for the treatment of brain metastases. Most patients are treated with whole brain radiotherapy (WBRT) because more than two-thirds have multiple metastases at diagnosis, which usually makes surgical or other focal treatment ineffective. Several large-scale, multiinstitutional trials conducted by the Radiation Therapy Oncology Group (RTOG) have shown that there is no significant difference in the frequency and duration of response for total radiation doses ranging from 2000 cGy over 1 week to 5000 cGy over 4 weeks. Regimens of 1000 cGy in a single dose or 1200 cGy in two doses were less effective and are no longer in use.

Currently, typical radiation treatment schedules for brain metastases consist of short courses (7–15 days) of whole brain irradiation with relatively high doses per fraction (150–400 cGy per day), with total doses in the range of 3000–5000 cGy. These schedules minimize the duration of treatment while still delivering adequate amounts of radiation to the tumor. Additional focal irradiation to the tumor site is not beneficial. Giving a boost dose to the tumor along with WBRT is no better than WBRT alone in preventing neurological recurrences or increasing survival.

Whole brain radiotherapy increases the median survival to 3–6 months. Data from large retrospective studies have shown that more than half of patients treated with WBRT die of progressive systemic cancer and not from their brain metastases. Retrospective studies on large numbers of patients treated in RTOG brain metastasis protocols have identified patient subgroups that were more likely to respond to WBRT. More favorable outcome is associated with Karnofsky performance scores of 70% or higher, absent or "controlled" primary tumor, patient age younger than 60 years, and metastatic spread limited to the brain. Building on these results, a recursive partitioning analysis (RPA) was applied to a combined group consisting of patients from several past RTOG radiotherapy studies. Three distinct prognostic groups were identified. The most favorable prognostic group was designated RPA class 1 and consisted of patients whose Karnofsky scores were 70% or higher, age was 65 years or less, primary tumors were controlled, and no extracranial metastases were present. RPA class 3 patients had the worst prognosis; these patients had Karnofsky scores less than 70% (with or without other unfavorable factors). RPA class 2 patients included patients who did not fit into class 1 or 3 (i.e., patients who had Karnofsky scores 70% or higher but also had one or more of the other unfavorable factors). Clearly, performance status at the time of treatment for brain metastases is the most important prognostic factor.

Radiotherapy has complications. Almost all patients experience a temporary loss of hair, but it can return 6–12 months after completing therapy. Also, in the short term, patients may have a transient worsening of neurological symptoms while receiving therapy. Many physicians believe that maintaining patients on steroids during radiotherapy minimizes complications, although conclusive proof is not available. During the initial days of treatment, mild symptoms, such as nausea, vomiting, headache, and fever, are common. This acute reaction may relate to distorted cerebrovascular autoregulation or increased capillary permeability induced by the radiotherapy. The long-term side effects of radiotherapy are usually not a significant issue for patients with brain metastases because of their relatively short survival. However, as many as 10% of long-term survivors (>12 months) may develop symptoms such as dementia, ataxia, and urinary incontinence caused by delayed radiation damage to the brain.

SURGERY

Surgical therapy is usually not an option for most patients with brain metastases because of multiple lesions or extensive systemic cancer. However, in the subgroup of patients who have isolated cerebral metastases, death is more likely due to the brain metastases than to progressive systemic disease. Therefore, in patients with controlled systemic cancer in whom brain metastases develop, treatment of the brain disease will determine survival. It is for this group that the question of more aggressive therapy, particularly surgery, for the brain metastasis is usually raised. Several advances during the past 20 years have decreased the risks associated with craniotomy. Safer anesthesia, the widespread use of corticosteroids, the development of modern noninvasive cranial imaging technology, and the introduction of stereotactic approaches have been foremost among these changes.

Three prospective randomized trials have assessed the value of surgical removal of single brain metastases. In a prospective randomized trial performed at the University of Kentucky, 48 patients with known systemic cancer were treated with either biopsy of the suspected brain metastasis plus WBRT or complete surgical resection of the metastasis plus WBRT. The radiation doses were the same in both groups and consisted of a total dose of 3600 cGy given as 12 daily fractions of 300 cGy each. There was a statistically significant increase in survival in the surgical group (40 vs 15 weeks). In addition, the time to recurrence of brain metastases, freedom from death due to neurological causes, and duration of functional independence were significantly longer in the surgical group. The 1-month mortality was 4% in each group, indicating that there was no extra mortality from surgery. An important finding was that despite screening with both contrast-enhanced MRI and computed tomography before entry into the study, 6 of 54 (11%) patients with known diagnoses of systemic malignancies were found not to have metastatic brain tumors when tissue was obtained at biopsy or attempted resection. The nonmetastatic lesions consisted of three astrocytomas, two abscesses, and one sterile inflammatory lesion.

A second randomized study, conducted as a multiinstitutional trial in The Netherlands, contained 63 evaluable patients. Patients were randomized to either complete surgical resection plus WBRT or WBRT alone. The WBRT schedules were the same for both treatment arms and consisted of 4000 cGy given in a nonstandard fractionation scheme of 200 cGy twice per day for 2 weeks (10 treatment days). Survival was significantly longer in the surgical group (10 vs 6 months). There was also a nonsignificant trend toward longer duration of functional independence in the surgically treated patients. No data concerning recurrence of brain metastases were provided. The 1-month mortality rates were 9% in the surgery group and 0% in the WBRT alone group; this was not a statistically significant difference.

Although diagnostic biopsies were not obtained in the WBRT alone group, 1 patient (out of 31) in this group was later found to have a malignant glioma after having surgery performed for progression of the presumed metastasis. All 32 patients in the surgery group had metastatic tumors verified pathologically at operation. Two additional patients were randomized into the study but excluded from the final analysis because they were found not to have metastases before the start of treatment. In all, 5% (3/65) did not have metastatic tumors.

A third randomized trial, conducted in Canada by Mintz *et al.*, failed to find a benefit from surgical treatment. In this study, 84 patients were randomized to receive radiotherapy alone (3000 cGy) or surgery plus radiotherapy. No difference was found in overall survival; the median survival was 6.3 months in the radiotherapy alone group and 5.6 months for the surgical group. There were also no differences in causes of death or quality of life. Only 1 patient of the 40 who had surgery had a lesion that was not a metastatic brain tumor; this patient had a glioblastoma.

It is unclear why the results from the Canadian study differed from those of the other two trials. In all three studies, the control arms (the radiation alone arms) had median survivals in the 3- to 6-month range—well within the expected range for patients treated with radiotherapy alone. The major difference in the studies was the poor outcome obtained in the surgical arm of the Canadian trial. That study contained a higher proportion of patients with extensive systemic disease and lower performance scores. Differences in patient selection in the Canadian trial may well have contributed to its failure to detect a significant benefit from the addition of surgical therapy. Also, the Canadian health care system sometimes discourages aggressive and expensive treatment for patients with disseminated cancer. It is possible that these factors (i.e., selection and philosophy) resulted in more patients dying of their systemic cancer before a long-term benefit of surgery was seen.

Although the data supporting surgery for single brain metastases were derived from relatively small randomized trials that were not uniformly positive, the results have generally been interpreted to show that surgical resection is beneficial in selected patients. Surgical therapy plus postoperative WBRT is now the treatment of choice for patients with surgically accessible single brain metastases.

The value of surgery in the management of multiple metastases remains to be demonstrated. It is difficult to draw firm conclusions regarding the efficacy of surgery for multiple metastases from the studies published to date. Current practice is to treat multiple metastases with WBRT alone. Surgery is sometimes performed on patients with multiple metastases who have one life-threatening brain lesion (e.g., a large compressive cerebellar lesion). The intent of surgery in these cases is to remove the single life-threatening lesion and to treat the remaining tumors with WBRT. Although this approach is speculative, long survival times have occasionally been achieved.

Despite the advantage of surgery in selected patients, WBRT alone remains the treatment for most patients with brain metastases. Single metastases occur in less than one-fourth of patients; unfortunately, approximately half of patients in this group are not surgical candidates due to inaccessibility of the tumor, extensive systemic disease, and other factors. Therefore, at most, only approxi-mately 10–15% of all patients with brain metastases will benefit from surgical resection. The rest should be treated with radiotherapy.

The best results from surgery are seen in those patients with a single surgically accessible lesion and either no remaining systemic disease (true solitary metastasis) or with controlled systemic cancer limited to the primary site only. Also, surgical treatment is indicated in those patients without known systemic cancer (to obtain a tissue diagnosis) and in patients with impending herniation due to pressure effects.

A point of controversy has been whether postoperative radiotherapy needs to be given as WBRT (as opposed to focal radiation) or whether radiotherapy is even necessary at all after a complete resection of a single metastasis. There is no doubt that radiation therapy, when given as the only treatment for brain metastases, results in longer survival. Postoperative WBRT is thought to be beneficial because there may be residual disease in the tumor bed or at distant microscopic sites in the brain. However, brain metastases tend to be discrete masses that are theoretically capable of being totally removed, and so postoperative WBRT may not be necessary.

Retrospective studies that examined the role of postoperative radiotherapy in the management of single brain metastasis failed to answer the question because of conflicting results. Only one randomized trial has addressed the question of postoperative radiotherapy. In this study, 95 patients who had single brain metastases that were completely resected (as determined by postoperative MRI scans) were randomized to postoperative WBRT (50.4 Gy) or to observation with no further treatment of the brain metastasis (until recurrence). Recurrence of tumor anywhere in the brain was significantly less frequent in the radiotherapy group than in the observation group (18 vs 70%). Postoperative radiotherapy prevented brain recurrence at the site of the original metastasis (10 vs 46%) and at other sites in the brain (14 vs 37%). As a result, patients in the radiotherapy group were less likely to die of neurological causes than patients in the observation group [6 of 43 died (14%) vs 17 of 39 (44%)]. However, there was no significant difference between the two groups in overall survival or the time during which patients remained functionally independent. The lack of difference in overall survival and quality of life may be explained by the fact that of the 32 patients in the observation group who had recurrence of brain metastases, 29 (91%) received WBRT at recurrence. This diluted the effect of WBRT given immediately postoperatively by most likely improving survival and quality of life in the observation group.

Several conclusions can be drawn from the randomized study. Radiotherapy prevents recurrence of tumor and reduces death from neurological causes. In addition, postoperative MRI scanning is relatively unreliable at detecting residual disease in the operative bed and at other sites in the brain. Postoperative WBRT reduced distant brain recurrences (outside the initial operative site); this shows that most of the micrometastases at distant sites were already present in the brain when radiotherapy was given. Radiotherapy would not have had an effect on metastases resulting from reseeding of the brain after completion of treatment. Therefore, although it is possible that a few recurrences were caused by reseeding, the major mechanism of metastasis to the brain appears to be a single event consisting of a shower of tumor emboli that become lodged at multiple sites in the brain. All these factors justify the routine use of WBRT, even after apparently complete resections.

RADIOSURGERY

Stereotactic radiosurgery, which is a method of delivering intense focal irradiation using a linear accelerator or multiple cobalt 60 sources (Gamma Knife), has been used with increasing frequency to treat single and multiple brain metastases. Radiosurgery does not replace conventional radiotherapy to the brain but may offer a substitute for surgical therapy in patients with lesions less than 3 cm in diameter.

To date, much of our information on radiosurgery comes from nonrandomized studies. For single metastases, the combined results of many retrospective reports suggest that radiosurgery prevents (or controls) local recurrence of 80–90% of treated metastases with approximately a 5–10% risk of radiation necrosis or new neurological deficits. Despite these apparently promising results, it is important to note that radiosurgery has not been established as an unequivocally effective treatment of single brain metastases. Prospective randomized clinical trials are still needed and are currently under way to determine the role of radiosurgery both in the initial treatment of patients with single metastases and in the management of recurrent brain metastases.

The role of radiosurgery in the treatment of multiple metastases has recently been the subject of three randomized trials. The first was reported by Kondziolka et al. This study contained only 27 patients and used nonstandard end points. As a result, it was uninterpretable. A second study reported by Chougule et al. contained methodological errors that made it impossible to draw firm conclusions from the data.

The RTOG reported the results of a randomized study involving patients with multiple brain metastases. This study (RTOG 9508) contained 144 patients with two or three brain metastases who were randomized to treatment with either WBRT (37.5 Gy) plus radiosurgery or WBRT (37.5 Gy) alone. There was no significant difference in failure rates in the brain: 21% in the radiosurgery arm and 37% in the WBRT alone arm. There was also no significant difference in survival of the two groups (median, 5.3 months for radiosurgery and 6.7 months for WBRT alone). Most noteworthy was the lack of difference between the percentages of patients in each group who died of neurological causes (33% radiosurgery vs 35% WBRT alone). Lower post-treatment Karnofsky scores and steroid dependence were more common in the WBRT alone patients. Nevertheless, this was a completely negative trial with regard to the major end points of tumor control in the brain, prevention of death due to neurological causes, and overall survival.

The results of RTOG 9508 have forced a major reevaluation of the use of radiosurgery in the treatment of brain metastases. This was the largest and best trial done to date, and it clearly failed to show a benefit of radiosurgery in the treatment of multiple brain metastases when radiosurgery was given in the management of newly diagnosed tumors. Treatment with WBRT alone now appears to be the treatment of choice in these circumstances. However, radiosurgery may still have a place as salvage treatment in patients who have recurrent brain tumors after WBRT, but this remains to be demonstrated. There have been no definitive randomized trials of radiosurgery in the upfront management of single brain metastases, but RTOG 9508 has a second ongoing study evaluating radiosurgery in these patients that it is hoped will further define the role of radiosurgery in the future.

CHEMOTHERAPY

Although chemotherapy has not emerged as a standard of therapy for patients with brain metastases, evidence has been accumulating that chemotherapy may have a role in the treatment of selected patients. Since more than half of patients with brain metastases who are treated with surgery or radiotherapy will subsequently die of systemic tumor progression, a chemotherapeutic agent that is effective against both systemic and brain disease is highly desirable. However, most systemically administered chemotherapeutic agents that are active against the primary cancer are ineffective against cerebral metastases from that primary tumor.

Chemotherapy has been used in the treatment of brain metastases from a variety of primary tumors, but results are generally modest. However, brain metastases from certain highly chemosensitive tumors (e.g., breast, small cell lung cancer, and germ cell tumors) have been treated effectively with chemotherapy. Recently, temozolamide, a new oral chemotherapeutic agent, has shown promise in the treatment of metastases. However, chemotherapy is rarely the primary therapy for most patients and is seldom the only therapy.

Currently, a reasonable use for chemotherapy for brain metastases is in those patients with small, asymptomatic tumors from primaries that are known to be chemosensitive. If progression occurs with the patient receiving chemotherapy alone, more definitive treatment with surgery, radiosurgery, or radiotherapy may be given.

—Roy A. Patchell

See also–Acoustic Neuroma; Brain Tumors, Biology; Brain Tumors, Clinical Manifestations and Treatment; Brain Tumors, Genetics; Central Nervous System Tumors; Childhood Brain Tumors; Glial Tumors; Meningiomas; Nerve Sheath Tumors; Pituitary Tumors; Spinal Cord Tumors, Biology of

Further Reading

Berk, L. (1995). An overview of radiotherapy trials for the treatment of brain metastases. *Oncology* 9, 1205–1219.

Delattre, J. Y., Krol, G., Thaler, H. T., *et al.* (1988). Distribution of brain metastases. *Arch. Neurol.* 45, 741–744.

Gaspar, L., Scott, C., Rotman, M., *et al.* (1997). Recursive partitioning analysis (RPA) of prognostic factors in three Radiation Therapy Oncology Group (RTOG) brain metastases trials. *Int. J. Radiat. Oncol. Biol. Phys.* 37, 745–751.

Glantz, M. J., Cole, B. F., Forsyth, P. A., *et al.* (2000). Practice parameter: Anticonvulsant prophylaxis in patients with newly diagnosed brain tumors. Report of the Quality Standards Subcommittee of the American Academy of Neurology. *Neurology* 54, 1886–1893.

Mintz, A. H., Kestle, J., Gaspar, L., *et al.* (1996). A randomized trial to assess the efficacy of surgery in addition to radiotherapy in patients with single cerebral metastasis. *Cancer* 78, 1470–1476.

Patchell, R. A., Tibbs, P. A., Walsh, J. W., *et al.* (1990). A randomized trial of surgery in the treatment of single metastases to the brain. *N. Engl. J. Med.* 322, 494–500.

Patchell, R. A., Tibbs, P. A., Regine, W. F., *et al.* (1998). Postoperative radiotherapy in the treatment of single metastases to the brain: A randomized trial. *J. Am. Med. Assoc.* 280, 1485–1489.

Sperduto, P. W., Scott, C., Andrews, D., *et al.* (2000). Preliminary report of RTOG-9508: A phase III trial comparing whole brain irradiation alone versus whole brain irradiation plus stereotactic radiosurgery for patients with two or three brain metastases. *Int. J. Radiat. Oncol. Biol. Phys.* 48, 113.

Vecht, C. J., Haaxma-Reiche, H., Noordijk, E. M., *et al.* (1993). Treatment of single brain metastasis: Radiotherapy alone or combined with neurosurgery. *Ann. Neurol.* 33, 583–590.

Methyl Alcohol

Encyclopedia of the Neurological Sciences
Copyright 2003, Elsevier Science (USA). All rights reserved.

METHYL ALCOHOL (methanol, wood alcohol) is used as a solvent, as a component of antifreeze, and as a frequent adulterant of alcoholic beverages. Although the compound is only mildly toxic, its oxidation products, formaldehyde and formic acid, induce a severe acidosis and account for the toxic signs related to methanol. The amount of methyl alcohol needed to cause serious effects varies with the individual. Some of this variation is attributed to a protective effect that ethyl alcohol may exert when consumed together with methanol. The two compounds share the same degradating enzyme, alcohol dehydrogenase, so that the competition by ethanol tends to diminish the rapid metabolism of methanol and the resultant production of toxic formaldehyde and formic acid.

In general, the breakdown and excretion of methyl alcohol is slow so that toxic symptoms do not develop for 12–48 hr and then may last for several days. When toxic symptoms and signs do appear, they involve the visual apparatus, the central nervous system, and the gastrointestinal and respiratory tracts. Clinical toxicity relates to metabolic acidosis as well as to the direct effects of the accumulation of toxic products. Early symptoms include nausea, vomiting, generalized weakness, severe abdominal pain, vertigo, and headache. Symptoms similar to severe ethyl alcohol toxicity appear, with restlessness and incoordination, and these may progress to delirium and hallucinations. Confusion and memory defects are common during intoxication. Increasing severity of the poisoning may lead to a depressed level of consciousness and coma, muscle jerks, and even seizures.

Visual disturbance and ocular abnormalities are frequent with methanol poisoning. Visual loss usually begins a few hours after consumption, although it may be delayed several days. Decreased vision, blind spots, or total blindness occur and may be the first disturbance noted. The pupils may be markedly dilated, causing light sensitivity and pain. After 3–6 days, pallor of the optic disks may be detected with an ophthalmological examination. The vision may improve after recovery from the acute intoxication, but permanent blind spots or total blindness often result. Profound nuchal rigidity may be present along with coma, resembling an acute meningitis.

In survivors of methanol intoxication, blindness and parkinsonian features are prominent. Bradykinesia or slowness, low voice volume, lack of facial expression, and tremor occur. Dementia and additional motor signs, with either increased or decreased reflexes, may accompany the clinical picture. Parkinsonian features may be associated with damage of the brain areas of the basal ganglia known to be involved in Parkinson's disease and other parkinsonian syndromes. Despite the similarity of signs with Parkinson's disease, methanol-intoxicated subjects do not respond well to the drugs generally used to treat Parkinson's disease, suggesting that primary targets of damage do not affect the cells that produce the chemical dopamine.

To manage acute intoxication, a three-part approach to treatment has been developed that involves the use of ethanol, bicarbonate, and, in severe cases, dialysis. Frequent measurements of methanol, CO_2, bicarbonate, and pH levels in the blood are essential. Ethyl alcohol administration saturates the alcohol dehydrogenase enzyme and thereby retards the conversion of methanol into its toxic by-products, formaldehyde and formic acid. Because methanol metabolism is slow, alkalinization must be carried out for several days to avoid relapses. Attention must be paid to the level of serum potassium, which tends to decrease with bicarbonate therapy. Dialysis is advocated when the methanol or formic acid blood concentrations are high.

—*Christopher G. Goetz*

See also–Alcohol-Related Neurotoxicity;
**Environmental Toxins; Intoxication; Lead;
Manganese; Mercury; Neuropathy, Toxic;
Neurotoxicology, Overview**

Further Reading

Goetz, C. G., Kompoliti, K., and Washburn, K. (1996). Neurotoxic agents. In *Clinical Neurology* (R. J. Joynt and R. C. Griggs, Eds.), Vol. 2, pp. 1–112. Lippincott–Raven, Philadelphia.

LeWitt, P. A., and Martin, S. D. (1988). Dystonia and hypokinesia with putaminal necrosis after methanol intoxication. *Clin. Neuropharmacol.* **2**, 161–167.

McLean, D. R., Jacobs, H., and Mielke, B. W. (1980). Methanol poisoning. *Ann. Neurol.* **8**, 161–167.

Mittal, B. V., Desai, A. P., and Khade, K. R. (1991). Methyl alcohol poisoning: An autopsy study of 28 cases. *J. Postgrad. Med.* **37**, 9–13.

Methylmalonic Acidurias
see Organic Acid Disorders

Mevalonic Aciduria
see Organic Acid Disorders

Meynert, Theodor Hermann

Encyclopedia of the Neurological Sciences

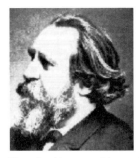

Theodor Hermann Meynert (reproduced with permission from the Louis D. Boshes archives at the University of Illinois at Chicago).

THEODOR MEYNERT (1833–1892) continues to emerge as an important figure in the history of neuroscience, recently labeled the founder of scientific brain research.

Meynert was born in Dresden, the son of a renowned historian and a well-known opera singer. He moved in influential Viennese social circles and taught some of the most notable figures in the history of neuroscience, including Sigmund Freud, James Jackson Putnam, and Carl Wernicke. He is perhaps best known as a neuroanatomist, with his name eponymically linked to at least seven areas of the brain, including the nucleus basalis of Meynert (made famous by its vulnerability to neurodegenerative pathology). Meynert also used his detailed anatomical studies to develop models of brain function that foreshadowed modern conceptions of relationships between cortical and subcortical structures, and he also attempted clinical pathological correlations. He described amentia as a form of what is now called delirium and the clinical features of aphasias related to damage in arcuate fasciculus, which he discovered with Wernicke, based on anatomical dissections.

Meynert's work was not universally esteemed by his contemporaries, some of whom were skeptical about the domination of biological methods and their relevance to the practical care for patients. However, during the past three decades, his contributions have drawn increased attention and have come to seem increasingly relevant. For example, in a 1985 review, I (PJW) pointed out the relevance of Meynert's work to ongoing discussions about the utility of concepts such as cortical and subcortical dementia. Other historical commentators have described Meynert as a pioneer methodologist and focused on the particular geographic origins of his concept of neuroscience.

Particularly interesting about Meynert are his forays out of the brain into mind and soul. Perhaps influenced by the artistic and humanities background of his parents, Meynert turned to other forms of intellectual expression beside science, such as poetry. Papez stated that Meynert put soul into the brain.

We have claimed that our abilities to treat diseases such as Alzheimer's will be enhanced by integrating approaches from the sciences and humanities. Thus, Meynert's creative engagement of both science and poetry is intriguing. Today, faced with continued growth in the number of older people, we find ourselves returning to issues of care and quality of life. Contemporary neuroscientists, deeply enamored of the technoscientific progress of the human mind, would do well to recall the limits Meynert seemed to finally confront. Meynert the poet and Meynert the one who tried to vitalize the fine aspects of our spirit should be remembered as well as Meynert the pioneer visionary of brain research.

Meynert was not a reductionist but sought to understand brain function holistically. For example,

he was interested in the biological and philosophical foundations of intentionality. He believed that the distribution of blood flow between cortical and subcortical structures resulted in different intellectual and affective states.

—*Peter J. Whitehouse and Jesse Ballenger*

See also–Freud, Sigmund; Wernicke, Carl (see Index entry Biography for complete list of biographical entries)

Further Reading

Marx, O. (1970). Nineteenth-century medical psychology: Theoretical problems in the work of Griesinger, Meynert, and Wernicke. *ISIS* **61**, 355–370.

Marx, O. (1971). Psychiatry on a neuropathological basis: Th. Meynert's application for the extension of his venia legendi. *Clio Med.* **6**, 139–158.

Pappenheim, E. (1975). History of medicine on Meynert's amentia. *Int. J. Neurol.* **9**, 311–326.

Seitelberger, F. (1997). Theodor Meynert (1833–1892): Pioneer and visionary of brain research. *J. Hist. Neurosci.* **6**, 264–274.

Whitehouse, P. J. (1985). Theodor Meynert: Foreshadowing modern concepts of neuropsychiatric pathophysiology. *Neurology* **35**, 389–391.

Whitehouse, P. J., Struble, R. G., Hedreen, J. C., Clark, A. W., and Price, D. L. (1985). Alzheimer's disease and related dementias: Selective involvement of specific neuronal systems. *CRC Crit. Rev. Clin. Neurobiol.* **1**, 319–339.

Whitrow, M. (1996). Theodor Meynert (1833–1892): His life and poetry. *Hist. Psychiatry* **7**, 615–628.

Microcephaly

Encyclopedia of the Neurological Sciences
Copyright 2003, Elsevier Science (USA). All rights reserved.

THE TERM MICROCEPHALY refers to a condition in which the occipitofrontal head circumference is more than two standard deviations below the mean adjusted for age, sex, and race. Microcephaly implies a small brain, or micrencephaly, which can result from a variety of conditions. In primary micrencepaly (micrencephaly vera), the cerebral configuration is essentially normal without evidence of any destructive process, whereas in secondary micrencephaly there can be evidence of a variety of migrational abnormalities, other malformations, or pathological changes secondary to genetic or chromosomal abnormalities, pre- or perinatal hypoxemic–ischemia, inflammation, traumatic, toxic, or teratogenic agents, or exposure to irradiation during

Table 1 COMMON CAUSES OF MICROCEPHALY/
MICRENCEPHALY

Genetic
Chromosomal karyotype abnormality
Prenatal hypoxia–ischemia
Congenital infections
Trauma
Metabolic/endocrine
Chemical agents (exogenous)
Irradiation
Malnutrition

the first two trimesters of gestation (Table 1). Although the majority of people included in the category of microcephaly are mentally retarded, approximately 2% appear to have normal mentality.

The genetic forms of microcephaly include those inherited as an autosomal dominant trait, autosomal recessive, X-linked recessive, and a familial type of undetermined inheritance. Those persons with microcephaly inherited as an autosomal dominant trait generally have a less severe form with normal facies and normal physical habitus, although associated abnormalities of the digits have been reported. The recessive forms usually have a normal face with notably sloping forehead and very small head, upward slanting palpebral fissures, and relatively large ears. The X-linked recessive form is less common but can be manifested in patients with Pelizaeus–Merzbacher disease or neuronal ceroid lipofucsinosis.

The evaluation of patients with an abnormally small head requires obtaining not only a careful history of the prenatal and perinatal course but also both maternal and paternal family histories with particular regard to family members with small heads and those with diabetes mellitus or any other metabolic disease. It is prudent to obtain the physical measurements of both parents, if possible, and the siblings because one generally cannot completely rely on the casual information regarding physical attributes of family members. The prompt investigation for potential physical findings suggestive of congenital infection such as chorioretinitis, cardiac abnormalities, and abnormal liver function should be carried out and followed up with appropriate diagnostic tests, including blood titers or cultures of the cerebrospinal fluid. Studies for inborn errors of metabolism should be completed as drug or toxicology screens, and patients with associated neurological

and dysmorphic findings should have a chromosomal karyotype completed. Some associated physical findings may appear syndromic, in which case one should consult recognized sources of dysmorphology. Neuroimaging studies are an essential part of the evaluation. For example, computerized tomography should provide evidence of craniosynostosis; however, magnetic resonance imaging is superior in demonstrating the details of cerebral structures as well as gray and white matter.

—*Bruce Berg*

***See also*–Brain Development, Normal Postnatal; Dysmorphology; Megalencephaly**

Further Reading

Dolk, H. (1991). The predictive value of microcephaly during the first year of life for mental retardation at 7 years. *Dev. Med. Child Neurol.* **33**, 974–983.
Dorman, C. (1953). A clinical and genetic study of microcephaly. *Am. J. Ment. Defic.* **57**, 620–637.
Dorman, C. (1991). Microcephaly and intelligence. *Dev. Med. Child Neurol.* **33**, 267–269.
Jones, K. L. (1997). *Microcephaly. Smith's Recognizable Patterns of Human Malformation*, pp. 776–777. Saunders, Philadelphia.
Nellhaus, G. (1968). Head circumference from birth to 18 years. *Pediatrics* **59**, 106–114.
Sells, C. J. (1977). Microcephaly in a normal school population. *Pediatrics* **59**, 262–265.
Tolmi, J. L., McNay, M., Stephenson, J. B., *et al.* (1987). Microcephaly: Genetic counselling and antenatal diagnosis after the birth of an affected child. *Am. J. Med. Genet.* **27**, 583–594.

Microglia

Encyclopedia of the Neurological Sciences
Copyright 2003, Elsevier Science (USA). All rights reserved.

MICROGLIA are highly ramified (Fig. 1) macrophage precursor cells that are resident to the central nervous system (CNS). They are ubiquitously distributed in nonoverlapping territories throughout the CNS and comprise between 10 and 20% of the glial population. Microglia are not coupled by gap junctions like other glia, and this may be a key reason why microglial cells are territorial in their reaction pattern. Microglial activation, as indicated by the new expression of immune response-associated molecules [e.g., major histocompatibility complex (MHC) antigens and complement receptors], is usually confined to the site of disease activity and thus permits the

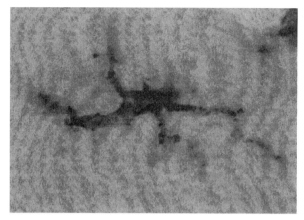

Figure 1
Human microglial cell immunoreactive for MHC class II antigen.

localization of disease processes. There appears to be no neuropathological condition without microglial participation because microglia respond even to slight alterations in their microenvironment. This includes remote lesioning of the CNS and even ionic disturbances. Microglia are now recognized as important "sensors" of threats to the CNS, a concept that is of great practical importance in diagnostic neuropathology as well as neuroimaging.

HISTORY

Microglial cells were discovered at the turn of the past century. Nissl's description of microglial rod cells (1899) represents the first mention of activated microglia. Robertson gave an independent account on microglial cells in 1900. The Spanish histologist Pio del Rio-Hortega, who invented a staining method for microglia and who named the cells, first conducted detailed studies on microglia in the 1920s. Microglial research was revived in the mid-1980s when new immunocytochemical and lectin markers became available. However, all microglia markers are only microglia specific in the sense that they do not label other glia or neurons, and most cross-react with peripheral macrophages.

MICROGLIAL ORIGIN

After an intense debate that lasted for decades, the developmental origin of microglia from monocytic cells is now widely accepted. Although microglia of the adult CNS form a very stable cell pool showing extremely little turnover and exchange with

peripheral bone marrow-derived cells under normal conditions, blood-derived monocytes/macrophages can enter lesioned CNS (trauma, infarct, and autoimmune inflammation) and transform into morphologically and immunophenotypically indistinguishable microglia cells.

MICROGLIAL ACTIVATION

Normal microglia of the healthy CNS are considered "resting" (i.e., they show a downregulated phenotype and are in a functionally quiescent mode). Upon stimulation through any type of insult to the CNS, microglia respond in a graded fashion. This response has been studied in detail in animal models that leave the blood–brain barrier intact, allowing the study of microglia in the absence of invading blood-derived cells. As a first reaction to pathological tissue change, microglia upregulate complement receptors and MHC antigens and may even undergo mitotic cell division. However, they do not necessarily become phagocytic. Instead, microglia can engage in the displacement of axon terminals (synaptic stripping). Following cell death occurring in their vicinity, however, microglia transform into full-blown brain phagocytes that secrete a number of factors including cytokines such as interleukin (IL)-1 and tumor necrosis factor-α (TNF-α). This transformation of microglia into cytotoxic effector cells appears to be under tight control *in vivo*. Stimuli that induce microglial activation and/or proliferation include interferon-γ, colony-stimulating factors such as macrophage colony-stimulating factor and granulocyte–macrophage colony-stimulating factor, changes in extracellular ATP levels, and ionic disturbances (spreading depression). In contrast, neurotrophins inhibit MHC class II expression by microglia, and β-adrenergic agonists may reduce IL-1 and TNF-α production by microglial cells.

MICROGLIAL CYTOTOXICITY

Microglial cytotoxicity to neurons, tumor cells, as well as infectious agents may be mediated by the large number of potentially cytotoxic products produced by these cells, including free oxygen intermediates, nitric oxide, proteinases, arachidonic acid derivatives, excitatory amino acids, and cytokines such as TNF-α. The massive invasion of ischemic or directly injured CNS parenchyma by microglia/macrophages has led some authors to hypothesize that these cells may cause more damage than is their contribution to tissue repair. As a result, it has been suggested that neuronal function can be rescued through suppression of microglial activity, but this idea must be viewed with caution. Given the great functional plasticity of microglia, it may be more effective to modify the neuroprotective and growth-promoting properties of these cells than to inhibit their response completely in order to support tissue recovery.

MICROGLIA AS ANTIGEN PRESENTING CELLS

A fundamental question in neuroimmunology concerns the identity of CNS cells that are capable of expressing MHC molecules *in vivo*. MHC class II antigens and costimulatory molecules such as B7 are required for effective presentation of antigen to specific T lymphocytes. Microglia are recognized as the key parenchymal cells that possess this capacity, whereas the ability of microglia to prime naive T cells is in doubt. Interestingly, microglial cells also upregulate MHC and other immune response-associated molecules in neurodegenerative diseases such as Alzheimer's, Parkinson's, and Creutzfeldt–Jakob disease, in which classic tissue inflammation (i.e., infiltration of lymphocytes and/or macrophages) is usually absent. Antigen presentation in the absence of costimulatory molecules, however, may shut down rather than stimulate T cell proliferation. Consequently, microglial inflammation may serve a protective function: MHC II-positive/B7-negative microglia could act as a firewall against unwanted immune attack. However, in classic immune conditions, microglia stimulate secondary T cell responses. The latter are of great importance in infectious diseases.

MICROGLIA AS A SENSOR OF TISSUE PATHOLOGY

Activated microglia are found in a large number of pathological conditions and, due to their low threshold of activation, have been proposed as a sensitive marker of early tissue damage. This can be exploited in diagnostic neuropathology and neuroimaging. Classic examples of microglial involvement in CNS diseases include the formation of rod-shaped microglia in the cerebral cortex in "general paralysis of the insane" (neurosyphilis) or subacute sclerosing panencephalitis and also the formation of "microglial nodules" by neuronophagic microglia clustering

around affected neurons in poliomyelitis and other neuronotropic viral infections. The pathological hallmark of HIV-1 encephalitis is the multinucleated giant cell, which may derive from microglia. In Alzheimer's disease, microglia are prominent not only in the core but also around the outer border of amyloid plaques. Some authors believe that microglial cells are actively involved in the formation of amyloid deposits. Demyelinating activity in multiple sclerosis and in its animal model, experimental autoimmune encephalomyelitis, is largely attributable to phagocytically active macrophages. Many of them are microglia derived. Macrophages in ischemic brain tissue actively remove tissue debris. However, the significance of the large number of microglia in some gliomas remains enigmatic.

OTHER CNS MACROPHAGES

It is of great importance to distinguish microglia from other macrophage precursors that are normally present within the bony confinements of the CNS. These include epiplexus and supraependymal macrophages (both located within the ventricles), meningeal macrophages, and perivascular cells (PVCs). Of all these, only microglia are true residents of the CNS parenchyma. PVCs are distinct from cells of the blood vessel wall proper as well as from perivascular microglia. PVCs are located in the perivascular space, where they are separated from the blood vessel wall and the CNS parenchyma by a basement membrane. In contrast to microglia, PVCs express several immune-associated molecules, such as MHC class II, B7, and certain myelomonocytic macrophage antigens including CD68. Due to their location at the blood–brain interface, PVCs represent the first line of CNS defense. In addition, they may be of great pathophysiological importance because they are continuously renewed from the bloodstream. They may thus function as a Trojan horse in CNS infections.

SUMMARY

Normal brain parenchyma with an intact blood–brain barrier does not contain macrophages but only resting microglia. Tissue surveillance is probably one of the most important functions of resting microglial cells (sensor of pathology). Resting microglia are characterized by a remarkable degree of alertness, as evidenced by their low threshold of expression for complement receptors and MHC molecules. They can respond to challenges in a graded manner. Upon appropriate stimulation, and without exerting classic macrophage functions, microglia have the ability to take on an active role in neural plasticity (e.g., by engaging in synaptic stripping). Tissue remodeling may be an important function of microglia in CNS repair and during development. In CNS infections and in response to injuries, microglia develop phagocytic and cytotoxic activity. However, the full potential of microglial cytotoxicity does not seem to be employed *in vivo* unless threats to the CNS need to be confined. Microglia are therefore best viewed as guardians, which are armed to defend but not to attack CNS tissue.

—*Manuel B. Graeber*

See also–Central Nervous System Infections, Overview; Glia; Glial Tumors; Measles Virus, Central Nervous System Complications of; Neuroimmunology, Overview; Neurosyphilis

Further Reading

Banati, R. B., Newcombe, J., Gunn, R. N., *et al.* (2000). The peripheral benzodiazepine binding site in the brain in multiple sclerosis: Quantitative in vivo imaging of microglia as a measure of disease activity. *Brain* **123**, 2321–2337.

Graeber, M. B., Blakemore, W. F., and Kreutzberg, G. W. (2001). Cellular pathology of the central nervous system. In *Greenfield's Neuropathology* (D. I. Graham and P. L. Lantos, Eds.), 7th ed. Arnold, London.

Kato, H., and Walz, W. (2000). The initiation of the microglial response. *Brain Pathol.* **10**, 137–143.

Kreutzberg, G. W. (1996). Microglia: A sensor for pathological events in the CNS. *Trends Neurosci.* **19**, 312–318.

Lawson, L. J., Perry, V. H., Dri, P., *et al.* (1990). Heterogeneity in the distribution and morphology of microglia in the normal adult mouse brain. *Neuroscience* **39**, 151–170.

Nakajima, K., and Kohsaka, S. (1998). Functional roles of microglia in the central nervous system. *Hum. Cell* **11**, 141–155.

Streit, W. J., and Graeber, M. B. (1996). Microglia—A pictorial. *Prog. Histochem. Cytochem.* **31**, 1–89.

Microneurography

Encyclopedia of the Neurological Sciences
Copyright 2003, Elsevier Science (USA). All rights reserved.

MICRONEUROGRAPHY is an electrophysiological technique for recording single or multiunit nerve traffic directly from human peripheral nerves. Approximately 30 years have passed since the initial successful introduction of this technique, which has provided novel information on physiological and pharmacological mechanisms as well as important insights into disease pathophysiology. This entry reviews the methods and applications of the microneurographic recording techniques of sympathetic nerve activity. Identification and quantification of the two components, muscle and skin sympathetic nerve activity (MSNA and SSNA), will be addressed. A brief overview of the demographic characteristics, reflex mechanisms, and disease conditions that substantially alter measurements of sympathetic nerve traffic will also be presented.

MICRONEUROGRAPHIC RECORDING TECHNIQUE

Selection and Identification of Nerve Recording Site

Although most accessible peripheral spinal nerves can be used for microneurographic recording of SNA, the peroneal nerve posterior to the fibular head and the tibial nerve at the popliteal fossa are most commonly used. Recordings have also been reported from cranial nerves (facial and trigeminal); median, ulnar, and radial nerves in the upper extremities; and sural nerves in the lower extremities. The double recording technique can be used to simultaneously record MSNA and SSNA from two different nerves or from two different points of the same nerve. Burst frequency is similar in SNA recorded simultaneously from two different peripheral nerves or from different position of the same nerve.

Electrode Placement and Recording Procedures

A 50- to 70-mm long tungsten or stainless-steel microelectrode with a shaft diameter of approximately 100–200 μm and a tip diameter of approximately 1 μm is used to record efferent SNA. The electrode must be insulated with epoxy resin, except for 5–25 μm near the tip, so that impedance is approximately 1–5 MΩ. Neural activities are recorded as a difference in electrical potential in millivolts between an intraneurally inserted recording electrode and a reference electrode inserted into the subcutaneous tissue near the recording electrode.

Complications of Microneurography and Strategies for Prevention

One study reported that only 3 of approximately 1000 healthy subjects experienced symptoms of local neuropathy, such as cutaneous hyperesthesia or partial muscle paresis. These symptoms disappeared within 6 months. A recent retrospective study based on a questionnaire of symptoms after human microneurography in 649 healthy subjects and 59 patients with polyneuropathy examined in multiple centers reported that only 63 subjects (9%) suffered from symptoms. According to the report, 95% of symptoms disappeared within 2 weeks, and in only 1 case did the symptoms persist longer. A low frequency of complications and resolution of symptoms within 6 months proved the technique to be relatively safe for human subjects if done with proper training and precautions. Several recommendations may help prevent or reduce the complications of microneurography. Probing should be limited to less than 1 hr to minimize any nerve fiber injury. Disposable electrodes should be used or the electrodes should be sterilized to prevent inoculation of infective agents into the subcutaneous tissue or nerve. Although long-term immobilization may be necessary, this should be limited, particularly in the elderly and in persons with a history of thrombosis or thromboembolism.

MUSCLE SYMPATHETIC NERVE ACTIVITY IN HEALTHY HUMANS

Identification and Evaluation of MSNA

MSNA is the vasoconstrictor message destined to muscle blood vessels and is recorded by the electrode tip being placed in the muscle nerve fascicle. MSNA may be evaluated quantitatively as burst rate (bursts per minute) and burst incidence (bursts per 100 heartbeats). Both are reasonably reproducible and may be suitable for evaluating inter- and intraindividual variations of SNA. In a single subject, the variations in resting MSNA in different sets of experiments are small and are remarkably constant even when recordings are repeated after a decade. However, resting MSNA burst rate between even healthy individuals varies markedly.

Regulation of Muscle Sympathetic Activity

Physical and Environmental Factors

Age: Age may be an important determinant of baseline SNA as measured by MSNA and plasma norepinephrine spillover. A positive correlation between age and MSNA was described in earlier studies. Later studies supported the age-dependent increase in MSNA, even though some studies have suggested that the age-related changes in MSNA may be linked to the increase in adiposity in older persons, particularly abdominal adiposity.

Gender and Genetics: Baseline levels of MSNA were higher in men than in women, in both young and older subjects. Effects of genetic factors on interindividual differences in MSNA have also been reported. A study of nine pairs of monozygotic male twins and eight pairs of age-matched male subjects without family relationships suggested that the degree of reproducibility between twins is similar to that reported previously between repeated recordings in the same subject.

Body Fat and Obesity: The sympathetic nervous system has been implicated in both the etiology and the pathophysiology of human obesity. Reduced sympathetic activity is linked to reduced metabolic rate and reduced energy expenditure that may result in weight gain. Although studies of obesity in animal models are consistent with regard to low sympathetic activity, studies in obese humans using microneurography have reported high MSNA. The increased MSNA in obese subjects may be related to the presence of symptomatic or occult obstructive sleep apnea. It has not been demonstrated unequivocally that human obesity per se is a cause of heightened MSNA.

Smoking and Drinking: During cigarette smoking in healthy subjects, blood pressure increases and MSNA is suppressed. However, if the increase in blood pressure is attenuated by a simultaneous infusion of sodium nitroprusside, MSNA and heart rate increase dramatically. Thus, the baroreflex response to the pressor effect of cigarette smoking inhibits the cigarette smoking-induced increase in MSNA. Cigarette smoking also increases skin SNA (Fig. 1). Oral alcohol ingestion of approximately 1.0 g/kg body weight also increases MSNA and heart rate.

Reflex Mechanisms

Central Command, Mental Stress, and Sleep: Cortical influences on MSNA are observed during static handgrip exercise before and after partial neuromuscular blockade by curare, presumably due to the effects of central command. Mental stress increases MSNA. The importance of changes in state of consciousness in the regulation of MSNA is further demonstrated by the striking effects of sleep.

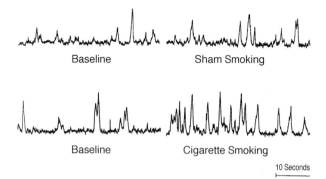

Figure 1

Recordings of skin sympathetic nerve activity at baseline and during placebo or sham smoking. The effect of actual cigarette smoking on skin sympathetic nerve traffic is striking. In studies of muscle sympathetic activity, increases in MSNA were only evident when the pressor effects of smoking were attenuated by nitroprusside infusion. In that situation, increases in MSNA also became apparent. Skin sympathetic nerve activity that is not under direct baroreflex control increases during cigarette smoking despite increases in blood pressure. Note the broad-based patterns of skin sympathetic activity that are unrelated to the cardiac cycle (reproduced with permission from Narkewicz *et al.*, 1998b).

Non-rapid eye movement (REM) sleep is associated with a decrease in MSNA as well as heart rate and blood pressure. However, REM sleep is associated with markedly increased MSNA (Fig. 2).

Baroreflex and Chemoreflex Influences: Simultaneous recordings of MSNA and systemic blood pressure clearly show that MSNA is enhanced when blood pressure is lowered and is suppressed when blood pressure is elevated. This response is mediated primarily by the arterial baroreflexes. Active standing or passive head-up tilt from the horizontal supine position markedly increase MSNA so as to prevent orthostatic hypotension and redistribute blood to vital organs, such as the brain. Lower body negative pressure (LBNP) has been used to simulate orthostasis without changing posture. The orthostatic increase in MSNA is mediated by the cardiopulmonary baroreflex, with additional contributions from the arterial baroreflex if blood pressure declines.

The chemoreflexes also exert a substantial influence on MSNA. Hypoxia increases MSNA. Elimination of the hyperventilatory response to hypoxia eliminates the sympathetic inhibitory effects of the thoracic afferents, potentiating the MSNA increase during hypoxia. Indeed, breath-holding has often been used as a potent stimulus to increase MSNA and differentiate it from SSNA.

SKIN SYMPATHETIC NERVE ACTIVITY

Identification and Evaluation of Skin Sympathetic Nerve Activity

When the electrode tip is placed in the skin nerve fascicle, multifiber SSNA can be recorded. Skin fiber traffic can be identified by the appearance of afferent discharges from peripheral skin receptors elicited by gentle touch of the skin area innervated by the impaled nerve. The following characteristics are used for identification of SSNA: The discharges are (i) pulse asynchronous, spontaneous, or induced; (ii) elicited and accentuated with almost constant latency of arousal and other sensory stimuli (sound, pain, electrical stimulation of the peripheral nerve trunk, etc.); (iii) followed by peripheral cutaneous vasoconstriction (vasoconstrictor fibers) or perspiration

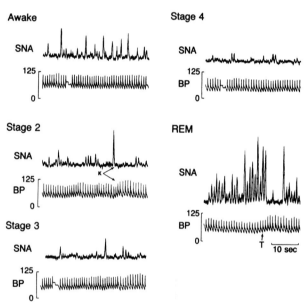

Figure 2

Recordings of muscle sympathetic nerve activity in a normal subject during wakefulness and stages 2–4 of non-REM sleep and during REM sleep. During non-REM sleep, there is a gradual reduction in MSNA with accompanying decreases in blood pressure and heart rate. During REM sleep, there is a dramatic increase in sympathetic traffic with intermittent surges in blood pressure and marked fluctuations in heart rate. During stage 2 sleep, K represents a K complex that is accompanied by increased MSNA and a subsequent pressor response. It is interesting that during wakefulness, arousal stimuli do not directly increase MSNA but do increase skin SNA. Thus, the response mechanisms appear to change during sleep. During REM, T represents an REM twitch that is linked to abrupt inhibitions and a surge in blood pressure, possibly due to interactions between the REM twitch and vascular control in the muscle vascular bed (reproduced with permission from Somers *et al.*, 1993).

(sudomotor fibers); and (iv) not apparently affected by changes in blood pressure, apnea, or the Valsalva maneuver. Simultaneous recordings of SSNA from upper and lower limb have shown similar discharge patterns, but measurements differ in hairy and glabrous skin.

Like MSNA, SSNA can be expressed as a burst rate and total activity. The SSNA bursts are recorded as a mixed activity of vasoconstrictor, sudomotor, piloerector, and possibly vasodilator impulses. Identification and evaluation of the different components are technically difficult. Therefore, for intra- or interindividual comparison it is often quantified as total SSNA rather than as the burst rate.

Regulation of Skin Sympathetic Nerve Activity

The skin is a thermoregulatory organ; therefore, SSNA plays an important role in thermoregulation, particularly since SSNA consists of vasoconstrictor impulses to the skin blood vessels, sudomotor impulses to sweat glands, and impulses to piloerector muscles. The SSNA leading to glabrous skin is regulated by central command that causes mental sweating, and SSNA leading to hairy skin is regulated by ambient temperature that causes thermal sweating.

Central Command: Central command has an influence on both vasoconstrictor and sudomotor components of SSNA. Spontaneous SSNA is enhanced by any stimulus that causes arousal. Therefore, sound, touch, pain, or electrical stimulation of peripheral nerve trunks produces short-lasting increases in spontaneous SSNA. An inspiratory gasp is also a strong stimulus for an increase in SSNA. Both decreased and unchanged SSNA have been reported during sleep. However, increased SSNA is seen during REM sleep and in association with K complexes in non-REM sleep. These differences illustrate the difficulties in quantification of the mixed vasoconstrictor and sudomotor traffic.

Peripheral Reflexes: SSNA changes with changes in ambient and local temperature on the skin to maintain the normal body core temperature. The vasoconstrictor component regulates heat loss through skin by increasing the activity at low temperatures and decreasing the activity at high ambient temperature. In contrast, the sudomotor component achieves the same function by decreasing activity at low temperatures and increasing activity at high ambient temperatures ($\pm 25^{\circ}$C). Hence,

vasoconstrictor activity increases at low temperature and sudomotor activity increases at high temperature.

SYMPATHETIC NERVE ACTIVITY IN CLINICAL CONDITIONS

Because of its potent pressor effects and its association with circulating catecholamine levels, MSNA has primarily been implicated in cardiovascular disease pathophysiology. Only a few of the many disease conditions in which MSNA may be directly involved in the pathophysiology are discussed here.

Hypertension

Increased sympathetic activity in both primary and secondary hypertension may be implicated in the etiology of hypertension, given the potent vasoconstrictor and pressor effects of increases in MSNA. Hypertensive patients have shown elevated MSNA at rest and in response to the cold pressor test, LBNP, apnea, hypoxia, and mental stress. Genetic factors in normotensive offspring of hypertensive patients may influence baseline MSNA and responses to mental stress. Earlier studies in essential and borderline hypertensive patients have shown not only an increase in baseline MSNA and responses to stressors but also a blunted baroreflex inhibition of MSNA compared to healthy subjects.

Patients with accelerated hypertension have been shown to also have high MSNA compared to subjects with benign hypertension. Matching age and adiposity between normal and borderline hypertensive groups also supports the concept of augmented MSNA in hypertension. Nevertheless, the association between heightened MSNA and hypertension remains controversial, with a number of studies noting no increased MSNA in hypertensive subjects.

Heart Failure

Increased sympathetic activity in heart failure may be related to a higher frequency of arrhythmia and mortality. Norepinephrine spillover and directly recorded MSNA are clearly increased in heart failure patients, even for mild heart failure. The mechanisms underlying sympathoexcitation in heart failure are not clear.

Sleep Apnea

Effects of sleep apnea on the sympathetic nervous system have been extensively documented. MSNA is markedly increased in sleep apneic patients, even when they are awake and breathing normally. During sleep, hypoxia and hypercapnia activate the chemoreflexes to further increase MSNA during sleep. Thus, the normal sleep stage-related control of MSNA is disrupted in patients with sleep apnea.

FUTURE PERSPECTIVES

The microneurographic technique has been used extensively to examine peripheral sympathetic activity and its effect on vascular resistance in healthy humans and in different clinical conditions. Only a few studies have used the single-unit recording technique due to the technical demands of this approach. However, this technique is providing new information regarding the physiology and burst-firing profile of single sympathetic nerve fibers.

Development of new methods for the evaluation of short-term variations of autonomic activity may also provide additional information. Power spectral analysis of heart rate variability is useful in evaluating autonomic control, providing certain well-defined caveats and limitations are recognized. A similar analytical technique has also been used for evaluating MSNA. Used simultaneously with other physiological measurements, including blood pressure and respiration, power spectral measures of MSNA are likely to complement the insights into neurocirculatory control in health and disease obtained by measurements of absolute MSNA.

—Abu S. M. Shamsuzzaman and Virend K. Somers

See also–Sympathetic System, Overview

Acknowledgments

ASMS is a recipient of an International Research John E. Fogarty Fellowship (5 F05 TW05463) and a Perkins Memorial Award from the American Physiological Society. VKS is an established investigator of the American Heart Association and is supported by National Institutes of Health Grants HL 65176 and HL 61560 and General Cardiovascular Research Center Grant M01-RR00585.

Further Reading

Bini, G., Hagbarth, K. E., Hynninen, P., *et al.* (1980). Thermoregulatory and rhythm-generating mechanisms governing the sudomotor and vasoconstrictor outflow in human cutaneous nerves. *J. Physiol.* **306**, 537–552.

Bini, G., Hagbarth, K. E., Hynninen, P., *et al.* (1980). Regional similarities and differences in thermoregulatory vaso- and sudomotor tone. *J. Physiol.* **306**, 553–565.

Bray, G. A., and York, D. A. (1998). The MONA LISA hypothesis in the time of leptin. *Recent Prog. Horm. Res.* **53**, 95–117.

Burke, D., Sundlof, G., and Wallin, B. (1977). Postural effects of muscle nerve sympathetic activity in man. *J. Physiol. (London)* **272**, 399–414.

Delius, W., Hagbarth, K. E., Hongell, A., *et al.* (1972). Manoeuvres affecting sympathetic outflow in human muscle nerves. *Acta Physiol. Scand.* **84**, 82–94.

Eckberg, D. L., Wallin, B. G., Fagius, J., *et al.* (1989). Prospective study of symptoms after human microneurography. *Acta Physiol. Scand.* **137**, 567–569.

Fagius, J., and Wallin, B. G. (1993). Long-term variability and reproducibility of resting human muscle nerve sympathetic activity at rest, as reassessed after a decade. *Clin. Auton. Res.* **3**, 201–205.

Grassi, G., Seravalle, G., Cattaneo, B. M., *et al.* (1995). Sympathetic activation and loss of reflex sympathetic control in mild congestive heart failure. *Circulation* **92**, 3206–3211.

Hagbarth, K. E. (1979). Exteroceptive, proprioceptive, and sympathetic activity recorded with microelectrodes from human peripheral nerves. *Mayo Clin. Proc.* **54**, 353–365.

Hara, K., and Floras, J. S. (1995). Influence of naloxone on muscle sympathetic nerve activity, systemic and calf haemodynamics and ambulatory blood pressure after exercise in mild essential hypertension. *J. Hypertens.* **13**, 447–461.

Hornyak, M., Cejnar, M., Elam, M., *et al.* (1991). Sympathetic muscle nerve activity during sleep in man. *Brain* **114**, 1281–1295.

Jones, P. P., Davy, K. P., Alexander, S., *et al.* (1997). Age-related increase in muscle sympathetic nerve activity is associated with abdominal adiposity. *Am. J. Physiol.* **272**, E976–E980.

Macefield, V. G., Wallin, B. G., and Vallbo, A. B. (1994). The discharge behaviour of single vasoconstrictor motoneurones in human muscle nerves. *J. Physiol.* **481**, 799–809.

Matsukawa, T., Gotoh, E., Uneda, S., *et al.* (1991). Augmented sympathetic nerve activity in response to stressors in young borderline hypertensive men. *Acta Physiol. Scand.* **141**, 157–165.

Matsukawa, T., Mano, T., Gotoh, E., *et al.* (1993). Elevated sympathetic nerve activity in patients with accelerated essential hypertension. *J. Clin. Invest.* **92**, 25–28.

Narkiewicz, K., van de Borne, P. J., Hausberg, M., *et al.* (1998a). Cigarette smoking increases sympathetic outflow in humans. *Circulation* **98**, 528–534.

Narkiewicz, K., van de Borne, P. J., Cooley, R. L., *et al.* (1998b). Sympathetic activity in obese subjects with and without obstructive sleep apnea. *Circulation* **98**, 772–776.

Ng, A. V., Callister, R., Johnson, D. G., *et al.* (1993). Age and gender influence muscle sympathetic nerve activity at rest in healthy humans. *Hypertension* **21**, 498–503.

Noll, G., Elam, M., Kunimoto, M., *et al.* (1994). Skin sympathetic nerve activity and effector function during sleep in humans. *Acta Physiol. Scand.* **151**, 319–329.

Pagani, M., Montano, N., Porta, A., *et al.* (1997). Relationship between spectral components of cardiovascular variabilities and direct measures of muscle sympathetic nerve activity in humans. *Circulation* **95**, 1441.

Scherrer, U., Randin, D., Tappy, L., *et al.* (1994). Body fat and sympathetic nerve activity in healthy subjects. *Circulation* **89**, 2634–2640.

Somers, V., and Narkiewicz, K. (1999). Sympathetic neural mechanisms in hypertension. In *Autonomic Failure* (C. Mathias and R. Bannister, Eds.), 4th ed., pp. 468–476. Oxford Univ. Press, Oxford.

Somers, V. K., Mark, A. L., Zavala, D. C., *et al.* (1989). Influence of ventilation and hypocapnia on sympathetic nerve responses to hypoxia in normal humans. *J. Appl. Physiol.* **67,** 2095–2100.

Somers, V. K., Dyken, M. E., Mark, A. L., *et al.* (1993). Sympathetic-nerve activity during sleep in normal subjects. *N. Engl. J. Med.* **328,** 303–307.

Somers, V. K., Dyken, M. E., Clary, M. P., *et al.* (1995). Sympathetic neural mechanisms in obstructive sleep apnea. *J. Clin. Invest.* **96,** 1897–1904.

Sundlof, G., and Wallin, B. G. (1978). Human muscle nerve sympathetic activity at rest. Relationship to blood pressure and age. *J. Physiol.* **274,** 621–637.

Takeuchi, S., Iwase, S., Mano, T., *et al.* (1994). Sleep-related changes in human muscle and skin sympathetic nerve activities. *J. Auton. Nerv. Syst.* **47,** 121–129.

Vallbo, A. B., Hagbarth, K. E., Torebjork, H. E., *et al.* (1979). Somatosensory, proprioceptive, and sympathetic activity in human peripheral nerves. *Physiol. Rev.* **59,** 919–957.

van de Borne, P., Mark, A. L., Montano, N., *et al.* (1997). Effects of alcohol on sympathetic activity, hemodynamics, and chemoreflex sensitivity. *Hypertension* **29,** 1278–1283.

Victor, R. G., Pryor, S. L., Secher, N. H., *et al.* (1989). Effects of partial neuromuscular blockade on sympathetic nerve responses to static exercise in humans. *Circ. Res.* **65,** 468–476.

Wallin, B. G., Kunimoto, M. M., and Sellgren, J. (1993). Possible genetic influence on the strength of human muscle nerve sympathetic activity at rest. *Hypertension* **22,** 282–284.

Young, J. (1980). Enhanced plasma norepinephrine response to upright posture and oral glucose administration in elderly human subjects. *Metabolism* **29,** 532–539.

Microneurosurgery

Encyclopedia of the Neurological Sciences

MICRONEUROSURGERY is surgery performed with the aid of magnification provided by the operating microscope (Fig. 1). Microoperative techniques require careful selection of the means of magnification and the accurate use of microinstruments to obtain optimal results. The application of microsurgery and microoperative techniques for the treatment of vascular and neoplastic disorders of the brain is among the major research advances in surgery in recent decades.

The advantages of microoperative techniques in neurosurgery were first demonstrated during removal

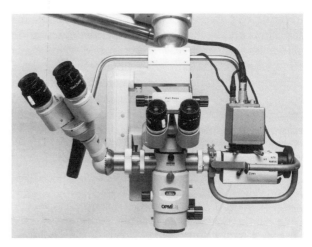

Figure 1
Zoom microscope with a TV camera attached on the right side and a binocular observer tube for the surgical assistant on the left [reproduced with permission from Rhoton, A. L., Jr. (1996). General and micro-operative techniques. In *Neurological Surgery* (J. R. Youmans, Ed.), 4th ed., pp. 724–756. W. B. Saunders, Philadelphia].

of acoustic neuromas. The benefits of magnified stereoscopic vision and intense illumination provided by the microscope were quickly realized in other neurosurgical procedures as well. Microsurgery has not only improved the technical performance of many standard neurosurgical procedures (e.g., brain tumor removal, aneurysm obliteration, neurorrhaphy, and even lumbar and cervical diskectomy) but also opened new dimensions that were previously unattainable for the neurosurgeon. With microsurgery, anastomoses of extracranial to intracranial arteries, trans-sphenoidal extirpation of sellar tumors with the preservation of pituitary gland, obliteration of previously inaccessible aneurysms, preservation of the facial and cochlear nerves during removal of acoustic neuromas, and numerous other successful interventions in areas of the brain and spinal cord are possible. Microsurgery improved operative results by permitting neural and vascular structures to be delineated with greater visual accuracy, deep areas to be reached with less brain retraction and smaller cortical incisions, bleeding points to be coagulated with less damage to adjacent neural structures, nerves distorted by tumor to be preserved with greater frequency, and anastomoses and suture of small vessels and nerves not previously possible. Its use has resulted in smaller wounds, less postoperative neural and vascular damage, better hemostases, more accurate nerve and vascular repairs, and operations for some previously inoperable lesions.

Microsurgery has introduced a new era in the education of surgeons by permitting the observation and recording, for later study and discussion, of minute operative details not visible to the eye.

Bringing the microscope to the operative field created the need for a deeper understanding of an entire array of anatomical knowledge that became known as microneuroanatomy and disclosed an increased necessity for designing and manufacturing new surgical instruments. Eventually, a new micro-technique was created, for which a specialized training period in a laboratory facility is recommended. Performing operations with loupes (magnifying lenses attached to eyeglasses) is a form of microsurgery. Loupes are an improvement over the naked eye, but even when combined with a headlight they lack many of the advantages of the microscope.

HISTORICAL ASPECTS AND MICROSURGICAL APPLICATIONS

In the late 1950s and 1960s, a relatively small group of pioneering neurosurgeons transformed microneurosurgery into the standard of care in modern neurosurgery. Theodor Kurze (1957) is considered the first neurosurgeon to use the microscope in the operating room. Following training received in William House's neurotological laboratory, he removed a neurilemoma of the seventh nerve in a 5-year-old patient. His contributions to microneurosurgery also include the creation of one of the first microneurosurgical laboratories, introducing many surgeons to the operating microscope. In 1961 and 1962, House, Kurze, and Doyle reported a subtemporal middle fossa approach to the internal auditory canal for removal of acoustic tumors, which was the first new approach to an intracranial lesion developed with the help of microtechniques. Kurze (1963) later applied microsurgical techniques in cordotomy, myelotomy, cerebellopontine angle tumors, en plaque meningiomas, rhizotomy, extracranial nerve anastomoses, and suboccipital operations for acoustic tumor with preservation of hearing and facial nerve function.

Peripheral nerve surgery profited tremendously from the use of magnification. As early as 1962, James Smith used the surgical microscope in a peripheral nerve reconstruction. In 1964, Chafee and Numoto demonstrated that a more complete return of function could be obtained in nerves sutured under magnification than in a controlled group in which magnification was not used. Using the microscope, Samii perfected cable grafting with sural nerve for nerve injury.

Many neurosurgical procedures already described or previously abandoned were reviewed or modified with the help of microsurgery. The original Gardner operation (developed following Dandy's work, as early as 1934) as a treatment for trigeminal neuralgia and hemifacial spasm was gradually improved with the advent of microneurosurgery. In 1966, Janetta and Rand published a famous series on microneurosurgery of the trigeminal nerve. Another example of a resurgence of an old technique is trans-sphenoidal surgery for pituitary tumors. This operation, almost completely abandoned by neurosurgeons after Cushing because of the deep, dark, and frequently blood-filled surgical field, experienced a rebirth after the introduction of the surgical microscope and became the standard procedure for sellar and selected suprasellar lesions.

In 1958, R. M. P. Donaghy established the world's first microsurgery research and training laboratory in Burlington, Vermont, which stressed the perfection of vascular anastomoses in small vessels. Donaghy's efforts, in close cooperation with Julius Jacobson, a vascular surgeon who advocated the use of microscope, culminated with the first published case of microneurovascular surgery in humans reporting the performance of a middle cerebral artery embolectomy. Jacobson is also credited to have positively influenced Carl Zeiss, Inc. to develop a two-person stereoscopic surgical microscope. This was only one of the many decisive changes that made the primitive monocular microscope more like the microscopes used in neurosurgery today.

The Yasargil–Donaghy operation of microvascular anastomoses of the superficial temporal artery to the middle cerebral artery, first performed in 1967, was developed in Donaghy's laboratory. In 1999, Yasargil was selected one of *Neurosurgery's* men of the century for his role in developing microneurosurgery. These bypass procedures were recently extended to the vertebral–basilar circulation using occipital artery anastomoses to the posterior inferior cerebellar artery or anterior cerebellar artery and superficial temporal artery to the superior cerebellar artery.

The use of microneurosurgical techniques in the treatment of aneurysms and arteriovenous malformations completely revolutionized the therapeutic approach to these lesions. J. Lawrence Pool (1965) was the first to publish a report on the use of the microscope for intracranial aneurysm surgery. Before the advent of microneurosurgery, aneurysm surgery was deemed a high-mortality procedure, and many neurologists opposed the surgical approach to these lesions. During the next few years, microsurgery became the accepted standard in the treatment of intracranial aneurysm. In 1975, the American College of Surgeons and the American Surgical Association ranked microsurgery in the treatment of cerebrovascular diseases among the first-order research advances between 1945 and 1970.

THE MICROSCOPE

The surgical microscope consists of a series of lenses, aligned to give a stereoscopic image, and a built-in illumination system. It is a low-power microscope capable of being adjusted to give stepwise increases in magnification between 3 and 40 times (Fig. 1).

The basic microscope consists of a set of eyepieces that can be adjusted to correct for myopia or hyperopia in either one or both of the surgeon's eyes, a binocular tube or head assembly into which the two adjustable eyepieces fit and that can be adjusted to accommodate the surgeon's interpupillary distance, a magnification changer of either a zoom or turret assembly type, and an objective lens that determines the working distances between the operative field and the microscope. The operating microscope should be equipped with coaxial lighting that provides an illuminated field that is concentric with the field of view and should have sufficient intensity to yield excellent stereoscopic vision in deep, narrow exposures. Accessories have been developed that allow the surgeon's assistants, the nurses, and others to observe the magnified image of the operation while it is in progress. A beam splitter attached between the head of the microscope and the binocular tube allows the use of observation tubes and still or TV cameras (Fig. 1).

A microscope for neurosurgery should provide (i) a clear stereoscopic view of the operative field without discomfort to the surgeon; (ii) ample illumination at the surgical field without transfer of heat, which might damage tissue; (iii) homogeneous illumination of the field; (iv) an interchangeable objective lens, which permits changes in working distance from surgical microscope to the operative field; (v) variable magnification; (vi) good balance and freedom in all axial motions, requiring minimal effort to position and allowing removal of the operative field without delay; (vii) a coaxial lamp assembly that is readily accessible in case of lamp failure, even though the surgical microscope is draped for sterility; and (viii) a microscope assembly with provision to accept accessories, including both film and electronic image formation, and an observation tube for direct view by an observer or assistant surgeon.

MICRONEUROSURGICAL INSTRUMENTATION

It was quickly realized that the instruments used in macroneurosurgery were unsuitable for the delicate tasks possible with microneurosurgery. Jacobson, Malis, Yasargil, Rhoton, and Spetzler made remarkable contributions, providing the concept that microinstruments should be the transition between the surgeons' hands and the tiny microneurosurgical field. The time-honored jeweler's forceps initially seemed to be an ideal tool, but it soon became clear that instruments needed to be longer in order to reach the target pathology in the deep, narrow exposure. In the past, instruments were often held in a pistol grip with the hand floating above the incision, but microneurosurgery demanded that they be held in a delicate pencil grip with the hand rested on the wound margin for stability and accuracy in dissection. The concept of instruments as prolongations of the surgeon's hands reached its peak with the introduction of the microdissectors, designed for completing microsurgical tasks varying from defining the neck of aneurysms to separating nerves and vessels from tumors (Fig. 2).

A major development in the microsurgical armamentarium was the introduction of bipolar coagulation. Monopolar coagulation was the first method applied for hemostasis in neurosurgery, but it proved inadequate for microprocedures because of the wide current and heat spread. Bipolar coagulation, developed by Greenwood and Malis, allowed fine coagulation of small vessels with a reduced current, caused less damage to adjacent tissues, and could be used under cooling saline irrigation. Bipolar coagulation could be used in areas where unipolar coagulation would be hazardous, such as near cranial nerves, within the ventricles, and around the brainstem and small vessels (Fig. 3). Suction tubes, used for aspirating cerebrospinal fluid and blood in the operative field, were also modified for the needs of microsurgery.

Because the operative site must be precisely maintained and firmly fixed, head fixation devices were developed consisting of a clamp to accommodate

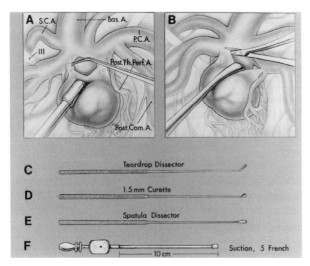

Figure 2

Instruments for aneurysm dissection. (A) The 40° teardrop dissector separates perforating branches and arachnoidal bands from the neck of the aneurysm of the basilar artery (Bas. A.). The blunt-tip suction of a 5-Fr tube provides suction and aids in the retraction of the aneurysm neck for dissection. Structures in the exposure include the superior cerebellar (S.C.A.), posterior communicating (Post. Com. A.), posterior cerebral (P. C. A.), and posterior thalamoperforating (Post. Th. Perf. A.) arteries and the oculomotor nerve (III). (B) The wall of the aneurysm is retracted with the spatula dissector, and the arachnoidal bands around the neck are divided with microscissors. (C) A 40° teardrop dissector defines the neck and separates perforating vessels from the neck of an aneurysm. (D) The angled microcurette with 1.5-mm cup is useful in removing the dura from the anterior clinoid process. (E) Spatula dissector for defining the neck and separating perforating vessels from the wall of an aneurysm. (F) Blunt-tip suction with a 10-cm shaft and a 5-Fr tip for suction and dissection around an aneurysm [reproduced with permission from Rhoton, A. L., Jr. (1996). General and micro-operative techniques. In *Neurological Surgery* (J. R. Youmans, Ed.), 4th ed., pp. 724–756. W. B. Saunders, Philadelphia].

the capsule may be removed with relatively little manipulation of adjacent normal structures. Laser (light amplification by the stimulated emission of radiation) is used for microneurosurgical procedures because it provides a more focal method for incision and coagulation. The carbon dioxide laser is the most commonly used laser in neurosurgery. It can be used free-hand but is more commonly linked to the operating microscope by means of a direct mechanical or electromechanical manipulator.

MICROOPERATIVE TECHNIQUES

Microoperative techniques have disadvantages. Training in the use of the microscope, microinstruments, and microsutures is required to adjust for the shift away from the tactile–manual technique using fingers to vision-oriented techniques. The equipment (microscope and microinstruments) is moderately expensive and requires additional space in the operating room, and care of the equipment places an added burden on the nursing staff. Only when the surgeon has acquired proficiency in the use of the microscope should operations be undertaken. The clinical microtechnique should be applied first to procedures with which the surgeon is entirely familiar, before expanding its use to new and technically difficult procedures. Early in one's experience with the microscope, one tends to use it in less demanding situations and to discontinue its use

three relatively sharp pins, which penetrate the scalp and are firmly seated on the outer table of the skull. After the clamp is secured to the head, it is attached to the headholder fixed to the operating table and final positioning is done.

Drills for delicate bone removal near arteries or nerves were also developed and are frequently used during removal of the sphenoid ridge, the clinoid process, the wall of the internal acoustic meatus, or protrusions of the cranial base. Ultrasonic aspirators and lasers for tumor removal are applied with a greater degree of accuracy when guided by the magnified vision provided by the operating microscope. The ultrasonic aspirator fragments unwanted tissue by high-frequency vibration of a titanium tip. It is used to debulk the center of a tumor, after which

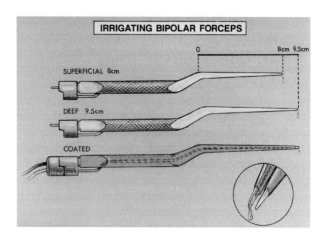

Figure 3

Bayonet bipolar forceps with combined irrigating system. Different lengths are required according to the depth of the operative field [reproduced with permission from Rhoton, A. L., Jr. (1996). General and micro-operative techniques. In *Neurological Surgery* (J. R. Youmans, Ed.), 4th ed., pp. 724–756. W. B. Saunders, Philadelphia].

when hemorrhage or problems of unusual complexity are encountered. However, with experience, bleeding is more accurately and quickly stopped under magnification and hemorrhage that occurs during operations performed under microscopes tends to be of lesser magnitude than that during operations without magnification.

Microsurgery requires that the surgeon be knowledgeable about the basic optical and mechanical principles of the operating microscope; the common types of electrical failure and how to correct them; the procedure of dismantling the microscope into its component parts and supporting couplings and rebuilding it; the technique of removing the microscope from its stand and modifying it for use with the patient in a variety of positions; selection of the lenses, eyepieces, binocular tubes, light sources, stands, and accessories for different operations; and the use of bipolar coagulators, air and electric drills, aneurysm clips and their appliers, self-retaining brain retractors, and other microsurgical instruments.

The surgical nurse plays an especially important role in microneurosurgery. During an operation, the surgeon is required to maintain their head and body in a relatively fixed position for prolonged periods because viewing of the operative field through the microscope necessitates continuous observation in order to coordinate hands and eyes. Hence, the nurse should make a constant effort to reduce the number of times the surgeon looks away from the microscope and to limit any distractions.

EDUCATION

Many neurosurgery training programs have incorporated microsurgery laboratories because laboratory training is fundamental to acquiring and developing microsurgical skills. Early in his career, Harvey Cushing developed a laboratory in which surgeons, using dogs, could practice and perfect their operative skills. Modern microsurgical laboratories, of which Donaghy's was the first of many, provide a place for experimentation, practice, testing of new instrumentation, and microneurosurgical educational programs.

Laboratories provide a setting in which the mental and physical adjustments required for microsurgery can be mastered. Laboratory training is essential before one undertakes microanastomotic procedures on patients (e.g., superficial temporal to middle cerebral artery anastomoses). Dissection under the microscope of tissues taken from cadavers or at autopsy may increase one's skill. Performance of

temporal bone dissection in the laboratory is an accepted component of microsurgical training for otological operations, and such exercises are of value to the neurosurgeon. A detailed microscopic exploration of the perforating branches of the circle of Willis and other common sites of aneurysm occurrence may improve one's technique. As the need arises, examination of selected other anatomic specimens may also increase the surgeon's familiarity with other operative sites (e.g., the jugular foramen, cavernous sinus, pineal region, or ventricles).

The availability of microscope accessories, such as observation tubes, 16- and 35-mm cameras, and closed-circuit color television, has turned the microscope into a valuable audiovisual means of training. Color television cameras mounted on the microscope are now commonly used to produce teaching cassettes or for transmitting the operative view directly to the classroom.

Although it has been recognized throughout the centuries that knowledge of anatomy is the basis of all surgery, the "new anatomical world" disclosed by the microscope was clearly beyond the imagination of the first microneurosurgeons. Refinement of classic neuroanatomical knowledge to accommodate the needs of microsurgery became an urgent need and led to many publications on the microanatomical aspects of varied cranial and spinal regions.

Microsurgery is the most spectacular advance in surgical techniques in modern times, and the application of microsurgery in neurosurgery has yielded a whole new level of neurosurgical performance and competence. Microsurgery has been applied in every neurosurgical subspecialty, resulting in new techniques and decisively improved outcomes. It is the foundation of modern neurosurgery and will serve as the basis for future advances in this field.

—*Carolina Martins and Albert L. Rhoton, Jr.*

***See also*–Aneurysms, Surgery; Cushing, Harvey; Endoscopic Microsurgery**

Further Reading
Donaghy, R. M. P. (1979). The history of microsurgery in neurosurgery. *Clin. Neurosurg.* **26**, 619–625.
Kriss, T. C., and Kriss, V. M. (1998). History of the operating microscope: From magnifying glass to microneurosurgery. *Neurosurgery* **42**, 899–908.
Lawton, M. T., Heiserman, J. E., Prendergast, V. C., *et al.* (1996). Titanium aneurysm clips. Part III: Clinical application in 16 patients with subarachnoid hemorrhage. *Neurosurgery* **38**, 1170–1175.

Malis, L. I. (1979). Instrumentation and techniques in micro-surgery. *Clin. Neurosurg.* **26**, 626–636.

Rand, R. W. (1985). *Microneurosurgery* (E. Klein, Ed.), 3rd ed. Mosby, St. Louis.

Rhoton, A. L., Jr. (1979). Improving ourselves and our specialty. Presidential address to the CNS meeting, Washington, DC, 1978. *Clin. Neurosurg.* **26**, xiii–xix.

Rhoton, A. L., Jr. (1995). General and micro-operative techniques. In *Neurological Surgery* (J. R. Youmans, Ed.), 4th ed., pp. 724–766. Saunders, Philadelphia.

Rhoton, A. L., Jr. (2000). The posterior cranial fossa: Microsurgical anatomy and surgical approaches. *Neurosurgery* **47**, 7–297.

Yasargyl, M. G. (1984). *Microneurosurgery.* Thieme Verlag, Stuttgart.

Yasargil, M. G. (1999). A legacy of microneurosurgery: Memoirs, lessons and axioms. *Neurosurgery* **45**, 1025–1091.

Micturition

Encyclopedia of the Neurological Sciences

MICTURITION, or urination, is the act of passing urine from the body. Normal micturition is a result of a complex system of reflexes involving the bladder, the internal sphincter, the external sphincter, the urethra, the peripheral nerves, spinal cord, and brain. Neurological disease can interfere with all or part of these elements of normal bladder function. This entry is a brief review of the anatomy, neuroanatomy, and physiology of the micturition reflex.

ANATOMY

The bladder is a hollow, muscular viscus in the pelvis composed of smooth muscle cells, interspersed with elastin and connective tissues, and lined with transitional epithelium. It lies immediately posterior to the symphysis pubis and anterior to the uterus and vagina in women. The ureters enter the bladder on its posteroinferior surface. The muscle fibers of the bladder condense into a funnel-like structure at the base, forming the bladder neck, also known as the internal sphincter. This structure is not a true circular sphincter but a coalescence of muscle as the bladder drains into the urethra. The female urethra is approximately 4 cm long and lies beneath the symphysis pubis, adjoining the anterior vaginal wall. Midway along the urethra is a true sphincter composed of striated muscle—the external sphincter. It is part of the pelvic floor musculature and surrounds the middle third of the urethra. The male urethra begins at the bladder neck and traverses the length of the prostate gland. Just distal to the prostate gland is the external sphincter. The remainder of the urethra extends the length of the penis and ends at the urethral meatus at the tip of the glans penis.

NEUROANATOMY

The micturition reflex is peripherally mediated by components of the somatic and the autonomic nervous systems. The bladder receives its motor innervation through the parasympathetic pelvic nerves. The principal nuclei innervating the urinary bladder of the cat consist of motor neurons located in the gray matter of the intermediolateral cell column of the sacral spinal cord and motor neurons in the ventral gray matter of the sacral spinal cord in the region of Onuf's nucleus. In humans, sacral nerve blocks have revealed that the detrusor nucleus has a rostral–caudal extension going from the S3 to S4 segment. The precise intramedullary location of detrusor motor neurons and their histological characteristics in the sacral spinal cord have not been described.

The bladder neck or internal sphincter is innervated by the hypogastric nerves, which are derived from T11–L2 (sympathetic). The external sphincter is the only structure in the lower urinary tract to receive somatic innervation, and this is via a branch of the perineal nerve, the second branch of the pudendal nerve. Its motor neurons are located in spinal segments S2–S4.

The areas of the central nervous system specifically defined in bladder innervation include the cerebral cortex, the pons, and the conus medullaris. The principal afferent and efferent spinal pathways from detrusor motor neurons in the conus medullaris have been identified in the posterior superficial portion of the lateral columns. The spinal pathways for innervation of the external urinary sphincter have not been identified in humans. However, they can be assumed to resemble the organization of skeletal muscle, with ascending pathways in the posterior columns and descending tracts in the corticospinal and reticulospinal pathways.

Areas near the nucleus locus ceruleus in the pons have been identified as crucial for the appearance of reflex detrusor contractions in certain quadriped animals. The location of the pontine nucleus responsible for detrusor contractions (also known as the pontine micturition center) in humans has not been identified but is presumed to be similar to that in animals, although reports of bladder dysfunction in humans with pontine lesions are limited. There are bilateral descending projections from homologous pontine nuclei to the intermediolateral cell column of the sacral spinal cord, through which efferent impulses travel to initiate a detrusor contraction.

The cerebral cortex, particularly areas of the prefrontal cortex, has been identified as regulatory influences on detrusor function. Patients with lesions of the prefrontal cortex are unable to suppress detrusor contractions (detrusor hyper-reflexia), suggesting that cortical (volitional) control of bladder function originates from this portion of the brain. Other areas of the central nervous system that have been demonstrated to influence bladder function in animals and humans include the basal ganglia, thalamus, limbic system, and cerebellum.

PHYSIOLOGY

The micturition cycle involves two phases: bladder filling/urine storage and bladder emptying. Bladder filling requires (i) accommodation of increasing volumes at low intravesical pressure (compliance) and appropriate sensation, (ii) the bladder outlet to be closed at rest and during increases in intra-abdominal pressure, and (iii) the absence of involuntary bladder contractions. Bladder emptying requires (i) coordinated contraction of the bladder of adequate magnitude and duration, (ii) lowering of resistance at sphincters, and (iii) the absence of obstruction (e.g., enlargement of the prostate gland in the aging male may result in bladder outlet obstruction, precluding efficient micturition). Bladder dysfunction can then be clinically identified as a problem of filling or emptying or a combination of both, and the site of dysfunction may be the bladder, the urethra, or both.

The normal function of the bladder is to store urine until it has reached capacity and until it is socially acceptable to evacuate urine. Urine storage is accomplished at low pressures, measured as compliance. Compliance is calculated as the change in volume over the change in pressure. Bladder compliance is a result of the viscoelastic properties of the bladder. The bladder wall contains elastin, which allows it to stretch without a subsequent increase in pressure. Typical adult bladder capacity is approximately 350–450 ml. Compliance is also facilitated by sympathetic discharge primarily mediated through the β-adrenergic receptors within the bladder wall. This sympathetic tone operates directly at the level of the bladder musculature to facilitate storage. There is

also sympathetic discharge at the level of the autonomic ganglia, which has an inhibitory effect on the parasympathetic postganglionic neurons, thus preventing detrusor contraction and facilitating urine storage. Loss of compliance may lead to renal insufficiency.

Continence is maintained through the action of the urinary sphincters. The internal sphincter, or the bladder neck, is richly innervated with α-adrenergic receptors. During bladder filling this structure remains closed through constant sympathetic discharge via the hypogastric plexus. The external sphincter, composed of striated muscle, also maintains a resting tone to maintain continence. It is believed that the fibers of the external sphincter are primarily of the slow twitch variety and thus can maintain tension for long periods of time. With rapid increases in intra-abdominal pressure, fast twitch fibers are recruited to contract and further increase the urethral resistance to avoid urinary leakage.

As the bladder fills, its visceral afferents travel through the peripheral nerves, ascending through the spinal cord to the pontine micturition center. It is at this level that a detrusor contraction is initiated. However, there are inhibitory signals from suprapontine centers (e.g., prefrontal cortex and basal ganglia) that prevent the generation of a detrusor contraction until the bladder is full. At normal bladder capacity (350–450 ml), sensations of fullness are transmitted through detrusor afferents, nerves that provide reflex excitation through the central nervous system to the motor innervation to the detrusor. The cortex releases its inhibition of the pontine micturition center. An efferent response travels through the spinal cord and through the pelvic nerves, and a detrusor contraction occurs. The contraction is coordinated with the opening of the internal and external sphincters to allow free egress of urine outside the body. A normal detrusor contraction is of adequate strength and duration to empty the bladder completely in one coordinated contraction. After urine evacuation, the sphincters return to their closed state and the cycle resumes.

—*Claire C. Yang*

***See also*–Bladder Disorders; Sphincter Disturbances**

Further Reading

Bradley, W. E., and Yang, C. C. (1997). Autonomic regulation of urinary bladder. In *Clinical Autonomic Disorders, Evaluation and Management* (P. A. Low, Ed.), 2nd ed., pp. 117–128. Lippincott–Raven, Philadelphia.

Ciba Foundation (1990). *Neurobiology of Incontinence*, Ciba Foundation Symposium No. 151. Wiley, Chichester, UK.

Krane, R. J., and Siroky, M. B. (Eds.) (1991). *Clinical Neuro-Urology*. 2nd ed. Little, Brown, Philadelphia.

Steers, W. D. (1998). Physiology and pharmacology of the bladder and urethra. *Campbell's Urology*, 7th ed., pp. 870–916. Saunders, Philadelphia.

Midbrain

Encyclopedia of the Neurological Sciences

THE MIDBRAIN, or mesencephalon, is the smallest of the five divisions of the brain. As its name implies, it is located anatomically in the middle of the head. It is caudal to the thalamus and hypothalamus and rostral to the pons. The mesencephalon lies at the junction of the posterior and middle cranial fossae, partly in both. Although it is only approximately 2.5 cm in length, the cells and nuclei contained within it serve many critical functions, including wakefulness, response to pain, coordination of motor function, eye movements, vision, and hearing. In addition, fiber tracts carrying all sensory input from the torso and extremities to the thalamus traverse the midbrain. The corticospinal tracts that relay voluntary motor commands from the motor cortex of the brain to the extremities pass through the midbrain in the cerebral peduncles. Despite its protected bony confines at the skull base, it may be affected by a variety of pathological logical entities, such as tumors, infections, hemorrhage, and trauma. This entry discusses the anatomy, physiology, and pathology of the midbrain.

EMBRYOLOGY

In addition to being the smallest division of the central nervous system (CNS), the midbrain is also the least differentiated. On approximately day 28 of development, the future brain is divided into three primary regions: the forebrain or prosencephalon, the midbrain or mesencephalon, and the hindbrain or rhombencephalon. By day 36, the prosencephalon divides into the telencephalon and diencephalon, which ultimately become the cerebral hemispheres, basal ganglia, thalamus, hypothalamus, olfactory system, and optic nerves. Also at this time, the rhombencephalon divides into the metencephalon and myelencephalon, which further develop into the pons, cerebellum, and medulla. The midbrain,

however, does not further subdivide as do the forebrain and hindbrain.

In the developing spinal cord, neurons become arranged such that the dorsal or alar plate is the site of sensory and coordinating neuronal cell bodies and the ventral or basal plate is the site of motor control neuronal cell bodies. This basic arrangement persists in the brainstem, including the midbrain. Thus, the sensory and coordinating nuclei of the midbrain (superior and inferior colliculi) develop from the alar (dorsal) plate and the motor nuclei of the midbrain (oculomotor and trochlear) develop from the basal (ventral) plate. However, there are exceptions throughout the brainstem to this arrangement. The most notable in the midbrain is the red nucleus. The red nucleus is involved in motor coordination and control. The neurons for this nucleus develop in the alar plate and migrate to the basal plate. One hypothesis for this is that the red nucleus has extensive interconnections with the cerebellum and basal ganglia and therefore monitors and coordinates muscle activity in relation to all types of sensory input and consequently serves both important sensory and motor functions.

ANATOMY AND PHYSIOLOGY

The midbrain can be separated into three transverse parts: the dorsal tectum or quadrigeminal plate, the central tegmentum, and the ventral cerebral peduncles (Fig. 1A). The cerebral aqueduct separates the tectum from the tegmentum, and the darkly pigmented substantia nigra separates the tegmentum from the cerebral peduncles. The midbrain is longitudinally divided into two main levels: the superior collicular level and the inferior collicular level.

The midbrain receives its blood supply from paramedian and short and long circumferential midbrain perforating vessels arising from the distal basilar, superior cerebellar, posterior cerebral, and posterior medial choroidal arteries. There is also a very small contribution to the upper midbrain from the anterior choroidal artery. Venous drainage is via the anterior pontomesencephalic and lateral mesencephalic veins that drain to the basal veins of Rosenthal, which ultimately anastomose with the internal cerebral veins to form the vein of Galen. The posterior mesencephalic veins also drain the midbrain. These veins may join the basal vein of Rosenthal or anastomose directly with the vein of Galen.

Like the rest of the brain, the midbrain is surrounded by cerebrospinal fluid (CSF). The cisterns

A

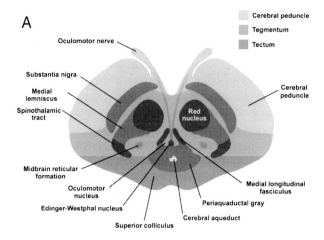

- Cerebral peduncle
- Tegmentum
- Tectum

Oculomotor nerve

Substantia nigra

Medial lemniscus

Spinothalamic tract

Red nucleus

Cerebral peduncle

Midbrain reticular formation

Oculomotor nucleus

Edinger-Westphal nucleus

Superior colliculus

Cerebral aqueduct

Periaquaductal gray

Medial longitudinal fasciculus

B

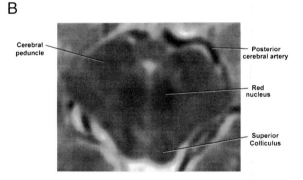

Cerebral peduncle

Posterior cerebral artery

Red nucleus

Superior Colliculus

Figure 1

(A) Artist rendition of the midbrain at the level of the superior colliculus. (B) Magnetic resonance imaging (MRI) scan of the midbrain at the level of the superior colliculus. The red nucleus is obviously visible, but the smaller, less discrete nuclei cannot be visualized on a MRI scan.

surrounding the midbrain are the interpeduncular cistern anteriorly, the ambient cisterns laterally, and the quadrigeminal cistern posteriorly. Separating the tectum from the tegmentum within the substance of the midbrain is the cerebral aqueduct. This ependymal-lined CSF space is usually only 3 or 4 mm in diameter and extends the length of the midbrain. It allows CSF to circulate from the third ventricle to the fourth ventricle and thus from the supratentorial to the infratentorial space. Compression or obstruction of the cerebral aqueduct result in noncommunicating hydrocephalus.

TECTUM

Superior Colliculus

The quadrigeminal plate or dorsal surface of the midbrain has four distinct protuberances: The paired

superior and inferior colliculi (Fig. 1). The superior colliculi are primarily involved in vision and visual reflexes. They receive input from the retina, the cerebral cortex (primarily from the frontal lobe eye fields—Brodmann's area 8), various brainstem nuclei, and the spinal cord. The superior colliculi project to the pulvinar and lateral geniculate body of the thalamus and to the visual cortex in the occipital lobes (areas 18 and 19). Some neurons in the superior colliculi also project to the paramedian pontine reticular formation (PPRF) and the rostral interstitial nucleus of the medial longitudinal fasciculus (RiMLF) involved in subcortical control of eye movements.

Physiological studies suggest that the superior colliculi play an important role in orienting the reactions that shift the head and eyes in order to bring an object of interest into the center of the visual field. Collicular neurons tend to respond best to interesting or moving stimuli. Stimulation of the superior colliculus results in contralateral conjugate deviations of the eyes, even though there are no direct projections to the nuclei of the extraocular muscles. This is probably mediated via the PPRF and the RiMLF. Medial regions of the colliculus are associated with upward eye movements, whereas lateral regions serve downward movements. The superior colliculi are also likely involved in the pupillary light reflex.

Damage to the superior colliculi results in the loss of the ability to visually fixate on an object and track it as it moves. Further damage results in the inability to orient the eyes, head, and body to visual signals. It does not seem to result in any visual field deficit or blindness per se. External pressure on the superior colliculi results in the inability to look upward, as is commonly observed in patients with large pineal region tumors (Fig. 2).

Inferior Colliculus

The inferior colliculi make up the caudal half of the quadrigeminal plate and serve as the main brainstem relay nuclei for auditory function. Auditory impulses traveling in the cochlear nerve synapse in the cochlear nuclei in the pons. They then travel to the superior olivary complex and then via the lateral lemnisci to the nuclei of the lateral lemnisci and the inferior colliculi. After synapsing in the inferior colliculi, auditory input travels to the medial geniculate bodies of the thalamus and from there to the primary auditory cortex in the temporal lobes (area 41).

A

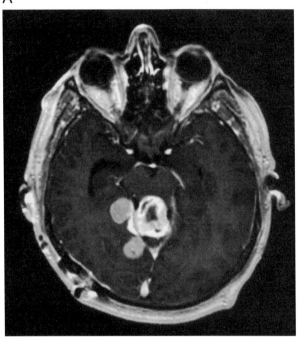

B

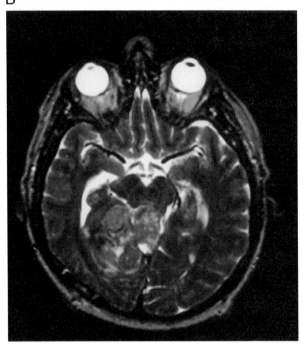

Figure 2
(A) T1 with gadolinium MRI scan shows a hemangiopericytoma of the pineal region compressing the dorsal midbrain. The patient presented with paralysis of upgaze and noncommunicating hydrocephalus. (B) T2 MRI scan showing the same tumor as in Fig. 2A with compression of the dorsal midbrain.

Neurons in the inferior colliculus are arranged in a laminar pattern that represents different frequency bands. This tonotopic arrangement is preserved throughout the auditory pathway. Each inferior colliculus appears to receive input from both ears. The inferior colliculus corresponds to wave V of the auditory brainstem response. Bilateral damage to the inferior colliculi results in deafness, whereas unilateral damage may result in the inability to localize sound.

TEGMENTUM

The tegmentum of the midbrain consists of ill-defined areas or nuclei that project to large regions of the CNS and assist with wakefulness, reproduction, analgesia, and behavior; very well defined nuclei responsible for controlling extraocular movements and extremity motor control and coordination; and passing fiber tracts relaying sensory input from the spinal cord to the thalamus (Fig. 1A).

Periaqueductal Gray

The midbrain periaqueductal gray surrounding the cerebral aqueduct contains many different nuclear groups that serve a wide range of functions. Primarily, however, the periaqueductal gray matter has been associated with central pain control mechanisms. Neurons in the periaqueductal gray contain and respond to enkephalins and endorphins that are the "endogenous opioids" and substance P, one of the primary neurotransmitters responsible for relaying painful stimuli. A stimulating electrode placed in the ventral lateral periaqueductal gray can produce profound analgesia. Also, microinjections of morphine in the ventral periaqueductal gray produce pronounced analgesia.

Reticular Activating System

The reticular formation that extends throughout the brainstem continues in the midbrain and is another ill-defined area of the tegmentum with critical function. Most of the neurons that make up the midbrain reticular formation lie dorsal and lateral to the red nuclei. Collectively, the brainstem reticular formation is involved in regulation of muscle reflexes, coordination of autonomic functions, modulation of pain sensation, and behavioral arousal. It is this last function for which the reticular formation has received the most attention. The ascending reticular activating system can be regarded as a system for conveying impulses of a nonspecific nature to the intralaminar nuclei of the thalami that are then transmitted to the cerebral cortex diffusely. The nonspecific sensory impulses ascending in the reticular activating system appear to sharpen the attentive state of the cortex and create optimal conditions for the conscious perception of classic sensory impulses (e.g., pain, temperature, and light touch). Animal experiments in the 1950s revealed that if the brainstem was sectioned directly caudal to the midbrain, the animals could not sleep. It was thus concluded that the rostral reticular activating system in the midbrain was responsible for wakefulness and the caudal reticular activating system in the pons and medulla was responsible for initiating and maintaining sleep. Since then, sleep has been shown to be a much more complex process, but the overall understanding of the reticular activating system has not changed greatly.

Red Nucleus

In contrast to the poorly defined reticular activating system, the red nucleus occupies a prominent, well-defined location in the midbrain (Fig. 1B). The red nucleus is a large, round mass of gray matter that occupies a central portion of the tegmentum on each side of the upper midbrain. Each red nucleus is grossly identifiable on cut section of the midbrain and appears somewhat red due to an extensive capillary network and a high iron content. The red nucleus is traversed by fibers of the oculomotor nerve rostrally and by fibers of the superior cerebellar peduncle caudally.

The red nucleus has extensive connections to the cerebellum, cortex, and spinal cord that allow participation in motor control and maintenance of tone. Fibers to the red nucleus arrive primarily from the cerebral cortex and the cerebellum. Projections from the cerebral cortex to the red nucleus arise from both the ipsilateral motor and premotor areas. Fibers arising from the dentate, globus, and emboliform nuclei of the cerebellum travel in the superior cerebellar peduncles, cross in the caudal midbrain, and terminate in the contralateral red nucleus. The main outflow from the red nucleus is via the rubrospinal tract to contralateral alpha motor neurons in the spinal cord. The main pattern of rubrospinal action is to excite limb flexor muscles and inhibit the corresponding extensor muscles, particularly involving the distal limb muscles. Thus, the red nucleus appears to act in close conjunction with the motor cortex and the cerebellum for the control of motor behavior. Lesions of the red nucleus usually result in contralateral tremor, ataxia, or choreiform movements. Complete interruption of

the rubrospinal tracts results in loss of flexor tone in the extremities such that the extremities become hyperextended in response to stimuli (decerebrate posture). The red nucleus is also integrated into motor function via connections to the ipsilateral ventrolateral nucleus of the thalamus, the rubrothalamic tract.

Substantia Nigra

The substantia nigra is also a distinct, deeply pigmented nucleus that is intimately involved in motor function. It forms the border of the tegmentum and cerebral peduncles (Fig. 1A). This nucleus can be further divided into the pars compacta (SNc) and the pars reticulata (SNr). The deep pigmentation is due to melanin-containing cells in the SNc. The pigmentation begins in approximately the fifth year of life and the amount of melanin in each cell increases with age. The pigmented neurons of the SNc give rise to the dopaminergic-rich projections that make up the nigrostriatal pathways that play an important role in the pathology of Parkinson's disease.

Afferents to the substantia nigra arise mainly from the caudate nucleus and putamen of the basal ganglia. These fibers are collectively known as the striatonigral fibers. In addition, the substantia nigra receives input from the external globus pallidus, subthalamic nuclei, cerebral cortex, and other brainstem nuclei. The majority of input to the substantia nigra is inhibitory, utilizing GABA as the primary neurotransmitter.

Efferent projections can be categorized as those arising from the SNc and those from the SNr. Nigrostriatal fibers arising from the SNc project to the caudate, putamen, globus pallidus, and thalamus, forming a closed feedback loop between the basal ganglia and the substantia nigra. As already mentioned, the majority of the output from the SNc utilizes dopamine as its neurotransmitter. Inhibitory GABA-rich projections of the SNr extend primarily to the ventral anterior and mediodorsal nuclei of the thalamus. These fibers constitute the only connections between the basal ganglia and the motor nuclei of the thalami. Also, the SNr has a major inhibitory projection to the superior colliculus.

Trochlear Nucleus (Fourth Cranial Nerve)

The trochlear nucleus and nerve innervate the superior oblique extraocular muscle. The nucleus is located ventral to the periaqueductal gray matter and caudal to the oculomotor nucleus. The fibers of the trochlear nerve exit the nucleus, travel dorsolaterally, and cross behind the tectum to emerge on the opposite side of the midbrain just below the inferior colliculus. The trochlear nerve then travels around the midbrain in the ambient cistern. It passes between the superior cerebellar and posterior cerebral arteries and courses toward the lateral wall of the cavernous sinus and the superior orbital fissure to ultimately enter the orbit. The trochlear nerve is unique among the cranial nerves for two main reasons: It is the only completely crossed cranial nerve, and it is the only cranial nerve to exit the dorsal brainstem.

Oculomotor Nucleus (Third Cranial Nerve)

The oculomotor nucleus is located at the level of the superior colliculus ventral to the periaqueductal gray matter (Fig. 1A). Thus, it can be considered as being in the center of the tegmentum. The fibers of the oculomotor nerve pass ventrally through the ipsilateral red nucleus and then exit the ventral midbrain along the medial cerebral peduncle. This nerve also passes between the superior cerebellar and posterior cerebral arteries, enters the lateral wall of the cavernous sinus, and passes through the superior orbital fissure to enter the orbit.

The oculomotor nerve innervates all the extraocular muscles except the superior oblique (trochlear nerve) and lateral rectus (abducens nerve). The extraocular muscles are the inferior oblique and the superior, medial, and inferior rectus muscles. In addition, it innervates the levator palpebrae muscles that open the eyelids and provides parasympathetic innervation to the eye. The actions of the individual extraocular muscles are detailed in Table 1. It should be noted that innervation to the superior rectus is crossed and innervation to the levator palpebrae is crossed and uncrossed. Thus, an isolated lesion involving the right oculomotor nucleus would result in paralysis of the right inferior oblique, medial, and

inferior recti; bilateral weakness of the levator palpebrae with bilateral ptosis; and bilateral weakness of the superior recti muscles. The superior rectus weakness is bilateral because the crossing takes place within the nucleus, such that with a right oculomotor lesion, the right superior rectus neurons and also axons from the left superior rectus neurons are involved. In fact, such lesions are extremely rare and most abnormalities of extraocular movement result from a lesion involving the nerve, such that all the deficits are restricted to one eye.

The subnucleus of the oculomotor nucleus that is responsible for parasympathetic innervation to the eye is the Edinger–Westphal nucleus. Its fibers travel with the oculomotor nerve as the long ciliary nerves. These fibers synapse in the ciliary ganglion behind the eyeball, and then postganglionic parasympathetic fibers innervate the pupilloconstrictor muscles. The action of the parasympathetic innervation is to constrict the pupil. The exact pathway of the pupillary light reflex is not completely known. Multiple nuclei in the midbrain are responsible for the pupils constricting in response to light shone on the retina. Impulses from the retina travel in the optic nerves, chiasm, and the optic tracts to nuclei in the region of the superior colliculi. Fibers then project to both Edinger–Westphal nuclei, which send impulses via the ciliary nerves to the eye to cause the pupils to constrict.

The medial longitudinal fasciculus (MLF) is a fiber tract located directly ventrolateral to the oculomotor nucleus that interconnects the oculomotor nucleus, trochlear nucleus, and abducens nucleus (Fig. 1A). It serves to coordinate conjugate eye movements, especially lateral gaze. Impulses relayed to the right abducens nucleus (for the right lateral rectus muscle) are also transmitted via the MLF to the left oculomotor nucleus (for the left medial rectus muscle) so the eyes look to the right in a conjugate

Table 1 EXTRAOCULAR MUSCLE FUNCTION AND INNERVATION

Muscle	Action	Innervation
Inferior oblique	Elevate eye when eye is adducted	Oculomotor, uncrossed
	Extort eye when eye is abducted	
Medial rectus	Adduct eye	Oculomotor, uncrossed
Inferior rectus	Depress eye when eye is abducted	Oculomotor, uncrossed
Superior rectus	Elevate eye when eye is abducted	Oculomotor, crossed
Levator palpebrae	Raise eyelids	Oculomotor, crossed and uncrossed
Superior oblique	Depress eye when eye is adducted	Trochlear, crossed
	Intort eye when eye is abducted	
Lateral rectus	Abduct eye	Abducens, uncrossed

fashion. A lesion of the MLF results in the inability of the eye on the affected side to adduct past midline and nystagmus of the abducting eye. Lesions of the MLF are most often seen in multiple sclerosis.

Sensory Pathways

Fiber tracts relaying important sensory information from the torso and extremities to the thalamus travel in the tegmentum of the midbrain. The most prominent of these is the medial lemniscus, which runs lateral and dorsal to the red nucleus (Fig. 1A). This fiber tract primarily carries light touch sensation, joint position sense, discriminative sensation, and vibration perception from the contralateral side of the body. Immediately dorsal to this prominent tract is the spinothalamic tract, which relays pain and temperature sensation, also from the contralateral side of the body. All these sensory fibers synapse in the ventral posterior lateral nucleus of the thalamus. Sensory fibers relaying facial sensation travel from the principal sensory trigeminal nuclei (touch and pressure) in the pons, and the spinal trigeminal nuclei (pain, temperature, touch, and pressure) in the more caudal brainstem and upper cervical spinal cord, to the ventral posteromedial nuclei of the thalamus. These fibers are relayed via the ventral (contralateral) and dorsal (ipsilateral) trigeminal lemnisci, which are contiguous with the medial lemnisci in the midbrain.

Cerebral Peduncles

The cerebral peduncles are the most ventral part of the midbrain (Fig. 1B). They consist of two paired, thick fiber tracts conveying motor fibers of the corticospinal and corticobulbar tracts. Fibers in the lateral cerebral peduncles are destined for the contralateral lower extremities, fibers in the middle peduncles serve the contralateral upper extremities, and fibers in the medial cerebral peduncles are associated with face and neck musculature, including the pharynx and larynx.

PATHOLOGY

A wide variety of pathologies can affect the midbrain. The most common are trauma, tumors, and vascular disorders, including hemorrhage and stroke. Various clinical syndromes related to lesions of the midbrain have been described, including Weber's, Benedikt's, Claude's, and Parinaud's syndromes (Table 2). However, because of the complex anatomy of the midbrain, discrete syndrome presentations are rare and usually a myriad of signs and symptoms result, many of which may be masked by a decreased level of consciousness.

Direct traumatic injury to the midbrain is rare because of its very protected location in the center of the head. However, it may be involved by the shifting of the brain in response to trauma. When there is unilateral significant injury to one hemisphere resulting in increased intracranial pressure (ICP) and brain shift, the ipsilateral temporal lobe may herniate over the tentorial edge and compress the midbrain and oculomotor nerve. This can result in an ipsilateral third nerve palsy with ptosis and an enlarging unreactive pupil and diplopia. This is usually a very ominous sign. If the shift and compression progress, the cerebral aqueduct can become kinked, resulting in obstructive hydrocephalus. This causes a further increase in ICP and more brain shift in a deleterious spiral of events that will quickly be fatal if not treated. Also, as the ipsilateral cerebral peduncle is compressed, a contralateral hemiparesis will ensue. If the shift and compression occur quickly, the contralateral cerebral peduncle and lateral tegmentum will become compressed against the contralateral tentorial edge, resulting in an ipsilateral hemiparesis. If this compression is

Table 2   MIDBRAIN SYNDROMES

Syndrome	Location	Findings
Weber's	Third nerve and corticospinal tract (cerebral peduncle)	Ipsilateral third nerve palsy and contralateral hemiparesis
Claude's	Third nerve and red nucleus	Ipsilateral third nerve palsy and contralateral cerebellar ataxia and tremor
Benedikt's	Third nerve, red nucleus, and corticospinal tract	Ipsilateral third nerve palsy and contralateral hemiparesis with tremor in the paralyzed limbs
Parinaud's	Midbrain tectum	Paralysis of upgaze, light—near dissociation, convergence–retraction nystagmus, lid retraction

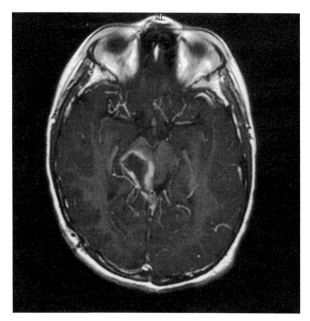

Figure 3
T1 with gadolinium MRI scan reveals a tumor involving much of the right side of the midbrain. The tumor started in the thalamus and extended into the midbrain.

severe enough, it will cause hemorrhage into the lateral midbrain (Duret's hemorrhage).

A variety of tumors may involve the midbrain, including meningiomas, pituitary macroadenomas, gliomas, and pineal region tumors. Pineal region tumors usually present by compressing the collicular plate, resulting in obstructive hydrocephalus and Parinaud's syndrome (Fig. 2). Gliomas usually reach the midbrain via the thalamus and the fiber tracts that traverse it (Fig. 3). Because of its very small size, it would be unusual for a tumor to be confined to the midbrain.

Hemorrhages, either spontaneous or secondary to a vascular malformation, may affect any of the structures in the midbrain (Fig. 4). The onset of symptoms is usually acute, with maximum neurological logical deficit resulting within minutes. A unique variant of subarachnoid hemorrhage related to the midbrain is the perimesencephalic hemorrhage. Patients usually present in the standard manner of a subarachnoid hemorrhage with very severe acute headache and possibly an oculomotor palsy. Computed tomography scan typically shows blood in the interpeduncular and ambient cisterns but no significant blood in any of the other subarachnoid spaces. Cerebral angiography searching for a cause of the hemorrhage is negative. The

patients almost always make a full recovery, and the risk of recurrent hemorrhage is extremely low. The etiology of the hemorrhage is uncertain but may be related to spontaneous bleeding from a tiny vascular malformation on the surface of the midbrain or from the spontaneous rupture of a small perimesencephalic vein.

SURGICAL APPROACHES

Surgical approaches to the midbrain can be categorized as anterior, lateral, and posterior approaches. Although slightly controversial, most surgeons agree that there are no "safe" entry zones into the midbrain. Surgery directed to the region of the midbrain is usually done to remove a tumor externally compressing the midbrain or to repair an aneurysm in the interpeduncular cistern. Only when a well-circumscribed lesion, such as a cavernous malformation, is presenting on the pial surface of the midbrain is an attempt made to actually remove an intra-axial lesion; even in this case, the surgery carries significant risk of new postoperative neurological logical deficits.

The anterior approach to the midbrain involves performing a frontotemporal craniotomy and opening

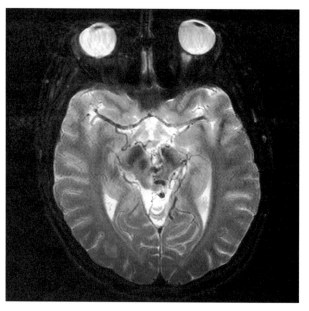

Figure 4
T2 MRI scan shows an arteriovenous malformation affecting the central and left tegmentum and tectum of the midbrain. The abnormal vessels obscure the left red nucleus. The patient presented with tremor, incoordination, and weakness of the right extremities.

the Sylvian fissure widely and identifying the origin of the posterior communicating artery and the oculomotor nerve as it runs along the tentorial edge. These structures are then followed to the posterior cerebral artery and proximal oculomotor nerve in the interpeduncular cistern. This is usually accomplished by working in the space between the internal carotid artery and the oculomotor nerve and retracting the temporal lobe laterally. The posterior clinoid may obscure the view of the anterior midbrain and basilar artery and its branches. The posterior clinoid may be removed with a high-speed drill to improve the exposure. This approach is commonly used to repair aneurysms arising from the basilar terminus or its proximal branches.

The lateral approach relies on a temporal craniotomy centered over the ear. The temporal lobe is gently elevated to provide a lateral view of the basilar artery and midbrain. The edge of the tentorium may be incised or retracted laterally with a stitch to improve the exposure. This approach is most commonly used for extra-axial tumors such as meningiomas arising from the tentorial edge, compressing the midbrain. It is also used to repair aneurysms of the basilar artery and its branches. It has the advantage that the posterior clinoid will not obstruct the view. However, if the basilar terminus is far superior in the interpeduncular cistern, excessive retraction of the temporal lobe may be necessary to achieve the exposure and thus an anterior approach would be preferable.

The posterior approach most commonly involves a suboccipital craniotomy and an infratentorial, supracerebellar approach to the quadrigeminal plate. This is commonly performed to decompress the posterior midbrain when there is a neoplasm arising from the pineal region. There are a wide variety of tumors that may occur in this location, including pinealcytoma, pinealoblastoma, meningioma, hemangiopericytoma, glioma, and germ cell tumors such as germinoma or teratoma (Fig. 2). This approach is commonly performed with the patient in the sitting position to allow gravity to retract the cerebellum inferiorly to facilitate the exposure. The choice of approach is dictated by the extent of the pathology in all cases.

CONCLUSION

The midbrain is the region of the CNS between the pons and the diencephalon. Its functions include extraocular muscle movements and coordination, motor function, vision, hearing, relaying sensory information, and controlling wakefulness and central response to pain. It has extensive connections to the rest of the CNS. Although it is well protected in the skull base, it may be affected by a variety of pathologies. When appropriate, the midbrain can be approached surgically from an anterior, lateral, or posterior route. However, entering the midbrain to directly remove a lesion is fraught with danger because of the critical neural and vascular structures contained in such a small area.

—*Michael J. Link and Catina Y. Sloan*

See also–Brain Anatomy; Brain Herniation, Surgical Management; Central Nervous System, Overview; Oculomotor Nerve (Cranial Nerve III); Trochlear Nerve (Cranial Nerve IV); Vertebrate Nervous System, Development of

Further Reading

Bradley, W. G., Daroff, R. B., Fenichel, J. M., *et al.* (Eds.) (2000). *Neurology in Clinical Practice*, 3rd ed., pp. 293–303, 1198. Butterworth-Heinemann, Boston.

Meyer, F. B. (1999). *Atlas of Neurosurgery*, pp. 170–177, 185–195, 199–207. Churchill Livingstone, Philadelphia.

Netter, F. H. (1991). *Ciba Collection of Medical Illustrations. Nervous System. Vol. 1, Part 1. Anatomy and Physiology* (A. Brass and R. Dingle, Eds.), pp. 31, 34, 35, 52, 53, 60, 61, 98, 99, 131–138, 166–168, 173, 177, 181, 192, 198. Ciba Foundation, West Caldwell, NJ.

Parent, A. (Ed.) (1996). *Carpenter's Human Neuroanatomy*, 9th ed., pp. 527–582. Williams & Wilkins, Baltimore.

Westmoreland, B. F., Benarroch, E. E., Daube, J. R., *et al.* (Eds.) (1994). *Medical Neurosciences*, 3rd ed., pp. 427–433. Little, Brown, Boston.

Migraine, Genetics of

Encyclopedia of the Neurological Sciences
Copyright 2003, Elsevier Science (USA). All rights reserved.

NUMEROUS clinical studies over the years have documented familial aggregation of migraine. The frequency of a positive family history varies from 40 to 90% compared with 5 to 20% in control populations. Migraine with aura appears to have a higher familial aggregation than migraine without aura. Twin studies also suggest a strong genetic component for migraine, particularly for migraine with aura. In a recent Danish study, of more than 2000 monozygotic and 3000 dizygotic same-sex twins, the concordance rate for migraine with aura was 34% in monozygotic twin pairs and 12% in dizygotic pairs. These findings emphasize the importance of genetic factors in migraine with aura but also suggest that environmental factors are important since the concordance rate is much less than 100% in the monozygotic pairs.

The prevalence of migraine in African and Asian populations is lower than that in European and North American populations. These differences among racial groups are probably due to genetic factors rather than cultural or environmental factors because they persist after migration to the United States. Furthermore, African Americans report a higher level of headache pain but are less likely to report nausea and vomiting with their attacks than Caucasians. African Americans are also less disabled by their attacks than Caucasians.

There is debate as to whether migraine with aura and migraine without aura are distinct syndromes, different manifestations of the same syndrome, or part of a continuum. Patients often have both types of attacks (with or without aura), and frequently both types of migraine run in the same family. Furthermore, the headache pain phases of both types of migraine are almost identical and the same treatments are usually effective for both types. On the other hand, certain epidemiological characteristics, overall familial aggregation, and varying pathophysiological findings suggest that these two types of migraine may be separate entities.

Several migraine syndromes have a clear autosomal dominant pattern of inheritance. Recently, an abnormal calcium channel gene was identified in families with familial hemiplegic migraine, an autosomal dominant syndrome characterized by headache attacks preceded by, or accompanied by, episodes of hemiplegia. Episodes of hemiplegia and migraine with aura may alternate within individuals and co-occur within families. The mode of inheritance is less clear for the more common syndromes of migraine with aura and migraine without aura. An autosomal dominant pattern with reduced penetrance has been suggested for both of these disorders, but the penetrance of the gene would have to be very low in most studies to support a simple autosomal dominant inheritance. A polygenetic cause seems more likely. Another problem with a simple autosomal dominant inheritance is the female-to-male preponderance with migraine of approximately 3:1. However, hormonal changes in women are well-known triggers for migraine symptoms, so different hormonal patterns could account for the increased penetrance in women compared to men.

Currently, the most likely candidate genes for migraine with aura and migraine without aura are those associated with ion channels and serotonin metabolism. With the finding of an abnormal voltage-gated calcium channel gene in familial hemiplegic migraine, mutations in other calcium channel genes are prime candidates for migraine syndromes, including migraine with aura and migraine without aura. These channels are remarkably diverse in their conductance and gating mechanisms, and most neurons express several subtypes that are characterized by different functional and pharmacological properties. Many of the well-known triggers for migraine symptoms, including stress and menstruation, could result from hormonal influences on a defective ion channel. Currently used prophylactic drugs for migraine, including beta blockers, calcium channel blockers, and tricyclic amines, might work by stabilizing an abnormal ion channel.

—*Robert W. Baloh*

See also–Brain Tumors, Genetics; Ion Channels, Overview; Migraine Mechanisms; Migraine, Menstrual; Migraine, Ophthalmoplegic and Retinal; Migraine, Transformed; Migraine Treatment; Migraine with Aura; Migraine without Aura; Serotonin

Further Reading

Baloh, R. W. (2000). Genetics of migraine. In *Neurogenetics* (S.-M. Pulst, Ed.), pp. 389–401. Oxford Univ. Press, New York.

Palotie, A., Baloh, R., and Wessman, M. (2001). Genetics of migraine. In *The Genetic Bases of Common Diseases* (R. E. King, J. I. Rotter, and A. Motulsky, Eds.). Oxford Univ. Press, New York.

Ulrich, V., Gervil, M., Kyvik, K. O., *et al.* (1999). Evidence of a genetic factor in migraine with aura: A population-based Danish twin study. *Ann. Neurol.* 45, 242–246.

Migraine Mechanisms

Encyclopedia of the Neurological Sciences
Copyright 2003, Elsevier Science (USA). All rights reserved.

THE PATHOPHYSIOLOGY of migraine is incompletely understood. Recent studies have shed light on the neuronal events mediating both the aura and the headache phases of migraine. Research has identified a cerebral cortical origin of migraine aura, and it has identified the trigeminovascular system and its central projections as the origin of headache.

INTERICTAL PHASE

The concept that the migraine attack originates in the brain and can be triggered by various factors under various conditions argues in favor of a threshold that governs the triggering of attacks. The nature of the final common pathway with which these factors interact probably constitutes the true cause of migraine. Neurophysiological, cerebral blood flow (CBF), and metabolic measurements have suggested neuronal and neurovascular instability between migraine attacks. One recently proposed model to explain these physiological shifts is transient or persistently exaggerated excitability of neurons in the cerebral cortex, especcially occipital. Although the pathways mediating headache pain may be the same in all individuals, these pathways may be more easily triggered in patients with episodic migraines. As an example of interictal differences in brain activity between normal people and migraine sufferers, transcranial magnetic stimulation to the occipital cortex required to produce phosphene generation was significantly lower in patients with migraines with aura between their headaches than it was in normal controls.

Differing cellular mechanisms may underlie increased central neuronal hyperexcitability in migraine. In a rare autosomal dominant subtype of migraine, familial hemiplegic migraine, mutation of a gene involved in the production of a brain-specific P/Q-type calcium channel was identified in approximately 50% of families. This indicates that at least this uncommon form of migraine results from a calcium channelopathy and possibly more typical migraine, at least in some families subsequently studied.

Other possible sources of neuronal hyperexcitability are a mitochondria defect or a disturbance in magnesium metabolism. Intracellular magnesium stores may be low in migraineurs; this deficiency could affect mitochondria function, or it could alter membrane stability by receptor gating or binding to membrane phospholipids. In support of this, Fig. 1 shows low magnesium in phosphorus-31 spectroscopic images of members of a family with hemiplegic migraine.

MECHANISM UNDERLYING AURA

One-fifth of migraine sufferers experience aura prior to headache onset that is predominantly visual. Cortical spreading depression, first observed by Leao in 1944, is considered the basis of the aura. Cortical

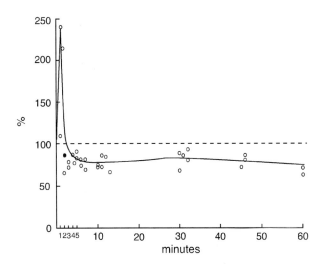

Figure 1
Phosphorus spectroscopic images of patients with familial hemiplegic migraine.

neuronal excitation followed by depression of normal neuronal activity spreads slowly from the site of initiation at rates between 2 and 6 mm/min. Spreading depression does not follow vascular boundaries, although pial arterial and venous dilation occur simultaneously with the first activated neural activity. A brief increase in regional cerebral blood flow (rCBF) is followed by decreased rCBF to oligemic values lasting approximately 1 hr after the passage of the wave of neuronal inhibition. Like spreading depression, this cortical oligemia does not follow vascular boundaries. Advances in brain imaging, including rCBF measured by Xe-133, diffusion/perfusion magnetic resonance imaging (MRI), functional MRI-BOLD, and magnetoencephalography, have allowed investigators to observe cortical spreading depression during migraine aura. Cao and colleagues, studying the properties of migraine attacks induced by visual stimulation using functional MRI, noted that transient activation followed by a spreading suppression of neuronal activity was accompanied by vasodilatation and hyperoxygenation.

The mechanism by which aura induces the headache of migraine is unclear. Spreading depression causes stimulation of the trigeminal nucleus caudalis, a region believed to be part of the central pathway mediating migraine pain. This might be secondary to involvement of cortical–subcortical connections to nociceptive centers recruited by the wave of cortical excitation/suppression. Alternatively, the wave of spreading depression may invade cortical trigeminal terminals, setting up a cascade of events leading to inflammation as a persistent source of trigeminal stimulation and headache. Recent evidence implicates both the trigeminal and parasympathetic systems, through brainstem connections, in causing vasodilatation and inflammatory change of the extracerebral circulation, particularly meningeal vessels, during and after cortical spreading depression.

Most studies of spreading depression in migraineurs have focused on the aura phase of migraine. Woods *et al.* observed spreading oligemia in association with spontaneous headache in a patient with migraine but no aura. Changes in rCBF resembled those observed during aura by other investigators. Cao and colleagues reported a spreading suppression of neural activity in the occipital cortex prior to headache in migraine patients with or without aura. These studies suggest that the same neuronal events may precede the initiation of migraine in all patients, although cortical spreading depression and changes in CBF remain clinically silent in migraine without aura. On the other hand, others have not observed changes in blood flow in migraine without aura, raising the possibility that the trigeminal system may be activated by noncortical mechanisms, such as changes in pain modulation.

HEADACHE MECHANISMS

Migraine headache may originate from dilation of the large cranial vessels and dura mater, innervated by the trigeminal nerve as part of the trigeminovascular system. Stimulation of trigeminal sensory neurons induces inflammation and plasma protein extravasation (PPE). The vasoactive peptides substance P and neurokinin A, released by the trigeminovascular system, cause PPE from the vessels, mast cell degranulation, platelet adherence and aggregation, and endothelial activation. The result is meningeal inflammation that persists for minutes to hours, possibly the principal mechanism for the prolonged intense headache pain. The antimigraine agents sumatriptan, ergotamine, dihydroergotamine, and methysergide have been shown to block this plasma extravasation, thereby reducing neurogenic inflammation. However, not all drugs that block PPE have an antimigraine effect, which is a point of controversy when attributing mechanisms of migraine headache since it is unclear whether PPE and meningeal inflammation occur in humans during migraine.

The vasodilator peptides calcitonin gene-related peptide (CGRP), substance P (SP), and neurokinin A are found in the cell bodies of trigeminal neurons. CGRP has been implicated most in the headache of migraine. CGRP is present in nonmyelinated fibers in the trigeminal ganglion, and CGRP-like immunoreactivity has been identified in regions of the trigeminal nuclei known to receive primary afferent terminals. The sensory role of CGRP in the trigeminal system is unclear but possibly involves vascular nociception. Electrical stimulation of the ganglion released CGRP in cat and humans, and CGRP was detected in jugular venous blood during a migraine attack but SP was not. The neurogenic inflammation theory of migraine proposed that CGRP released from trigeminal sensory afferents causes vasodilatation and plasma extravasations from dural vessels. Triptans, acting as 5-HT1B/D agonists, block these responses. Infusion of CGRP to susceptible individuals can elicit migraine-like headache.

NOVEL ASPECTS OF MIGRAINE MECHANISMS

The brainstem may play a pivotal role in the pathophysiology of migraine. In a study of acute migraine without aura using positron emission tomography, an area of the contralateral rostral brainstem covering the dorsal pons and midbrain (particularly the periaqueductal gray matter, dorsal raphe nucleus, and the locus ceruleus) was activated during the attack and after effective treatment by sumatriptan. Furthermore, iron levels were abnormal in the midbrain periaqueductal gray matter (PAG) of patients with episodic and chronic migraine. These areas, especially PAG, may produce migraine-like headache when stimulated or triggered by certain structural pathologies. Thus, episodic dysfunction of brainstem neurons may have a key role in migraine pain, either through aberrant activation or through impaired modulation of impulse flow in the trigeminal system. Since the PAG is the center of a powerful antinociceptive system in the brain, this offers new approaches to acute migraine drugs acting as neuromodulators via this system.

Evidence for central neuronal hyperexcitability was obtained in a study of cutaneous allodynia during migraine in humans; the findings indicated central sensitization at a second- or third-order neuronal level. Abnormal supraspinal pain modulation is in keeping with PAG dysfunction and aberrance of its balanced nociceptive facilitatory or inhibitory functions.

—*K. M. A. Welch*

See also–Migraine, Genetics of; Migraine, Menstrual; Migraine, Ophthalmoplegic and Retinal; Migraine, Transformed; Migraine Treatment; Migraine with Aura; Migraine without Aura; Stroke, Migraine-Induced

Further Reading

Aurora, S. K., Ahmad, B. K., Welch, K. M. A., *et al.* (1998). Transcranial magnetic stimulation confirms hyperexcitability of occipital cortex in migraine. *Neurology* **50**, 1111–1114.

Bolay, H., Reuter, U., Dunn, A. K., *et al.* (2002). Intrinsic brain activity triggers trigeminal meningeal afferents in a migraine model. *Nature Med.* **8**, 136–142.

Burstein, R., Yarnitsky, D., Goor-Aryeh, I., *et al.* (2000). An association between migraine and cutaneous allodynia. *Ann. Neurol.* **47**, 614–624.

Cao, Y., Welch, K. M. A., Aurora, S., *et al.* (1999). Functional MRI-bold of visually triggered headache in patients with migraine. *Arch. Neurol.* **56**, 548–554.

Goadsby, P. J. (2001). The pathophysiology of headache. In *Wolff's Headache and Other Head Pain* (S. D. Silberstein, R. B. Lipton, and S. Solomon, Eds.), 7th ed., pp. 57–72. Oxford Univ. Press, Oxford.

Goadsby, P. J. (2002). Neurovascular headache and a midbrain vascular malformation—Evidence for a role of the brainstem in chronic migraine. *Cephalalgia* **22**, 107–111.

Goadsby, P. J., and Hoskin, K. L. (1999). Differential effects of low dose CP122,288 and eletriptan on Fos expression due to stimulation of the superior sagittal sinus in the cat. *Pain* **82**, 15–22.

Goadsby, P. J., Edvinsson, L., and Ekman, R. (1988). Release of vasoactive peptides in the extracerebral circulation of man and the cat during activation of the trigeminovascular system. *Ann. Neurol.* **23**, 193–196.

Hadjikhani, N., Sanchez del Rio, M., Wu, O., *et al.* (2001). Mechanisms of migraine aura revealed by functional MRI in human visual cortex. *Proc. Natl. Acad. Sci. USA* **98**, 4687–4692.

Hoskin, K. L., Zagami, A., and Goadsby, P. J. (1999). Stimulation of the middle meningeal artery leads to bilateral FOS expression in the trigeminocervical nucleus: A comparative study of monkey and cat. *J. Anat.* **194**, 579–588.

Leao, A. A. P. (1944). Spreading depression of activity in cerebral cortex. *J. Neurophysiol.* **7**, 359–390.

Millan, M. J. (2001). Descending monoaminergic modulation of pain: Basic principles, novel insights from receptor multiplicity, and therapeutic perspectives. *Neurosci. News* **4**, 19–34.

Moskowitz, M. A., and Cutrer, F. M. (1993). Sumatriptan: A receptor-targeted treatment for migraine. *Annu. Rev. Med.* **44**, 145–154.

Nyholt, D. R., Lea, R. A., Goadsby, P. J., *et al.* (1998). Familial typical migraine: Linkage to chromosome 19p13 and evidence for genetic heterogeneity. *Neurology* **50**, 1428–1432.

Ophoff, R. A., Terwindt, G. M., Vergouwe, M. N., *et al.* (1996). Familial hemiplegic migraine and episodic ataxia type-2 are caused by mutations in the Ca^{2+} channel gene CACNLA4. *Cell* **87**, 543–552.

Roon, K. I., Olesen, J., Diener, H. C., *et al.* (2000). No acute antimigraine efficacy of CP-122,288, a highly potent inhibitor of neurogenic inflammation: Results of two randomized double-blind placebo-controlled clinical trials. *Ann. Neurol.* **47**, 238–241.

Russel, M. B., Rassmussen, B. K., Fenger, K., *et al.* (1996). Migraine without aura and migraine with aura are distinct clinical entities: A study of four hundred and eight-four male and female migraineurs from the general population. *Cephalalgia* **16**, 239–245.

Schoenen, J., Jacquy, J., and Lenaerts, M. (1997). High-dose riboflavin is effective in migraine prophylaxis: Results from a double blind, randomized, placebo-controlled trial. *Neurology* **48**, A86–A87.

Veloso, F., Kumar, K., and Toth, C. (1998). Headache secondary to deep brain implantation. *Headache* **38**, 507–515.

Welch, K. M. A., Nagesh, V., Aurora, S. K., *et al.* (2001). Periaqueductal gray matter dysfunction in migraine: Cause or the burden of illness? *Headache* **41**, 629–637.

Woods, R. P., Iacoboni, M., and Mazziotta, J. C. (1994). Bilateral spreading cerebral hypoperfusion during spontaneous migraine headache. *N. Engl. J. Med.* **331**, 1689–1692.

Migraine, Menstrual

Encyclopedia of the Neurological Sciences
Copyright 2003, Elsevier Science (USA). All rights reserved.

THE PREVALENCE of migraine in children shows no sex difference until the early teen years, corresponding with the time at which young women begin menarche. Menstrually related migraine begins at menarche in 33% of susceptible women. For many women, migraine continues to occur primarily at the time of menses. True menstrual migraine, seen exclusively with menses, is less common but is an important entity because it may merit different therapeutic management. Menstrually related migraine and true menstrual migraine are differentiated on the basis of occurrence. Menstrually related migraine may be seen at the time of menses, but women who experience it also have migraine at other times of the month. True menstrual migraine is limited to the perimenstrual period (within 2 days of the menstrual cycle) according to MacGregor's definition.

The controversy regarding the treatment of menstrual migraine and whether it should be differentiated from that of migraine in general has existed for some time. Many authors believe that menstrual migraine management should be differentiated because the underlying pathophysiology may be different. Whether menstrual attacks are resistant to treatment has been a topic of continued debate. The predictable recurrence of attacks allows for "burst" prophylactic therapy. For many women, the so-called miniprophylaxis may be an ideal approach and is well suited to predictably recurrent attacks of migraine. Management of migraine triggers in the presence of the premenstrual decrease of estrogen or change in the progesterone:estrogen ratio may be particularly challenging and of significant clinical importance. Lastly, comorbidity with the premenstrual syndrome may require therapies that treat both.

PATHOGENESIS

Menstrual migraine may be associated with other somatic complaints related to changes in sex hormones levels. Comorbidities include the premenstrual syndrome (late luteal dysphoric disorder) and, as women enter the fifth and sixth decades, perimenopause.

The decrease in estrogen that occurs during the luteal phase of the menstrual cycle is thought to be the critical trigger in the development of menstrual migraine. In particular, the decrease in estradiol on the day prior to menstrual flow correlates with migraine onset for many patients. Ovulatory headache is described less often in the literature, but based on a review of patient diaries it appears to be another common pattern.

The mechanisms of migraine development in relationship to cyclical fluctuations in estrogen levels have not been completely delineated. It appears that multiple neurotransmitter systems are involved. Withdrawal of estrogen correlates with prostaglandin release, changes in opioid tone, increased sensitivity of dopamine receptors, increased serotonergic transmission, and reactivity of the cerebral vasculature to serotonin. In addition, there are menstrual-related changes in melatonin secretion. Melatonin, a hormone produced by the pineal gland, regulates the sleep–wake cycle. Its concentration is elevated during darkness and suppressed by light. In humans, melatonin produces sleep. In women with menstrual migraine (unlike control subjects), melatonin secretion does not increase in the luteal phase, leading to sleep fragmentation, which in turn may exacerbate menstrual migraine.

OBSTACLES TO TREATMENT OF MENSTRUAL MIGRAINE

Several factors interfere with effective treatment of menstrual migraine. Failure to make the diagnosis is probably the most common problem. Not recognizing or appreciating the amount of disability associated with migraine can also limit treatment initiation. Together, these factors highlight the need for physician awareness of menstrual migraine, the role of hormonal fluctuations in its development, and the consequences of untreated menstrual migraine. Lack of patient awareness is also a significant problem that may keep women from seeking medical attention. Many affected individuals do not realize that they have migraines. They may rule menstruation out as a cause of their headache based on their own self-diagnosis, or they may attribute their headaches to other causes, such as changes in weather or even sinus congestion. Unless they are asked to keep diaries, few patients recognize that their headaches have a hormonally influenced pattern. Even those who do recognize a cyclical pattern to their headaches may call them hormone headaches and not migraines. Sometimes, menstrual migraine may not be diagnosed until the woman becomes perimenopausal or menopausal. Some patients may even overlook their headaches if they are not severe enough to be disabling or if they have developed a habit of using NSAIDs for other menstrual-related discomfort. Others with classic features of migraine simply may not make the connection that would lead them to seek medical attention.

Many patients are unaware that they are experiencing a prodrome, for example, or they may be hesitant to report prodromal symptoms because they are fearful that the physician will think that the symptoms are psychiatric. Prodrome as the first stage in a migraine attack needs to be explored during history taking. Rather than relying on patient self-reporting, the history should include questions that will elicit information about prodromal symptoms: Does the patient yawn excessively, have specific food cravings (such as chocolate), experience fluctuations in mood, or become overwhelmingly tired or fatigued? The questions should be framed in a way that will make the patient feel comfortable about responding.

Even after diagnosis, migraineurs tend to have low expectations for successful treatment. In one survey of patients who had been treated unsuccessfully, 10% responded that they were satisfied with their treatment. This suggests that buried within our population are thousands or even millions of women who continue to suffer without complaint because they are unaware that effective treatments are available. Therefore, in addition to increasing physician awareness about menstrual migraine, it is important to make patients aware that effective treatment is available.

MIGRAINE, MENSTRUAL   165

MANAGEMENT

A cornerstone of menstrual migraine management is identifying the relationship between the menstrual cycle and migraine. In the clinical setting, being able to establish this relationship is dependent on a thorough history and an accurate patient diary. Women will repeatedly state that their headaches bear no relationship to menstrual periods or to ovulation or other hormonal fluctuations; however, clinical experience consistently shows that women who keep diaries accurately and record both ovulation and menstrual periods can frequently begin to identify a menstrual association with their migraine. Patient education in regard to the importance of keeping a diary is critical to management. One strategy for encouraging patients to keep diaries is to emphasize that if they can identify, for example, menstrual migraine, their pharmacological therapy may be limited to the time of menstrual cycle. They may also be able to take less medication and may benefit from miniprophylaxis as opposed to prophylaxis on a daily basis. Reassuring patients that migraine is a biological disorder is also crucial to their management. Many women have been made to believe that headache is a part of the premenstrual syndrome and that they are condemned to have headache during "certain times of the month"; thus, they often do not believe that headache in this setting merits treatment. It is important for them to recognize that triggering factors that may make their menstrual migraine more severe can be managed. In particular, in regard to management of migraine triggers during times of hormonal vulnerability, patients may need to be particularly careful regarding sleep hygiene, avoid alcohol, avoid specific food triggers, and/or preemptively treat any altitudinal changes or barometric pressure changes that occur during the time in which their estrogen levels are declining. Strategies for management should include both acute treatment for the onset of menstrual migraine and/or prodrome and prophylactic therapy on the basis of disability and headache duration. Patients should be encouraged to have adequate trials of prophylaxis and/or miniprophylaxis at full or reasonable dosages, and they should be encouraged to take medications for 3 months, particularly if hormonal strategies are being employed, to be certain that efficacy has been obtained and that they have had adequate time to respond to therapy.

Abortive therapy should be prescribed to achieve pain-free status and restore function to patients.

Migraine-specific therapy includes the triptans and hydroergotamines, which offer impressive efficacy for all menstrual migraine end points, including pain relief, pain-free status, control of nausea and vomiting, and relief of functional disability. Several studies have shown sumatriptan, both subcutaneous and oral, to be as effective in the treatment of menstrual migraine as it is for nonmenstrual migraine. The efficacy of rizatriptan and zolmitriptan has been established in menstrual migraine as well.

Cyclical or miniprophylaxis with a nonsteroidal antiinflammatory agent or triptan beginning 2 or 3 days before menses and lasting for up to 1 week may also be a useful strategy for patients who have predictable menstrual headaches. Hormonal therapies for menstrual migraine prophylaxis may include the use of oral contraceptives. Migraine has been shown to improve in one-third of patients in whom oral contraceptives are used, worsen in one-third of patients, and remain unchanged in the remaining patients. Thus, predictability of improvement for management is challenging. Strategies may include continuous oral contraceptives, where a patient is asked to take three consecutive pill packs, and during the week of placebo miniprophylaxis can be added, including migraine-specific therapy for breakthrough attacks. With regard to determining patient response, careful diary information is particularly useful once oral contraceptives are added.

Prophylactic approaches have also included percutaneous estradiol gel given for menstrual migraine. Two studies by de Lignieres and Dennerstein, employing a double-blind, placebo-controlled design, showed a reduction in migraine frequency, severity, and duration when patients were given percutaneous estradiol gel prior to the onset of menstrual migraine. Transdermal estrogen has also been given for menstrual migraine prophylaxis, and Pradalier showed a reduction in migraine frequency and use of rescue medications in an open-label trial of high-dose treatment. Other miniprophylaxis regimens that have been successful include naprosen given 7 days before menses and continued for 6 days after onset of menstruation. Thirty-three percent of patients in this trial were free of headache with naprosen dosed in this manner, whereas no patients were free of headache in the placebo group. Ergotamine tartrate can be used for miniprophylaxis dosed at 1 mg twice a day for the 3- to 5-day menstrual period. Naratriptan is the only triptan that has been shown to reduce menstrual headache when given as a miniprophylactic agent. In the naratriptan miniprophylactic study, 23%

of patients receiving 1 mg of naratriptan twice daily for 2 days before their period and continuing into the third day of the menstrual cycle were without menstrual headache during three menstrual periods.

Anticonvulsant therapy may also be beneficial for menstrual migraine prophylaxis, and gabapentin and levetiracetam have the advantage of not interfering with birth control pills, although recent data suggest that topirimate in doses ranging from 100 to 400 mg has no effect on oral contraceptive efficacy. Cyclical oral magnesium supplementation of 360 mg a day has been compared to placebo in women with menstrual migraine. Reduction was reported both in menstrual migraine and in premenstrual syndrome symptomatology.

Other hormone manipulations have been reported to be effective, including dopamine agonists, synthetic androgens, and antiestrogens. Although these continue to be discussed in the headache literature, in clinical practice they have not proven to be widely useful.

GENERAL TREATMENT APPROACHES

The relationship between migraine and hormonal changes should be discussed with the patient and established. A headache diary is critical for documentation of headaches and evaluation of the effectiveness of therapy and to guide medication dosages as well as allow for add-on therapy. Patients with menstrual migraine should avoid any additional triggers under their control.

Abortive therapy should be an initial approach with the goals of achieving pain-free status within 2 hr, returning to full function, and no recurrence. If ineffective, patients should be switched to other triptans and polytherapy for abortive treatment that can be expanded to include a nonsteroidal agent or COX-2 inhibitor as well as an antiemetic. Patients should be taught how to redose their abortive medications. In particular, triptan therapies should be redosed and used at maximum dosage if patients do not achieve headache-free status.

If patients are on preventive therapy for menstrual and nonmenstrual attacks, preventive therapies can be boosted during the time of anticipated ovulatory or menstrual migraine. Patients who continue to have longer duration menstrual migraine or recurrence or who are unable to achieve pain-free status may benefit from miniprophylaxis. Initiation with prostaglandin inhibitors may be most cost-effective, and these have been shown to be effective and well tolerated. They can be initiated 1 or 2 days before the day of onset of the headache and continued throughout the patients' vulnerable period. If one antiinflammatory agent is not affective, another can be tried, and if gastrointestinal disturbances occur, the patient may be switched to a COX-2 inhibitor.

If NSAIDs or COX-2 inhibitors are ineffective or only partially affective, hormonal manipulation may be initiated. This may include oral contraception, as mentioned previously. Short-term but sustained estrogen may be given in the form of transdermal patches or estradiol gels during the period of highest risk and may be useful as supplemental therapy during the placebo days of oral contraceptives. Lastly, miniprophylaxis may be beneficial using triptan therapy dosed at 1 mg bid naratriptan, and ergotamine tartrate may also be considered, although it limits the use of a triptan for breakthrough attack.

CONCLUSION

Menstrual migraine may be extremely disabling and challenging to treat. Manipulation of the menstrual cycle and stabilization of estrogen levels may prove key in preventing menstrual migraine attacks, and therapy directed at those triggers may be of most benefit in patients who have severe menstrual migraine. Abortive therapy may be highly successful in patients with milder menstrual migraine. For patients with more severe and disabling attacks, therapy can include acute polytherapy, miniprophylaxis, and/or hormonal therapies.

—*Jan Lewis Brandes*

See also–Migraine, Genetics of; Migraine Mechanisms; Migraine, Ophthalmoplegic and Retinal; Migraine, Transformed; Migraine Treatment; Migraine with Aura; Migraine without Aura

Further Reading

Davies, G. M., Santanello, N. C., Kramer, M., *et al.* (1998). Determinants of patient satisfaction with migraine treatment. *Headache* **38**, 380.

Epstein, M. T., Hockaday, J. M., and Hockaday, T. D. (1975). Migraine and reproductive hormones throughout the menstrual cycle. *Lancet* **1**, 543–548.

Faccinetti, F., Bonellie, G., Kangasniemi, P., *et al.* (1995). The efficacy and safety of subcutaneous Sumatriptan in the acute treatment of menstrual migraine. The Sumatriptan Menstrual Migraine Study Group. *Obstet. Gynecol.* **85**, 911–916.

Granella, F., Sances, G., Zanferrari, C., *et al.* (1993). Migraine without aura and reproductive life events: A clinical epidemiological study in 1300 women. *Headache* **33**, 385–389.

Gross, M. L. P., Barrie, M., Bates, D., *et al.* (1995, September). The efficacy of oral sumatriptan in menstrual migraine–A prospective study. Poster presented at the Seventh Annual Headache Congress, Toronto.

Johannes, C. B., Linet, M. S., Stewart, W. F., *et al.* (1995). Relationship of headache to phase of the menstrual cycle among young women: A daily diary study. *Neurology* **45**, 1076–1082.

Lipton, R. B., Stewart, W. F., and Simon, D. (1995). Medical consultation for migraine: Results from the American Migraine study. *Headache* **38**, 87–96.

Silberstein, S. (1998). Sex hormones and headache. *Semin. Headache Manage.* **3**, 1–8.

Silberstein, S., Norman, B., Jiang, K., *et al.* (1999). Rizatriptan is effective in menstrual migraine. *Neurology* **52**, A208.

Solbach, M. P., and Wayner, R. S. (1993). Treatment of menstruation-associated migraine headache with subcutaneous sumatriptan. *Obstet. Gynecol.* **82**, 769–772.

Vliet, E. (1996, November/December). An approach to perimenopausal migraine. *Menopause Manage.* 25–33.

Welch, K. M. A. (1997). Migraine and ovarian steroid hormones. *Cephalalgia* **17**, 12–16.

Migraine, Ophthalmoplegic and Retinal

Encyclopedia of the Neurological Sciences

OPHTHALMOPLEGIC MIGRAINE is defined as repeated attacks of headache associated with paresis of one or more ocular cranial nerves in the absence of demonstrable intracranial lesion.

Ocular migraine and ophthalmic migraine have been used to describe this condition, but usually these terms describe situations in which the visual complaints are prominent, such as in migraine with aura. The condition is rare, estimated to occur in less than 2% of migraineurs, with onset usually before age 10. Attacks may occur in infancy or be painless. It appears to be more common in males. There is no clear genetic pattern. Reports have shown abnormalities of the oculomotor nerve using magnetic resonance imaging (MRI) in children with recurrent painful ophthalmoplegia fulfilling the criteria for ophthalmoplegic migraine. It is now believed that all modern cases show MRI enhancement of the third nerve which may represent a type of inflammation and, therefore, ophthalmoplegic migraine is going to be taken out of the official Classification of Headache of the International Headache Society.

The pathophysiology of ophthalmoplegic migraine remains obscure. Microvascular constriction with peripheral cranial nerve ischemia is a possible cause or a recurrent idiopathic inflammation similar to that occurring in peripheral seventh nerve palsy. Because many attacks leave some residual effects and the ophthalmoplegia tends to become worse after repeated attacks, it seems likely that repeated episodes produce progressive third nerve injury. The headaches usually precede the ophthalmoplegia by 3 or 4 days. The headache is usually unilateral and may be throbbing or constant but is occasionally bilateral or alternating. It is often of the crescendo type, lasting hours to days. The ophthalmoplegia usually follows, affecting one or more nerves and possibly alternating sides in subsequent attacks. Extraocular muscle paralysis may occur with the first attack of headache or, rarely, may precede it. However, the paralysis usually appears subsequent to an established migraine pattern. The pupillomotor fibers are usually involved, producing a mydriatic and poorly responsive pupil. The sixth and fourth nerves are less commonly involved.

The following is a typical clinical syndrome: A child or young adult with periodic headache has ophthalmoplegia involving all functions of the third nerve, beginning at the height of an attack of cephalgia. The pain is primarily unilateral and in the orbital region. The ocular motor dysfunction lasts for days to weeks following the cessation of headaches; recovery is gradual and tends to be less complete after repeated attacks. Standard migraine prophylactic therapy, including beta blockers or calcium channel blockers, is recommended.

Retinal migraine describes repeated attacks of monocular scotoma or blindness lasting less than 1 hr and associated with headache. Ocular or structural vascular disorder must be ruled out. Other terms include ocular migraine, anterior visual pathway migraine, and ophthalmic migraine. This condition occurs more frequently than ophthalmoplegic migraine. The frequency of strictly monocular visual phenomena occurring in conjunction with migraine is estimated to be 1 in 200 migraine sufferers.

Ten of 24 patients reported by Tomsak and Jergens described concentric contraction of vision, and only 5 patients had an altitudinal or quadratic visual change consistent with spasm of retinal artery branch. In some cases, retinal migraine may be due to a primary neuronal event such as retina spreading depression. Permanent unilateral visual loss from retinal migraine is well documented but uncommon. In addition to arterial or venous retinal vascular occlusions, central serous retinopathy, vitreous hemorrhage, retinal hemorrhage, and ischemic optic neuropathy have been noted. A typical history is that of a young adult with a pattern of common or classic migraine who has recurrent episodes of monocular visual loss or monocular scintillating scotomas. The visual loss is often one-sided and stereotyped in nature and tends to affect the entire monocular visual field, although any of the visual patterns described in migraine with aura may occur on a monocular basis in retinal migraine. Approximately one-third of patients have a prior history of migraine. In general, the prognosis for retinal migraine is similar to that for migraine headache with typical aura.

I believe that all patients with retinal migraine should be placed on prophylactic antimigrainous therapy, such as calcium channel-blocking and beta-blocking agents or anticonvulsants.

—*B. Todd Troost*

See also–Migraine, Genetics of; Migraine Mechanisms; Migraine, Menstrual; Migraine, Transformed; Migraine Treatment; Migraine with Aura; Migraine without Aura; Oculomotor Nerve (Cranial Nerve III); Ophthalmoplegia; Progressive External Ophthalmoplegia (PEO); Stroke, Migraine-Induced

Further Reading

Durkan, G. P., Troost, B. T., Slamovits, T. L., *et al.* (1981). Recurrent painless oculomotor palsy in children: A variant of ophthalmoplegic migraine. *Headache* **21**, 58.

Ostergaard, J. R., Moller, H. U., and Christensen, T. (1996). Recurrent ophthalmoplegia in childhood: Diagnostic and etiologic considerations. *Cephalalgia* **16**, 276–279.

Straube, A., Bandmann, O., Buittner, U., *et al.* (1993). A contrast enhanced lesion of the III nerve on MR of a patient with ophthalmoplegic migraine as evidence for a Tolosa–Hunt syndrome. *Headache* **33**, 446–448.

Tomsak, R. L., and Jergens, P. B. (1987). Benign recurrent transient monocular blindness: A possible variant of acephalgia migraine. *Headache* **27**, 66–69.

Wong, V., and Wong, W. C. (1997). Enhancement of oculomotor nerve—A diagnostic criterion for ophthalmoplegic migraine. *Pediatr. Neurol.* **17**, 70–73.

Woody, R. C., and Blaw, M. E. (1986). Ophthalmoplegic migraine in infancy. *Clin. Pediatr.* **25**, 82–84.

Migraine, Transformed

Encyclopedia of the Neurological Sciences
Copyright 2003, Elsevier Science (USA). All rights reserved.

TYPICAL MIGRAINE is an episodic disorder. In other words, it periodically occurs for a day to several days and then terminates. Its key features may include moderate to severe headache, nausea and vomiting, light sensitivity, worsening on exertion, and a variety of other neurological and nonneurological symptoms. Headaches often occur on one side and have a pulsating quality, but these features are not universal. Many patients with migraine will experience symptoms that precede the primary headache event, which can include neurological or constitutional symptoms.

Some patients who have typical, periodic attacks undergo an evolution of their headache pattern. Headaches that were at one time occasional can insidiously increase in frequency until a headache is experienced daily or almost daily. The initial observation is credited to Dr. John R. Graham, who described the phenomenon in 1968, suggesting that migraine could progress from intermittent to daily. Often, but not always, this evolution is prompted by the overuse of certain medications that cause rebound headache. The term transformational migraine was credited to Mathew (1982) after other authors, including Graham and Saper, previously described the evolutive nature of migraine. Recently the term chronic migraine has been used as an alternate term for what has previously been called transformed migraine. It is one of the four headache categories under the umbrella term chronic daily headache.

The key clinical features of transformational migraine include:

• Intermittent migraine by ages 20–30
• A gradual increase in headache frequency between ages 25 and 40
• Daily or almost daily mild to moderate head, neck, or face pain
• Periodically acute, severe attacks of migraine, superimposed on the milder day-to-day headaches
  • Frequent coexistent conditions that include:
    Sleep disturbance
    Overuse of analgesics, triptans, or ergotamine tartrate
    Anxiety/depressive states
    Reduction in quality of life and activities of daily living

In general, after 5–10 years of intermittent headaches, and usually between the ages of 25 and 40, vulnerable individuals begin to experience an increased frequency of headaches. Medication overuse may or may not be a causative factor. Increasingly frequent headaches may prompt the superimposed medication overuse, which then compounds the dilemma.

The daily or almost daily headaches will generally be mild to moderate in severity. Head, neck, or face pain may dominate. A sense of tight muscles and tenderness in the neck and shoulder muscles are common. Periodically, superimposed severe attacks of migraine will occur at varying frequencies, ranging from two or more per week to monthly or even less. Neuropsychiatric symptoms commonly accompany this progressive form of migraine, and include sleep disturbance, anxiety and depressive states, as well as medication overuse and a general deterioration in quality of life. A family history of headaches, medication or alcohol overuse in a parent, and depression are often found. As with migraine in general, a female predominance exists in this evolutive form.

There are no diagnostic studies to establish the diagnosis of this condition. The diagnosis is made by careful chronicling of the headache pattern over time, accompaniments, and medication usage. Because daily headache could reflect a condition other than migraine, it is essential that other more serious disorders that can cause daily pain are ruled out by appropriate testing.

The treatment for daily chronic headache is often difficult and challenging. Research and clinical experience suggest that patients often require one or more of a variety of migraine preventive medications, including antidepressants, migraine-helpful anticonvulsants, beta blockers, and calcium channel blockers. Acute attacks of migraine are treated with conventional migraine treatments. If rebound or excessive medication usage are concurrent problems, detoxification and withdrawal are essential. Because patients with this condition are often affected by coexisting neuropsychiatric conditions, such as depression, sleep disturbance, anxiety, and panic disorders, these too must be addressed by medication treatment and appropriate behavioral and psychotherapeutic treatment. Biofeedback, stress management, relaxation training, and a variety of other interventions useful for migraine and headache in general are advisable. Healthful activities, such as regular exercise, discontinuing smoking, performing day-to-day activities at regular times each day, and a variety of other self-help interventions, are recommended for most patients.

Patients with more resistant cases require aggressive and more advanced treatment, and some patients require referral to advanced care centers or even specialized hospital programs to help terminate the daily pain, discontinue offending medications, if present, and establish effective preventive interventions. Aggressive behavioral and psychotherapeutic treatments may also be required. A careful diagnostic review for cervical, trigeminal (dental, sinus, etc.), and intracranial pathology is required. Also recommended is a strategic consideration of metabolic, toxic, infectious/inflammatory, malignant, endocrinopathic, and behavioral disorders, among others, which may likewise provoke/enhance daily headache and may mimic a primary headache disorder.

CONCLUSION

Some patients with migraine will evolve from intermittent pain to daily or almost daily pain. This evolution may be prompted by a variety of factors, including genetic predisposition, psychological influences, or medication overuse. Coexisting neuropsychological conditions, such as depression, obsessive–compulsive disorders, sleep disturbances, anxiety, and panic states, are frequently present. Treatment is often difficult and directed at terminating the frequently occurring headaches, establishing preventive treatment, and treating coexistent and confounding problems such as medication overuse. Appropriate testing to rule out physical (organic) illness that can mimic this primary headache condition is necessary.

—*Joel R. Saper*

See also–Headache, Medication Abuse; Migraine, Genetics of; Migraine Mechanisms; Migraine, Menstrual; Migraine, Ophthalmoplegic and Retinal; Migraine Treatment; Migraine with Aura; Migraine without Aura

Further Reading

Bartsch, T., and Goadsby, P. J. (2001). Stimulation of the greater occipital nerve (GON) enhance responses of dural responsive convergent neurons in the trigeminal cervical complex in the rat. *Cephalagia* **21**, 401–402.

Mathew, N. T. (1997). Transformed migraine, analgesic rebound, and other chronic daily headaches. *Neurol. Clin.* **15**, 167–186.

Mathew, N. T., Stubbits, E., and Nigam, M. R. (1982). Transformation of episodic migraine into daily headache: An analysis of factors. *Headache* **22**, 66.

Saper, J. R. (2002). Chronic daily headache: A clinician's perspective. *Headache* **42**, 538–542.

Saper, J. R., Silberstein, S. D., Gordon, C. D., *et al.* (1999). *Handbook of Headache Management*, 2nd ed. Lippincott Williams & Wilkins, Baltimore.

Welch, K. M., Nagash, V., Aurora, S. K., *et al.* (2001). Periaqueductal gray matter dysfunction in migraine: Cause or the burden of illness. *Headache* **41**, 629–637.

Migraine Treatment

Encyclopedia of the Neurological Sciences
Copyright 2003, Elsevier Science (USA). All rights reserved.

HEADACHE is the most common neurological disorder, and migraine is the recurrent headache syndrome most commonly encountered in clinical practice. Approximately one-tenth of the general population actively suffers from migraine, and on any given day approximately 150,000 Americans are functionally disabled by an acute migraine attack. The financial burden imposed by migraine is estimated to be as high as $18 billion annually in the United States, almost as much as the cost attributed to all cerebrovascular disease. Thus, migraine is common, costly, and a significant source of at least short-term physical disability that demands effective treatment.

WHAT IS MIGRAINE?

The International Headache Society (IHS) has provided a relatively simple and objective list of criteria for the clinical diagnosis of migraine (Table 1). If one has suffered five or more attacks of unprovoked headache lasting 4–72 h, with those headaches sufficiently severe to prohibit or at least inhibit routine physical activity and accompanied by nausea or light and sound sensitivity or both, then (presuming the physical examination is normal) the diagnosis is migraine. A more complete history will be required to exclude coexisting disorders that also may generate headache, but at the very least the individual has migraine. As per management guidelines recently provided by the U.S. Headache

Table 1   INTERNATIONAL HEADACHE SOCIETY DIAGNOSTIC CRITERIA FOR MIGRAINE

At least five attacks fulfilling the following
  Headache attacks lasting 4–72 hr (untreated or successfully
    treated)
  Headache has at least two of the following characteristics
    Unilateral location
    Pulsating quality
    Moderate or severe intensity
    Aggravation by walking stairs or similar routine physcial
      activity
  During headache at least one of the following
    Nausea and/or vomiting
    Photophobia and phonophobia
  No evidence of "organic" disorder causing chronic headaches

Consortium, a headache syndrome with historical features meeting the IHS criteria and accompanied by a normal examination establishes the diagnosis as migraine, and further neurodiagnostic intervention is typically not required. At this point, adequate treatment—not diagnosis—becomes the primary management issue. Defining and diagnosing migraine thus is a relatively simple process. More daunting is the question: What causes migraine?

To comprehend migraine's source, it is necessary to understand how head pain generally is produced and anatomically conducted. The brain is insensate, and receptors for head pain are located on meningeal arteries and veins. These receptors receive their sensory innervation primarily through the ophthalmic division of the trigeminal nerve. Trigeminal sensory fibers eventually enter the brainstem and descend southward to synapse on cell bodies located within the inferior region of the trigeminal nucleus (trigeminal nucleus caudalis). Fibers conveying head pain then ascend to terminate within the sensory nuclei of the thalamus, and the thalamus in turn projects to parietal sensory cortex, the cingulate gyrus, and other cortical and subcortical regions. What distinguishes migraine is an instability (presumably genetic) within this anatomical system, and it appears that migraineurs may generate headache attacks in the absence of any extrinsic stimulation of the trigeminovascular system. In other words, migraine attacks may progress from inside-out, arising within the central nervous system and traveling counter to the usual flow of incoming sensory input. This retrograde activation of the trigeminal sensory nerve afferents may provoke the release of vasoactive neuropeptides at the trigeminovascular junction within the meninges. These neuropeptides provoke changes in the caliber and permeability of the blood vessels they bombard, producing a sterile perivascular inflammation that in turn may further sensitize the trigeminal nerve endings. A to-and-fro, mutually reinforcing process is set into motion (inside-out, outside-in), and the clinical result is a constellation of headache and associated symptoms termed migraine.

TARGETS OF OPPORTUNITY

Contemplating this scenario, one can envision a number of sites at which the migraine process may be vulnerable to therapeutic intervention. If, for example, an individual's attacks are initiated by an electrical event (spreading depression) that originates in biogenetically electrosensitive occipital cortex, then therapies that prevent spreading depression should reduce attack frequency. Gamma-aminobutyric acid (GABA) inhibits spreading depression, and many of the newer agents used for migraine prophylaxis or acute migraine treatment are promoters of GABA. At the peripheral endpoint of the migraine process, agents that block neuropeptide release within the trigeminovascular junction or otherwise reduce perivascular inflammation may alleviate acute migrainous pain. There are 5-HT_{1D} receptors located on the trigeminal nerve endings that, once stimulated, inhibit neuropeptide release and consequent perivascular inflammation. The triptan class of drugs are selective for these inhibitory, presynaptic receptors. At the anatomical midpoint, agents that penetrate the blood–brain barrier and block pain transmission at the caudal end of the trigeminal nucleus would be expected to abort headache. Inhibitory, antinociceptive 5-HT_{1D} receptors reside in that region and triptans with sufficient access may exert their therapeutic action at that site. Thus, site-specific and receptor-specific pharmacotherapy for migraine is now a reality, and further refinements in migraine theory are likely to yield more targets of opportunity.

ACUTE THERAPY

For patients with episodic migraine that is relatively infrequent, effective control of the headache syndrome may be achieved with abortive therapy only.

With few exceptions, abortive therapies generally are most effective when utilized early in the course of an attack, and this is especially true of the simple analgesics and nonsteroidal antiinflammatory drugs (NSAIDs). Patients should be instructed to take an adequate dose of the agent or agents chosen; 975 mg of aspirin taken early in an attack may be more effective than a narcotic administered long after the head pain has become intense. The gastroparesis often associated with acute migraine may preclude adequate absorption of oral medications, and this can be overcome by simultaneous administration of caffeine or metoclopramide.

Patients should be provided with a multitiered strategy for acute treatment of migraine in which the agent administered is matched to headache intensity. NSAIDs and simple analgesics are reasonable choices for migraine headaches that are mild in intensity, whereas a triptan or dihydroergotamine (DHE) typically will be more effective for moderate to severe head pain. Reliable patients may be provided with an opiate or opioid analgesic to use as a last resort for headaches that are particularly severe and refractory. Migraine-associated nausea should be treated with a dopamine antagonist, and at least four of these (prochlorperazine, chlorpromazine, droperidol, and metoclopramide) may also be effective in treating the headache.

Although polytherapy is often advisable in treating acute migraine, patients should be instructed regarding potentially adverse drug–drug interactions. In particular, an excessive dose of an individual serotonin agonist or concomitant administration of two agonists may provoke clinically significant arterial vasospasm. To prevent this or other complications, use of a triptan should be followed by treatment with an ergotamine preparation for at least 6 hr; conversely, use of ergotamine precludes treatment with a triptan for a period of at least 24 hr.

Finally, patients should be instructed to avoid frequent use of an abortive agent on a chronic basis. Virtually all the abortive medications, including the simple analgesics, reputedly have the potential for provoking rebound headaches if they are administered in excess. What constitutes "excess" remains in question, but as a rule one should consider the possibility of a rebound component in any patient with pervasive migraine who takes a given abortive agent more than 3 days per week. Rebound should especially be suspected if these patients are experiencing headaches that awaken them from sleep or are present upon awakening; they also may exhibit a tendency to administer the abortive agent in anticipation of headache. Drugs considered to have particularly high rebound potential include the butalbital and caffeine-containing compounds, ergotamine tartrate, the opioid analgesics, and, increasingly, the triptans. Drugs considered less likely to provoke rebound include the NSAIDs and DHE.

Specific Drugs

The classes of medications most commonly used for acute treatment of migraine are the simple analgesics (e.g., acetaminophen), NSAIDs, dopamine antagonists, serotonin agonists, and opioid analgesics.

As noted previously, the simple analgesics and NSAIDs are most beneficial when used during the early phase of a migraine attack, when the headache has not yet escalated to become severe. Especially when administered with metoclopramide, aspirin may be effective in treating acute migraine. Naproxen has been reported to be effective both for acute treatment and for migraine prophylaxis, and other NSAIDs (ibuprofen, flurbiprofen, and ketorolac) have also been shown to be beneficial in clinical trials involving acute migraine. Based on the available data, there seems to be little choice among the various NSAIDs; thus, it may be most sensible to prescribe according to cost. Although its cost is higher than that of certain of its brethren, naproxen sodium represents a reasonable option; it may be more rapidly absorbed than naproxen and tends to induce less gastrointestinal intolerance.

Several agents are useful for treating moderate to severe migraine. Sumatriptan (Imitrex), a serotonin agonist with particular affinity for the 5-HT_{1D} receptor, has proven its worth in multiple well-designed clinical trials, and injectable (subcutaneous), intranasal, and oral formulations of this agent are available. The subcutaneous formulation is the most rapidly acting but also the most likely of the three to produce the typical array of triptan side effects (neck/chest/jaw tightness or pressure, paresthesias, nausea, and dysphoria). In addition, early recurrence of headache (not to be confused with rebound) may occur in up to 40% of treated patients. Safety data from a large prospective study of subcutaneously administered sumatriptan indicate that clinically significant cardiac complications or stroke are exceedingly rare if treatment is restricted to the appropriate patient population. Interestingly, subcutaneous administration of sumatriptan during the aura phase of a "classic" migraine attack neither shortens the aura's duration nor prevents the ensuing headache. Subcutaneous therapy is best rendered later in an attack, when the headache has become moderate to severe in intensity, and it may be effective up to 72 hr following headache onset. The oral formulation is initially less effective than the subcutaneous and also less likely to provide significant relief. Also, side effects are less common or intense with oral administration. Two strengths of oral sumatriptan are currently available (25 and 50 mg), and evidence suggests a strong patient preference and greater efficacy for the higher prescribed doses (i.e., 50–100 mg). The intranasal formulation may be considered intermediate between the oral and subcutaneous in terms of its clinical utility. Its onset of action is typically faster than that of the oral formulation and slower than that of the subcutaneous, and its side effects profile approximates that of the oral. The incidence of significant headache relief 2 hr following intranasal administration of 20 mg sumatriptan was 63% in one study.

The next generation of triptans has been developed. Zolmitriptan (Zomig) is available in 2.5- and 5-mg oral formulations. More lipophilic than sumatriptan, zolmitriptan may penetrate the blood–brain barrier more readily and thus activate centrally located inhibitory receptors that modulate transmission of pain. Zolmitriptan's clinic benefit has consistently been demonstrated in placebo-controlled clinical trials, and there is evidence that it may be effective for patients who have responded poorly to ergots, aspirin, NSAIDs or sumatriptan. Rizatriptan (Maxalt) is a third triptan that is available in 5- and 10-mg tablets and in a 10-mg "melt" wafer; propranolol, the only beta blocker used, increases serum levels of rizatriptan, and the 5-mg dose is intended for patients concomitantly taking that agent. Currently, data from comparator studies that would allow ranking of the relative effectiveness of these three oral triptans are lacking, and it is unclear whether an alternative triptan may offer relief to migraine patients whose headaches fail to respond to the first triptan chosen. Naratriptan (Amerge) is a fourth triptan currently available for clinical use. Its onset of action is slower than that of sumatriptan, rizatriptan, and zolmitriptan, but its side effects profile and early headache recurrence rate are more favorable. Additional triptans will soon be available.

Dihydroergotamine, also a serotonin agonists, lacks the cache of being "new" but nonetheless offers some potential advantages over sumatriptan and, perhaps, the newer triptans. Administered intravenously in conjunction with prochlorperazine or metoclopramide, DHE long has been used to treat acute migraine headache and status migrainosus and to assist in withdrawing a patient with rebound headache from the offending agent. Although a device specifically intended for subcutaneous injection of DHE has not been developed, as one was for sumatriptan, many patients have been trained to self-administer DHE subcutaneously with a simple syringe. In one published trial, subcutaneously administered DHE was compared directly with subcutaneously administered sumatriptan for the treatment of acute migraine headache. Although very early headache relief occurred more often with sumatriptan, by 3 hr post-treatment the response rates were similar for the two drugs (86% for DHE vs 90% for sumatriptan). Of even more potential relevance to clinical practice and cost containment, recurrence of headache within 24 hr of treatment occurred at 2.5 times greater frequency with sumatriptan than with DHE (45 vs 17.7%).

Dihydroergotamine is available in a 3-mg nasal formulation (Migranal), and in one published study 70% of patients using this drug reported resolution of headache within 4 hr; the incidence of early recurrent headache was only 14%.

Orally, sublingually, or rectally administered ergotamine tartrate is demonstratively superior to placebo in treating acute migraine headache, but the advent of the triptans and the availability of DHE have reduced the relevance of this agent. Combined with persisting concerns regarding ergotamine tartrate's tendency to produce arterial vasoconstriction (and potentially vasospastic complications) and to provoke rebound headaches if used in excess, the presence of attractive alternatives for acute migraine treatment leaves this drug in search of a therapeutic niche.

What should be the first-line agent for patient-administered treatment of acute migraine headache that moderate to severe in intensity? Without data from clinical trials comparing two or more active agents directly, any attempt to answer this question must, of necessity, depend on indirect comparisons from active versus placebo trials that have involved different study populations and methods. If rapid onset of relief is a primary concern, subcutaneously administered sumatriptan or DHE are most likely to produce this effect. If early recurrent headache is the concern, DHE or naratriptan are reasonable choices. When the subcutaneous formulation of sumatriptan is effective but produces intolerable side effects, intranasal formulation of the agent or oral triptan or DHE (subcutaneous or intranasal) should be considered. If an oral triptan with relatively rapid therapeutic effect is desired, zolmitriptan, sumatriptan, and rizatriptan all deserve consideration. Newer triptans that will soon become available may alter or expand these management suggestions, as will emerging evidence that early treatment with an oral triptan (i.e., when the headache is mild to moderate in intensity) is more effective clinically than treating when the pain is severe.

PROPHYLACTIC THERAPY

Once a patient's migraine headaches have become sufficiently pervasive, presumably reflecting increased instability within an inherently disordered biological system, an attempt may be made to restore stability through a course of prophylactic therapy. However, this may prove frustrating for both patient and clinician. Currently, no given agent prescribed for migraine prophylaxis has more than a 50% chance of significantly reducing headache frequency, and there exist no reliable means of predicting the drug to which a given patient is likely to respond. Consequently, a stepwise trial-and-error approach is required, which is a time-consuming process that is further aggravated by treatment-induced side effects, a latency between initiation of treatment and onset of therapeutic benefit that may last months, and, depending on the drug, the frequent need to start treatment with a low, subtherapeutic dose and then gradually increase the dose. Thus, it is not surprising that compliance with prophylactic therapy is very low.

To reduce noncompliance and increase the likelihood of a positive treatment response, patients should be informed carefully and prospectively of the intended management plan, potential side effects of the drug to be prescribed, and response latency. Especially during the first weeks of prophylactic therapy, patients should have available to them an appropriate means of dealing with "breakthrough" headaches. Finally, noncompliance may be reduced by maintaining frequent patient contact and specifically by encouraging the patient to report any perceived adverse reaction to therapy.

SPECIFIC AGENTS

Although many drugs are currently prescribed for migraine prophylaxis, few can boast solid credentials for such use; those most commonly prescribed, their recommended doses, and their most common side effects are listed in Table 2. Propranolol, amitriptyline, and divalproex sodium are the drugs for migraine prophylaxis that have received the highest rating from the U.S. Headache Consortium. Each has been tested extensively in clinical trials, has proved to be efficacious in all or at least a substantial number of those trials, and is generally recognized to be useful in clinical practice. However, each is imperfect and, at best, will provide significant net benefit to 50% or fewer patients for which it is prescribed. Commonly employed alternative agents, such as verapamil or the SSRIs, are believed to be of even less potential value in migraine treatment, and newer therapies such as gabapentin, topiramate, and botulinin toxin injections are either still under investigation or have performed inconsistently in clinical trials.

Amitriptyline's modest efficacy in reducing migraine attack frequency appears to be independent of its antidepressant effect. Side effects are dose related

Table 2 DRUGS COMMONLY PRESCRIBED FOR MIGRAINE PROPHYLAXIS

Drug	Recommended maximum daily dose (mg)	Side effects
Propranolol	320	Fatigue, nausea, depression, insomnia
Nadolol	240	Same as for propranolol
Atenolol	100	Same as for propranolol
Amitriptyline	150	Sedation, weight gain, dry mouth
Verapamil	480	Constipation, peripheral edema
Divalproex sodium	1500	Nausea, weight gain, alopecia
Methysergide	8	Muscle cramps, insomnia, fibrosis
Naproxen sodium	1650	Dyspepsia, diarrhea, fluid retention

and occur at a frequency high enough that initiation of treatment at a low dose (e.g., 10 mg nightly) is often required, with gradual dose escalation thereafter to a maximum of 150 mg daily. Even then, many patients will not tolerate chronic treatment with amitriptyline.

Divalproex sodium arguably represents the best choice for migraine prophylaxis. Its performance in clinical trials has been consistently good, and the response latency associated with its use appears to be relatively short; most patients can determine whether they are responders or nonresponders within 4 weeks following initiation of treatment. In clinical trials, effective total daily doses have ranged between 500 and 1500 mg, and there is no convincing evidence of a dose–response relationship within this range. When required, dose escalation with divalproex sodium is typically a rapid and simple process. To its disadvantage, divalproex sodium produces side effects (mainly gastrointestinal disturbance, tremor, weight gain, and alopecia) in a significant proportion of patients, and concerns regarding potential hepatic toxicity have led to the recommendation that blood studies be obtained regularly.

A rational basis for prophylactic treatment of migraine is emerging but much more slowly than is the case for acute treatment. Of necessity, clinical management is often based largely on empiricism and the individual's prior experience. Confronted with this bleak therapeutic environment, it is probably wisest for the clinician to know two or three prophylactic agents well, to prescribe them appropriately, and to look forward to scientifically derived evidence that will allow an increase in the number of available therapeutic options.

—*John F. Rothrock*

***See also*–Analgesics, Non-Opioid and Other; Migraine, Genetics of; Migraine Mechanisms; Migraine, Menstrual; Migraine, Ophthalmoplegic and Retinal; Migraine, Transformed; Migraine with Aura; Migraine without Aura; Pain, Neurobiology of; Pain, Overview**

Further Reading

Lipton, R. B., and Stewart, W. F. (1993). Migraine in the United States: A review of epidemiology and health care use. *Neurology* **43**, S6–S10.

Noack, H., and Rothrock, J. (1996). Migraine: Definitions, mechanisms, and treatment. *J. South. Med. Assoc.* **89**, 762–769.

O'Guinn, S., Davis, R., Gutterman, D., *et al.* (1999). Prospective large-scale study of the tolerability of subcutaneous sumatriptan for acute treatment of migraine. *Cephalalgia* **19**, 223–231.

Parsons, A. (1998). Recent advances in mechanisms of spreading depression. *Curr. Opin. Neurol.* **11**, 227–231.

Ramadan, N., Schultz, L. L., and Gilkey, S. J. (1997). Migraine prophylactic drugs: Proof of efficacy, utilization and cost. *Cephalalgia* **17**, 73–80.

Rothrock, J. (1997). Clinical studies of valproate for migraine prophylaxis. *Cephalalgia* **17**, 81–83.

Silberstein, S. D., and Rosenberg, J. (2000). Multispecialty consensus on diagnosis and treatment of headache. *Neurology* **54**, 1553.

Welch, K. (1993). Drug therapy of migraine. *N. Engl. J. Med.* **329**, 1476–1483.

Migraine with Aura

Encyclopedia of the Neurological Sciences

MIGRAINE is classified by using the International Headache Society (IHS) classification of headache disorders. The IHS calls common migraine "migraine without aura" and classic migraine "migraine with aura," with the aura being the complex of focal neurological symptoms that precedes or accompanies an attack. At most, only 30% of migraine headaches are classic. The same patient may have migraine headache without aura, migraine headache with aura, and migraine aura without headache.

To establish a diagnosis of IHS migraine with typical aura, at least two attacks fulfilling the criteria

Table 1 DIAGNOSTIC CRITERIA FOR TYPICAL AURA WITH MIGRAINE HEADACHE (CLASSIC MIGRAINE)

A. At least two attacks fulfilling criteria B–E

B. Fully reversible visual and/or sensory and/or speech symptoms but no motor weakness

C. At least two of the following:
  Binocular hemianopic symptoms including excitation (flickering lights and pins-and-needles) and/or inhibition (scotoma and numbness)
  At least one symptom developing gradually over 5 min and/or different symptoms occur in succession
  Each symptom lasts ≥5 and ≤60 min

D. Headache, which meets criteria for migraine without aura, begins during the aura or follows aura within 60 min

E. Not attributed to another disorder

---

in Table 1 are required. Migraine with aura is subdivided into typical aura with migraine headache, typical aura with nonmigraine headache (such as cluster or tension-type headache), typical aura without headache, hemiplegic migraine, basilar-type migraine, retinal migraine, and childhood periodic syndromes. Ophthalmoplegic migraine is believed to be a recurrent cranial neuralgia and not migraine.

Most migraine-with-aura sufferers also have attacks without aura. The aura usually lasts 20–30 min and typically precedes the headache, but occasionally it overlaps with the headache or occurs only during the headache. In contrast to a transient ischemic attack (TIA), the aura of migraine evolves gradually and consists of both positive (e.g., scintillations and tingling) and negative (e.g., scotoma and numbness) features. Almost any symptom or sign of brain dysfunction may be a feature of the aura, but the most common aura is a visual phenomenon.

Focal symptoms and signs of the aura may persist beyond the headache phase. Formerly termed complicated migraine, the IHS classification has introduced two more specific labels. If the aura lasts for more than 2 weeks with normal magnetic resonance imaging, the term persistent aura without infarction is applied. If a neuroimaging procedure demonstrates a stroke, a migrainous infarction has occurred. Particularly in mid- or late life, the aura may not be followed by the headache (typical aura without headache).

CLINICAL FEATURES OF MIGRAINE

The migraine attack may be divided into four phases: the premonitory (or prodrome) phase, which occurs hours or days before the headache; the aura, which immediately precedes the headache; the headache; and the postdrome. Migraine without aura consists of at least the headache and possibly the postdrome. Migraine with aura consists of at least the aura and the headache. If the headache is absent, it is migraine aura without headache. Both may be associated with premonitory symptoms.

Premonitory Phase (Prodrome)

Premonitory phenomena occur hours to days before headache onset in approximately 60% of migraineurs and may consist of psychological, neurological, or general (constitutional and autonomic) symptoms. Psychological symptoms include depression, euphoria, irritability, restlessness, mental slowness, hyperactivity, fatigue, and drowsiness. Neurological phenomena include photophobia, phonophobia, and hyperosmia. General symptoms include a stiff neck, a cold feeling, sluggishness, increased thirst, increased urination, anorexia, diarrhea, constipation, fluid retention, and food cravings.

Aura

The migraine aura is composed of focal neurological phenomena that precede or accompany an attack. Most aura symptoms develop over 5–20 min and usually last less than 60 min. The typical aura may be characterized by visual or sensory phenomena and may also involve language or brainstem disturbances (Table 2). Motor weakness is not regarded as typical. The headache, if it occurs, usually begins within 60 min of the end of the aura. In one prospective study, headache followed the aura in only 80% of cases. The headache may begin before or simultaneously with the aura, or the aura may occur in isolation.

Table 2 TYPICAL AURA SYMPTOMS

Visual
  Scotoma; photopsia or phosphenes; geometric forms; fortification spectra; objects may rotate, oscillate, or shimmer; brightness appears often very bright
Visual hallucinations or distortions
  Metamorphopsia, macropsia, zoom or mosaic vision
Sensory
  Paresthesias, often migrating, often lasting for minutes (cheiro-oral), and can become bilateral; olfactory hallucinations
Motor
  Ataxia, apraxia, chorea
Language
  Dysarthria or aphasia
Delusions and disturbed consciousness
  Déjà vu, multiple conscious trance-like states

Rarely, auras may occur repeatedly (migraine aura status). Structural causes must be considered. Patients may experience more than one type of aura, with a progression from one symptom to another. Most patients with a sensory aura also have a visual aura.

Visual aura is the most common of the neurological events; it occurs in 99% of patients who have an aura and often has a hemianopic distribution. The aura may consist of photopsia (the sensation of unformed flashes of light before the eyes), scotoma (circumscribed area of blurring, dimness, or darkness in the visual field), or the almost diagnostic aura of migraine—the fortification spectrum.

Auras vary in complexity. Elementary visual disturbances include scotomata, simple flashes (phosphenes), specks, or geometric forms. They may move across the visual field, sometimes crossing the midline. Shimmering or undulations in the visual field may also occur and may be described by patients as "heat waves." More complicated auras include teichopsia (Greek for town wall and vision) or fortification spectrum, the most characteristic visual aura of migraine. An arc of scintillating lights, usually but not always beginning near the point of fixation, may form into a herringbone-like pattern that expands to encompass an increasing portion of a visual hemifield. It migrates across the visual field with a scintillating edge of often zigzag, flashing, or occasionally colored phenomena. The visions of Hildegard of Bingen, an 11th-century Abbess, have been attributed in part to her migrainous auras. Characteristic of the visions that she and other visionary prophets, including Ezekiel, experienced were lights that shimmered and moved, often in a wave-like manner.

Visual distortions and hallucinations, speculated to represent Lewis Carroll's descriptions in *Alice in Wonderland*, may occur. These phenomena are more common in children, usually followed by a headache, and characterized by a complex disorder of visual perception that may include metamorphopsia, micropsia, macropsia, and zoom or mosaic vision. Nonvisual symptoms may occur and include complex difficulties in the perception and use of the body (apraxia and agnosia); speech and language disturbances; states of double or multiple consciousness associated with déjà vu or jamais vu; and elaborate dreamy, nightmarish, trance-like, or delirious states. Olfactory hallucinations may also occur.

Paresthesias are the second most common aura and occur in approximately one-third of migraineurs with aura. They are typically cheiro-oral, with numbness starting in the hand, migrating up the arm, and then involving the face, lips, and tongue. The leg is occasionally involved. As with visual auras (with positive followed by negative symptoms), paresthesias may be followed by numbness and, in a few cases, loss of position sense. Paresthesias begin bilaterally or become bilateral in half of patients. Sensory auras rarely occur in isolation and usually follow a visual aura.

Hyperkinetic movement disorders, including chorea, have been reported. Aphasic auras have been reported in 17–20% of patients. However, since patients are rarely examined during an aura, many of the reported cases may be dysarthria and not aphasia.

Migraine Aura without Headache

Periodic neurological phenomena may occur in isolation. These phenomena (scintillating scotoma and recurrent sensory, motor, and mental phenomena) must be differentiated from TIAs and focal seizures, and they are diagnosed as migraine only after full investigation and reasonable follow-up. Transient visual disturbances, with flickering or scintillating phenomena, also occur with numerous other conditions, including blood cell diseases, retinal detachment, cluster headaches, trauma, and syncope, but they are not generally associated with cerebrovascular embolic or thrombotic disease. Headache occurring in association with the symptoms of aura will help confirm the diagnosis but does not exclude TIA. Approximately half of the patients who have had headache with aura have also had aura without headache at some time.

Transient neurological loss was found in 32% of Cornell neurologists; visual symptoms (field cuts, obscurations, and scotomata) were most common, and nonvisual symptoms (hemiparesis, clumsiness, paresthesias, and dysarthria) were less common. Migraine was more commonly reported in those with transient central nervous system dysfunction. None developed any residual deficit or chronic neurological disorder at 5-year follow-up, suggesting that these are benign migrainous accompaniments.

Fisher was the first to carefully describe transient neurological phenomena not characteristically associated with headaches (late-life migrainous accompaniments or transient migrainous accompaniments) in patients older than age 40; 60% were men and 57% had a history of recurrent headache. The attacks of episodic neurological dysfunction lasted from 1 min to 72 hr and had variable recurrence rates (1 attack, 27%; 2–10 attacks, 45%; more than 10 attacks, 28%). Scintillating scotoma was considered to be diagnostic of migraine even when it occurred in isolation, whereas other episodic neurological symptoms (paresthesias, aphasia, and sensory and motor symptoms) needed more careful evaluation (Table 3).

In the Framingham study, migrainous visual aura symptoms were reported by 14% of those with visual symptoms, with a prevalence of 1.23% overall (1.33% in women and 1.08% in men). They lasted 15–60 min in 50% of subjects. In 65% of subjects, the episodes were stereotypical. They began after age 50 in 77%. The pattern of visual manifestations varied widely among subjects. The episodes were never accompanied by headaches in 58% of subjects, and 42% had no headache history. Only in 19% of subjects did the migrainous visual episodes meet the IHS criteria for migraine aura, usually because one of the criteria (i.e., at least one aura symptom develops gradually over more than 4 min) could not be reliably ascertained.

Three subjects had a stroke 1 or more years later: One had a subarachnoid hemorrhage 1 year later, one had a brainstem infarct 3 years later, and one had a cardioembolic stroke secondary to atrial fibrillation 27 years later. The stroke incidence rate of 11.5% was significantly lower than the stroke incidence rate of 33.3% in subjects with TIAs in the same cohort (these usually occurred within 6 months) and did not differ from the stroke incidence rate of 13.6% of those without migrainous phenomena or TIAs.

Table 3   MIGRAINE EQUIVALENTS

Scintillating scotoma
Paresthesias
Aphasia
Dysarthria
Blindness
Blurring of vision
Hemianopia
Transient monocular blindness
Ophthalmoplegia
Oculosympathetic palsy
Mydriasis
Confusion, stupor
Cyclical vomiting
Diplopia
Deafness
Chorea

In another study, the lifetime prevalence of transient visual disturbances of possible migraine origin was 37% in migraine patients and 13% in the general population. There were no differences in the transient visual disturbances characteristics between the groups. Slightly less than half of each group had a gradual onset of 5 min or more. Headache following transient visual disturbances had more migrainous features in patients than in controls. The transient visual disturbances that did not fulfill the IHS criteria for migraine with aura probably represented abortive migraine phenomena.

Visual migrainous phenomena are not rare; they occurred in 1.33% of women and 1.08% of men in a general population sample and were usually benign. Transient migrainous accompaniments (scintillating scotomata, numbness, aphasia, dysarthria, and motor weakness) may occur for the first time after the age of 45 and be easily confused with TIAs of cerebrovascular origin. Diagnosis in all but the most classic cases is still by exclusion.

Postdrome

Following the headache, the patient may have impaired concentration or feel tired, washed out, irritable, and listless. Some people feel unusually refreshed or euphoric after an attack. Muscle weakness and aching and anorexia or food cravings may occur.

MIGRAINE VARIANTS

Basilar-type Migraine

Basilar-type migraine, originally called basilar artery migraine, basilar migraine, or Bickerstaff's syndrome, was believed to be mainly a disorder of adolescent girls. However, it affects all age groups and both sexes, with the usual migraine female predominance. The aura generally lasts less than 1 hr and is usually followed by a headache that may be occipital. The headache may be associated with nausea and even projectile vomiting. A typical hemianopic field disturbance may rapidly expand to involve both visual fields, occasionally leading to temporary blindness. A distinguishing characteristic of basilar migraine is the bilateral nature of many of the associated neurological events, which helps differentiate it from more typical migraine with aura. The visual aura is usually followed by one or more of the following symptoms: dysarthria, vertigo, tinnitus, decreased hearing, diplopia, ataxia, bilateral paresthesia, and impaired cognition that, when marked, defines confusional migraine. The IHS criteria for basilar migraine require the presence of two or more of the preceding aura symptoms. Motor weakness excludes basilar-type migraine and is designated hemiplegic migraine when associated with recurrent headaches.

Confusional Migraine

Confusional migraine occurs more commonly in boys than in girls, with a frequency of approximately 5%. It is characterized by a typical aura, a headache (which may be insignificant), and confusion (which may precede, occur with, or follow the headache). The confusion is characterized by inattention, distractibility, and difficulty maintaining speech and other motor activities. Agitation, memory disturbances, obscene utterances, violent behavior, and sedation or a drugged feeling may occur. The electroencephalogram may be abnormal during the attack. Single attacks are most common, multiple attacks are rare, and attacks may be triggered by mild head trauma. If the level of consciousness is more profoundly disturbed, migraine stupor lasting 2–5 days may occur.

Familial Hemiplegic Migraine

Familial hemiplegic migraine (FHM) is an autosomal dominant, genetically heterogeneous form of migraine with aura, with variable penetration. The aura is characterized by motor weakness of variable intensity. The syndrome also includes attacks of migraine without aura, migraine with typical aura, and severe episodes with prolonged aura (up to several days or weeks), fever, meningismus, and impaired consciousness ranging from confusion to profound coma. Headache may precede the hemiparesis or be absent. The onset of the hemiparesis may be abrupt and simulate a stroke. Most patients have associated paresthesias. In one study, 88% had visual auras, and 44% had speech disturbances. Weakness lasted less than 1 hr in 58% of patients; however, it lasted 1–3 hr in 14%, 3–24 hr in 12%, and between 1 day and 1 week in 16% of patients. The syndrome may change in an affected individual over his or her lifetime. A person who has FHM in adolescence may develop migraine with aura as an adult and migraine without aura later in life.

The headache may be generalized (29%), contralateral (47%), or ipsilateral (22%) to the hemiparesis (2% are inconspicuous). Attacks may vary from a single neurological episode to more than seven attacks. The longer lasting episodes are often associated with more profound weakness and tend to be less frequent in recurrence.

In 20% of unselected FHM families, patients may have fixed cerebellar symptoms and signs, such as nystagmus and progressive ataxia. Cerebellar ataxia may occur before the first hemiplegic migraine attack and progress independently of the frequency or severity of hemiplegic migraine attacks. All these families have been shown to be linked to chromosome 19. Mutations within CACNA1A also cause episodic ataxia type 2. Another gene has been mapped to chromosome 1.

Sporadic Hemiplegic Migraine

Sporadic hemiplegic migraine, like the familial form, typically begins in childhood. The average age of onset may be earlier than that of migraine without aura, and the attacks are frequently precipitated by minor head injury. Changes in consciousness ranging from confusion to coma are a feature, especially in childhood. The prevalence of hemiplegic migraine is uncertain. The differential diagnosis of hemiplegic migraine includes focal seizures, stroke, homocystinuria, and MELAS syndrome.

—Stephen D. Silberstein

See also–Migraine, Genetics of; Migraine Mechanisms; Migraine, Menstrual; Migraine, Ophthalmoplegic and Retinal; Migraine, Transformed; Migraine Treatment; Migraine without Aura; Stroke, Migraine-Induced

Further Reading

Amery, W. K., Waelkens, J., and Caers, I. (1986). Dopaminergic mechanisms in premonitory phenomena. In *The Prelude to the Migraine Attack* (W. K. Amery and A. Wauquier, Eds.), pp. 64–77. Bailliere Tindall, London.
Bickerstaff, E. R. (1994). Migraine variants and complications. In *Migraine: Clinical and Research Aspects* (J. N. Blau, Ed.), pp. 55–75. Johns Hopkins Univ. Press, Baltimore.
Blau, J. N. (1980). Migraine prodromes separated from the aura: Complete migraine. *Br. Med. J.* **281**, 658–660.
Ducros, A., Joutel, A., and Vahedi, K. (1997). Mapping of a second locus for familial hemiplegic migraine to 1q21–q23 and evidence of further heterogeneity. *Ann. Neurol.* **42**, 885–890.
Fisher, C. M. (1980). Late life migraine accompaniments as a cause of unexplained transient ischemic attacks. *Can. J. Neurol. Sci.* **7**, 9–17.
Gardner, K., Barmada, M. M., Ptacek, L. J., *et al.* (1997). A new locus for hemiplegic migraine maps to chromosome 1q31. *Neurology* **49**, 1231–1238.

Hachinski, V. C., Porchawka, J., and Steele, J. C. (1973). Visual symptoms in the migraine syndrome. *Neurology* **23**, 570–579.

Headache Classification Committee of the International Headache Society (1988). Classification and diagnostic criteria for headache disorders, cranial neuralgia, and facial pain. *Cephalalgia* **8**, 1–96.

Hosking, G. (1988). Special forms: Variants of migraine in childhood. In *Migraine in Childhood* (J. M. Hockaday, Ed.), pp. 35–53. Butterworth, Boston.

Hupp, S. L., Kline, L. B., and Corbett, J. J. (1989). Visual disturbances of migraine. *Surv. Ophthalmol.* **33**, 221–236.

Jensen, K., Tfelt-Hansen, P., Lauritzen, M., *et al.* (1986). Classic migraine, a prospective recording of symptoms. *Acta Neurol. Scand.* **73**, 359–362.

Kuritzky, A., Ziegler, K. E., and Hassanein, R. (1981). Vertigo, motion sickness and migraine. *Headache* **21**, 227–231.

Lance, J. W., and Anthony, M. (1966). Some clinical aspects of migraine. *Arch. Neurol.* **15**, 356–361.

Levy, D. E. (1988). Transient CNS deficits: A common, benign syndrome in young adults. *Neurology* **38**, 831–836.

Manzoni, G., Farina, S., Lanfranchi, M., *et al.* (1985). Classic migraine—Clinical findings in 164 patients. *Eur. Neurol.* **24**, 163–169.

Mattsson, P., and Lundberg, P. O. (1999). Characteristics and prevalence of transient visual disturbances indicative of migraine visual aura. *Cephalalgia* **19**, 479–484.

O'Connor, P. S., and Tredici, T. J. (1981). Acephalgic migraine: Fifteen years experience. *Ophthalmology* **88**, 999–1003.

Olesen, J. (1978). Some clinical features of the acute migraine attack. An analysis of 750 patients. *Headache* **18**, 268–271.

Ophoff, R. A., Terwindt, G. M., and Vergouwe, M. N. (1996). Familial hemiplegic migraine and episodic ataxia type-2 are caused by mutations in the Ca^{2+} channel gene CACNLA4. *Cell Tissue Res.* **87**, 543–552.

Russell, M. B., and Olesen, J. (1996). A nosographic analysis of the migraine aura in a general population. *Brain* **119**, 355–361.

Sacks, O. (1985). *Migraine. Understanding a Common Disorder.* Univ. of California Press, Berkeley.

Selby, G., and Lance, J. W. (1960). Observation on 500 cases of migraine and allied vascular headaches. *J. Neurol. Neurosurg. Psychiatr.* **23**, 23–32.

Silberstein, S. D., and Young, W. B. (1995). Migraine aura and prodrome. *Semin. Neurol.* **45**, 175–182.

Silberstein, S. D., Saper, J. R., and Freitag, F. (2001). Migraine: Diagnosis and treatment. In *Wolff's Headache and Other Head Pain* (S. D. Silberstein, R. B. Lipton, and D. J. Dalessio, Eds.). Oxford Univ. Press, New York.

Stewart, W. F., Shechter, A. L., and Lipton, R. B. (1994). Migraine heterogeneity: Disability, pain intensity, attack frequency, and duration. *Neurology* **44**, S24–S39.

Tournier-Lasserve, E. (1999). Hemiplegic migraine, episodic ataxia type 2, and the others. *Neurology* **53**, 3–4.

Whitty, C. W. M. (1967). Migraine without headache. *Lancet* **2**, 283–285.

Whitty, C. W. M. (1986). Familial hemiplegic migraine. In *Handbook of Clinical Neurology* (F. C. Rose, Ed.), pp. 141–153. Elsevier, New York.

Wijman, C., Wolf, P. A., Kase, C. S., *et al.* (1998). Migrainous visual accompaniments are not rare in late life: The Framingham Study. *Stroke* **29**, 1539–1543.

Migraine without Aura

Encyclopedia of the Neurological Sciences
Copyright 2003, Elsevier Science (USA). All rights reserved.

MIGRAINE is characterized by attacks consisting of various combinations of headache and neurological, gastrointestinal, and autonomic symptoms. The International Headache Society (IHS) classification of headache disorders attempts to diagnose the headache attack rather than headache syndromes. In epilepsy, headache syndromes may be associated with different seizure types. The IHS examines only headache types, not the spectrum of headaches occurring in any syndrome, such as familial hemiplegic migraine. Migraine headaches are classified as migraine without aura and migraine with aura, with the aura being the complex of focal neurological symptoms that precedes or accompanies an attack. At most, only 30% of migraine headaches are with aura. The same patient may have migraine headache without aura, migraine headache with aura, and migraine aura without headache.

To establish a diagnosis of migraine under the IHS classification, structural disease must be excluded and certain clinical features must be present. The criteria for diagnosing migraine without aura include five attacks of headache (each lasting 4–72 hr) and two of the following characteristics: unilateral location, pulsating quality, moderate to severe intensity, and aggravation by routine physical activity. In addition, the attacks must have at least one of the following: nausea, vomiting, photophobia, and phonophobia (Table 1). No single associated feature is mandatory for diagnosing migraine, although recurrent episodic attacks must be documented.

Table 1 DIAGNOSTIC CRITERIA FOR MIGRAINE WITHOUT AURA

A. At least five attacks fulfilling criteria B–D

B. Headache lasting 4–72 hr (untreated or unsuccessfully treated)

C. Headache has at least two of the following characteristics:
   Unilateral location
   Pulsating quality
   Moderate or severe intensity (inhibits or prohibits daily activities)
   Aggravation by walking stairs or similar routine physical activity

D. During headache, at least one of the following:
   Nausea and/or vomiting
   Photophobia and phonophobia

E. Not attributed to another disorder

A patient who has pulsatile pain aggravated by routine activity, photophobia, and phonophobia meets the criteria, as does the more typical patient with unilateral throbbing pain and nausea. If one of the criteria is missing, the headache, called migrainous in the 1988 IHS classification, will be designated "probable migraine" in the 2003 classification.

A migraine attack usually lasts less than 1 day; when it persists for more than 3 days, the term status migrainosus is applied. Although migraine often begins in the morning, sometimes awakening the patient from sleep at dawn, it can begin at any time of the day or night. The frequency of attacks is extremely variable, from a few in a lifetime to several a week. The median attack frequency is 1.5 attacks per month; 10% of migraineurs have one attack per week.

CLINICAL FEATURES OF MIGRAINE

The migraine attack can be classified into four phases: premonitory (prodrome), which occurs hours or days before the headache; the aura, which immediately precedes the headache; the headache; and the postdrome. Migraine without aura consists of at least the headache and possibly the postdrome. Migraine with aura consists of at least the aura, the headache (if absent, it is migraine aura without headache), and the postdrome. Both may be associated with premonitory symptoms.

Headache

A migraine headache is typically unilateral, pulsatile, moderate to marked in severity, and aggravated by routine physical activity. Not all of these features are required by the IHS: Pain may be bilateral and pulsatile or unilateral and nonpulsatile. The pain onset is usually gradual; the pain peaks and then subsides and usually lasts less than 24 hr, with a range of 4–72 hr in adults and 2–48 hr in children. The headache is bilateral in 40% and unilateral in 60% of cases; it consistently occurs on the same side in 20% of patients. Migraineurs whose headaches alternate sides do not develop more consistently lateralized headache with the passage of time.

The pain varies greatly in intensity, ranging from annoying to incapacitating, although most migraineurs report at least moderate pain. The pain has a throbbing quality, particularly when severe, but it can be tight or band-like. During an attack, pain may move from one part of the head to another and may radiate down the neck into the shoulder. The pain is commonly aggravated by physical activity or simple head movement. Patients prefer to lie down in a dark, quiet room. Scalp tenderness occurs in many patients during or after the headache. This tenderness may involve the head and neck and prevent the patient from lying on the affected side.

Many migraineurs have headache profiles that do not meet the IHS criteria for migraine. Some are "migrainous" (probable migraine), missing one criterion, whereas others are shorter and less severe and often meet the IHS criteria for episodic tension-type headache (TTH). Some patients note that their headache begins as a TTH and builds into a "migraine." I believe that these phenomenological TTHs are all migrainous in nature, have more migraine features than TTH features, and, unlike typical TTH occurring in nonmigraineurs, respond to specific migraine drugs.

Migraineurs may also experience short-lived jabs of pain, lasting for seconds, occurring between more characteristic migraine attacks (so-called idiopathic stabbing headache). The pain is described as an "ice pick," "needle," "nail," "jabs and jolts," or "pinprick" headache, and it occurs in approximately 40% of migraineurs.

Associated Phenomena

Migraine attacks are characteristically accompanied by other associated symptoms that often contribute to migraine-related disability. Gastrointestinal disturbances are often the most distressing symptoms. Anorexia is common, but food cravings can occur; nausea occurs in 90% of patients and vomiting in approximately one-third. Gastroparesis contributes to gastrointestinal distress and poor absorption of oral medication. Diarrhea occurs in approximately 16% of patients. Many migraineurs have enhanced sensory perception or sensitivity manifested by photophobia, phonophobia, and osmophobia, and they seek a dark, quiet room. Others have lightheadedness and vertigo. Premonitory symptoms, such as exhilaration, agitation, fatigue, lethargy, disorientation, hypomania, anger, rage, or depression, can continue into the headache. Constitutional, mood, and mental changes are almost universal. Blurry vision, nasal stuffiness, pallor or redness, and sensations of heat, cold, or sweating may occur. Fluid retention can develop hours to days before the headache. Frank edema may precede, accompany, or follow the headache with resolution of the fluid retention, often with polyuria, after the headache is over.

The frequency of associated symptoms is higher in clinic-based than in population-based studies, probably because more effective interviewing techniques and more definitive criteria are used in the clinic. In addition, a selection bias toward patients with more severe headache may result in more symptoms being reported. Studies grading the severity of nausea, photophobia, and phonophobia improved the differentiation of migraine from TTH; by definition, these symptoms were more prevalent and more severe in migraineurs.

A population-based telephone interview was used to estimate the prevalence of severe headaches in adolescents and young adults. Symptoms usually considered diagnostic of migraine (nausea and/or vomiting, visual disturbances, and photophobia) were significantly associated with prolonged duration and more severe pain. Although these symptoms were reported relatively infrequently in the study population, they were associated with headaches that caused the greatest impairment.

The frequency of migraine-associated symptoms, particularly nausea and vomiting, has also been estimated by placebo-controlled drug studies. Chabriat *et al.* found that 45–100% of patients had nausea prior to treatment, similar to frequency rates observed in other studies of adult migraineurs. The frequency of vomiting was much lower but varied dramatically from study to study. Photophobia occurred in 86–97% of patients, whereas phonophobia was rarely studied.

A telephone interview survey of 500 self-reported migraine sufferers found that the most common symptoms associated with migraine, in addition to pain, were nausea, visual problems, and vomiting. Nausea occurred in more than 90% of all migraineurs; approximately one-third of these experienced nausea during every attack. Vomiting occurred at least once in approximately 70% of all migraineurs; approximately one-third of these vomited in the majority of attacks. Approximately 30% of those who experienced nausea and 42% of those with vomiting indicated that the symptom interfered with their ability to take their oral migraine medication. Visual problems were also reported to occur in most attacks by 32% of respondents. The only other symptom that occurred in more than 20% of respondents in a majority of attacks was sound sensitivity or auditory problems. Some symptoms that were reported by 10% or less of respondents (light sensitivity, dizziness, and neck pain) occurred in a high percentage of their attacks, suggesting that

these symptoms may be specific but not sensitive indicators of migraine. Most of the commonly associated symptoms were usually rated as moderate to severe, consistent with the increased severity expected with the more severe headaches in this study (as a result of selection criteria).

Nausea and/or vomiting, photophobia, and phonophobia are important criteria for migraine diagnosis, particularly if the headache is not accompanied by aura.

STATUS MIGRAINOSUS

The IHS defines status migrainosus as an attack of migraine, the headache phase of which lasts more than 72 hr whether it is treated or not. The headache is continuous throughout the attack. Relief during periods of sleep or by medication is disregarded. No clear distinction is made between transformed migraine and prolonged status migrainosus because no time limit is given to status migrainosus. Factors responsible for triggering status migrainosus include emotional stress, depression, abuse of medications, anxiety, diet, hormonal factors, and multiple nonspecific factors. Status migrainosus may be secondary to an acute neurological disorder. However, acute central nervous system events can trigger an otherwise typical migraine.

—*Stephen D. Silberstein*

See also–Migraine, Genetics of; Migraine Mechanisms; Migraine, Menstrual; Migraine, Ophthalmoplegic and Retinal; Migraine, Transformed; Migraine Treatment; Migraine with Aura; Stroke, Migraine-Induced

Further Reading

Anthony, M., and Rasmussen, B. K. (1993). Migraine without aura. In *The Headaches* (J. Olesen, P. Tfelt-Hansen, and M. A. Welch, Eds.), pp. 255–261. Raven Press, New York.

Cady, R. K., Gutterman, D., Saiers, J. A., *et al.* (1997). Responsiveness of nonIHS migraine and tension-type headache to sumatriptan. *Cephalalgia* **17**, 588–590.

Chabriat, H., Joire, J. E., Danchot, J., *et al.* (1994). Combined oral lysine acetylsalicylate and metoclopramide in the acute treatment of migraine: A multicenter double-blind placebo-controlled study. *Cephalalgia* **14**, 297–300.

Drummond, P. D. (1986). A quantitative assessment of photophobia in migraine and tension headache. *Headache* **26**, 465–469.

Drummond, P. D., and Lance, J. W. (1984). Clinical diagnosis and computer analysis of headache symptoms. *J. Neurol. Neurosurg. Psychiatry* **47**, 128–133.

Headache Classification Committee of the International Headache Society (1988). Classification and diagnostic criteria for headache disorders, cranial neuralgia, and facial pain. *Cephalalgia* **8**, 1–96.

Lipton, R. B., Cady, R. K., O'Quinn, S., *et al.* (1999). Sumatriptan treats the full spectrum of headache in individuals with disabling IHS migraine. *Neurology* **52**, A256.

Olesen, J. (1978). Some clinical features of the acute migraine attack. An analysis of 750 patients. *Headache* **18**, 268–271.

Rasmussen, B. K., Jensen, R., and Olesen, J. (1991). A population-based analysis of the diagnostic criteria of the international headache society. *Cephalalgia* **11**, 129–134.

Silberstein, S. D. (1995). Migraine symptoms: Results of a survey of self-reported migraineurs. *Headache* **35**, 387–396.

Silberstein, S. D., Saper, J. R., and Freitag, F. (2001). Migraine: Diagnosis and treatment. In *Wolff's Headache and Other Head Pain* (S. D. Silberstein, R. B. Lipton, and D. J. Dalessio, Eds.). Oxford Univ. Press, New York.

Stewart, W. F., Shechter, A. L., and Lipton, R. B. (1994). Migraine heterogeneity: Disability, pain intensity, attack frequency, and duration. *Neurology* **44**, S24–S39.

Tfelt-Hansen, P. (1993). Sumatriptan for the treatment of migraine attacks—A review of controlled clinical trials. *Cephalalgia* **13**, 238–244.

Tfelt-Hansen, P., and Olesen, J. (1984). Effervescent metoclopramide and aspirin (Migravess) versus effervescent aspirin or placebo for migraine attacks: A double-blind study. *Cephalalgia* **4**, 107–111.

Volans, G. N. (1978). Research review: Migraine and drug absorption. *Pharmacokinetics* **3**, 313–318.

Ziegler, D., Ford, R., Kriegler, J., *et al.* (1994). Dihydroergotamine nasal spray for the acute treatment of migraine. *Neurology* **44**, 447–453.

Mills, Charles Karsner

Encyclopedia of the Neurological Sciences
Copyright 2003, Elsevier Science (USA). All rights reserved.

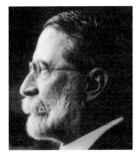

Charles Karsner Mills (courtesy of the National Library of Medicine).

CHARLES KARSNER MILLS (1845–1931) was a founder of the Philadelphia School of Neurology, an eminent neuroscientist, and author of most authoritative 19th-century textbooks of neurology.

Mills fought for the Union with his high school classmates at the battles of Antietam and Gettysburg. He received a MD degree in 1869 and a Ph.D. in 1871 from the medical department of the University of Pennsylvania, Philadelphia.

In 1874, Mills was appointed chief of the Neurology Clinic at the University of Pennsylvania Hospital. From 1891 to 1902, he was professor of neurology at the Women's Medical College of Pennsylvania, now called the Medical College of Pennsylvania. Mills served as professor of neurology at the University of Pennsylvania from 1903 until his retirement in 1915. The American Neurological Association honored Mills by twice electing him president.

Among Mills' many substantial contributions to neuroscience were the localization of functions in human brain and spinal cord ablation of seizure foci, aphasia, medical jurisprudence, and the publication of *The Nervous System and Its Diseases*. Mills conclusively proved by electrical stimulation of human cerebral cortex exposed during operations that the cortex controlling discrete movements of limbs lay anterior to the Rolandic fissure and the prefrontal cortex controlled eye movements. This information provided landmarks for neurosurgeons to avoid damage to these critical structures. Mills assisted neurosurgeon William W. Keen, Jr. (1837–1932) in finding the site in a young woman's cerebral cortex where her epileptic seizures began. Her seizures began as a strange feeling in her left arm, followed by jerking of this arm and her head toward her right shoulder. Mills and Keen electrically stimulated the motor cortex of her right hemisphere and reproduced the seizure. They determined that the motor neurons representing shoulder and leg muscles lay superior to the hand region, presaging by 40 years Wilder Penfield's (1891–1976) similar report.

Mills showed that neurosurgeons could predict prior to surgery that a tumor in the cervical spinal canal was inside the dura but not in the substance of the spinal cord by noting that these patients had "root symptoms" of pain radiating from the center of the spine into the shoulder or hand. Patients with tumors within the spinal cord (intramedullary) initially had loss of fine, discrete movements of the hand (pyramidal signs and symptoms) with loss of power in the limb and exaggeration of the (tendon) reflexes on the side of the body below the level of the tumor.

Mills was a pioneer in the rehabilitation of patients who had lost the ability to speak (aphasia), and he believed strongly in the value of speech therapy. Mills made an extensive study of patients with alterations of their emotions due to tumors or strokes. He described a patient who suffered irrepressible weeping and laughing following a stroke that affected the red nucleus in the right half of the midbrain.

Mills was a founder of the Philadelphia School of Neurology. He was trained by Silas Weir Mitchell (1829–1914). Mills collaborated with William G. Spiller (1863–1940) in neuropathological research through the William Pepper Laboratory at the University of Pennsylvania. Spiller succeeded Mills as professor of neurology at the University of Pennsylvania in 1914.

The Nervous System and Its Diseases was the American rival of the British William Richard Gowers' *A Manual of Diseases of the Nervous System*. Both authors meticulously described the history and physical findings of patients, often their own. Mills provided more annotated references to literature than Gowers, but Gower's text was exquisitely illustrated by his etchings.

—Edward J. Fine

See also–Gowers, William Richard; Mitchell, Silas Weir; Penfield, Wilder (see Index entry Biography for complete list of biographical entries)

Further Reading

Frazier, C. H., Spiller, W. G., Burr, C. W., *et al.* (1932). Charles Karsner Mills. Memorial Meeting of the Philadelphia Neurological Society. *Arch. Neurol. Psychiatry* **28**, 1390–1410.

Gowers, W. R. (1888). *A Manual of Diseases of the Nervous System*. Blakiston, Philadelphia.

Lloyd, J. H. (1931). Obituary. Charles Karsner Mills, MD. *J. Nerv. Ment. Dis.* **74**, 685–686.

Mills, C. K. (1898). *The Nervous System and Its Diseases*. Lippincott, Philadelphia.

Mills, C. K. (1910). Tumors and cysts of the spinal cord with a record of two cases. *J. Nerv. Ment. Dis.* **37**, 529–546.

Mills, C. K. (1912). The cerebral mechanism of emotional expression. *Trans. Coll. Physicians Philadelphia* **34**, 147–185.

Mills, C. K., and Frazier, C. H. (1905). The motor area of the human cerebrum, its position and subdivisions, with some discussion of the surgery of this area. *Univ. Penn. Med. Bull.* **18**, 134–137.

Mills, C. K., and Keen, W. W. (1891). Jacksonian epilepsy, trephining, removal of a small tumor and excision of cortex. *Am. J. Med. Sci.* **102**, 587–600.

Mills, C. K., and Spiller, W. G. (1907). The symptomatology of lesions of the lenticular zone with discussion of the pathology of aphasia. *J. Nerv. Ment. Dis.* **35**, 558–587.

Weisenburg, T. (1931). Obituaries: Charles Karsner Mills. *Arch. Neurol. Psychiatry* **26**, 170–178.

Mitchell, Silas Weir

Encyclopedia of the Neurological Sciences
Copyright 2003, Elsevier Science (USA). All rights reserved.

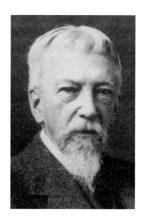

SILAS WEIR MITCHELL (1829–1914) was born in Philadelphia, the son and grandson of physicians. Mitchell's early educational career was less than inspired. Later in life, he recalled that he loathed lessons and had no cheerful memories of the schools he had attended. Enrolled at the University of Pennsylvania at the age of 15 in 1844, he was reprimanded on several occasions for disorderly conduct. He left the university after 3 years without obtaining his degree. He chose a medical career, undoubtedly influenced by his father's example. There is no indication that the young Mitchell felt any particular early fervor or inspiration for this calling. His father was at first surprisingly dubious, telling the young Mitchell, "You have no appreciation of the life. You are wanting in nearly all the qualities that go to make success in medicine. You have brains enough, but no industry." Despite these parental misgivings, Mitchell enrolled in Jefferson Medical College in 1848 and graduated in 1850.

Mitchell decided to pursue a career in general medicine and followed the conventional career route of the time by traveling to Europe for postgraduate studies. During this trip, he had an opportunity to meet many of the leading physicians of the day, including James Paget and William Jenner. He also attended courses in physiology given by Claude Bernard. He credits Bernard with telling him, "Why think, when you can experiment." Upon his return to Philadelphia, his microscope would become the first in the city used for medical investigations.

After his return from Europe, Mitchell applied for an internship at the Pennsylvania Hospital but was unexpectedly turned down; instead, he took a position at a local dispensary and assisted his father in general medical practice. During the subsequent decade, he published regularly in the medical literature. These papers spanned a wide variety of subjects, from reports of unusual cases to studies of medicinal chemistry (e.g., the generation of uric acid). Toward the later part of this period, he began his classic experimental studies on the venom of rattlesnakes (*Crotalus*)—a subject to which he would repeatedly return throughout his career. He tried to characterize the chemical composition of venom, the method by which it was formed and ejected, and the nature of the disease it produced.

Mitchell had a lifelong interest in venoms, toxins, poisons, and the animals that produced them. His studies in this area included investigations not only of snake venoms but also of Gila monster toxin, South American arrow poisons, and curare. With his friend William Hammond, he performed self-experimentation with the "ordeal poison" used by natives of the West African coast. This poison was used in native ceremonies in which the guilt or innocence of the accused was ascertained based on whether the subject was able to retain the infusion (a sign of guilt) or regurgitated it (a sign of innocence). Mitchell performed self-experimentation, which led him to believe that the poison had both emetic and mildly narcotic-like properties. A similar spirit of self-experimentation led him to try mescal buttons. Astonishingly, Mitchell took the drug on a busy afternoon and maintained his usual patient schedule, all the while making observations on the visual hallucinations he was experiencing.

In addition to time spent at his medical practice, Mitchell maintained a physiology laboratory in the building of the Philadelphia Association for Medical Instruction, gave lectures on physiology to students and interested colleagues, and published an important critical review on the state of physiological research in America (1858). Mitchell actively campaigned for the chair in physiology at the University of Pennsylvania (1863), but to his great chagrin he did not receive the appointment. He later wrote, "I have lost my election. It ought to satisfy me as it did not turn upon the question of science or ability to teach but on such outside influences as age—church connections—and social pressure." This rejection prompted the following famous reply from Mitchell's friend Hammond: "I am disgusted with everything and can only say that it is an honor to be rejected by such a set of apes." Despite this setback, at the time

of the onset of the Civil War, Mitchell was probably America's leading experimental physiologist.

In was during the Civil War that Mitchell's interest in diseases of the nervous system developed. Although he would never completely abandon his earlier interest in experimental physiology, it would be in the area of nervous diseases that Mitchell's would make his most historically significant contributions. His goal of obtaining a professorship would forever elude him. The man who would become America's greatest neurologist, and the acknowledged peer of his great European contemporaries Charcot, Gowers, and Jackson, would never hold a major academic position.

In October 1862, Mitchell became acting assistant surgeon at the Filbert Street Hospital, no doubt prompted by his close friend Hammond. Mitchell's position enabled him to maintain his private practice and the income it generated. At the Filbert Street Hospital, Mitchell became interested in "cases of nervous disease and wounds of nerves, about which little was then known. In consequence, other men who did not like these cases began to arrange transfers to my ward." There is surprisingly little in Mitchell's medical career prior to his Civil War experiences that foreshadowed his almost miraculous turning to neurology.

Soon after Mitchell began his work at Fibert Street, a larger specialized hospital for nervous diseases was established, and Mitchell and his medical classmate Dr. George Reed Morehouse (1829–1905) were put in charge. Following the battle of Gettysburg in July 1863, which resulted in more than 27,000 casualties, the overcrowded Christian Street Hospital was enlarged to 400 beds and moved to new quarters at Turner's Lane. Mitchell and Morehouse were joined by the younger William Williams Keen (1837–1932), who, although officially an assistant surgeon, functioned more in the capacity of a resident physician. At Mitchell's request, and with the approval of his friend Surgeon General Hammond, the three were freed of virtually all administrative duties, which permitted them to devote all available time to their cases.

The tragedy of war brought with it a treasure trove of neurological cases. As Mitchell noted, the wards were filled with patients with epilepsy, chorea, palsies, "stump disorders," and "every kind of nerve wound." Mitchell recalled the number of cases was enormous, representing virtually every imaginable type of disease and injury to the nervous system. Among these were a vast collection of wounds and contusions of nerves, including all the rarest forms of nerve lesion of almost every great nerve in the human body. The three colleagues kept meticulous notes of the history of each case, the findings on examination, and the effects of therapy including the use of electricity (which was "constantly employed"), and the effects of medications. The latter included enormous amounts of morphine given by the then novel route of hypodermic administration. Mitchell later referred to Turner's Lane as a "Hell of Pain," noting that 40,000 morphine injections per year were administered.

The hell of Turner's Lane would become the birthplace of American neurology. At Turner's Lane, Mitchell became America's first real full-time neurologist, a preeminent position he would retain for the remainder of his life. Mitchell would become to American neurology what Charcot was to French neurology and Hughlings Jackson was to British neurology. He was the first American neurologist whom these eminent contemporaries would have regarded as a peer and a colleague.

At Turner's Lane, Mitchell took on the primary responsibility for compiling medical experiences concerning traumatic nerve injuries. The results of the first 18 months' experience at Turner's Lane with nerve injuries were presented in what became one of the classic monographs in American neurological history, *Gunshot Wounds and Other Injuries of Nerves* (1864). The original edition was only 164 pages in length, lacked illustrations, and had few references. It was later expanded into a definitive version as *Injuries of Nerves and Their Consequences* (1872). These monographs filled a tremendous gap because there was virtually nothing of a comprehensive nature in the literature on the symptoms, signs, treatment, and outcome of nerve injuries. Mitchell noted that he had "endeavored to present in as concise a form as possible the history of lesions of nerve trunks and their consequences" based on his own experience. *Injuries of Nerves and Their Consequences* was a greatly expanded version of Mitchell's original monograph. The book was divided into 14 chapters. Initial chapters covered the anatomy of nerves, their neurophysiology, and the physiological pathology of nerve lesions. Subsequent chapters covered in a logical sequence the varieties of mechanical injuries of nerves, the symptomatology of nerve lesions, remote symptoms, sensory lesions, and the diagnosis and prognosis of injuries of nerves. Three chapters were devoted to treatment, and the final chapters dealt with lesions of special nerves and the "neural maladies of stumps."

Regarding symptomatology, Mitchell noted that the character of symptoms varied only slightly in the different forms of nerve injury. He divided the symptoms into local and general categories. Among the earliest local symptoms, experienced at the onset of injury, were a sensation as if being struck by a stick or stone, instant and intense pain, and a feeling of numbness or tingling pain. Mitchell noted that slight injuries of mixed nerves were more likely to be associated with abnormalities or loss of sensory rather than motor function, although in graver injuries both sensation and motion were lost. General symptoms were primarily those of "shock." Mitchell was unsure to what extent this was due to associated injury of muscle and bone and to what extent it was the result of a "reflex effect of the injury of nerves."

In the chapter on remote symptoms, he described chorea, referring to movements that would today be called fasciculations. He noted that complete injuries of great nerves to a limb can be associated with dramatic atrophic changes in which "muscles waste away, the areolar tissue disappears, the skin becomes dry, ragged, yellowish or brown, and rough; the nails and hair degenerate." Atrophic muscles were noted to have "lost tension" so that they felt "flabby and relaxed." He noted the tendency of nerve injuries to result in cutaneous eruptions that were "herpetic, vesicular, or in the shape of bullae." Trauma and pressure were more likely to lead to late ulceration in areas in which the nerves had been totally divided.

Mitchell, Morehouse, and Keen gave the first descriptions of causalgia (a term originally coined by Mitchell in 1867), to which later depictions have added little. The pain was "burning" or "mustard red-hot" and often felt like a "hot file rasping the skin." Causalgia was described as

the most terrible of all the tortures that a nerve wound may inflict. The affected part was exquisitely hyperesthetic, and a finger tap, a light touch, or even exposure to air could induce an intense burning sensation. The affected extremity, often the palmar surface of the hand or the dorsum of the foot, often underwent "nutritive skin changes" and was always found to be warmer in temperature than surrounding parts. At times the skin of the involved extremity became "tapering, smooth, hairless, almost void of wrinkles, glossy, pink." These glossy surfaces often became devoid of hair, and the nails underwent "remarkable alterations."

They became curved in their long axis, at times producing extreme lateral arching. Although occasionally seen in association with nerve injuries of many types, these nutritive changes were most profound in patients with causalgia. Mitchell would later speculate that causalgia was a "reflex phenomena" in which the irritation or injury of a nerve would induce "changes in the circulation and nutrition of parts in its distribution, and that these alterations might be themselves of a pain-producing nature."

The sensory functions of nerves might be "lessened, exalted, or perverted" as a consequence of wounds. Hyperaesthesia was only rarely seen as an immediate effect of injury but tended to develop later. Hyperaesthesia for pain was often associated with a lessened or lost sense of tactile appreciation. Loss of tactile impressions was common and might occur instantly and be of any degree of severity. Mitchell used several tests. For rough examination, the touch of a pencil point on the surface or, in dubious cases, the tip of a feather were used. The most delicate test of all was to touch the tips of single hairs on the skin. He recorded the results on previously prepared drawings of the parts being examined. Second, an aesthesiometer, consisting of two compass points covered with small rounded balls and with a distance scale showing their separation, was used to ascertain the smallest distance at which the separated points were clearly felt as double. Third, the patient was asked to localize exactly where the touch had occurred. Finally, pain sense was tested with a needle or, if needed, an electrical stimulus.

Treatment of nerve injuries usually consisted of electrical stimulation and manipulation (shampooing, rubbing, massage, etc.) of the involved muscles. Eventually, the treatment of the terrible pains of traumatic neuralgia often required hypodermic injections of narcotics. Occasionally, "it was almost the only plan of treating severe neuralgic pain." As noted previously, Mitchell estimated that at least 40,000 doses of various narcotics were administered per year, with some patients receiving 500 or more injections. Finally, when other means of relieving pain had failed, he resorted to neurotomy. He believed that simple division should be avoided, that "not less than 2 in. of its [the nerve's] length ought to be removed," and that a piece of muscle or fascia should be interposed between the cut nerve ends to preclude their reunion.

In the chapter on lesions of special nerves, Mitchell gave an excellent description of sympathetic palsy, which antedated Horner's description of miosis, ptosis, and enophthalmos. He noted that, "My own attention was first drawn to the man by accidentally observing as he passed me in the wards that one pupil was contracted." The patient was a 24-year-old man who had been wounded at Chancellorsville by a rifle ball that had entered his right neck just behind the ramus of the jaw at the anterior edge of the sterno-cleidomastoid muscle. Mitchell noted that the pupil of the man's right eye was very small, that there was "slight but very distinct ptosis of the right eye," and that "the ball of the right eye looks smaller than that of the left." When the patient's face was exposed to heat, it became flushed on the right side and pale on the left.

The final chapter of the book on nerve injuries, titled Neural Maladies of Stumps, is a classic. Mitchell notes, "No history of the physiology of stumps would be complete without some account of the sensorial delusions to which persons are subject in connection with their lost limbs." He called these hallucinations vivid and strange and noted that little was written about the subject in the medical literature. He noted that "nearly every man who has lost a limb carries about with him a constant or inconstant phantom of the missing member; a sensory ghost" and in fact found this to be true in 86 of 90 patients he examined. Patients rarely felt the limb as a normal whole as it had existed premorbidly; they more typically felt its distal extremity (i.e., the hand or the foot). A curious consequence of this perceptual bias was that the phantom limb often appeared abnormally short compared to its normal counterpart, with the hand or foot feeling closer to the stump than they did on the normal side. Patients with phantom limbs frequently had "subjective sensations referred to the absent limb" including pain or itching. Frequently, the phantom limb seemed to move in coordination with the movements of the stump.

One of Mitchell's most remarkable short stories, *The Case of George Dedlow* (1866), dramatically portrayed the symptoms of phantom limbs for the lay public and prompted an outpouring of donations and public sympathy for the imaginary protagonist. Mitchell noted that he began writing this story after becoming intrigued when a friend inquired, "How much of a man would have to be lost in order that he should lose any portion of his sense of individuality?" The unfortunate protagonist and narrator of this tale was a fictional Army physician who had all four of his limbs amputated after a series of wartime injuries. Using Dedlow's voice, Mitchell clearly describes the horrible pains of causalgia that Dedlow, a Union officer, suffered after receiving a wound involving his right arm during one of the skirmishes of the western campaign. Following his wound, Dedlow noted that "I felt as if the hand was caught and pinched in a red-hot vice [sic]." Later he described the hand as "red, shining, aching, burning, and as it seemed to me, perpetually rasped with hot files … The pain became absolutely unendurable … I screamed, cried, and yelled in my torture." No morphia was available, and the only relief came from covering the hand with a wetted handkerchief. Dedlow ultimately agreed to have the affected limb amputated near the shoulder joint, which was done without the benefit of ether. Released from Confederate prison in a prisoner exchange in the summer of 1863, Dedlow returned to serve with the Union forces at Chickamauga. He was hit by artillery fire in both legs, which were amputated by field surgeons. Upon awakening from chloroform anesthesia, Dedlow became "suddenly aware of a sharp cramp in my left leg. I tried to get at it to rub it with my single arm, but, finding myself too weak hailed an attendant." The attendant, being requested to rub Dedlow's left calf, tells him, "You ain't none [sic], pardner. It's took off." Dedlow remarks, "I know better, said I. I have pain in both legs. Wall, I never! said he. You ain't got nary leg. As I did not believe him, he threw off the covers, and, to my horror, showed me that I had suffered amputation of both thighs, very high up." Dedlow's remaining limb, his left arm, is later lost to gangrene, leaving him a limbless torso: "Against all chances I recovered, to find myself a useless torso, more like some strange larval creature than anything of human shape. Of my anguish and horror of myself I dare not speak." During this period, Dedlow experiences recurrent phantom limb sensations and describes these and other similar experiences of fellow inmates of the "Stump Hospital" in vivid detail. Dedlow's story ends when he is taken to a spiritualist seance at which he is reunited with his missing limbs. After the story was published, Mitchell noted, "The unfortunate George Dedlow's sad account of himself proved so convincing that people raised money to help him and visited the Stump Hospital to see him."

From a modern perspective, Mitchell's work on injuries of nerves must surely rate as his greatest contribution to neurology. Mitchell's contemporaries also recognized his contributions in the area of "reflex paralysis" and the "rest cure" as major accomplishments, although the luster of both have dimmed over time. In 1864, Mitchell, Morehouse, and Keen wrote a small circular of 23 pages titled Reflex Paralysis. The common theme of the 7 cases included in this short pamphlet was that localized injury at a specific anatomic site might cause distant neurological signs and symptoms. Mitchell noted that this report included "very infrequent cases, in which paralysis

of a remote part or parts has been occasioned by a gunshot wound of some prominent nerve." Although Mitchell called these cases rare and very infrequent, he was able to find 7 among approximately 60 well-studied cases of nerve wounds. Examples of these phenomena included wounds in one thigh causing paralysis of the arm, paralysis of the arm and opposite leg, and paralysis of the opposite thigh. Mitchell speculated that perhaps a very severe injury or violent excitement of a nerve trunk might result in an exhaustion of the irritability and power of the nerve centers to which it was connected, resulting in a loss in function. He speculated that local injuries typically produced only local effects, much like the local results of electrically stimulating a nerve trunk. However, severe injuries might produce remote effects, just as being hit by lightening produces dramatic systemic effects compared to the lesser effects of localized electrical stimulation. He suggested that since this exhaustion of the higher centers was not associated with their permanent injury or destruction, these remote effects should eventually resolve as the higher centers' irritability and power are replenished. Although it is perhaps tempting to suggest that some of Mitchell's ideas represented a nascent version of the concept of diaschisis, rereading Mitchell's cases suggests that many were examples of hysterical paralysis or malingering.

Mitchell's contemporaries clearly regarded his elucidation of the "rest cure" for neurological diseases as one of his seminal contributions. Osler noted, "What brought his greatest reputation in the profession was the introduction of the so-called rest treatment." Mitchell had been particularly impressed with the effects that rest had engendered in his patients with locomotor ataxia. In 1871, he prepared a "little sermon" for popular consumption titled Wear and Tear; Or Hints for the Overworked. In this book, he suggested that an increase in nervous diseases had been caused by the stress of excessive mental work and emphasized the potential of ill health triggered by "mental fatigue." Exercise, vacations, and reduction in academic stress all had beneficial effects on mental fatigue. He noted that women seemed particularly at risk, and that problems engendered by mental fatigue might "decrease their future womanly usefulness." Later he wrote,

The women's desire to be on a level of competition with man and to assume his duties is, I am sure, making mischief, for it is my belief that no length of generations of change in her education and modes of activity will ever really alter her characteristics.

Mitchell's forays into writing medical literature for the lay public continued with his equally popular books *Fat and Blood and How to Make Them* (1877), *Nurse and Patient and Camp Cure* (1877), and *Doctor and Patient* (1888). These books were enormously popular and were the 19th-century equivalent to the best-selling medical self-help books that often figure so prominently on nonfiction best-seller lists today.

By 1875, Mitchell had formulated all of the key components of his rest cure in a paper titled "Rest in Nervous Disease: Its Use and Abuse." The subjects of the rest care were typically, but not exclusively, women belonging to the upper classes of society. Their illnesses would today probably be classified among various forms of depression, although in some cases there was an uncanny resemblance to what is today called chronic fatigue syndrome and what was then often referred to by Mitchell and his contemporaries as neurasthenia. In its full form, the rest cure entailed secluding the patient from all contact with the outside world except for medical attendants, who included the physician, a skilled nurse, and a trained physical therapist. As Mitchell noted, "You [the physician] are her whole audience, and this with a hysterical girl gives you great power."

To seclusion was added rest. Rest was to be so complete as to exclude all potential sources of fatigue—both physical and mental. The goal was the total "absence of all possible use of brain and body." Care was taken that letters brought no worrying news from the outside world. The patient was not allowed to write and was forbidden to read, although the patient could listen as a nurse read aloud. Initially, the patient was not even allowed to feed herself, this duty being given to the nurse. Mitchell frequently regulated the diet, emphasizing the initial importance of skim milk and bland foods. Such absolute rest was not without its complications. Mitchell included among these enfeebled circulation, weakened digestion, lessened appetite, and constipation. Two additional components of the rest cure, massage and electrotherapy, were designed to counteract these problems.

Another key component of the rest cure was the gradual reduction in the restrictions and severity of the regimen as the patient's condition improved. This program was at the sole discretion of the physician, and any decline brought with it a corresponding reinstitution of the full rest cure treatment. The patient in essence earned the ability to feed herself, embellish her diet, write or read, see visitors, or take walks or even trips outside by showing improvement in her condition.

In addition to his major contributions on nerve injuries and his writings on reflex paralysis and the rest cure, Mitchell was constantly contributing to the medical literature during the period following the Civil War. Other notable papers included "Researches on the Physiology of the Cerebellum"(1869), in which he described the results of 87 ablative and 260 irritative cerebellar lesions in a variety of birds and animals. The paper is perhaps most notable for showing Mitchell's continuing interest in experimental physiology rather than for the novelty of any of its findings. Mitchell was among the first American neurologists to study the tendon reflexes. He wrote on the "Diagnostic Significance of the Tendon Reflex" (1878) and studied the effects of voluntary acts, patient position, time of day, and repeated elicitation on the intensity of the knee jerks. He devised a system for recording the activity of the knee jerk using a series of " + " marks for exaggerated activity and "−" notations for depressed activity.

Mitchell also described an unusual condition, erythromelalgia, sometimes referred to as Mitchell's disease. He derived the name by combining the Latin terms for redness, extremity, and pain. He originally described this condition in 1872, but he did not use the term erythromelalgia until 1884 when he described cases in various medical journals. He discussed the disorder more fully in *Clinical Lessons on Nervous Diseases* (1897). Of the 27 cases Mitchell had encountered by 1897, all but 2 were men. The involved extremity, typically the foot, appeared normal until placed in a dependent position, when it became "rose red"—a feature he illustrated with two color plates in his book. The involved foot ached or burned continually and was tender to pressure. In more severe cases, even the touch of a feather could produce pain, which at times became unendurably intense. This could be relieved by removing the limb from its dependent position and allowing the patient to elevate it. The arteries of the involved foot throbbed when it was dependent, and the veins were prominent. He called erythromelalgia a "chronic disease in which a part or parts—usually one or more extremities—suffer with pain, flushing, and local fever, made far worse if the parts hang down." Since Mitchell's time, the existence of erythromelalgia as a distinct clinical entity has been controversial, and the diagnosis is rarely made or encountered in modern neurological settings.

Mitchell, like Hammond, developed an interest in disorders of sleep. He wrote on the subject in 1876 and covered the topic more extensively in *Lectures on Diseases of the Nervous System—Especially in Women* (1881). The subject was also extensively reviewed in *Clinical Lessons on Nervous Disease* (1897). He described hypnagogic hallucinations, noting that these predormital visions reminded him of the hallucinations brought on by mescal. He noted that the hallucinations that occurred between waking and sleep could involve both sight and hearing. Related cases involved predormital sensations of fear or terror. He subsequently described patients who experienced sleep numbness, nocturnal paresis, or paralysis. He described cases of "sleep jerks" and "chorea." including various types of myoclonus, periodic leg movements of sleep and restless legs.

Although Mitchell's goal of obtaining a professorial chair eluded him, he life was filled with numerous honors and accolades. His friend Keen would write of him that he was the most versatile American since Benjamin Franklin. Osler considered him "one of the foremost neurologists of his time" and noted "he also held a leading place among American writers of fiction in the later half of the 19th century." Osler referred to him as the "leading authority" on the subject of nervous diseases in America. He was elected, but declined to serve, as the founding president of the American Neurological Association in 1875 (an oversight he remedied in 1909). He received numerous honorary degrees, including doctorates from Harvard and Princeton, and was elected to virtually all the major scientific and medical societies of the day. He achieved great recognition as both a poet and a popular novelist during his lifetime. He wrote approximately 19 novels, 7 books of poetry containing over 150 poems, a biography of George Washington, and a children's Christmas story (*Kris Kringle*). Contemporary literary critics favorably compared his historical novel *Hugh Wynne* (1897) to Thackeray's best works and one of his best poems ("Ode on a Lycian Tomb," 1898) to Keat's "Ode on a Grecian Urn." Mitchell had no difficulty getting his poetry publishing in the *Atlantic Monthly* and other leading literary journals when those same journals were regularly rejecting Emily Dickinson's work and refusing to publish Walt Whitman's poetry because it was considered obscene. After "Ode on a Lycian Tomb" appeared in *Century Magazine*, no less an authority than Charles Eliot Norton told Mitchell it represented "the high tide of American verse." *Hugh*

Wynne alone reportedly sold more than 500,000 copies.

Mitchell died at age 84 of complications of influenza. Osler's obituary tribute is worth repeating: "He was a man of commanding presence and personality. He was a pioneer in neurology, and the influence of his work is writ large in the history of the development of that branch of medical science."

—Kenneth L. Tyler

***See also*–Nerve Injury; Neuropathic Pain Syndromes; Osler, William; Phantom Limb and Stump Pain (see Index entry Biography for complete list of biographical entries)**

Further Reading

Burr, A. R. B. (1929). *Weir Mitchell, His Life and Letters.* Duffield, New York.

DeJong, R. N. (1982). *A History of American Neurology,* pp. 14–21. Raven Press, New York.

Earnest, E. (1950). *Silas Weir Mitchell, Novelist and Physician.* Univ. of Pennsylvania Press, Philadelphia.

Fye, W. B. (1983). S. Weir Mitchell, Philadelphia's "lost" physiologist. *Bull. Hist. Med.* 57, 188–202.

Goldner, J. C. (1971). S. Weir Mitchell: Nerves, peripheral and otherwise. *Mayo Clin. Proc.* 46, 274–281.

Haymaker, W. (1970). Weir Mitchell (1829–1914). In *The Founders of Neurology* (W. Haymaker and F. Schiller, Eds.), 2nd ed., pp. 479–484. Thomas, Springfield, IL.

LaFia, D. J. (1955). S. Weir Mitchell on gunshot wounds and other injuries of nerves. *Neurology* 5, 468–471.

McHenry, L. C., Jr. (1959). Silas Weir Mitchell. *N. Engl. J. Med.* 260, 712–714.

Metzer, W. S. (1989). The experimentation of S. Weir Mitchell with mescal. *Neurology* 39, 303–304.

Mills, C. K. (1914). Silas Weir Mitchell—His place in neurology. *J. Nerv. Ment. Dis.* 41, 65–74.

Mitchell, S. W. (1866). The case of George Dedlow. *Atl. Mon.* 18, 1–11.

Mitchell, S. W. (1871). *Wear and Tear.* Lippincott, Philadelphia.

Mitchell, S. W. (1872). *Injuries of Nerves and Their Consequences.* Lippincott, Philadelphia.

Mitchell, S. W. (1877). *Fat and Blood and How to Make Them.* Lippincott, Philadelphia.

Mitchell, S. W. (1881). *Lectures on Diseases of the Nervous System—Especially in Women.* Lea, Philadelphia.

Mitchell, S. W. (1888). *Doctor and Patient.* Lippincott, Philadelphia.

Mitchell, S. W. (1895). *Remote Consequences of Injuries of Nerves and Their Treatment.* Lea, Philadelphia.

Mitchell, S. W. (1897). *Clinical Lessons on Nervous Diseases.* Lea, Philadelphia.

Mitchell, S. W., Morehouse, G. R., and Keen, W. W. (1864). *Gunshot Wounds and Other Injuries of Nerves.* Lippincott, Philadelphia.

Mitchell, S. W., Morehouse, G. R., and Keen, W. W. (1864). Reflex paralysis (circular #6). Surgeon-General's Office, Washington, DC.

Walker, R. D. (1971). *S. Weir Mitchell, M.D.–Neurologist. A Medical Biography.* Thomas, Springfield, IL.

Walter, R. D. (1975). Silas Weir Mitchell (1829–1914). In *Centennial Anniversary Volume of the American Neurological Association (1875–1975)* (D. Denny-Brown, Ed.), pp. 129–133. Springer, New York.

Mitochondrial Encephalomyopathies, Overview

Encyclopedia of the Neurological Sciences
Copyright 2003, Elsevier Science (USA). All rights reserved.

MITOCHONDRIAL MYOPATHIES have been known since the early 1960s, when systematic ultrastructural and histochemical studies revealed excessive proliferation of normal- or abnormal-looking mitochondria in muscle of patients with weakness or exercise intolerance. Because with the modified Gomori trichrome stain the areas of mitochondrial accumulation looked like purplish blotches (Fig. 1), the abnormal fibers were dubbed ragged-red fibers (RRFs) and came to be considered the pathological hallmark of mitochondrial disease. It soon became apparent, especially to pediatric neurologists, that in many patients with RRFs, the myopathy was overshadowed by diverse symptoms and signs of brain involvement, and the term mitochondrial encephalomyopathies was introduced.

According to the widely accepted endosymbiotic hypothesis, mitochondria are the remnants of protobacteria that populated anaerobic nucleated cells and endowed them with the precious gift of oxidative metabolism. Thus, mitochondria are the main source of energy for all human tissues and contain many metabolic pathways, only some of which (e.g., pyruvate dehydrogenase complex, the carnitine cycle, the β-oxidation "spirals," and the Krebs cycle, also known as the tricarboxylic acid cycle) are shown in Fig. 2.

Although defects in all these pathways are by definition mitochondrial diseases, the term mitochondrial encephalomyopathy indicates disorders due to defects in a single mitochondrial metabolic pathway, the respiratory chain. This is the "business end" of oxidative metabolism, where ATP is generated. The reducing equivalents produced in the Krebs cycle and in the β-oxidation spirals are passed along a series of protein complexes embedded in the inner mitochondrial membrane (the electron transport

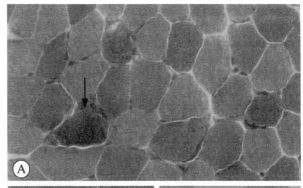
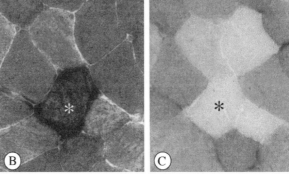

Figure 1

(A) Ragged-red fibers (RRFs) revealed by the modified Gomori trichrome stain. Abnormal accumulations of mitochondria appear as reddish blotches, mostly at the periphery of muscle fibers. (B and C) Serial cross sections from the muscle biopsy of a patient with Kearns–Sayre syndrome. In B, an RRF (asterisk) is highlighted by the histochemical stain for succinate dehydrogenase, which is entirely encoded by nuclear DNA. In C, the same RRF (asterisk) shows no activity for cytochrome *c* oxidase, an enzyme that contains three subunits encoded by mtDNA. (See color plate section.)

chain). The electron transport chain consists of four multimeric complexes (I–IV) and two small electron carriers, coenzyme Q (or ubiquinone) and cytochrome *c*. The energy generated by these reactions is used to pump protons from the mitochondrial matrix into the space between the inner and outer mitochondrial membranes. This creates an electrochemical proton gradient, which is utilized by complex V (or ATP synthase) to produce ATP in a process known as oxidation/phosphorylation coupling.

A unique feature of the respiratory chain is that it is controlled by two distinct genomes, the nuclear DNA (nDNA) and the mitochondrial DNA (mtDNA). Of the approximately 80 proteins that make up the respiratory chain, 13 are encoded by mtDNA and all others are encoded by nDNA. As indicated by the different shadings in Fig. 2, complex II, coenzyme Q, and cytochrome *c* are exclusively encoded by nDNA. In contrast, complexes I and

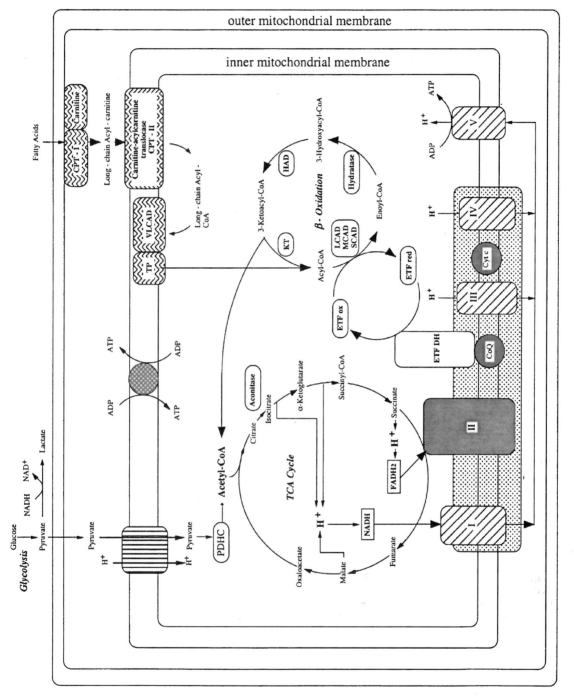

Figure 2

Schematic representation of mitochondrial metabolism. ADP, adenosine diphosphate; ATP, adenosine triphosphate; CoA, coenzyme A; TCA, tricarboxylic acid; FADH2, flavin adenine dinucleotide, reduced form; CPT, carnitine palmitoyltransferase; I–V, complexes of the respiratory chain (stippled, complexes containing both subunits encoded by nuclear DNA and subunits encoded by mitochondrial DNA; solid, complexes encoded entirely by nuclear DNA); NADH, nicotinamide adenine dinucleotide, reduced form; CoQ, coenzyme Q; Cyt c, cytochrome c; PDHC, pyruvate dehydrogenase complex.

III–V contain some subunits encoded by mtDNA: 7 for complex I, 1 for complex III, 3 for complex IV, and 2 for complex V.

Human mtDNA (Fig. 3) is a 16.569-kb circular, double-stranded molecule that contains 37 genes: 2 rRNA genes, 22 tRNA genes, and 13 structural genes encoding the respiratory chain subunits listed previously. In the course of evolution, mtDNA has lost much of its original autonomy and now depends heavily on the nuclear genome for the production of

factors needed for mtDNA transcription, translation, and replication. Since 1988 (when mutations in mtDNA were first associated with human disease), the circle of mtDNA has become crowded with pathogenic mutations, and the following principles of mitochondrial genetics should therefore be familiar to the practicing physician:

- *Heteroplasmy and the threshold effect*: Each cell contains hundreds or thousands of mtDNA copies

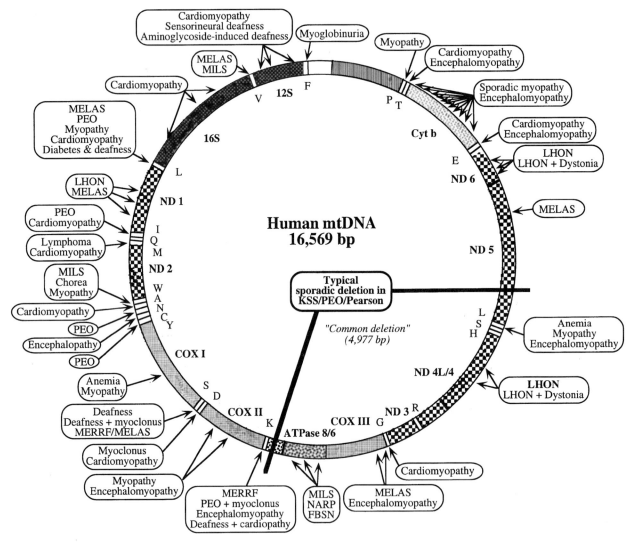

Figure 3

Morbidity map of the human mitochondrial genome as of January 1, 2000. The two mutations described in 1988 are shown in bold. The map of the 16.569-kb mtDNA shows differently shaded areas representing the protein-coding genes for the seven subunits of complex I (ND), the three subunits of cytochrome oxidase (COX), cytochrome *b* (Cyt *b*), and the two subunits of ATP synthetase (ATPase 6 and 8); the 12S and 16S ribosomal RNAs (rRNA); and the 22 transfer RNAs (tRNA) identified by one-letter codes for the corresponding amino acids. FBSN, familial bilateral striatal necrosis; KSS, Kearns–Sayre syndrome; LHON, Leber's hereditary optic neuropathy; MELAS, mitochondrial encephalomyopathy, lactic acidosis, and stroke-like episodes; MERRF, myoclonic epilepsy with ragged-red fibers; MILS, maternally inherited Leigh syndrome; NARP, neuropathy, ataxia, retinitis pigmentosa; PEO, progressive external ophthalmoplegia.

that, at cell division, distribute randomly among daughter cells. In normal tissues, all mtDNA molecules are identical (homoplasmy). Deleterious mutations of mtDNA usually affect some but not all mtDNAs within a cell, a tissue, and an individual (heteroplasmy), and the clinical expression of a pathogenic mtDNA mutation is largely determined by the relative proportion of normal and mutant genomes in different tissues. A minimum critical number of mutant mtDNAs is required to cause mitochondrial dysfunction in a particular organ or tissue and mitochondrial disease in an individual (threshold effect).

• *Mitotic segregation*: At cell division, the proportion of mutant mtDNAs in daughter cells may shift and the phenotype may change accordingly. This phenomenon, called mitotic segregation, explains how certain patients with mtDNA-related disorders may actually shift from one clinical phenotype to another as they grow older.

• *Maternal inheritance*: At fertilization, all mtDNA derives from the oocyte (Fig. 4). Therefore, the mode of transmission of mtDNA and of mtDNA point mutations (single deletions of mtDNA are usually sporadic events) differs from Mendelian inheritance. A mother carrying an mtDNA point mutation will pass it on to all her children (males as well as females), but only her daughters will transmit it to their progeny. A disease expressed in both sexes but with no evidence of paternal transmission is strongly suggestive of a mtDNA point mutation.

The best way for the clinician to chart a course toward a diagnosis in the jungle of mitochondrial encephalomyopathies is to use a classification that combines genetic and biochemical criteria. From the genetic standpoint, there are two major categories: disorders due to defects of mtDNA and disorders due to defects of nDNA.

DISORDERS DUE TO DEFECTS OF mtDNA

These disorders include rearrangements (single deletions or duplications) and point mutations.

mtDNA Rearrangements

Single deletions of mtDNA have been associated with three sporadic conditions. First, Pearson syndrome is usually a fatal disorder of infancy characterized by sideroblastic anemia and exocrine pancreas dysfunction. Second, Kearns–Sayre syndrome (KSS) is a

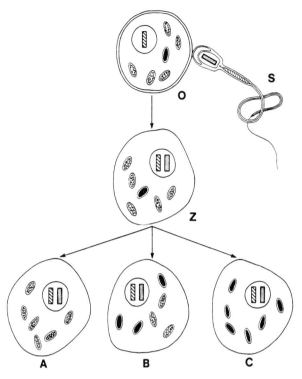

Figure 4

Drawing illustrating maternal inheritance of mitochondrial genomes and the random distribution of normal and mutant genomes in daughter cells of the zygote (Z). For simplicity, the relative sizes of the oocyte (O) and the sperm (S) have not been respected, and it has been assumed that individual mitochondria contain either a single copy of mtDNA or a uniform population of mutant (filled mitochondria) or normal (open mitochondria) genomes. Stem cells of different tissues are labeled A–C. In A, cells are homoplasmic for normal mtDNA; in B, cells are heteroplasmic; and in C, cells are homoplasmic for mutated mtDNA.

multisystem disorder with onset before age 20 of impaired eye movements [progressive external ophthalmoplegia (PEO)], pigmentary retinopathy, and heart block. Frequent additional signs include ataxia, dementia, and endocrine problems (diabetes mellitus, short stature, and hypoparathyroidism). Lactic acidosis, elevated cerebrospinal fluid (CSF) protein (>100 mg/dl), and RRFs in the muscle biopsy are typical laboratory abnormalities. The third condition is PEO with or without proximal limb weakness, often compatible with a normal lifespan. Deletions vary in size and location, but a "common" deletion of 5 kb is frequently seen in patients and in aged individuals (Fig. 3).

Duplication of mtDNA can occur in isolation or together with single deletions and has been seen in patients with KSS or with diabetes mellitus and deafness. Duplications and duplications/deletions (as well as the associated phenotypes) are transmitted by maternal inheritance.

Point Mutations

More than 100 pathogenic point mutations have been identified in mtDNA from patients with a variety of disorders, most of which are maternally inherited and multisystemic, but some are sporadic and tissue specific (Fig. 3). Among the maternally inherited encephalomyopathies, four syndromes are most common. The first is MELAS (mitochondrial encephalomyopathy, lactic acidosis, and stroke-like episodes), which usually presents in children or young adults after normal early development. Symptoms include recurrent vomiting, migraine-like headache, and stroke-like episodes causing cortical blindness, hemiparesis, or hemianopia. Magnetic resonance imaging of the brain shows "infarcts" that do not correspond to the distribution of major vessels, raising the question of whether the strokes are vascular or metabolic in nature. The most common mtDNA mutation is A3243G in the tRNA$^{Leu(UUR)}$ gene, but approximately 12 other mutations have been associated with MELAS.

The second syndrome is MERRF (myoclonus epilepsy with ragged red fibers), characterized by myoclonus, seizures, mitochondrial myopathy, and cerebellar ataxia. Less common signs include dementia, hearing loss, peripheral neuropathy, and multiple lipomas. The typical mtDNA mutation in MERRF is A8344G in the tRNA^{Lys} gene.

The third syndrome has two types: (i) NARP (neuropathy, ataxia, retinitis pigmentosa) usually affects young adults and causes retinitis pigmentosa, dementia, seizures, ataxia, proximal weakness, and sensory neuropathy, and (ii) maternally inherited Leigh syndrome (MILS) is a more severe infantile encephalopathy with characteristic symmetrical lesions in the basal ganglia and the brainstem.

The fourth syndrome, LHON (Leber's hereditary optic neuropathy), is characterized by acute or subacute loss of vision in young adults, more frequently males, due to bilateral optic atrophy. Approximately 12 different mtDNA point mutations in structural genes (mostly genes encoding subunits of complex I) have been associated with LHON, but only three appear to be pathogenic, even when present in isolation (primary mutations), and all three affect genes of complex I (ND genes): G11778A in ND4, G3460A in ND1, and T14484C in ND6.

Not surprisingly, syndromes associated with mtDNA mutations can affect every system or organ in the body, including the eye (optic atrophy, retinitis pigmentosa, and cataracts), hearing (neurosensory deafness), the endocrine system (short stature, diabetes mellitus, and hypoparathyroidism), the heart (familial cardiomyopathies and conduction blocks), the gastrointestinal tract (exocrine pancreas dysfunction, intestinal pseudo-obstruction, and gastroesophageal reflux), and the kidney (renal tubular acidosis). Any combination of the symptoms and signs listed previously should raise suspicion of a mitochondrial disorder, especially if there is evidence of maternal transmission.

On the other hand, point mutations in mtDNA protein-coding genes often do not follow the rules of mitochondrial genetics in that they affect single individuals and single tissues, most commonly skeletal muscle. Thus, patients with exercise intolerance, myalgia, and, sometimes, recurrent myoglobinuria may have isolated defects of complex I, complex III, or complex IV due to pathogenic mutations in genes encoding ND subunits, cytochrome *b*, or cytochrome oxidase (COX) subunits. The lack of maternal inheritance and the involvement of muscle alone suggest that mutations arose *de novo* in myogenic stem cells after germ-layer differentiation (somatic mutations).

DISORDERS DUE TO DEFECTS OF nDNA

These are all transmitted by Mendelian inheritance and include three major subgroups.

Mutations in Genes Encoding Subunits or Ancillary Proteins of the Respiratory Chain

As noted previously, mtDNA encodes only 13 subunits of the respiratory chain, whereas nDNA encodes all subunits of complex II, most subunits of the other four complexes, as well as coenzyme Q10 (CoQ10) and cytochrome *c*. Although most of the progress in the past decade has been in our understanding of the molecular bases of mtDNA-related disorders, attention is shifting toward Mendelian defects of the respiratory chain. These can affect respiratory chain complexes directly or indirectly.

Direct "hits" are mutations in gene-encoding respiratory chain subunits, including subunits of complex I and complex II. These have been associated with autosomal recessive forms of Leigh syndrome. Apparently, primary CoQ10 deficiency can cause three major syndromes—a predominantly myopathic disorder with recurrent myoglobinuria, a predominantly encephalopathic disorder with ataxia and cerebellar atrophy, and a generalized form. Presumably, the different presentations reflect mutations in different biosynthetic enzymes, but this remains to be documented. Diagnosis is important because all patients with CoQ10 deficiency respond to CoQ10 supplementation.

Indirect hits are mutations in gene-encoding proteins that are not components of the respiratory chain but are needed for the proper assembly and function of respiratory chain complexes. This "murder by proxy" scenario is best illustrated by Mendelian defects of COX (complex IV). Mutations in four ancillary proteins—SURF1, SCO2, COX10, and SCO1—have been associated with COX-deficient Leigh syndrome or other multisystemic fatal infantile disorders in which encephalopathy is accompanied by cardiomyopathy (SCO2), nephropathy (COX10), or hepatopathy (SCO1).

This is a burgeoning field of research with important theoretical and practical implications. From an investigative standpoint, these disorders are teaching researchers much about the structural and functional complexity of the respiratory chain. At a more practical level, identification of mutations in these genes renders prenatal diagnosis available to young couples that have usually lost one or more infants to intractable diseases.

Defects of Intergenomic Signaling

As noted previously, the mtDNA is highly dependent for its proper function and replication on numerous factors encoded by nuclear genes. Mutations in these genes cause Mendelian disorders characterized by qualitative or quantitative alterations of mtDNA. Examples of qualitative alterations include autosomal dominant or autosomal recessive multiple deletions of mtDNA, usually accompanied clinically by PEO and a variety of other symptoms and signs. Two of these conditions have been characterized at the molecular level. Mutations in the gene for thymidine phosphorylase (TP) are responsible for an autosomal recessive multisystemic syndrome called MNGIE (mitochondrial neurogastrointestinal encephalomyopathy). Mutations in the gene for one isoform of the adenine nucleotide translocator (ANT1) have been identified in some, but not all, patients with autosomal dominant PEO. Interestingly, both types of mutations affect mitochondrial nucleotide pools and may have similar pathogenic mechanisms.

Examples of quantitative alterations of mtDNA include severe or partial expressions of mtDNA depletion, usually characterized clinically by congenital or childhood forms of autosomal recessively inherited myopathy or hepatopathy. The molecular basis (or bases) of mtDNA depletion remains unknown. An iatrogenic form of mtDNA depletion may follow treatment with nucleoside analogs such as zidovudine.

Indirect Causes of Respiratory Chain Dysfunction

These include mutations in nuclear genes that do not affect directly respiratory chain subunits or ancillary proteins nor mtDNA structure or copy number. For example, the function of the respiratory chain can be impaired by alterations in the lipid composition of the inner mitochondrial membrane or by defective importation of one or more subunits. The first situation is exemplified by Barth syndrome, an X-linked recessive disorder characterized by mitochondrial myopathy, cardiopathy, and leukopenia. The gene responsible for this disorder encodes a family of proteins ("tafazzins") involved in the synthesis of phospholipids, and biochemical analysis has shown altered amounts and composition of cardiolipin, the main phospholipid component of the inner mitochondrial membrane.

—Salvatore DiMauro and Eduardo Bonilla

***See also**–Mitochondrial Encephalopathy, Lactic Acidosis and Stroke (MELAS); Progressive External Ophthalmoplegia (PEO); Myopathy, Metabolic; Myopathy, Overview; Oxidative Metabolism; Respiratory Chain Disorders*

Acknowledgments

This work was supported by National Institutes of Health Grants NS11766 and P01HD32062 and by a grant from the Muscular Dystrophy Association.

Further Reading

Chinnery, P. F., and Turnbull, D. M. (2000). Mitochondrial DNA mutations in the pathogenesis of human disease. *Mol. Med. Today* 6, 425–432.

DiMauro, S. (ed.) (2000). Symposium on mitochondrial encephalomyopathies. *Brain Pathol.* 10, 419–472.

Schon, E. A. (2000). Mitochondrial genetics and disease. *Trends Biochem. Sci.* 25, 555–560.

Smeitink, J., van den Heuvel, L., and DiMauro, S. (2001). The genetics and pathology of oxidative phosphorylation. *Nat. Rev. Genet.* 2, 342–352.

Mitochondrial Encephalopathy, Lactic Acidosis, and Stroke (MELAS)

Encyclopedia of the Neurological Sciences
Copyright 2003, Elsevier Science (USA). All rights reserved.

MELAS is a mitochondrial encephalomyopathy caused by an inherited mutation in a mitochondrial gene. The classic MELAS syndrome consists of mitochondrial encephalopathy, lactic acidosis, and stroke-like episodes. Variability in the clinical and genetic features of this syndrome present many difficulties for clinicians.

CLINICAL AND LABORATORY FEATURES

Recurrent focal neurological deficits that resemble strokes are a hallmark of this disorder (Table 1). The stroke-like episodes commonly result in hemianopia, cortical visual loss, or hemiparesis. Focal or generalized seizures, dementia, short stature, recurrent headaches, or vomiting also may occur. Lactic acidosis may be present. Ragged red fibers are seen in muscle biopsies. Brain lesions usually involve the cortex and subcortical white matter. There may be low-density lesions on head computed tomography corresponding with hyperintense signal on T2-weighted magnetic resonance imaging scans. The lesions are most common in the parietal–occipital areas, but they may occur anywhere and they may not respect the boundaries of major arterial territories. Age of onset varies from infancy to late adulthood, with the average age of onset in most studies ranging from 10 years to the early 20s. The clinical course is also highly variable, ranging from asymptomatic carriers of a MELAS-associated mutation to patients with severe and progressive deficits leading to death within a few years. The progressive course generally is punctuated by acute cerebral lesions with variable resolution. Mutational burden (the percentage of mitochondrial DNA molecules that harbor a particular mutation) may be a factor in both the age of onset and the prognosis of MELAS.

GENETICS

Mitochondria, and therefore mitochondrial DNA, almost always are inherited entirely from one's mother. Therefore, like other mitochondrial genetic diseases, MELAS is inherited through the maternal lineage. Both men and women can be affected by the disease, but only women can pass it on to their offspring. At least 80% of patients with the classic MELAS phenotype have an A-to-G point mutation at nucleotide position 3243 in the mitochondrial transfer RNA-Leu(UUR) gene (the numbering is based on the originally published human mitochondrial DNA sequence; Anderson *et al.*, *Nature*, 1981). Other mutations can also present with the MELAS phenotype.

Genetic testing for MELAS is complicated by the frequency of heteroplasmy and tissue mosaicism. Heteroplasmy refers to a situation in which there is a mix of DNA species within the same tissue or within the same cells. Some mitochondrial DNA molecules harbor the mutation, whereas others do not. Since each cell can have hundreds of mitochondria, and

Table 1 CLINICAL AND LABORATORY FEATURES

Clinical features	Imaging	Laboratory features	Treatments tried (no controlled trials)
Stroke-like episodes	Parietal–occipital lesions	Lactic acidosis (blood)	Coenzyme Q10
Hemianopia	Computed tomography: low density	Ragged red fibers (muscle)	Creatine
Cortical visual loss	Magnetic resonance imaging: high T2		Dichloroacetate
Hemiparesis			Riboflavin
Seizures			Steroids
Dementia			
Myopathy			
Short stature			
Headaches			
Vomiting			
Hearing loss			
Diabetes mellitus			
Ataxia			
Dystonia			

each mitochondrion may have several copies of the genome, virtually any percentage of mitochondrial DNA may be mutant. The MELAS 3243 mutation is always heteroplasmic, presumably because a homoplasmic tRNA mutation would not be compatible with life. Mosaicism refers, in this case, to differences in the mutational burden between different tissues within an individual. Leukocytes tend to have relatively low mutational burdens, whereas the mutational burden in muscle and brain tends to be higher. Along with selective vulnerability, this helps to determine the clinical features associated with the MELAS mutation and other mitochondrial DNA mutations. Genetic background and environmental features are also likely to play important roles.

CLINICAL HETEROGENEITY

The 3243 MELAS mutation, like many mitochondrial DNA mutations, is associated with clinical heterogeneity, meaning that the clinical features associated with this mutation vary across individuals. For example, patients with the 3243 MELAS mutation have been reported to present with progressive external ophthalmoplegia, optic atrophy, sensorineural hearing loss, dystonia, or cardiomyopathy. The 3243 MELAS mutation is also found in approximately 1 to 2% of patients with non-insulin-dependent diabetes mellitus.

GENETIC HETEROGENEITY

MELAS also exhibits genetic heterogeneity, meaning that the same clinical syndrome can be associated with distinct mutations in different individuals. The classic MELAS phenotype has been reported in association with mitochondrial DNA mutations at several sites in the tRNA-Leu(UUR) gene as well as in several other mitochondrial genes (Table 2). These reports must be interpreted cautiously because the pathogenicity of the reported mutations is uncertain for several of these mutations.

DIAGNOSIS

The diagnosis of MELAS is based on the presence of typical clinical features of the disease (see Table 1). A maternal pattern of inheritance also is supportive, although this may not always be apparent due to incomplete penetrance. Investigations that may support the diagnosis include CNS imaging, blood or cerebrospinal fluid analysis for lactic acidosis, and a muscle biopsy for ragged red fibers. A definitive

Table 2 MITOCHONDRIAL DNA MUTATIONS REPORTED IN ASSOCIATION WITH CLINICAL FEATURES OF MELAS

Nucleotide position	Base pair change	Gene
1642	G to A	TRNA-Val
3243	**A to G**	**TRNA-Leu(UUR)**
3243	A to T	TRNA-Leu(UUR)
3252	A to G	TRNA-Leu(UUR)
3271	T to C	TRNA-Leu(UUR)
3291	T to C	TRNA-Leu(UUR)
3308	T to C	NDI (complex I)
8993	T to G	ATPase 6
9957	T to C	COX III (complex IV)
11084	A to G	ND4 (complex I)
13513	G to A	ND5 (complex I)
14787	CTCC deletion	Cytochrome *b*

diagnosis may be possible through genetic studies to identify the 3243 or another MELAS-associated mitochondrial DNA mutation. Blood is usually sufficient for the genetic studies, but muscle is better as the mutational burden often is higher in muscle.

PATHOPHYSIOLOGY

The precise mechanism by which the A3243G mutation causes MELAS is unknown. The A3243G mutation is associated with impaired mitochondrial protein synthesis, possibly related to impairment in the rate of synthesis of mitochondrial proteins or mistranslation of leucine residues. The result is an impairment of oxidative phosphorylation, a decreased rate of ATP production, and an increase in susceptibility to oxidative stress, which may represent common downstream mechanisms for most pathogenic mitochondrial DNA mutations.

TREATMENT

MELAS is sufficiently rare and variable in its clinical and genetic features that controlled clinical trials of therapeutic agents have not been conducted. There are anecdotal reports of treatments with dichloroacetate, riboflavin, prednisone, dexamethasone, creatine, and coenzyme Q10. Although no treatment has consistently been associated with clinical improvement, several of the anecdotal reports of coenzyme Q10 treatment, each involving a single patient, indicated clinical improvement or a slowing of deterioration. Doses of coenzyme Q10 used in these patients ranged from 90 to 300 mg per day.

—*David K. Simon*

See also—Acute Hemorrhagic Encephalopathy; Anoxic–Ischemic Encephalopathy; Charcot–Marie–Tooth Disease; Mitochondrial Encephalomyopathies, Overview; Myopathy, Metabolic; Sepsis-Associated Encephalopathy; Toxic Encephalopathy; Uremic Encephalopathy; Wernicke's Encephalopathy

Further Reading

Anderson, S., Bankier, A. T., Barrell, B. G., *et al.* (1981). Sequence and organization of the human mitochondrial genome. *Nature* 290, 457–465.

Ciafaloni, E., Ricci, E., Shanske, S., *et al.* (1992). MELAS: Clinical features, biochemistry, and molecular genetics. *Ann. Neurol.* 31, 391–398.

Fadic, R., and Johns, D. R. (1997). Treatment of the mitochondrial encephalomyopathies. In *Mitochondria and Free Radicals in Neurodegenerative Diseases* (M. F. Beal, Ed.), pp. 537–555. Wiley-Liss, New York.

Goto, Y., Nonaka, I., and Horai, S. (1990). A mutation in the tRNA(Leu) (UUR) gene associated with the MELAS subgroup of mitochondrial encephalomyopathies. *Nature* 348, 651–653.

Pavlakis, S. G., Phillips, P. C., DiMauro, S., *et al.* (1984). Mitochondrial myopathy, encephalopathy, lactic acidosis, and strokelike episodes: A distinctive clinical syndrome. *Ann. Neurol.* 16, 481–488.

Schon, E. A., Bonilla, E., and DiMauro, S. (1997). Mitochondrial DNA mutations and pathogenesis. *J. Bioenerg. Biomembr.* 29, 131–149.

Simon, D. K., and Johns, D. R. (1999). Mitochondrial disorders: Clinical and genetic features. *Annu. Rev. Med.* 50, 111–127.

Monakow, Constantin von

Encyclopedia of the Neurological Sciences
Copyright 2003, Elsevier Science (USA). All rights reserved.

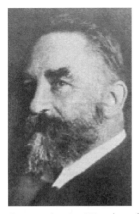

Constantin von Monakow [from W. Haymaker and F. Schiller (Eds.), *Founders of Neurology*, 2nd ed., 1997. Courtesy of Charles C. Thomas, Publisher, Ltd., Springfield, IL].

CONSTANTIN VON MONAKOW, son of a Russian nobleman and a Polish mother, was born in 1853 on the family country estate Bobretzovo, located in Vologda, just north of Moscow. His father, Iwan Monakow, was a wealthy and well-educated nobleman who served as a censor of the political press during the reigns of Nicolas I and Alexander II. The family moved to Zurich in 1867 after brief stays in Dresden and Paris. With the exception of intervals of training, Constantin was to spend the rest of his life in Zurich and regarded Switzerland as his intellectual "cradle."

Disappointing performance in his studies and unruly behavior prompted the elder Monakow to cast his contentious 17-year-old son out of the home. Young Monakow's subsequent decision, to study medicine in Zurich, was against his father's wishes. There, he fell under the influence of another very contentious individual, Eduard Hitzig, who in addition to his university post served as director of the important local psychiatric asylum. Hitzig's epochal paper on the electrical excitability of cortex had been published just 6 years earlier. His mapping of cortical motor functions by electrical stimulation helped deal a lethal blow to the "holistic" theories of brain function that had previously been ascendant.

Monakow was to tread a careful path between the holistic and localizationist theories of brain function, just as would Hughlings Jackson and others. Whether or not they might be assigned to discrete brain loci, Hitzig's belief that complex intellectual and emotional functions were proper subjects for scientific study undoubtedly profoundly inspired the young Monakow. At Hitzig's urging, Monakow visited German psychiatric asylums in order to gather such new scientific and clinical information as might prove beneficial in Zurich. He attended lectures by Westphal, Virchow, du Bois-Reymond, Oppenheim, and Munk in Berlin and visited the clinics of Meynert in Vienna.

Among the most important destinations of this tour was the Kreis-Irrenanstalt in Munich, where von Gudden introduced him to the histological methods of Reil, Hannover, Klebs, and Gerlach and the Wallerian technique of studying neurological pathways by the degeneration of fibers connected to an extirpated neurological landmark. Monakow learned the theory and application of these methods of research to neuroscience. Monakow learned the use of von Gudden's large mechanical microtome, which permitted whole brains to be sectioned. Upon his departure from

Munich, he was thus equipped with the techniques on which his life's experimental work in brain anatomy would be based.

After the completion of his medical studies, Monakow completed a voyage to Brazil as ship's doctor in order to replenish his funds. He then served as ward physician in the Psychiatric Asylum of St. Pirminsberg, located near the resort of Bad Ragaz in St. Gallen, Switzerland. Here, he independently employed Waller/Gudden techniques in order to describe for the first time the connections of occipital lobes to the lateral thalamus. In 1885, he returned to Zurich to assume a position at the Burghölzli Psychatric Asylum and a position in the Brain Anatomy Institute and the University of Zurich. Little remained of the student who had caroused late into the night. In fact, Monakow quickly joined his colleagues August Forel and Eugen Bleuler in an earnest campaign against the use of alcohol, which many in that era perceived as a vehicle of personal and social degeneration.

Monakow worked arduously in the laboratory. Critical to his success was his capacity to keep newborn rabbits alive for as much as 2 years after the surgical removal of their occipital lobes. Carl Wernicke thought that Monakow's revelations concerning the thalamocortical pathways of the visual system, published in the 1880s, were among the most noteworthy and comprehensive neuroanatomical achievements of the era. In the 1890s, Monakow achieved similarly important results in his investigation of the pathways of the auditory system. He would subsequently apply himself to the anatomical explanations for various forms of aphasia or apraxia. Having proven himself one of the most gifted neuroanatomists and conceptual neurobiologists of his age, Monakow's investigations and his deep knowledge of the entire field of neuroanatomical and neuropathological investigation permitted him to publish his landmark textbook, *Brain Pathology*, in 1897. This work contained more than 3000 references, which was highly unusual for that era, reflecting his omnivorous reading.

From his particular vantage point, one that he shared with experimental physiologists such as George Coghill and C. J. and C. L. Herrick, but few others, Monakow developed an almost unequaled appreciation for the complex interconnectedness of areas in which particular functions were housed. It was natural for him to dwell upon the manner in which these interconnections exerted modifying influences on the interpretation of sensory information and the carrying out of such responses as that information might require.

The "hard wiring" that could be demonstrated for specific tasks did not explain the use to which such tasks could be put or the influence of sensations and actions on the evolution of an individual or a species. It did not explain the complex functions of which humans were capable or the complex dysfunctions exhibited by patients who sought von Monakow's opinion at the Burghölzli. The elicitation of simple functions by electrical stimulation did not begin to address such complex issues as human unpredictability or adaptation. At the same time, it could readily be observed that functions lost apparently due to damage to discrete brain centers had a natural history that entailed variable courses of loss or recovery of function. As important, they entailed change of function, a phenomena that proved that various aspects of human behavior were variously housed, whether in discrete loci or, more likely, in some complex nexus of functional aggregates.

Monakow fostered and actively engaged in the discussions of psychiatry in a group that would come to be called the Psychiatric–Neurological Society. Together with his colleagues August Forel, Eugene Bleuler, and Carl Jung, theoretical and practical questions of neurology and psychiatry were entertained in an era that was remarkable for the epochal tensions that had been generated by the work of Sigmund Freud. It is quite clear that von Monakow viewed psychiatric and neurological questions to be one and the same, both deriving from the complex activities of brain, and that he regarded the continued integrated conceptualization of these disciplines as essential to the progress of investigation of complex brain function.

Monakow was profoundly influenced by Darwin and other contemporaries. His neuropsychiatric theories grew more complex through the first decade of the 20th century and provided a synthesis of what he found to be best in the theories of localization and those of disseminated function. To these he added the dimension that would so fundamentally alter biology and physics: time. Monakow conceived the individual mind as containing intrinsic information, to which experience made additional contributions. The intrinsic information represented the memory of the species, acquired during the course of evolution. The experience of the individual added to this store. Each addition of information, whether recorded in the experience of the species or of the individual, might modify or obscure prior knowledge. Over time, the accumulation represented adaptation, sophistication, and alternation of function, all of which would be tried against the changing circumstances of life for the individual and for the species.

The discovery of the sites within which such information might be stored and processed and the manner in which it was used were all worthy subjects for scientific investigation, as was the important question of the manner in which these various forms of information influence each other. Here was a new dimension for cerebral localization, which Monakow termed chronogenic localization. Although the substrate and process whereby such stratified individual or species memories might be laid down was not clear, the concept was pertinent to a number of pressing questions that other schools of localization had not effectively addressed.

Thus, the puzzling problem of loss of function and the subtler question of emergence of different types of function could be explained by the changes that injury produced on conglomerates of modifying influences or the emergence of more primitive functions in place of the subsequently acquired or developed functions. Higher achievements, whether of the individual or of the species, were more vulnerable and more fragile, possibly because they entailed more widespread representation. Interconnectedness was subject to the deleterious propagated effects of injury or shock and could result in temporary loss of function in uninjured regions or conglomerates distant from a given site of brain injury. This concept Monakow termed diaschisis, an intriguing explanation for the recovery of brain function after injury. The term designated different forms of physiological effect at several different levels of nervous system organization and had relevance both to nervous system development and to acute physiological function.

Monakow's theories also enabled him to retain his sense of the integral nature of psychiatry and neurology. The partly or completely hidden experiences of the early stages of development—of the individual and of the species—were in the manner of a subconscious. It does not appear that Monakow regarded these primitive memories to be as readily available for study as Freud and others suggested. He thought that they helped to form behavior and that various elements were likely to emerge in times of brain injury or other forms of stress. Monakow's theories provided intriguing explanations for such human traits as unpredictability, adaptability, and

unexpected uniformities of human behavior under various stressful circumstances, especially where these unexpected patterns of behavior were shockingly primitive.

Monakow wrote a dazzling second edition of *Brain Pathology* in 1914. Among many other important anatomical contributions in this work, he may have first characterized the classic triad of anterior choroidal artery occlusion: total hemiplegia, hemianesthesia, and hemianopia contralateral to the side of the occlusion with sparing of higher cortical functions. Hemiplegia is the most constant finding and hemianopia the most variable because the blood supply to the posterior limb of the internal capsule is from the distal geniculate body and that to the optic tract from the lateral geniculate body, and the origin of the optic radiation is more proximal along the course of the anterior choroidal artery. The triad was long designated Monakow's (or von Monakow's) syndrome, although the term has fallen into obscurity.

He published the full extent of his theories of brain localization in *Localization in the Cortex and Breakdown of Function through Cortical Lesions*. This brilliant exposition of the theory of integration of brain functions and disachisis was overshadowed by the outbreak of World War I, which had profound effects on Monakow. His resulting depression caused him to retreat into the Swiss mountains, where, as he would do each subsequent autumn of the war, he would live simply with peasants and contemplate the sudden deterioration of civilization. He abandoned a revision of *Brain Pathology*, his enthusiasm for discussion of neurological theories, and his devotion to the laboratory. He became an unexpected presence in the clinic, where he engaged in long discussions with his neurotic patients concerning their feelings and thoughts.

Monakow retired at age 75 in 1928 and died on October 19, 1930, of complications of uremia due to an enlarged prostate. He had declined medical care and died while resting in the midst of preparing a manuscript titled *The Value of Life*. His request that his spinal cord be investigated for the explanation of long-standing atrophy of his thenar eminence was neglected. His had been a highly influential career, especially insofar as he served as a bridge between the early and subsequent important traditions of brain pathology, exemplified by the link he provided between von Gudden and Kurt Goldstein and Paul Yakovlev. In addition to his fundamental contributions to the anatomy of the visual and auditory systems, his elaborate conceptions of diaschisis and chronogenic memory are fundamental to the study of the developmental aspects of brain function. His pupil, Maria Waser, portrayed his colorful life in a doting biographical novel, *Evening Encounter*.

—*Robert S. Rust*

See also–Diaschisis; Forel, August-Henri; Goldstein, Kurt; Localization; Wernicke, Carl (see Index entry Biography for complete list of biographical entries)

Further Reading

Kesselring, J. (2000). Constantin von Monakow's formative years in Pfafers. *J. Neurol.* 247, 200–205.
Koehler, P. J., and Jagella, C. (2002). Constantin von Monakow (1853–1930). *J. Neurol.* 249, 115–116.

Mononeuropathy Multiplex

MONONEUROPATHY MULTIPLEX (MM) is a type of peripheral neuropathy characterized by involvement of two or more individual nerves. MM is synonymous with multifocal mononeuropathies and is distinguished from polyneuropathy.

MM is caused by inflammation, infiltration, infarction, or physical injury to peripheral nerve at two or more anatomical sites. Among human peripheral neuropathies, MM is much less common than polyneuropathy, which diffusely affects peripheral nerve usually due to metabolic, toxic, or hereditary mechanisms. MM is often used to suggest the possibility of vasculitic neuropathy. However, although vasculitic neuropathy is the most serious disease that may be manifest as MM, many other diseases may present as MM. Compression or entrapment of nerve at two or more sites (e.g., an ulnar neuropathy at the elbow and carpal tunnel syndrome) or inflammatory demyelination at two or more sites (e.g., multifocal motor neuropathy) may be described as presenting with MM.

—*Richard K. Olney*

See also–Neuropathies, Iatrogenic; Vasculitic Neuropathy

Monro, Alexander

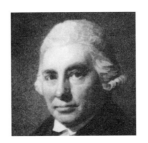

ALEXANDER MONRO (1733–1817), styled *secundus* to distinguish him both from his celebrated father and from his son, was professor of anatomy and surgery at the University of Edinburgh from 1754 to 1808. During that time, he carried on his father's tradition of charismatic teaching, anatomical and physiological investigation, and civic leadership. The three Monros played an important part in establishing the University of Edinburgh as an international center of medical education and research in the 18th century. Alexander Monro *secundus* described the foramen between the lateral and third cerebral ventricle, now known as the foramen of Monro.

Monro's paternal grandfather, John Monro, was a prominent physician and citizen of Edinburgh at the turn of the 18th century. John Monro's son, Alexander Monro *primus* (1697–1767), was professor of anatomy and surgery at the University of Edinburgh from 1719 to 1758. He studied under Cheselden in London and was a favorite of Boerhaave in Leiden. He was one of two professors who, in 1720, gave the first organized course of lectures on medicine at the University of Edinburgh. Monro *primus* was renowned for speaking extemporaneously rather than reading a prepared lecture, and his anatomy course attracted students from many nations. He was instrumental in founding the Edinburgh Royal Infirmary as a teaching hospital. Alexander Monro *primus* was an able administrator, a leading citizen in the city of Edinburgh, and a careful and imaginative anatomist.

His youngest son, Alexander *secundus*, was born in Edinburgh in 1733. He was a student in his father's anatomy class at age 11, entered the University of Edinburgh at age 12 studying a general curriculum including Latin, and became a medical student at the University of Edinburgh at age 17. His father's internationally famous anatomy class attracted an ever-increasing audience, and in 1753

Alexander *secundus* began teaching his father's evening anatomy session. This was so successful that in 1754 he was appointed joint professor of anatomy and surgery along with his father, who held the chair. He received a medical degree for a thesis on the anatomy of the testis and the nature of semen. He studied in London under William Hunter, a student and scientific adversary of Alexander *primus*. He then proceeded to Paris, and thence to Berlin and Leiden. In January 1758, he took possession of his father's chair of anatomy and surgery upon his return to the University of Edinburgh, where his lectures on anatomy, physiology, and surgery became tremendously popular. He was socially prominent and intellectually ambitious, being joint secretary of the Philosophical Society of Edinburgh with David Hume and sole secretary of this society upon its incorporation as the Royal Society of Edinburgh. Monro *secundus* seems to have had an attractive personality and was celebrated for his convivial spirit, although he wrote scathing and argumentative defenses of his priority of discovery. He retired at age 75 in 1808 and died in 1817. His son, Alexander Monro *tertius*, succeeded him as professor of anatomy at the University of Edinburgh.

The early writings of Alexander Monro *secundus* were devoted to rancorous exchanges with William Hunter and William Hewson concerning each man's claim to the priority of discovery of thoracic paracentesis and of the anatomy and physiology of the lymphatic system. His first major treatise, published in 1783, was titled *Observations on the Structure and Functions of the Nervous System*. In this work, he first described the connection between the lateral ventricle and the third ventricle and made an early observation on the partial decussation of nerve fibers in the optic chiasma. He described the association of the dorsal root ganglion with the posterior spinal root and the union of the anterior and posterior spinal roots distal to the ganglion. He also noted that if the two ends of a frog's nerve were transected and then reconnected, the two ends grow together but nerve function does not return.

In 1785, Monro *secundus* published a book on comparative anatomy that served as an aid to students of anatomy. His 1788 text on bursae contained the exceptional observation that the risk of infection in an open wound is mainly due to exposure to the air. Although he had no knowledge of microorganisms, this observation was an important innovation in the development of aseptic surgical technique. In 1793, he published *Experiments on the*

Nervous System, with Opium and Metalline Substances; Made Chiefly with the View of Determining the Nature and Effects of Animal Electricity. In this work, he demonstrated that stimulation of a nerve in a number of ways, including galvanic stimulation and mechanical irritation with a ligature, evoked a muscular contraction. This observation is not usually accorded priority for discovering electricity as the motive force in nerve conduction because he distinguished between external electrical stimulation and the energy contained within the nerve rather than seeing an identity between the two. Even so, his scientific scope and his influence on the development of scientific medicine throughout the world mark Alexander Monro *secundus* as a leading figure in 18th-century medicine.

—George K. York

See also–Galvani, Luigi (see Index entry Biography for complete list of biographical entries)

Further Reading

Guthrie, D. (1956–1957). The three Alexander Monros and the foundation of the Edinburgh Medical School. *J. R. Coll. Surgeons Edinburgh* **2**, 24–34.

Monro, A. (1783). Observations on the Structure and Functions of the Nervous System. William Creech *et al.*, Edinburgh, UK.

Monro, A. (1785). The Structure and Physiology of Fishes Explained, and Compared with Those of Man and Other Animals. C. Elliot *et al.*, Edinburgh, UK.

Monro, A. (1788). A Description of All the Bursae Mucosae of the Human Body; Their Structure Explained, and Compared with That of the Capsular Ligaments of the Points; and of Those Sacs which Line the Cavities of the Thorax and Abdomen; with Remarks on the Accidents and Diseases which Affect Those Several Sacs, and on the Operations Necessary for Their Cures. C. Elliot *et al.*, Edinburgh, UK.

Monro, A. (1793). Experiments on the Nervous System, with Opium and Metalline Substances; Made Chiefly with the View of Determining the Nature and Effects of Animal Electricity. A. Neill *et al.*, Edinburgh, UK.

Simon, S. W. (1927). The influence of the three Monros on the practice of medicine and surgery. *Ann. Med. Hist.* **9**, 244–266.

Wright-St. Clair, R. E. (1964). *Doctors Monro: A Medical Saga*. Wellcome Historical Medical Library, London.

Mood Disorders, Biology

Encyclopedia of the Neurological Sciences
Copyright 2003, Elsevier Science (USA). All rights reserved.

THE PRIMARY mood disorders (major depression and bipolar-spectrum disorders) have long been suspected to arise from abnormalities of brain biology. Biological origins are suggested by the familial nature of mood disorders and by their broad array of signs and symptoms (e.g., dramatically increased or decreased psychomotor activity, altered or impaired cognition, psychotic symptoms, and sleep and appetite changes). However, prior to the publication of the fourth edition of the *Diagnostic and Statistical Manual of Mental Disorders* (*DSM-IV*) in 1994, the term "organic mood disorder" was used only to describe mood disorders with known biological causes (e.g., depression due to hypothyroidism or amphetamine-induced mania). In contrast, major depression and bipolar disorder were viewed as "functional mood disorders," with implied origins more in the psychosocial realm than the biological. With improved understanding of the genetics and neurochemistry of primary mood disorders, and with the advent of functional brain imaging techniques, the "organic" underpinnings of the primary mood disorders are now being deciphered. It remains true, however, that in addition to biological determinants, mood disorders arise to varying degrees from psychological and social factors (e.g., a history of childhood trauma, the stress of a new job, or the death of a spouse) impacting the susceptible individual over time.

MOLECULAR GENETICS

The tendency for mood disorders to run in families could reflect genetic or environmental factors or both. Although genetic factors are implicated for both major depression and bipolar-spectrum disorders, bipolar I disorder is the most clearly genetic of the mood disorders. The rate of mood disorders (both major depression and bipolar disorder) is increased several-fold in the family members of individuals with bipolar disorder. The heritable risk for bipolar disorder is higher for genetically closer relatives. For example, the concordance rate for identical twins is several-fold higher than that for fraternal twins. Adoption studies also suggest that genetic factors largely account for the familial transmission of bipolar disorder. Nevertheless, among approximately 40% of affected identical twin pairs, only one twin has bipolar disorder. This implies that the inheritance of susceptibility gene(s) does not guarantee expression of the disease. Psychosocial and/or other environmental factors must play a role in the pathogenesis of bipolar disorder.

The patterns of inheritance for mood disorders are complex. Epidemiological studies do not support classic Mendelian recessive or dominant modes of inheritance. This makes the genetic study of mood disorders difficult. Identifying a gene for bipolar disorder, for example, is complicated by factors such as incomplete penetrance (i.e., not all genetically susceptible individuals develop the illness) and genetic heterogeneity (mutations in several different genes may produce the same or very similar clinical pictures). It is also possible that mutations in several genes are required for the disease to be expressed, making the identification of any one of them difficult. The current model is thus one in which the phenotypes of bipolar disorder and major depression each result from a combination of one or more susceptibility genes plus the influence of environmental and psychosocial factors.

Despite the genetic complexity of mood disorders, some consistent findings are beginning to emerge. Replicated genetic linkage findings suggest susceptibility genes for bipolar disorder may exist on chromosomes 18, 21, and X. Once identified, susceptibility genes will greatly enhance our understanding of the biology of mood disorders. In addition, identifying individuals at genetic risk will lead to greater understanding of the environmental and psychosocial factors that contribute to illness expression.

NEUROCHEMISTRY

It is likely that the clinical phenomena of major depression and bipolar disorder can each arise from several different abnormalities of brain biology. Thus, for example, the same cluster of signs and symptoms in a group of depressed patients may stem from several different causes, confounding efforts to identify a single pathological mechanism. Nevertheless, several consistent findings have emerged from the study of patients with major depression. Of the various neurotransmitters that may play a role in the neurochemistry of depression, the monoamines norepinephrine (NE), serotonin (5-hydroxytryptamine; 5-HT), and dopamine (DA) have been most clearly implicated. Figure 1 depicts the major noradrenergic, serotonergic, and dopaminergic neuronal pathways and the findings supporting the involvement of each neurotransmitter system in the pathophysiology of depression. In addition to the monoamines, certain neuropeptide neurotransmitters and neurotrophic factors have also been implicated in the biology of depression.

Norepinephrine

The noradrenergic system has been studied extensively and was the first to be implicated in the

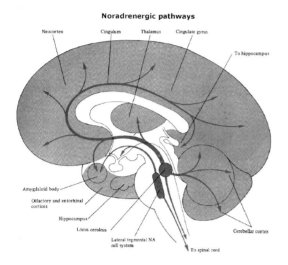

Noradrenergic pathways

Findings Implicating Noradrenergic Dysfunction In the Pathophysiology of Depression

α-methylparatyrosine, an inhibitor of tyrosine hydroxylase that depletes central NE stores, results in depression relapse in antidepressant-treated patients

Depletion of monoamine stores by reserpine results in depressive symptoms

NE reuptake inhibitors are antidepressants

Monoamine oxidase inhibitors are antidepressants

Low NE metabolites in bipolar depression

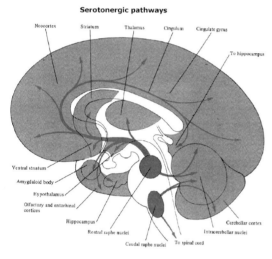

Serotonergic pathways

Findings Implicating Serotonergic Dysfunction In the Pathophysiology of Depression

Tryptophan depletion results in depression relapse in antidepressant-treated patients

Depletion of monoamine stores by reserpine results in depressive symptoms

Lithium, which enhances 5-HT release, augments antidepressant action

5-HT reuptake inhibitors are antidepressants

Monoamine oxidase inhibitors are antidepressants

Low 5-HT metabolites in CSF of patients prone to violent suicide

5-HT$_2$ receptor antagonists are antidepressants

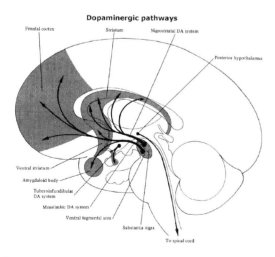

Dopaminergic pathways

Findings Implicating Dopaminergic Dysfunction In the Pathophysiology of Depression

Depletion of monoamine stores by reserpine results in depressive symptoms

Depression comorbid with Parkinson's disease

L-DOPA relieves mood symptoms in Parkinson's patients

Stimulants (which increase DA release) elevate mood

DA reuptake inhibitors are antidepressants

Monoamine oxidase inhibitors are antidepressants

Increased DA metabolites in CSF of manic patients

Typical antipsychotics (D$_2$ receptor antagonists) induce apathy, anhedonia, and avolition

Figure 1

Three lateral views of the brain showing the major noradrenergic, serotonergic, and dopaminergic neuronal pathways. Listed to the right of each view are the major findings that implicate each neurotransmitter system in the pathophysiology of depression [views of the brain are reprinted from Heimer, L. (1983). *The Human Brain and Spinal Cord*, pp. 232–234. Springer-Verlag, New York; lists of findings are adapted from Garlow *et al.*, 1999].

pathophysiology of depression. Noradrenergic neurons originate in the locus ceruleus of the brainstem and project rostrally to the cerebral cortex, limbic system, basal ganglia, hypothalamus, and thalamus and caudally to the adrenal medulla (the principal source of NE in the peripheral blood circulation). The noradrenergic system is involved in initiating and maintaining limbic and cortical arousal. The acute response to stress and novel stimuli, for example, appears to be mediated through an increase in the activity of the locus ceruleus. In contrast, vegetative functions (e.g., eating and sleeping) decrease locus ceruleus activity. Pharmacological interventions that decrease or increase central NE levels have been correlated with depression relapse or antidepressant effect, respectively (Fig. 1). For example, when remitted depressed patients are given α-methylparatyrosine (AMPT), a tyrosine hydroxylase inhibitor that depletes central NE stores, they experience a return of depressive symptoms. Interestingly, giving AMPT to depressed patients worsens the anergia and fatigue associated with depression, consistent with the role of NE in maintaining limbic and cortical arousal. Conversely, pharmacological agents that increase synaptic NE levels, such as NE reuptake inhibitors and monoamine oxidase inhibitors, are effective antidepressants. Additional evidence that noradrenergic dysfunction is involved in the pathogenesis of depression is the finding that levels of 3-methoxy-4-hydroxyphenylglycol, the principal metabolite of NE, are decreased in bipolar depression.

Serotonin

Several lines of evidence have correlated abnormalities in the serotonergic system with the depressed state and have lead to a serotonin hypothesis of depression. Serotonergic neurons have their cell bodies in the dorsal raphe nuclei of the brainstem and project to the cerebral cortex, hypothalamus, thalamus, basal ganglia, septum, and hippocampus (Fig. 1). Consistent with these diffuse neuronal projections, the serotonergic system has been implicated in a wide array of behavioral and physiological processes, including the regulation of sleep, appetite, libido, circadian rhythms, goal-directed motor activity, the inhibition of aggressive behavior, and the response to stress. As observed when central NE levels are perturbed, interventions that decrease or increase central 5-HT levels result in depression relapse or remission, respectively (Fig. 1). For example, when remitted depressed patients are placed on a diet deficient in the essential amino acid

L-tryptophan (from which 5-HT is synthesized), they experience a rapid return of depressed mood and the cognitive and neurovegetative symptoms of depression. Conversely, agents that increase synaptic 5-HT levels, such as 5-HT reuptake inhibitors and monoamine oxidase inhibitors, are effective antidepressants. Also supporting the serotonin hypothesis of depression is the finding that 5-hydroxyindoleacetic acid (5-HIAA) (a metabolite of 5-HT) is reduced in the cerebral spinal fluid (CSF) of patients who attempted or committed suicide using violent means. Reduced CSF 5-HIAA levels in these patients presumably reflect decreases in central serotonergic activity. Interestingly, there are also reports linking low CSF 5-HIAA levels with violent criminal behavior and fire setting.

Dopamine

The dopaminergic system has classically been implicated in the pathophysiology of schizophrenia, but several lines of evidence implicate it in the pathophysiology of mood disorders as well. Of the four major DA pathways (Fig. 1), the mesolimbic and mesocortical pathways are the most likely to play a role in the biology of depression. Mesolimbic neurons have their cell bodies in the ventral tegmentum and project to most limbic regions. They regulate emotional expression, learning and reinforcement, and hedonic capacity. Mesocortical neurons also originate in the ventral tegmentum and project to the orbitofrontal and prefrontal cortex. They regulate motivation, concentration, and executive cognitive functions. As observed with central NE and 5-HT level changes, perturbations that decrease or increase central DA levels tend to correlate with depression and antidepressant effect, respectively (Fig. 1). For example, patients with Parkinson's disease often have depressive symptoms that develop before or along with the motor symptoms of the disease. Moreover, treatment with L-DOPA (which is metabolized centrally to DA) has been reported to improve the depressive symptoms of Parkinson's disease in a subset of patients, even before the physical symptoms have improved. Other findings implicating DA in the biology of depression include the mood-elevating effect of stimulants (e.g., amphetamine and methylphenidate), which increase DA release, and the antidepressant effect of DA reuptake inhibitors (e.g., bupropion), which increase synaptic DA levels. Measurements of CSF levels of homovanillic acid (HVA), the major metabolite of DA, also implicate DA in the biology of depression. Changes in CSF HVA levels are presumed to reflect changes in presynaptic dopaminergic function. Several studies have found CSF HVA levels to be decreased in depressed patients and increased in agitated and manic patients. Finally, typical antipsychotics, which are antagonists at dopamine receptors, have been associated with side effects (e.g., apathy, anhedonia, and avolition) that resemble depression.

Neuropeptides

Certain neuropeptide neurotransmitters have been implicated in the pathogenesis of depression, including corticotropin-releasing factor (CRF), somatostatin, and thyroid-releasing hormone (TRH). CRF is a key regulator of the hypothalamic–pituitary–adrenal (HPA) axis and appears to coordinate the endocrine, autonomic, immune, and behavioral components of the response to stress. Levels of CRF tend to be elevated in the CSF of untreated depressed patients and then normalize after treatment with ECT or antidepressants. CRF dysregulation is also suggested by the elevated cortisol levels, the dexamethasone suppression test nonsuppression, and the stress intolerance found among patients suffering from depression. As with the elevated CSF levels of CRF, these findings also tend to normalize with effective treatment. Somatostatin, which inhibits the secretion of growth hormone and also acts centrally as a neurotransmitter, has been shown to affect sleep, eating behavior, activity, memory, and cognition. CSF levels of somatostatin are decreased in depressed patients and, as with CRF, tend to normalize with effective treatment. In addition, elevated levels of CSF somatostatin have been observed in mania. Altered CSF somatostatin is not specific to mood disorders, however. Decreased levels have been reported among patients with Alzheimer's disease, Parkinson's disease, and multiple sclerosis, and increased levels have been found among patients with meningitis, encephalitis, and head injury. Abnormalities in the hypothalamic–pituitary–thyroid (HPT) axis have also been found among depressed patients. The clinical picture of hypothyroidism, for example, can be identical to that of major depression, with depressed mood, prominent neurovegetative symptoms, and impaired cognition. However, even among depressed patients who are clinically euthyroid, subtle abnormalities in the HPT axis have been detected. CSF levels of TRH are increased in some depressed patients and 25–30% of euthyroid depressed patients do not have the expected level of increase in thyroid-stimulating hormone in response to a TRH challenge. Although these findings appear to be specific to depression, the role of HPT axis alterations in the pathophysiology of depression remains unknown.

Neurotrophic Factors

Neurotrophic factors are proteins expressed throughout the central nervous system that are involved in neuronal differentiation, development, functioning, and survival. Brain-derived neurotrophic factor (BDNF) is the most abundant and widely distributed of these factors. BDNF has been implicated in the stress response and in the action of antidepressants. It may play an important role in the pathophysiology of depression. In animal models, exposure to stress causes a rapid and long-lasting decrease of BDNF expression in the hippocampus. Treatment with glucocorticoids also causes a smaller but significant decrease in BDNF expression in the hippocampus; therefore, part of this response to stress may be mediated through adrenal steroid production. In addition, exposure to either chronic stress or glucocorticoids causes atrophy of hippocampal CA3 pyramidal neurons. This effect has been observed both in rodents exposed to physical stress and in nonhuman primates exposed to psychosocial stress. Decreased expression of BDNF may contribute to this stress-induced neuronal atrophy. A possible clinical correlate of these findings is the result of brain imaging studies showing decreased hippocampal volume among patients with either depression or post-traumatic stress disorder. This has led to the hypothesis that hippocampal atrophy, possibly resulting from decreased BDNF expression, may account for some of the emotional and cognitive deficits seen in depression. Further support for this neurotrophic hypothesis of depression is the finding that chronic antidepressant treatment increases BDNF expression in rat hippocampus and enhances the growth and survival of cortical neurons as well as 5-HT and NE neurons. Antidepressant pretreatment can prevent the decrease in BDNF that occurs in response to stress and may also prevent the stress-induced atrophy of hippocampal CA3 neurons. Finally, BDNF infusion has been found to have antidepressant-like effects in the forced swim and learned helplessness animal models of depression. Thus, greater understanding of the biology of neurotrophic factors may further our understanding of the mechanism of antidepressant action and may eventually help to explain how psychosocial stress interacts with genetic and other biological factors to produce depression in the vulnerable individual.

NEUROIMAGING

The application of structural and functional neuroimaging technology to the study of normal and pathological emotional states is providing clues to the anatomy and biology of mood disorders. Computed tomography and magnetic resonance imaging (MRI) scans provide a sensitive, noninvasive way of visualizing brain structural lesions and regional volume changes that correlate with specific mood disorders. Positron emission tomography (PET) scans and the results of other functional imaging methods provide a means for identifying specific brain regions in which changes in either metabolic activity or neurotransmitter receptor binding correlate with specific mood disorders.

Structural Lesions

The most consistent finding from structural neuroimaging studies of patients with mood disorders is the increased frequency of MRI signal hyperintensities in the deep and periventricular white matter of elderly patients with major depression. These white matter lesions appear from histopathological studies to represent the consequence of cerebrovascular disease. They are particularly common among patients who have risk factors for atherosclerosis and have their first episode of major depression in late life. In addition to late-onset depression, the MRI signal hyperintensities have been observed in some patients with bipolar disorder and are common in both multi-infarct and Alzheimer's-type dementia. The frequency of deep and periventricular white matter hyperintensities is similar among patients with dementia and age-matched depressed patients, although cortical atrophy is much more common among patients with dementia. It has been proposed that a subset of patients with late-onset depression may thus have a form of poststroke depression, in which white matter lesions have compromised neuronal pathways important to emotional processing and the maintenance of mood.

Cerebral Metabolic Changes

Functional neuroimaging of depressed patients using PET scanning has identified metabolic abnormalities within the prefrontal cortex (PFC) and related subcortical and limbic structures that appear to correlate with the depressed state. The most consistent findings seen in depressed patients are increased metabolic activity in the ventral PFC, medial orbital cortex, and amygdala and decreased metabolic activity in the dorsal PFC, particularly on the left. Effective antidepressant treatment tends to normalize metabolism in the ventral PFC and orbital cortex. It has been suggested that the increased metabolic activity seen in these regions in the depressed state reflects their role in emotional processing and/or obsessive rumination. Consistent with this hypothesis, metabolic activity in these regions also increases during experimentally induced sadness or anxiety in healthy subjects and in anxious or obsessional states in subjects with anxiety disorders. Studies of the increased metabolic activity in the amygdala have found that it correlates with the severity of depression and with the risk of relapse. During antidepressant treatment that is both effective and protects against relapse, amygdala metabolism decreases toward normal. Elevated amygdala metabolism also correlates with elevated plasma cortisol levels, suggesting that increased amygdala activity may play a role in the increase HPA axis activity seen in depression.

CONCLUSION

It is likely that the clinical phenomena of major depression and bipolar disorder can each arise from a variety of pathophysiological mechanisms. Although this diagnostic heterogeneity confounds attempts to define the biology of these disorders, progress is being made on a variety of fronts. Genetic studies are identifying patterns of inheritance and genetic linkage for bipolar disorder and will likely soon lead to the identification of susceptibility genes for this disorder. A growing understanding is emerging of the key neurotransmitter systems, neuropeptides, and neurotrophic factors implicated in the neurochemistry of depression. Neuroimaging studies are identifying the structural and functional brain abnormalities that correlate with the depressed state and are beginning to link neuroanatomical, neurochemical, and clinical insights into the biology of mood disorders. Together, all these approaches hold great promise for the rational development of more effective strategies for treating and preventing mood disorders in the future.

—*Adam Travis*

See also–Bipolar Disorder; Depression; Dopamine; Mood Disorders, Treatment; Mood Stabilizer Pharmacology; Neuropeptides, Overview; Neurotransmitters, Overview; Neurotrophins; Norepinephrine; Serotonin

Further Reading

American Psychiatric Association (1994). *Diagnostic and Statistical Manual of Mental Disorders*, 4th ed. American Psychiatric Association, Washington, DC.

Bertelsen, A., Harvald, B., and Hauge, M. A. (1977). A Danish twin study of manic–depressive disorders. *Br. J. Psychiatry* **130**, 330–351.

Drevets, W. C., Gadde, K. M., and Krishnan, K. R. R. (1999). Neuroimaging studies of mood disorders. In *Neurobiology of Mental Illness* (D. S. Charney, E. J. Nestler, and B. S. Bunney, Eds.), pp. 394–418. Oxford Univ. Press, Oxford.

Duman, R. S. (1999). The neurochemistry of mood disorders: Preclinical studies. In *Neurobiology of Mental Illness* (D. S. Charney, E. J. Nestler, and B. S. Bunney, Eds.), pp. 333–347. Oxford Univ. Press, Oxford.

Garlow, S. J., Musselman, D. L., and Nemeroff, C. B. (1999). The neurochemistry of mood disorders: Clinical studies. In *Neurobiology of Mental Illness* (D. S. Charney, E. J. Nestler, and B. S. Bunney, Eds.), pp. 348–364. Oxford Univ. Press, Oxford.

Linnoila, M., and Virkkunen, M. (1992). Aggression, suicidality and serotonin. *J. Clin. Psychiatry* **53**, 46–51.

Maes, M., and Meltzer, H. Y. (1995). The serotonin hypothesis of major depression. In *Psychopharmacology: The Fourth Generation of Progress* (F. E. Bloom and D. J. Kupfer, Eds.), pp. 933–944. Raven Press, New York.

Mendlewicz, J., and Rainer, J. D. (1977). Adoption study supporting genetic transmission in manic–depressive illness. *Nature* **268**, 326–329.

Miller, H. L., Degado, P. L., Salomon, R. M., *et al.* (1996). Effect of alpha-methyl-paratyrosine (AMPT) in drug-free depressed patients. *Neuropsychopharmacology* **14**, 151–157.

Nurnberger, J. I., Jr., Goldin, L. R., and Gershon, E. S. (1994). Genetics of psychiatric disorders. In *The Medical Basis of Psychiatry* (G. Winokur and P. J. Clayton, Eds.), pp. 459–492. Saunders, Philadelphia.

Sanders, A. R., Detera-Wadleigh, S. D., and Gershon, E. S. (1999). Molecular genetics of mood disorders. In *Neurobiology of Mental Illness* (D. S. Charney, E. J. Nestler, and B. S. Bunney, Eds.), pp. 299–316. Oxford Univ. Press, Oxford.

Siuciak, J. A., Lewis, D. R., Wiegand, S. J., *et al.* (1996). Antidepressant-like effect of brain derived neurotrophic factor (BDNF). *Pharmacol. Biochem. Behav.* **56**, 131–137.

Smith, K. A., Fairburn, G. G., and Cowen, P. J. (1997). Relapse of depression after rapid depletion of tryptophan. *Lancet* **349**, 915–919.

Mood Disorders, Treatment

Encyclopedia of the Neurological Sciences
Copyright 2003, Elsevier Science (USA). All rights reserved.

MOOD DISORDERS cause untold suffering for the afflicted and their loved ones. Societal stigma and pervasive lack of awareness of what constitutes effective treatment are major problems. Family and friends may unwittingly turn a blind eye to the illness in a misguided attempt to avoid causing their loved one feelings of shame. Many physicians fail to screen for, diagnosis, and treat depression because they harbor the erroneous belief that depression cannot be effectively treated. This entry focuses on the treatment of depression.

Treatment can be divided into three phases: acute, maintenance (remission), and relapse. Each requires a different focus. In the acute phase, the practitioner must assess the patient's safety regarding suicide and focus on developing a therapeutic relationship and a collaborative treatment plan aimed at reducing symptoms of depression. During remission, addressing risk factors for relapse is essential. This phase often focuses on developing a healthier perspective on psychologically stressful events, elaborating new patterns of thinking and behavior to replace maladaptive ones, and monitoring the medication's side effects, its therapeutic effects, and patient compliance. Treating relapse is similar to treating the acute episode but our formulation of the patient (how we understand the patient and their illness) must be reviewed and often revised. Long-term treatment is often complicated by comorbid conditions, such as substance use disorders, personality disorders, and anxiety symptoms.

Mood disorders are common and are best conceptualized as a heterogeneous set of ailments with multiple etiologies. This entry provides a conceptual framework for individuals interested in the treatment of mood disorders and for practitioners who want a broad overview to guide initial treatment of a particular patient. Clinical skills such as assessing suicidality and developing an optimal patient–doctor relationship are not discussed. This entry briefly reviews current treatment guidelines and reviews selected treatment developments.

CURRENT TREATMENT GUIDELINES

Treatment plans must be tailored to the individual patient's needs. Most treatment involves medication and psychotherapy. Antidepressants are the most commonly used medications for depression. Medications for mood stabilization are often added if patients suffer from symptoms consistent with bipolar disorder or fail to respond to antidepressants alone. Other pharmacological augmentation strategies are primarily the province of psychiatrists.

Many types of psychotherapy are used to treat depression. Proponents of specific approaches, such as Aaron Beck and followers of Gerald Klerman for cognitive and interpersonal psychotherapy, respectively, have written treatment manuals that can be purchased and used to effectively treat mood disorders. Other forms of psychotherapy, such as the psychodynamic approach, rely on different principles. These comprehensive conceptual frameworks may provide clinicians with new tools for understanding but also require that clinicians tailor treatment using detailed data to understand the patient's personality and problems. Medications and time-limited psychotherapies are easiest to study, most studied, and therefore best supported by research. Nonetheless, many people seek out and pay for other types of psychotherapy.

Pharmacological treatment for depression has changed a great deal in the past 15 years. Fluoxetine, the first of a new class of antidepressants called selective serotonin reuptake inhibitors (SSRIs), was the harbinger of a new era in treating depression. SSRIs are more tolerable and safer than the previously available agents, tricyclic antidepressants and monoamine oxidase inhibitors. Other SSRIs have also been developed, each with slightly different pharmacological properties and side effect profiles. These differences lead to differential response, with some patients responding to one SSRI and not to another. Recently, venlafaxine was developed. Venlafaxine blocks reuptake of both serotonin and noradrenaline. It works faster than SSRIs and has a similar side effect profile. Buproprion, nefazadone, and mirtazapine all have different side effect profiles from those of each other and from SSRIs. Buproprion is a complete non-SSRI. Nefazadone, although a serotonin reuptake inhibitor, also blocks serotonin 2a receptors and weakly inhibits norepinephrine reuptake. Mirtazapine, an α_2 antagonist, acts primarily at the presynaptic receptor to increase net serotonergic and noradrenergic transmission. Mirtazapine also minimizes side effects by blocking several serotonin receptors subtypes.

Most doctors initially prescribe a single agent to treat a patient's depression. Together, patient and doctor must consider which medication is most likely to work, which will cause the fewest side effects, and problems with compliance. Unfortunately, matching patients to medications is still in its infancy. If a patient or their family member has responded positively to a particular agent, then starting with that one is best. If there are no clear best choices, then discussing side effect profiles and the dosing regimens can help in choosing an antidepressant. For example, a suicidal patient who reports that sexual dysfunction would be an intolerable side effect might want to avoid SSRIs. One who reports a history of difficulty remembering to take medications might be better off avoiding agents that require more than one dose per day.

Once started on medication, patients must be titrated up to therapeutic doses and remain at those doses for at least 4 weeks in order to determine if their illness improves with that medication. Sleep and appetite usually improve first. Improved mood and relief from anhedonia occur later and may take more than 6–8 weeks. The most common errors in treating depression pharmacologically are insufficient doses for insufficient periods. Up to 70% of patients will get better from their first trial of an antidepressant. Many doctors switch to another class of agents if the patient does not benefit from the first agent despite an adequate trial (appropriate dose for appropriate time). One increases the dose if there is a partial response and no difficulty with side effects. Primary care doctors can change agents or refer patients for augmentation if they have a partial response at the maximum dose. Augmentation can be either pharmacological or psychological.

Most mental health practitioners draw on a mixture of psychotherapy techniques. Supportive therapy helps patients recognize and mobilize their available resources. Resources include relationships and coping strategies that have worked for them in the past. Cognitive therapy techniques are also popular. Most people prone to depression routinely distort their perception of the world. Thinking patterns, such as catastrophizing, can be identified and replaced by new thinking patterns, such as consciously estimating the likelihood of a catastrophic outcome. Behavioral therapy also offers easily implemented suggestions for treating depression. Planning pleasurable activities and social outings will hasten recovery from depression even if the person feels pessimistic about enjoying themselves. Interpersonal and psychodynamic therapies can help identify stressful events that contributed to the depression. Familiarity with one's liabilities can improve management of similar challenging circumstances in the future. Some studies show that manualized therapies (cognitive, behavioral, and interpersonal) are as effective as medication but require well-trained clinicians and motivated patients whose depressions are mild to moderate. Components of these manualized treatments can add to and enhance any pharmacological treatment plan.

Ideally, the patient's pharmacological and psychological treatments enhance one another. Medications usually require less motivation and are easiest to start. As the medications begin to work, psychotherapy becomes more productive because the patient can more effectively discern maladaptive patterns of behavior and thinking and can even begin applying new solutions to old problems. When the depressive symptoms remit, patients can continue to practice their new skills at combating depressive relapses. The process of acute stabilization, development of new coping skills, and consolidation of those skills usually takes longer than patients realize. The American Psychiatric Association recommends that patients continue treatment for 2 years after their first episode.

EVALUATION

A thorough initial evaluation is essential to a successful outcome. It should include all the components of the biopsychosocial framework. Even after the initial assessment, providers will continue to receive new information and will have to modify the diagnosis and treatment plan. Major depression may eventually develop into recurrent depression or bipolar disorder.

In addition to biological precipitants, one must also address psychological factors. New information leading to a change in diagnosis may also shed new light on how the patient is likely to view themselves. For example, a patient who has functioned at extremely high levels professionally while hypomanic may have unrealistic expectations of themselves. Although psychological formulation is challenging, the ramifications are important for helping the patient come to terms with their illness and improve compliance with the treatment plan.

Last, as patients recover from their mood disorder, other aspects of their personality may become apparent. In some instances, what appeared to be a personality disorder will remit. In other instances, a retarded depression will give way to a more energized state that may have many stigmata of a personality disorder. In both cases, the treatment plan needs to be adjusted. Mood disorders combined with personality disorders are more complicated to treat. Primary care doctors may want to refer such patients to psychiatrists.

Treatment should decrease suffering associated with illness. Amelioration of symptoms is often straightforward, but addressing occupational and interpersonal dysfunction is essential and may not be adequately treated by antidepressants. Quantifying improvement on a few target activities can maintain

the focus on a functional recovery providing both a sensitive metric for improvement and an early warning system for detecting relapse. Such a system can include asking the patient

1. On a scale of 1 to 10, where is your mood now?
2. What activities are important to you?
3. What would a 10 in that activity be, 10 being the best imaginable?
4. How would you recognize a low level of "1"?
5. How would rate yourself in that activity in the past week?

For somebody interested in performing arts, a 10 might be seeking out, auditioning for, and getting a desired role, and a 1 might be not even looking to see what parts are available and not attending acting classes. The scale provides a starting point for the patient's ongoing assessment of their illness and a personalized shorthand for the doctor and patient to use.

TREATMENT DEVELOPMENTS

Most people suffering from mood disorders initially seek help from their primary care physician or from a nonpsychiatrist mental health professional. Often, these frontline practitioners are the only providers of treatment. The former often relies on medication alone and the latter on counseling or psychotherapy as the sole treatment.

The dichotomization of treatment for mood disorders into mutually exclusive pharmacological or psychological categories reflects an old, flawed heuristic. Although there are important differences, psychotherapies change patients' brain chemistry just as medications do, and many patients experience pharmacotherapy as "opening up their true personality." Treatments are arbitrarily categorized as pharmacological, electrical, and psychological but are not in any way mutually exclusive. Indeed, the best treatment often employs multiple approaches.

Despite the high prevalence of depression in primary care settings, it is underaddressed. Unfortunately, the consequences of delayed treatment appear to be greater than previously thought. Even partially treated depression does not prevent a chronic deteriorating course. More aggressive approaches for acute depression appear essential. Delays stem not only from provider factors but also from patient factors. More work needs to be done to improve treatment retention rates. Innovative approaches such as medication-support groups and automated reminders are being investigated.

SELECTED REVIEW OF TREATMENT DEVELOPMENTS

The development of new antidepressant medications is continuing at an increasing pace. Snyder and Ferris suggest that a new explosion of agents is on the horizon. Each advance in our understanding of brain biochemistry and in the roles of newly discovered "neurotransmitters" suggests whole new sets of treatment possibilities. Who knows what role brain chemicals such as neuropeptides and trophic factors elaborated by glial cells will play in the future treatment of depression?

New approaches based on how they change neuro-amine levels in the synaptic cleft have been successfully developed. Investigators predicted and then went on to show clinically that the combining of norepinephrine and serotonin reuptake inhibition should cause a more rapid downregulation of β-adrenergic receptors. Fluoxetine and desipramine administered together resulted in a treatment response 1 to 1.5 weeks quicker than that of either agent alone. Manipulations in the synaptic cleft are merely one of many possible interventions in the long chain of neurophysiological events that ultimately result in remission of a mood disorder. Our ability to carefully intervene simultaneously at several points in the anabolic and catabolic pathways as well as at multiple locations on and in neurons should continue to increase.

Patient–treatment matching is improving. Gender appears to influence antidepressant response. A study comparing response to imipramine and sertraline found that men respond better to imipramine and women to sertraline and that the ratio of higher female to male responders for sertraline does not hold for postmenopausal women.

Electrical treatments may soon take their place alongside office-based pharmacological and psychological interventions. ECT is already well established, albeit not office based. Early experimental data obtained from using repetitive transcranial magnetic stimulation as a treatment for depression are promising. It could be a useful alternative after failed medication trials and before ECT because of its lower cost and benign side effect profile. Vagal nerve stimulation is another electrical treatment, and it is currently approved by the Food and Drug Administration as an "effective long-term, adjunctive treatment for partial seizures." The vagal nerve stimulator

provides access to limbic structures with known projections to several areas thought to be relevant to the pathogenesis of depression. Although more rigorous trials are essential, results from an open trial of 30 patients indicated an initial response rate of 40% and a remission rate of 17%, and the follow-up study showed that 10 of 11 responders maintained their response at 9 months and 6 of the 16 nonresponders became responders.

Pregnancy and mood disorders in women deserve special mention. One of 11 pregnant women meet research diagnostic criteria for depression. Investigators have effectively used interpersonal psychotherapy to treat postpartum depression. This offers an important alternative to medications. Many antidepressant medications (in contrast to mood stabilizers) may be as safe as other pharmacological agents identified as nonteratogens. However, one must review the current data on an agent, consider the individual case, and explain the risks and benefits of treatment options to the patient. Communication is essential, and documentation of informed consent including risks and alternatives is a must. It is important to discuss the dangers of no treatment, such as poor nutrition and the risk of self-harm and impulsive behavior. Succinctly stated by Wisner, "Depression is a disease state that affects fetal and infant health."

Other exciting developments include more sophisticated use of genetics and the potential to stimulate nerve growth in the central nervous system. Pharmacogenomics is an extension of the family history. In the near future, we may be able to screen patients' genetic material for genes that predict medication response and side effects. Cytogenesis may provide novel ways to address structural deficits, such as those associated with post-traumatic stress disorder. Neuroscience is exploding with possibilities to help people suffering from mood disorders.

—*Paul Damian Cox, Martin H. Leamon, and Catherine S. Brennan*

***See also**–Antianxiety Pharmacology; Antidepression Pharmacology; Antipsychotic Pharmacology; Bipolar Disorder; Depression; Mood Disorders, Biology; Mood Stabilizer Pharmacology; Norepinephrine; Serotonin*

Further Reading

American Psychiatric Association (2000). *American Psychiatric Association Practice Guidelines for the Treatment of Psychiatric Disorders: Compendium 2000.* American Psychiatric Association, Washington, DC.

Clark, D. A., Beck, A. T., and Alford, B. A. (1999). *Scientific Foundations of Cognitive Theory and Therapy of Depression.* Wiley, New York.

Jefferson, J. W., and Griest, J. H. (1996). In *Synopsis of Psychiatry* (R. E. Hales and S. C. Yudofsky, Eds.), 2nd ed. American Psychiatric Press, Washington, DC.

Klerman, G. L., Weissman, M. M., Chevron, E. S., *et al.* (1984). *Interpersonal Psychotherapy of Depression.* Basic Books, New York.

Stahl, S. M. (2000). *Essential Psychopharmacology, Neuroscientific Basis and Practical Applications,* 2nd ed. Cambridge Univ. Press, New York.

Wisner, K. L., Zarin, D. A., Holmboe, E. S., *et al.* (2000). Risk–benefit decision making for treatment of depression during pregnancy. *Am. J. Psychiatry* 157, 1933–1941.

Mood Stabilizer Pharmacology

Encyclopedia of the Neurological Sciences
Copyright 2003, Elsevier Science (USA). All rights reserved.

THE IDEAL MOOD STABILIZER would be an agent that is effective not only in treating mania but also in preventing depression and that continues to do so indefinitely. No current mood stabilizer fits this ideal completely, although for some patients a particular medication may be associated with remission. Currently, only four agents have a Food and Drug Administration (FDA) indication for treating mania: lithium carbonate, divalproex sodium, chlorpromazine, and olanzapine. In practice, many medications are used, often in combination. Besides lithium, the most frequently used drugs for bipolar disorder are antiepileptics and, increasingly, atypical antipsychotics.

When treating bipolar disorder, clinicians may be guided by a variety of principles. Monotherapy, although often difficult to achieve, is optimal for a variety of reasons. Patients are better able to adhere to the treatment regimen, costs are lower, and the potential for drug–drug interactions is lessened. In order to successfully employ monotherapy, health care providers must be accomplished diagnosticians since one key to providing monotherapy is to simultaneously treat comorbid conditions, such as psychosis or a comorbid anxiety disorder.

There are other important considerations. Some agents are best at targeting certain symptoms and syndromes. Some may interact with drugs taken for other medical conditions at the level at the cytochrome P450 system, causing unintended iatrogenic harm. The patients' health may dictate treatment:

Some agents are metabolized by the liver, whereas others are excreted by the kidneys. Finally, those agents that have best treated first-degree relatives may be the drugs of first choice.

LITHIUM

Lithium carbonate is perhaps the best studied mood stabilizer, shown to be effective in treating both the manic and depressive phases of illness and in maintaining a patient in long-term euthymia. Lithium is also used for treating depression, mainly as an adjunctive agent. Its mechanism of action remains unknown, and among the many theories are that lithium affects the sodium/potassium balance within the neuron, slows intracellular second messenger systems, and increases brain levels of the inhibiting neurotransmitter γ-aminobutyric acid (GABA). Lithium is excreted from the kidney and has a half-life of 24 hr. Dosing typically starts at 600–900 mg/day and can be given in a divided or single dose. Typical effective serum concentrations are 0.5–1.2 mEq/liter.

Lithium appears to work more effectively in patients with euphoric rather than mixed or dysphoric mania. In addition, the following attributes are associated with a successful course of treatment: non-rapid cycling, a lack of substance abuse, a family history of mania, and few lifetime episodes. Conversely, dysphoric, rapidly cycling mania in the presence of substance abuse predicts a poor response to lithium. Significantly, lithium is the only mood stabilizer that has been associated with a reduction in suicide risk.

Lithium toxicity is avoided by periodic serum monitoring. Serum lithium levels in excess of 1.5 mEq/ml are associated with toxicity. Lithium use has also been associated with hypothyroidism and kidney failure, and both organ systems should be routinely monitored. Routine side effects include cognitive dulling, tremor, weight gain, diarrhea, excessive urination, and acne. Lithium serum levels increase with concurrent medications that reduce its renal clearance, such as thiazide diuretics, NSAIDs, and ACE inhibitors; agents that increase its renal clearance reduce its serum levels. Examples of the latter are acetazolamide, aminophylline, theophylline, and caffeine.

ANTIEPILEPTICS

Valproate

Valproate, or divalproex sodium, is FDA approved for the treatment of acute mania, epilepsy, and migraine prophylaxis. It is also used in the prophy-lactic treatment of bipolar disorder. Its mechanism of action is unknown, but divalproex sodium use is thought to cause an increase in brain GABA through a variety of mechanisms and to block neuronal sodium channels. Sodium channel blockade appears to cause a reduction in glutamine release, an activating neurotransmitter.

Valproate has a half-life of 6–16 hr and is highly protein bound (>90%). Valproate is especially useful as a mood stabilizer because it can be delivered as a 20- to 30-mg/kg loading dose. A therapeutic window of 50–125 µg/ml is often used, but in clinical practice the patient's condition is often a better guide than serum concentration.

The more serious adverse events associated with valproate are hepatotoxicity, teratogenicity, and pancreatitis. The following common side effects are considered dose related: asthenia, gastrointestinal upset, sedation thrombocytopenia, tremor, and weight gain. Alopecia may or may not reverse with cessation of treatment, and zinc and selenium are commonly recommended as palliation. Whether women who take valproate are more likely to develop polycystic ovarian syndrome is controver-sial. Oral contraceptives suppress the development of polycystic ovaries and may mask valproate's poten-tial to cause this syndrome. Valproate is also associated with fetal neural tube defects.

Valproate is a weak inhibitor of certain P450 enzymes and, as such, medications metabolized by these enzymes will increase in the serum if coadmi-nistered, with potentially harmful consequences. These enzymes include aspirin, carbamazepine, lamotrigine, rifampin, tricyclic antidepressants, and diazepam.

Carbamazepine

Carbamazepine is widely used to treat bipolar disorder and, along with lithium and valproate, considered one of the major mood stabilizers. It is thought to provide mood stabilization by blocking sodium channels. It is also used for the acute and prophylactic treatment of bipolar disorders and as an adjunct to other mood stabilizers. Carbamazepine induces its own metabolism and, as such, has half-lives and doses that vary during the time course of treatment. Its initial half-life is 25–65 hr, but with repeated doses this decreases to 12–17 hr.

Because carbamazepine reduces its own serum concentration, dosing is typically increased over time. Initially, the drug is started at 200–400 mg/day in divided doses and often increased after 2 weeks to 1200 mg/day. The usual maintenance serum concen-tration is 8–12 µg/ml. Serious side effects include aplastic anemia and agranulocytosis (both occurring in 1/100,000 patients). Because these rates are low and the conditions reversible, some clinicians re-commend periodic white blood cell counts, whereas others counsel their patients to contact them if they develop an unusual number of infections. Another rare but serious side effect is Stevens–Johnson syndrome, a potentially lethal rash. Other side effects include sedation, lightheadedness, ataxia, blurred vision, and gastrointestinal distress.

Clinicians must be cautious when valproate is augmented with carbamazepine since valproate inhibits P450 3A4, the enzyme that metabolizes carbamazepine, but both drugs compete for the same protein binding site. Therefore, both medications increase each other's serum levels, and the principal metabolite of carbamazepine (10,11-epoxide) is elevated and can cause toxicity. Drugs that also inhibit P450 3A4 include fluoxetine, cimetidine, isoniazid, varapamil, and ketoconazole.

OTHER ANTICONVULSANTS

Lamotrigine

Lamotrigine has been the subject of several clinical trials, and its efficacy in treating mania has not been determined. However, the compound has been shown to be effective in bipolar depression, long-term prophylaxis against mania, and rapid-cycling bipolar disorder. It is thought to work as a sodium channel blocker and to inhibit the release of activating amino acids such as glutamate. In addi-tion, lamotrigine has serotonin reuptake inhibition activity. Lamotrigine has a half-life of 23–37 hr. Lamotrigine is extensively metabolized by the liver. Drugs that induce the P450 3A4 enzyme, such as carbamazepine and phenytoin, decrease lamotrigine levels; those that inhibit it, such as valproate, increase lamotrigine levels.

Serious rash, including Stevens–Johnson syn-drome, can occur in 1% of pediatric patients and 0.3% of adults. Approximately 5% of patients may experience a benign rash. The risk of rash is greatest during the first 8 weeks of treatment. The potential for rash is reduced by slow upward titration, usually 25 mg/day for 2 weeks and gradually increasing by 25- to 50-mg increments each week. The typical effective maintenance dose is 200–500 mg/day in divided doses. When lamotrigine is added to a drug that inhibits P450 3A4, such as valproate, the dose is reduced by half. More common side effects include dizziness, visual problems, ataxia, and nausea, especially early in the course of treatment.

Gabapentin

Gabapentin is an unusual compound in many ways. Although structurally similar to GABA, it does not interact with GABA receptors and its mechanism of action in treating mood disorders is unknown. Nevertheless, central nervous system GABA levels increase in a dose-dependent fashion with gabapentin use. As might be expected from a compound that increases brain GABA, gabapentin also appears to have anxiolytic qualities. Although gabapentin has become widely used, it has not been shown to be effective in the treatment of acute mania, either in monotherapy or as an adjunct. Gabapentin has a serum half-life of 5–7 hr and is entirely excreted by the kidneys. Side effects include somnolence, ataxia, fatigue, nystagmus, nausea, and, over time, weight gain. Dosing begins at 300 mg/day in divided doses to minimize these side effects, and it can be increased to 3600 mg/day or more as tolerated.

Topiramate

Topiramate is another antiepileptic agent that shows promise in treating bipolar disorder. The drug has been shown to be useful in several open-case series and is the subject of clinical trials. Topiramate is notable because it is associated with weight loss (an average of 7 kg in one study). Topiramate's antimanic activity is also thought to be related to sodium channel blockade. Topiramate has a half-life of 21 hr and is weakly protein bound; it is mainly excreted by the kidney. Dosing is started slowly at 25 mg/day and increased to a maintenance level of 50–400 mg. In addition to weight loss, other side effects include sedation, confusion, cognitive dysfunction, paresthesias, and renal calculi.

Oxcarbazepine

Oxcarbazepine is an antiepileptic agent with a molecular structure nearly identical to that of carbamazepine. However, oxcarbazepine does not undergo autoinduction. Its mechanism of action is also thought to be due to sodium channel blockade. Oxcarbazepine is FDA indicated for the treatment of epilepsy, but it is increasingly used to treat bipolar disorder. Oxcarbazepine has a half-life of 2 hr, and its principal active metabolite has a half-life of 9 hr. Dosing begins at 300 mg/day in divided doses and increases by 300–600 mg/day each week. In general, 1 mg of carbamazepine is equivalent in potency to 1.5 mg of oxcarbazepine. More frequent side effects include dizziness, sedation, blurred vision, and gastrointestinal distress. Hyponatremia, defined as serum sodium < 125 mmol/liter, can occur in 2.5% of patients.

ANTIPSYCHOTICS

Neuroleptics have been a mainstay of acute mania treatment for 30 years. Chlorpromazine, the only neuroleptic FDA approved for the treatment of mania, is no longer widely used for its acute treatment or maintenance. However, high-potency neuroleptics such as haloperidol are frequently used for acute management, particularly because they can be given intramuscularly. Atypical antipsychotics are increasingly used for the treatment of bipolar disorder and offer the opportunity for monotherapy in patients with bipolar disorder with psychosis.

Atypical Antipsycotics

Although olanzapine is currently the only atypical antipsychotic drug to be FDA approved for the treatment of bipolar disorder, every atypical antipsychotic available in the United States has demonstrated some antimanic activity: clozaril, risperidone, quetiapine, and ziprasidone. The atypical antipsychotics' mechanism of action is unknown but is thought to involve a relation, as yet poorly understood, between their ability to block the serotonin 5-HT_2 receptors more effectively than the dopamine D_2 receptor. This also confers on them a measure of antidepressant activity lacking in the neuroleptics. Atypical antipsychotics are also far less likely than the older antipsychotics to cause tardive dyskinesia. This is of particular importance since this movement disorder is thought to occur more frequently among people with mood disorders treated with antipsychotics.

Several large clinical trials have demonstrated the efficacy of olanzapine in both acute treatment and prophylaxis against mania. Doses are usually approximately 15 mg/day. Case series have suggested that olanzapine may be started at higher doses (e.g., 40 mg/day) to effect sedation acutely and then reduced to typical doses as needed. Common adverse effects include somnolence, dry mouth, dizziness, weight gain, and weakness. The weight gain associated with olanzapine has been linked in some case series with higher rates of new-onset diabetes. An evolving clinical practice is to obtain periodic serum glucose levels.

CONCLUSION

Bipolar disorder is difficult to treat. The illness manifests itself in many ways, and no single agent is reliably effective for any given patient; as for recurrent depression, patients must take medication for an extended period, perhaps for life. In addition, numerous factors particular to the illness impede the patients' ability to take a mood stabilizer: the concentration difficulties inherent in the illness, an unwillingness to take medication during a manic episode, and family and friends who may be exhausted by the patient's illness and no longer able to provide support.

Certainly, the current pharmacological treatment of bipolar disorder is increasingly promising. A wide array of compounds have been put into use in a few short years, and it is hoped that the field of FDA-approved mood stabilizers will rapidly expand from the current four. Being able to offer patients and their health care providers a greater number of choices will no doubt increase the likelihood of treatment adherence and success.

—Mark H. Townsend

See also–Antianxiety Pharmacology; Antidepression Pharmacology; Antipsychotic Pharmacology; Antiepileptic Drugs; Bipolar Disorder; Depression; Lithium Carbonate; Mania; Mood Disorders, Biology; Mood Disorders, Treatment; Paranoia

Further Reading

Bloom, F. E., and Kupfer, D. J. (Eds.) (1995). *Psychopharmacology: The Fourth Generation of Progress.* Raven Press, New York.
Bowden, C. L. (1995). Treatment of bipolar disorder. In *The American Psychiatric Press Textbook of Psychopharmacology* (A. F. Schatzberg and C. B. Nemeroff, Eds.). American Psychiatric Press, Washington, DC.
Manji, K. M., Bowden, C. L., and Belmaker, R. H. (Eds.) (2000). *Bipolar Medications: Mechanisms of Action.* American Psychiatric Press, Washington, DC.
Stahl, S. M. (2000). *Essential Psychopharmacology of Depression and Bipolar Disorder.* Cambridge Univ. Press, Cambridge, UK.
Tohen, M., Sanger, T. M., McElroy, S. L., *et al.* (1999). Olanzapine versus placebo in the treatment of acute mania. *Am. J. Psychiatry* **156**, 702–709.

Moro Reflex

Encyclopedia of the Neurological Sciences

THE MORO REFLEX is a normal developmental or primitive reflex best elicited by raising the head of a supine infant approximately 30° from the cot and then suddenly dropping it to the level surface while supporting it with the examiner's hand to avoid impact. The hands are opened and the arms are briskly extended and abducted, followed by flexion (embracing response), adduction, and hand closure. This primitive reflex is generally symmetric, but in cases of asymmetry one must consider the possibility of a fractured clavicle, brachial plexus palsy, or hemiparesis.

The reflex is fragmentary at 24 weeks of gestation and well developed at 28 weeks, but it is not fully developed until 38 weeks. In normal infants, it will gradually disappear by the age of 3–5 months. It may persist in infants with chronic, nonprogressive motor disabilities of cerebral origin (static encephalopathies).

—Bruce Berg

See also–Anencephaly; Brain Development, Normal Postnatal; Grasp Reflex

Further Reading

Paine, R. S., Brazelton, T. B., and Donovan, D. E. (1964). Evolution of postural reflexes in normal infants and in the presence of chronic brain syndromes. *Neurology* **14**, 1036–1048.
Prechtl, H. F. R., and Beintema, D. (1964). *The Neurological Examination of the Full-Term Newborn Infant.* Heinemann, London.
Saint-Anne Dargiessies, S. (1977). *Neurological Development in the Full-Term and Premature Neonate.* Excerpta Medica, New York.

Motion and Spatial Perception

Encyclopedia of the Neurological Sciences

WHILE MANY INSECTS have retinal-based mechanisms for motion perception, primates have evolved a sophisticated network of cortical and subcortical processes for visual motion analysis. Motion information can serve many purposes. An obvious one is the analysis of the trajectory of a moving object.

Also, the pattern of motion of large stationary portions of the environment during the movement of the observer, called optic flow, is a potent source of information about self-motion and the direction of heading. Differences in motion of near and far objects as an observer moves sideways are important monocular depth cues called motion parallax. Motion can also provide data about object form, a point of interaction between the different spatial and form pathways in visual cortex. The boundaries and surfaces of a moving object can be revealed through differences in the patterns of motion of the object versus its background. The different patterns of motion of different surfaces of an object as either the object or the observer move provide vivid cues to its three-dimensional structure.

A large portion of naturally encountered motion signals can be considered as positional changes of luminant patterns across space and time. These spatiotemporal gradients are potentially subject to Fourier analysis and are termed first-order motion. However, movement of stimuli other than luminant edges can also be detected, including texture, flicker, stereodisparity, and color. These non-Fourier motions are variously labeled as second- or even third-order motion. At least some of them, such as color, appear to depend on an attention-based motion system that relies on positional rather than velocity information and may use different cortical networks than that used for luminance-based motion perception.

At a retinal level, some have referred to the magnocellular (M) stream as a motion pathway. M retinal ganglion cells give transient responses to the onset and offset of a luminant stimulus and have large axons with rapid conduction times—properties thought advantageous for detecting a motion signal. Indeed, lesions of the M layers of the lateral geniculate nucleus (LGN) in monkeys have a profound effect on the motion responses of the middle temporal (MT) area, whereas lesions of the P (parvocellular) layer have little effect. However, a few MT neurons do have significant P system input. In monkeys the M system terminates in the C-alpha part of layer IV in striate cortex, which in turn has a dominant projection to layer IVB and then to the thick stripes of V2. Neurons with responses selective for motion direction are first encountered in striate cortex.

V5, also known as MT, is the main extrastriate region with predominantly motion-selective responses. Its neurons are selective for both the direction and the speed of moving signals. Adjacent to MT is another region, V5a or MST (medial superior temporal area), which has more complex motion responses. The ventral portion of MST may have specific responses to a target moving against a background, whereas the dorsal portion of MST prefers large optic flow patterns that are generated by observer motion through the environment. In humans, functional imaging also shows optic flow-related signals in medial parieto-occipital cortex, and responses to motion-defined contours (kinetic boundaries) in a region called KO, which is between V5 in the lateral occipitotemporal region and V1 at the occipital pole. These motion-defined boundaries can be utilized by the inferotemporal cortex in form perception. Another point of convergence between form and motion lies in the anterior superior temporal polysensory area, which has responses selective for complex body motions, such as hand actions and gait.

In addition to this cortical network, motion-selective regions in the brainstem exist. These have been especially well studied in the rabbit. The nucleus of the optic tract and the accessory optic system in the midbrain have selective optic flow responses that are aligned along the axes of the semicircular canals and project to brainstem regions involved in generating optokinetic responses. They thus provide a visual supplement to vestibular information about head motion. The degree to which these brainstem regions are superseded in humans by cortical areas such as MST is not clear.

Tests of motion perception involve complex computerized animation sequences. These can be designed to test almost any aspect of motion perception, including global signal averaging, motion segmentation, form from motion, speed or direction discrimination, heading judgments, and attention-based motion perception. Detailed anatomical information about these from human lesion studies is only beginning to emerge.

Some data support a relatively greater impact of glaucoma on retinal ganglion cells of the M system. In keeping with this, several studies have found subclinical impairments of motion perception in primary open-angle glaucoma. This does not appear to have any bearing on the functioning of the patient, and its sensitivity as an index of disease status is being investigated.

Studies of patient series have shown that motion perception is impaired by lesions of lateral occipitotemporal cortex, near the junction of Brodmann areas 19 and 37. This location is more ventral than the location of V5 in monkeys, but it accords with functional imaging studies of motion perception in humans. Unilateral lesions of this region do not cause symptoms and do not impair the perception of coherent first-order motion. Rather, impairments are found with more complex analyses, such as the perception of second-order motion and global first-order motion averaging from a noisy signal. This too is consistent with the data from monkeys. Lesions that impair the analyses of first-order and second-order motion information overlap each other. Bilateral lesions are rare, but two such cases have shown significant symptoms and more profound defects on motion tests. Attention-based motion perception is disrupted more by lateral parietal lesions than by lateral occipitotemporal lesions.

SPACE PERCEPTION

Space and time are the fundamental dimensions of vision, and coding of this information is integral to a variety of visual processes. For example, changes in spatial position over time constitute motion, which has an elaborate processing network as described previously. Likewise, the spatial arrangement of luminant, texture, and color patterns is a key component of form perception in both two and three dimensions. However, once visuospatial data have been analyzed to generate static or moving forms, objects, and backgrounds, information about the spatial location of these items with respect to the observer is another vital aspect of the visual percept. Furthermore, it provides key input to systems involved in preparing and guiding ocular motor, manual, and other actions in response to the environment. These include reaching movements and saccades.

Visual localization in two dimensions is present at virtually every anatomical level. The retina is a "place code" for vision in that the location of light-induced activity on the retinal map indicates the position of the light in space. (Contrast this with hearing, where the location of sound-induced activity in the cochlea indicates frequency, not spatial location.) This retinotopic coding of visual information is preserved in transmission through the retinal ganglion cells, optic radiations, and striate cortex. The system is characterized by greater emphasis on central vision (cortical magnification factor), with an inverse nonlinear correlation of spatial resolution and spatial accuracy with retinal eccentricity. Although still present in early extrastriate regions such as V2–V5, retinotopic location tends to become coarser at more specialized cortical levels. Neurons

develop very large receptive fields and many cells develop specific responses to complex stimuli that are location invariant. This is found in the object-processing regions of inferotemporal cortex and the optic flow processing portion of area MST.

In monkeys, area 7a of the parietal lobe has been considered a "command area" for the preparation of visually guided responses. Within the inferior parietal lobe there are important functional subregions that use visual location data in sensorimotor transformations. The lateral intraparietal area is involved in saccadic targeting, and the adjacent parietal reach area performs a similar function for manual reaching movements. These areas project to frontal motor cortices and subcortical regions involved in motor programming, many of which eventually code the motor response as a vector in space.

In addition to the vertical and horizontal dimensions of a visual scene, there is the third dimension of depth, or distance away from the observer. Stereopsis refers to the cues about relative distance of an object given by the disparity in the location of its images on the two retinas (only if the object is at the same distance as the location of current fixation is there no sense of disparity; this region is known as Panum's plane). However, stereopsis is only one cue to depth perception. Monocular cues also exist. With distance, objects become smaller and decrease in saturation: Our innate sense of these rules is exploited in some classic visual illusions. Also, the patterns of visual motion as the observer shifts his or her head slightly to the side provide vivid depth cues known as motion parallax. Motion parallax is also evident when looking out the window of a moving vehicle: Objects in the foreground move by at a much faster rate than objects in the distance.

There are some anatomical data regarding stereopsis but little concerning the representation of monocular depth cues. Regions with neurons selective to stereodisparity are found mainly in the dorsal pathway, such as area MT. Whether this information in MT is used to code for depth or simply to assist the grouping and segmentation of motion signals is not clear.

Spatial defects in vision exist at every level. The effects of retinal, optic nerve, optic radiation, and striate damage are typified by visual field defects, in which all or nearly all visual data are lost from a specific retinotopic location in the visual map. It is possible that some spatial localization may be spared with striate lesions because of surviving projections either to the superior colliculus, which also has a retinotopic map for location in two dimensions, or to extrastriate visual cortex. However, although these are spatial defects in perception, they are not truly defects in spatial perception. In humans, the latter have generally been described under the rubric of Bálint's syndrome.

Bálint's syndrome consists of a loosely associated triad of visuospatial dysfunctions, which are traditionally considered to be simultanagnosia, optic ataxia, and ocular motor apraxia. Patients with simultanagnosia can identify single objects but cannot identify multiple items or describe their relation to each other coherently. It is considered a problem of spatially distributing visual attention. The "cookie theft picture" of the Boston Diagnostic Aphasia Examination battery is typical of a test picture for simultanagnosia. Impaired judgment of object location in three dimensions has been called visual disorientation and likely contributes to optic ataxia, which is defective reaching under visual guidance despite normal strength and position sense. Misreaching may represent failure of a multimodal rather than just a visual targeting mechanism since some patients cannot touch parts of their own body accurately. Acquired ocular motor apraxia is difficulty in initiating saccades to visual targets, particularly to command, although some patients can make saccades reflexively to a suddenly appearing object or sound. Saccades may also be very inaccurate, with the eyes performing a wandering series of saccades searching for the target. Not all elements of Bálint's syndrome are present in a given patient, indicating that although closely situated, the anatomical substrates for manual targeting, saccadic targeting, and spatial attention are distinct from each other. Most patients with Bálint's syndrome have bilateral parietal lesions, and some have additional bifrontal pathology.

The perception of depth has been seldom tested in patients with Bálint's syndrome. However, there have been a few reports of astereopsis, the loss of stereoscopic depth perception, in patients with bilateral occipitoparietal lesions and similar but milder deficits in some patients with unilateral lesions. Tests of stereopsis require special cards in which the two eyes see images of the same object from slightly different viewpoints, with the different images segregated to each eye by means of glasses with lenses polarized or colored differently for each eye. Most eye clinics have examples of these at hand, such as the Titmus Fly test.

A different deficit of spatial perception may cause some forms of topographagnosia, the failure to recognize and navigate through familiar surroundings. One type of topographagnosia is associated with prosopagnosia and achromatopsia and represents the inability to identify familiar landmarks and buildings. The demarcation by functional imaging of a parahippocampal place area near the fusiform face area provides anatomical support for this conclusion. A second type, however, may be due to disruption of the spatial processing needed to describe, follow, or memorize routes, usually described with right parietotemporal lesions.

—*Jason J. S. Barton*

See also–Balint's Syndrome; Memory, Spatial; Occipital Lobe; Perception and Perceptual Disorders; Perceptual-Motor Integration; Retina; Vision, Color and Form; Visual Fields; Visual System, Central

Further Reading

Farah, M. (1990). *Visual Agnosia*. MIT Press, Cambridge, MA.

Hécaen, H., and de Ajuriaguerra, J. (1954). Bálint's syndrome (psychic paralysis of visual fixation) and its minor forms. *Brain* 77, 373–400.

Husain, M., and Stein, J. (1988). Rezsö Bálint and his most celebrated case. *Arch. Neurol.* 45, 89–93.

Luria, A. R. (1959). Disorders of simultaneous perception in a case of bilateral occipito-parietal brain injury. *Brain* 82, 437–449.

McCarthy, R., Evans, J., and Hodges, J. (1996). Topographic amnesia: Spatial memory disorder, perceptual dysfunction, or category specific semantic memory impairment? *J. Neurol. Neurosurg. Psychiatry* 60, 318–325.

Rizzo, M. (1993). Bálint's syndrome and associated visuospatial disorders. In *Bailliere's International Practice and Research* (C. Kennard, Ed.), pp. 413–437. Saunders, Philadelphia.

Rizzo, M., and Barton, J. J. S. (1998). Central disorders of visual function. In *Walsh and Hoyt's Neuro-Ophthalmology* (N. R. Miller and N. J. Newman, Eds.), 5th ed., pp. 387–483. Williams & Wilkins, Baltimore.

Sekuler, R., Anstis, S., Braddick, O., *et al.* (1990). The perception of motion. In *Visual Perception: The Neurophysiological Foundations* (L. Spillman and J. S. Werner, Eds.), pp. 205–230. Academic Press, London.

Tootell, R., and Taylor, J. (1995). Anatomical evidence for MT and additional cortical visual areas in humans. *Cereb. Cortex* 5, 39–55.

Ungerleider, L., and Mishkin, M. (1982). Two cortical visual systems. In *The Analysis of Visual Behaviour* (D. J. Ingle, R. J. W. Mansfield, and M. S. Goodale, Eds.), pp. 549–586. MIT Press, Cambridge, MA.

Vaina, L. (1998). Complex motion perception and its deficits. *Curr. Opin. Neurobiol.* 8, 494–502.

Zeki, S. (1991). Cerebral akinetopsia (visual motion blindness). A review. *Brain* 114, 811–824.

Zihl, J., von Cramon, D., and Mai, N. (1983). Selective disturbance of movement vision after bilateral brain damage. *Brain* 106, 313–340.

Motor Control, Peripheral

IN A NORMAL HUMAN skeletal muscle, the individual muscle fiber components are organized into functional groups called motor units. The term motor unit was first used by Liddell and Sherrington in 1929 and refers to a single alpha motor neuron and the muscle fibers it innervates by way of its motor axon (Fig. 1). Alpha motor neurons are the most common among a population of motor neurons in the anterior gray matter of the spinal cord, and they are the principal neurons innervating muscle fibers (the muscle fibers that move joints, also called extrafusal muscle fibers). Medium- (beta) and small-sized (gamma) motor neurons also innervate muscle, but the latter supply specialized muscle fibers, so-called intrafusal fibers, that are found in tiny structures called muscle spindles whose function is to regulate muscle tone and reflex activity. One alpha motor neuron innervates multiple muscle fibers, but each muscle fiber is innervated by only one motor neuron. The average number of muscle fibers in a motor unit determines the innervation ratio (muscle fibers per motor neuron) of the muscle. This ratio varies greatly from one muscle to another and is related to the degree of dexterity required of that muscle. For instance, the external ocular muscles requiring very fine motor control have an innervation ratio of 10:1; the ratio for a small hand muscle is approximately 100:1. In muscles in which precise control is not needed, the ratios are higher: The ratio for a muscle in the upper arm (biceps) is 500:1,

whereas in a leg muscle (gastrocnemius) the ratio is 2000:1.

The muscle fibers belonging to a single motor unit are not grouped together but rather are dispersed over a limited area in the skeletal muscle. This area is known as the motor unit territory and in the biceps, for example, reaches a span of $20\,\mathrm{mm}^2$. This overlapping arrangement of the territories of many motor units within a muscle allows the muscle to contract smoothly and evenly.

HISTOLOGY AND CONNECTIONS OF THE PERIPHERAL NERVOUS SYSTEM

Alpha Motor Neurons

As noted previously, motor axons are extensions of alpha motor neurons that reside in the anterior horn gray matter of the spinal cord. These anterior horn cells are clustered in nuclei or motor neuron pools, forming longitudinal columns extending from one to four spinal segments. Alpha motor neurons are influenced directly by motor neuron projections from the motor cortex via descending corticospinal fibers and by spinal interneurons. (In an analogous fashion, brainstem motor neurons are influenced by projections from the motor cortex via descending corticobulbar fibers and by brainstem interneurons.) Accordingly, alpha motor neurons are the lowest in the hierarchy of motor control and are thereby designated lower motor neurons.

The alpha motor neuron is among the largest in the nervous system. It has a single axon extending to its innervated muscle fibers and a number of large dendrites that sometimes are more than 1 mm in width and extend well into the white matter of the spinal cord, providing an extensive receptive field. Many synaptic endings or boutons (approximately 10,000) contact the dendritic surface (Fig. 2). Excitatory inputs are located at the proximal portion of the dendrites or at the cell body or soma; inhibitory synapses are found along the proximal portion of the axon. Acetylcholine is the excitatory transmitter released by the alpha motor neuron's axon at the junction between the nerve terminal and the muscle fiber (neuromuscular junction).

The anterior horn cell determines the characteristic physiology of muscle contraction in the motor unit and the biochemical characteristics of muscle fibers belonging to that motor unit. Functionally, there are three types of motor units: slow fatigable, fast fatigable, and intermediate. Proximal

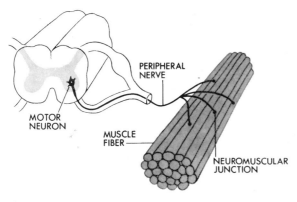

Figure 1
The motor unit. Note the motor neuron, its axon, and the many muscle fibers that are innervated by it [reproduced with permission from Layzer, R. (1975). *Primary Care* **2**, 235].

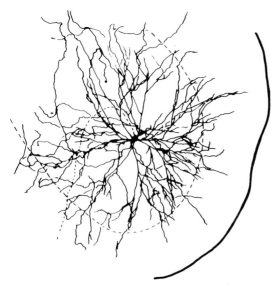

Figure 2
Alpha motor neuron. This is a transverse section of the spinal cord showing the extensive dendritic system, some of which extends into the white matter. The thick dotted line indicates an axon arising from the cell body. A gray and white matter junction is shown by the thin dashed line [reproduced with permission from Brown, A. G. (1981). *Organization in the Spinal Cord*, p. 199. Springer-Verlag, Berlin].

and axial muscles that sustain posture contain predominantly slow-twitch, nonfatigable motor units. Their slow-twitch, fatigue-resistant muscle fibers are known as type 1 fibers. Due to a high concentration of myoglobin, these fibers appear red (in animals); such muscle fibers are rich in oxidative enzymes and poor in glycolytic enzyme activity. Extremity muscles involved in fast phasic or ballistic contractions that generate large forces quickly possess mainly fast fatigable motor units. Their fast fatigable muscle fibers are known as type 2 fibers. They are low in myoglobin and appear white (in animals); such muscle fibers have abundant glycolytic enzyme activity but little oxidative enzyme activity. With a specific histochemical stain, myosin ATPase (at pH 9.4), these muscle fibers may be visualized using light microscopy (Fig. 3): Type 1 stain darkly and type 2 appear dark. Finally, type 2a fibers belong to the intermediate motor units. These muscle fibers are more aerobic and have more oxidative enzyme activity than type 2 fibers; they are therefore relatively fatigue resistant compared to type 2 fibers. Although individual animal muscles may be composed of a single fiber type, each human muscle contains a random arrangement of these fiber types.

Motor Axon and Neuromuscular Junction

The motor axons of the motor unit are heavily myelinated. As a myelinated motor fiber enters a muscle, it breaks into a number of solitary branches that lose their myelin sheaths. Each branch ends as a naked axon, expanded slightly at its terminal portion that comes to lie in a groove on the surface of a muscle fiber (Fig. 4). The axon terminal–muscle fiber association is known as the neuromuscular junction. The plasma membrane of the axon is separated from the plasma membrane of the muscle fiber by 20–50 nm. Thus, the neuromuscular junction consists of pre- and postsynaptic components. Within the former, the axon terminal, there are abundant vesicles and mitochondria. The vesicles, filled with molecules of acetylcholine (ACh), congregate at the presynaptic membrane around structures called dense bars corresponding in their placement to junctional peaks of the postsynaptic membrane. The postsynaptic membrane is highly folded, with ACh receptors concentrated at the peaks. The sarcoplasm immediately beneath the membrane is filled with numerous mitochondria. Acetylcholine esterase, an enzyme that degrades ACh and thereby terminates its physiological action, is present in the gap between axon and muscle fiber.

Muscle Fibers

Muscle fibers in adults are approximately 50 μm in diameter. They are polygonal in shape and are bundled into fascicles (Fig. 5). Individual fibers are invested by connective tissue, which forms the boundary of the endomysial compartment, and are

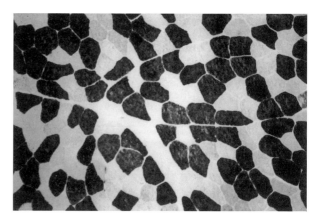

Figure 3
Normal muscle cross section stained with myosin ATPase (pH 9.4) demonstrating the normal arrangement of light (type 1) and dark (type 2) fibers.

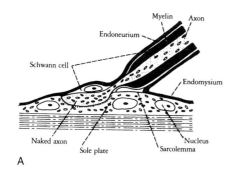

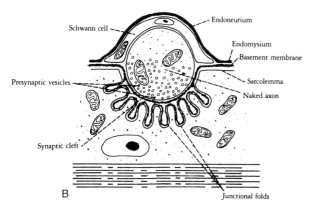

Figure 4
(A) A skeletal muscle neuromuscular junction. (B) Enlarged view
of muscle fiber showing the terminal axon lying in the surface
groove of muscle fiber (reproduced with permission from Snell,
1992, p. 135).

bordered by capillaries. Denser perimysial connective
tissue and blood vessels separate fascicles. Groups of
fascicles are surrounded by adipose tissue, blood
vessels, and loose connective tissue forming the
epimysium. Nuclei number in the hundreds per
muscle cell and are positioned eccentrically. Satellite
cells capable of aiding in regeneration are also
present at the periphery of the cell beneath the
basement membrane. The cytoplasm or sarcoplasm
contains the contractile apparatus, lipid and glycogen stores, and organelles such as mitochondria.

Each fascicle contains approximately 20–60 muscle
fibers and each muscle fiber consists of 50–100
myofibrils (Fig. 6). Each myofibril is longitudinally
divided into sarcomeres, which are the smallest
contractile units (Fig. 7). The sarcomere is that
portion of the myofibril that extends from Z band
to Z band. The sarcomere consists of two filaments—
thick (myosin) filaments alternating with thin (actin)
filaments. The four major contractile proteins that are
present in a myofilament are actin, myosin, troponin,
and tropomyosin. Within the sarcomere, thick

myosin alternates with thin actin filaments. Thin
filaments attach at the Z band and form the I (lighter
or isotropic) band. The thick filaments are located
within the A (darker or anisotropic) band, and thin
filaments also extend into this region except at the H
zone, where there is no overlap of thick and thin
filaments. The transverse or T tubules are located
near the junction of the A and I bands and transmit
the initial depolarization at the motor end plate
(Fig. 8). On either side of the T tubule is a terminal
cistern of the sarcoplasmic reticulum. The terminal
cisterns act as the storage space for calcium ions. This
sarcoplasmic reticulum–T tubule–sarcoplasmic reticulum complex is called the triad and is responsible
for converting electrical signals (membrane action
potentials) to chemical signals (calcium release).

Gamma Motor Neurons and Intrafusal Muscle Fibers

Among the motor axons contained in peripheral
nerve are those derived from the gamma motor
neurons, also known as fusimotor neurons, and they
constitute up to one-third of the lower motor
neurons of the spinal cord. These fusimotor neurons
innervate the intrafusal muscle fibers by way of
thinly myelinated axons. Intrafusal muscle fibers are
contained within muscle spindles, which are structures that are 1–4 mm in length and surrounded by a
fusiform capsule of connective tissue. Approximately
6–14 intrafusal muscle fibers reside inside this

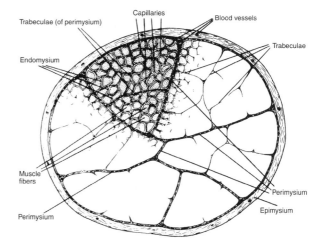

Figure 5
Schematic diagram of the connective tissue sheaths of muscle.
Muscle fibers are bundled into fascicles bordered by perimysial
connective tissue [reproduced with permission from DeGirolami,
U., and Smith, T. W. (1982). Pathology of skeletal muscle. *Am. J.
Pathol.* 107, 235–276].

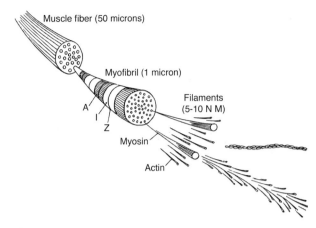

Figure 6
Ultrastructure of muscle fiber. Each fiber is made up of many myofibrils containing filaments of actin and myosin organized in bands A, I, and Z. NM, nanometers (reproduced with permission from Westmoreland *et al.*, 1994).

capsule. (Muscle fibers discussed previously that are innervated by alpha motor neurons are termed extrafusal because they are situated outside the muscle spindles.) Muscle spindles are numerous in any given muscle but are especially abundant toward the tendinous attachment of the muscle (Fig. 9). Intrafusal fibers are of two types—nuclear bag and nuclear chain fibers (Fig. 10). In the former, numerous muscle nuclei are present in an expanded equatorial region of the fiber where cross-striations are absent. In the latter, the muscle nuclei form a row or chain in the center of each fiber at the equatorial region. Nuclear bag fibers are larger in diameter than chain fibers, and they extend beyond the capsule at each end to attach to the endomysium of the extrafusal fibers. Intrafusal fibers are innervated by the gamma motor neurons via small end plates (neuromuscular junctions) situated at both ends of the muscle fibers.

Westmoreland *et al.* noted that an important role of the gamma motor neurons is to "activate the intrafusal fibers leading to contraction and shortening of these fibers on either end of the central noncontractile region." The result is to stretch the central region of the intrafusal fibers and activate sensory receptors and the afferent nerve terminals (vide infra). The functional role of the spindles is discussed later.

Sensory Neurons and the Simple Reflex Arc

The alpha motor neurons are influenced not only by upper motor neurons in the motor cortex and motor control neurons in the brainstem but also by sensory inputs from the periphery. In fact, the peripheral pathway that serves as the foundation for the generation of spontaneous muscle contraction in the resting state (also known as muscle tone) is the simple reflex arc. It is composed of a sensory or afferent limb [the heavily myelinated axon originating in the muscle spindle (known as Ia afferent fiber, the largest among all nerve fibers) whose unipolar cell body resides in the sensory or dorsal root ganglia] and a motor or efferent limb (the myelinated axon extending from the lower motor neuron). The afferent limb directly stimulates the efferent lower motor neuron via a single synapse; hence, the reflex arc is designated monosynaptic (Fig. 9). The specialized unipolar structure of the sensory neuron cell body allows for its axon to bifurcate after leaving the cell body: One process passes to the muscle spindle in the periphery, whereas the other travels into the spinal cord to make its monosynaptic contact with the lower motor neuron.

With regard to the sensory innervation of the muscle spindle, the large-diameter myelinated axon (Ia) pierces the capsule of the spindle, loses its myelin sheath, and becomes a naked axon that winds spirally around the equatorial regions of the nuclear bag or chain portions of the intrafusal fibers (Fig. 10). A slightly smaller diameter myelinated axon, arising from a smaller dorsal root ganglion

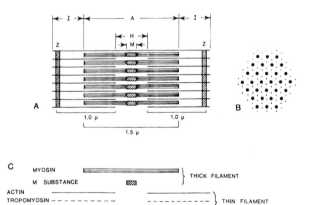

Figure 7
Organization of protein filaments in a myofibril. (A) Longitudinal section through one sarcomere (Z disk to Z disk) showing the overlap of actin and myosin. (B) Cross section through the A band, where the thin actin filaments interdigitate with the thick myosin filaments in a hexagonal formation. (C) Location of specific proteins in the sarcomere (reproduced with permission from Westmoreland *et al.*, 1994).

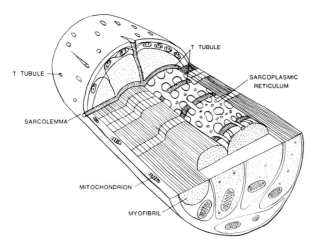

Figure 8
Structure of a single muscle fiber cut both horizontally and longitudinally. Individual myofibrils are surrounded and separated by sarcoplasmic reticulum. T tubules are continuous with extracellular fluid and interdigitate with sarcoplasmic reticulum. Note the regular association of the T tubule with the sarcoplasmic reticulum to form membranous triads. Also note the location of myonuclei at the periphery of the muscle fiber and the presence of many mitochondria (reproduced with permission from Westmoreland *et al.*, 1994).

neuron, also pierces the muscle spindle capsule, loses its myelin sheath, and forms a naked axon that branches terminally and ends as varicosities, resembling a spray of flowers. These endings are situated mainly on the nuclear chain fibers and some distance away from the equatorial region.

Golgi Tendon Organs

These are neurotendinous spindles that are located in tendons at the junction of the tendon and the muscle (Fig. 9). They consist of fibrous capsules that surround bundles of collagen fibers. Like the sensory innervation of the muscle spindle described previously, myelinated sensory fibers pierce the capsule and end in club-shaped endings. These fibers are less thickly myelinated and are designated Ib fibers.

Interneurons

The interneurons are distributed in the anterior horn of the spinal cord and the brainstem and play a major role in determining the final common output of the motor neurons. Inputs to the interneurons derive from descending tracts originating in the brainstem, motor cortex, and limbic motor system. Additionally, interneurons receive direct or indirect information from peripheral sensory fibers. These inputs comprise both excitatory and

inhibitory influences that in turn modulate the overall excitability of the motor neurons, whose motor axons form the final common pathways for innervation of skeletal muscle.

Interneurons form intricate neuronal circuits that form the anatomical substrate for a variety of neurophysiological functions, including automatic and stereotyped spinal reflexes that continue to function even when the spinal cord has been separated from the brain and protective and postural reflexes triggered by unpleasant cutaneous stimuli. The interneuronal circuitry also coordinates timing for the integrated activation of synergist muscles and inhibition of antagonist muscles to allow for highly skilled voluntary movements.

Among the interneurons is the Renshaw cell. When anterior horn cells are activated and initiate action potentials along their motor axons, collateral branches terminate on Renshaw cells, which in turn send axonal projections to connect with anterior horn cells (Fig. 11). The result is that activation of the Renshaw cells causes inhibition of anterior horn cells (the chemical inhibitory neurotransmitter is amino acid in nature—glycine or taurine). This "recurrent inhibition" or negative feedback serves to stabilize the discharge frequency of pools of anterior horn cells and prevent them from discharging at excessive rates.

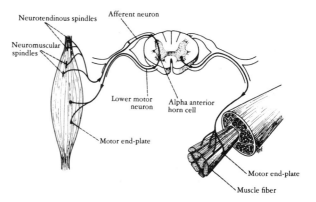

Figure 9
Schematic overview of the peripheral motor control system. To the right of the spinal cord section, note the alpha motor neuron innervating seven muscle fibers, representing a motor unit. Also to the right of the spinal cord section, note the sensory afferents from the muscle spindles (designated neuromuscular spindles) and the Golgi tendon organs (neurotendinous spindles). The afferent fiber (originating in the muscle spindle) makes a monosynaptic connection with the alpha motor neuron, which in turn projects to the muscle ending as the motor end plate (reproduced with permission from Snell, 1992, p. 134).

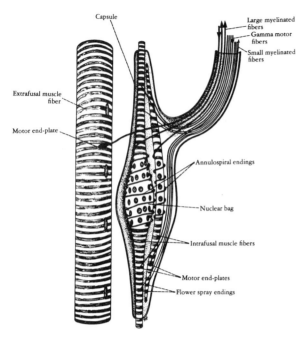

Figure 10
A neuromuscular spindle showing two types of intrafusal fibers: the nuclear bag fiber and the nuclear chain fiber (to the right of the nuclear bag fiber and characterized by a longitudinal row of nuclei in the shape of a chain). The extrafusal fiber (shown on the left of the intrafusal fibers) is innervated by a heavily myelinated fiber (from an anterior horn cell) terminating in a motor end plate. The intrafusal fibers are innervated by the gamma motor fibers. Large afferent myelinated fibers originate in annulospiral endings on the nuclear bag fiber (reproduced with permission from Snell, 1992, p. 130).

PHYSIOLOGICAL EVENTS LEADING TO MUSCLE CONTRACTION

Neuromuscular Transmission

Muscle contraction occurs as a result of a series of steps beginning with activation of the lower motor neuron (Fig. 12). The process starts with an action potential traveling along its axon toward the muscle to be activated. The arrival of an action potential at the axon terminal triggers an influx of calcium ions and the release of hundreds of quanta of acetylcholine simultaneously, producing an end plate potential (EPP) in the muscle. If the EPP reaches sufficient amplitude (threshold response), it leads to further muscle membrane depolarization that opens another class of channels—the voltage-gated sodium channels in the muscle cell—resulting in the current needed to generate a muscle fiber action potential (Fig. 13). In the resting state, small fluctuations in membrane potential occur at the end plate region of a given muscle fiber and are called miniature end

plate potentials (MEPPs). The MEPPS are produced by the spontaneous release of quanta of acetylcholine from the motor nerve ending and are not of sufficient amplitude to produce a muscle fiber action potential.

Muscle Fiber Excitation Contraction Coupling

The muscle fiber action potential propagates at a rate of 3–5 m/sec along the muscle membrane (the sarcolemma) and into the T tubules (located at the junction of the A and I bands) (Fig. 8). The latter, flanked by the sarcoplasmic reticulum and forming a triad complex, transmits the action potential inside the muscle fiber; this action potential causes signal transduction through ryanodine receptors releasing calcium ions. The calcium ions then bind to the troponin subunits, causing a conformational change in the tropomyosin and the actin helix configuration. In another calcium-dependent process that requires ATP, cross-bridges are formed between thick and thin filaments. Sliding of the thin actin filaments over the thick myosin filaments produces muscle contraction. The shortening of the sarcomeres and the I band during contraction is not due to a change in the absolute length of the filaments but rather to the sliding of the filaments. Contraction ceases when calcium is removed from the sarcoplasmic reticulum by active transport.

SPINAL CONTROL MECHANISMS FOR MUSCLE CONTRACTION

Here, I return to the muscle spindles and the motor neuron and interneuron populations of the spinal

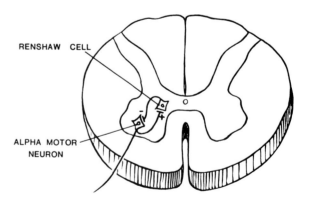

Figure 11
Note the recurrent collateral branch of the alpha motor neuron (arrow) making an excitatory synaptic contact with a Renshaw cell. Excitation of the Renshaw cell in turn produces inhibition of the alpha motor neuron (reproduced with permission from Westmoreland et al., 1994).

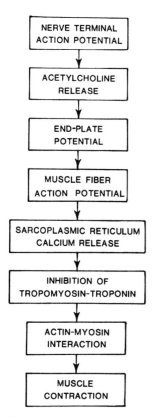

Figure 12
Sequence of events leading to muscle contraction [reproduced with permission from Daube, J. R., Reagan, T. J., Sandok, B. A., and Westmoreland, B. E. (1986). *Medical Neurosciences. An Approach to Anatomy, Pathology and Physiology by Systems and Levels.* Little, Brown, Boston].

inhibition is brought about by these same Ia afferents that simultaneously stimulate inhibitory interneurons that inhibit the alpha motor neurons for the antagonist extensor, the triceps. The biceps alpha motor neurons that have been excited also send collateral impulses to the inhibitory interneurons (the Renshaw cells), thereby regulating their own excitation. The mechanical contraction

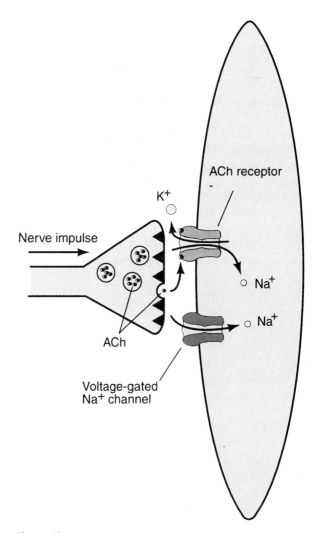

Figure 13
The binding of acetylcholine (ACh) at transmitter-gated channels opens channels permeable to both Na^+ and K^+. The flow of these ions in and out of the cell depolarizes the cell membrane, producing the end plate potential. This depolarization opens neighboring voltage-gated Na^+ channels. To elicit an action potential, the depolarization produced by the end plate potential must open sufficient Na^+ channels to reach the threshold for initiating the action potential [reproduced with permission from Kandel, E. R., Schwartz, J. H., and Jessell, T. M. (1995). *Essentials of Neural Science and Behavior.* Appleton & Lange, Stamford, CT].

cord and examine how their anatomical connections and physiological interrelationships allow for the integrated activation of agonist and antagonist muscles. We can explore the role of the component parts of the peripheral motor control system by closely examining the sequence of physiological events that follow the stretch of a flexor muscle (e.g., the activation of the biceps muscle by tapping on the biceps tendon to elicit a reflex biceps contraction).

First, following the tendon tap, excitatory signals are transmitted from the annulospiral endings of the nuclear bag intrafusal fibers that are stretched by tendon tap along the Ia afferents to activate the motor neurons, which in turn activate the extrafusal muscle fibers and lead to the biceps monosynaptic muscle contraction (Fig. 14). So that the biceps may contract without resistance, the motor neurons innervating the antagonist triceps muscle are inhibited (designated reciprocal inhibition). This

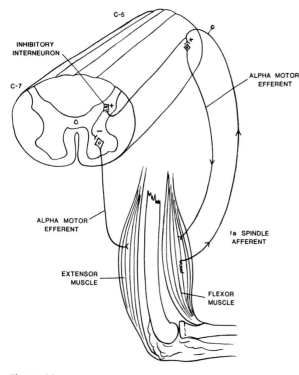

Figure 14
Pathways for the monosynaptic reflex and for reciprocal
inhibition. An Ia afferent fiber is shown making monosynaptic
contact with a flexor (biceps) motor neuron and an inhibitory
interneuron. The latter sends a projection to an extensor (triceps)
motor neuron, providing the pathway for reciprocal inhibition
(reproduced with permission from Westmoreland *et al.*, 1994).

(flexion) of the biceps exerts tension on the IIb
sensory fibers of the Golgi tendon organ that project
to the spinal cord. These Golgi tendon organ
afferents have an inhibitory effect on alpha motor
neurons (via inhibitory interneurons), thereby preventing too much tension from being generated by
the biceps, and they stimulate excitatory interneurons that activate alpha motor neurons innervating
the antagonist triceps muscle. This antagonist
contraction inhibits further flexor contraction and
restores the flexor muscle (biceps) to its original
position. Finally, biceps contraction loosens the
intrafusal fibers, which stimulates a feedback system
that activates the gamma motor neurons to contract
the intrafusal fibers. In effect, the gamma motor
neurons cause the intrafusal fibers to shorten (or
adjust) and this stretches the equatorial region of the
fibers, thereby stimulating the annulospiral and
flower spray endings and once again restoring the
stretch sensitivity of the muscle spindle.

—David A. Chad

See also–Motor System, Overview; Motor Unit
Potential; Muscle Contraction, Overview;
Neurons, Overview

Further Reading

Mitsumoto, H., Chad, D. A., and Pioro, E. P. (1998). *Amyotrophic
Lateral Sclerosis, Contemporary Neurology Series.* Oxford
Univ. Press, New York.
Snell, R. S. (1992). *Clinical Neuroanatomy for Medical Students,*
3rd ed. Little, Brown, Boston.
Westmoreland, B. E., Benarroch, E. E., Daube, J. R., *et al.*
(1994). *Medical Neurosciences. An Approach to Anatomy,
Pathology and Physiology by Systems and Levels.* Little,
Brown, Boston.

Motor Cortex

Encyclopedia of the Neurological Sciences
Copyright 2003, Elsevier Science (USA). All rights reserved.

HUGHLINGS JACKSON was one of the first physicians
to speculate that the cortex around the central sulcus
contained an organized representation of body
movements. He observed that motor epilepsies often
began with small twitches in the hand or the corner
of the mouth and then spread to involve adjacent
muscles and finally the whole body. In a small
number of cases that came to pathology, he saw that
there was limited damage to part of the cerebral
cortex around the central sulcus. He suggested that
this indicated that there was a discrete representation
of movements of different body parts in this area,
and that "irritation" could produce movements of
the corresponding part of the contralateral body. He
further noted that some parts were likely to have a
larger or more excitable effect than others, explaining the propensity for twitches to begin in the hands
or face. His ideas were later confirmed by Fritsch and
Hitzig and David Ferrier in the 1870s, who showed
that electrical stimulation of the central area in dogs
and monkeys could produce movements of the
opposite side of the body. Movements of different
parts of the body were produced by different
locations of the stimulating electrode, with the
lowest threshold effects observed in the distal limbs.
Bartholow first stimulated the human motor cortex
only a few years later in a patient whose cortex was
exposed by a large ulcer on her scalp.

These experiments defined the motor cortex as the
area from which movements could be elicited at
lowest intensity. Within this area there was a map of
the body in which movements of the legs were

represented medially, with the trunk, arms, and face progressively more lateral. As predicted by Hughlings Jackson, movements of the lower face and hands were much more readily evoked, and from a wider area of cortex, than movements of other parts of the body. This arrangement was later popularized in the familiar motor "homunculus" drawn by Penfield and coworkers.

ANATOMICAL AND ELECTROPHYSIOLOGICAL DEFINITIONS OF THE MOTOR AREAS OF CORTEX

Neurophysiologists now recognize that there are several representations of the body in the "motor areas" of the cerebral cortex. Anatomically, these occupy Brodmann's areas 4 and 6 on the lateral and medial surfaces of the hemispheres anterior to the central sulcus, together with areas 23 and 24 in the cingulate gyrus. Electrical stimulation over these areas can evoke contralateral body movements. To date, seven different representations, each with a somatotopic representation of part or all of the body, have been identified in studies on monkey.

The primary motor cortex has been studied in most detail. This occupies area 4 of Brodmann, which is mostly buried in the anterior bank of the central sulcus. It is distinguished from adjacent sensory areas by its lack of a pronounced cortical layer IV (agranular cortex). It differs from area 6 by the presence of large pyramidal neurons in layer V (Betz cells). The primary motor cortex has a lower threshold for electrical stimulation than any other motor area and produces twitch-like movements of a small number of muscles in the contralateral body, such as a flick of the fingers or a twitch of biceps or the corner of the mouth depending on the point of stimulation. The location of the primary motor cortex is frequently mapped during neurosurgical operations in man. Patients are often awake during such operations, and they state that the movements feel involuntary, as if imposed by an external force. The implication is that awareness of the effort of a voluntary movement must arise in other areas of cortex. Patients also note that during stimulation they feel unable to move that part of the body. Presumably, activation of the cortex by electrical current prevents patients from using that area in voluntary movements. Approximately one-third of the primary motor cortex is devoted to control of the hand. Magnetic resonance images show that in most subjects, this region is marked by folding of the

central sulcus into an "omega" shape when viewed from the surface. It is a rare example of an anatomical marker for a specific cortical function.

In the monkey, two additional representations of the body are found anterior to area 4 in the lateral part of area 6 around the arcuate sulcus. These are known as the dorsal and ventral premotor areas. Stimulation of these areas has a higher threshold and provokes more complex movements than stimulation of area 4, often involving more than one part of the body simultaneously. This area has not been extensively studied in humans. One problem is that the limits of human premotor areas must be defined. The precentral sulcus is thought to be the human analog of the arcuate sulcus, but human area 6 extends further anterior to this point than it does in the monkey. Another problem is that there are no detailed mapping studies to compare with the monkey work. In fact, in the original somatotopic maps of human cortex this region is part of the trunk representation.

The medial portion of area 6 anterior to the leg representation in the primary motor cortex comprises the supplementary area (SMA). This is organized with the legs posterior, adjacent to the primary leg area, and the arms and face anterior. The effects of stimulation are relatively well described in humans. The threshold is higher than for the primary motor cortex, and the movements are more complex, often involving combined turning of the head and extension of the arm. Bilateral movements and vocalization can also be produced.

In the past 10 years, three more motor representations have been described around the cingulate gyrus, approximately ventral to the SMA. These lie in parts of areas 6, 23, and 24 of Brodmann and are called the dorsal, ventral, and rostral cingulate motor areas, respectively. The main evidence for these representations initially derived from anatomical studies that showed they had direct projections to spinal cord. Electrical stimulation studies are rare, although it has been confirmed in humans that at least one similar representation of the body lies in the cingulate gyrus at this level. Stimulation produced tonic extension of the arm or the leg.

OUTPUT OF CORTICAL MOTOR AREAS

All cortical motor areas have a direct output to the spinal cord. This is composed of axons from pyramidal neurons in cortical layer V, which run in the corticospinal (or pyramidal) tract and innervate all levels of the contralateral spinal cord. In humans, there are approximately 500,000 fibers in the corticospinal tract on each side, 2% of which are large diameter and conduct impulses rapidly at speeds of up to 80 m/sec. They are probably the axons of the large Betz cells of primary motor cortex. The majority of corticospinal fibers are smaller diameter and slower conducting (10–30 m/sec).

The fibers run in the lateral and anterior columns, with the majority traveling in the former. Most of the projection is contralateral, although a small percentage (approximately 10%), particularly fibers in the anterior columns, run ipsilaterally. Terminations are mostly onto interneurons in the gray matter of the intermediate zone. However, especially in primates and man, there are extensive monosynaptic projections directly to spinal motoneurons in lamina IX. This projection is particularly prominent to distal muscles of the forearm and hand, and it is thought to contribute to the increased dexterity of humans compared with that of other species.

Although the corticospinal tract is large, it is important to remember that motor cortical areas also communicate with spinal motoneurons via projections to nuclei in the brainstem. Some of these are collaterals of corticospinal fibers, whereas some project to the brainstem only. These brainstem nuclei have descending fibers that form the reticulospinal tracts and innervate all segments of the cord, sometimes bilaterally. The density of these corticoreticulospinal projections is higher from premotor, SMA, and cingulate motor areas than it is from the primary motor cortex.

The relative roles of corticospinal and noncorticospinal pathways are illustrated by experiments in which the corticospinal fibers are surgically cut. This has been performed several times in monkey by lesioning the pyramids in the medulla; in man, corticospinal fibers have been cut for relief of involuntary movements by lesioning the middle third of the cerebral peduncle. In both cases, the loss of approximately 1 million fibers is accompanied by little evidence of gross movement deficit. There is no spasticity and little weakness. The main deficit is in control of manipulative movements of the hands: The fingers are no longer used independently and precision grip is lost. The implication is that although the corticospinal system is important for fine distal movement, the noncorticospinal projections are of equal or even greater importance for other types of movement. When projections from cortex to the brainstem nuclei are lesioned, as occurs in a capsular stroke, these noncorticospinal projections lose their input from the cerebral cortex. The resulting movement deficit is much greater than that seen after pure pyramidal lesions.

Motor areas of the cortex also send projections to pontine nuclei that innervate the cerebellum and to the ascending sensory systems in the gracile and cuneate nuclei (in both cases, often as collateral of corticospinal fibers). The cerebellar projection provides a copy of the motor command that could potentially be used to update movement more quickly than by relying on sensory feedback. The projection to sensory nuclei is important in controlling the flow of sensory information during movement.

INPUTS TO CORTICAL MOTOR AREAS

The motor areas are also distinguished by differences in the inputs that they receive from other parts of the brain. The nature of these inputs is presumably an important factor in determining the contribution of each area to specific types of movement. The primary motor cortex receives input mainly from sensory cortex and from areas of thalamus that receive input from the cerebellum and, to a lesser extent, the basal ganglia. There are also extensive connections both to and from the other motor areas. The premotor areas receive a major input from regions of the posterior parietal cortex that are involved in the combined processing of visual and somatosensory input as well as input from cerebellum via the thalamus. The SMA receives a large input from parietal cortex and from thalamic nuclei that receive input from basal ganglia. Cingulate motor areas are thought to have extensive connections with regions in the frontal lobes.

ACTIVITY OF MOTOR CORTICAL NEURONS

The pattern of input is reflected in the way in which neurons in each area contribute to different parts of the preparation and execution of movement. Neurophysiological recordings of cell discharge in behaving animals show that neurons in primary motor cortex change their firing rate just before and during a movement. Neurons with monosynaptic connections to motoneurons tend to behave much like the muscles that they drive, being active just before and during contraction. The relation of cortical interneurons or pyramidal neurons without direct connections to spinal motoneurons tends to be more complex. Their activity may reflect stages in cortical processing or the input to spinal interneurons rather than motoneurons. In general, activity in these neurons occurs at approximately the time of movement and tends to be related to parameters such as the force of muscle contraction or the direction of the movement.

The activity of neurons in SMA and premotor areas is more likely related to preparation, rather than execution, of movement. The neurons may discharge well before a movement as if they were specifying what movement is to be made next rather than the nature of the movement currently under way. There appear to be few differences in the contribution of SMA and premotor cortex to simple tasks, such as pushing a button when a light comes on. However, activity in these two areas differs substantially in more complex tasks, such as those requiring a sequence of movements. Premotor neurons are more likely to change their activity when visual cues are used to guide the sequence of movements, whereas SMA activity is more intense when the sequence is made from memory, without visual cues. Examples include pointing at a series of lights as they are illuminated in random order or pointing to the same positions from memory. The former is an externally guided movement and involves activity in premotor cortex; the latter is an internally generated movement and involves activity in the SMA.

The main input that drives externally guided movements comes from parietal cortex. It can be hypothesized that processed sensory input from this area can help the premotor regions select appropriate movements from a set of stored commands. Indeed, some neurons in this area have been labeled "mirror" neurons because they discharge both when a monkey makes a particular movement and also when it observes another animal make the same movement. Such neuronal types could obviously help us to learn movements by observing them.

EFFECT OF LESIONS OF MOTOR CORTICAL AREAS

Small lesions of the primary motor cortex produce transient weakness that often resolves, presumably because neighboring areas of cortex can compensate for the lost function of the damaged area. Larger lesions, particularly if they involve premotor areas, result in permanent weakness and spasticity. The latter is thought to be a consequence of removal of input to reticular centers of the brainstem that influence muscle tone. Pure lesions of the premotor

areas and SMAs are rare in humans but have been studied extensively in monkey. Lesions of premotor areas affect the ability of the monkey to retrieve the correct movement on the basis of external cues, whereas SMA lesions affect the ability of monkeys to perform a series of movements from memory (internally guided movements). SMA lesions also affect coordination in actions involving object manipulation in both hands.

In humans, rare patients with limited lesions of presumed premotor areas also have difficulty associating visual cues with particular movements. For example, they cannot learn to produce different hand postures when they view particular visual symbols. Lesions of the SMA in humans are most commonly associated with difficulty in initiating or maintaining speech, a feature that is not evident in the monkey data. In addition, patients with larger midline lesions may exhibit the "alien hand" sign, a condition in which the hand contralateral to the lesion behaves independently of the subject's will and may reach out to grasp objects within reach. This can be interpreted as a possible uncoupling of the externally guided premotor system from the internally guided SMA system. Finally, the movements of patients with SMA lesions, even after apparently good recovery, are often slower than normal. Interestingly, bradykinesia is a principal symptom of Parkinson's disease, and since the SMA is an important output target of the basal ganglia, slowness of movement after a lesion may be due to lack of basal ganglia input to the motor system.

PLASTICITY OF PRIMARY MOTOR CORTEX

It has been known for many years that electrical stimulation at the same site in primary motor cortex does not always produce exactly the same movement on every occasion over a period of several hours. However, this capacity of the cortex to change its organization, even in the adult, has only been investigated in detail in the past 10–20 years. The majority of studies have analyzed the somatosensory system and the postcentral cortex; relatively few have examined the motor system, but in those that have, the data are remarkably similar to those expected from sensory cortex.

For example, in rats there is a large representation of the whiskers in the primary motor cortex. If the seventh nerve is lesioned, the rats can no longer use the whiskers. At the motor cortex, stimulation of sites that previously evoked whisker movement now gives rise to movements of the periocular or arm muscles, which previously had been represented in adjacent areas of cortex. These changes occur so rapidly that they cannot involve growth of new connections or synapses. Instead, it is thought that they rely on changes in horizontal connections between cortical areas. Thus, after seventh nerve section, the excitability of connections from the whisker area to other regions becomes more excitable. They are activated by electrical stimulation and evoke movements of the arm or periocular muscles indirectly via adjacent cortex. The excitability of the horizontal connections that are involved in this remodeling of cortical representation is controlled by GABAergic inhibition. This inhibitory system in turn is regulated by sensory information about the state of the peripheral motor apparatus.

Similar remodeling occurs if the damage is in the motor cortex rather than the periphery. After small lesions, healthy surrounding areas can evoke movements previously elicited by stimulation of the damaged part. It is particularly interesting that such reorganization is enhanced if animals undergo training of the affected part of the body. The implication is that physiotherapy may have an important influence in outcome from cortical damage. The situation with larger lesions is unexplored. However, horizontal connections in the cortex are short (~2 mm) and often do not cross boundaries between cortical areas. Thus, recovery from large lesions may require a different form of reorganization.

Finally, there is good evidence for similar patterns of reorganization in human primary motor cortex. The technique of transcranial magnetic stimulation, in which a magnetic field is used to induce electrical stimulating currents in the brain, allows coarse mapping of the motor cortex to be carried out in intact conscious subjects. Mapping the cortex of amputees, for example, shows that stimulation of the area previously controlling movements of the lost limb can evoke movement in immediately adjacent parts of the body. As in rat experiments, it seems that the pattern of representation of the body on the cortex can change after injury.

—*John C. Rothwell*

See also–Betz Cells; Brain Anatomy; Corticospinal/Corticobulbar Tracts; Electrostimulation; Frontal Lobes; Jackson, John Hughlings; Plasticity

Further Reading

Passingham, R. (1993). *The Frontal Lobes and Voluntary Action.* Oxford Univ. Press, Oxford.

Porter, R., and Lemon, R. N. (1993). *Corticospinal Function and Voluntary Movement.* Oxford Univ. Press, Oxford.

Rizzolatti, G., and Luppino, G. (2001). The cortical motor system. *Neuron* **31**, 889–901.

Rothwell, J. C. (2001). First studies of the organisation of the human motor cortex. In *Classics in Movement Science* (M. L. Latash and V. M. Zatisiorsky, Eds.), pp. 273–288. Human Kinetics, Champaign, IL.

Sanes, J. N., and Donoghue, J. P. (2001). Plasticity and primary motor cortex. *Annu. Rev. Neurosci.* **23**, 393–415.

Motor System, Overview

Encyclopedia of the Neurological Sciences

THE MOTOR system controls the initiation, execution, and coordination of all movements that occur in health and disease. The motor system generates three general types of movements: Reflex movements are rapid, involuntary movements elicited by stimuli that require a quick, unconscious reaction, such as withdrawal of the hand that has touched a hot kitchen burner; rhythmical movements are stereotyped sequences of muscle activation, best typified by walking or running; and voluntary movements are goal-directed and require conscious direction until well learned. They may be simple or elaborate and complex. Through practice, skilled movements such as typing or playing a musical instrument require lessconscious effort and become more automatic.

The motor system is anatomically organized in a hierarchical manner to execute and integrate the three types of movements. The spinal cord contains the circuits for most reflex responses and some rhythmical motor sequences. The brainstem system contains the circuits for more complex rhythmic and automatic patterns of motor movements. The cortex is necessary for the effective planning and initiation of volitional movements and uses additional inputs, including the reflex and patterned responses of the brainstem and spinal cord, to generate and refine movement. Most cells in the cortex that relate directly to motor systems are in the frontal and parietal lobes. The frontal lobe neurons most directly involved in volitional movement are in a well-organized band (the motor strip) located in the region called the precentral gyrus. Because these important cells are shaped like a pyramid, they are called pyramidal cells. The projections or axons of cells travel from the cortex downward through the lower regions of the brain (subcortex and brainstem) and cross to the other side of the spinal cord in the well-delineated pathway known as the lateral corticospinal tract to end in the spinal cord at the level that is appropriate for control of given muscle groups. This system is called the pyramidal system, and the hallmark of damage to this system is weakness.

In addition to the three hierarchical levels that interplay to affect the pyramidal system, there are two other parts of the motor system that regulate movement. The cerebellar system, which includes the cerebellum or hindbrain along with its fiber pathways that connect it to the cortex, brainstem, and spinal cord, regulates the coordination and accuracy of movement by comparing the sensory feedback from the periphery with the descending motor commands. When patients have damage to this part of the motor system, they are not weak, but they perform tasks with sloppy, uncoordinated movements and often have severe balance problems during walking (gait ataxia). The second motor system that influences the pyramidal function involves the basal ganglia, a series of subcortical and brainstem nuclei and pathways that receive inputs from both motor and sensory cortical regions and project to the motor regions of the thalamus and frontal lobe. This system has historically been called extrapyramidal, although its function is intimately integrated with the pyramidal pathways. Like patients with cerebellar damage, patients with basal gangliar system motor deficits have no weakness, but they are abnormally slow (hypokinesia) or have involuntary movements, such as shaking, jerking, or twisting (hyperkinesia).

The motor system cannot function in isolation and requires a continual sensory input to produce accurate and appropriate movements. A common and clear-cut example of the importance of sensory input for normal motor function is the slurred speech that patients develop transiently after receiving local anesthesia to the mouth during dental procedures.

Ultimately, all the descending motor pathways converge to terminate collectively on a set of cells in the spinal cord called the alpha motor neurons or the lower motor neurons. These cells give rise to the motor nerves that innervate skeletal muscle and produce movement. As such, with the combined influences of the pyramidal, cerebellar, basal gangliar, and sensory systems, these cells form the final common pathway for all neurally driven motor activation. In contrast, the motor neurons that generate voluntary, rhythmical, and reflex responses are collectively the upper motor neurons. In fact, most of the control signals coming from the upper motor neurons do not act directly on the lower motor neurons but use networks of interspersed, tiny neurons known as interneurons or the internuncial pool of neurons. These neurons are essential for integrating patterns of movements.

The final effector of movement, skeletal muscle, responds to stimulation with either tonic, slow contractions or phasic, rapid contractions. Back and trunk muscles primarily respond tonically to support posture, whereas the extremities have a high proportion of muscles that are phasic in their contractions. The relative density and innervation of tonic and phasic muscles largely dictate the functions that can be executed by any set of muscles.

Based on the anatomical details of the motor system, five types of prototypic movement syndrome develop in neurological disease. In the upper motor (pyramidal) neuron syndrome, there is damage of the frontal lobe cells or their descending projections (axons) as they travel through the subcortex, brainstem, and spinal cord to activate volitional movement. In strokes or tumors affecting these regions, weakness develops with increased deep tendon reflexes and spasticity. In the basal gangliar syndromes, in which there is damage in the nuclei and pathways of these subcortical areas that influence the pyramidal system, patients experience no weakness, but hypokinesia or hyperkinesia predominate along with changes in muscle tone. Examples include Parkinson's disease, Huntington's disease, and dystonia. In the cerebellar syndromes, damage affects the cerebellum and its pathways that interconnect with the pyramidal upper motor neurons; patients have no weakness, but when they move they are unstable, poorly coordinated, and can fall from imbalance. Causes include multiple sclerosis and tumors of the cerebellum. The lower motor neuron syndrome is caused by damage of the spinal cord alpha motor neuron or its projections out to the muscles. Patients with damage to this final motor pathway are weak, and the muscles degenerate or atrophy from denervation and develop rippling movements called fasciculations. Peripheral nerve compression, inflammation, or degeneration can provoke this syndrome and be localized to one area of the nervous system (mononeuropathy) or be diffuse (polyneuropathy). Involvement may be selective to the motor nerves (motor neuron disease), or both sensory and motor components of peripheral nerves may be involved. The muscle or myopathy syndrome occurs when the muscle fibers are damaged by infection, inflammation, or degeneration; in these cases, patients experience widespread weakness, often with muscle tenderness and cramps. Muscular dystrophies, infections, and drug reactions are among the causes of myopathies.

—*Christopher G. Goetz*

See also–Learning, Motor; Lower Motor Neuron Lesions; Motor Control, Peripheral; Motor Cortex; Movement Disorders, Overview; Muscle Contraction, Overview

Further Reading

Evarts, E., and Wise, S. P. (1985). *The Motor System in Neurobiology*. Elsevier, Amsterdam.
Georgopoulos, A. (1995). Current issues in directional motor control. *Trends Neurosci.* **18**, 506–510.
Hammerstad, J. P. (1998). Strength and reflexes. In *Textbook of Clinical Neurology* (C. G. Goetz and E. J. Pappert, Eds.), pp. 225–284. Saunders, Philadelphia.
Leigh, P. N., and Swash, M. (1995). *Motor Neuron Disease*. Springer-Verlag, Basel.

Motor Unit Potential

Encyclopedia of the Neurological Sciences

THE CONCEPT of motor unit (MU) was put forth by Sherrington as consisting of the spinal alpha motor neuron and the muscle fibers innervated by its axon. Motor unit potential (MUP) represents temporal and spatial summation of all single muscle fiber action potentials (MFAPs) within a motor unit. Needle electrode examination of a muscle is the standard procedure for recording MUP and is an integral part of clinical electromyography (EMG).

MORPHOLOGICAL CHARACTERISTICS

MUP is usually a bi- or triphasic response. Its duration is the time interval from onset of initial deflection to its return to baseline. MUP amplitude is measured between the largest negative and positive peaks. A phase is part of the MUP between two baseline crossings. A peak that does not cross the baseline is called a turn and it imparts a serrated appearance to the MUP (Fig. 1).

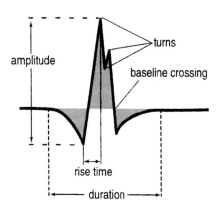

Figure 1
Features of the motor unit action potential [reproduced with permission from Aminoff, M. J. (1998). General aspects of needle electromyography. In *Electromyography in Clinical Practice*. Churchill Livingstone, New York].

ANATOMICAL AND PHYSIOLOGICAL BASIS

Muscle fibers of an MU are widely scattered within the muscle, interspersed with fibers belonging to other motor units. Electrically recorded MUP represents activity only from muscle fibers within the recording area of the needle electrode. Morphological features of MUP are related to spatial distribution of end plates on muscle fibers and impulse propagation in terminal nerve endings and muscle fibers. MUP duration depends on the number and density of muscle fibers and the delay in arrival of earliest and latest single MFAPs. Peak-to-peak amplitude of the MUP is markedly influenced by proximity of the electrode to muscle fibers. Optimal placement of the needle electrode is reflected by rise time of MUP—that is, the time interval from onset of major negative deflection to its peak. The number and density of muscle fibers closest to the recording electrode and synchronicity of their firing are directly correlated with the amplitude of MUP.

Changes in the shape of MUP occur due to the presence of multiple phases and turns, as a result of temporal dispersion of single muscle fiber potentials. MUPs with five or more phases are termed polyphasic potentials and may constitute up to 15% of MUPs in a normal muscle. Occasionally, one or more muscle fibers within a motor unit may have a long or slow conducting terminal nerve branch, resulting in a small delayed potential that is time locked with the major MUP waveform and is called a satellite potential. The size of a normal MUP varies in different muscles and is also affected by age and muscle temperature. Lower intramuscular temperature is associated with an increase in the duration and amplitude of MUPs. Quantitative study of MUP requires isolation of at least 20 MUPs and determination of mean duration, amplitude, and other parameters. Computer-assisted techniques based on template matching, signal decomposition, and so on may facilitate quantitative analysis.

RECRUITMENT/INTERFERENCE PATTERN

MU recruitment involves rate modulation of individual MUPs and activation of additional motor units. With weak voluntary effort, a low-threshold, small motor unit is recruited at 4 or 5 Hz. With increasing effort, MU firing frequency increases, and successively higher threshold, larger units are activated (Henneman's size principle). On relaxation, derecruitment occurs in reverse order. The size principle of MU recruitment is retained in steady/ramp as well as rapid/ballistic movement. In general, small, low-threshold MUs are type 1, fatigue-resistant units, and large, higher threshold units are type 2 fast fatigable motor units. Therefore, individual MUPs studied at low effort during EMG belong to small type 1 motor units. With strong contraction, an increased number and firing frequency of motor units result in overlap of MUPs, described as interference pattern. A decrease in the number of recruitable MUs produces a mixed pattern, also termed reduced or incomplete pattern. A "discrete" or single-unit pattern corresponds to severe loss of motor units.

MUP IN PATHOLOGICAL STATES

Neuropathic Disorders

Peripheral nerve and anterior horn cell lesions are associated with an increase in MU territory and muscle fiber density due to collateral axonal sprouting and reinnervation by surviving motor neurons. MUP from such a motor unit has a high amplitude, prolonged duration, and may be polyphasic in shape (Fig. 2). However, the altered morphology evolves over time. During earlier stages of reinnervation, immature slow-conducting nerve endings result in temporal dispersion with prolonged duration, low amplitude, and polyphasic and unstable (nascent) MUPs. The addition of more muscle fibers and maturation of nerve endings complete the MU remodeling, with resultant large and stable MUPs. Such changes are most prominent in anterior horn cell lesions (e.g., in

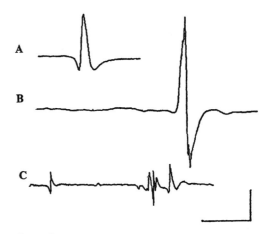

Figure 2
Characteristics of (A) normal, (B) neurogenic, and (C) myopathic motor unit potentials. Calibration: horizontal, 10 msec; vertical, 200 µV (A and C) and 1 mV (B).

old poliomyelitis in which giant MUPs of more than 10 mV amplitude may be seen). The recruitment pattern in neurogenic lesions is characterized by a reduced number and increased firing frequencies of MUPs.

Myopathic Disorders

Primary muscle disorders are associated with random atrophy and loss of muscle fibers, and thereby a smaller size but normal number of MUs. Consequently, the MUPs have a short duration, low amplitude, and marked polyphasia (Fig. 2). Force production by small MUs is reduced; therefore, MUs are recruited in increasing numbers for the given level of voluntary effort. The interference pattern is full but of low amplitude. The neurogenic and myopathic patterns do not always distinguish between primary nerve or muscle disorders. Advanced myopathy may be associated with loss of motor units, whereas low-amplitude, polyphasic MUPs are seen during early reinnervation. Terminal axonopathy may also produce a myopathic pattern.

Central Nervous System Disorders

Upper motor neuron syndromes may not produce any change in MUP morphology; however, the number of MUPs at maximum effort is reduced, and their rate of firing remains low. Analysis of single MU discharge patterns shows decreased variability of consecutive interspike intervals and slow random fluctuations over time, indicating impaired central motor control.

—Upinder K. Dhand and Bhagwan T. Shahani

See also–Action Potential, Generation of; Electromyography (EMG); Membrane Potential; Motor Control, Peripheral; Motor System, Overview

Further Reading

Buchthal, F., Pinelli, P., and Rosenfalck, P. (1954). Action potential parameters in normal human muscle and their physiological determinants. *Acta Physiol. Scand.* **32**, 219–229.

Fang, J., Shahani, B. T., and Bruyninckx, F. (1997). Study of single motor unit discharge patterns using 1/F process model. *Muscle Nerve* **20**, 293–298.

Fang, J., Agarwal, G. C., and Shahani, B. T. (1999). Decomposition of multiunit electromyographic signals. *IEEE Trans. Biomed. Eng.* **64**, 685–697.

Henneman, E., Shahani, B. T., and Young, R. R. (1976). Voluntary control of human motor units. In *The Motor System* (M. Shahani, Ed.), pp. 73–78. Elsevier, Amsterdam.

Shahani, B. T., and Young, R. R. (1985). Clinical electromyography. In *Clinical Neurology* (A. B. Baker and R. J. Joynt, Eds.), Vol. 1, pp. 1–52. Harper & Row, Philadelphia.

Movement Disorders, Overview

Encyclopedia of the Neurological Sciences
Copyright 2003, Elsevier Science (USA). All rights reserved.

MOVEMENT DISORDERS are defined as neurological disorders in which there is either an excess of abnormal involuntary movements (hyperkinesias or dyskinesias) or a paucity of voluntary and automatic movements (hypokinesia) (Table 1). Most movement disorders are associated with pathological alterations in the basal ganglia, a group of gray matter nuclei lying deep within the cerebral hemispheres (caudate, putamen, and pallidum), the diencephalon (subthalamic nucleus), and the mesencephalon (substantia nigra). The basal ganglia integrate with the primary pyramidal motor system and cerebellar system. The basal ganglia are sometimes called the extrapyramidal system because they are distinct from the pathways related to volitional motor control (pyramidal system). The basal ganglia act as modifying influences on the pyramidal system to control and alter the speed of movement. Myoclonus and many forms of tremors do not appear to be related primarily to basal ganglia pathology but are due to brainstem abnormalities that influence the motor system. Likewise, deep brain structures called the limbic system that are technically outside the basal ganglia may influence or generate tic movements that are part of a classic movement disorder, Tourette's syndrome.

The maintenance of normal movement by the basal ganglia nuclei is ensured by a continual coordination between excitatory and inhibitory neurochemical signals that travel the pathways connecting these nuclei. There are several neurotransmitters involved in the basal ganglia functions, including GABA, one of the major inhibitory neurotransmitters in the basal ganglia; acetylcholine, which plays an important role in memory, autonomic nervous system, and motor system control; dopamine, the main neurotransmitter affected in Parkinson's disease and also involved in hyperkinetic movements, such as chorea and dystonia; glutamate, a neuroexcitatory neurotransmitter that can have excitotoxic effects. An excess of glutamate may produce toxic effects resulting in neuronal damage, and glutamate is believed to play a role in neurodegenerative process, such as in Huntington's disease and amyotrophic lateral sclerosis, and in dopaminergic drugs side effects in Parkinson's disease; serotonin, which also plays an important role in depression, hallucinations, and hyperkinetic movements such as myoclonus; and norepinephrine, a catecholamine neurotransmitter synthesized from dopamine. This chemical plays an important role in the autonomic nervous system and also enhances dopamine effects in some systems.

The first question to be answered when seeing a patient for the possible presence of abnormal movements is whether the movements are hyperkinetic or hypokinetic. The patient should be observed at rest

Table 1   MOVEMENT DISORDERS

Parkinson's disease

Symptomatic parkinsonism
  Drug-induced
  Hemiatropy/hemiparkinsonism
  Infectious
  Tumor
  Vascular
  Toxins including carbon monoxide, manganese, MPTP
    (1-methyl-4-phenyl-1,2,3,6-tetrahydropyridine), etc.

Parkinsonism-plus syndrome
  Cortico basal ganglionic degeneration
  Multiple system atropy
  Progressive supranuclear palsy

Wilson's disease

Juvenile Huntington's disease

Neuroacanthocytosis

Hallervorden–Spatz disease

Table 2 DIFFERENTIAL DIAGNOSIS OF HYPERKINESIAS THAT ARE PRESENT AT REST OR WITH ACTION

At rest only (disappears with action)
  Akathitic movements
  Paradoxical dystonia
  Resting tremor
  Restless legs
  Orthostatic tremor (standing)
With action only
  Tremor: postural, action, intention
  Action dystonia
  Action myoclonus
At rest and continues with action
  Athetosis, ballism, chorea, rest dystonia, moving toes/fingers,
    rest myoclonus, tics

and during activity. In hypokinetic disorders, there is a paucity of movement, including lack of normal gesturing and spontaneous movements (Table 2). The face is hypomimetic (lack of expression), and there is reduced rate of blinking. Rest tremor, if present, is elicited when the hands and feet are completely relaxed. In hyperkinesias, key information is obtained by observing the patient at rest in complete repose without talking. Many hyperkinesias are present at rest, such as athetosis, ballism, chorea, moving digits, myokimia, and tics. Patients with akathisia resist sitting quietly because their restlessness increases. In dystonia, the abnormal movements are often absent during rest and activate with a maintained posture. Importantly, tics are highly influenced by environment, and patients are usually able to suppress their tics at least partially in the presence of the observer. If myoclonus or a heightened startle reflex is suspected, the investigator should suddenly clap his or her hands or drop a book on the floor to surprise the patient in order to document it in the neurological examination.

The patient should also be observed during the maintenance of a posture. Postural tremor is maximized when the patient assumes and attempts to maintain a posture. In the case of a patient with hand tremor, there may be no tremor at rest, but when the hands are outstretched a fine, coarse tremor develops. Patients with myoclonus or dystonia are also unable to maintain a posture because of the presence of lightning-like jerks or tremor. One of the clinical hallmarks of chorea is motor impersistence, and patients are also unable to maintain a posture without the superimposition of the random choreic movements [e.g., when the subject tries to grip the examiner's hand or finger with steady pressure,

there is uncontrolled squeezing and release (milk-maid grip)].

Execution of tasks is also interrupted by hypokinesia and hyperkineisa. Finger tapping is slow and cramped in hypokinesia and sloppy and overridden with additional movements in chorea or cerebellar incoordination. Speech is a particularly valuable task to evaluate because it allows the examiner to detect dysarthria (slurred speech), hypophonia (decrease amplitude of speech), and other language disorders such as voice dystonia.

Tone should be also assessed. Unlike spasticity, cogwheel rigidity is the hallmark of hypokinesia. Dystonic patients also have increascd tone when the dystonia is active. In chorea, the tone is often reduced (hypotonia). In patients with tics, the tone is normal.

Gait integrates numerous anatomical systems, including pyramidal, extrapyramidal, cerebellar, visual, vestibular, and cognitive. Hyperkinetic and hypokinetic disorders may cause gait disturbances.

With this information, the category of the involuntary movement, such as chorea, dystonia, myoclonus, tics, and tremor, can be determined. To do so, one evaluates features such as rhythmicity, speed, duration, pattern (e.g., repetitive, flowing, continual, diurnal, paroxysmal, or intermittent), induction (e.g., stimuli induced, such as noises and touch, or action induced by movements), complexity of the movements (simple versus several movements), suppressibility by volitional attention or by sensory tricks (e.g., touching the involved area or adjacent body part can often reduce the muscle contractions), and whether the movements are accompanied by sensations such as restlessness or the urge to make a movement that can release a built-up tension. In addition, it must be determined which body parts are involved.

Once the movement disorder is classified, the next step is to determine the etiology of the disorder. As a general rule, the etiology can be ascertained on the basis of the history and selected laboratory tests when needed. Neuroimaging, including magnetic resonance imaging (MRI) and computed tomography (CT) scans of the brain, is usually normal. However, in Huntington's disease, there may be focal atrophy of the caudate nucleus. Similarly, in multiple system atrophy of the olivopontocerebellar type, localized atrophy of the brainstem and cerebellum may be prominent and iron deposits can be seen in the basal ganglia. MRI and CT scans are particularly useful in disclosing nondegenerative causes of movement disorders. Strokes, brain abscesses, and tumors can be identified, as can calcium deposit that may suggest parathyroid disease, old hemorrhage, or infection. Hypokinesia caused by carbon monoxide intoxication likewise has a characteristic pattern of degeneration of the globus pallidus. Other neuroimaging techniques may prove useful, particularly single photon emission computed tomography in corticobasal ganglionic degeneration in which focal parietal lobe hypoactivity can be detected. Positron emission tomography is usually used in research centers and not in the regular clinical setting. Electrophysiological studies including electroencephalography (brain waves) are also used when seizures are suspected, for example, in paroxysmal dyskinesias and myoclonus. Electromyography studies are usually used in characterizing tremor frequency and evaluating dystonic patients. Few blood and urine tests are of primary interest in the characterization of movement disorders. In specific cases including Wilson's disease, acanthocytosis, blood, and urine tests can be diagnostic.

Neuropsychological tests are important to document cognitive and affective dysfunction that can be useful in determining diagnosis such as Huntington's disease and also in guiding potential decisions regarding medical therapy. Some movement disorders commonly coexist with specific types of behavioral patterns (e.g., Tourette's syndrome and attention deficit disorder and obsessive–compulsive disorder and also Parkinson's disease and depression).

The final question is how best to treat the movement disorder. Treatment of movement disorders focuses first on replacement of the chemical systems that are imbalanced. For disorders with overactivity of a chemical system, drugs that deplete the neurotransmitter or block its receptor sites are useful. Examples include the use of anticholinergic drugs in Parkinson's disease to block overactive cholinergic receptors in the striatum, and the use of antidopaminergic drugs to block dopamine receptors in Huntington's disease. In disorders with deficits of neurotransmitters such as dopamine in Parkinson's disease, replacement therapy with its precursor, levodopa, has shown excellent results. When the movement disorder is severe and unresponsive to pharmacological treatment, surgery in the basal ganglia can be considered. Deep brain stimulation is used to treat some cases of essential tremor, Parkinson's disease, and dystonia. Chronic high-frequency stimulation is applied to different targets, including the thalamus, subthalamic nucleus, and globus pallidus. The best target is chosen based on the disease and the symptoms to be controlled. Pallidotomy or thalamotomy (in either case, the thalamus or globus pallidus are lesioned) have also been used, but potential side effects, such as visual field deficits and other focal neurological deficits, have been reported.

Physical therapy programs are aimed at improving motor function, increasing range of motion, and building endurance. These programs include therapeutic exercises, gait training, and psychosocial support, and they are especially useful in hypokinetic disorders. Likewise, occupational therapy is useful in task-specific dystonias to instruct patients how to avoid specific postures that may exacerbate the dystonia. Attention to weight and nutrition is important in hyperkinetic patients because they may be hypermetabolic and use an unexpectedly large amount of calories and fluids. If swallowing is affected by either hypokinesia or hyperkinesia, attention must be directed to proper nutrition. In some patients with advanced diseases, feeding tubes are required.

—Esther Cubo and Christopher G. Goetz

See also–Akinesia; Basal Ganglia, Diseases of; Dyskinesias; Gilles de la Tourette's Syndrome; Huntington's Disease; Motor System, Overview; Parkinson's Disease; Tremors

Further Reading

Brooks, D. J. (1995). The role of the basal ganglia in motor control. Contributions from PET. *J. Neurol. Sci.* **128**, 1–13.

Fahn, S. (1998). Hypokinesia and hyperkinesia. In *Parkinson's Disease and Movement Disorders* (J. Jankovic and E. Tolosa, Eds.), pp. 267–284. Lippincott Williams & Wilkins, Baltimore.

Levy, R., Hazrati, L. N. G., and Herrero, M. T. (1997). Reevaluation of the functional anatomy of the basal ganglia in normal and parkinsonian states. *Neuroscience* **76**, 335–343.

Mercuri, N. B., Calabresi, P., and Bernardi, G. (1996). Basal ganglia disorders. An electrophysiologic approach. *Adv. Neurol.* **69**, 117–121.

Parent, A., and Hazrati, L. N. (1995). Functional anatomy of the basal ganglia. The cortico-basal-ganglia-thalamo-cortical loop. *Brain Res.* **20**, 91–127.

Weeks, R. A., and Brooks, D. J. (1994). Positron emission tomography and central neurotransmitter systems in movement disorders. *Fundam. Clin. Pharmacol.* **8**, 503–517.

Moyamoya Disease

Encyclopedia of the Neurological Sciences
Copyright 2003, Elsevier Science (USA). All rights reserved.

MOYAMOYA DISEASE is named for its classic angiographic appearance—likened to a "puff of smoke"—produced when an injected contrast agent passes through enlarged collateral blood vessels at the base of the skull. This collateral blood flow is established in response to progressive stenosis of the internal carotid artery (ICA) as it passes through and above the skull base. The cause of the disease is unknown. The entity has also been referred to as basal telangiectasia, cerebral artery rete, idiopathic progressive arteriopathy of childhood, and basal cerebral mirabile.

Most of the literature on moyamoya disease originates from Japan, which has the highest incidence of the disease. There, it is believed to affect approximately 1/100,000 persons annually. There is a juvenile peak of occurrence below the age of 10 years; an adult peak occurs in the second and third decades of life. Moyamoya disease most often affects women. Although its etiology remains elusive, other conditions may be associated with it: cerebral aneurysms, arteriovenous malformations, fibromuscular dysplasia, Down's syndrome, neurofibromatosis, syndactylia, primitive trigeminal arteries, immune deficiency, pulmonary hypertension, Shy–Drager syndrome, renovascular hypertension, polycystic kidney disease, tuberosclerosis, retinitis pigmentosa, pseudoxanthoma elasticum, and Fanconi's anemia. It also follows radiation treatment for skull base tumors.

Microscopic examination of the involved arteries shows enlargement of the cells lining the lumen of the vessel, but arteritis or atheromatous plaque is absent. The vessels through which collateral blood flow develops show no characteristic pathological changes compared to normal vessels.

Typically, juvenile patients become symptomatic with transient neurological deficits, such as arm and leg weakness on one side of the body. Other presentations include seizures, headache, abnormal mental development, and visual defects. The severity of the disease in juveniles is believed to be inversely related to the age of onset. Adult onset usually involves hemorrhage into the brain. Aneurysmal dilations or weakening of blood vessels are thought to cause the hemorrhage.

Moyamoya disease can be diagnosed with magnetic resonance (MR) imaging and MR angiography, but conventional cerebral angiography is the gold standard. The latter typically shows bilateral stenosis and/or occlusion of the intracranial ICA after it enters the skull, with dilation of collateral blood vessels coursing through the brain. The findings can include collateral blood flow from the external carotid artery (ECA).

Contemporary treatment includes medical therapy and surgical treatment to increase blood flow distal to the narrowed portion of the ICA. Medications include steroids, vitamin C, antiplatelet agents, antiepileptics, and calcium-channel blockers. The best surgical treatment is controversial. Superficial temporal artery-to-middle cerebral artery bypass (extracranial-to-intracranial) has been performed with success in patients with focal ischemia.

There are several variations in the technical aspects of the distal portion of the bypass. Some surgeons perform a direct bypass, opening the recipient artery and suturing the donor vessel to provide immediate blood flow. A disadvantage of this approach is that the brain, supplied by the recipient vessel, lacks blood flow during the procedure because it must be interrupted to suture the vessels. Other techniques do not interrupt blood flow. Encephalomyosynangiosis is a treatment that applies muscle with an intact blood supply to the surface of the brain and thereby facilitates the flow of collateral blood from the ECA. Some concerns have been raised that these techniques have the potential to induce seizures. Yet another technique involves suturing a scalp artery (superficial temporal artery) to the brain adjacent to a blood vessel.

The death rate for the pediatric form of moyamoya is approximately 3%. The adult form has a worse prognosis, with a mortality rate of approximately 11%. In both groups, death is usually caused by intracranial hemorrhage. Although it is believed that ischemic manifestations are addressed by revascularization procedures, whether these techniques lower the chance of subsequent hemorrhage is controversial.
—*Paul W. Detwiler, Randall W. Porter, and Robert F. Spetzler*

See also–Angiography, Cerebral; Carotid Artery; Revascularization, Cerebral; Stenosis

Further Reading
Karasawa, J., Kikuchi, H., Furuse, S., *et al.* (1978). Treatment of moyamoya disease with STA-MCA anastomosis. *J. Neurosurg.* 49, 679–688.
Maki, Y., and Enomoto, T. (1988). Moyamoya disease. *Childs Nerv. Syst.* 4, 204–212.

Mucopolysaccharidoses

Encyclopedia of the Neurological Sciences
Copyright 2003, Elsevier Science (USA). All rights reserved.

IN 1917, HUNTER described two brothers with clinical symptoms and signs of the X-linked form of the mucopolysaccharidoses. In 1919, Hurler described clinical findings of a disease in two unrelated boys with similar characteristics as the cases of Hunter but with autosomal recessive mode of inheritance. The term mucopolysaccharidosis was given to this group of diseases upon discovery of excessive amounts of mucopolysaccharides (glycosaminoglycans) in the tissues and urine. The idea that the mucopolysaccharidoses were caused by defects of lysosomal hydrolases was proposed in 1964 by van Hoof and Hers. The first hydrolase, α-L-iduronidase, deficient in Hurler's disease, was described by Matalon and Dorfman in 1972. This discovery was followed by the identification of all the hydrolases deficient in the mucopolysaccharidoses.

MANIFESTATION OF THE MUCOPOLYSACCHARIDOSES

The mucopolysaccharidoses diseases are inherited as autosomal recessive conditions with the exception of Hunter's disease, which is X-linked recessive. Each disease is caused by a different enzyme deficiency and there is a spectrum of severity. As a group, the clinical findings include coarse facial features, chronic rhinorrhea, and the joints are stiff in most patients. Some patients have corneal clouding and vision problems. The main feature of these storage diseases is hepatosplenomegaly where the glycosaminoglycans are stored within lysosomes.

The mucopolysaccharidoses have characteristic skeletal findings that on radiographs are referred to as dysostosis multiplex. These characteristics include a large, dolicocephalic-shaped skull; a thickened calvarium with hyperostosis of the cranium; a large, boot-shaped sella tursica; thickened clavicles, especially in the midportion; and ovoid vertebral bodies with beak-like projections. The ribs are flared distally and the iliac bones have shallow acetabulae and hip deformities. The head of the femur has features similar to aseptic necrosis. The hands show tapering of the terminal phalanges and tapering of the proximal ends of the metacarpals. The long bones show cortical thinning, and the distal end of the radius curves toward the ulna.

HURLER'S DISEASE

Hurler's disease, caused by α-L-iduronidase deficiency, leads to the accumulation of dermatan sulfate and heparan sulfate and urinary excretion of these glycosaminoglycans. The infant with Hurler's disease

appears normal at birth, but after 6 months coarse facial appearance can be noted. Hepatosplenomegaly can be detected, and umbilical and inguinal hernias may appear. Chronic rhinorrhea may suggest frequent colds or allergies. Recurrent upper airway infection, otitis media, and hypertrophy of tonsils and adenoids may persist beyond early childhood. Hearing impairment may be secondary to such events. When these children attempt to sit, very mild kyphosis can be noticed, which will progress as the child grows older to the gibbus appearance, typical of Hurler's disease. Vision is impaired because of clouding of the corneas that can be detected in the first year of life. Children with Hurler's disease may sit, walk, and develop early language skills, but soon these skills are lost. Severe mental retardation becomes apparent, and affected children become bedridden (Fig. 1).

HURLER–SCHEIE SYNDROME

Prior to the discovery of iduronidase, patients with Hurler–Scheie syndrome were thought to have a

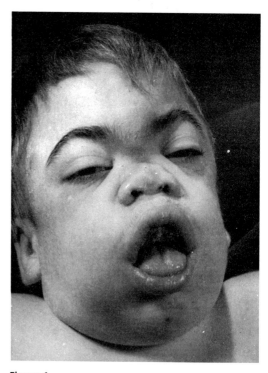

Figure 1
A 3-year-old boy with Hurler's disease. Note the coarse facial appearance, prominent glabella, depressed nasal bridge, chronic rhinorrhea, gingival hypertrophy, and severe mental retardation. He also had corneal clouding.

different disease. Iduronidase deficiency in these patients, however, is milder than in Hurler's disease. Patients have severe joint limitations, small stature, hepatosplenomegaly, and corneal clouding but are not mentally impaired. The glycosaminoglycans in urine is composed primarily of dermatan sulfate. These patients live longer than those with Hurler's disease and as adults may develop cardiac disease, such as aortic regurgitation or mitral insufficiency, to which they may succumb.

SCHEIE SYNDROME

This is the mildest form of iduronidase deficiency, with urinary excretion of dermatan sulfate. Such individuals usually attain normal height and have mild hepatosplenomegaly. The stiffness of joints may not be recognized early in life because these children are not retarded and they do not have coarse features. The dysostosis multiplex is very mild. These patients may present to the physician due to carpal tunnel syndrome or joint stiffness. More commonly, ocular involvement such as corneal clouding and retinal degeneration may lead to the suspicion of a mucopolysaccharide disorder. Usually, the diagnosis is not made before age 10 years and frequently not until after age 20 years.

The gene for α-L-iduronidase has been localized to the short arm of chromosome 4 (4p16.3), in close proximity to the Huntington gene. Mutation analysis indicates that a common allele leading to Hurler's disease is the substitution of the amino acid tryptophan to a stop codon (Trp$_{402}$→Ter). Other mutations are associated with severe or milder phenotypes.

HUNTER'S SYNDROME

The diagnosis of Hunter's syndrome is confirmed by iduronosulfatase deficiency with urinary excretion of dermatan and heparan sulfate. Hunter's syndrome is the only X-linked recessive disease among the mucopolysaccharidoses. Phenotypically, there are two forms of Hunter's syndrome: one with mental retardation and one with no retardation. This disease also has a spectrum of severity of clinical manifestations. The facial features in both forms are similar, with slightly less coarseness in the form without mental retardation. In general, children with Hunter's syndrome look similar to patients with Hurler's disease, with a few exceptions. The corneas are not involved in Hunter's syndrome and hearing rapidly deteriorates. The gibbus in patients with Hunter's syndrome is usually very mild, and patients have skin rash over the arms, shoulders, and thighs. Patients without mental retardation develop severe hearing problems, carpal tunnel syndrome, and progressive upper airway obstruction. Death may occur from upper airway obstruction and heart failure. Some patients with Hunter's syndrome have survived beyond the fifth or sixth decade of life.

The gene for iduronosulfatase has been localized to the Xq28 region close to the fragile X site. Southern blot analysis of genomic DNA from Hunter patients suggests that a significant number of patients have gross deletions in the iduronosulfatase gene. Patients with complete deletion, partial deletion, or gross rearrangements of the gene all have the severe phenotype. Other mutations are associated with Hunter's syndrome without mental retardation.

SANFILIPPO SYNDROMES

There are four types of Sanfilippo syndrome, all of which include mild dysostosis multiplex, mild coarse facial features, and mild hepatosplenomegaly. As children with this disease grow older, the liver and spleen may be only slightly enlarged and hepatosplenomegaly can be missed. Hyperactivity, speech delay, and frank mental retardation are symptoms of this syndrome. By the end of the first decade, patients undergo rapid neurological deterioration and become bedridden, and they die in their middle teens. Few Sanfilippo patients live beyond the second decade.

The mucopolysacchariduria is characterized by increased levels of heparan sulfate. Enzyme assays must be performed to determine the type of Sanfilippo syndrome. Sanfilippo A is the most common, with deficiency of sulfamidase. Sanfilippo B syndrome is second most common, and the enzyme deficiency in this syndrome is α-N-acetylhexosaminidase. Sanfilippo C is probably the mildest of the Sanfilippo syndromes, and the enzyme defect is acetyl-CoA:α-glucosamide N-acetyltransferase. Sanfilippo D is the rarest of the Sanfilippo syndromes, with deficiency of N-acetylglucosamine-6-sulfate sulfatase. Sanfilippo D patients excrete not only heparan sulfate but also N-acetylglucosamine-6-sulfate.

The gene for sulfamidase (Sanfilippo A) has been cloned and localized to the long arm of chromosome 17 (17q25.3). The most common mutation among those of European ancestry is ARG$_{245}$→HIS. Other mutations have been detected among other ethnic groups. The common mutation $Arg_{245} \rightarrow His$ has been described in the Cayman Islands, indicating a founding father effect in a genetic isolate.

The gene for α-N-acetylglucosaminidase deficiency (Sanfilippo B) has been isolated and localized to chromosome 17q21. Some mutations have been identified, but there is no predominant mutation. The gene for acetyl-CoA:α-glucosaminide N-acetyl-transferase (Sanfilippo C) has not been cloned. The gene for N-acetylglucosamine-6-sulfatase (Sanfilippo D) has been cloned and localized to the long arm of chromosome 12 (12q14).

MORQUIO SYNDROME

There are two types of Morquio disease: type A, caused by deficiency of N-acetylgalactosamine-6-sulfate sulfatase, and type B, caused by deficiency of β-galactosidase. Patients with type A have enamel hypoplasia, whereas those with type B usually lack enamel hypoplasia. In both types, there is skeletal dysplasia and keratan sulfaturia. The skeletal dysplasia is often severe, but mild forms of Morquio syndrome have been observed. Patients with Morquio syndrome usually lack mental impairment, but there is joint laxity, shortness of stature, and pectus carinatum. Skeletal abnormalities include shortened vertebrae (platyspondyly universalis), short neck, genu valgum, pes planus, and large joints. There is usually midfacial hypoplasia and protrusion of the mandible, which makes these children appear as if they have a permanent grin. The neck is short, and there is underdevelopment of the odontoid process of the cervical spine that may lead to atlantoaxis subluxation. Corneal clouding is present in 50% of cases. Hepatomegaly may be present, but it is not as prominent as in the other mucopolysaccharidoses. Cardiac involvement includes aortic regurgitation. Tooth enamel is severely affected and is usually very thin. Patients with Morquio syndrome usually survive until middle age. Because of the pectus carinatum and kyphoscoliosis, however, cor pulmonale may develop.

The gene for galactosamine-6-sulfate sulfatase (Morquio type A) has been cloned and localized to the long arm of chromosome 16 (16q24.3). More than 100 mutations have been reported in Morquio type A patients. The gene for β-galactosidase (Morquio type B) has been cloned and assigned to the short arm of chromosome 3 (3p21.33), and several point mutations have been reported.

MAROTEAUX–LAMY SYNDROME

Maroteaux–Lamy syndrome is caused by deficiency of N-acetylgalactosamine-4-sulfate sulfatase (arylsulfatase B), with urinary excretion of dermatan sulfate. The clinical features are similar to those of Hurler's disease but without mental retardation. Maroteaux–Lamy syndrome also has a spectrum of severity of clinical manifestations; in the severe form of the disease, children die from constricted chest and upper airway obstruction.

The gene for N-acetylgalactosamine-4-sulfatase (arylsulfatase B) has been cloned and localized to chromosome 5 (5q13–5q14). Mutations have been identified that cause severe, moderate, and mild forms of Maroteaux–Lamy syndrome, so genotype and phenotype may be correlated.

β-GLUCURONIDASE DEFICIENCY

β-Glucuronidase deficiency (Sly disease) has a spectrum of clinical manifestations with mild and severe forms. Often, these patients cannot be distinguished from patients with Hurler's disease. The coarse facial features are usually milder, and the gibbus formation is not as pronounced. The mucopolysacchariduria consists mainly of chondroitin-4/6-sulfate.

The gene for β-glucuronidase has been cloned and localized to the long arm of chromosome 7 (7q 21.11). A variety of mutations have been identified, including two resulting in hydrops fetalis.

TREATMENT

Symptomatic treatment is needed to relieve hydrocephalus, cardiac disease, corneal clouding, and upper airway obstruction. Medication for hyperactivity can be helpful. An experimental treatment using bone marrow transplantation, reported by Hobbs et al. in 1981, resulted in improvement of the coarse facial appearance, corneal clouding, hepatosplenomegaly, and mucopolysacchariduria. The mental function of these patients also seemed to improved. Subsequent bone marrow transplantation studies performed on a larger scale in the United States support the earlier findings of Hobbs. It seems that the best results can be obtained when bone marrow therapy is done early in life before patients' intelligence deteriorates. Unfortunately, bone marrow therapy has not been successful in patients with Sanfilippo syndrome or Hunter's or Morquio diseases. Enzyme replacement therapy has been attempted in a mild form of iduronidase deficiency, mostly Hurler–Scheie syndrome, and the treatment has been effective in reducing mucopolysacchariduria and hepatosplenomegaly, but the skeletal tissues have not shown improvement with this treatment method. Clinical trials are under way. Experiments with gene therapy have not reached human clinical trials. Animal studies have been used for this type of therapy and for early stem cell treatment.

—*Reuben Matalon and Kimberlee Michals Matalon*

***See also*–Lysosomal Storage Disorders**

Further Reading

Matalon, R. (1983). In *Musculoskeletal Diseases of Children* (M. E. Gershwin and D. L. . Robbins, Eds.), pp. 381–445. Grune & Stratton, New York.

Matalon, R., and Michals-Matalon, K. (2002). In *The Molecular and Genetic Basis of Neurological Disease* (R. N. Rosenberg, S. B. Prusiner, S. DiMauro, and R. L. Barchi, Eds.), 3rd ed. Butterworth-Heineman, Boston.

Matalon, R., Kaul, R., and Michals, K. (1995). In *Pediatric Neuropathology* (S. Duckett, Ed.), pp. 525–544. Williams & Wilkins, Baltimore.

Neufeld, E. F., and Muenzer, J. (2001). In *The Metabolic and Molecular Bases of Inherited Disease* (C. R. Scriver, A. L. Baudet, W. S. Sly, and D. Valle, Eds.), 8th ed., pp. 3421–3452. McGraw-Hill, New York.

Multiple Sclerosis (MS), Basic Biology

Encyclopedia of the Neurological Sciences
Copyright 2003, Elsevier Science (USA). All rights reserved.

MULTIPLE SCLEROSIS (MS) is a common neurological disease, mainly affecting young adults. The clinical course of the disease is highly variable, but most patients present with relapsing remitting neurological deficit, which at later stages may convert into steady disease progression. Variants of the disease include benign forms, fulminate acute lethal forms, and a primary progressive disease manifestation. Although a strong genetic contribution is evident, this genetic risk is mediated by multiple genes with only moderate individual influence. In addition, an exogenous factor, possibly of infectious origin, seems to contribute to the precipitation of the disease. It is thus likely that MS is a complex chronic disease in which many different pathogenetic factors contribute to its development.

In pathology, MS is defined as a chronic inflammatory disease that is associated with widespread primary demyelination, defined by loss of myelin with relative sparing of axons. However, axons are also affected within the demyelinated lesions and the progressive degeneration and loss of axons is a major correlate of permanent functional deficit. Chronic plaques of MS show pronounced glial scarring, with the demyelinated axons embedded in a dense network of astroglial cell processes. Finally, the lesions may also show signs of spontaneous remyelination, which in some patients results in large confluent remyelinated plaques—the so-called shadow plaques. Although most of these features of MS lesions have been extensively described, only recently have we obtained a better insight into the biological mechanisms that are responsible for their formation.

THE IMMUNOLOGY OF THE INFLAMMATORY PROCESS

The inflammatory infiltrates in MS lesions are mainly composed of T lymphocytes and activated macrophages or microglia cells. Both CD4 and CD8-positive T cells are present within the lesions, and their relative contribution to the inflammatory process is controversial. Although the disease association with certain HLA-DR haplotypes and the close similarity between MS lesions and those in TH1 T cell-mediated autoimmune encephalomyelitis strongly supports a major role of CD4-restricted cells, numerically CD8 cells dominate the lesions in MS and clonal expansion of T cells within the lesions is mainly found within the CD8 T cell population. Thus, class I MHC-restricted T cells may play an important role at least in a subset of MS patients.

The dominant cells within actively demyelinating MS lesions are activated macrophages and microglia cells. These cells are closely attached to myelin sheaths at sites of active myelin destruction and are instrumental in the uptake and degradation of myelin fragments. In addition, the density of activated macrophages within the lesions is the best correlate of acute axonal injury in demyelinated plaques.

This T cell and macrophage-dominated inflammatory reaction is also reflected by the local expression of respective cytokines, adhesion molecules, chemokines, MHC class I and II molecules, and costimulatory molecules, which is most prominent in acutely demyelinating lesions but also present in chronic plaques without recent demyelinating activity. A plethora of different pro- and anti-inflammatory cytokines is present within the lesions, and studies on the lesional level have not revealed clear stage-dependent expression patterns. However, studies of cytokine levels in sera and cerebrospinal fluid (CSF) of MS patients suggest that proinflammatory TH1 cytokines dominate in active exacerbations, whereas TH2 and immunoregulatory cytokines are more prominent during remission of the disease.

Thus, the inflammatory response in MS is consistent with a chronic T cell-mediated immunological process mediated by both CD4 and CD8 T lymphocytes expressing a TH1-like cytokine response. However, there are exceptions to this rule. In fulminate acute MS, particularly in Devic's neuromyelitis optica, extensive deposition of immunoglobulins (both IgG and IgM) and activated complement components are present at sites of active myelin destruction. This is associated with a pronounced infiltration of the lesions by granulocytes and even eosinophils. This raises the possibility that in a subset of MS cases additional TH2 T cell responses may contribute to the formation of the lesions and may potentiate tissue damage. Obviously, this has profound consequences for the design of immunomodulatory therapies.

RELATION BETWEEN INFLAMMATION AND DEMYELINATION OR TISSUE DAMAGE IN MS

Active demyelination as well as acute axonal injury in MS invariably occur in the background of the previously described inflammatory response. However, there is not a simple relation between inflammation and demyelination or tissue damage. The degree of inflammation at very early stages of demyelination is frequently very mild in comparison to that present at later stages of lesion formation or even in inactive lesions. In addition, inflammation in MS brains is a widespread process that is not restricted to areas of active demyelination. Thus, particularly in chronic MS, profound inflammation is also present in inactive lesions, the periplaque white matter, the normal white matter far distant from plaques, and the gray matter as well as in areas that are completely devoid of myelin, such as the peripheral retina. Obviously, this widespread and diffuse inflammation in the brain may contribute to the diffuse changes in the normal white matter, observed in MRI studies, and it may also lead to

progressive tissue damage in plaques or the so-called "normal" white matter, even at stages in which the formation of new demyelinated plaques has ceased. Alternatively, this widespread inflammatory reaction may also contribute to remyelination and repair through leukocyte secretion of neurotrophic factors, such as nerve growth factor or brain-derived neurotrophic factor.

PATTERNS AND MECHANISMS OF DEMYELINATION

The hallmark of MS pathology is primary demyelination with relative sparing of axons. The demyelination occurs in a segmental manner. Thus, in established plaques myelin sheaths terminate at a node of Ranvier and the axon can be traced devoid of myelin into the lesion. It is clearly established that removal of myelin from the axons and its degradation are accomplished by activated macrophages. The events that initiate demyelination appear to be heterogeneous between different MS patients.

A recent investigation of a large sample of actively demyelinating MS lesions, mainly from patients in the early stages of the disease, revealed four distinctly different patterns of myelin destruction, which all occurred in the background of the previously described chronic inflammatory process. In the first pattern, demyelination occurred in areas with massive infiltration of activated macrophages, but there was no further indication of involvement of antibodies or complement and no signs of oligodendrocyte dystrophy. This pattern is closely reflected in some mouse models of T cell-mediated autoimmune encephalomyelitis. The second pattern showed a similar T cell and macrophage-dominated inflammatory reaction. At the site of active demyelination, however, the disintegrating myelin sheaths were coated by massive deposition of immunoglobulins and activated complement components. A similar pattern of demyelination has been shown in models of autoimmune encephalomyelitis, which are induced by a synergistic action of T cell-mediated inflammation and demyelinating antibodies. The third pattern of demyelination was characterized by changes of myelin protein expression and oligodendrocyte apoptosis. In particular, a selective loss of myelin-associated glycoprotein and an enhanced expression of myelin oligodendrocyte glycoprotein are characteristic features of these lesions. Such lesions have never been found in models of autoimmune encephalomyelitis, but they are prominent in human virus-induced diseases of the white matter. The fourth pattern of demyelination, which has only been found in a small subset of patients with primary progressive MS, revealed degeneration and DNA fragmentation of oligodendrocytes in a small rim of periplaque white matter, closely adjacent to the site of active myelin breakdown. This pattern, which has not been seen in any experimental model or any other human white matter disease, suggests a primary oligodendrocyte degeneration followed by demyelination.

With the exception of the last pattern, there is little correlation between these patterns of pathology and the clinical course or variant of the disease. However, some pathological subtypes are strictly related to these patterns of demyelination. Thus, all cases with Devic's neuromyelitis optica follow the pattern of antibody and complement deposition (the second pattern). On the contrary, concentric lesions of Balo's sclerosis are always associated with loss of myelin-associated glycoprotein and oligodendrocyte apoptosis at sites of active myelin destruction (the third pattern).

These studies further show that the mechanisms of demyelination are different among MS patients but are uniform within multiple lesions occurring at the same time in a single MS patient. This could mean either a true interindividual heterogeneity of MS or that the disease may be initiated through different starter lesions, which later in the course of the disease may converge into a more common pattern of autoimmunity. These possibilities will have to be clarified in future prospective clinicopathological studies.

THE FATE OF OLIGODENDROCYTES AND REMYELINATION

A reduction of oligodendrocyte density is found in all demyelinating MS lesions. The extent of oligodendrocyte loss, however, is highly variable between different lesions, particularly between lesions of different patients. It at least in part depends on the mechanisms of demyelination discussed previously. Thus, when demyelination occurs secondarily to oligodendrocyte dystrophy, oligodendrocytes are lost to a greater extent compared to lesions with antibody and/or macrophage-mediated demyelination. A similar heterogeneity is also noted in the degree of remyelination. In some MS patients, during the early stages of the disease, remyelination can be extensive and large shadow plaques are common. In contrast, in patients with long-standing disease shadow

plaques are infrequent, and remyelination in these cases is mainly restricted to a small rim at the periphery of the plaques.

The source of remyelinating oligodendrocytes in MS lesions is a matter of debate. They may be derived from undifferentiated progenitor cells, which seem to be abundant within the normal central nervous system tissue as well as in demyelinated MS plaques and may increase in number in demyelinating lesions. Alternatively, remyelinating cells could also be derived from mature oligodendrocytes that have escaped the destructive process during the acute stage of demyelination. Several explanations have been proposed for the observation that in some MS patients the lesions remyelinate effectively, whereas in others they do not. In the course of repeated demyelinating episodes within the same brain area, the pool of progenitor cells, necessary for generating remyelinating oligodendrocytes, can be exhausted. On the other hand, oligodendrocytes as well as their progenitors may effectively be destroyed during the phase of acute demyelination. Finally, lack of a proper supply of growth factors or the presence of specific remyelination-inhibiting antibodies or inflammatory mediators may block myelin repair.

AXONAL PATHOLOGY IN MS

Despite inflammation and demyelination being the hallmark of MS lesions, axonal pathology within the lesions is of utmost clinical importance. The functional consequences of both inflammation and demyelination can be reversed by clearance of the inflammatory process, by redistribution of ion channels along demyelinated axons, as well as by remyelination. In contrast, when axons are destroyed within the demyelinated plaques, the functional consequences are irreversible.

Multiple sclerosis is an inflammatory demyelinating disease with relative sparing of axons. However, as noted previously, emphasis must be placed on the term relative. In fact, axons are always injured and destroyed within MS lesions, although to a variable degree. Massive acute axonal injury occurs during the stage of active myelin destruction. The extent of axonal loss and injury correlates well with the density of activated macrophages and CD8[+] T lymphocytes within the actively demyelinating lesions. Thus, at this stage of lesion formation, freshly demyelinated axons seem to be highly susceptible to injury through inflammatory mediators.

In addition to the axonal damage in acute plaques, there is also a chronic, slowly progressive axonal injury and loss in established demyelinated plaques. This too occurs in the background of persistent inflammation but is independent from acute myelin destruction. This progressive axonal injury does not occur in remyelinated shadow plaques, despite a similarly persistent inflammatory reaction. It is not clear whether the low burning axonal destruction in inactive lesions is still accomplished through inflammatory mediators or whether the lack of trophic support of axons through the lack of myelin/oligodendrocyte ensheathment is the main culprit for this destructive process. In clinical terms, this slow axonal degeneration in chronic inactive demyelinated plaques may at least in part explain disease progression in secondary progressive MS that can occur despite the absence of newly developing demyelinating plaques.

CONCLUSION

The basic pattern of pathology that is present in all MS brains is demyelination, which occurs secondarily to a chronic T cell-mediated inflammatory process. The demyelinated axons in part degenerate both during the acute phase of myelin destruction and (in a slowly progressive manner) in inactive chronic lesions. This results in tract degeneration and then profound changes and tissue atrophy far distant from the original lesions. This process is counteracted by a variable degree of remyelination.

This basic scheme is modified by several different factors, resulting in a profound interindividual heterogeneity of the disease. Variable factors include the fine-tuning of the inflammatory reaction, the mechanisms of demyelination, the extent of remyelination and repair, and the degree of axonal destruction. For each of these variables, several different mechanisms may be responsible. This highly complex pathogenetic situation is not surprising in a disease that is controlled by multiple different genes and environmental factors.

—*Hans Lassmann*

See also–Demyelinating Disease, Pathology of; Multiple Sclerosis, Diagnosis; Multiple Sclerosis, Epidemiology; Oligodendrocytes

Further Reading

Becher, B., Prat, A., and Antel, J. P. (2000). Brain immune connection: Immunoregulatory properties of CNS resident cells. *Glia* 29, 293–304.
Gay, F. W., Dryce, T. J., Dick, G. W., *et al.* (1997). The application of multifactorial cluster analysis in the staging of plaques in early multiple sclerosis. Identification and characterization of primary demyelinating lesions. *Brain* 120, 1461–1483.
Keirstead, H. S., and Blakemore, W. F. (1999). The role of oligodendrocytes and oligodendrocyte progenitors in CNS remyelination. *Adv. Exp. Med. Biol.* 468, 183–197.
Kornek, B., and Lassmann, H. (1999). Axonal pathology in multiple sclerosis: A historical note. *Brain Pathol.* 9, 651–656.
Lassmann, H. (1998). Pathology of multiple sclerosis. In *McAlpine's Multiple Sclerosis* (A. Compston, Ed.), 3rd ed., pp. 323–358. Churchill Livingstone, London.
Lucchinetti, C., Brück, W., Parisi, J., *et al.* (1999). A quantitative analysis of oligodendrocytes in multiple sclerosis lesions. A study of 113 cases. *Brain* 122, 2279–2295.
Lucchinetti, C. F., Brück, W., Parisi, J., *et al.* (2000). Heterogeneity of multiple sclerosis lesions: Implications for the pathogenesis of demyelination. *Ann. Neurol.* 47, 707–717.
Trapp, B. D., Peterson, J., Ransohoff, R. M., *et al.* (1998). Axonal transsection in the lesions of multiple sclerosis. *N. Engl. J. Med.* 338, 278–285.

Multiple Sclerosis, Diagnosis

Encyclopedia of the Neurological Sciences

MULTIPLE SCLEROSIS (MS) is primarily a disease of young adults. The mean age of onset is approximately 30 years. Age of onset is slightly younger for females than for males. It is rare for patients to present under the age of 15 or after the age of 50. Most patients have an onset between 25 and 35 years of age. The age of onset is consistent in studies from different areas of the world. MS affects females more than males at a ratio of between 2:1 and 3:1.

The typical onset of a patient younger than 40 years of age begins with subacute attacks of neurological dysfunction with spontaneous remission. Subsequent relapses over time then occur with variable frequency and eventually most patients develop a permanent neurological deficit. At older ages of onset (older than age 40), relapsing and remitting disease is less common and a chronic progressive spinal form of the disease is the most common presentation. Older patients usually present diagnostic problems because of the monosymptomatic nature of their disease. An additional problem is that paraclinical studies such as evoked potentials and magnetic resonance imaging (MRI) both become less specific and reliable with advancing age. Therefore, in older patients, investigation usually must be more extensive than in the typical younger patient with relapsing disease. Recent developments in imaging, particularly the use of MRI, have increased the degree of clinical accuracy in making a diagnosis. MRI has also opened a window on the brain for understanding the evolution of the pathology over time. However, there is no unequivocal diagnostic test for MS and the goal standard for the diagnosis remains a clinical one.

A detailed and painstakingly documented history is of utmost importance. Usually when patients are seen, they do not have a specific neurological deficit, although there may be some neurological findings. Therefore, the history is extremely important, and a careful history is irreplaceable.

HISTORY OF THE DIAGNOSIS OF MULTIPLE SCLEROSIS

The first pathological description for MS was by Ollivier in 1842. However, the clinical diagnosis was made apparent by Charcot, who established the disease as a clinical/pathological entity in 1866. Following Charcot, Bourneville wrote the first monograph on MS that reflected many discussions between Charcot and Bourneville concerning their new observations. MS is also a disease seen most commonly in people of northern European descent. There is a striking geographic variation in frequency. Therefore, when a young female is seen in the clinic setting who is blond haired, blue eyed, and fair skinned, the suspicion for MS must immediately be very high.

TYPICAL INITIAL SYMPTOMS

Sensory Symptoms

More than 50% of patients initially have sensory symptoms at onset (Table 1). Sensory symptoms include numbness, tingling, loss of vision, or a combination of these. The most frequent onset is an abnormal sensation in the distal portion of the limb that gradually spreads proximally over several days. The numbness may then extend across the trunk to involve the opposite side. Symptoms usually reach their maximum extent in the first week. Occasionally, the symptoms can be purely radicular and sometimes painful. The sensory symptoms may not be associated with any functional abnormality of the limbs or bladder, even though they are clearly of spinal cord origin. The majority of such patients with acute sensory symptoms improve spontaneously and the symptoms usually resolve completely. In the Optic Neuritis Treatment Trial (ONTT), in patients who presented with optic neuritis as the first "clear-cut" symptom of MS, a careful history suggested that minor sensory symptoms frequently preceded the optic neuritis. Those minor symptoms were considered nonspecific and nondiagnostic at the time. However, the presence of such symptoms predicts the diagnosis of MS. When MS sensory symptoms begin in a radicular distribution, the lesion is probably an acute one at the sensory root entry zone into the spinal cord or brainstem. In fact, some of these acute radicular sensory syndromes suggest compression of nerve roots. It is not unusual to find an MS patient who has had previous spinal surgery for attempted relief of a suspected root compression syndrome.

One sensory symptom that is very typical of MS is the sensory "useless hand" syndrome. This patient usually has loss of discriminatory sensations, such as vibratory sense, two-point discrimination, and proprioception. The symptoms can become so severe that the hand becomes functionally useless even though there is no actual motor involvement. The sensory useless hand in MS is usually unilateral but

Table 1 INITIAL SYMPTOMS OF MS AND THEIR FREQUENCY

Symptom	Central nervous system site or origin	Frequency (%)
Sensory symptoms (numbness, tingling)	Spinal cord	40
Optic neuritis (visual loss)	Optic nerve	<16
Diplopia (double vision)	Brainstem	<10
Gait disturbance (spasticity and/or ataxia)	Spinal and/or cerebellum	<10
Ataxia of limb (clumsiness and/or intention tremor)	Cerebellum	<5
Bladder symptoms (frequency, urgency, hesitancy or retention and/or incontinence)	Spinal cord	<5
Dementia (cognitive changes)	Cerebral hemisphere	<5
Paroxysmal symptoms (various)	Various	<1

has occasionally been described as bilateral. It can be identified by apparent hand weakness seen when tested with the eyes closed but not seen when the hand is under visual control.

Another typical MS-related symptom is the L'hermitte phenomenon. L'hermitte first described a tingling sensation like an electric current going down the back and legs brought on by flexion of the neck. The symptom was first seen in patients with traumatic diseases of the cervical spinal cord. However, L'hermitte pointed out that the symptom occurred most frequently in patients with MS. It is a frequent symptom in spinal-onset MS patients, and occasionally the symptom can be brought on by any kind of spinal movement. Sometimes, the symptom can become quite distressing and disabling on its own.

Optic Neuritis

A sensory symptom that is of particular importance in the diagnosis of MS is acute loss of vision in one eye. This loss of vision is usually due to retrobulbar neuritis (optic neuritis). Optic neuritis (ON) is very closely associated with MS and is the initial symptom in 16% of patients. It is important to note that in the follow-up of the ONTT, those patients with anterior ON involving papillitis and edema of the retina did not have an increased risk for MS. Anterior ON may be a separate disease since the risk of developing MS in anterior ON patients was much lower than that in the typical retrobulbar neuritis patients. In the adult, retrobulbar neuritis typically affects only one eye, although it can occasionally be bilateral. The typical symptom is a central scotoma that is characterized by visual loss in the central field. In severe retrobulbar neuritis visual loss can be complete.

There is usually associated pain on eye movement that can precede, accompany, or follow the visual loss. The discomfort is usually maximum on eye movement, but there may also be tenderness of the globe. Most patients with ON recover normal functional vision over 6 months. Examination will typically show an afferent pupillary defect (APD) using the swinging light test. Some conservative physicians will not make a diagnosis of ON without an APD.

Careful follow-up of patients with ON has shown that at least 50% will develop MS within 5 years. The risk is highest in females. The interval between the first onset of ON and the second attack allowing diagnosis of clinically definite MS can be as long as 30 years.

An accompanying abnormality with ON is loss of the retinal nerve fiber layer. Approximately one-half of patients with MS will have defects in the retinal nerve fiber layer. Only in the retina can one clinically see the manifestations of axonal loss following acute inflammatory disease.

Acute Partial Transverse Myelopathy

A combination of motor and sensory symptoms occurring in a subacute fashion is very typical for MS. It is rare to have the acute onset of motor symptoms without some accompanying sensory symptoms. Complete inflammatory cord transection with the syndrome of acute transverse myelitis (ATM) is unusual. The risk of developing MS after complete ATM is quite low in comparison to the risk following partial acute transverse myelopathy.

Acute Onset of Brainstem or Cerebellar Syndromes

A less common type of onset, but a very important one, is an acute syndrome involving brainstem or cerebellar dysfunction. Acute brainstem dysfunction can be ataxia alone, but usually there is associated double vision. The typical brainstem onset of MS is due to a bilateral internuclear ophthalmoplegia in which there is bilateral adduction impairment causing horizontal diplopia on lateral gaze in both directions. These patients will typically not have diplopia when the eyes are in primary position but will develop horizontal double vision on lateral gaze in either direction. In the analysis of such diplopia, using a red glass over one eye, it must be remembered that the image from the impaired eye is displaced furthest in the direction of gaze.

When this particular acute symptom is associated with cerebellar ataxia of limb or gait, the diagnosis of MS is very likely. In fact, an acute spontaneously resolving bilateral internuclear ophthalmoplegia is almost pathognomonic for the diagnosis of MS.

Acute Hemispheric Lesions

Less common than spinal cord, brainstem, or optic nerve lesions is the acute onset of a cerebral syndrome with hemisensory loss, hemiparesis, or a combination of the two. Occasionally, MS patients can present with a large hemispheric lesion that causes an acute onset of combined contralateral motosensory symptoms. Most of these patients will eventually recover. Unfortunately, many such patients present with an imaging appearance that suggests an acute malignant brain tumor. Therefore, brain biopsy in this situation is not unusual. An MRI scan in the early course of such patients can sometimes reveal additional lesions as well as the suspected tumor-like lesion, making the diagnosis of MS much more likely and helping to avoid biopsy. If oligoclonal banding is also seen in the cerebrospinal fluid and/or the visual evoked potential is characteristically prolonged, the diagnosis of MS is assured.

CLINICAL PRESENTATIONS

Acute Relapses

As mentioned previously, the typical young adult with MS will initially have attacks of motor and/or sensory disturbance with complete or near complete recovery. More than 70% of MS patients initially have relapses and remissions. However, the factors related to resolution of dysfunction are not well understood. Resolution of inflammation and restoration of conduction are obvious factors. Some patients initially have minimal symptoms that are nonspecific and difficult to interpret. However, at the time of the initial clear-cut relapse, an MRI scan will usually show more than four white matter lesions in patients who are destined to develop clinically definite MS (CDMS) within 5 years.

Chronic Onset of Symptoms

Less common than relapsing onset, some patients (usually older ones) initially have a slow evolution of motor and/or sensory abnormalities. The insidious onset of motosensory spinal cord symptoms, in the absence of a tumor or other evidence of spinal cord injury, is often due to MS presenting in an atypical way. Unfortunately, in these patients with a slow, chronic onset of neurological dysfunction (chronic myelopathy), the prognosis is clearly worse than that in patients with the relapsing form of MS.

Other Unusual but Not Rare Presentations of MS

Other presentations of MS include the following:

• *Pain:* Various radicular or diffuse pain syndromes can occur, such as trigeminal neuralgia.
• *Paroxysmal symptoms:* These symptoms include visual loss, diplopia, dysarthria, general sensory disturbances, weakness, incoordination, and painful tonic spasms.
• *Dementia and various psychiatric syndromes:* Cognitive and behavioral changes are commonly seen in chronic MS but can be the presentation

feature. Dementia in a young adult must be considered as possibly due to MS.
• *Fatigue:* Fatigue is a common symptom in established MS, but it is occasionally seen as the onset symptom.
• *Chorea, seizures, aphasia, hemiopsia, and various autonomic disturbances:* These are rare in MS and difficult to diagnose.

Physical Examination

At the onset of MS, despite persistent symptoms, the physical examination can be completely normal.

Various subtle disturbances of sensory function are common. Hyperactive deep tendon reflexes especially with asymmetries and extensor plantar responses are a convincing sign of corticospinal tract damage. The asymmetry may actually be the opposite of that indicated by the patient's symptoms. Occasionally, a deep tendon reflex will be lost. A single lost deep tendon reflex (presumably due to a dorsal root entry zone lesion) in a patient with otherwise generalized hyper-reflexia both above and below the lost reflex is highly suggestive of MS. Abdominal reflexes usually are lost, but this sign is nonspecific and not very helpful.

The most subtle physical examination abnormality may be loss of smooth pursuit on lateral eye movements. This finding might be missed if one examines pursuit movements either too fast or too slowly. Nystagmus is also quite common. Another subtle finding of internuclear ophthalmoplegia is a delay in adduction when combined with nystagmus that is greatest in the abducting eye. Unusual and atypical features that can occasionally be seen include amyotrophy.

When focal muscle wasting is seen, one must be very careful to ensure that an entrapment neuropathy, such as an ulnar entrapment, is not the cause of the muscle wasting. Amyotrophy in the hand is usually seen in more advanced patients. However, amyotrophies can occasionally be seen as part of the initial presentation. Facial myokymia can also be seen. It is usually seen in more advanced patients, but it can be seen early. Although quite alarming to the patient, it is a benign finding. Myokymia can occasionally be associated with hemifacial spasms and facial nerve palsies.

Table 2 lists the important conditions to be ruled out in the differential diagnosis of MS. Note that many MS patients have an abnormal antinuclear antibody test; therefore, distinguishing between lupus and MS may be difficult.

Table 2   DIFFERENTIAL DIAGNOSIS OF MS: CONDITIONS THAT MIMIC MS BY SIMILAR SYMPTOMS WITH DISSEMINATION IN TIME/SPACE[a]

Condition	Tend to disseminate in time	Tend to disseminate in space	Comments
Multiple cerebral emboli	+	+	Usually seen in patients with a known source of embolus
Cardiolipin antibody (CLA)	+	+	Serology can detect the CLA
Cerebral vasculitis	+	+	Usually seen in patients with other autoimmune diseases
Acute disseminated encephalomyelitis (ADEM)	−	+	ADEM can look just like MS–only time will distinguish the difference with clear-cut dissemination in time
Hypertensive cerebrovascular disease (CVD)	+	+	Prolonged hypertension is unusual in MS; cerebrospinal fluid and visual evoked potential will be normal in CVD; CVD is also usually seen in older patients
Cerebral lymphoma	+	+	CSF will not show oligoclonal banding (OB)
Lupus erythemotosus	+	+	CSF will not show OB

[a]There are many other disorders with multifocal central nervous system disease with lesions that may seem to develop clinically at different times (e.g., syphilis, AIDS, hereditary spastic paraplegia, spinocerebellar degenerations, and vitamin B_{12} deficience). These disorders have been mistaken for MS both clinically and electrophysiologically.

Prognosis Based on Early Symptoms and Findings

There are some initial symptoms in MS that carry a relatively poor prognosis (Table 3). For example, the chronic onset of nonresolving motor symptoms, especially in an older male, is a poor prognostic sign. The early onset of a permanent neurological deficit, especially ataxia of limb, is a poor prognostic sign. In contrast, young females with resolving sensory symptoms tend to have a relatively good prognosis.

USE OF PARACLINICAL STUDIES

Dissemination in Space

Evoked potentials were developed in the 1960s as a way of measuring neurological function in demyelinated fibers. The pattern evoked potential is very important in helping to establish optic nerve dysfunction. It is particularly helpful in young adults with neurological symptoms suggesting spinal, brainstem, or cerebellar lesions to demonstrate asymptomatic lesions in the optic nerve in support of the concept of dissemination in space. The typical abnormality in the visual evoked potential is a delay in the latency of the P100 impulse. When such a delay is seen in one eye of a young adult presenting with an acutely evolving spinal cord syndrome, the diagnosis of MS is very likely. If oligoclonal banding is present, a diagnosis of laboratory-supported definite MS can be made. Somatosensory evoked potentials have also been helpful in the same way but are not nearly as specific for MS as are unilateral abnormal visual evoked potentials.

Evoked potentials, which can show evidence for demyelination in central nervous system tracts, can also be used as evidence for dissemination in space. For example, if a patient with ON can be shown to have abnormal spinal cord somatosensory evoked potentials, then the concept of dissemination in space would be supported. In contrast, if a patient presents with spinal cord symptoms and signs and there is an abnormal visual evoked potential, dissemination in space would then also be confirmed.

Table 3   EARLY PROGNOSTIC VARIABLES IN MS

Variable	Those with a relatively poor prognosis	Those with a relatively good prognosis
Sex	Male	Female
Age	Older	Younger
Type of onset	Chronic nonremitting	Acute remitting
System involved	Motor and coordination	Sensory
Number of relapses in the first 2 years	Many	Few
Number of lesions on the diagnostic MRI scan	Many	Few

In the 1980s, MRI became available and revolutionized the ability to show dissemination in space. MRI has an exquisite sensitivity for revealing MS lesions. A number of studies have shown very clearly that there are multiple preexisting asymptomatic MRI lesions present in the majority of patients who will eventually develop CDMS. Studies have shown that at the time of an initial symptom suggestive of MS (an isolated neurological symptom), an abnormal MRI scan (particularly with more than four lesions) is a strong predictor for the development of CDMS within 5 years.

There have been a number of approaches to the MR examination in MS. The most useful approach is to do a proton density/T2 axial and sagittal series of slices. The appearance of oval or flame-like lesions in the white matter above the corpus callosum can be very specific for the diagnosis of MS (Fig. 1). The following characteristics are required to identify a scan as strongly suggestive of MS in a patient younger than the age of 45:

- White matter lesions >3 mm in diameter.
- At least three such lesions, if one is periventricular. Otherwise, four individually identified white matter lesions are required.
- Specificity features that may increase the likelihood of the development of CDMS, are as follows:
- Corpus callosum location
- Oval appearance, particularly in those lesions that appear to be rising off the corpus callosum seen on the parasagittal view
  - Intratentorial location
  - Lesions >6 mm in diameter
  - Enhancement in some but not all of the lesions

Unfortunately, a standard proton density, T2-weighted or FLAIR MR scan cannot distinguish between the various states of abnormal water and pathology in the brain. They are also not able to distinguish between acute and chronic MS lesions. However, if systematic repeated studies are done, new lesions can be seen to develop at an average rate of approximately four per year. When these new lesions develop, they usually appear in an area of previously normal-appearing white matter.

Specific MR techniques are being developed to identify, in life, specific pathological changes in MS (Table 4). Breakdown in the blood–brain barrier is show by gadolinium enhancement, new lesions are easily seen on proton density/T2, FLAIR, or unenhanced T1 scans. Inflammation changes can be

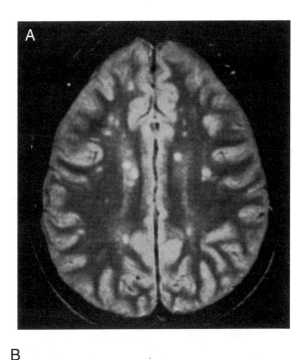

Figure 1
(A) An axial view of proton density showing several typical MS lesions above the level of ventricles. (B) A parasagittal view of proton density showing several lesions above the level of the corpus callosum.

seen by dynamic changes in the size of proton density lesions, active demyelination can be detected by spectroscopy evidence for breakdown products of myelin, and demyelination overall can be detected by evidence of diminished myelin concentration on T2 relaxation studies. Gliosis is perhaps T1 sensitive.

Table 4 MAGNETIC RESONANCE TECHNIQUES HELPFUL IN IDENTIFYING SPECIFIC PATHOLOGIES DURING LIFE

MR technique	Pathology
Gadolinium enhancement on T1-weighted scan	Breakdown of the blood–brain barrier
Proton density, T2-weighted, or FLAIR scan	When found to be new or dynamic, mostly inflammation
	When stable over time contains mixed pathologies
Hypointensities on T1 nonenhanced scan	When acute and dynamic, mostly inflammation
	When chronic, the most severe pathologies including axonal loss
Magnetization transfer imaging	Most severe destructive pathologies
Magnetic resonance spectroscopy	In acute lesions, can detect breakdown products of myelin (neutral fat peaks)
	In both acute and chronic lesions, or normal appearing white matter, N-acetyl aspartate (NAA) reveals axonal injury or loss

Axonal damage or loss can be measured by MR spectroscopy for decrease in N-acetyl aspartate (NAA) concentration. Systematic imaging over time has shown that there is a very dynamic pathological process occurring in MS that does not, for the most part, produce specific neurological symptoms.

Standard diagnostic MRI does not necessarily require the use of gadolinium enhancement. However, gadolinium enhancement, a sign of breakdown in the blood–brain barrier, is generally considered a sign of active inflammation. Therefore, if some but not all lesions seen on proton density enhance at the time of initial symptoms, the lesions may be of a different age, some acute (enhancing) and some chronic (unenhancing), seen at the same time. This finding (supporting the idea that the lesions are of different ages) would confirm dissemination in time as well as dissemination in space. In fact, new diagnostic criteria say that new or enhancing lesions at 3 months after clinical onset will allow the diagnosis of MS.

Figures 2–4 show several of the different kinds of lesions that can be seen in MS. The most practical use of MRI in MS for diagnostic purposes uses a summation of the information to support the concept of dissemination in space and perhaps dissemination in time. Recently, an international group of neurologists and radiologists have proposed a standard protocol for initial and follow-up scans in both suspected and proven cases of MS (see Consortium of MS Centers Web site: http://www.mscare.org).

In clinical practice, it is not unusual to perform a set of appropriate evoked potentials and an MRI scan to support the diagnosis of MS. As with clinical evaluation, it is the pattern with which dissemination in time and space is shown that supports the diagnosis of MS. Clinical judgment that the pattern matches MS is better than a rigid approach to the concept of dissemination. For example, several small strokes due to emboli associated with mitral stenosis and/or anti-cardiolipin antibody can closely mimic MS on MRI with dissemination in time and space.

Evidence for an Immune Response in the Central Nervous System

Immunological evidence for abnormal immune responses in the central nervous system can also be used to support the diagnosis of MS. For example, if

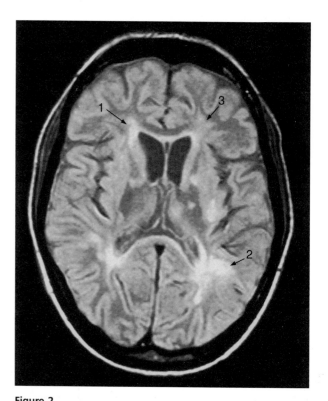

Figure 2

Several lesions are seen on an axial view. Note the subtle lesions indicated by the arrows.

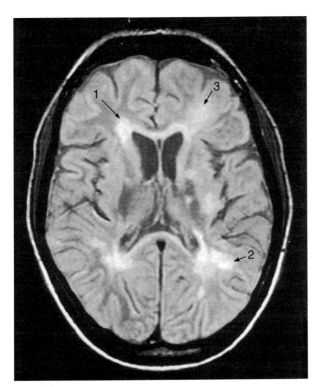

Figure 3
Lesions 1 and 3 have enlarged from 1 month previously (Fig. 2). Lesion 2 has not changed in the interim.

there is clear-cut dissemination in space and the presence of oligoclonal banding in the cerebrospinal fluid, the diagnosis of laboratory-supported definite MS (LSDMS) can be made. Follow-up studies of LSDMS have shown that this diagnostic category is as accurate as an initial diagnosis of CDMS. In addition to cerebrospinal fluid analysis, blood evaluation for circulating cytokines can also be helpful. Elevated levels of tumor necrosis factor, γ-interferon, and other cytokines suggest that an active immune response is occurring.

Caveat

Often, the diagnosis of MS can be a primary one, when all of the criteria are present. However, all diagnostic schemes must have the qualifying statement that the clinical syndrome is not better explained by a process other than MS. Even in the most expert hands, diseases with symptoms similar to those of MS can fool the clinician. Therefore, in the follow-up of patients, even those with a prior diagnosis of CDMS, one must be alert for other conditions with symptoms similar to those of MS.

Recently, a category of magnetic resonance-supported definite MS (MRDMS) has been proposed. A patient with an initial isolated clinical syndrome suggestive of MS and an MRI with the following abnormalities could be diagnosed as MRDMS:

- Four white matter lesions > 3 mm in diameter or three white matter lesions if one is periventricular
- One or more of the following specificity features:
- Nine lesions
- Corpus callosum (CC) and/or oval lesions above the CC
- Infratentorial lesions
- Lesions > 6 mm in diameter
- At least some but not all lesions enhancing

PROGNOSIS BASED ON INFORMATION AVAILABLE AT ONSET

Every patient when first seen and given the diagnosis of MS wants to know what the future will bring. As mentioned previously, in the early stages of relapsing and remitting MS it is very difficult to assign a prognosis. However, the early development of secondary progressive disease is generally a poor prognostic sign. The following are other relatively

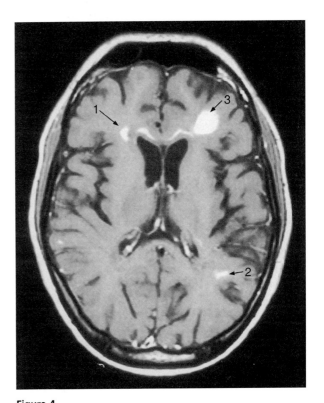

Figure 4
An enhanced scan performed at the same time as Fig. 3. Note that all three lesions enhance as an indication of fresh activity.

poor prognostic signs identifiable early in the course of the disease:

- Incomplete resolution from initial relapses, especially those with many relapses (>5 in 2 years)
- Male sex
- Number and extent of MRI lesions at onset and within the first few years

WHAT TO TELL THE PATIENT CONCERNING THE DIAGNOSIS?

Most patients at the onset want to know as much as possible about their prognosis for conversion to CDMS as well as their prognosis for neurological disability. For many years, it was common neurological practice to "protect" patients from knowledge of the suspicion of MS. Today, it is necessary to provide patients with all the data that are available (full disclosure). However, recent studies have shown that as soon as the diagnosis is communicated to the patient, the quality of life declines (probably due to emotional and social factors rather than neurological ones). Such factors are probably related to the uncertainty and the incurable nature of the disease. Therefore, physicians must be very careful not only to provide patients with factual information but also to provide them with overall education about the disease. Emotional and social adjustment is difficult and patients need both information and support. One must remember that MS is a disease of young adults. Adjustment to a chronic neurological disease is very difficult for young people. MS patients are usually just beginning to develop plans for themselves and their children and are in a stage of life in which the diagnosis of MS can be a very devastating emotional blow.

Today, it is common practice to do an MRI scan in people who have had an initial symptom suggestive of MS. If the MRI scan is clearly abnormal as described previously, it is appropriate to tell the patient of the likelihood of MS. However, it is also appropriate to tell the patient that an accurate prognosis is not going to be available until after several years of follow-up. If the head and spine MRI are normal at onset, patients with an initial symptom suggestive of MS can be reassured with a high degree of certainty that they are not likely to develop MS within 5 years.

Recently, there has been a move toward simplifying the categories in the diagnosis of MS to the following:

I. *Proven MS:* Autopsy proven
II. *MS:* This all-inclusive category includes the following:
- Clinically definite MS
- Laboratory-supported definite MS [possibly included in this category]
- Magnetic resonance-supported definite MS
- Others
III. *Suspected MS:* This category includes what previously had been called
- *Probable MS:* Investigated and supported but not yet considered as MS
- *Patients that cannot meet the criteria noted for MS, including possible MS:* Those patients with symptoms suggestive of MS but where the investigation is negative or has not been done

—*Donald W. Paty*

***See also**–Brainstem Syndromes; Multiple Sclerosis, Basic Biology; Multiple Sclerosis, Epidemiology*

Further Reading

Brex, P. A., Ciccarelli, O., O'Riordan, J. I., et al. (2002). A longitudinal study of abnormalities on MRI and disability from multiple sclerosis. *N. Engl. J. Med.* **345**, 158–164.

Confavreux, C., Aimard, G., and Devic, M. (1980). Course and prognosis of multiple sclerosis assessed by the computerized data processing of 349 patients. *Brain* **103**, 281–300.

Ebers, G. C., and Paty, D. W. (1980). CSF electrophoresis in one thousand patients. *Can. J. Neurol. Sci.* **7**, 275–280.

Fazekas, F., Barkhof, M., Filippi, M., et al. (1999). The contribution of magnetic resonance imaging to the diagnosis of multiple sclerosis. *Neurology* **58**, 448–456.

McDonald, W. I., Compston, A. S., Edan, G., et al. (2001). Recommended diagnostic criteria for multiple sclerosis: Guidelines from the International Panel on the Diagnosis of Multiple Sclerosis. *Ann. Neurol.* **50**, 121–127.

O'Riordon, J. I., Thompson, A. J., Kingsley, D. P. E., et al. (1998). The prognostic value of brain MRI in clinically isolated syndromes of the CNS: A 10-year follow-up. *Brain* **121**, 495–503.

Paty, D. W., and Li, D. K. B. (1999). Diagnosis of multiple sclerosis 1998: Do we need new diagnostic criteria? In *Frontiers in Multiple Sclerosis* (A. Sira, J. Kesselring, and A. Thompson, Eds.), Vol. 2, pp. 47–50. Dunitz, London.

Poser, C. M., Paty, D. W., Scheinberg, L., et al. (1983). New diagnostic criteria for multiple sclerosis: Guidelines for research protocols. *Ann. Neurol.* **13**, 227–231.

Schumacher, G. A., Beebe, G., Kibler, R. F., et al. (1965). Problems of experimental trials of therapy in multiple sclerosis: Report by the panel on the evaluation of experimental trials of therapy in multiple sclerosis. *Ann. N. Y. Acad. Sci.* **122**, 552–568.

Weinshenker, B. G., and Ebers, G. C. (1987). The natural history of multiple sclerosis. *Can. J. Neurol. Sci.* **14**, 255–261.

Weinshenker, B. G., Bass, B., Rice, G. P. A., *et al.* (1987). The natural history of multiple sclerosis: A geographically based study. IV. Applications to planning and interpretation of clinical therapeutic trials. *Brain* **114**, 255–261.

Weinshenker, B. G., Bass, B., Rice, G. P., *et al.* (1989). The natural history of multiple sclerosis: A geographically based study. I. Clinical course and disability. *Brain* **112**, 133–146.

Weinshenker, B. G., Bass, B., Rice, G. P., *et al.* (1989). The natural history of multiple sclerosis: A geographically based study. II. Predictive value of the early clinical course. *Brain* **112**, 1419–1428.

Weinshenker, B. G., Bass, B., Rice, G. P. A., *et al.* (1991). The natural history of multiple sclerosis: A geographically based study. III. Multivariate analysis of predictive factors and models of outcome. *Brain* **114**, 1045–1056.

Multiple Sclerosis, Epidemiology

Encyclopedia of the Neurological Sciences
Copyright 2003, Elsevier Science (USA). All rights reserved.

MULTIPLE SCLEROSIS (MS) is an inflammatory demyelinating disease of the central nervous system. It affects approximately 300,000 persons in the United States and up to 2 million worldwide. MS is the most common progressive neurological disorder of young adults. Despite intensive research efforts during the past century, no specific cause has been identified. Nonetheless, epidemiology has been a powerful tool to help unravel some of the basic determinants of MS and better focus research into its pathophysiology and treatment.

Epidemiology can be defined as the study of the natural history of disease. The epidemiological unit is a person with a diagnosed disorder. The basic question, after diagnosis, is how common is the disease, and this in turn is delineated by measures of the number of cases (numerator) within defined populations (denominator). These ratios, with the addition of the time factor to which they pertain, are referred to as rates.

EPIDEMIOLOGY IN MULTIPLE SCLEROSIS

In virtually all studies of MS we are dealing with a clinical diagnosis without recourse to a pathognomonic diagnostic test or to pathological verification. Several schemes for diagnostic criteria have been put forth, none with universal acceptance.

In almost all of these, there are several grades relating to the degree of confidence in the correctness of the label. If we limit attention to the classes considered the better ones and discard "possible MS" and "uncertain MS," we have defined groups that are quite similar in time and space. Thus, the assessments of morbidity data that follow are based on series of cases variously labeled "definite," "clinically definite," and "probable" MS. The major clinical criteria in current use for a diagnosis of MS are those of Poser and coworkers and Schumacher and colleagues. An earlier categorization still used in some surveys is that of Allison and Millar: probable, early probable or latent, and possible MS.

The relative influences of genes and environment are the backdrops used to explain the population patterns of MS. The geographic distribution of MS has been the subject of many mortality and morbidity surveys as well as the topic of several symposia. Recent overviews of the epidemiology of MS should be consulted for interpretations that may differ, often drastically, from the views presented in this entry.

DISTRIBUTION FROM PREVALENCE SURVEYS

Prevalence studies provide the best information on the distribution of disease but are expensive in terms of money, time, and people. Despite this, there are well over 300 such surveys for MS. Almost all of them have been performed since World War II. To epitomize distributions, prevalence rates of 30 or more per 100,000 were considered high frequency, those of 5–29 were called medium frequency, and rates under 5 per 100,000 were classified as low-frequency MS regions. This trichotomy, made in the early 1960s, still provides a valid overview.

Prevalence in Europe

Prevalence rates for Europe and the Mediterranean basin as of 1980 are shown in Fig. 1, correlated with geographic latitude. The distribution then comprised two clusters, one for high prevalence rates and one for medium rates. Taking only the best studies, the high prevalence zone extended from 44 to 64° north latitude. The medium zone extended from 32 to 47° north, plus two sites (numbers 11 and 12) from the west coast of southern Norway. The only high rate below 44° was that for a small survey of Enna, Sicily

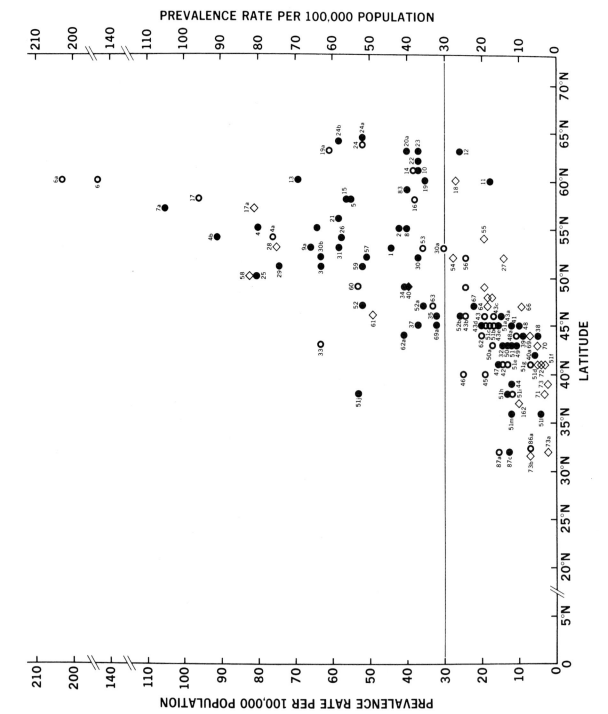

Figure 1

Prevalence rates per 100,000 population as of 1980 for probable MS in Europe and the Mediterranean area, correlated with geographic latitude. Numbers identify studies as indicated in Kurtzke (1980). ●, best (class A) surveys; ○, good (class B); ◇, poor (class C); ◆, estimates from ALS:MS case ratios (class E).

(No. 51j). However, southern Europe and western Norway are now high-frequency regions. Figure 2 shows the recent situation. Both Portugal and Greece are also now high, with prevalence rates in the 40s.

Boiko of Moscow University recently summarized a large literature on the distribution of MS in the former Soviet Union, but his study is still unavailable in the West. Much of northwestern Russia down past Kiev and Moscow appears to be high prevalence, surrounded to the north, east, and south by medium prevalence areas. Overall, the Ukraine and the Caucasus seem to average in the medium range. The Asian part of his work will be discussed later in this entry.

Prevalence in the Americas

Prevalence rates from the Americas as of 1974 are distributed in all three risk zones: high frequency from 37 to 52°, medium frequency from 30 to 33°, and low frequency from 12 to 19° and from 63 to 67° north latitude. The prevalence rates for the northern United States and Canada are quite similar to the high frequency rates of western Europe. Recent works confirm all of Canada and the northern United States as high-frequency regions, with prevalence rates mostly in the range of 60–120.

There were then no studies from South America. There are now several MS ratio estimates for

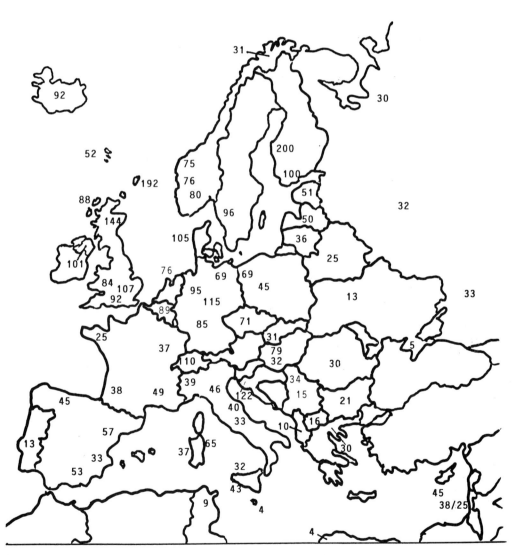

Figure 2
Prevalence rates per 100,000 population for MS in Europe and the Mediterranean area based on publications from 1980 to 1994 (modified with permission from Lauer, 1994).

Argentina and Uruguay and for Lima, Peru, that indicate that these are medium frequency areas. Similar material for Venezuela and Brazil apparently allots these regions to the low-frequency zone. Studies from the 1997 World Congress of Neurology in Argentina provide additional data for Latin America, with evidence that Mexico, Costa Rica, and Cuba are medium prevalence areas.

Prevalence Elsewhere

In general, Australia and New Zealand comprise high prevalence areas for 44° to 34° south latitude and medium frequency for 33° to 13° south. This high zone includes all New Zealand and southeastern Australia with Tasmania.

In Asia and Africa, earlier assessments provided low prevalence rates throughout, except for English-speaking whites of South Africa. Rates are still low in Japan, Korea, China, and Southeast Asia but not in the former Soviet Union.

Boiko indicated that in the southern regions of the Ukraine, the Volga area, the Caucasus, and into Novosibirsk and Kazakhstan, rates were generally in the medium prevalence range, whereas Uzbekistan, Samarkand, Turkistan, and Turkmenistan areas were low. In the Far East, medium prevalence again appeared, and rates were indeed in the high range in the central and western parts of the Amur region, which abuts the Pacific Ocean north of China and includes Vladivostok. In all these areas, rates were higher for Russian-born or those of Russian parentage than for the indigenous population.

The northern African shores of the Mediterranean are now of medium prevalence, and this extends into the Near East, with Israel of high frequency. South Africa is now of medium prevalence for all whites.

Worldwide Distribution

The general worldwide distribution of MS thus seems well described by a division into high prevalence (>30 per 100,000), medium prevalence (5–29 per 100,000), and low prevalence (<5 per 100,000) regions, as proposed years ago. A "super high" class for prevalence of more than, e.g., 90 does not seem to be indicated. Figure 2 shows how scattered such regions would be in Europe. The most recent distribution is shown in Fig. 3.

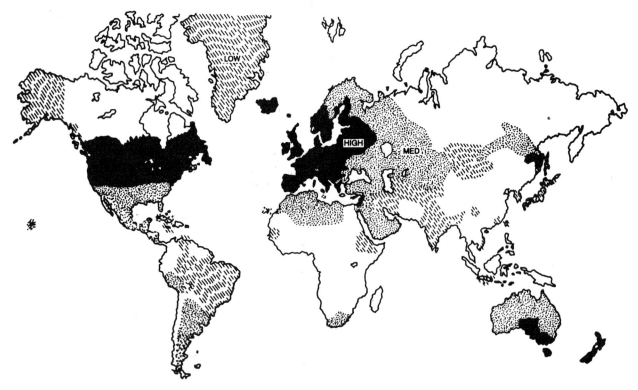

Figure 3
Worldwide distribution of MS as of 1998, with high (prevalence 30+; solid), medium (prevalence 5–29; dotted), and low (prevalence 0–4; dashed) regions defined. Blank areas are regions without data or people (reproduced with permission from Kurtzke and Wallin, 2000).

SEX AND RACE

The prevalence of MS in whites from North America and Europe is more than an order of magnitude greater than that in African blacks and Asians. All the high-risk and medium-risk areas for MS have predominantly white populations. Regardless of residence, in a United States veteran series of 5305 cases matched to preillness military peers, blacks or African Americans had only half the risk of white males (Table 1). Young white females had nearly twice the risk of MS as white males. The group of nonwhites and nonblacks suggested a paucity as well in Native Americans and Asians. An apparent deficit found among Hispanics would seem more a reflection of geography than of race. This is borne out with comparisons by race among foreign-born veterans. Japanese and possible Polynesians from Hawaii were low, as were Filipinos in the Philippines.

Therefore, MS is predominantly a white person's disease. However, it is clear that, where there are good data, the less susceptible racial groups do share the geographic gradients of the whites, with higher frequencies in high-risk areas than in low-risk areas.

SURVIVAL

Survival is a fundamental measure of disease severity. Ideally, it is best measured prospectively from disease onset within a defined population. The study of a male World War II Army hospital cohort showed a 25-year survival after onset of 69%. The survival curves were similar to those observed in a Mayo Clinic study (25-year survival, 74%) and a Lower Saxony study (25-year survival, 63%). Results of our U.S. veteran cohort showing median survival by sex and race ranging from 30 to 43 years are in line with results of other recent incident studies of MS survival.

Regarding risk factors for survival, all studies but one showed that later age of onset and male sex were associated with shorter survivals. Other risk factors that were in agreement across studies and predicted worse survival were early high initial disability scores and progressive disease course.

FAMILY STUDIES AND GENETICS

Family studies in MS have provided a means of assessing environmental factors against a set genetic background. Such studies have shown that the risk for MS is 3 or 4% for primary relatives and 20–30% for monozygotic twins. This is in contrast to the general population prevalence of approximately 0.1%. The increased family frequency might be related to shared environment as opposed to shared genetic factors because close relatives would be expected to share similar environmental influences. However, the following evidence indicates that MS is under some genetic control:

1. Twin studies, most of which show an excess of concordant monozygous twins: The difference in concordance rates between monozygotic and dizygotic twins is primarily attributable to genetic factors.
2. Higher rates in children of MS patients than in adoptees of such patients.
3. The association of human leukocyte antigen (HLA) alleles and MS and the higher frequency of HLA sharing in affected sibling pairs.
4. Population groups relatively resistant to MS in high-frequency areas (Asians and Native Americans in North America, Lapps in Scandinavia, and Gypsies in Hungary)

Although the fourth observation may be true, many of these groups have not been systemically

Table 1   CASE/CONTROL RATIOS BY TIER OF RESIDENCE AT ENTRY INTO ACTIVE DUTY (EAD) FOR MAJOR SEX AND RACE GROUPS[a]

Sex and race	Control ratio by tier of residence at EAD[b]			
	North	Middle	South	Total
White male	1.41	1.02	0.58	1.04
White female	2.77	1.71	0.80	1.86
Black male	0.61	0.59	0.31	0.45
Total	1.41	1.00	0.53	1.00

[a] United States veteran series of 5305 cases of World War II and the Korean Conflict and matched military controls from Kurtzke *et al.* (1979).

[b] States north of 41 or 42° comprised the north tier, and those south of 37° comprised the south tier.

studied and their true risk for MS is not clear. Moreover, these groups not only differ genetically but also have substantially different lifestyles and environmental exposures compared with the majority populations in the countries in which they live. Interestingly, recent population studies in Finland and Jordan have shown two racially similar groups sharing similar geography can have a very different risk for developing MS.

A search for candidate genes has been unrewarding. Evidence from family and genetic studies suggests a complex inheritance pattern. The HLA region was positive in some studies and chromosome 5 was another locus of interest. Nevertheless, no single chromosome locus was clearly identified as a risk factor.

MIGRATION

The fate of migrants who move into regions of differing risk of MS is critical to our understanding of the nature of the disease. If migrants retain the risk of their birthplace, then either the disease is innate or it is acquired early in life. However, if upon moving, their risk does change, then clearly there is a major environmental cause or precipitant active in this disorder. If such altered risk is also dependent on age at migration, we can define not only external cause but also internal (personal) susceptibility. Furthermore, if an age of susceptibility can be delineated in this manner, there may also be found a duration of exposure needed for acquisition and an "incubation" period between acquisition and clinical onset.

There is considerable evidence that migrants' risk for MS does change. In migrants who move from a country of origin in which MS is common to a country in which it is less common, there is a decrease in the rate of disease; the few studies of low to high migration show the reverse effect.

For the veteran series, Table 1 described three geographic tiers for state of residence at entry into military service: a northern tier of states above 41° and 42° north latitude; a middle tier; and a southern tier below 37°, including California from Fresno south. Migrants are those born in one tier who entered service from another tier. In Table 2, the marginal totals provide the ratios for birthplace and residence at service entry for whites of World War II or Korean service. The major diagonal (north–north, middle–middle, and south–south) gives the case–control ratios for nonmigrants, and cells off this diagonal define the ratios for the migrants.

All ratios decrease as one goes from north to south. The nonmigrant ratios are 1.48 north, 1.03 middle, and 0.56 south. For the migrants, those born north and entering service from the middle tier have a ratio of 1.27; if they enter from the south, their ratio is 0.74—half that of the nonmigrants. Birth in the middle tier is marked by an increase in the MS:C ratio for northern entrants to 1.40 and a decrease to 0.73 for the southern ones. Migration after birth in the south increases the ratios to 0.65 (middle) and 0.70 (north). The migrant risk ratios are intermediate between those characteristics of their birthplace and their residence at entry.

In a study of European immigrants to South Africa, the MS prevalence rate, adjusted to a population of all ages, was 13 per 100,000 for immigration younger than age 15, which is the same medium prevalence rate as that for the native-born English-speaking white South Africans. However, for age groups older at immigration, the prevalence was 30–80 per 100,000, the same as expected from their high-risk homelands. This change was major and occurred exactly at age 15. This indicates that natives of high-risk areas are not very susceptible to MS acquisition before age 15 and that there is a long period between acquisition and onset of symptoms.

Table 2   CASE/CONTROL RATIOS FOR ALL WHITE VETERANS OF WORLD WAR II OR THE KOREAN CONFLICT BY TIER OF RESIDENCE AT BIRTH AND AT ENTRY INTO ACTIVE DUTY (EAD)[a]

Birth tier	Control ratio by EAD tier			
	North	Middle	South	Birth total
North	1.48	1.27	0.74	1.44
Middle	1.40	1.03	0.73	1.04
South	0.70	0.65	0.56	0.57
EAD total	1.46	1.03	0.58	1.06

[a] Coterminous United States only (From Kurtzke et al., 1985).

Inferences regarding the opposite migration, low to high, were afforded by north African migrants to France. Among approximately 7500 respondents with known place of birth who had completed a nationwide questionnaire survey for MS in France in 1986, 260 were born in former French North Africa (Morocco, Algeria, and Tunisia). They had migrated to France between 1923 and 1986, but 66% came between 1956 and 1964. Two-thirds were from Algeria, where virtually the entire European population had emigrated in 1962 at the end of the Algerian war for independence. The 225 migrants with onset more than 1 year after immigration presumably acquired MS in France. They had an age-adjusted (U.S. 1960) MS prevalence rate 1.54 higher than that for all of France. If the latter is taken at 50 per 100,000 population, their estimated adjusted rate is 76.8. The other 27 with presumed acquisition in north Africa had an estimated adjusted prevalence of 16.6 per 100,000. For those migrants with acquisition in France, there was a mean interval of 13 years between immigration or age 11 and clinical onset, with a minimum of 3 years. The oldest patient at immigration was the only one to enter France in the fifth decade of life.

EPIDEMICS

In the past, there has been little reason to consider that MS occurred in the form of epidemics. All known geographic areas that had been surveyed at repeated intervals until 1980 provided either stable or increasing prevalence rates, the latter compatible with both better case ascertainment and perhaps improved survival. Epidemics of MS would serve to define the disease as not only an acquired one but also perhaps a transmittable one. We have encountered separate epidemics of MS, which in fact may have common precipitants and which have occurred in the ethnically similar lands of the Faroe Islands, the Shetland–Orkney Islands, and Iceland. The experience in the Faroes is the best studied.

The Faroe Islands are a semiindependent unit of the Kingdom of Denmark located in the North Atlantic Ocean between Iceland and Norway. As of 1999, 54 native nonmigrant resident Faroese had onset of MS in the 20th century. There were none before 1943, but between 1943 and 1949, 17 patients had symptom onset in a populace of less than 30,000. All had been at least 11 years old in 1941 and thus had 2 years "exposure" before first onset. Another 4 were also at least age 11 then; these 21 cases comprise

a type 1 epidemic of clinical MS. Recall that an epidemic may be defined as disease occurrence clearly in excess of normal expectancy and derived from a common or propagated source. Epidemics are divisible into two types: Type 1 epidemics occur in susceptible populations, exposed for the first time to a virulent infectious agent, whereas type 2 epidemics occur in populations within which the virulent organism is already established. If the entire populace is exposed to a type 1 epidemic, the ages of those affected clinically will define the age range of susceptibility to the infection. Type 2 epidemics will tend to have a young age at onset because the effective exposure of the patients will be greatest for those reaching the age of susceptibility.

We found that Faroese migrant MS patients required 2 years' exposure in a high-risk area from age 11 to acquire MS, so the same criteria were applied to the resident Faroese (the 2 years before 1943 being 1941 and 1942). Epidemic I was followed by three later epidemics with peaks at 13-year intervals (Fig. 4), comprising 10, 10, and 13, cases, respectively.

We concluded that the disease was introduced to the Faroes by British troops that had occupied the islands for 5 years beginning in April 1940. We believe that an infection was introduced that was transmitted during the war to the Faroese population at risk, of whom the epidemic I cases of clinical MS were a part. We called this infection the primary MS affection (PMSA), which we defined as a single, specific, widespread, systemic but unknown infectious disease (that might be totally asymptomatic). PMSA produces clinical neurological MS (CNMS) in only a small proportion of the affected after an incubation period averaging 6 years in virgin populations and perhaps 12 years in endemic areas. Using this hypothesis, transmissibility is limited to part or all of the systemic phase, which ends by the usual age of onset of MS symptoms. The PMSA cases from the first cohort of Faroese transmitted the disease to the next Faroese population cohort, those who reached age 11 in the period in which the first cohort was transmissible. Included in the second Faroese cohort were the epidemic II cases of CNMS, and this cohort similarly transmitted PMSA to the third population cohort with its own (epidemic III) cases and from there to the fourth cohort with epidemic IV.

Two years of exposure for those between ages 11 and 47 were required to acquire PMSA in such a virgin but susceptible population. We believe that PMSA is a specific, but unknown, age-limited infection that can

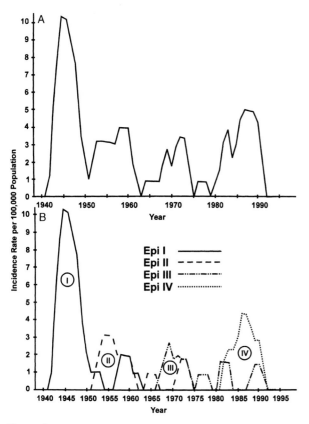

Figure 4
Annual incidence rates per 100,000 population for clinical MS in native resident Faroese, 1998, calculated as 3-year centered moving averages. (A) Total series. (B) Rates for each of four epidemics (reproduced with permission from Kurtzke and Heltberg, 2001).

be acquired only during these hormonally active years and that only rarely leads to clinical MS.

CONCLUSION

The best measures of geographic distribution in MS come from prevalence studies, of which there are currently more than 300. These works indicate that, geographically, MS is distributed throughout the world within three zones of high, medium, and low frequency. High-frequency areas, with prevalence rates of 30 or more per 100,000 population, include most of Europe, Israel, Canada and the northern United States, New Zealand, and southeastern Australia. This also seems to include the easternmost part of Russia.

In MS there is a female preponderance, which appears to be increasing. There is also a clear predilection for whites, but other racial groups share the geographic distributions of the whites but at lower levels. Thus, location, sex, and race are independent risk factors for this disease.

Regarding migration and MS, a number of studies show that migration from high- to low-risk areas in early life results in a decreased risk of MS. A few studies have shown the reverse: Migration from low- to high-risk regions increases one's risk for MS. Migrant studies from high-risk to low-risk areas indicate that the age of adolescence is critical for risk retention: Those migrating when they are older than age 15 retain the MS risk of their birthplace; those migrating when they are younger than age 15 acquire the lower risk of their new residence. Low-to-high-risk migration studies have shown that those migrating from birth to approximately age 45 do in fact increase their risk of MS, but symptoms begin 3 years after age 11 or migration if older. The migrant data support the idea that MS is ordinarily acquired in early adolescence, with a lengthy latent period between disease onset and symptom onset, and young children are not susceptible to this illness. However, susceptibility extends to approximately age 45.

Recent epidemics of MS have been described—one (definite) in the Faroe Islands, the others (probable) in Iceland and the Shetland–Orkneys. We have been able to identify on the Faroe Islands 54 cases of MS among native-born resident nonmigrant Faroese during the 20th century. They comprised four successive epidemics, with peaks at 13-year intervals and with clinical onset for the first patient in 1943. The 21 cases included in the first epidemic met all criteria for a type 1 point-source epidemic. Current evidence regarding a source for the epidemic points to British troops that occupied the Faroes in large numbers for 5 years beginning in April 1940 and that were stationed where the patients lived.

The etiological debate in MS has historically been divided between the contributions of genetics and the environment. The distinction between these opposing views has recently become blurred because many in the field hold that MS is likely related to both nature and nurture. We agree but argue that the environment is the overwhelming driving force in the etiology of MS. First, there is now good evidence for the existence of geographic variations in the United States, Australia, and Europe. Diffusion of high-risk areas over one or two generations has also been reported—a pace too rapid for genetic influences to be effective. Second, studies of migration and the epidemics (Faroes, Iceland, and Shetland–Orkneys) lend further support to an environmental hypothesis.

Opponents cite the observation that MS is rare not only in the Orient but also in the aboriginal populations of Australia and New Zealand and in certain groups in North America and Hungary as evidence that these groups lack genes that confer susceptibility to the disease. Although this may be true, these groups living outside Asia have not been systematically studied and their true risk for MS is not clear. More important, these groups not only differ genetically but also have substantially different lifestyles and environmental exposures compared with populations at high risk of MS. Lastly, because identical twins are discordant for MS 70% of the time, the maximum genetic loading for MS is approximately 30%. These points argue for influences beyond one's genetic lineage that define the cause(s) of this disease.

—Mitchell T. Wallin and John F. Kurtzke

***See also*—Epilepsy, Epidemiology; Multiple Sclerosis, Basic Biology; Multiple Sclerosis, Diagnosis; Neuroepidemiology, Overview; Parkinson's Disease, Epidemiology; Stroke, Epidemiology**

Further Reading

Anderson, D. W., Ellenberg, J. H., Leventhal, C. M., *et al.* (1992). Revised estimate of prevalence of multiple sclerosis in the United States. *Ann. Neurol.* 31, 333–336.

Boiko, A. N. (1994). Multiple sclerosis prevalence in Russia and other countries of the USSR. In *Multiple Sclerosis in Europe. An Epidemiological Update* (W. Firnhaber and K. Lauer, Eds.), pp. 219–230. LTV, Darmstadt.

Kurtzke, J. F. (1980). Geographic distribution of multiple sclerosis: An update with special reference to Europe and the Mediterranean region. *Acta Neurol. Scand.* 62, 65–80.

Kurtzke, J. F. (1997). The epidemiology of multiple sclerosis. In *Multiple Sclerosis: Clinical and Pathogenetic Basis* (C. S. Raine, H. McFarland, and W. W. Tourtellotte, Eds.), pp. 91–139. Chapman & Hall, London.

Kurtzke, J. F., and Heltberg, A. (2001). Multiple sclerosis in the Faroe Islands: An epitome. *J. Clin. Epidemiol.* 54, 1–22.

Kurtzke, J. F., and Wallin, M. T. (2000). Epidemiology. In *Multiple Sclerosis: Diagnosis, Medical Management, and Rehabilitation* (J. S. Burks and K. P. Johnson, Eds.), pp. 49–71. Demos, New York.

Kurtzke, J. F., Beebe, G. W., and Norman, J. E., Jr. (1979). Epidemiology of multiple sclerosis in United States veterans: I. Race, Sex and geographic distribution. *Neurology* 29, 1228–1235.

Kurtzke, J. F., Beebe, G. W., and Norman, J. E., Jr. (1985). Epidemiology of multiple sclerosis in United States veterans: III. Migration and the risk of MS. *Neurology* 35, 672–678.

Kurtzke, J. F., Delasnerie-Lauprêtre, N., and Wallin, M. T. (1998). Multiple sclerosis in North African migrants to France. *Acta Neurol. Scand.* 98, 302–309.

Lauer, K. (1994). Multiple sclerosis in the Old World: The new old map. In *Multiple Sclerosis in Europe. An Epidemiological Update* (W. Firnhaber and K. Lauer, Eds.), pp. 14–27. LTV, Darmstadt.

Martyn, C. N., and Gale, C. R. (1997). The epidemiology of multiple sclerosis. *Acta Neurol. Scand.* 95, 3–7.

Najim Al-Din, A. S., Kurdi, A., Mubaidin, A., *et al.* (1996). Epidemiology of multiple sclerosis in Arabs in Jordan: A comparative study between Jordanians and Palestinians. *J. Neurol. Sci.* 136, 162–167.

Sadovnick, A. D., Yee, I. M. L., Ebers, G. C., *et al.* (1998). Effect of age at onset and parental disease status on sibling risks for MS. *Neurology* 50, 719–725.

Sumelahti, M. L., Tienari, P. J., Wikström, J., *et al.* (2000). Regional and temporal variation in the incidence of multiple sclerosis in Finland 1979–1993. *Neuroepidemiology* 19, 67–75.

Wallin, M. T., Page, W. F., and Kurtzke, J. F. (2000). Epidemiology of multiple sclerosis in US veterans VIII. Long-term survival after onset of multiple sclerosis. *Brain* 123, 1677–1687.

Wynn, D. R., Rodriguez, M., O'Fallon, W. M., *et al.* (1990). A reappraisal of the epidemiology of multiple sclerosis in Olmsted County, Minnesota. *Neurology* 40, 780–786.

Multiple Sleep Latency Test (MSLT)

Encyclopedia of the Neurological Sciences
Copyright 2003, Elsevier Science (USA). All rights reserved.

THE COMPLAINT of excessive daytime sleepiness (EDS) requires thorough evaluation due to its important potential consequences. EDS leads to impaired performance and diminished intellectual capacity, and it can be a major cause of accidents and other catastrophes.

The measurement of daytime sleepiness has evolved into a major tool for diagnosing and describing sleep disorders. A number of methods have been proposed for assessing sleepiness. Pupillometry was first described by Yoss *et al.* as an indication of level of sleepiness. It is based on the fact that the size of the pupil is an indication of autonomic activity, which is related to states of arousal, excitation, and sleep. Patients with EDS were found to have an unstable pupillary diameter while sitting in the dark, with frequent oscillations of pupillary size. However, this technique did not achieve widespread use due to its limitation by ocular or autonomic lesions, dependence on the patient's cooperation, difficulties in data interpretation, and an inability to identify an underlying cause for the phenomenon.

Performance tasks, specifically those that are long, repetitive, and simple, have been used to assess the effect of sleepiness on the patient's performance. However, the stimulating circumstances of the performance setting may offset the impact of the sleep tendency.

Subjective measures of sleepiness were proposed, depending on the patient's own rating of his or her condition. The Stanford Sleepiness Scale, proposed by Hoddes *et al.*, consists of a 7-point rating scale describing the patient's self-assessment of sleepiness. However, it was found that patients with chronic sleepiness lose their ability to accurately assess their level of impairment. The Epworth Sleepiness Scale, introduced by Johns, is a commonly used questionnaire by sleep specialists. It assesses the patient's likelihood of falling asleep in eight different situations. The score ranges from 0 to 24, and a score of 10 or higher usually warrants further investigation. Recent evidence, however, indicates that there is no correlation between the subjective Epworth Sleepiness Scale and the objective Multiple Sleep Latency Test (MSLT), suggesting that subjective and objective methods may assess different aspects of sleepiness.

The technique most commonly used to evaluate daytime sleepiness, both experimentally and clinically, is the MSLT. It has achieved widespread acceptance because of its simple, intuitive approach to sleepiness (i.e., the greater the level of sleepiness, the more rapid the sleep onset), and because it provides several opportunities to test for sleep-onset rapid eye movement (REM) episodes, the primary diagnostic sign of narcolepsy. The physiological sleepiness measured by the MSLT cannot be reliably assessed by most subjects.

MSLT METHODOLOGY

A well-controlled and consistent procedure facilitates interpretation of test results as well as retest comparisons. The MSLT technique is well standardized according to the published American Academy of Sleep Medicine guidelines. Subjects should withdraw any medication that might affect sleep latency (e.g., sedatives, hypnotics, and antihistamines) or REM latency (e.g., tricyclic antidepressants) 2 weeks before the study. A urine drug screen on the morning of the MSLT is helpful in identifying patients in whom drug effects are suspected. It is recommended to perform an overnight polysomnogram (sleep study) the night before the MSLT to examine both the quality and the quantity of the night's sleep, which can influence the MSLT results. The patient should complete sleep diary forms for 1 or 2 weeks before the MSLT since the MSLT may be influenced by sleep for up to 7 nights before the test.

The MSLT is routinely performed at 2-hr intervals, beginning 1.5–3 hr after awakening from nocturnal sleep, and it consists of four or five naps. In general, subjects should be prohibited from taking caffeine and alcohol the day of the study; however, acute withdrawal from high doses of caffeine may affect test results. Subjects should be in bed 5 min before the scheduled start of the test to allow for calibrations of the recorded parameters and to establish a standard lead-in into the test. This is an important step because different levels of activity before the nap affect the nap's latency. The naps should be carried out in a sleep-inducing environment; thus, the rooms must be dark and quiet and the temperature adjusted to a comfortable level. The subject is instructed to try to sleep and not to resist sleeping, with the same instructions given for each nap. The wording of the instruction, however, seems to have only minor effects on sleep latency. Bedroom lights are then turned off, signaling the start of the test, from which sleep latency is calculated. The test is ended after 20 min if there has been no sleep or after 15 min from the beginning of sleep.

The recording montage includes the standard Rechtschaffen and Kales technique: central electroencephalogram (EEG), horizontal electro-oculogram (EOG), and chin electromyogram electrodes. Strongly recommended additions to this montage are occipital EEG, vertical EOG, and electrocardiogram electrodes. In patients known to snore, measures of respiratory flow and respiratory sounds may be helpful to identify occasions when snoring affects the sleep onset.

INTERPRETING THE MSLT

For each nap, sleep-onset latency and stages of sleep are recorded according to the standard criteria of sleep scoring, and the mean latency of all the naps is calculated. The MSLT can sometimes be difficult to interpret, and different raters may vary in their findings of whether a patient has sleep-onset REM periods, but less so for the sleep-onset latency. Controversy also exists regarding whether the median sleep latency should be used rather than the mean, but there seems to be little difference between the two measures. The criteria used for sleep onset are also variable, with some preferring to score sleep onset by the first 30-sec epoch of sleep, whereas others require three 30-sec epochs to determine sleep onset. Although this produces minor differences, it is recommended to follow the guidelines and score sleep onset by the first single 30-sec epoch.

The basic approach of the MSLT is that lower scores indicate greater sleepiness and vice versa. It is accepted that a mean score of less than 5 min indicates a pathological level of daytime sleepiness. This level is associated with impaired performance in patients and in sleep-deprived normal subjects. Adult normal controls usually range from 10 to 20 min. Scores between 5 and 10 min indicate moderate sleepiness and may or may not be pathological.

Abnormal sleep-onset REM periods, which occur within 15 min of sleep onset, are of major importance in the diagnosis of narcolepsy. However, other causes of sleep-onset REM periods must be excluded, such as sleep deprivation or other sleep disorders (e.g., obstructive sleep apnea).

The MSLT recognizes episodes of sleep only if they last at least 15 sec (more than half of a 30-sec epoch), but episodes of sleep lasting 5–10 sec, termed microsleeps, have also been associated with impaired performance.

APPLICATIONS OF THE MSLT

Using the MSLT as an objective laboratory assessment of the clinical symptom of sleepiness, as well as abnormal sleep structure, has greatly facilitated the diagnosis, differentiation, and treatment of various disorders of EDS. A brief review of its applications is as follows.

Narcolepsy

Sleepiness is the main symptom of narcolepsy, and it often precedes the other well-known symptoms of the disease—namely cataplexy, periodic sleep paralysis, and hypnagogic hallucinations. Evaluation of the MSLT of narcoleptic patients has demonstrated a short sleep latency (<5 min) and more than one sleep-onset REM period (SOREMP). The more specific finding in the MSLT of narcoleptic patients is more than two SOREMPs, presumed to reach a specificity of 99%, which further increases to 99.2% if three SOREMPs are recorded. However, other studies have questioned this high specificity and have shown that more than one SOREMP can occur in nonnarcoleptic patients as in sleep apnea, sleep deprivation, depression, periodic limb movements, circadian rhythm disruption, and withdrawal from REM-suppressing medications such as tricyclic antidepressants. Thus, the findings of the MSLT, which is always performed for suspected narcoleptic patients, must be interpreted with caution and in view of the clinical history.

Diagnosis of Various Disorders of EDS

The differential diagnosis of EDS includes narcolepsy, sleep apnea syndrome, sleep deprivation, periodic limb movement disorder, idiopathic central nervous system (CNS) hypersomnia, psychiatric diseases, and sedating medications. Attempts have been made to reach a differential diagnosis using the MSLT. Reynolds *et al.* and Zorick *et al.* carried out the MSLT for groups of patients with various disorders of EDS. They found that the narcoleptics and sleep apnea patients had the shortest sleep latency (<5 min), whereas patients with psychiatric disorders showed the longest latency (>10 min), reaching values similar to those of normals. Patients with idiopathic CNS hypersomnia, periodic limb movement disorder, or sleep deprivation occupied a middle position (5–10 min). REM latency was significantly shorter in narcolepsy than in apnea. More than 70% of the naps were SOREMP positive in narcolepsy, whereas less than 20% were positive for the other disorders. Sleep percentage was gradually reduced during the day in depressives, paralleling improvement in mood and energy levels. In contrast, sleep percentages increased and sleep latencies decreased during the day in narcoleptic and apneic groups.

In one study, 100 sleep apnea-free patients with EDS due to other prediagnosed disorders underwent the MSLT and nocturnal polysomnograph (PSG). The results were compared to the established diagnosis in an attempt to verify the MSLT's ability to classify patients into their own categories. Using regression analysis, it was found that the use of the mean sleep latency alone correctly classified 82% of narcoleptics in a group of patients with EDS. In addition, the MSLT mean sleep latency value and the sleep latency on the nocturnal PSG objectively differentiated between different groups with EDS.

These findings illustrate the value of the MSLT as a clinical tool in the differential diagnosis of complaints with EDS. Previous studies have shown that the MSLT differentiates normals from patients with pathological sleepiness. These data show that the MSLT effectively differentiates patients with various disorders of EDS. Consistent differences in the degree of sleepiness and in the nature of the sleep obtained during the naps were found among these patients.

Insomnia

A different clinical application of the MSLT is the assessment of patients with insomnia. One might expect that, as in sleep-deprived individuals, patients with insomnia would have a short sleep latency on the MSLT. However, in a study by Siedel and Dement, only 7% of insomniacs were in the pathological range on MSLT (<5 min), whereas 17% were in the "gray area" (510 min) and 41% had scores >15 min. These data suggest that insomniacs are a heterogeneous population and that many abnormally respond to restricted nocturnal sleep. The unexpected recorded latencies led to the hypothesis that the insomniac patients may be suffering from a state of chronic activation that disturbs night sleep but prevents EDS from occurring in the morning, or that these patients are naturally "short sleepers" whose sleep need is fulfilled with relatively short sleep at night. The diurnal sleep tendency of insomniac patients as measured by the MSLT may eventually yield clues to underlying pathologies in these groups.

Effect of Treatment

Different lines of treatment for sleep disorders associated with EDS, such as continuous positive airway pressure or airway surgery, were evaluated using the MSLT. In comparing pre- and post-treatment symptoms, a subject may perceive an improvement of awareness as very substantial, whereas the MSLT may reveal that the vulnerability remains. Hence, the objective assessment of the response is offered by the MSLT. The alerting effect of caffeine has been proven by its ability to increase the sleep latency on the MSLT of normal sleep-deprived subjects.

Hypnotic drug efficacy depends not only on its action on improving the quality of nocturnal sleep but also on the diurnal effects of the drug. The ideal sleeping pill would increase the amount and consolidation of nocturnal sleep, which should improve waking alertness or at least not further compromise it. Carskadon compared two groups of insomniacs treated with a short-acting (e.g., triazolam) and a long-acting (e.g., flurazepam) benzodiazepine. Both compounds increased nocturnal sleep by 1 hr; however, the flurazepam group had shorter sleep latencies on the MSLT with the drug than on baseline, whereas the triazolam group had a longer sleep latency with treatment. These findings were attributed to a carryover of sedating effects of the long-acting compounds and improvement of daytime alertness with short-acting compounds due to improved nocturnal sleep.

The MSLT has also been used for assessment of other types of compounds that may affect diurnal somnolence. Antihistamines, for example, are commonly associated with subjective sleepiness. Roehrs et al. showed that certain types of antihistamines increase sleepiness, with the MSLT used as the objective measure, whereas other types do not.

These studies highlight the potential of the MSLT as a valuable tool for assessing many types of compounds—not just those in which the primary action is sleep inducing. The assessment of various drug regimens using a sensitive measure of diurnal somnolence may aid in the determination of appropriate treatment strategies while minimizing sleepiness-inducing side effects.

—*Lamia Afifi and Clete A. Kushida*

See also—Drowsiness; Excessive Daytime Sleepiness; Fatigue; Insomnia; Jet Lag; Narcolepsy; Sleep Disorders; Sleep–Wake Cycle

Further Reading

Benbadis, S. R., Mascha, E., Perry, M. C., et al. (1999). Association between the Epworth Sleepiness Scale and the Multiple Sleep Latency Test in a clinical population. *Ann. Intern. Med.* **130**, 289–292.

Carskadon, M. A., and Dement, W. C. (1987). Daytime sleepiness: Quantification of a behavioural state. *Neurosci. Biobehav. Rev.* **11**, 307–317.

Hoddes, E., Dement, W. C., and Zarcone, V. (1972). The development and use of the Stanford Sleepiness Scale (SSS). *Psychophysiology* **1**, 150–157.

Johns, M. W. (1991). A new method of sleepiness: The Epworth Sleepiness Scale. *Sleep* **14**, 540–545.

Lagarde, D., and Bategate, D. (1994). Evaluation of drowsiness during prolonged sleep deprivation. *Neurophysiol. Clin.* **24**, 35–44.

Murphy, T., Ogilvie, R., Snow, T., et al. (1995). Inadvertent versus purposeful sleep onset: The effect of intention on sleep onset latencies. *J. Sleep Res.* **24**, 107–112.

Parkes, J. D. (1993). Daytime sleepiness. *Br. Med. J.* **306**, 772–775.

Rechtschaffen, A., and Kales, A. (1968). *A Manual of Standardised Terminology, Techniques and Scoring System for Sleep Stages of Human Subjects.* UCLA Brain Information Service/Brain Research Institute, Los Angeles.

Reynolds, C. F., Coble, P. A., Kupfer, D. J., et al. (1982). Application of multiple sleep latency test in disorders of excessive sleepiness. *Electroencephalogr. Clin. Neurophysiol.* **53**, 443–452.

Roehrs, T., Tietz, E., Zorick, F., et al. (1984). Daytime sleepiness and antihistamines. *Sleep* **7**, 137–141.

Yoss, R. E., Moyer, N. J., and Ogle, K. N. (1969). The pupillogram and narcolepsy: A method to measure decreased levels of wakefulness. *Neurology* **19**, 921–928.

Zorick, F., Roehrs, T., Koshorek, G., et al. (1982). Patterns of sleepiness in various disorders of excessive daytime somnolence. *Sleep* **5**, S165–S174.

Multisystem Atrophy (MSA)

MULTISYSTEM ATROPHY is a neurological disorder that includes degeneration in the extrapyramidal, pyramidal, autonomic, and cerebellar systems. Formerly, it was divided into conditions known as striatonigral degeneration, Shy–Drager syndrome, and olivopontocerebellar atrophy. Currently, these names are collapsed into multisystem atrophy. The clinical hallmark features of multisystem atrophy are parkinsonism and varying degrees of hypotension, sexual impotency, ataxia, and weakness with spasticity.

—*Esther Cubo and Christopher G. Goetz*

See also–**Parkinsonism; Shy–Drager Syndrome**

Further Reading

Quinn, N. (1994). Multiple system atrophy. In *Movement Disorders* (C. D. Marsden and S. Fahn, Eds.), pp. 263–281. Butterworth, Oxford.

Münchausen by Proxy

FACTITIOUS disorder by proxy (FDP), popularly known as Münchausen by proxy (MBP), is a condition in which a parent or caretaker on multiple occasions falsifies symptoms or actually induces illness in an infant or older child, frequently while in a hospital setting. First described in England by Roy Meadow in 1977, it is one of the most perplexing disorders in all of medicine. There have been more than 400 reports of it in the international scientific literature and much popular attention to it in the media. The disorder is overwhelmingly one of women, who appear as very caring and selfless mothers but at the same time are repeatedly causing grave harm to their children. Because there are several other conditions in which a parent may fabricate symptoms or directly harm a child, the motivation for this behavior is an essential part of the diagnosis, important in evaluating prognosis for treatment of the mother, and crucial in planning for the current and future disposition of the child. Many case studies indicate that this disorder involves persistent or compulsive behavior that causes grave harm either directly or through the ministrations of physicians. Horrific consequences not infrequently leading to death (6% in the McClure *et al.* study) are the norm. Usually this occurs in only one child, but cases involving more than one at a time and up to 9 children serially have been reported. Most alarming is the high rate of recidivism when children are returned to these parents.

Typically, as a result of the mother's elaborate production of symptoms or illness, the child is hospitalized and harmed through invasive procedures related to attempts by the child's doctors to understand and treat a confusing clinical picture. The aim of this "perverse" behavior on the part of these mothers involves a need to be close to and in a relationship with medical staff and/or be the center of attention. This relationship is one of needy dependency that involves manipulation, but in some cases it also appears to contain elements of cruelty not only toward the child but also toward the people whose life work is to cure and protect children.

Case analyses repeatedly find difficulties in suspecting the mother's activities, which go well beyond our inability to think that anyone, especially a mother, could repeatedly (with premeditation) suffocate, starve, or poison an infant. Detection is difficult even when these otherwise seemingly competent women leave glaring clues to their actions. Their skills resemble those seen in impostors (in this case, impostoring, caring mothers), coupled with the kind of abilities that have been described in the male psychopath and a kind of object relations found in female forms of perversion. However, those with these skills may be overrepresented in the cases uncovered. Others may be much less active in their abuse and have not yet been found.

When examined carefully, the interpersonal dynamics suggest that a group of individuals, those who are seen as powerful in society, are targeted and may be especially susceptible to the manipulations of these women. These include people in the professions who have a need to be seen as smart, caring, and able to function independently to solve complicated problems. Despite training aimed at developing an ability to adopt a neutral and inquisitive stance toward patients, professionals, including psychiatrists, are often not proficient at detecting lying, especially the kind these women are capable of simulating. Some have argued persuasively that to understand this phenomenon, we must view at it as a dyadic (mother and doctor) or triadic (and infant) interactional disorder. In this schema, the physician plays an active role in the continuance of the process.

A common misperception fostered by the media is that MBP is rare. Extrapolating from a carefully designed study done in England by McClure *et al.* concerning two of the myriad of conditions involved in MBP suggests that at least 1200 new cases of MBP presenting with just the two conditions, acute life-threatening events (apnea) and nonaccidental poisoning, would be expected to occur each year in the United States. Though clearly representing the more serious cases, we found a death rate of 9% in an informal survey of pediatric neurologists. In suffocation cases, it is frequently found that one or more siblings have died previously of sudden infant death syndrome (SIDS), or unexpectedly of mysterious causes, or have been abused. There are several cases involving the murder of more than seven children by one woman, and recently a mother was tried and convicted of suffocating all five of her natural children, 25 years after the fact. Some number of deaths from suffocation in the past were incorrectly attributed to SIDS and may have erroneously fostered the risk of familial SIDS.

In 1995, the American Professional Society on the Abuse of Children published a set of definitional guidelines (revised in 2002) to address some of the confusion in the field, including some of the problems with the definition in the *Diagnostic and Statistical Manual of Mental Disorders*, fourth edition (*DSM-IV*), for factitious disorder by proxy. The society put forth that Münchausen by proxy consists of two components. The first is the identification of the victimization of the child. The second relates to the identification of the psychological motivations for the abuse. In addition, the committee noted that the family often plays a role in MBP "either through passive support or directly [through] participation in the deception that is at the core of the child's victimization." There are two terms used. In addition to FDP, the society coined the term pediatric condition (illness, impairment, or symptom production) falsification (PCF), which is "child maltreatment in which an adult falsifies physical and/or psychological signs and/or symptoms in a victim causing that person to be regarded as ill or impaired by others." Examples include directly causing a condition, over- or underreporting signs or symptoms, creating a false appearance of signs and symptoms, and coaching the victim or others to misrepresent the victim as ill. The presence of a valid

illness does not preclude concurrent exaggeration or falsification. PCF through psychological neurobehavioral (e.g., Tourettes' syndrome, attention deficit hyperactivity disorder, and temporal lobe epilepsy "rages") or developmental symptoms (autism and learning disabilities) has been described but appears to be less common. Neurological conditions (seizures, apnea, and recently mitochondrial encephalopathy), gastrointestinal problems (pseudo-bowel obstruction), infectious diseases, and endocrinological disorders as well as various poisonings are the most common conditions involved in a FDP process. Often, a child will present with an array of disorders that are unlikely to be related, which should arouse more suspicion on the part of physicians than is usually evidenced in the chart notes. It must be recognized that a child victimized by abuse through PCF, regardless of the motivation of the abuser, requires immediate protection.

Persons who intentionally falsify history, signs, or symptoms in a child to meet their own self-serving psychological needs should be diagnosed with FDP. However, not all illness falsification is FDP. The other cases in which a parent may fabricate illness (PCF) in his or her child that are not FDP (or MBP) include the following: overwhelmed or overly anxious parents who blatantly falsify symptoms to get assistance for their child, typically only on one or two occasions, and children who are "school-refusers" secondary to anxiety disorders in them and/or their parents. They only infrequently present to the doctor, usually because they need excuse notes for school. Missed school and its ramifications comprise the harm done in this disorder.

Other conditions that are not MBP are pseudoseizure and other conversion disorders with psychological motivation that is unconscious and the source of the problem symptom is the child. These situations do not involve ongoing deception, nor motivation to manipulate the doctors. Also, when a parent cannot cope with or fails to feed the child causing him to fail to thrive, this is not FDP. Failure to thrive is not uncommonly found in cases of FDP, but the FDP diagnosis should be reserved for cases where the motivation is as described herein. Another category of parents who may confuse the diagnosis of FDP are those of chronically ill children because they have their own psychological issues or because they disagree with the medical staff and may be "difficult" and appear to interfere with treatment. Parents may appear difficult or noncompliant out of frustration or they are aggressive in their advocacy for their children. Psychotic delusion of illness in one's child may be mistaken for FDP, but if these delusions are the source of the illness falsification, then the correct diagnosis is delusional disorder, somatic type. None of these latter three conditions—inability to care for a child, chronically ill children, or psychotic delusions—involve illness falsification or the usual motives of MBP, and they are neither PCF nor FDP.

It needs to be emphasized that there is no particular psychological profile or checklist of behavior that definitively confirms or excludes the diagnosis of MBP. Rather, there are common patterns that should raise suspicion but should be examined on a case-by-case basis.

On testing, personality problems in the parent are quite common but perpetrators may appear relatively healthy on the usual psychological tests and in interviews, especially to the uninformed examiner. Up to 75% of mothers exhibited somatizing problems when younger and approximately one-third have had factitious disorders.

Regarding motivation, it should be noted that contrary to the DSM-IV definitions, external incentives such as monetary gain or seeking revenge on an abandoning spouse may be present along with the dynamics described previously and do not preclude the diagnosis.

Parents who "doctor shop" when the motivation is not to get help for the child but to subject the child to the abuse of repeated investigations in order to gain attention, maintain relationships and manipulate powerful figures (doctors), and/or evade suspicion because of their behavior with former doctors should be diagnosed with MBP. Physicians and others health care providers may have long-term relationships with the children being victimized and indeed may be supportive of the mother even after falsification at the mother's hand is uncovered.

Last, it is important to note that the immediate physical consequence of the abuse is not necessarily representative of the seriousness of the MBP condition or of the potential for future harm to the child. Perpetrators have been known to switch from seemingly mild to life-threatening forms of abuse, and the characteristics of those more likely to commit the latter behavior are not well understood. In 31 cases of factitious epilepsy, Meadow reported the fate of 34 siblings: 5 had nonaccidental injuries, 7 were SIDS deaths, 1 was brain damaged, and 10 were also said to have suffered seizures. Furthermore, studies indicate that there is a high recidivism rate of abuse in MBP. Mothers have been known to continue their harm-inducing behavior even during supervised visits while the child is in protective custody.

—Herbert A. Schreier

***See also*—Child Abuse, Head Injuries; Delusions; Factitious Disorder; Münchausen Syndrome; Somatoform Disorders; Sudden Infant Death Syndrome (SIDS)**

Further Reading

Ayoub, C., Alexander, R., and Schreier, H. (2002). Special focus section: Münchausen by proxy. Child Maltreat. 7, 103–169.
Meadow, R. (1984). Factitious epilepsy. Lancet 2, 25–28.
Eminson, M., and Postlehwaite, R. (1999). Münchausen Syndrome by Proxy Abuse: A Practical Approach. Butterworth-Heinemann, Oxford.
Levin, A., and Sheridan, M. (1995). Münchausen Syndrome by Proxy. Issues in Diagnosis and Treatment. Lexington, New York.
Parnell, T., and Day, D. (1997). Münchausen by Proxy Syndrome. A Misunderstood Child Abuse. Sage, Thousand Oaks, CA.
Schreier, H. (1997). Factitious presentation of psychiatric disorder: When is it Münchausen by proxy? Child Psychol. Psychiatr. Rev. 2, 108–115.
Schreier, H., and Libow, J. (1993). Hurting for Love: Münchausen by Proxy. Guilford, New York.

Münchausen Syndrome

Encyclopedia of the Neurological Sciences
Copyright 2003, Elsevier Science (USA). All rights reserved.

MÜNCHAUSEN syndrome is a psychiatric condition in which patients wander from hospital to hospital, feigning illness in order to receive medical care. It is the most severe form of factitious disorder and, as such, there are three key criteria: an intentional production or feigning of physical or psychological symptoms, a desire to assume the sick role, and an absence of external incentives (such as monetary gain, shelter, or avoiding jail).

In addition to these criteria, patients with Münchausen syndrome exhibit several other features that are not commonly found in most cases of factitious disorder. Patients with Münchausen syndrome present at many different hospitals, wandering across the country for years in succession. They fabricate grandiose, spectacular tales about their lives and their illness, a phenomenon known as pseudologia fantastica. The vast majority of these patients manifest some form of antisocial behavior.

HISTORY

The term Münchausen syndrome was introduced in 1951 by Richard Asher. The syndrome takes its name from Baron Karl Friederich von Münchausen (1720–1791), a German cavalry officer who served with the Russian army against the Turks. The baron was known as an eager raconteur of extraordinary tales about his life and the war. The tales were ultimately written as a popular children's book, *The Amazing Travels and Adventures of Baron Von Münchausen.* When Asher coined the term, he was referring to both the fantastic stories of these patients and their chronic travels from hospital to hospital. Alternative names have been used, such as Van Gogh's syndrome, peregrinating problem patients, and hospital hoboes, but these names are no longer found in the literature. Although the *Diagnostic and Statistical Manual of Mental Disorders*, fourth edition, uses the term factitious disorder to refer to these patients, the colorful Münchausen eponym has remained in the literature, and the two terms are often inaccurately used interchangeably.

EPIDEMIOLOGY

Prevalence

Due to the deceptive and wandering nature of patients with Münchausen syndrome, the exact prevalence of the disorder is not known. Standard epidemiological techniques are not applicable, and data have been discerned from case reports and studies about factitious disorder in general. Recent studies have found that approximately 0.5–1% of patients seen by psychiatric consultation–liaison services are diagnosed with factitious disorder. However, only a small fraction (approximately 10%) of these patients have characteristics consistent with Münchausen syndrome. Some experts argue that the disorder is underdiagnosed because patients attempt to conceal it, whereas other experts argue that it is overdiagnosed because the same patient will present at multiple hospitals.

PATIENT CHARACTERISTICS

Patients are more commonly male, with a mean age of 35 years at the time of initial diagnosis. They are usually unemployed and estranged from their families. A disproportionate number have worked in the health care system, and they are found more often in urban areas. Many patients have criminal records, and nearly all have interpersonal relationship problems. The majority have a comorbid psychiatric diagnosis, including personality disorders, substance abuse, and mood disorders.

CLINICAL FEATURES

Presentation

Patients typically present to a hospital emergency department at night or on the weekend. They simulate a disease process in a dramatic fashion, supported by an elaborate and fascinating history of how they became afflicted. In most cases of Münchausen syndrome, the disease fabricated (or self-inflicted) has predominantly physical symptoms, including diseases such as myocardial infarction, pulmonary embolus, renal stones, gastrointestinal bleeding, stroke, seizure, nonhealing skin ulcers, and a variety of infectious diseases such as tuberculosis or acquired immunodeficiency syndrome. In some cases of Münchausen syndrome, the illness feigned has predominantly psychological symptoms, such as auditory hallucinations, delusions, suicidal ideation, amnesia, posttraumatic stress disorder, and feigned bereavement.

In addition to the fabricated medical history, patients create false personal histories, which are designed to arouse the interest of the medical staff. In this pseudologia fantastica, the patient might claim to be a war hero, a famous athlete, or a former congressman. When these patients are in the hospital setting, the inconsistency between their alleged famous personal histories and the lack of visitors or phone calls one would expect of a celebrity can be observed.

They readily submit to all diagnostic procedures and therapies and are especially interested in invasive procedures. They appear to be model patients who follow all recommendations and seem to idealize their doctors until doubts arise as to the authenticity of their disease. If confronted with these doubts, there is an abrupt severing of the doctor–patient relationship. The patient responds with anger, disruptive behavior, threats of litigation, or self-discharge from the hospital. The patient will then present at another hospital often in a different city, and the cycle will continue.

Course and Prognosis

Münchausen syndrome is a chronic illness with an unremitting course that can span more than a decade of a patient's life. Some case reports have uncovered patients with as many as 400 successive hospital stays over an extended period of time. There can be significant morbidity and mortality associated with the disease, either from self-inflicted injury or from unnecessary surgeries, procedure, or therapies. As a general rule, patients with Münchausen syndrome do not accept psychiatric treatment, and full remissions are rare. It is important to note that sound data regarding long-term prognosis are difficult to collect due to the surreptitious nature of the illness.

ETIOLOGY

A number of psychological theories have been proposed to explain the motivations underlying the behavior of patients with Münchausen syndrome. Often, these patients have had abusive, emotionally deprived backgrounds. It is hypothesized that by assuming the sick role, they satisfy the longing for attention, caring, and nurturance. Moreover, narcissistic needs may be met through the phenomenon of pseudologia fantastic. Other interpretations of the behavior include a need to suffer (masochism), a need for mastery, denial of failure, and cheating authority figures. Although patients are conscious of their behavior, they are seldom if ever aware of the underlying motivations.

Recently, a few small studies have found abnormalities on brain imaging of patients with Münchausen syndrome, particularly in the frontal and temporal lobes. Neuropsychological testing has revealed deficits in conceptual organization, judgment, and information processing.

TREATMENT AND MANAGEMENT

There is no specific, well-established treatment for Münchausen syndrome. Management techniques have ranged from supportive but direct confrontation to face-saving measures in which the diagnosis is not completely disclosed. The only consistent treatment strategy is to safeguard the patient against further invasive procedures.

Because the disease is fundamentally psychiatric in nature, the primary treatment falls within the purview of mental health specialties. However, only a small minority of patients will accept either a psychiatric diagnosis or therapy. Some success has been obtained by offering less "threatening" interventions, such as physical therapy or hypnosis. These techniques provide both attention and a face-saving

mechanism for the patient to abandon his or her behavior. Although no specific pharmacotherapy is recommended for Münchausen syndrome, comorbid psychiatric diagnoses (such as depression) should be treated aggressively. In some cases, an extended psychiatric hospitalization or the appointment of a public guardian have been useful, but patients seldom meet legal criteria for these approaches.

—*Lee A. Rawitscher*

See also–Anosognosia; Conversion Disorder and Other Somatoform Disorders; Delusions; Factitious Disorder; Malingering; Münchausen by Proxy

Further Reading

Murray, J. B. (1997). Münchausen syndrome/Münchausen syndrome by proxy. *J. Psychol.* **131,** 343–353.
Plassmann, R. (1994). Münchausen syndrome and factitious diseases. *Psychother. Psychosom.* **62,** 7–26.
Robertson, M., and Cervilla, J. (1997). Münchausen syndrome. *Br. J. Hosp. Med.* **58,** 308–312.
Sadock, and Sadock (Eds.) (2000). *Comprehensive Textbook of Psychiatry*, pp. 1533–1543. Lippincott Williams & Wilkins, Baltimore.

Munk, Hermann

Encyclopedia of the Neurological Sciences

Copyright 2003, Elsevier Science (USA). All rights reserved.

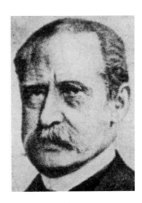

THE GERMAN physiologist Hermann Munk (1839–1912) was a famous proponent of the theory of localization of cortical function. He was born in Posen, Germany. He studied in Berlin and Göttingen and earned his doctorate in 1859. In 1862, he qualified as a university lecturer, and he became a professor in 1869 at the University of Berlin. In 1876, he became a lecturer in physiology and head of the physiological laboratory at the Veterinary High School of Berlin. Munk became a member of the Academy of Science in 1880 and became honorary professor of the University of Berlin in 1897.

Munk was a prolific writer whose papers covered such diverse subjects as the reproduction of nematodes, the physiology of the nervous system, the mechanisms of nervous excitation, the anatomy of cardiac and laryngeal nerves, and, most significantly, the function and physiology of the cerebral cortex. To explore the origin of nervous function, Munk investigated the effects of focal ablation of the cerebral cortex. His lesion experiments in dogs provided strong experimental support for the localization of vision within the occipital lobes. Later, he distinguished between forms of blindness following bilateral destruction of the calcarine cortex (*Rindenblindheit*) and blindness (optic agnosia) following lesions to visual association cortex (*Seelenblindheit*, literally, blindness of the soul). Much of his work on cerebral localization was summarized in his two monographs, *Über die Funktionen der Großhirnrinde* (*About the Functions of the Cerebral Cortex*) (1881, second edition 1890) and *Erfahrungen zu Gunsten der Lokalisation* (*Experiences Supporting Localization*) (1887). Unfortunately, only short excerpts of these works have been translated into English. Munk died in 1912.

—*Rolf Malessa*

See also–Localization (see Index entry Biography for complete list of biographical entries)

Further Reading

Munk, H. (1881). *Ueber die Functionen der Grosshirnrinde.* Hirschwald, Berlin.
Munk, H. (1887). Erfahrungen zu Gunsten der Localization. *Verh. Physiol. Ges. Berlin* **16**.
Munk, H. (1890). *Über die Functionen der Großhirnrinde Gesammelte Mitteilungen. Zweite vermehrte Auflage.* Hirschwald, Berlin.

Muscle Biopsy

Encyclopedia of the Neurological Sciences
Copyright 2003, Elsevier Science (USA). All rights reserved.

A MUSCLE BIOPSY is performed when neurological examination, laboratory tests, and electrodiagnostic studies indicate a neuromuscular disorder, mainly a peripheral neuropathy or a primary muscle disease (myopathy). The microscopic examination can help to distinguish neurogenic from myogenic disorders. The result usually confirms the findings of the nerve conduction studies and electromyogram. The pathology can also help to subclassify myopathies. Lymphocytic infiltration strongly suggests an acquired, potentially treatable myopathy and distinguishes it from other acquired myopathies and muscular dystrophy. Less commonly, the biopsy renders a specific diagnosis. Necrotizing arteritis and amyloidosis in a neuropathy may be identified in muscle as well as nerve using routine histology of formalin fixed tissue. A definitive diagnosis more often requires analysis of rapidly frozen muscle tissue using enzyme histochemistry, immunohistochemistry, and molecular analysis. Occasionally, electron microscopic examination may be helpful to narrow the diagnostic possibilities.

In the past decade, advances in molecular genetics have resulted in the rapid transfer of technology from research laboratories to commercial enterprises. As a consequence, practicing clinicians can order DNA analysis of a blood sample as part of the workup to identify gene defects without recourse to muscle biopsy. For example, in the infantile form of spinal muscular atrophy (Werdnig–Hoffmann disease), deletions of the survival motor neuron gene occur in 98% of patients. In other inherited disorders, muscle biopsy may still be required when DNA analysis fails to document a mutation. In Duchenne's muscular dystrophy, approximately 30% of patients have point mutations or other minor rearrangements of the dystrophin gene that cannot be detected because of limitations of methodology. In these patients, immunohistochemical stains of a muscle biopsy can establish the diagnosis based on the absence of dystrophin.

BIOPSY

The decision to biopsy should be made only after a careful neurological evaluation that includes a family history, determination of serum creatine kinase activity, and electrodiagnostic studies. The clinical diagnosis obviates the biopsy in typical cases of amyotrophic lateral sclerosis, diabetic neuropathy, Guillain–Barré syndrome, myasthenia gravis, myotonic dystrophy, dermatomyositis, and others. If muscle biopsy is necessary, then the clinician should provide information to the pathologist to direct analysis of the muscle efficiently. The minimum should include a clinical diagnosis or the major complaint, such as limb weakness, progressive external ophthalmoplegia, infantile hypotonia, myalgia, cramps, or exercise tolerance. Those with myoglobinuria triggered by exercise should have the biopsy performed 6–8 weeks later to allow muscle to recover. These patients have a potential inherited disorder of metabolism, and interpretation of morphological and biochemical analysis is more reliable when the acute changes in muscle have subsided.

Many muscle biopsies are not fruitful, but the yield of an informative diagnosis can be improved by careful selection of a muscle that is guided by clinical information and electrodiagnostic studies. The yield is higher in a moderately weak muscle than in an unaffected one as it may have a normal histology. On the other hand, a severely weak muscle may be largely replaced by adipose tissue, precluding a diagnosis. If possible, the clinician should select a commonly biopsied muscle. The vastus lateralis and biceps are the muscles of choice for biopsy when proximal limb weakness predominates, and the gastrocnemius muscle is preferred in patients with distal weakness, often in conjunction with a sural nerve biopsy for peripheral neuropathy.

Four separate pieces of muscle are submitted to the laboratory for each biopsy. One is placed in formalin for routine histology, another is frozen for enzyme histochemistry, and a third is fixed in glutaraldehyde for electron microscopy. A fourth sample must be frozen immediately at the time of the surgical procedure and stored in a freezer in case the biopsy or clinical information indicate biochemical or DNA analysis is necessary.

The amount and the quality of the tissue for enzyme histochemistry are critical to achieving a diagnosis. The sample should be at least 0.5 cm in diameter and 1.5 cm in length. The surgeon should try to avoid the use of electrocautery near the site of the biopsy. A muscle clamp can be used to minimize contraction of the excised muscle. Alternatively, the physician can dissect out a cylinder of muscle and tie it *in situ* to a small splint (e.g., a segment of a Q-tip stick) with a suture at each end of the sample (Fig. 1). The surgeon then cuts the muscle just outside the sutures. This maneuver tends to minimize artifacts induced by twisting or hacking out of the tissue with scissors. The method leaves a 1.0-cm length of muscle that is free of compression between the sutures. The specimen must never be exposed to excess fluid, in contrast to the common treatment of

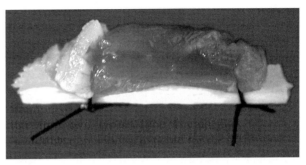

Figure 1
A muscle biopsy specimen for enzyme histochemistry. The surgeon carefully dissected out a cylinder of muscle *in situ*. Sutures are passed around each end of the sample and tied to a Q-tip stick securely but without severing it. Then the cylinder is transected just outside each suture to excise it.

biopsy tissue by surgeons, who excise a piece of tumor and drop it into a jar of saline for frozen section diagnosis. Instead, the sample should be wrapped in a piece of gauze or similar material that has been slightly moistened with physiological solution to prevent drying. The physician or assistant then places it into a tightly capped vial, and the sample is transported over ice to keep it cool.

The specimen used for enzyme histochemistry should optimally arrive at the laboratory within 30–60 min. (The specimen for biochemical analysis requires immediate freezing.) Those received after 1 hr or overnight are not ideal but can be useful, as long as the tissue is handled flawlessly and kept cold. The tissue must be frozen rapidly to eliminate ice crystal artifacts, preferably using isopentane cooled to the freezing point with liquid nitrogen.

NORMAL MUSCLE

Each muscle fiber contains many nuclei, and most are located at the myofiber surface. The muscle fibers appear to be nearly uniform in composition in the hematoxylin and eosin stain (Fig. 2A) but differ in function, biochemical properties, and histochemistry. In frozen sections, the myosin ATPase stain (preincubation of pH 9.4–10.3) distinguishes two major histochemical types (Fig. 2C). Pale fibers are designated type 1. These fibers have slow-twitch properties and are rich in mitochondria. The type 2, dark fibers are fast twitch and poor in mitochondria. The type 1 and type 2 fibers are distributed throughout the muscle in a nearly random fashion. Some laboratories subdivide type 2 fibers into types 2a–2c using a modified preincubation of the ATPase reaction at

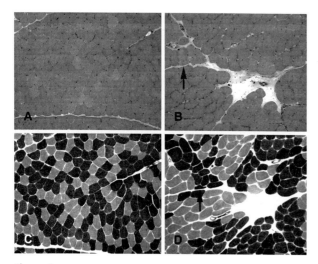

Figure 2
Normal muscle (A and C) compared to muscle in a patient with peripheral neuropathy (B and D). The cryosections in the neurogenic disorder are nearly normal in the section stained by hematoxylin and eosin (B) except for a rare atrophic fiber (arrow) and thick perimysial septa. However, the ATPase stain (D) of the same field shows pronounced grouping of muscle fibers of the same histochemical type (arrow). This fiber type grouping is diagnostic of a neurogenic disorder. The finding contrasts with the seemingly random pattern of type 1 and type 2 myofibers of normal muscle (C).

pH 4.6 and 4.3. Fast-twitch and slow-twitch fibers each express a different myosin heavy chain and can be recognized by an immunohistochemical stain.

The modified Gomori trichrome method produces a dark reddish (fuchsinophilic) stain of organelle membranes, appearing as fine granules that contrast with the greenish-blue sarcoplasm. The major components are mitochondria, sarcoplasmic reticulum, and transverse tubules. Mitochondria are distinguished from other organelles by the histochemical stains of NADH dehydrogenase or tetrazolium reductase (NADH-TR; complex I of the electron transport chain), succinate dehydrogenase (complex II), and cytochrome c oxidase (complex IV). Mitochondria are distributed throughout the sarcoplasm but are clustered together in the subsarcolemmal zone next to capillaries, myonuclei, and motor end plates. Lysosomes are sparse and small; they are identified by the histochemical stain for acid phosphatase.

NEUROGENIC DISORDERS

There are three major diagnostic criteria of a neurogenic disorder in muscle: groups of abnormally small (atrophic) myofibers, fiber type grouping, and target fibers. These alterations can occur in peripheral neuropathy as well as in plexopathy, radiculopathy, and motor neuron disease. The changes develop only weeks or months following the onset of disease. Large groups of atrophic fibers are virtually diagnostic of neurogenic disorders and may be easily recognized by paraffin histology. In contrast, small groups of atrophic fibers may occur in myogenic disorders. A selective atrophy of type 2 fibers is the most common cause of small groups. It is the only abnormality in a variety of neuromuscular disorders, including inactivity or disuse of muscle, collagen vascular diseases, cancer, glucocorticoid treatment, polymyalgia rheumatica, hyperparathyroidism, and starvation. It also occurs during the first weeks of acute denervation.

Fiber type grouping is defined by the ATPase stain and consists of an abnormally large group of fibers of the same histochemical type (Fig. 2D). Target fibers typically consist of a central zone that displays myofibrillar disorganization and a lack of mitochondria. Histochemical stains for mitochondrial oxidative stains, particularly NADH-TR, are the most sensitive method for identifying the central pallor in targets.

MYOGENIC DISORDERS

Acute myopathies exhibit segmental necrosis of myofibers as the most severe form of cell injury. Examples of these diseases include acute alcoholic myopathy and the muscle breakdown in McArdle's disease following vigorous exercise. The fiber damage provokes recruitment of monocytes largely from the circulation. These cells pass into the tissue and penetrate the surface of necrotic fibers, where they engulf or phagocytize cytoplasmic debris. Satellite cells are normally located next to muscle fibers, and they begin to proliferate and differentiate to form myoblasts. These cells subsequently fuse to form a basophilic regenerating fiber, and it eventually replaces the necrotic fiber segment. Fiber regeneration can completely restore muscle structure and function within 1 or 2 months in humans, providing the disorder is episodic.

In other disorders, the injury to fibers is less severe. The myopathy of critical illness demonstrates atrophy of type 2 myofibers and disorganization of myofibrils, often with selective loss of myosin thick myofilaments. The prognosis is good if the patient responds to treatment for the underlying disease, with recovery of strength within a few weeks.

Subacute and chronic myopathies may have necrotic and regenerating fibers but also exhibit signs of chronic disease, including increased variation of myofiber size, increased central myonuclei, and fibrosis of the endomysium. These myopathic features occur in chronic alcoholism, myotoxic side effects of certain medications, malignancies, muscular dystrophies, and others. They also occur in muscle biopsies of polymyositis (PM), inclusion body myositis (IBM), and dermatomyositis with or without lymphocytic infiltration of the tissue. Fiber necrosis and regeneration often become sparse or absent with increasing duration of disease. The pathological findings in a long-standing chronic myopathy can share many features of a chronic neurogenic disorder, making the distinction difficult or impossible. Many central nuclei and prominent endomysial fibrosis support a myopathy in the absence of clear neurogenic abnormalities.

Muscular dystrophies can be indistinguishable from noninflammatory, acquired myopathies based on routine histology, but immunohistochemical stains can identify deficiency of the gene product. Duchenne's muscular dystrophy shows a near or complete absence of dystrophin in muscle fibers. The finding is virtually diagnostic of the disorder. Mutations should be documented by DNA analysis of the patient and family members to have the option for prenatal diagnosis. In some instances, immunohistochemistry detects a mosaic pattern of dystrophin deficiency in women who are carriers of the mutant gene. In addition, weak staining or discontinuities of dystrophin may be detectable at the fiber surface in Becker's dystrophy, a slowly progressive disorder that is allelic to Duchenne's dystrophy. Because the result can also be an artifact due to technical deficiencies, the diagnosis must be confirmed by DNA analysis or immunoblot to detect a protein that is reduced in size or abundance. Mutations of an increasing number of genes have been linked to muscular dystrophy, including those that encode sarcoglycans (α-, β-, γ-, and δ-sarcoglycan), merosin, dysferlin, emerin, caveolin, and others. Deficiency of these proteins can be identified in muscle biopsies by immunohistochemistry.

Many other inherited myopathies do not exhibit necrotic fibers or fibrosis but are recognized pathologically by a distinctive structural abnormality of the muscle fibers. Examples include mitochondrial myopathies (ragged red fibers), lipid storage myopathies, glycogen storage diseases, congenital myasthenic syndrome (CMS), and congenital myopathies such as central core disease, nemaline myopathy, and myotubular or centronuclear myopathy. Histochemical stains can demonstrate a genetic deficiency of a limited number of enzymes, including phosphorylase, phosphofructokinase, myoadenylate deaminase, and cytochrome c oxidase. A deficiency of acetylcholine esterase or acetyl choline receptor (using α-bungarotoxin as a marker) is found at motor end plates in two forms of CMS. The genes responsible for many of the inherited diseases have been identified, and DNA analysis can often establish a diagnosis by identifying a mutation.

Most inflammatory myopathies are subclassified into three distinct groups based on clinical and pathological findings. PM and IBM share pathological features, including single fiber necrosis, fiber regeneration, and T cell infiltration of mainly the endomysium. IBM displays greater chronic changes than polymyositis, and it displays rimmed vacuoles, eosinophilic hyaline inclusions, and sparse intracellular amyloid inclusions. These findings can be clearly defined only in frozen sections. The amyloid inclusions are weakly congophilic and require a fluorescence microscope using rhodamine optics to identify them. These abnormalities are not completely specific, but they strongly support the diagnosis of IBM in the context of an inflammatory myopathy. Electron microscopy displays abnormal filaments near rimmed vacuoles, but these are not required for diagnosis. The recognition of IBM is important because the disorder does not respond to immunosuppressive agents as a rule.

Although muscle biopsy is not necessary in typical dermatomyositis, it is important to recognize the disorder in patients with an indistinct or atypical rash. Current treatment of dermatomyositis does not differ substantially from that of PM, but dermatomyositis in adults has a greater risk for malignancy than that for the normal population. Hence, it may require a costly workup for a clinically silent neoplasm. The characteristic histological picture includes atrophy of muscle fibers along the edge of muscle fascicles (perifascicular atrophy) and lymphocytic infiltration of predominantly the perimysium. The lymphocytes include B cells as well as T cells. Some biopsies may have few or no abnormalities by routine histology, but immunohistochemical stains of frozen sections may be diagnostic as indicated by immune complexes in the walls of capillaries. Moreover, electron microscopy usually exhibits endothelial tubuloreticular aggregates during active disease. These inclusions support the diagnosis but may be seen in certain other collagen vascular diseases and in human immunodeficiency virus type 1 infection.

—Arthur P. Hays

See also–Motor Control, Peripheral; Muscle Strength, Assessment of; Muscle Tone; Muscular Dystrophy: Limb–Girdle, Becker's, and Duchenne's; Myopathy, Overview; Stereotactic Biopsy

Further Reading

Carpenter, S., and Karpati, G. (2001). *Pathology of Skeletal Muscle*, 2nd ed. Oxford Univ. Press, New York.
Engel, A. G., and Franzini-Armstrong, C. (1994). *Myology*, 2nd ed. McGraw-Hill, New York.

Muscle Contraction, Overview

Encyclopedia of the Neurological Sciences

THE QUESTION of how skeletal muscle acts to contract and result in movement of a living organism has long been considered by physiologists. Prior to the mid-1600s, it was thought that the nerve supplied the muscle with a spiritus liquor that accompanied the apparent increase in muscle bulk during contraction. In the 17th century, Swammerdan demonstrated that contracting muscle maintained a constant volume, leading to the conclusion that conformational changes of muscle fibers were sufficient to cause movement. In 1782, Luigi Galvani showed that electrical energy was an integral component of muscle contraction. The relationship between conformational change and electrical activity remained obscure until the mid-1950s, when Hodgkin and Huxley demonstrated that ionic currents through membrane channels were the trigger for contractile activity and theorized that sliding filaments were the intrinsic apparatus underlying the contractile force of the muscle. Since then, details of the processes whereby muscle tissue and individual muscle fibers convert neurochemical signals, through electrochemical propagation, to generate mechanical force have been elucidated. This entry focuses on basic mechanisms of contraction of the individual skeletal muscle fibers and highlights illustrative examples of disease states produced by abnormalities of either the electrical or the contractile apparatus.

MEMBRANE PROPAGATION OF ELECTRICAL ACTIVITY

As is true for neural tissue, a resting membrane potential renders the interior of the muscle fiber negative with respect to the extracellular space. At the neuromuscular junction, ion channels open in response to acetylcholine binding to specific receptors and a depolarizing electric current is produced. This depolarization spreads from the synaptic region to areas of muscle membrane possessing different ion channels that open in response to voltage changes in the membrane, in which a muscle action potential is generated. The muscle action potential spreads in all directions along the muscle fiber membrane by a regenerative process involving differential ion permeabilities governed by transmembrane channels.

The three main channels responsible for generation of the muscle action potential are the voltage-gated sodium, potassium, and chloride channels. Channels are composed of transmembrane proteins that form pores in the muscle membrane and, triggered by depolarization, change conformation, thus altering their respective ion conductances. When activated, the voltage-gated sodium channels open, allowing the rapid influx of extracellular sodium down its electrochemical gradient and producing a depolarizing electrical current. Activation of voltage-gated potassium channels permits efflux of potassium ions that produces an opposing repolarizing electrical current. Voltage-gated chloride channels are predominantly open at rest but close in response to hyperpolarization; the resulting decrease in chloride conductance acts to stabilize the resting membrane potential. Subsequent conformational changes are responsible for inactivation and resetting of these channel proteins. The sequence and differential kinetics of these channel activations and voltage shifts lead to the generation of an action potential that is brief, self-limited, and regenerative.

The voltage-gated sodium channels open quickly, and the sodium current leads to rapid depolarization of local areas of membrane. This depolarization spreads as additional voltage-gated sodium channels open in neighboring areas of the membrane. These channels then rapidly inactivate, become temporarily refractory to further opening, and require repolarization to reset and be available for reactivation. The deactivation of these sodium channels limits the depolarizing phase of the action potential. Voltage-gated potassium channels activate and inactivate more slowly than sodium channels, allowing the repolarizing potassium current to bring the local membrane potential back toward the resting voltage. The delayed inactivation causes a brief hyperpolarization that temporarily inhibits further depolarization.

The action potential spreads as a wave of depolarization followed by repolarization along the exterior muscle membrane and then to specialized tubular invaginations of sarcolemma called T tubules. This extensive tubular system of membrane distributes the muscle action potential to the interior of the muscle fiber so that the resultant contraction occurs nearly simultaneously throughout the muscle fiber. This produces a more efficient muscle contraction than would occur otherwise. In the T tubule system, the same ions, channels, and currents are responsible for propagation of the action potential. However, the extracellular volume within the T tubule system is quite limited. With this decreased volume for equilibration of ions, the relatively small ionic shifts during action potential propagation can accumulate and alter the voltage characteristics of the membrane. In normal muscle, the stabilizing role of chloride channels is critical for maintaining the appropriate membrane potential. Within the T tubule system, this is particularly important because the inward rectifying chloride currents help repolarize the membrane and inhibit afterdepolarization in circumstances of localized potassium accumulation that may occur following repeated contractions. Abnormalities in chloride conductance can result in certain disease states, as discussed later in this entry.

EXCITATION/CONTRACTION/RELAXATION CYCLE

The muscle action potential triggers a sequence of actions that ultimately results in the contraction and relaxation of the muscle fiber. This sequence is called the excitation/contraction/relaxation cycle. An early step in this cycle is the release of stored calcium from an intracellular membrane complex called the sarcoplasmic reticulum (SR). This is mediated through the activation of a specialized membrane protein complex that binds the drug dihydropyridine and has been called the dihydropyridine receptor (DHPR). The DHPR is a tetrameric complex located in the sarcolemmal membrane of the T tubules at the junctional region between the T tubules and the terminal cisternae of the SR. Each DHPR is believed to represent a functional unit in the transduction of sarcolemmal depolarization and sarcoplasmic calcium release. The transmembrane portions of the

DHPR constitute the voltage-sensitive elements and are believed to change conformation in response to depolarization similar to the voltage-gated channels described previously. Although the DHPR has also been shown to have the properties of a slowly activating, voltage-sensitive, calcium channel *in vitro*, entry of extracellular calcium is not required for either signal detection or transmission. It has been shown that a cytoplasmic loop portion of the DHPR is the critical element for transmission of the external membrane depolarization to the intracellular SR calcium release channels.

The SR calcium release channels consist of four identical monomers that bind a plant alkaloid ryanodine and therefore have been called ryanodine receptors (RyRs). These channels are located in the SR, with a cloverleaf pattern of protein constituents forming a central pore that branches in four radially arranged canals. Interestingly, although each tetrad of DHPRs faces one RyR at the junctional region with the T tubules, this only accounts for half of the RyRs, and it is not known how the rest of these channels are activated.

On the cytoplasmic face of the SR, the calcium release channels are associated with several small proteins whose functions are not as clear. Calsequestrin is a low-affinity calcium-binding protein in the SR membrane. Another small protein, triadin, is believed to either anchor calsequestrin in the membrane or provide a direct link between calsequestrin and the SR calcium release channels. A small cytoplasmic protein that binds the immunosuppressive drug FK506, called FK506-binding protein (FKBP), has been found to stabilize the full calcium conductance of the RyRs. In addition, the activity of the RyRs is modulated by several endogenous cytoplasmic factors, ATP, Mg^{2+}, H^+, inorganic phosphate, and different phosphorylation states of the RyR, but the most important appears to be a very strong inhibitory association with Mg^{2+}.

Several lines of evidence support the following model for the mechanism of coupling excitation and contraction proposed by Stephenson *et al.* Depolarization of the T tubule membrane triggers conformational changes in the DHPR that, through interaction between cytoplasmic loop portions of the DHPR complex and the FKBP, lead to changes in the RyRs complex that lower its affinity for Mg^{2+} binding. Dissociation of ionic magnesium releases the RyRs from the inhibited state, and sarcoplasmic calcium is released into the cytoplasm. This is accompanied by further Ca^{2+}-activated calcium release that results in a rapid increase in cytoplasmic calcium. It is the interaction of this intracellular calcium with the contractile apparatus that ultimately leads to contraction.

Once depolarization, activation, and contraction cease, relaxation of the muscle fiber proceeds by more well-understood mechanisms. Relaxation is achieved when the cytoplasmic Ca^{2+} concentration is decreased to its resting state. This is partially accomplished by resequestration of Ca^{2+} by the sarcoplasmic calcium pump. This membrane protein is widespread in the SR, except at the junctional region with the T tubules, and it couples the active transport of Ca^{2+}, against its concentration gradient, with hydrolysis of Mg/ATP. The observed decrease in cytoplasmic calcium concentration, however, precedes full activation of the SR calcium pump and therefore must also be mediated by other cytoplasmic binding sites. The balance of calcium release and sequestration is modulated by the frequency of sarcoplasmic depolarization. Higher frequencies of nerve action potentials as well as pathological depolarization lead to greater calcium release and subsequent contraction.

CONTRACTILE APPARATUS AND NONCONTRACTILE STRUCTURAL COMPLEXES

The contractile apparatus consists of the many striated myofibrils that make up each myosite (Fig. 1). The change in length of the myofibril during forge generation is accompanied by a change in the banding pattern observed on light microscopy. This was determined to be the result of shifting overlap of the thin and thick filaments of the myofibrils and, in the 1950s, led Huxley to propose the sliding filament theory as the structural basis of muscle contraction. The interactions of other proteins, nucleotides, and ions have been shown to be essential for both regulation of contraction and anchoring of the contractile apparatus in the cell membrane and the extracellular matrix in order to ensure orderly contraction and functional transmission of force at the tissue level.

The sarcomere is the functional unit of contraction and contains thick and thin filaments bound on either end by Z disks, which form a cross-sectional structure that spans the myofibril at repeated intervals. Thin filaments are made up of two helically arranged filamentous polymers of the protein actin together with a long filamentous protein tropomyo-

sin that lies in the grooves of the helix as well as an associated globular protein troponin, found at intervals along the filament. Thin filaments are anchored at the Z disks and extend in both directions along the long axis of the myofibril. The thick filaments are formed by approximately 250 myosin molecules, in which the long filamentous "tail" portions are intertwined along most of their length and globular "head" subunits on flexible stems are arranged radially in a staggered array that covers most of the length of the filament. These thick filaments overlap the thin filaments and are held in the center of the sarcomere by thin proteins called connectins. Contractile force is produced by the formation of cross-bridges between filaments and conformational changes that cause adjacent thin and thick filaments to slide past each other.

The thin filaments mediate the onset of contraction in response to the increase in intracellular calcium. The released intracellular calcium is bound by troponin and through interaction with tropomyosin leads to conformational changes in the thin filaments that expose actin binding sites for myosin. The myosin heads then bind to actin, forming a multitude of cross-bridges between the filaments. This interaction leads to a conformational change whereby the flexible neck portions of individual myosin molecules bend, providing the force that slides the thin filaments in respect to the thick filaments. If sufficient ATP is present, the myosin heads dissociate and are reset; if binding sites on the thin filaments remain exposed, cyclical interaction and the generation of force continue. In this way, the Z disks are thus drawn closer together, the sarcomeres shorten, and the fibril contracts. During relaxation, free intracellular calcium is resequestered and the thin filaments return to their previous conformation where myosin binding sites are unavailable.

The myosin head subunits mediate the conversion of chemical energy to mechanical work through the hydrolysis of ATP. Binding of ATP by the multiple myosin head subunits is required for dissociation of the cross-bridges. Hydrolysis of ATP is accompanied by a conformational change in the myosin heads that have stored mechanical energy and reset its position with respect to the thin filaments. The subsequent interaction between the myosin head units and the thin filaments is very energetically favorable so that the contraction that results from the formation of cross-bridges and sliding of thick filaments across thin filaments requires little energy expenditure.

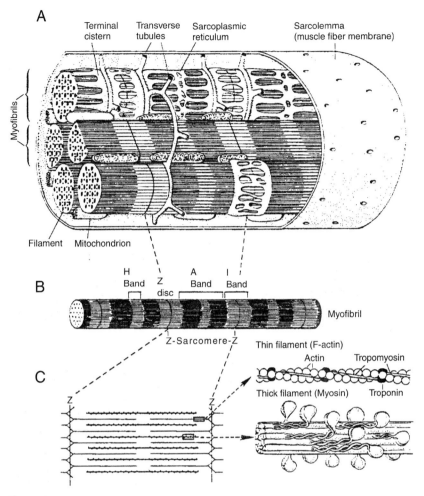

Figure 1
Alternating light and dark bands within the myofibrils give skeletal muscle its characteristic striated appearance. (A) Three-dimensional reconstruction of a sector of muscle fiber showing the relationships of the membrane and tubular systems to the myofibrils. (B) Individual myofibril showing light and dark bands. Individual sarcomeres are separated by thin Z disks. The dark bands correspond to regions of overlap of thin and thick filaments. (C) Schematic cross section of an individual sarcomere. The thin filaments are composed principally of polymerized actin, whereas the thick filaments are made up of arrays of myosin molecules. The myosin molecule includes a stem and a globular double head that protrudes from the stem (reproduced with permission from Kandel *et al.*, p. 549, Fig. 36-1).

The contractile apparatus is connected to the extracellular matrix by interactions with a host of structural proteins. These proteins play a crucial role in the conversion of mechanical force generated by the contracting sarcomeres and individual myofibrils into the coordinated action of the myosites and ultimately contraction of the muscle tissue. The structural proteins that connect the contractile apparatus to the sarcoplasmic membrane and ultimately to the extracellular matrix are found in the intra- and extracellular space in addition to spanning the membrane (Fig. 2). On the cytoplasmic side, the large dystrophin molecule runs parallel to the sarcolemma; one end binds filamentous actin,

whereas the other binds to dystroglycan. Utrophin is another large protein that binds actin and dystroglycan and is widespread under the sarcolemma, but after birth it is restricted to end plate regions. Other proteins are also involved with linking filamentous actin to dystroglycan, but after birth dystrophin is the most extensive and important. Syntrophins are another group of intracellular proteins that in different tissues bind dystroglycan and in skeletal muscle are abundant at the neuromuscular junction.

Embedded in the membrane is the sarcoglycan complex, which is a tightly associated collection of five glycoproteins that are believed to interact with

Dystrophin Associated Protein Complex

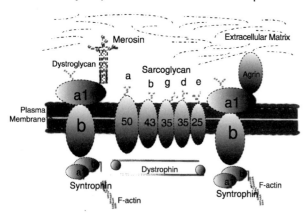

Figure 2
Structural proteins of the sarcolemmal membrane showing syntropin and f-actin complexed with dystrophin on the intracellular face bound through dystroglycan to the membrane-spanning sarcoglycan complex. On the extracellular face, merosin, a subunit of the extracellular matrix protein laminin, is bound to this complex through dystroglycan (reproduced with permission from Brown, 1997).

dystrophin and dystroglycan. Dystroglycan is an integral membrane protein that has two subunits. The beta subunit spans the sarcolemmal membrane, whereas the alpha subunit interacts with the extracellular matrix. On the extracellular side of the sarcolemma, the matrix protein laminin is composed of a heterotrimer in which the α_2 subunit, also called merisin, binds to dystroglycan. A direct link from the contractile apparatus to the extracellular matrix is postulated as follows: Filamentous actin through dystrophin interacts with dystroglycan that is stabilized by the sarcoglycan complex. In turn, dystroglycan, through merosin, binds the extracellular matrix.

DISEASES OF MUSCLE EXCITATION AND CONTRACTION

It is clear that many of the muscular dystrophies are caused by mutations in the genes encoding dystrophin and the dystrophin-associated proteins. In 1987, the gene defect responsible for Duchenne's muscular dystrophy (DMD) was identified on the X chromosome; both deletions and point mutations in the dystrophin gene were shown to result in the near or complete absence of synthesis of the dystrophin protein. Becker's muscular dystrophy was later shown to be the result of several different mutations in the same dystrophin gene causing either reduced concentrations of normal dystrophin or synthesis of

abnormal protein. The limb–girdle muscular dystrophies (LGMDs) are a collection of diseases that in their most severe form present similar to DMD but in autosomal dominant and recessive patterns as well as in boys and girls. Kindred and genetic linkage analyses have led to the identification of several genes and defects concerning the components of the sarcoglycan complex as the abnormalities in many of the LGMDs. The sarcoglycan complex appears to be sensitive to defects in any of its components. Immunostaining of muscle from many LGMD patients shows a severe reduction in staining for the sarcoglycan complex, regardless of which component is affected, and relatively normal dystrophin staining, whereas muscle from DMD patients shows a near absence of dystrophin staining and significant reduction in sarcoglycan complex staining. α_2 laminin or merosin deficiency has been linked to a congenital muscular dystrophy. Mutations in genes for the contractile proteins myosin and tropomyosin have been found to cause central core and nemoline rod diseases, which are characterized by slowly progressive, lifelong muscle weakness.

In contrast to the diseases discussed previously in which either point mutations or DNA deletions result in reduced or abnormal protein products, the genetic abnormality producing myotonic dystrophy (MD) is one of increased genetic material. In normal circumstances, the gene for myotonin contains up to 30 identical repeats of the sequence CTG. When there are more than 50 repeats, however, MD is the result. In general, as the number of repeated sequences increases, so does the severity of the disease. Myotonic dystrophy is the second most common muscular dystrophy behind DMD and is a multisystem disorder characterized by subtle muscle stiffness due to electrical irritability, facial and distal limb muscle wasting and weakness, dysarthria, frontal balding, atypical cataracts, and cardiac conduction system defects. Despite detailed knowledge of the genetic abnormality underlying MD, the physiological and pathophysiological role of myotonin is not known, but it is believed to code for a ubiquitous protein kinase.

Defects in other structural, membrane, and channel proteins have been linked to specific muscle diseases. An abnormality in the Ryanodine receptor gene has been linked to malignant hyperthermia as well as one type of central core disease. Mutations in genes encoding voltage-dependent ion channels have been identified; patients with diseases that result from such mutations have specific symptoms that can be ascribed to abnormal channel function. Approximately 19 different mutations of the same sarcolemmal chloride channel genes, named ClC-1, have been associated with both dominantly and recessively inherited myotonia. The muscle membrane irritability and prolonged contraction characteristic of Thomsen's myotonia congenita and Becker's autosomal recessive myotonia are due to mutations in voltage-sensitive chloride channels that buffer potassium accumulation in the T tubule system; abnormal chloride channel function leads to afterdepolarizations and continued contraction. Several mutations of the voltage-gated sodium channel have been linked to both hereditary hyperkalemic periodic paralysis and paramyotonia congenita as well as atypical myotonias. Defects in sodium channel deactivation allow small persistent or brief repeated influx of sodium, causing depolarization of the resting membrane and inactivation of the same sodium channels that has been observed during attacks of periodic paralysis. Late and prolonged openings due to similar failure of deactivation states are thought to cause myotonia. In hypokalemic periodic paralysis, membrane depolarization is also associated with paralysis, and associated mutations have been found in the DHPR gene. Although these mutant DHPR channels expressed in other cells have been shown to have reduced calcium conductance, entry of extracellular calcium is not required for the detection of the depolarizing signal in the T tubules or transmission to the SR calcium release channels. The pathophysiological mechanism linking the abnormal DHPRs to membrane depolarization is unknown.

—*Michael L. Vertino and Jeremy M. Shefner*

See also–Action Potential, Generation of; Motor Control, Peripheral; Motor System, Overview; Muscle Strength, Assessment of; Muscle Tone; Muscular Dystrophy: Limb–Girdle, Becker's, and Duchenne's; Neuromuscular Disorders, Overview

Further Reading

Barchi, R. B. (1997). Ion channel mutations and disease of skeletal muscle. *Neurobiol. Dis.* **4**, 254–264.

Brown, R. H. (1997). Dystrophin-associated proteins and the muscular dystrophies. *Annu. Rev. Med.* **48**, 457–466.

Cooke, R. (1997). Actomyosin interactions in striated muscle. *Physiol. Rev.* **77**, 671–697.

Cooper, E. C., and Jan, L. Y. (1999). Ion channel genes and human neurological disease: Recent progress, prospects, and challenges. *Proc. Natl. Acad. Sci. USA* **96**, 4759–4766.

Ghez, C. (1996). Muscles: Effectors of the motor systems. In *Principles of Neural Science* (E. R. Kandell, J. H. Schwartz, and T. J. Jessel, Eds.), 3rd ed., pp. 548–563.

Stephenson, D. G., Lamb, G. D., and Stephenson, G. M. M. (1998). Events of the excitation–contraction–relaxation cycle in the fast and slow twitch mammalian muscle fibers relevant to fatigue. *Acta Physiol. Scand.* **162**, 229–245.

Muscle Strength, Assessment of

Encyclopedia of the Neurological Sciences
Copyright 2003, Elsevier Science (USA). All rights reserved.

STRENGTH affords independence in daily activities, allows the artistic movement of dance and the physical prowess of athletics. When the dancer, athlete, or retiree complains of functional weakness, the only tool that may be available for a physician to assess strength loss is manual muscle testing (MMT). MMT may show normal strength when quantitative strength measures show a 50% decrease in strength.

Up to one-third of motor neurons may die before functional problems occur. Many quantitative tests assess maximal isometric strength, but many important functional tasks, such as ambulation and speech, do not require maximal isometric strength.

Quantitating and tracking strength can be done in numerous ways. Strength can be expressed by comparison to a norm. The caveat is that it takes a significant body of data to adequately determine norms. Strength can be measured and plotted over time to assess change, which means a sensitive, reliable way of measuring force must be used. A simple way to test strength is by observation of function, such as the patient demonstrating Gowers' sign (walking the hands up the legs from a bent-over position) when attempting to stand up. As technology has advanced, clinicians have been able to choose from more sensitive quantitation tools. Early detection of weakness can lead to early diagnosis, treatment, and monitoring of disease progression.

SELECTION OF ASSESSMENT TOOLS

Several criteria should be considered when selecting a strength assessment tool. Are data needed for clinical or research purposes, and how sensitive need the assessment be? Will the strength data be used to assess efficacy of a treatment, and how small is the treatment effect that the clinician wishes to detect?

Quick and meaningful clinical testing can be done in the office with only hands, pen, and paper. To document subtle changes in strength, more sensitive mechanized tools are needed. Cost-effectiveness, training needs, and availability must be accounted for in the selection of strength assessment tools.

MANUAL MUSCLE TESTING

For clinical use, there are several cost-effective ways to measure strength. The most common technique is MMT as described by Kendall and Kendall. Manual resistance by the examiner and the patient's ability to move a limb against gravity are used to grade muscles from 0 (no muscle contraction detectable) to 5 (able to move against gravity and give strong resistance). A notable shortcoming of this technique is its relative insensitivity to subtle changes in strength in strong muscles. The patient may complain of strength changes that the clinician is unable to detect. In a comparison study of MMT and isokinetic testing in 108 subjects, it was noted that MMT could not distinguish patients without weakness from those categorized as having 75% of normal strength. Studies have demonstrated a wide distribution of quantitative strength values within each MMT grade, with the widest distribution found in grades 4 and 5. MMT produces ordinal data with uneven intervals between grades. Muscles in grades 4 and 5 may lose up to 40% of their strength before dropping one muscle grade, whereas muscles in grades 1 and 2 drop a full grade with a loss of 2–5% of strength. When documentation of mild weakness is paramount, a more sensitive measure should be chosen.

MMT has been used successfully in research under the following circumstances: the evaluators are all health care clinicians, large numbers of muscles are tested, a single rater follows each patient, and the examiner is stronger than the patient. MMT grades also give an approximate clinical impression of the functional difficulties a patient may be facing and therefore may elucidate an opportunity for rehabilitative or orthotic intervention. Using MMT, the clinician is less likely to be able to detect a small strength change that may hamper high-performance activities such as athletics. Overall, MMT is easily performed and is a good general indicator of both strength and the likelihood of notable functional impairment.

HANDHELD DYNAMOMETRY

Handheld dynamometry (HHD) is an efficient, objective, sensitive, and affordable alternative for strength quantitation. A small portable device is held by the examiner and placed against the patient's limb during a maximal isometric contraction. The device can be used to test both proximal and distal muscles in all extremities. Specific dynamometers are used to test grip strength. The testing positions are standardized to reduce variance of serial measures. This strength measure is more sensitive to change than MMT and correlates well with fixed dynamometry up to 30-kg force.

As with MMT and fixed dynamometry, variability of test results increases when multiple raters are used in longitudinal assessments. In 18 studies reviewed by Bohannon, inter-rater (variability between different raters) reliability coefficients for HHD ranged from −0.19 to 0.99, with the majority surpassing 0.70. Goonetilleke found that HHD readings obtained by multiple raters may be up to 53% more variable than those obtained by a single rater. In contrast, he found low intrarater variability (variability between tests performed by a single rater), with a coefficient of variation of 5.4%. In most studies that assessed upper and lower extremities, the reliability coefficients for the upper extremity tests were greater.

Another notable source of variability in HHD is the strength of the examiner. Strong muscles may be underestimated by clinicians whose strength is less than that of the patient due to the clinician's inability to immobilize the HHD when the subject exerts a force greater than the examiner is able to resist.

MAXIMAL VOLUNTARY ISOMETRIC CONTRACTION WITH FIXED DYNAMOMETRY

Fixed computerized dynamometry minimizes some of the drawbacks seen in other means of maximal isometric strength testing. Examiner strength is a less significant variable due to the use of straps between the limb and metal bars, which attach to an examination table. This mechanism aids the examiner in holding the limb in a standard position. Maximal Voluntary Isometric Contraction (MVIC) has been used increasingly for over 10 years in more than 50 academic centers in the United States. It is more practical to acquire this system for use in research, although the equipment can be used for clinical purposes as well. Software is now available to produce strength reports that express results in kilograms, percentage-predicted strength, and percentage change since the previous evaluation. A normal database was developed using cross-sectional data from 440 normal subjects aged 20–90. Percentage predicted strength provides more clinically meaningful data than other statistical expressions of strength. MVIC results can also be expressed in kilograms or in megascores.

To allow comparison of raw MVIC scores from different muscles, megascores represent grouped data after they have been standardized. To standardize MVIC data, a z-score transformation relates each piece of raw data to the mean value for a similar function of a reference population (z score = raw score−mean of reference population/standard deviation of reference population). Thus, a value of 1 indicates that a particular score is one standard deviation above the mean of the reference population. The megascore improves the efficiency of data analysis by summarizing large numbers of data points (megascore = z score No. 1−z score No. 2/2). The reliability of the composite measure is greater than that of any single measure due to balancing of measurement errors and reducing erroneous significant findings by decreasing the number of statistical comparisons. Although statistically useful, these scores are not as readily understood in clinical terms as percentage of predicted strength (e.g., pulmonary function is usually expressed as percentage of predicted). Megascores are not the best means of evaluating intra-rater (test–retest by the same examiner) and inter-rater (test–retest by different examiners) reliability since the grouping of many data points may mask excess variability in some measurements.

The MVIC equipment consists of aluminum uprights fixed around a hydraulic table, a strain gauge (force transducer) interfaced with a computer, and specialized software. Many different software packages are in use throughout the United States. There are standard positions for the patient's joint, for stabilization of the limb, for strap placement, and for coaching. The results are sensitive and can document changes in strength that are not detectable clinically. In a 9-month study comparing manual muscle testing and MVIC in 20 patients with amyotrophic lateral sclerosis, it was shown that MMT overestimated strength at the first visit by an average of 24% compared to MVIC. This study highlights the advantage of MVIC over MMT in detecting mild isometric weakness (Fig. 1).

As seen in other quantitative strength measures, variability between different raters (inter-rater) is much greater than test–retest for the same rater (intra-rater). When testing both upper and lower

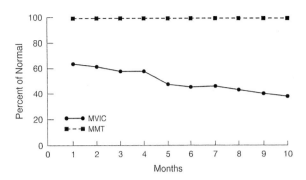

Figure 1

Comparison of MMT measurement of quadriceps decline with MVIC measurement of quadriceps decline during a 10-month period [reproduced with permission from Munsat, T. L., *et al.* (1990). Therapeutic trials in amyotrophic lateral sclerosis: Measurement of clinical deficit. In *Amyotrophic Lateral Sclerosis* (F. C. Rose, Ed.), p. 70. Demos, New York].

extremity muscles, intra-rater reliability ranges from 6.5% mean absolute percentage variation (data obtained from experienced rehabilitation professionals) to 10.4% (data obtained from trained examiners with varied professional backgrounds). Inter-rater variability ranges from 7.6% (few evaluators and many test–retests performed) to 13.1% (many evaluators and few test–retests). Adequate training is critical to minimizing errors due to the rater. Small changes in joint testing angle, strap placement (lever length), and coaching by the examiner can affect the strength outcome. The best reliability outcomes have been shown in small groups of health care professionals who have become rigorously standardized as evaluators. The MVIC system costs several thousand dollars. The major flexor and extensor muscle groups of all extremities (shoulder, elbow, hip, and knee) can be tested with this system (Fig. 2). Sanjak *et al.* at the University of Wisconsin developed and published a method for testing neck extensors and flexors. Small, handheld, specialized MVIC equipment also exists for lingual and lip strength testing.

ISOKINETIC DYNAMOMETRY

Isokinetic dynamometry assesses maximal torque production at a specified velocity of limb movement. Isokinetic tests may reveal weakness before isometric tests indicate any strength loss. In a study comparing isokinetic dynamometry and MMT (ankle and knee flexors and extensors), muscles graded as normal by MMT were represented by isokinetic values as low as 48.5% of predicted. These isokinetic data show that

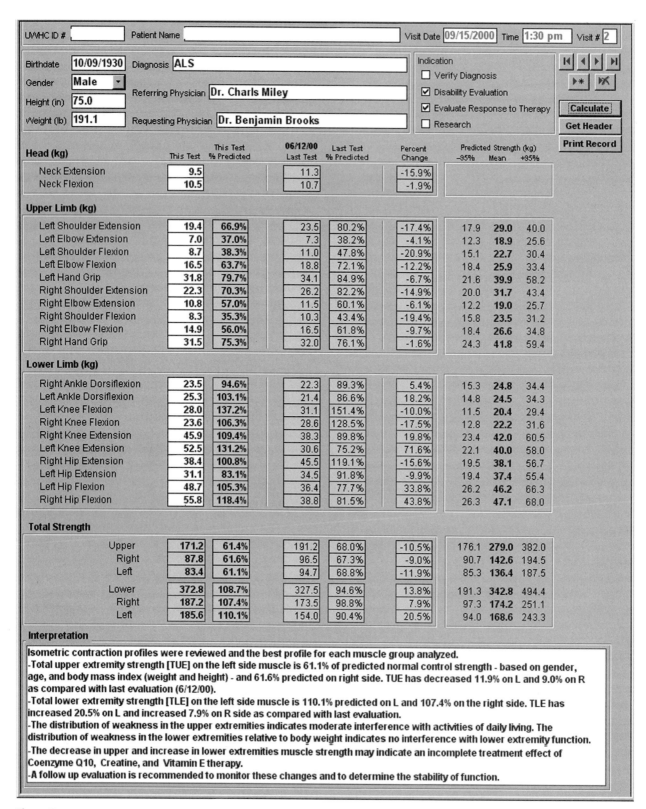

		This Test	06/12/00	Last Test	Percent	Predicted Strength (kg)		
UWHC ID #	Patient Name				Visit Date 09/15/2000	Time 1:30 pm	Visit # 2	

UWHC ID # | **Patient Name** | Visit Date 09/15/2000 | Time 1:30 pm | Visit # 2

Birthdate 10/09/1930 Diagnosis ALS
Gender Male
Height (in) 75.0 Referring Physician Dr. Charls Miley
Weight (lb) 191.1 Requesting Physician Dr. Benjamin Brooks

Indication
☐ Verify Diagnosis
☑ Disability Evaluation
☑ Evaluate Response to Therapy
☐ Research

Calculate
Get Header
Print Record

Head (kg)	This Test	This Test % Predicted	06/12/00 Last Test	Last Test % Predicted	Percent Change	Predicted Strength (kg) -95%	Mean	+95%
Neck Extension	9.5		11.3		-15.9%			
Neck Flexion	10.5		10.7		-1.9%			

Upper Limb (kg)								
Left Shoulder Extension	19.4	66.9%	23.5	80.2%	-17.4%	17.9	29.0	40.0
Left Elbow Extension	7.0	37.0%	7.3	38.2%	-4.1%	12.3	18.9	25.6
Left Shoulder Flexion	8.7	38.3%	11.0	47.8%	-20.9%	15.1	22.7	30.4
Left Elbow Flexion	16.5	63.7%	18.8	72.1%	-12.2%	18.4	25.9	33.4
Left Hand Grip	31.8	79.7%	34.1	84.9%	-6.7%	21.6	39.9	58.2
Right Shoulder Extension	22.3	70.3%	26.2	82.2%	-14.9%	20.0	31.7	43.4
Right Elbow Extension	10.8	57.0%	11.5	60.1%	-6.1%	12.2	19.0	25.7
Right Shoulder Flexion	8.3	35.3%	10.3	43.4%	-19.4%	15.8	23.5	31.2
Right Elbow Flexion	14.9	56.0%	16.5	61.8%	-9.7%	18.4	26.6	34.8
Right Hand Grip	31.5	75.3%	32.0	76.1%	-1.6%	24.3	41.8	59.4

Lower Limb (kg)								
Right Ankle Dorsiflexion	23.5	94.6%	22.3	89.3%	5.4%	15.3	24.8	34.4
Left Ankle Dorsiflexion	25.3	103.1%	21.4	86.6%	18.2%	14.8	24.5	34.3
Left Knee Flexion	28.0	137.2%	31.1	151.4%	-10.0%	11.5	20.4	29.4
Right Knee Flexion	23.6	106.3%	28.6	128.5%	-17.5%	12.8	22.2	31.6
Right Knee Extension	45.9	109.4%	38.3	89.8%	19.8%	23.4	42.0	60.5
Left Knee Extension	52.5	131.2%	30.6	75.2%	71.6%	22.1	40.0	58.0
Right Hip Extension	38.4	100.8%	45.5	119.1%	-15.6%	19.5	38.1	56.7
Left Hip Extension	31.1	83.1%	34.5	91.8%	-9.9%	19.4	37.4	55.4
Left Hip Flexion	48.7	105.3%	36.4	77.7%	33.8%	26.2	46.2	66.3
Right Hip Flexion	55.8	118.4%	38.8	81.5%	43.8%	26.3	47.1	68.0

Total Strength								
Upper	171.2	61.4%	191.2	68.0%	-10.5%	176.1	279.0	382.0
Right	87.8	61.6%	96.5	67.3%	-9.0%	90.7	142.6	194.5
Left	83.4	61.1%	94.7	68.8%	-11.9%	85.3	136.4	187.5
Lower	372.8	108.7%	327.5	94.6%	13.8%	191.3	342.8	494.4
Right	187.2	107.4%	173.5	98.8%	7.9%	97.3	174.2	251.1
Left	185.6	110.1%	154.0	90.4%	20.5%	94.0	168.6	243.3

Interpretation

Isometric contraction profiles were reviewed and the best profile for each muscle group analyzed.
-Total upper extremity strength [TUE] on the left side muscle is 61.1% of predicted normal control strength - based on gender, age, and body mass index (weight and height) - and 61.6% predicted on right side. TUE has decreased 11.9% on L and 9.0% on R as compared with last evaluation (6/12/00).
-Total lower extremity strength [TLE] on the left side muscle is 110.1% predicted on L and 107.4% on the right side. TLE has increased 20.5% on L and increased 7.9% on R side as compared with last evaluation.
-The distribution of weakness in the upper extremities indicates moderate interference with activities of daily living. The distribution of weakness in the lower extremities relative to body weight indicates no interference with lower extremity function.
-The decrease in upper and increase in lower extremities muscle strength may indicate an incomplete treatment effect of Coenzyme Q10, Creatine, and Vitamin E therapy.
-A follow up evaluation is recommended to monitor these changes and to determine the stability of function.

Figure 2

Reproduction of MVIC printout [reproduced with permission from Sanjak, M., Konopaki, R., Belden, D., *et al.* (2000). *Computerized Isometric Muscle Strength Test Report Generation Software*, Version 2. University of Wisconsin Hospital and Clinic, Neurology Department, Madison].

muscles may lose more than 50% of predicted strength while having an MMT grade of normal. This highlights the greater sensitivity of isokinetic testing compared with MMT to detect early strength loss. Gleeson and Mercer noted a coefficient of variation of 13% in lower extremity isokinetic testing. Other studies of knee and ankle isokinetic testing show test–retest variability between 4.8 and 14%, with higher variability in very weak muscles and with eccentric testing. Isokinetic testing may not be the first choice for strength assessment in severely impaired neurological patients due to both the necessity of antigravity strength (MMT grade 3) to move the dynamometer arm the full range required and the labor intensity of testing multiple joints. Test results include peak torque, force decrement with repeated tests, the ratio of agonist to antagonist strength, and average power. The limb can be tested at different angular velocities, from very slow movement to high-speed repetitive movement. Although these devices are expensive for general use, patients can be referred to qualified physical therapy clinics for testing. In practice, quantitative isometric muscle testing (HHD or MVIC) is more practical for tracking several muscle groups over time.

ERGOMETRIC TESTS

Other ergometric tests, such as those used in cardiac and sports rehabilitation, can be used to assess muscle endurance. Muscular endurance refers to the ability of muscles to sustain either repeated contractions or a prolonged isometric contraction. For example, the number of times a patient can step up and down in a set amount of time is a simple endurance assessment tool [work (kg/min) = body weight × step height × number of steps per minute]. For some patients with progressive neurological impairments, this type of test may be unsafe due to the risk of falling. Stationary bicycles and treadmills can be used to assess muscular endurance as well, and the rate of oxygen consumption during standardized work can be measured. When a subject exercises to the level of exhaustion, cardiovascular and muscular endurance capacity, as indicated by the highest attainable oxygen consumption (VO_2 max), can be recorded. With endurance training, VO_2 max can increase. These tests are usually performed by exercise physiologists in cardiac laboratories. The VO_2 max tests require a relatively high functioning patient who has enough strength, balance, and endurance to safely perform the tests.

FUNCTIONAL TESTS

Functional tests are useful benchmarks for clinicians and patients to track strength changes. Functional baseline data elicited by query or by observation (such as the ability to rise from a chair with or without use of arms and the ability to go up and down stairs) is a basic but meaningful way to monitor a patient's progress. When queried, a patient may offer a range of functional deficits related to strength. Although these data are clinically valuable, they are less useful as research tools. In research these functions are timed or rated, numbered, and validated as a functional scale. The clinician should also note that functional tests, although meaningful, are insensitive to early strength changes that antedate functional changes.

FUNCTIONAL SCALES

Functional scales have been developed to measure the effects of disease processes on patients' functional capabilities and to assess the efficacy of therapeutic intervention. The clinician questions the patient regarding his or her functional status or observes the patient's function and rates the subject's performance. These scales often include several sections based on, for example, upper extremity activities of daily living, ambulation status, oral motor function, respiratory function, writing, or eating. There are general disability scales and disease-specific scales with varying merits based on their sensitivity to short-term and long-term changes and their relevance to the disease process. Since strength loss antedates functional loss, scales are insensitive to these preclinical changes. Although ordinal data are produced, scales are cost-effective and useful in both the clinical and research setting. Some scales, such as the amyotrophic lateral sclerosis functional rating scale (ALSFRS), are quick to perform, sensitive to change, and correlate with measures such as computer-based isometric testing.

RESPIRATORY MUSCLE STRENGTH

Patients may lose up to 50% of their limb strength prior to a clinician being able to detect strength loss, and studies have shown that patients who are strong may be steadily losing strength without noticing any functional changes. Similarly, changes in respiratory function, as detected by pulmonary tests, may not be accompanied by functional complaints such as dyspnea. Also, patients may not mention other symptoms of respiratory muscle weakness, such as somnolence, frequent nocturnal arousals, decreased voice intensity, failure to feel rested after sleeping, and ineffective cough. Schiffman and Belsh noted that 86% of their patients with ALS had signs of respiratory muscle weakness at enrollment in a pulmonary function study, whereas only a small percentage of these patients had complaints of respiratory symptoms. Others have confirmed that respiratory muscle weakness can precede both symptomatic complaints and reduction in vital capacity.

Maximal respiratory strength is not required to fully inflate or deflate lungs, so one would not expect high sensitivity in detecting early respiratory strength loss using volume measures such as the forced vital capacity (FVC). One may have a high FVC but have early weakness of the respiratory muscles. In contrast, maximal inspiratory pressures (MIP), or negative inspiratory force (NIF), and expiratory pressures have been shown to be a more sensitive indicator of early loss of respiratory muscle strength. However, variability is greater in MIP measurements than in FVC measurements, and some authors suggest that there is a learning effect that does not carry over between patient visits. If the patient uses intraoral pressure when performing the test, this can falsely inflate the values. Some clinicians have suggested the use of more than five test repetitions and the use of masks during testing to limit error from intraoral pressures. The MIP or NIF is a useful early indicator of reduced inspiratory muscle strength, although more studies on reliability and appropriate testing methods are needed.

VARIANCE AND RELIABILITY

With all these methods for tracking strength, attention to accuracy of testing is essential. Errors can occur due to the tester, the patient, or the equipment. Guiloff estimated that raters contributed 37% of the total variability in HHD, and data derived by three different raters had 53% greater variability than intrarater data. These errors decrease sensitivity of the method to reliably detect change. Measures such as dynamometry and MMT require thorough training and rigid attention to detail. Variables such as joint position during the test, lever length (where the strap or the examiner's hand is placed for resistance), coaching, stabilization of proximal joints, biofeedback, the number

of test repetitions, and rest intervals must be standardized. Many studies have shown that reliability decreases with multiple testers. If multiple testers are used, inter-rater reliability should be assessed, and thorough training in the standard protocol should be arranged. Reliability testing for single raters is also advisable. Equipment should be calibrated daily.

VARIABILITY DUE TO THE PATIENT

When the goal of testing is to elicit a maximal voluntary muscle contraction, the examiner must attend to emotional and intellectual patient variables. Since subject performance in strength measurement is effort dependent, mood states such as depression can adversely affect test outcome. The patient must also fully understand both how to perform the test and the goal of the test. Expectations for patient performance must be understood by the patient for the results to be reliable. The tenor of the clinician's coaching also has an effect on patient performance and motivation. For maximal strength testing, the patient should be encouraged to give his or her best effort. Meek or indecisive coaching may adversely affect the subject's effort. In the presence of pain, an accurate strength test is unlikely and should not be forced. The patient should be advised to inform the clinician of any unusual strenuous activity in the days prior to the test or any other pertinent variables, such as a recent cold or flu. This information should be recorded and may become useful in explaining outlier data. Attention to these details helps to minimize unexplainable variation due to patient performance.

CONCLUSION

The selection of an appropriate quantitative strength measure is critical to the clinician's ability to detect muscular weakness. There may be significant strength and motor neuron loss prior to the presentation of functional problems, but the clinician may be able to detect weakness in asymptomatic muscles when using sensitive strength measures. Strength quantitation can be a powerful tool in the monitoring of disease progression and therapeutic intervention.

—*Michelle Mendoza and Robert G. Miller*

***See also*–Muscle Biopsy; Muscle Contraction, Overview; Muscle Tone**

Further Reading

Andersen, H., and Jakobsen, J. (1997). A comparative study of isokinetic dynamometry and manual muscle testing of ankle dorsal and plantar flexors and knee extensors and flexors. *Eur. Neurol.* **37**, 239–242.

Andres, P., Finison, L. J., Conlon, T., *et al.* (1988). Use of composite scores (megascores) to measure deficit in amyotrophic lateral sclerosis. *Neurology* **38**, 405–408.

Andres, P., Skerry, L., Thornell, B., *et al.* (1996). A comparison of three measures of disease progression in amyotrophic lateral sclerosis. *J. Neurol. Sci.* **139**, 64–70.

Bohannon, R. W. (1999). Intertester reliability of hand-held dynamometry: A concise summary of published research. *Percept. Mot. Skills* **88**, 899–902.

Brinkman, J., Andres, P., Sanjak, M., *et al.* (1996). Muscular weakness assessment: Use of normal isometric strength database consortium. *Arch. Phys. Med. Rehab.* **77**, 1251–1255.

Brinkmann, J. R., Andres, P., Mendoza, M., *et al.* (1997). Guidelines for the use and performance of quantitative outcome measures in ALS clinical trials. *J. Neurol. Sci.* **147**, 97–111.

Cedarbaum, J. M., and Stambler, N. (1997). Performance of the amyotrophic lateral sclerosis functional rating scale (ALSFRS) in multi-center clinical trials. *J. Neurol. Sci.* **152**, S1–S9.

Goonetilleke, A., Modarres-Sadeghi, H., and Guiloff, R. (1994). Accuracy, reproducibility, and variability of hand-held dynamometry in motor neuron disease. *J. Neurol. Neurosurg. Psychiatry* **57**, 326–332.

Hoagland, R., Mendoza, M., Armon, C., *et al.* (1997). Reliability of maximal voluntary isometric contraction testing in a multi-center study of patients with amyotrophic lateral sclerosis. *Muscle Nerve* **20**, 691–695.

Kendall, F., and McCreary, E. (1983). *Muscle Testing and Function*, 3rd ed. Williams & Wilkins, Baltimore.

Sanjak, M., Belden, D., Armon, C., *et al.* (1996). Muscle strength measurement. In *Handbook of Muscle Disease* (R. J. Lane, Ed.), pp. 19–31. Dekker, New York.

Muscle Tone

ASSESSMENT of muscle tone is an essential part of every neurological examination because alteration in muscle tone may indicate the presence of structural or biochemical lesions at many levels of the neuraxis. Muscle tone is the resistance, felt by the examiner, to passive movement of a joint when a patient is relaxed. As such, the characteristics and intensity of resistance to passive movement are a subjective assessment based on the examiner's experience. Most often, resistance to movement of a limb is assessed but occasionally evaluation of axial tone is performed. Resistance to passive movement of a joint represents the summation of multiple resistances arising from the joint, the intrinsic viscoelastic physical properties of muscle, the ability of the patient to consciously relax, and compensatory responses to resist passive stretching of muscle that are mediated by neural reflexes. In practice, the latter two factors (conscious relaxation and neural reflexes) are predominant and provide the most pathophysiological information.

Muscle tone may be increased or decreased from normal or paroxysmally altered as indicated in Table 1. In addition, alterations in muscle tone may be a generalized phenomenon or restricted in distribution to specific muscle groups. Recognizing the type of alteration in muscle tone is important since diagnostic and therapeutic decisions are based on these observations.

NEUROPHYSIOLOGICAL REGULATION OF MUSCLE TONE

Muscle tone is regulated by local spinal cord reflexes at the segmental level innervating that muscle and also by suprasegmental influences. The neural circuits subserving the spinal reflex are illustrated in Figs. 1 and 2. The afferent limb of the circuit consists of three elements: (i) Annulospiral mechanoreceptors (nuclear bag fibers) and their myelinated type Ia axons, (ii) flower-spray mechanical stretch receptors (nuclear chain fibers) and their type II axons, and (iii) Golgi tendon organ mechanoreceptors and their type Ib myelinated axons. The annulospiral and flower-spray receptors are interposed between flanking intrafusal muscle fibers that collectively form the

Table 1   CLINICAL CONDITIONS EXHIBITING ALTERED MUSCLE TONE

Increased	Decreased	Paroxysmal
Spasticity	Acute "upper motor neuron" (UMN) lesion	Cataplexy
Rigidity		Epileptic drop attacks
Cogwheel rigidity		
Decerebrate/ decorticate rigidity	"Lower motor neuron" (LMN) lesion	Paroxysmal kinesogenic dystonia
Gegenhalten (paratonia)		
Cramp	Cerebellar hypotonia	Periodic paralyses
Tetanus, tetany		
Physiological contracture		
Dystonias		
Stiff-person syndrome		

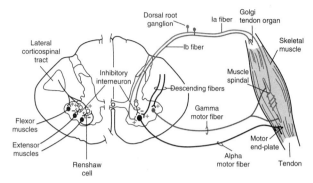

Figure 1
(Right) Reflex circuits organized at the spinal cord level involving afferents from the muscle spindle and the α-motoneuron. (Left) The relationship of inhibitory interneurons and Renshaw cells with α-motoneurons. Interneurons provide the basis for inhibition of antagonist muscles during contraction.

muscle spindle. The muscle spindle is oriented in parallel with the extrafusal skeletal muscle fibers and together they merge into a common tendonous attachment to bone. The parallel arrangement allows these receptors to encode the event of muscle stretch (flower-spray receptors and type II axons) as well as the rate of passive elongation (annulospiral receptors and type Ia axons) of the extrafusal muscle fibers. In contrast, Golgi tendon organs are aligned in series with the entire mass of the muscle by virtue of its localization within the tendonous attachment of muscle. In this way, the Golgi tendon organ encodes the stretch on the tendon generated by the total force of a given muscle during contraction.

α-Motoneurons have long been recognized as the final common efferent pathway for voluntary movement. These large neurons receive widespread synaptic input via 20,000–50,000 synaptic sites, including direct excitatory contacts from Ia and II afferents from the muscle spindle. Important inhibitory contacts arise from interneurons driven by type Ib afferents from the Golgi tendon organ, interneurons interposed between the corticospinal projections and the α-motoneuron, and from Renshaw cells (Fig. 1, left). Thus, inhibitory interneurons play an important role in coordinated movements by inhibiting α-motoneurons innervating antagonist muscles (a phenomenon termed reciprocal inhibition).

Descending fibers originating from the reticulo-, vestibulo-, rubro-, and corticospinal tracts converge on α-motoneurons and excite them. These supraspinal excitatory pathways also converge on γ-motoneurons that innervate the muscles in the intrafusal muscle spindle and cause their contraction and

stretch of the annulospiral mechanoreceptors. Therefore, the effect of γ activation is stimulation of the Ia afferents and secondary reflex contraction of extrafusal muscle via α-motoneuron activation. This has been termed the gamma loop, and it results in shortening of the muscle due to supraspinal influences as opposed to reflex contraction initiated by passive stretch of the muscle. Coordinated coactivation of the γ and α motor systems is essential in maintaining a sustained voluntary muscle contraction against a load.

Therefore, the overall impression of muscle tone is dependent on a multiplicity of voluntary and reflex, excitatory and inhibitory influences on the basic segmental arrangement of motor units.

CLINICAL SYNDROMES OF ALTERED MUSCLE TONE

With the rich interplay of reflex and supraspinal influences on muscle tone, it might be anticipated that altered muscle tone is frequently a manifestation of disease in the central and peripheral nervous systems. As can be appreciated, a lesion involving the posterior afferents would interfere with reflex

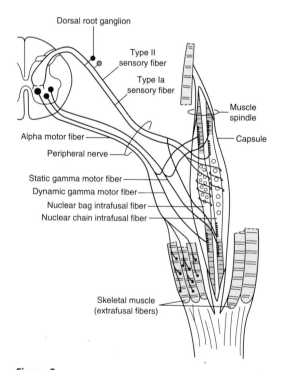

Figure 2
Detailed illustration of the muscle spindle afferents and the gamma motor efferent innervation of intrafusal fibers.

tone and cause hypotonia by abolishing the detection of muscle stretch. Hypotonia is also a manifestation of the lower motor neuron syndrome due to a lesion in the efferent motor unit. Lesions involving descending suprasegmental pathways that directly activate α-motoneurons initially cause hypotonia (e.g., spinal shock).

Spasticity is considered to result from facilitation of γ-motoneuron activation of intrafusal muscles. Lance provided the following widely quoted definition of spasticity: "a motor disorder characterized by a velocity-dependent increase in tonic stretch reflexes with exaggerated tendon jerks, resulting from hyperexcitabilty of the stretch reflex, as one component of the upper motor neuron syndrome. In addition, the hypertonia due to spasticity does not affect extensor and flexor muscles equally. Finally, one observes the "clasp-knife" phenomenon, a sudden release of the reflex contraction of muscle with continued stretch. Hypertonia caused by a lesion in the extrapyramidal system is conventionally termed rigidity. Rigidity is distinguished from spasticity inasmuch as rigidity is a constant resistance to movement during both passive flexion and extension. This is best appreciated in Parkinson's disease, in which one encounters "lead pipe" rigidity and cogwheel rigidity, the latter of which is a combination of rigidity and tremor. Other movement disorders (e.g., torticollis and oromandibular dystonias) may occasionally give the appearance of increased tone.

The complexity of supraspinal influences on muscle tone and their selective influence on extensor vis-à-vis flexor muscles is best illustrated by the clinical examples of decorticate and decerebrate rigidity seen as part of the progressive rostrocaudal deterioration during central or uncal herniation. These clinical findings closely mimic the experimental results of Sherrington on cats, with transections of descending cortical projections either rostral or caudal to the red nucleus. Hence, these syndromes reflect varying degrees of disconnection of descending corticospinal, corticoreticular, and corticorubral fibers and their targets in the midbrain and pons, causing an imbalance of excitatory and inhibitory influences on the spinal reflex arc. Sustained resistance to movement in demented or confused patients is termed gegenhalten and is indicative of an inability to relax during the examination, which is frequently a sign of frontal lobe dysfunction.

Physiological contracture is seen after exercise in patients with inborn errors of metabolism such as McArdle's disease and must be distinguished from physical contracture of muscle due to irreversible shortening. The rare stiff-person syndrome is characterized by continuous motor unit activity that is thought to be due to dysfunction of GABAergic inhibitory interneurons. Finally, toxic and metabolic processes, such as tetanus and tetany, may result in hypertonia.

MANAGEMENT OF ALTERED MUSCLE TONE

In general, conditions of hypertonia are more amenable to therapy than those of hypotonia with the possible exception of paroxysmal loss of muscle tone, for which treatment of the underlying condition (e.g., epilepsy) may be efficacious. Therapy of hypertonia is based on treatment of the underlying pathophysiological mechanisms that sustain the increase in muscle tone, perhaps best appreciated in the case of Parkinson's disease. Many focal dystonias are successfully treated with botulinum toxin injections to reduce the efferent limb of the motor response. Spasticity may be reduced or abolished by administering oral baclofen, gabapentin, diazepam, or tizanidine in conjunction with physical therapy. In selected refractory patients, botulinum toxin, intrathecal baclofen, or selective posterior rhizotomy may be indicated.

—*Edward J. Kasarskis*

See also–Cramps, Muscle; Lower Motor Neuron Lesions; Muscle Biopsy; Muscle Contraction, Overview; Muscle Strength, Assessment of; Rigidity; Spasticity

Further Reading

Burke, R. E. (1990). Spinal cord: Ventral horn. In *The Synaptic Organization of the Brain* (G. M. Shepard, Ed.), pp. 88–132. Oxford Univ. Press, New York.
Kuypers, H. G. J. M. (1981). Anatomy of the descending pathways. In *Handbook of Physiology*. (V. B. Brooks, Ed.), Vol. 2, pp. 597–666. American Physiological Society, Bethesda, MD.
Lance, J. W. (1980). Symposium synopsis. In *Spasticity: Disordered Motor Control* (R. G. Feldman, R. R. Young, and W. P. Doella, Eds.), pp. 485–494. Ciba-Geigy, Basel.
Matthews, P. B. C. (1981). Muscle spindles: Their messages and their fusimotor supply. In *Handbook of Physiology*. (V. B. Brooks, Ed.), Vol. 2, pp. 189–228. American Physiological Society, Bethesda, MD.
Sherrington, C. S. (1898). Decerebrate rigidity and the reflex coordination of movements. *J. Physiol. London* 22, 319–322.

Muscular Dystrophy: Emery–Dreifuss, Facioscapulohumeral, Scapuloperoneal, and Bethlem Myopathy

Encyclopedia of the Neurological Sciences
Copyright 2003, Elsevier Science (USA). All rights reserved.

THIS ENTRY discusses several of the regional muscular dystrophies, including facioscapulohumeral muscular dystrophy (FSHD), scapuloperoneal muscular dystrophy, Emery–Dreifuss muscular dystrophy, and Bethlem myopathy. Although each of these disorders is typically characterized by a distinct distribution of muscle weakness, there is considerable phenotypic overlap between both FSHD and scapuloperoneal muscular dystrophy as well as between Emery–Dreifuss muscular dystrophy and Bethlem myopathy. The significant advances that have been made in genetics and molecular biology are enabling more precise classifications of these dystrophies, as in many others. It is hoped that as research further defines the molecular basis for these diseases, we will better understand the pathogenesis, eventually leading to the development of improved treatments.

FACIOSCAPULOHUMERAL MUSCULAR DYSTROPHY

Clinical Features

FSHD is inherited in an autosomal dominant manner and has a prevalence of 1 in 20,000. Penetrance is variable and up to 30% of affected family members are unaware of their deficits. Onset of symptoms is typically in adolescence or early adulthood but can occur throughout the life span, including infancy.

As the name suggests, the muscles involved at onset include those of the face, particularly orbicularis oculi, orbicularis oris, and zygomaticus, as well as muscles used to fixate and rotate the scapula and the biceps and triceps, with initial relative sparing of the deltoids. Characteristic findings include a relatively expressionless face with weakness of eye and mouth closure and scapular winging. The sternocostal head of pectoralis major is also affected early. Wrist extensors are weaker than wrist flexors. As the disease progresses, patients demonstrate weakness of tibialis anterior leading to foot drop and eventually

the pelvic musculature may become involved, resulting in hyperlordotic posture and a waddling gait. Involvement may be asymmetrical. As noted previously, the disease exhibits variable penetrance and not all affected patients progress to this point. In fact, some manifest with only scapular winging. Bulbar, extraocular, and respiratory muscles are typically spared.

The disease exhibits slow progression and long periods of relative stability occur. However, approximately 20% of patients eventually become wheelchair dependent. Although cardiac or other system involvement is unusual, there have been rare reports of patients with FSHD manifesting cardiac conduction defects. There is also an association between FSHD and Coats' syndrome (retinal telangiectasias), both with and without hearing loss.

The infantile-onset FSHD tends to be more severe, with most patients requiring a wheelchair by age 9 or 10. These patients present with symptoms in the first 2 years of life.

Occasionally, a diagnostic dilemma arises in patients with a scapuloperoneal syndrome and mild facial weakness or in patients with an autosomal dominant limb–girdle dystrophy and mild facial weakness. In both entities, facial weakness tends to be much milder than that seen with FSHD and tends to occur late in the disease, unlike in FSHD.

Laboratory Features

As with the other myopathies, laboratory findings are nonspecific. The serum creatine kinase (CK) levels can be normal or mildly elevated. Electromyography demonstrates changes consistent with a chronic myopathy. Muscle biopsy is also nonspecific, although it can confirm the myopathic origin of the signs and symptoms. Interestingly, mononuclear infiltrates are seen more often in FSHD biopsies than in other types of muscular dystrophy. Despite this, there is no evidence that it is a primary inflammatory disorder. Genetic testing can confirm the diagnosis by demonstrating a deletion in chromosome 4q35.

Molecular Genetics

FSHD is linked to a deletion in the long arm of chromosome 4 in the 4q35 region. DNA analysis demonstrates a "short fragment" in this region, which is usually less than 35 kb in length, compared with 300 kb in unaffected individuals. A short fragment is detected in 85–95% of patients with clinical evidence of FSHD, and approximately 98% of patients with a short fragment have clinical evidence of FSHD. Several studies have shown an inverse association between fragment size and severity of disease. However, fragment size is clearly not the sole predictor of severity because some families have shown increased symptom severity as the disease is passed from one generation to the next, despite a stable fragment size. Despite the identification of this linkage, the gene or genes affected by this deletion have not been identified.

Treatment

No treatment is available to slow or reverse progression of symptoms in FSHD. Several medications have been studied, including prednisone, albuterol, and creatine. Although a very modest increase in strength was seen in the patients treated with creatine for 8 weeks, none of these studies enrolled a sufficient number of patients or followed patients for a sufficient time period to demonstrate a clinically significant benefit.

As with other dystrophies, occupational, physical, and speech therapy may be beneficial to help optimize functional status. Surgery to fix the scapula to the thorax may help increase upper extremity function in some patients. This procedure is only indicated in patients with relatively preserved deltoid function.

SCAPULOPERONEAL DYSTROPHY

Clinical Features

Scapuloperoneal dystrophy, although clinically similar to FSHD, is a distinct entity. Characteristic features described in scapuloperoneal syndromes include weakness of scapular stabilizer muscles with associated scapular winging, weakness of arm flexors and extensors (biceps and triceps), and anterior tibial and peroneal weakness resulting in foot drop. Three distinct etiologies have been described in the literature: a primary myopathic process, a motor neuronopathy, and a peripheral neuropathy. The latter presents with sensory symptoms as well as muscle weakness and wasting. Unfortunately, it is often difficult to differentiate these etiologies clinically, even after electrophysiological studies and muscle biopsy. The advent of genetic testing for FSHD may help to distinguish this entity from a scapuloperoneal syndrome. Recently, Felice et al. demonstrated the 4q35 deletion in 10 of 14 unrelated patients with facial-sparing scapular myopathy, indicating that differentiation cannot be made on phenotype alone.

Evidence that scapuloperoneal dystrophy is a distinct entity is supported by genetic studies by Wilhelmsen et al., who demonstrated a linkage to chromosome 12 in a large kindred with an autosomal dominant scapuloperoneal myopathy, and by Tawil et al., who were unable to demonstrate a linkage to chromosome 4q35 in two large kindreds with scapuloperoneal syndromes.

As in FSHD, the symptoms may begin at any age but generally start in adolescence or early adulthood. Muscle weakness progresses slowly, with years of relative stability being common. The weakness generally progresses from the shoulder girdle to the anterior tibial muscles and then to the pelvic girdle. Unlike FSHD, facial weakness occurs later in the disease and is usually mild.

Laboratory Features

Serum creatine kinase may be normal or mildly elevated. Most reports indicate nonspecific chronic myopathic findings on electromyography and on muscle biopsy.

Molecular Genetics

Our understanding of the molecular genetics is also limited by unclear classification of the scapuloperoneal syndromes in the literature. Autosomal dominant, autosomal recessive, and sporadic cases have been reported; however, it is likely that not all these cases are myopathic in etiology. Linkage to chromosome 12 has been demonstrated in one large autosomal dominant family. A common gene or abnormal gene product has not been identified.

Treatment

No treatment is available to slow progression of the disease. Ankle–foot orthoses are beneficial in patients with foot drop and, occasionally, surgery to stabilize the scapula improves upper extremity function.

EMERY–DREIFUSS MUSCULAR DYSTROPHY

Clinical Features

Emery–Dreifuss muscular dystrophy (EDMD) is characterized by early onset contractures (often preceding weakness), initial humeroperoneal distribution of weakness, and cardiac conduction defects. The most common form of EDMD demonstrates an X-linked mode of inheritance and is associated with an abnormality of the nuclear membrane protein emerin. A less common form of the disease is inherited in an autosomal dominant pattern and is associated with abnormalities of the nuclear membrane proteins lamins A and C. An autosomal recessive form (affecting lamins A and C) has also been reported. All forms are phenotypically very similar. Onset is usually in childhood and the progression is slow, with patients often remaining ambulatory into the third decade, although more severe forms do occur. Initial manifestations include contractures of the heel cords, elbows, and posterior cervical muscles. Later, weakness develops, initially affecting the biceps brachii, triceps, and anterior tibial and peroneal muscles and then progressing over time to involve the proximal limb–girdle musculature. Calf hypertrophy is not seen, which also helps to differentiate EDMD from the dystrophinopathies. Potentially lethal cardiac conduction abnormalities develop by the time the patient reaches the late teenage years or early 20s. These range from sinus bradycardia to complete heart block. Patients may also develop progressive cardiac failure. Although female carriers of the X-linked form of EDMD do not manifest contractures or muscle weakness, they may develop cardiac conduction defects. Isolated cardiac conduction defects may also be seen as the sole manifestation of both the X-linked and autosomal dominant forms of the disease.

Laboratory Features

Serum CK may be normal to moderately elevated. Electromyography demonstrates nonspecific myopathic changes, as does routine muscle histology. Immunohistochemistry of muscle biopsy tissue, fibroblasts, leukocytes, skin, or exfoliative buccal cells for emerin can confirm the diagnosis of X-linked EDMD. A mosaic pattern of emerin expression can be seen in nonaffected carriers. Chorionic villus tissue can also demonstrate abnormalities in emerin expression and can be used for prenatal diagnosis. There is currently no commercially available genetic test. There is also no commercially available immunohistochemical or genetic test for autosomal dominant EDMD due to mutations of lamins A and C.

Molecular Genetics and Pathogenesis

The X-linked EDMD locus has been mapped to the emerin gene STA on chromosome Xq28, and more than 90 mutations have been identified. Emerin is expressed in the inner nuclear membrane of skeletal, cardiac, and smooth muscle. However, its function is unknown.

Autosomal dominant EDMD has been mapped to the nuclear lamin A/C (LMNA) gene on chromosome 1q11–q23. Lamins A and C are also inner nuclear membrane proteins, which interact with other lamina-associated proteins (LAPs) and emerin. The exact function of lamins A and C is also unknown.

Treatment

Therapy is focused on maintaining and maximizing function as well as on preventing cardiac complications. Thus, all patients should be referred to physical and occupational therapy. It is unlikely that bracing or surgery will prevent contractures because these occur early and are not the result of immobility. Cardiac monitoring is very important. Electrocardiograms should be obtained annually, both on patients and on possible female carriers. Cardiac consultations are recommended if any significant abnormalities are found and/or if the patient demonstrates signs or symptoms of cardiac disease. Some patients will require prophylactic implantation of cardiac pacemakers.

BETHLEM MYOPATHY

Clinical Features

The characteristic features of this myopathy include contractures, relatively mild weakness, autosomal dominant inheritance, and childhood onset, although occasional adult-onset cases have been reported. Signs in infancy may be absent or are nonspecific, including hypotonia, torticollis, flexion contractures of the ankles, and/or delayed motor milestones. However, most patients do not become fully symptomatic before 5 years of age. Nearly all patients exhibit flexion contractures of the fingers, wrists, elbows, and ankles. Knees, hips, and shoulders may also be involved. Weakness is mild and involves predominantly proximal and extensor muscles, except in the hip. There is absence of cranial and cardiac muscle involvement. Sensory exam is normal.

After presentation, muscle weakness appears to remain relatively stable throughout childhood. However, there may be deterioration in walking due to tight heel cords. Other contractures do not appear to lead to functional disability. Patients report an improvement in strength at puberty with resolution of the Gowers' sign. However, very slow deterioration in strength and function occurs starting in middle age, with approximately two-thirds of patients requiring a wheelchair for outside ambulation after age 50. However, most patients remain ambulatory within the home. Contractures do not appear to progress during adulthood. Neonatal hypotonia does not predict severity of adult disease. Life expectancy is normal.

Laboratory Features

Serum CK may be highly elevated in young patients (up to 15 times the upper limit of normal), although it may also be normal or only slightly elevated. Motor and sensory nerve conduction studies are normal. Electromyography demonstrates features consistent with a chronic myopathy (absent or rare abnormal spontaneous activity and often a mixture of small-amplitude, short-duration polyphasic motor unit action potentials with large-amplitude, long-duration ones). Muscle biopsy demonstrates non-specific myopathic changes. There is variability in fiber size, increased splitting, and central nuclei and mild endomysial fibrosis. Cardiac evaluation, including electrocardiogram, Holter monitor, and echocardiogram, is normal.

Pathogenesis

Collagen type VI is the defective protein complex in Bethlem myopathy. Different families have shown linkage to COL6A1 and COL6A2 genes on chromosome 21q and to the COL6A3 gene on chromosome 2q. These genes encode the three subunits of type VI collagen, the α_1–α_3 collagen chains. Collagen type VI is widely expressed and demonstrates cell adhesive properties. However, the actual pathophysiology of this disorder remains unknown.

Treatment

Physical and occupational therapy are indicated. They can provide range of motion exercises that may prevent progression of contractures and also assess the need for adaptive equipment or techniques to improve function. Surgery to improve contractures should only be considered if the contractures cause functional disability. Although often initially successful, contractures may recur after surgery.

—*Hannah R. Briemberg and Anthony A. Amato*

See also–Leukodystrophy; Muscle Contraction, Overview; Muscular Dystrophy: Limb–Girdle, Becker's, and Duchenne's; Myotonic Dystrophy; Neuromuscular Disorders, Overview; Oculopharyngeal Muscular Dystrophy

Further Reading

Amato, A. A., and Dumitru, D. (2002). Hereditary myopathies. In *Electrodiagnostic Medicine* (D. Dumitru, A. A. Amato, and M. J. Zwarts, Eds.), 2nd ed., pp. 1284–1290. Hanley & Belfus, Philadelphia.

Bonne, G., Di Barletta, M. R., Varnous, S., et al. (1999). Mutations in the gene encoding lamin A/C cause autosomal dominant Emery–Dreifuss muscular dystrophy. *Nat. Genet.* **21**, 285–288.

Ellis, J. A. (2001). 81st ENMC International Workshop: 4th Meeting on Emery–Dreifuss muscular dystrophy, 7th and 8th July 2000, Naarden, The Netherlands. *Neuromusc. Disord.* **11**, 417–420.

Emery, A. E. H. (2000). Emery–Dreifuss muscular dystrophy—A 40 year retrospective. *Neuromusc. Disord.* **10**, 228–232.

Felice, K. J., North, W. A., Moore, S. A., et al. (2000). FSH dystrophy 4q35 deletion in patients presenting with facial-sparing scapular myopathy. *Neurology* **54**, 1927–1931.

Jobsis, G. J., Boers, J. M., Barth, P. G., et al. (1999). Bethlem myopathy: A slowly progressive congenital muscular dystrophy with contractures. *Brain* **122**, 649–655.

Kissel, J. T. (1999). Facioscapulohumeral dystrophy. *Semin. Neurol.* **19**, 35–43.

Kuo, H.-J., Maslen, C. L., Keene, D. R., et al. (1997). Type VI collagen anchors endothelial basement membranes by interacting with type IV collagen. *J. Biol. Chem.* **272**, 26522–26529.

Laforet, P., de Toma, C., Eymard, B., et al. (1998). Cardiac involvement in genetically confirmed facioscapulohumeral muscular dystrophy. *Neurology* **51**, 1454–1456.

Lunt, P. W., Jardine, P. E., Koch, M. C., et al. (1995). Correlation between fragment size at D4F104S1 and age of onset or at wheelchair use, with possible generation effect, accounts for much phenotypic variation in 4q35-facioscapulohumeral muscular dystrophy (FSHD). *Hum. Mol. Genet.* **4**, 951–958.

Manilal, S., Sewry, C. A., Man, N., et al. (1997). Diagnosis of X-linked Emery–Dreifuss muscular dystrophy by protein analysis of leucocytes and skin with monoclonal antibodies. *Neuromusc. Disord.* **7**, 63–66.

Mechut, M. P., Zdonczyk, D., and Gujrati, M. (1990). Cardiac transplantation in female Emery–Dreifuss muscular dystrophy. *J. Neurol.* **237**, 316–319.

Merlini, L., Villanova, M., Sabatelli, P., et al. (1999). Decreased expression of laminin β1 in chromosome 21-linked Bethlem myopathy. *Neuromusc. Disord.* **9**, 326–329.

Mohire, M. D., Tandan, R., Fries, T. J., et al. (1988). Early onset benign autosomal dominant limb–girdle myopathy with contractures (Bethlem myopathy). *Neurology* **38**, 573–580.

Munsat, T. L. (1994). Facioscapulohumeral disease and the scapuloperoneal syndrome. In *Myology* (A. G. Engel and C. Franzini-Armstrong, Eds.), 2nd ed., pp. 1220–1232. McGraw-Hill, New York.

Pepe, G., Bertini, E., Giusti, T., et al. (1999). A novel de novo mutation in the triple helix of the COL6A3 gene in a two-generation Italian family affected by Bethlem myopathy. A diagnostic approach in the mutations' screening of type VI collagen. *Neuromusc. Disord.* **9**, 264–271.

Sabatelli, P., Squarzoni, S., Petrini, S., et al. (1998). Oral exfoliative cytology for the non-invasive diagnosis in X-linked Emery–Dreifuss muscular dystrophy patients and carriers. *Neuromusc. Disord.* **8**, 67–71.

Somer, H., Laulumaa, V., Paljarvi, L., et al. (1991). Benign muscular dystrophy with autosomal dominant inheritance. *Neuromusc. Disord.* **1**, 267–273.

Tawil, R., Myers, G. J., Weiffenbach, B., *et al.* (1995). Scapuloperoneal syndromes. Absence of linkage to the 4q35 FSHD locus. *Arch. Neurol.* **52,** 1069–1072.

Tawil, R., Forrester, J., and Griggs, R. C. (1996). Evidence for anticipation and association of deletion size with severity in facioscapulohumeral muscular dystrophy. *Ann. Neurol.* **39,** 744–748.

Vohanka, S., Vytopil, M., Bednarik, J., *et al.* (2001). A mutation in the X-linked Emery–Dreifuss muscular dystrophy gene in a patient affected with conduction cardiomyopathy. *Neuromusc. Disord.* **11,** 411–413.

Walter, M. C., Lochmuller, H., Reilich, P., *et al.* (2000). Creatine monophosphate in muscular dystrophies: A double-blind, placebo-controlled clinical study. *Neurology* **54,** 1848–1850.

Wilhelmsen, K. C., Blake, D. M., Lynch, T., *et al.* (1996). Chromosome 12-linked autosomal dominant scapuloperoneal muscular atrophy. *Ann. Neurol.* **39,** 507–520.

Muscular Dystrophy: Limb–Girdle, Becker's, and Duchenne's

Encyclopedia of the Neurological Sciences

RECENT ADVANCES in molecular genetics have significantly enhanced the understanding of the pathogenesis of muscular dystrophies. This entry focuses on the dystrophinopathies and other types of limb–girdle muscular dystrophies. Prior to discussing these myopathies, the constituents of the sarcolemmal membrane are reviewed because many of these proteins when aberrantly produced lead to one of the forms of muscular dystrophy.

DYSTROPHIN–GLYCOPROTEIN COMPLEX

Dystrophin

Duchenne's and Becker's muscular dystrophies are caused by mutations in the dystrophin gene. Dystrophin is a large protein that localizes to the cytoplasmic face of skeletal and cardiac muscle membranes. Dystrophin binds to filamentous actin at the amino terminus and to β-dystroglycan at the carboxy terminus. Dystrophin is also present in the brain at the postsynaptic density (PSD), a disk-shaped structure beneath the postsynaptic membrane in chemical synapses. The PSD may play an important role in synaptic function by stabilizing the synaptic structure, anchoring postsynaptic receptors, and transducing extracellular matrix cell signals.

Dystrophin-Associated Proteins/Glycoproteins

Dystrophin is tightly associated with a large oligomeric set of sarcolemmal proteins in a complex referred to as the dystrophin–glycoprotein complex (DGC) (Fig. 1). The DGC is composed of dystrophin, the syntrophin complex, the dystroglycan complex, and the sarcoglycan complex. The dystroglycan complex is composed of a transmembrane glycoprotein, β-dystroglycan, which binds to dystrophin and an extracellular glycoprotein, α-dystroglycan, which binds to α-laminin in the basement membrane. The sarcoglycan complex includes four membrane spanning proteins: α-sarcoglycan, previously known as adhalin; β-sarcoglycan; γ-sarcoglycan; and δ-sarcoglycan. In addition, there is a transmembrane protein, sarcospan, that colocalizes with the sarcoglycan complex. The sarcoglycan complex associates with the cysteine-rich domain or the first half of the carboxy terminal of dystrophin directly or indirectly via the dystroglycan complex. The exact relationship between the sarcoglycan complex and the dystrophin–dystroglycan complex is unclear. Mutations in the various genes that encode for the different proteins of the DGC are now known to be responsible for most forms of muscular dystrophy (Table 1).

Merosin/Laminin

Laminin is a large basement membrane polypeptide composed of three different but homologous α, β, and γ chains held together by disulfide bonds. The major isoform of laminin heavy chains in muscle is laminin-2, which is composed of α_2, β_1, and γ_1 chains. Merosin is the collective name for laminins that share a common α_2 chain. α-Dystroglycan binds specifically to the α_2 chain of laminin-2 or merosin (Fig. 1).

Merosin, α-dystroglycan, and β-dystroglycan are also expressed in the endoneurial basement membrane surrounding the myelin sheath of peripheral nerves. These proteins are expressed on the Schwann cell's outer membrane abutting the endoneurium, but they are not present in the inner membrane or on compact myelin. This complex appears to have a role in peripheral myelinogenesis. Mutations involving the merosin gene are responsible for most cases of classic congenital muscular dystrophy (CMD) and are also associated with mild demyelinating sensorimotor polyneuropathy.

Integrins

Integrins are transmembrane, heterodimeric (α/β) receptors that link the extracellular matrix with the

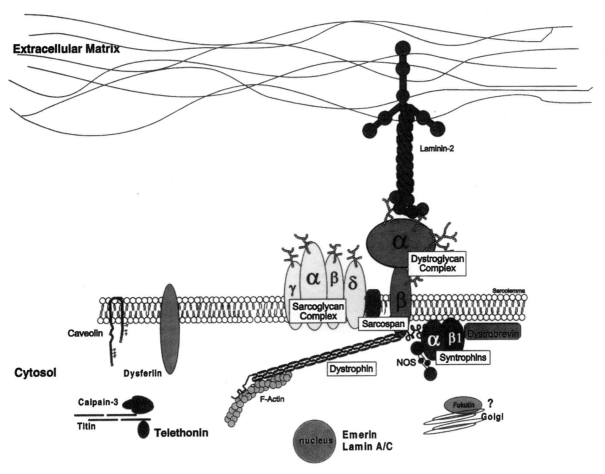

Figure 1

The dystrophin–glycoprotein complex and related proteins. The dystrophin–glycoprotein complex and related proteins are important in the structural integrity of the sarcolemmal membrane. Mutations in the genes that encode for various subunits of the complex are responsible for many forms of muscular dystrophy. SG, sarcoglycan; DG, dystroglycan (reproduced with permission from Cohn and Campbell, 2000).

cytoskeleton and also help transduce extracellular matrix cell signals. Integrins play important roles in the regulation of adhesion, migration, differentiation, proliferation, and cytoskeletal organization. The major integrin expressed in muscle membranes is $\alpha_7\beta_1D$. Similar to α-dystroglycan, $\alpha_7\beta_1D$ integrin also binds to merosin in skeletal muscle and serves to enhance the structural stability of the muscle membrane (Fig. 1). Mutations in the α_7 gene are responsible for some forms of merosin-positive CMD.

Function of the DGC

The DGC is a transsarcolemmal complex of proteins and glycoproteins that links the subsarcolemmal cytoskeleton to the extracellular matrix. The complex appears to be essential in providing structural support to the sarcolemma during muscle contraction. Mutations affecting various components of the

DGC result in the loss of integrity of the sarcolemma and subsequent muscle fiber damage.

OTHER SARCOLEMMAL PROTEINS

Dysferlin

Dysferlin is a cytoskeletal protein located predominantly on the subsarcolemmal surface on the muscle membrane, but it has a small transmembrane spanning tail (Fig. 1). The protein is not directly connected to the DGC. Dysferlin is present in skeletal and cardiac muscle but its function is not known, although it may have a role in membrane fusion, stabilizing the sarcolemmal membrane, or signal transduction.

Caveolins

Caveolins are located in caveolae membranes (invaginations in the sarcolemma), in which they act as

Table 1 MOLECULAR DEFECTS OF MUSCULAR DYSTROPHIES[a]

Disease	Chromosome	Protein
X-linked recessive dystrophies		
DMD/BMD	Xp21	Dystrophin
EDMD	Xq28	Emerin
Autosomal dominant dystrophies		
LGMD 1A	5q22–31	Myotilin
LGMD 1B with cardiopathy/AD-EDMD	1q11–12	Nuclear lamin A/C
LGMD 1C	3p25	Caveolin-3
LGMD 1D	6q23	?
LGMD 1E	7q	?
Myotonic dystrophy	19q13.2	Myotonin protein kinase
Myotonic dystrophy type 2/PROMM	3q	DM2
FSHD	4q35	?
Oculopharyngeal dystrophy	14q	Polyalanine binding protein-2
Bethlem myopathy 1	21q22.3	Collagen type VI (α_1 or α_2 subunits)
Bethlem myopathy 2	2q37	Collagen type VI (α_6 subunits)
Autosomal recessive dystrophies		
LGMD 2A	15q15	Calpain-3
LGMD 2B/Miyoshi myopathy	2p13	Dysferlin
LGMD 2C	13q13	γ-Sarcoglycan
LGMD 2D	17q21	α-Sarcoglycan
LGMD 2E	4q12	β-Sarcoglycan
LGMD 2F	5q33	δ-Sarcoglycan
LGMD 2G	17q11–12	Telethonin
LGMD 2H	9q31–q33	E3-ubiquitine ligase (TRIM-32)
LGMD 2I	19q13.3	Fukutin-related protein, *FKRP1*
Congenital muscular dystrophy		
Merosin-negative classic type (CMD1)	6q21–22	Merosin (α_2 subunit)
CMD2	12q13	α_7 Integrin
CMD3	19q13.3	Fukutin-related protein, *FKRP1*
Fukuyama type	9q31–33	Fukutin
Walker–Warburg type	9q31–33	?
MEB	1p32–p34	POMGnT1
CMD with rigid spine syndrome	1p35–36	Selenoprotein

[a]Abbreviations used: DMD, Duchenne's muscular dystrophy; LGMD, limb–girdle muscular dystrophy; BMD, Becker's muscular dystrophy; FSHD, facioscapulohumeral muscular dystrophy; EDMD, Emery–Dreifuss muscular dystrophy, MEB, muscle–eye–brain disease; AD, autosomal dominant; POMGnT1, D-mannose β-1,2-N-acetylglycosaminyl transferase.

scaffolding proteins to organize and concentrate caveolin-interacting lipids and proteins (Fig. 1). Caveolin-3 is localized by immunostaining to the sarcolemma at caveolae. It cofractionates with the DGC, but is thought to be part of a discrete complex. Mutations in the gene encoding for caveolin-C are responsible for causing limb–girdle muscular dystrophy (LGMD) 1C.

MUSCULAR DYSTROPHIES

The muscular dystrophies specifically refer to a group of hereditary, progressive intrinsic muscle disorders in which there is destruction of muscle tissue and replacement by connective and fatty tissue. Muscular dystrophies traditionally have been classi-fied according to their pattern of weakness (e.g., limb–girdle, facioscapulohumeral, and scapuloperoneal) and mode of inheritance. Recent advances in genetics have led to the classification of muscular dystrophies based on the responsible gene defect. The following sections concern those dystrophies with a limb–girdle pattern of weakness: the dystrophinopathies and the limb–girdle muscular dystrophy.

THE DYSTROPHINOPATHIES: DUCHENNE'S AND BECKER'S MUSCULAR DYSTROPHY

Duchenne Muscular Dystrophy

Clinical Features: Duchenne's muscular dystrophy (DMD) is an X-linked recessive disorder with an incidence of approximately 1 per 3500–5600 male births and a mean prevalence of approximately 63/100,000 approaching 1 per 18,000 (ranging from 19.5 to 95/100,000) males. Weakness is worse proximally than distally and more so in the lower compared to upper limbs. Most affected boys appear normal at birth and achieve the motor milestones of sitting, standing, and walking normally or with only slight delay. Affected boys have difficulty with jumping and running and in this regard are noted to be slower than their peers. By the ages of 2–6 years, children begin to have more difficulty ambulating and start having falls. They have a wide-based gait and waddle, and there is a tendency to walk on the toes. Around this time, patients also have difficulty rising from the floor, and they employ the so-called Gower's maneuver (rising from a squatting position by marching their hands up their legs) to help them rise to a standing position. By 8 years of age, they have difficulty climbing stairs. Weakness progresses and affected children are confined to a wheelchair by 12 years of age. Respiratory function gradually declines and even minor colds become significant life-threatening events late in the disease. Pulmonary insufficiency combined with chronic infections eventually result in death by the early twenties.

Cardiac muscle is also affected, although most patients are asymptomatic. However, dysrhythmias and congestive heart failure can occur late in the disease. Smooth muscle involvement may lead to gastroparesis and intestinal pseudo-obstruction. The average IQ of affected children is one standard deviation below the normal mean, perhaps related to the loss of dystrophin at the postsynaptic densities in the brain.

Laboratory Features: The serum creatine kinase (CK) levels are markedly elevated (50–100 times normal or greater) at birth and peak at approximately 3 years of age. Subsequently, serum CK levels decrease approximately 20% per year due to the loss of muscle, although CK levels always remain elevated. Motor and sensory nerve conduction studies (NCS) are normal. Needle electromyography (EMG) demonstrates increased insertional and spontaneous complex repetitive discharges, positive sharp waves, and fibrillation potentials. As muscle tissue is progressively replaced with both adipose cells and connective tissue, the amount of electrical activity noted following needle movement declines. There is early recruitment of both short- and long-duration

motor unit action potentials, reflecting the chronicity of the myopathic process.

Histopathology: Muscle biopsies reveal considerable fiber size variation, with hypertrophic and hypercontracted fibers in addition to small, rounded, regenerating fibers, scattered necrotic fibers, and increased endomysial connective tissue. Endomysial inflammatory cells consisting mainly of cytotoxic T lymphocytes and macrophages are present to a variable degree and phagocytize necrotic fibers. Fiber splitting and central nuclei may be seen but are less frequent than in other muscular dystrophies. Immunohistochemistry demonstrates diminished dystrophin staining on the muscle membrane (Fig. 2). Approximately 60% of DMD patients have some faint staining of the sarcolemma utilizing antibodies directed against the amino terminal or rod domain of dystrophin. Antibodies directed against the carboxy terminal of dystrophin are more sensitive, with less than 1% of muscle fibers demonstrating sarcolemmal staining in DMD. These few dystrophin-positive fibers are known as revertants and arise secondary to spontaneous subsequent mutations that restore the "reading frame" and allow transcription of dystrophin, albeit of abnormal size and shape. Immunohistochemistry also demonstrates a reduction of dystroglycan, dystrobrevin, and all the sarcoglycan proteins, including sarcospan (Fig. 2). Interestingly, utrophin, which is normally restricted to the neuromuscular junction, is overexpressed in DMD and is present throughout the sarcolemma. Western blot of muscle tissue demonstrates a significantly reduced size or quantity of the dystrophin.

Becker's Muscular Dystrophy

Clinical Features: Becker's muscular dystrophy (BMD) is a milder form of dystrophinopathy, with an incidence of 1/18,450 male births and a prevalence of approximately 3–524 per 100,000. As with DMD, there is preferential involvement of the hip and shoulder girdle muscles. There is a wide spectrum of clinical severity depending on the degree to which dystrophin is altered as well as intrafamilial variability. Patients remain ambulatory past the age of 15 years, with the mean age of losing the ability to ambulate independently in the fourth decade. Exertional myalgias or cramps occur in more than 90% of patients and are the presenting symptom in 28%. The life expectancy is reduced (mean, 42 years). With the advent of molecular genetics, some patients manifesting with only myalgias, myoglobinuria,

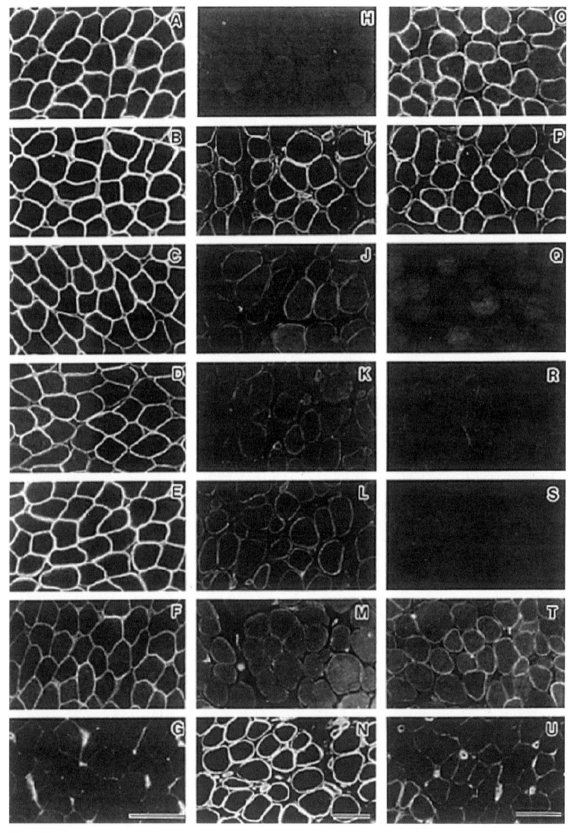

Figure 2

cardiomyopathy, and asymptomatic hyper-CK-emia have been demonstrated to have mild forms of dystrophinopathy.

Cardiac abnormalities are similar to those described for DMD. Some patients manifest with a cardiomyopathy with little or no skeletal muscle weakness. Mental abilities have not been investigated as thoroughly as in DMD, but some series have demonstrated a borderline or mildly impaired IQ in BMD patients.

Laboratory Features: Serum CK levels are elevated up to 200 times normal. Patients with mild BMD may have asymptomatic hyper-CK-emia. EMG and NCS are similar to those noted for DMD.

Histopathology: The histological features are similar to those observed for DMD but are less severe. BMD may be distinguished histologically from DMD with dystrophin immunostaining. Most patients with BMD demonstrate the presence of dystrophin utilizing carboxy-terminal antibodies on muscle membranes. In contrast, immunostaining with antibodies directed against the carboxy terminal of dystrophin is usually negative in DMD. However, the degree and intensity of the dystrophin staining are usually not normal in BMD. The staining pattern may be uniformly reduced or can vary between and within fibers. Immunoblot reveals an abnormal quantity and/or size of dystrophin.

Outliers

This is an older term referring to children who have a clinical phenotype in between that of DMD and BMD. These children continue to ambulate after the age of 12 but are confined to a wheelchair by the age of 15. Prior to age 12, outliers may be distinguished from DMD by their ability to completely flex their neck while lying supine. Children with DMD are unable to flex their necks fully against gravity (MRC grade <3). Immunological studies on muscle tissue usually reveal the presence of some dystrophin, although often reduced in amount and/or size.

Female Carriers

The daughters of males with BMD (males with DMD are usually infertile) and the mothers of affected children who also have a family history of DMD or BMD are obligate carriers of the mutated dystrophin gene. Mothers and sisters of isolated DMD or BMD patients are at risk for being carriers; therefore, it is essential to determine the carrier status of at-risk females because there is a 50% chance that males born to carrier females will inherit the disease, whereas 50% of the daughters born will be carriers of the mutated gene. Carrier females are usually asymptomatic, but approximately 8% of carriers have mild muscle weakness. These cases may be explained by the Lyon hypothesis, in which there is a skewed inactivation of the normal X chromosome resulting in increased transcription of the mutated dystrophin gene. In addition, females with translocations at the chromosomal Xp21 site or Turner's syndrome (XO genotype) may also develop dystrophinopathies.

Usually, manifesting female carriers have a mild limb–girdle phenotype similar to that of BMD. Prior to the recent advances in molecular genetics, these females were often diagnosed with limb–girdle muscular dystrophy, particularly when there was no family history of DMD or BMD. Rarely, females can manifest severe weakness as seen in DMD.

Serum CK levels are elevated in manifesting female carriers. However, serum CK levels are frequently normal in nonsymptomatic carriers. Muscle biopsies of manifesting carriers reveal dystrophic features. Immunostaining for dystrophin demonstrates an absent, decreased, or mosaic pattern of staining in manifesting carriers. However, immune staining is usually normal in asymptomatic carriers. Thus, immunostaining and Western blot analysis are not very sensitive in identifying carrier status of asymptomatic females.

Figure 2

Immunofluorescent staining for components of the dystrophin–glycoprotein complex in a normal patient (A–G), a child with Duchenne's muscular dystrophy (H–N), and a patient with γ-sarcoglycanopathy (O–U). These muscles were stained for dystrophin (A, H, and O), β-dystroglycan (B, I, and P), α-sarcoglycan (C, J, and Q), β-sarcoglycan (D, K, and R), γ-sarcoglycan (E, L, and S), and δ-sarcoglycan (F, M, and T). Note the characteristic diffuse sarcolemmal localization of dystrophin, the sarcoglycans, and β-dystroglycan in the normal patient (A–F) and restriction of utrophin to the neuromuscular junction (G). The patient with DMD demonstrates absent dystrophin staining and reduction of all the sarcoglycans and to a lesser extent β-dystroglycan (H–M), whereas utrophin is abnormal, expressed diffusely along the sarcolemma (N). The patient with γ-sarcoglycanopathy demonstrates not only diminished γ-sarcoglycan staining but also reduced staining of all the sarcoglycans (Q–T). Dystrophin and β-dystroglycan stains were normal, although they can occasionally be reduced in sarcoglycanpathies (O and P). A slight increased expression of utrophin is seen along the sarcolemma (U) (reproduced with permission from Ozawa et al., 1998).

DNA analysis for mutations in the dystrophin gene is the most reliable method of detecting carrier status. First, DNA analysis should be performed on affected male relatives. A detectable mutation in affected DMD/BMD males makes carrier detection of at-risk female relatives much easier and also allows for subsequent prenatal detection in at-risk fetuses. If a mutation is demonstrated in an affected male relative, at-risk females can be screened for the same mutation. Carrier status of a mother of a sporadic DMD case must be interpreted cautiously because of the potential for germline mosaicism. In a germline mosaic, the mutation involves only a percentage of the germ cells (i.e., oocytes) but is not present in the leukocytes in which DNA analysis is performed. In such a situation, the affected child may have an identifiable mutation on DNA analysis; however, the mother could still be a carrier but have no demonstrable mutation in the leukocytes. The recurrence rate in germline carriers has been estimated to be as high as 14%. Prenatal diagnosis can be performed with DNA analysis of chorionic villi or amniotic fluid cells when there is an identifiable mutation in the family. When mutations are not evident in affected DMD cases, carrier detection depends on the less reliable linkage analysis of many family members using restriction fragment length polymorphisms.

Molecular Genetics and Pathogenesis of the Dystrophinopathies

Dystrophin is bound to the sarcolemma, where it provides structural integrity to the muscle membrane (Fig. 1). Lack of dystrophin results in loss of membrane integrity and segmental necrosis. The dystrophin gene is located on chromosome Xp21 and is composed of approximately 2.4 mb of genomic DNA; it includes 79 exons that code for a 14-kb transcript. The large size of the gene accounts for the high spontaneous mutation rate (one-third of new cases of DMD and 10% of BMD). Large deletions (several kilobases to more than 1 million base pairs), are demonstrated in approximately two-thirds of dystrophinopathy patients. Another 5–10% of DMD cases are caused by point mutation resulting in premature stop codons, whereas duplications are evident in another 5% of cases. Smaller mutations, which are not readily detectable, account for the remainder. Mutations are not random in location but rather occur primarily in the center (80%) and near the amino terminal (20%) of the gene. "Out-of-frame" mutations disrupt the translational reading of

the gene and result in near total loss of dystrophin and a DMD clinical phenotype. In contrast, "in-frame" mutations result in the translation of semi-functional dystrophin of abnormal size and/or amount, typically leading to outlier or BMD clinical phenotypes. Although there are exceptions to the "reading-frame rule," 92% of phenotypic differences are explained by in-frame and out-of-frame mutations. The sarcoglycans are also reduced by immunohistochemical studies of DMD and BMD, suggesting that normal dystrophin is important for the integrity of the sarcoglycan complex (Fig. 2).

Treatment of the Dystrophinopathies

Steroids: Prednisone (0.75 mg/kg/day) increases strength and function (peaking at 3 months) and subsequently slows the rate of deterioration in children with DMD. These beneficial effects are noted as early as 10 days and are sustained for at least 3 years. Lower doses of prednisone (<0.75 mg/kg/day) are not as effective. These clinical benefits are accompanied by an increase in muscle mass and a decline in the rate of muscle catabolism. An analog of prednisone, deflazacort (at doses of 0.9 and 1.2 mg/kg/day), appears to be as effective as prednisone and associated with less side effects. In addition, a pilot study of oxandrolone, an anabolic steroid, given for 3 months to 10 boys with DMD reportedly led to improved strength. There have been no large, double-blinded, placebo-controlled studies assessing the efficacy of steroids in BMD, although small series suggest a possible benefit.

Creatine monohydrate (5–10 g/day) has been reported to modestly improve strength in a small number of patients with DMD and BMD. Creatine supplementation may increase the muscle supply of phosphocreatine and increase the ATP resynthesis. Furthermore, creatine may have a cytoprotective effect.

Gene Therapy: Myoblast transfer has been attempted in several trials without any significant benefit. Direct gene replacement therapy involves the introduction of artificially engineered dystrophin gene constructs into plasmid or viral vectors. A double-blind, placebo-controlled trial of gene therapy utilizing a adenovirus vector is currently under way.

Supportive Therapy: Physical therapy is a key component in the treatment of patients with muscular dystrophy. Contractures develop early in the disease, particularly at the heal cords, iliotibial bands, and the hips; therefore, stretching exercises must also be started early in the disease. Long leg braces may be useful in prolonging ambulation. Scoliosis is a universal complication of DMD and results in patient pain, aesthetic damage, and perhaps respiratory compromise. Spinal fusion is considered in children with 35° scoliosis or more and who are in significant discomfort. Ideally, forced vital capacity (FVC) should be greater than 35% to minimize the risk of surgery. Quality of life seems to be improved following spinal stabilization; however, scoliosis surgery does not appear to increase respiratory function.

LIMB–GIRDLE MUSCULAR DYSTROPHY

The LGMDs are a heterogeneous group that clinically resembles DMD and BMB except that these myopathies occur equally in males and females (Table 1). The incidence of LGMD is approximately 6.5 per 100,000 and prevalence is 2 per 100,000. The LGMDs may be inherited in an autosomal recessive or, less commonly, autosomal dominant fashion. In the past, patients with a clinical phenotype similar to DMD were labeled as having severe childhood autosomal recessive muscular dystrophies (SCARMD), whereas patients with milder phenotypes resembling BMD were labeled as having LGMD. Electrophysiology and routine histology of muscle biopsies are not distinguishable between DMD and BMD.

Recent advances in molecular genetics have demonstrated that there are several distinct forms of LGMD/SCARMD and that the mild and severe phenotypes can be allelic (Table 1). Autosomal dominant LGMDs are classified as type 1 (e.g., LGMD 1), whereas recessive forms are termed type 2 (e.g., LGMD 2). Further alphabetical subclassification has been applied to these disorders as they have become genotypically distinct (e.g., LGMD 2A and LGMD 2B).

Sarcoglycanopathies (LGMD 2C–2F)

Approximately 40% of muscular dystrophies have normal dystrophin. Of these, 10% are due to mutations in one of the sarcoglycan genes (α-sarcoglycan, 6.6%; β-sarcoglycan, 3.1%; γ-sarcoglycan, 1.5%; δ-sarcoglycan, <1%). The clinical, laboratory, and histological features of the sarcoglycanopathies are similar to those of the dystrophinopathies. Patients may manifest with early onset of severe weakness resembling DMD or have a later

onset and much milder course as seen in BMD. In contrast to the dystrophinopathies, there is no significant intellectual impairment or significant cardiac abnormalities in the sarcoglycanopathies. Serum CK levels are markedly elevated. Muscle biopsies demonstrate normal dystrophin; however, each sarcoglycan is absent or diminished on the sarcolemma, regardless of the primary sarcoglycan mutation.

LGMD 2C: LGMD 2C is caused by mutations in the γ-sarcoglycan gene located on chromosome 13q12. The age of onset of LGMD 2C ranges from 3 to 12 years. There is variability in severity and progression of the disease, even within affected families members. The glutei, iliopsoas, thigh adductors, pectoralis, and trapezius muscles are the earliest muscles involved. Approximately 20–25% of patients are confined to a wheelchair by 10–15 years, and 55% are wheelchair bound by 20 years.

LGMD 2D: LGMD 2D is caused by mutations in the α-sarcoglycan (adhalin) gene located on chromosome 17q21. The age of onset typically ranges from 2 to 15 years and progression is variable. The clinical phenotypes appear to correlate with the expression of α-sarcoglycan. Patients who are homozygous for null mutations and therefore expressing no α-sarcoglycan have severe phenotypes. Patients with missense mutations have varying levels of α-sarcoglycan expression and are less severely affected.

LGMD 2E: LGMD 2E is caused by mutations in the β-sarcoglycan gene located on chromosome 4q12. The age of onset and progression are variable, even within families.

LGMD 2F: LGMD 2F was linked to mutations in the δ-sarcoglycan gene located on chromosome 5q33. Age of onset and progression can be variable, even within families.

Congenital Fibrosis of the Extraocular Muscles: Mutations in the sarcospan gene located on chromosome 12p11.2 are associated with congenital fibrosis of the extraocular muscles, a rare form of autosomal dominant muscular dystrophy.

Pathogenesis of the Sarcoglycanopathies: The proteins of the sarcoglycan complex function as a unit (Fig. 1). Mutations involving any of the sarcoglycans destabilize the entire complex, leading to reduced expression of all the sarcoglycan proteins (Fig. 2). Dystrophin is usually present at a normal physiological level in the sarcoglycanopathies, but a slight reduction, in addition to a mild increase in utrophin, is sometimes observed. As apparent with the dystrophinopathies, the clinical severity of the sarcoglycanopathies may correlate with the type of mutation (i.e., whether the reading frame is preserved) and subsequent level of functional protein expression.

OTHER AUTOSOMAL RECESSIVE LIMB–GIRDLE MUSCULAR DYSTROPHIES

LGMD 2A

Clinical Features: The earliest reports of this dystrophy came from affected families on Reunion Island in the Indian Ocean, but subsequently this dystrophy has been reported throughout the world. The mean age of onset is 13.5 years, with a range of 3–30 years. Pelvic girdle muscles are clinically affected first. Periscapular weakness and atrophy predominantly affecting the latissimus dorsi, serratus magnus, rhomboids, and the pectoralis major occur 2–5 years later. The deltoid, biceps brachii, and brachioradialis are less severely affected, whereas the supra- and infraspinati, triceps, brachialis, and forearm muscles are relatively spared. Only mild weakness of neck muscles can be detected. Progression is steady but variable between different affected kinships. However, there appears to be little variability within families. For the most part, the earlier onset of symptoms and signs correlates with a faster evolution of the disease process. Approximately 50% of patients are confined to a wheelchair by the age of 20, but some are able to walk late in life. Respiratory function is only moderately affected. Similar to the sarcoglycanopathies, cardiac function is normal and there is no intellectual impairment. However, calf hypertrophy is rare.

Laboratory Features: Serum CK levels are increased up to 20 times normal early in the disease but decrease to approximately the normal range later when patients become wheelchair bound.

Molecular Genetics and Pathogenesis: LGMD 2A is caused by mutations in calpain-3 located on chromosome 15q15. Molecular and biochemical studies suggest that calpainopathies account for approximately 20–26% of dystrophies with normal dystrophin and sarcoglycans. Approximately 69% of patients with calpainopathy manifest with a BMD-like phenotype, 11% present early similar to DMD, and 6% have asymptomatic hyper-CK-emia.

The mutations result in an absence or reduction of calpain-3, a muscle-specific, calcium-dependent, non-lysosomal, proteolytic enzyme present in muscle. The pathophysiological mechanism by which mutations involving this enzyme result in a dystrophic process is unknown. Calpain-3 is present in the cytosol and nuclei of skeletal muscle fibers (Fig. 1). It may be involved in the activation of another enzyme important in muscle metabolism. Dysfunction of calpain-3 may lead to the accumulation of toxic substances in muscle cells. Alternatively, calpain-3 may play a role in gene expression by regulating turnover or activity of transcription factors or their inhibitors. Importantly, prenatal diagnosis of LGMD 2A is possible through DNA analysis of fetal cells obtained by amniocentesis or chorionic villus sampling.

LGMD 2B

Clinical Features: The age of onset of LGMD ranges from 13 to 35 years (mean, 21 years). Patients have slowly progressive weakness initially affecting the pelvic girdle followed by glutei, hamstrings, and quadriceps with involvement of the shoulder girdle 2–10 years later. Progression and severity are variable. Some patients are rendered nonambulatory by their mid-20s, whereas many remain ambulatory until late in life. Calf hypertrophy is rare. Some patients have early involvement of the gastrocnemius and soleus muscles with contractures at the ankles. This is particularly interesting given the recent colocalization of LGMD 2B and Miyoshi myopathy to the same gene on chromosome 2p13. Miyoshi myopathy is associated with early involvement of the posterior compartment of the distal lower extremities. Still other patients have early, prominent involvement of the anterior tibial muscles. Of note, there is intra- and interfamilial variability in disease progression and pattern of muscle involvement.

Laboratory Features: Serum CK levels are markedly elevated (usually 35–200 times normal).

Molecular Genetics and Pathogenesis: Mutations within the dysferlin gene on chromosome 2p13 have been identified in patients with Miyoshi myopathy, LGMD 2B, and distal myopathy with anterior tibial weakness linked to chromosome 2p13, thus proving that these phenotypically different disorders are indeed allelic. In a study of 372 muscle biopsies from patients with unclassified myopathies (normal dystrophin and sarcoglycan), 7% had abnormal dysferlin by Western blot and immunostaining.

Dysferlinopathy accounted for 1% of patients with an unknown limb–girdle syndrome and 34% of patients with a distal myopathy. In the patients with dysferlinopathy, 68% manifested with distal weakness, 12% had a LGMD phenotype, and 20 presented with asymptomatic hyper-CK-emia.

Dysferlin shares amino acid sequence homology with *Caenorhabditis elegans* spermatogenesis factor FER-1. Dysferlin is localized to the sarcolemma (Fig. 1) and is absent on immunohistochemistry in patients with LGMD 2B/Miyoshi myopathy. Dysferlin does not appear to have a significant interaction with the DGC, and immunostaining for dystrophin, dystroglycans, merosin, and the sarcoglycans is normal.

LGMD 2G

Clinical Features: LGMD 2G is a rare myopathy with a mean age of onset of muscle weakness of 12.5 years in the one reported kinship. The presenting symptoms include difficulty walking, running, and climbing stairs. Affected individuals also have significant distal weakness, legs worse than arms.

Laboratory Features: Serum CK levels are elevated 3- to 17-fold.

Histopathology: Muscle biopsy demonstrates nonspecific dystrophic features. Muscle fibers may contain one or more rimmed vacuoles. Dystrophin and sarcoglycan staining are normal.

Molecular Genetics and Pathogenesis: LGMD 2G is caused by mutations in the telethonin gene located on chromosome 17q11–12. Telethonin is a 19-kDa sarcomeric protein that is present in skeletal and cardiac muscle and is among the most abundant proteins in muscle. Telethonin localizes with titin to the Z disk of human myotubes. It also overlaps with myosin. The interaction of telethonin with titin may be important in myofibrillogenesis.

LGMD 2H

Clinical Features: This genetically distinct LGMD was described in 15 individuals from four related families of Manitoba Hutterite origin. Age of onset of weakness ranged from 8 to 27 years. The majority of affected individuals were still walking without assistance in the fourth decade of life; one patient was in a wheelchair at the age of 61 years.

Laboratory Features: Serum CKs ranged from 250 to 3130 IU/liter. Electromyography was reported as "myopathic."

Histopathology: Muscle biopsies demonstrated typical dystrophic features. Dystrophin and sarcoglycan immunostaining were normal.

Molecular Genetics and Pathogenesis: LGMD 2H is linked to chromosome 9q31–q33 and is caused by mutations in E3-ubiquitine ligase (TRIM-32).

LGMD 2I

Clinical Features: The first cases of LGMD 2I were reported from a large consanguineous Tunisian family with 13 affected members. The age of onset ranged from 1.5 to 27 years (mean, 11.6 years) and the course was variable. Affected individuals had proximal weakness that was worst in the pelvic muscles. Some, but not all, patients became wheelchair dependent in their 30s. Overall, the severity was believed to be milder than that of most sarcoglycanopathies.

Laboratory Features: Serum CK levels were increased up to 5696 IU/liter but were normal in some of the older affected patients.

Histopathology: Nonspecific dystrophic features were evident on muscle biopsy. Dystrophin, dystroglycan, sarcoglycan, and sarcospan staining were normal.

Molecular Genetics and Pathogenesis: LGMD 2I links to chromosome 19q13.3 and is caused by mutations in the gene encoding for fukutin-related protein.

AUTOSOMAL DOMINANT LIMB–GIRDLE MUSCULAR DYSTROPHIES

LGMD 1A

Clinical Features: This autosomal dominant inherited LGMD has an age of onset ranging from late teens to the late 60s (mean, 24.8 years). Affected individuals have proximal greater than distal weakness, with the legs more affected than the arms. Distal weakness is evident in a few patients. Rare patients develop dysarthria secondary to palatal muscle involvement and mild facial weakness.

Laboratory Features: Serum CK levels are normal or elevated up to nine times normal. Muscle biopsies are notable for the frequent occurrence of rimmed vacuoles. Marked disorganization and streaming of the Z disk are apparent on EMG.

Molecular Genetics and Pathogenesis: LGMD 1A l is caused by mutations in the gene that encodes for myotilin located on chromosome 5q22.3–31.3. Myotilin is a sarcomeric protein that colocalizes with α-actinin on the Z disk. Mutations in myotilin do not appear to affect its binding with α-actinin but may perturb the normal structure of the Z disk.

LGMD 1B with Cardiomyopathy

Clinical Features: The nonchromosome 5q-linked autosomal dominant LGMD represents a heterogeneous group of disorders. One subgroup is associated with severe cardiac conduction defects leading to sudden death. These patients often require insertion of a pacemaker. Affected individuals develop proximal weakness in childhood or early adult life. Some patients have early contractures and predilection for the humerol–peroneal muscle weakness similar to that in Emery–Dreifuss muscular dystrophy (EDMD). Thus, this disorder was also reported as autosomal dominant EDMD until the two disorders were found to be allelic.

Laboratory Features: Serum CK levels can be normal or elevated up to 25 times normal.

Histopathology: Muscle biopsies demonstrate variation in fiber size, increased endomysial connective tissue, and normal dystrophin, sarcoglycan, and emerin staining. Occasionally, rimmed vacuoles are evident on muscles biopsy similar to those seen in other autosomal dominant LGMDs. Lamin A/C expression on nuclear membranes may be reduced or normal in autosomal dominant EDMD.

Molecular Genetics and Pathogenesis: Autosomal dominant EDMD and LGMD 1B with cardiomyopathy are caused by mutations in lamin A/C on chromosome 1q11–21. The nuclear lamina is a complex of intermediate-sized filaments (e.g., lamin A/C) associated with the nucleoplasmic surface of the inner nuclear membrane. These lamins bind to the inner nuclear membrane by interacting with various lamina-associated protein (LAPs), including LAP1 and LAP2, as well as lamin B receptor. LAP2, lamin B receptor, and the lamins are known to bind to chromatin and promote its attachment to the nuclear membrane. Of note, X-linked EDMD is caused by mutations in the emerin gene. Emerin also localizes to the inner nuclear membranes of skeletal, cardiac, and smooth muscle fibers as well as skin cells. Emerin is a member of the nuclear LAP family. Thus, mutations in emerin or lamin A/C may result in the disorganization of the nuclear lamina and heterochromatin.

LGMD 1C

Clinical Features: This rare autosomal dominant LGMD was described in two families. The affected patients met early motor milestones, but noticeable weakness occurred at approximately 5 years of age. Weakness primarily affected the proximal muscles. Some patients experienced exercise-induced myalgias. Calf hypertrophy was usually evident. Sporadic LGMD 1C was reported in two children ages 4 and 6 years. They had asymptomatic mild hyper-CK-emia without objective weakness on examination at the time of evaluation.

Laboratory Features: Serum CK was elevated 3- to 25-fold.

Histopathology: Muscle biopsies demonstrated nonspecific myopathic features, with normal dystrophin, sarcoglycan, and merosin staining. In contrast, there is reduced caveolin-3 staining along the sarcolemma.

Molecular Genetics and Pathogenesis: LGMD 1C links to mutations in the caveolin-3 gene located on chromosome 3p25. Caveolins play a role in the formation of caveolae membranes (Fig. 1). The mechanism by which mutations in caveolin-3 lead to the myopathy is not known. Mutations in the caveolin-3 gene are also responsible for autosomal dominant rippling muscle disease.

Histopathology of the LGMD

There are no specific muscle biopsy findings suggestive of LGMD or histological abnormalities that distinguish one type of LGMD from another or even from one of the other forms of muscular dystrophy. Muscle biopsies reveal prominent muscle fiber size variation, increased endmysial connective tissue, muscle fiber splitting, fiber atrophy and hypertrophy, and variable degrees of muscle fiber degeneration, phagocytosis, and regeneration. Mononuclear inflammatory infiltrate is seen in some patients. Muscle fibers with rimmed vacuoles have been noted in LGMD 2B, LGMD 1A, LGMD 1C, and other LGMD syndromes. Rimmed vacuoles are a nonspecific myopathic feature but are characteristically present in inclusion body myositis (IBM), hereditary

IBM, oculopharyngeal dystrophy, several of the distal myopathies, and myofibrillar myopathy. Dystrophin is usually normal, although a mild reduction may occasionally be seen in the sarcoglycanopathies. The sarcoglycan proteins are absent or diminished in the sarcoglycanopathies, which may distinguish them from other forms of dystrophy.

Treatment of the LGMD

Treatment is largely supportive. Physical and occupational therapy are important to prevent contractures and improve function. Whether or not corticosteroids can improve strength and delay progression similar to that observed in DMD is not known, although some patients with LGMD reported benefit from such treatment. Modest improvement in strength has been reported in a small number of patients with LGMD treated with short courses of creatine monohydrate (5–10 g/day). Advances in molecular genetics may lead to better forms of treatment in the future. Currently, gene therapy trials are being conducted in some forms of LGMD.

—*Anthony A. Amato*

See also–Dystrophin and Dystrophin-Associated Proteins; Muscle Contraction, Overview; Muscular Dystrophy: Emery–Dreifuss, Facioscapulohumeral, Scapuloperoneal, and Bethlem Myopathy; Myotonic Dystrophy; Neuromuscular Disorders, Overview; Oculopharyngeal Muscular Dystrophy

Further Reading

Angelini, C., Fanin, M., Freda, M. P., *et al.* (1999). The clinical spectrum of sarcoglycanopathies. *Neurology* **52**, 176–179.
Bonifati, M. D., Ruzza, G., Bonometto, P., *et al.* (2000). A multicenter, double-blinded, randomized trial of deflazacort versus prednisone in Duchenne muscular dystrophy. *Muscle Nerve* **23**, 1344–1347.
Bushby, K. M. D. (1999). Making sense of the limb–girdle muscular dystrophies. *Brain* **122**, 1403–1420.
Bushby, K. M. D., and Gardner-Medwin, D. (1993). The clinical, genetic and dystrophin characteristics of Becker muscular dystrophy. I. Natural history. *J. Neurol.* **240**, 98–104.
Bushby, K. M. D., Thambyayah, M., and Garnder-Medwin, D. (1991). Prevalence and incidence of Becker muscular dystrophy. *Lancet* **337**, 1022–1024.
Cohn, R. D., and Campbell, K. P. (2000). Molecular basis of muscular dystrophies. *Muscle Nerve* **23**, 1456–1471.
Comi, G. P., Prelle, A., Bresolin, N., *et al.* (1994). Clinical variability in Becker muscular dystrophy. Genetic, biochemical, and immunohistochemical correlates. *Brain* **117**, 1–14.

Duggan, D. J., Gorospe, J. F., Fanin, M., *et al.* (1997). Mutations in the sarcoglycan genes in patients with myopathy. *N. Engl. J. Med.* **336**, 618–624.
Emery, A. E. H. (1991). Population frequencies of inherited neuromuscular diseases—A world survey. *Neuromusc. Disord.* **1**, 19–29.
Fenichel, G., Pestronk, A., Florence, J., *et al.* (1997). A beneficial effect of oxandrolone in the treatment of Duchenne muscular dystrophy: A pilot study. *Neurology* **48**, 1225–1226.
Griggs, R. C., Moxley, R. T., Mendell, J. R., *et al.* (1993). Duchenne dystrophy: Randomized, controlled trial of Prednisone (18 months) and Azathioprine (12 months). *Neurology* **43**, 520–527.
Hoffman, E. P., Brown, R. H., and Kunkel, L. M. (1987). Dystrophin: The protein product of the duchenne muscular dystrophy locus. *Cell* **51**, 919–928.
Hoffman, E. P., Arahata, K., Minetti, C., *et al.* (1992). Dystrophinopathy in isolated cases of myopathy in females. *Neurology* **42**, 967–975.
Mendell, J. R., Sahenk, Z., and Prior, T. W. (1995). The childhood muscular dystrophies: Diseases sharing a common pathogenesis of membrane instability. *J. Child Neurol.* **10**, 150–159.
Ozawa, E., Noguschi, S., Mizuno, Y., *et al.* (1998). From dystrophinopathy to sarcoglycanopathy: Evolution of a concept of muscular dystrophy. *Muscle Nerve* **21**, 421–438.

Musculocutaneous Nerve

Encyclopedia of the Neurological Sciences
Copyright 2003, Elsevier Science (USA). All rights reserved.

THE MUSCULOCUTANEOUS NERVE supplies three upper arm muscle that produce flexion of the arm at the elbow (biceps, brachialis, and coracobrachialis) and a sensory branch that supplies the skin of the lateral side of the anterior forearm.

The musculocutaneous nerve is a branch of the lateral cord of the brachial plexus. More proximally, the sensory and motor nerve fibers traverse the C5 and C6 cervical nerve roots and the upper trunk of the brachial plexus. After the musculocutaneous nerve arises from the lateral cord, it supplies the corachobrachialis at the level of the axilla. It then pierces this muscle and runs between the brachialis and biceps muscles, where it innervates them in the mid-arm. It continues distally just lateral to the biceps tendon as a terminal sensory branch—the lateral cutaneous branch of the forearm. This supplies sensation to the skin over the lateral side of the forearm from the elbow to the wrist.

Due to the limited motor and sensory distribution of the musculocutaneous nerve, the clinical manifestations of an injury to the nerve are straightforward.

A lesion in the proximal arm results in weakness of elbow flexion, a reduced or absent biceps reflex, and sensory loss in the lateral half of the anterior forearm. There may be mild weakness of supination, a partial action of the biceps muscle, but this movement is primarily subserved by the supinator. Even in complete lesions there may be some preserved elbow flexion from the action of the brachioradialis and pronator teres muscles. A lesion distal to the mid-arm results in only sensory loss in the distribution of the lateral cutaneous nerve of the forearm. The extent of the sensory loss can be quite variable, from a broad patch over the lateral half of the forearm extending to the back of the forearm to a tiny band.

An upper cervical root (C5 or C6) or brachial plexus (upper trunk) injury usually produces more widespread weakness, generally in the deltoids, brachioradialis, and infraspinatus muscles. The sensory disturbance in such lesions is usually more prominent in the hand (thumb and index finger). Weakness in elbow flexion due to a ruptured biceps muscle or tendon may resemble a nerve lesion. However, with such a mechanical rupture there is local pain with swelling, a palpable abnormality in the contracted biceps muscle, and no sensory loss in the forearm.

Isolated musculocutaneous neuropathy is not common and is usually due to trauma. It can be seen as a mononeuropathy with shoulder dislocations, but more often it is associated with injury to other large nerves of the shoulder girdle, such as the suprascapular and axillary nerves. It may also occur with fractures of the humerus, as a surgical injury during axillary node dissection, or during shoulder arthroscopy.

Occasionally, blunt trauma to the shoulder can produce injury limited to this nerve. Injury to the musculocutaneous nerve has been reported after strenuous exercise, particularly heavy weightlifting. It may occur after extension of the forearm during a fall or a similar forceful hyperextension injury. It has been suggested that the nerve is relatively fixed as it passes through the coracobrachialis muscle, making it susceptible to injury with such vigorous maneuvers.

The distal sensory branch, the lateral antebrachial cutaneous nerve, may be injured near the lateral aspect of the biceps tendon or more distally. This has been reported after venipuncture, catheterization, and other local needle injuries. Rare cases of compression by the biceps tendon as the nerve pierces the fascia to become subcutaneous occur.

Electrodiagnostic studies (nerve conduction studies and electromyography) not only allow confirmation of a musculocutaneous nerve injury but also give information on any associated nerve injuries. They also provide important prognostic information that generally allows a good estimate of the timing and extent of recovery after a traumatic nerve injury. Magnetic resonance imaging may occasionally be helpful. The management of an acute injury depends on the extent of the nerve injury. With severe injuries, the important management decision involves whether to perform surgery, intraoperative nerve recordings, and possible nerve graft.

—Shawn J. Bird

See also–Neck and Arm Pain; Nerve Injury; Neuropathy, Axillary

Further Reading

Bird, S. J., and Brown, M. J. (1996). Acute focal neuropathy in male weight lifters. *Muscle Nerve* **19**, 897–899.

Braddom, R. L., and Wolfe, C. (1978). Musculocutaneous nerve injury after heavy exercise. *Arch. Phys. Med. Rehab.* **59**, 290–293.

Davidson, J. J., Bassett, F. H., and Nunley, J. A. (1998). Musculocutaneous nerve entrapment revisited. *J. Shoulder Elbow Surg.* 7, 250–255.

De Laat, E. A., Visser, C. P., Coene, L. N., *et al.* (1994). Nerve lesions in primary shoulder dislocations and humeral neck fractures: A prospective clinical and EMG study. *J. Bone Jt. Surg. Br.* **76**, 381–383.

Liveson, J. A. (1984). Nerve lesions associated with shoulder dislocation: An electrodiagnostic study of 121 cases. *J. Neurol. Neurosurg. Psychiatry* **47**, 742–744.

Quan, D., and Bird, S. J. (1999). Nerve conduction studies and electromyography in the evaluation of peripheral nerve injury. *Univ. Pennsylvania Orthop. J.* **12**, 45–51.

Stanish, W. D., and Peterson, D. C. (1995). Shoulder arthroscopy and nerve injury. *Arthroscopy* **11**, 458–466.

Young, A. W., Redmond, D., and Belandres, P. (1990). Isolated lesion of the lateral cutaneous nerve of the forearm. *Arch. Phys. Med. Rehab.* **71**, 251–252.

Mushroom Toxicity

Encyclopedia of the Neurological Sciences

MUSHROOM poisoning has been described since ancient history; the wife and children of Euripides and Emperor Claudius were probable victims of lethal intoxication. Poisonous mushrooms may be divided into two groups—those causing toxic signs early (within 6 hr after ingestion) and those causing toxic signs late (6–40 hr).

Mushrooms with early signs of toxicity induce a variety of clinical disorders. Based on its concentrations of ibotenic acid, muscazon, and muscimol, *Amanita* (*A. muscaria* and *A. pantherina*) has strong anticholinergic effects. Agitation, muscle spasms, incoordination or ataxia, large pupils, jerking body movements called myoclonus, and convulsions develop. The action of these compounds on the neurochemical γ-aminobutyric acid accounts for part of the psychoactive response encountered. No specific antidote is available, and atropine, a drug used to counteract toxicity with other mushrooms, is contraindicated. *Amanita pantherine* carries a mortality rate of 10–20% after ingestion.

The genera *Inocybe* and *Clitocybe* contain muscarine, a compound that stimulates nerve endings of the parasympathetic nervous system in a manner mimicking the chemical acetylcholine. Atropine, a drug that blocks receptor site proteins for acetylcholine, has decreased mortality and the recommended starting dose is 2 mg. *Coprinus atramentarius*, generally considered edible, contains coprine, an amino acid that inhibits the enzyme acetaldehyde dehydrogenase. When consumed in combination with alcohol, this mushroom causes facial flushing, paresthesias or strange tingling sensations, and severe nausea and vomiting. *Psilocybe*, a mushroom often consumed for psychoactive effects, contains psilocybin and psilocin, two compounds with strong hallucinogenic properties. Furthermore, the presence of phenylethylamine may be responsible for the adverse effects, such as rapid heart rate.

Two major groups of mushrooms cause intoxication with late neurological responses. *Gyromitra* causes neurological symptoms probably as a result of direct neurotoxic effects, and *G. esculenta*, or false Morel, results in fatality rates ranging from 15 to 35%. When neurotoxic signs accompany electrolyte imbalance, pyridoxine hydrochloride treatment is important. Some *Aminita* mushrooms cause neurological symptoms as a result of primary liver damage. These mushrooms are responsible for approximately 95% of fatalities associated with mushroom ingestion, and there are several hundred fatalities per year globally. The clinical course begins 6–8 hr after ingestion. Symptoms include massive vomiting and bloody cholera-like diarrhea. Although patients often die during this phase from electrolyte imbalance, the most dangerous phase of hepatorenal failure does not occur until 3–5 days following mushroom ingestion.

Secondary neurological manifestations include a gradual decline of mental status with confusion, asterixis or a jerking movement that occurs when patients try to hold their hands outstretched as if stopping traffic, and eventually coma and death. Treatment is mainly supportive and includes careful regulation of fluid status and electrolyte balance, correction of low blood glucose levels (hypoglycemia), and monitoring of coagulation, renal, and liver function.

—*Christopher G. Goetz*

See also–Ergotism; Neurotoxicology, Overview

Further Reading
Beck, O., Helander, A., Karlson-Stiber, C., *et al.* (1998). Presence of phenylethylamine in hallucinogenic *Psilocybe* mushroom: Possible role in adverse reactions. *J. Anal. Toxicol.* 22, 45–49.
de Wolff, F. A., and Pennings, E. J. M. (1995). Mushrooms and hallucinogens: Neurotoxicological aspects. In *Handbook of Clinical Neurology* (P. J. Vinken and G. W. Bruyn, Eds.), pp. 35–60. Elsevier, Amsterdam.
Goetz, C. G. (1997). Biological toxins. In *Clinical Neurology* (R. J. Joynt and R. C. Griggs, Eds.). Lippincott Williams & Wilkins, Philadelphia.
Hanrahan, J. P., and Gordon, M. A. (1984). Mushroom poisoning. Case reports and a review of therapy. *J. Am. Med. Assoc.* 251, 1057–1061.

Myasthenia Gravis

Encyclopedia of the Neurological Sciences
Copyright 2003, Elsevier Science (USA). All rights reserved.

MYASTHENIA GRAVIS (MG) is a disease causing weakness in the arms and legs and in the muscles responsible for eye movement, facial expression, speech, swallowing, and respiration, affecting 1 in 10,000 people. These symptoms are the result of an immunological abnormality in which the patient's antibodies attack the acetylcholine receptor (AChR) at the muscle end plate, interfering with the normal transmission of signals from the peripheral nerve to the muscle. Although MG has been recognized as a distinct disease for well over a century, its cause remained obscure until the early 1970s, when experimental procedures enabled the production of antibodies directed against the AChR in animals. Serendipitously, these animals soon developed a disease that closely resembled human MG, and subsequent studies confirmed AChR antibodies as the cause of MG in humans. These discoveries generated great excitement in the neurological and immunological communities and spawned an entire field of neuroscientific investigation that continues unabated to this day.

Armed with these insights, neurologists soon applied immunological therapies to combat the disease with dramatic and often life-saving results. Consequently, the prevalence of MG has increased during the past 50 years, reflecting increased patient survival as effective therapies have been applied. Thus, a rate of 1 in 10,000 is more accurate for the modern era. It can strike at almost any age but is most common in either younger females (15–30 years) or older males (60–75 years). Natural history studies performed prior to the advent of contemporary therapies and advances in intensive care reported a significant mortality rate of 20–30% in the first 3 years after disease onset, most commonly the result of primary respiratory failure. Another 20% of patients had stable symptoms with no significant worsening or improvement, whereas 20–25% experienced improved but persistent symptoms and 20–25% had a spontaneous clinical remission.

CLINICAL FEATURES

Initially, MG may affect the eye muscles, the muscles of facial expression, speech, swallowing, or respiration, or the muscles of the arms or legs, either alone or in combination. Double vision (diplopia) and drooping of the eyelids (ptosis) are common early symptoms in 50–60% of patients; an additional 30% of patients will eventually develop these symptoms. In contrast, 90% of patients presenting with symptoms isolated to the eyes, such as diplopia and ptosis (pure ocular MG), will eventually develop more widespread weakness (generalized MG). The odds of permanent pure ocular disease increase the longer symptoms remain isolated to the eyes, such that those patients without progression for at least 2 years have only a 10% chance of developing generalized MG. Although occasionally only one extraocular muscle (EOM) may be weakened, more commonly combinations of EOMs are affected and may mimic a variety of neuro-ophthalmological syndromes due to other causes, such as stroke and multiple sclerosis. However, prominent fatigability and recovery with rest by history and on physical examination (with fluctuating diplopia and ptosis) is frequently present in MG, helping to distinguish it from other diseases. Instructing the patient to maintain upward gaze for more than 30 sec while looking at a fixed target will

often provoke visibly worsening ptosis and dysconjugate gaze in MG patients, with clear improvement following brief eye closure and rest. When asked, many patients may also report a mild degree of photophobia due to fatigability of the constrictor muscles of the pupil.

Although ocular symptoms are common, weakness of the facial musculature may also appear. This weakness may manifest as a paucity of the facial expression (which sometimes mimics depression), poor eye closure, and difficulty whistling or blowing up a balloon. In more severe cases, an attempted smile may result in decreased horizontal movement of the lips, with more prominent vertical movement resulting in a facial expression termed the myasthenic snarl. Some patients may also report difficulty with chewing or closing of the mouth, and others may keep the jaw closed with one hand propped under the chin. Posterior neck stiffness and cramping especially toward the end of the day may also be present. Speech changes are also relatively frequent and include progressive slurring of speech with sustained conversation (dysarthria) as well as increased nasality and, less commonly, hoarseness. Difficulty with swallowing, especially large portions of solid food such as steak, may also appear and, in some patients, aspiration, pneumonia, or substantial weight loss may be initial symptoms.

In generalized MG, the arms and legs are also typically affected, with weakness of the extensor muscles of the arms (especially the triceps and finger extensors) and weakness of the hip flexors. Extremity weakness also classically worsens with repetitive or prolonged exercise, such as extended ambulation. Generalized weakness, more prominent in the upper extremities and the extensor muscles (especially the triceps and finger extensors), is common and typically worsens with repetitive exercise. The most serious, and potentially fatal, complication of myasthenia is respiratory muscle weakness. Dyspnea on exertion may appear initially, progressing to dyspnea at rest and, in some cases, respiratory failure and death if intubation and mechanical ventilation are not instituted. In some cases, these symptoms may appear acutely and progress rapidly over a matter of hours, necessitating careful attention to pulmonary function during such exacerbations. Patients with respiratory involvement must frequently be hospitalized for observation and serial measurements of pulmonary function and may ultimately require intubation and mechanical ventilation until immunotherapy results in substantial improvement in respiratory function.

Transient neonatal MG is a unique form of myasthenia occurring in 12–54% of newborn children of myasthenic mothers due to transplacental transfer of AChR antibodies from mother to child. Symptoms may appear within hours to days after birth and range from poor suck and swallow to generalized weakness and respiratory depression. Arthrogryposis (joint contracture due to decreased fetal movement during gestation) may also be present in some cases. Although there is a direct correlation between maternal and newborn antibody levels, there is no direct relationship between symptoms in the mother and those in her offspring, and some cases may be negative with currently available AChR antibody assays (likely because not all AChR antibodies are detectable with current methods). Ventilatory support may be required initially, but the prognosis is usually excellent, with full recovery in nearly all patients within a relatively short period of time.

Other autoimmune diseases may also be found more frequently in MG patients, appearing in 2.3–24.2% of cases. Thyroiditis with hyperthyroidism is most common, affecting 2–17% of patients, and thyroid dysfunction may worsen associated MG or produce additional neuromuscular disease, causing more severe symptoms. Rheumatoid arthritis is the second most common, affecting 0–10.3% of patients. Other less common associations include systemic lupus erythematosus, Sjogren's syndrome, sarcoidosis, scleroderma, polymyositis, and Lambert–Eaton myasthenic syndrome (LEMS). Although central nervous system disease is not believed to be associated with MG, a possible increased incidence of multiple sclerosis has been reported in a few studies.

NORMAL NEUROMUSCULAR TRANSMISSION

The neuromuscular junction (NMJ) is a functional unit consisting of highly specialized structures at the nerve terminal (presynapse) and at the muscle end plate (postsynapse) as well as the gap between them (synapse), across which electrochemical communication occurs. As individual motor axons within a peripheral nerve approach the muscle, they branch repeatedly, ultimately forming single lightly myelinated nerve fibers, each of which loses its insulating myelin just before dividing into several smaller branches known as the terminal spray. Each of these branches then terminates in a bulbous swollen tip (the terminal bouton), just above the specialized portion of an individual muscle fiber membrane known as the end plate zone. Each terminal bouton contains an abundance of small, rounded, membrane-enclosed vesicles arranged for quick release, each containing 5000–12,000 molecules of the chemical neurotransmitter ACh (Fig. 1). Following vesicle fusion, ACh molecules are released and passively diffuse across the synaptic cleft toward the muscle fiber end plate.

Following their arrival at the end plate, the ACh molecules within each vesicle successfully activate an average of 1000–2000 AChR ion channels in a given muscle fiber. The subsequent influx of sodium into the muscle fiber results in a localized area of electrical depolarization around the receptor site known as a miniature end plate potential (MEPP). During actual contraction, a large number of simultaneous MEPPs summate, creating a larger, global EPP that eventually reaches the muscle fiber's threshold for propagating a depolarization wave. This wave then travels over the entire muscle fiber, igniting a chain of events ultimately resulting in contraction of the fiber. Following completion of depolarization, the ACh molecules are released from their receptors and hydrolyzed by synaptic acetylcholinesterase, preventing further receptor activation until the next wave of ACh is released.

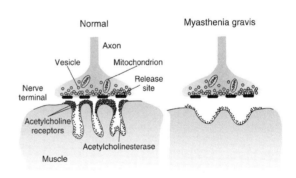

A   B

Figure 1

Cross section of a normal (A) and a myasthenic (B) neuromuscular junction. The normal end plate is convoluted, with acetylcholine receptors concentrated on the shoulders of its crests. The myasthenic end plate demonstrates significant flattening due to sustained autoimmune attack, with loss of the normal convolutions, decreased numbers of acetylcholine receptors, and widening of the synapse (reprinted with permission from Drachman, 1994).

IMMUNOLOGY

The idea that neurotransmitter release at the NMJ could cause muscle contraction was proposed as early as 1904, and specific release of ACh at the NMJ was demonstrated in 1934. A number of thymic abnormalities were described in the tissue of myasthenic patients, and symptomatic improvement following thymectomy was reported during this same period, ultimately prompting further study and recommendation of thymic resection as primary therapy. In 1973, rabbits immunized with solubilized membranes from the electric organs of the torpedo electric fish in an attempt to create AChR antibodies developed a syndrome that closely paralleled human MG. Finally, AChR antibodies were identified in the serum of patients with MG, further supporting an immunological cause for this disorder.

Acetylcholine Receptor

The nicotinic AChR is a transmembrane protein with five subunits, designated alpha, beta, gamma, delta, and epsilon, arranged radially around a central ion channel. Two alpha subunits and one beta, delta, and epsilon subunit are present in adult muscle AChRs, whereas the gamma subunit is found embryonically and following denervation but is ultimately replaced by the epsilon subunit in adult development. The larger portion of the receptor extends toward the extracellular space, and binding sites for ACh are found on both alpha subunits in this area. Only when both sites are occupied does the central channel open, initiating muscle membrane depolarization and the cascade ultimately leading to muscle contraction. In MG, antibodies to multiple sites on the extracellular portion of the AChR are generated, but antibodies directed against the alpha subunit predominate. Many of the anti-alpha subunit antibodies appear to bind to a specific epitope consisting of a hydrophobic, negatively charged decapeptide within the alpha subunit designated the main immunogenic region (MIR). The MIR is separate and distinct from the ACh binding site and is highly conserved between species; antibodies against it readily crossreact to AChRs from different animals. Anti-MIR antibodies mediate AChR loss in cell culture, initiate compliment fixation, and induce disease following passive transfer to animals. These are the most extensively studied epitopes, but a growing amount of data support a significant heterogeneity of antibodies directed against the AChR in myasthenic sera.

The NMJ in acquired MG is structurally altered by both the binding of antibodies to AchRs at the end plate and the subsequent immune-mediated attack such binding provokes. Functionally, autoantibodies may induce MG through a number of mechanisms. Antibodies binding at or near the ACh binding site may prevent neurotransmitter docking by directly covering the site or via stearic hindrance. Alternatively, antibodies against other portions of the receptor may interfere with ion flux through other, less clear mechanisms. Finally, autoantibodies can increase receptor degradation and/or complement-mediated focal lysis. It is unclear why pure or disproportionately severe ocular weakness occurs in some patients, but the persistence of the gamma subunit within the AChR of EOMs may provide unique epitopes for relatively selective autoimmunity to EOM NMJs, thereby producing relatively restricted ocular symptoms.

Thymus

The thymus is located in the fat pad immediately beneath the sternal bone. It is covered by a connective tissue capsule that penetrates internally to form septa, dividing it into incomplete lobules approximately 0.5–2.0 mm in diameter. An internal thymic primordial epithelial cell network is invaded in early development by lymphocyte-forming cells that intensely proliferate throughout early life and childhood, pushing the epithelial cells apart to form a reticular pattern. Each lobule consists of a peripheral cortex of densely packed lymphocytes and a central medulla containing a large number of epithelial reticular cells. These cells sometimes aggregate, creating epithelial collections known as Hassall's corpuscles. Other medullary cells include dendritic cells and myoid cells (muscle-like cells containing the nicotinic AChR and MIR epitopes). With age, the thymus involutes, shrinking from 30–40 g at puberty to 10–15 g in the elderly, although it retains significant proliferative capability. The cortex is the active site of T cell differentiation. Prototypic stem cells first enter this region and begin maturation, followed by central migration. Initially, genetic rearrangement of the T cell receptor locus produces antigen specificity and dendritic cells may play a role in the antigen presentation in this process. Functional T cells develop both CD4 and CD8 surface antigens, then lose one or the other with further maturation to become $CD4^+CD8^-$ or $CD4^-CD8^+$. Epithelial reticular cells also contribute to T lymphocyte development via thymic hormone and lymphokine elaboration. This process of "positive selection" includes the restriction of these T cells to the recognition of specific antigens only in the presence of certain types of major histocompatibility complex (MHC) molecules. This phase of maturation is designated MHC restriction. The next critical step involves the induction of self-tolerance, during which those T cells with high affinity for self-antigens are eliminated (negative selection), although some survive to migrate to the peripheral lymph system, where further selection occurs. Mature T cells then move toward the medulla, which contains only 5% of the total thymic lymphocyte population at any given time, and exit the thymus via venules and the lymph system, migrating to other lymphoid organs.

The myasthenic thymus demonstrates frequent abnormalities. Ten to 15% of myasthenics have a lymphoepithelial tumor and 70% of those without tumor demonstrate lymphoid follicular hyperplasia (LFH). In LFH, active germinal centers form between the cortex and the medulla, distending and sometimes disrupting the boundaries of the perivascular spaces. These patients demonstrate an increased percentage of mature T lymphocytes as well as an increased percentage of thymic B cells. Tumors of the thymus can be classified as lymphomas and epithelial, carcinoid, and mesenchymal tumors according to their cells of origin. The epithelial thymic tumor is the classic "thymoma" and is often referred to as a lymphoepithelial tumor. It is graded according to lymphocytic infiltration (although the epithelial cell is the neoplastic element) or classified by cortical, medullary, or mixed cell type. Noncancerous collections of lymphoctes between muscle fibers (lymphorrhages) may also be seen in up to two-thirds of patients with myasthenia, whether or not thymoma is also present. Thymoma epithelial cells demonstrate numerous AChR epitopes. Patients with thymoma and myasthenia also demonstrate heterogeneous antibodies cross-reacting to striated skeletal muscle, cardiac muscle, and thymic myoid cells that do not react to AChR epitopes (anti-striational antibodies).

As mentioned previously, approximately 10–15% of patients with MG also have a thymoma, but 40% of patients with thymoma also have myasthenia. The average age for all patients with thymoma is 50 years, with a 1:1 male-to-female ratio. Ninety percent are easily treated with resection, whereas 10% are malignant, spreading beyond the thymic capsule to local mediastinal tissue, the lymphatic system, or the blood. However, only 1–5% metastasize distantly. Recurrence of benign tumors is rare, but patients with malignancies that have spread to the pleura or elsewhere have a 5- to 10-year average survival despite surgical and radiotherapy. Most patients with both MG and thymoma have severe generalized weakness (with a much lower incidence of pure ocular disease) and cardiac involvement, which is not seen in other forms of MG (herzmyasthenia). Hertzmyasthenia may include arrhythmia, bundle branch block on electrocardiograph, and/or cardiac failure with focal myocarditis. MG is most commonly associated with thymoma, but a low incidence of other autoimmune and neurological diseases has also been reported, including motor neuropathy, LEMS, and giant cell polymyositis. MG associated with thymoma diagnosed at a later stage is typically more severe, with more frequent exacerbations and a higher mortality rate, whereas MG associated with thymoma diagnosed at an early stage has a slightly better prognosis than MG without tumor.

The precise role of the thymus in the pathogenesis of MG remains controversial. Myoid cells having AChR and MIR epitopes are near mature lymphocytes and interdigitating dendritic cells in the thymic medulla. The embryonic gamma subunit (not normally expressed in adult skeletal muscle) may also be found within the thymus. The myoid and dedritic cells (which have a role in antigen presentation) may provide both an AChR antigen and an antigen presenting cell. In addition, persistence of the embryonic gamma AChR subunit in the thymus might encourage loss of self-tolerance, with subsequent generation of wider autoimmunity against the receptor. AChR epitopes may also be found in the neoplastic epithelial thymoma, which in the altered microenvironment accompanying tumor growth might result in loss of self-tolerance and autoimmunity. The frequency of additional antibodies with cross-reactivity to myoid cells and other striated muscle components in this patient group suggests a similar mechanism of autosensitization.

DIAGNOSIS

AChR Antibody Assays

A number of AChR antibodies are serological markers for acquired myasthenia. Three have been adopted for routine screening: binding, blocking, and modulating antibodies. The binding antibody assay indirectly measures antibodies binding to the AChR binding site and is also positive in nonmyasthenic patients with thymoma. The blocking antibody assay measures those antibodies blocking access to the binding site. Because these are found only in 1% of myasthenic patients who do not have detectable binding antibodies, it is not useful as a first-line screening test, and false-positive results may occur after surgery if curare-like muscle relaxants are used. In contrast, the modulating antibody assay measures antibodies promoting endocytosis and degradation of the AChR, although blocking antibodies will also hide intact receptors and contribute to the observed value. This test is most useful when the AChR binding antibody assay is negative. It may be more sensitive in patients with early, mild disease or pure ocular disease but carries a greater risk of false positivity from disruption of the assay and other extraneous sources. Sensitivity and specificity vary with each assay and the clinical presentation of the patient (i.e., generalized vs ocular). A positive result is up to 99% specific for myasthenia. However, sensitivities range from 59% (AChR blocking antibody) to 90% (binding and modulating antibody assays) in generalized and 30% (blocking antibody) to 70% (binding and modulating antibody) in ocular MG. Correlation between AChR antibody titers and disease severity in individual patients at initial diagnosis is poor, but mean antibody titers increase with worsening disease severity in large groups of patients. However, high titers may be found in early onset disease and in patients with thymoma, and decreased titers following therapy correlate with symptomatic improvement in some patients.

A minority of patients with symptomatic disease do not have detectable antibodies by routine assay (seronegative MG). Such apparent seronegativity has several possible causes. Processing by a reputable, well-recognized laboratory with extensive experience in AChR assays is critical because a variety of technical inadequacies can render unacceptably high false-negative results. In some patients, only one of the available assays (typically the binding antibody assay) is performed with a negative result, whereas other assays may be positive. In other patients, high-affinity antibodies may aggressively adhere to their respective antigens *in vivo*, rendering standard assays negative due to very low serum levels. Immunosuppression, especially when administered for more than 1 year, may reduce antibody production to undetectable levels. Seronegative patients appear to respond to immunosuppression, and increasing evidence suggests significant heterogeneity among antibodies in these patients.

Other Antibody Assays

Anti-striated muscle antibodies react against thymic myoid cells as well as the contractile elements of skeletal muscle and are present in 27% of all MG patients. Particularly high levels may be noted in up to 90% of patients with both MG and thymoma. Progressive increases in titers may be the first indication of thymic tumor recurrence. They may be also be positive when AChR antibody assays are negative, making them a useful adjunctive test. Other antibodies may also be found in a significant percentage of MG patients, including anti-nuclear (20–40%), thyroid (15–40%), rheumatoid factor (10–40%), gastric parietal cell (10–20%), lymphocyte (40–90%), and platelet (5–50%) antibodies as well as anti-smooth muscle, mitochondrial, red blood cell, and squamous epithelial antibodies, often without additional disease.

Electrodiagnosis

Two major electrodiagnostic tests are available to assess NMJ function. Repetitive nerve stimulation (RNS) involves repeated supramaximal stimulation of a selected peripheral nerve (typically at a frequency of 1, 2, 3, or 5 Hz) while recording the electrical waveforms produced by the resulting, recurrent muscle contractions (CMAPs) of a selected muscle innervated by that nerve (Fig. 2). Trains of these CMAPs (5–10 waveforms) are then recorded at baseline and following 30–60 sec of maximal voluntary contraction and at variable intervals (30–60 seconds apart) for several minutes after exercise. The amplitudes and areas of the first and one of the later waveforms of a given train are then compared to assess whether there is a decrementing or incrementing response within each train. Myasthenic patients typically demonstrate significant decrementing in excess of 10–15% as increasing numbers of NMJs fail (due to antibody-mediated AChR blockade) with the demands of repeated activation. In addition, the amplitude of the first waveform of the first train following exercise may be increased by 10–50% when compared to the amplitude of the first waveform of the baseline preexercise train in the MG patient. The baseline decrement within each train may also transiently improve following exercise. This phenomenon, known as postexercise facilitation, may be due to a temporarily enhanced concentration of ACh in the NMJ following a brief maximal contraction. A decay of this transient improvement in waveform

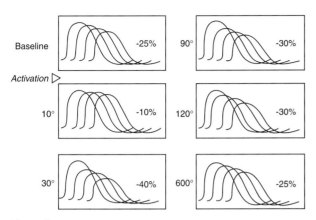

Figure 2
Repetitive nerve stimulation in myasthenia gravis. A baseline train of repetitive nerve stimulation at rest demonstrates significant decrement by the fourth stimulus. A second train, performed 10 sec after sustained voluntary contraction, demonstrates improvement, with reduced decrement ("repair" of decrement, due to postexercise potentiation, as acetylcholine release transiently increases). A third train, 30 sec after exercise, demonstrates worsening, with decrement exceeding baseline levels (due to postexercise exhaustion as acetylcholine vesicles are depleted). During the next few minutes, interval recordings demonstrate a gradual return to baseline decrement as the system returns to its resting state [reprinted with permission from Sanders, D. B. (1993). Clinical neurophysiology of disorders of the neuromuscular junction. *J. Clin. Neurophysiol.* 12, 169].

amplitude and train decrement occurs during the next 3 or 4 min, often declining below baseline levels (postactivation exhaustion) as junctional and reserve ACh levels decline.

A second, more sophisticated test of NMJ function is single-fiber electromyography (SFEMG). This technique, developed by Eric Stalberg, involves placement of a specially engineered needle, designed to record the discharges of single muscle fibers, between two or more muscle fibers of the same motor unit that are then voluntarily activated by the patient. A certain variability in the interval between the firing of these fibers, resulting from variation in the time required for neuromuscular transmission across the NMJ, can be recorded in the healthy patient and is called jitter. In the myasthenic patient, jitter is considerably increased and may be associated with some blocking of neuromuscular transmission, in which complete failure of NMJ transmission results in failure of contraction in one of the muscle fibers intermittently. Analysis of jitter by various mathematical and computerized methods enables quantitation of this phenomenon in any given patient and comparison of findings to normative values. A less widely utilized method involves electrical axonal stimulation of the motor nerve and recording of jitter from a single NMJ. The sensitivity and specificity of RNS and SFEMG differ considerably. RNS in a hand or shoulder muscle has a sensitivity of approximately 75% in generalized MG and less than 50% in ocular disease, whereas SFEMG has a sensitivity of 95% or higher in generalized and 90% or higher in ocular MG when appropriate muscles are tested. Because of its high sensitivity, SFEMG has its greatest diagnostic utility in cases of mild generalized, ocular, or seronegative MG. Because jitter may be increased in a variety of neuromuscular diseases, the specificity of this technique is limited and other conditions must be appropriately excluded prior to SFEMG studies.

Other Diagnostic Tests

Edrophonium (Tensilon), an AChE inhibitor, administered intravenously to a suspected MG patient may transiently improve certain symptoms, providing supportive evidence for the diagnosis. For an appropriate examination, a markedly affected, easily testable and/or observable muscle should be selected (frequently the deltoid or an upper extremity extensor). Two 1-ml tuberculin syringes should be prepared: one as a placebo injection (1 ml normal saline) and one as an injection of 10 mg of edrophonium in 1 ml of solution. The placebo is usually administered first, with observation for improvement for a few minutes. The edrophonium is administered next with an initial dose of 2 mg, with observation and/or strength testing for 1 min. If no improvement is noted, the remaining 8 mg is given and the process is repeated. If no effect is noted following the second dose, the test is negative. Any symptomatic improvement in responsive patients is short lived, lasting no longer than 30 min. Ideally, the patient should not take any AChE inhibitor for at least 24 hr prior to the test. Several cholinergic side effects may appear following intravenous edrophonium, including asystole, bradycardia, syncope nausea, and excessive lacrimation and salivation, and the examiner must be aware of these risks, which in certain patients are relative contraindications for this test. Reported sensitivities and specificities for this test are 90–95% and 80–95%, respectively, in generalized and 80–95% and 80–90% in ocular MG, but these data depend greatly on a carefully performed and judiciously interpreted examination and are subject to significant error in the hands of a careless examiner.

THERAPY

Acetylcholinesterase Inhibitors

Nonimmunological therapy has traditionally emphasized AChE inhibitors, beginning with Mary Walker's use of physostigmine in 1934. These agents have their greatest utility in pure ocular disease, early mild generalized disease, or as an adjunct in relatively stable but symptomatic disease following an appropriate course of immunosuppressive therapy. AChE inhibitors are purely symptomatic therapy and do not effect lasting changes in the primary disease process. Pyridostigmine is most commonly utilized in the United States. Most patients initially respond to doses of 30–60 mg administered every 3–6 hr. Pyridostigmine typically takes effect within 20–30 min and peaks at approximately 2 hr in most patients. Doses in excess of 120 mg every 3 hr may produce paradoxical increases in weakness, resulting in cholinergic crisis. A slow-release form of this drug is sometimes used before bedtime to decrease weakness on awakening. It may be particularly useful in reducing early morning dysphagia in patients with weakness of the pharyngeal muscles, making it easier for them to take their first morning dose of standard oral pyridostigmine. Intravenous acetylcholinesterase inhibitors, such as neostigmine, are also available for use in the hospital when the patient is no longer able to swallow the oral preparation. These agents were primary therapy for decades, prior to the application of the much more successful immunosuppressive measures discussed later in this entry. However, management of significant MG exacerbations with acetylcholinesterase inhibitors alone can be precarious, and aggressive primary immunotherapy is usually needed to restore and/or preserve respiratory function.

Thymectomy

In 1911, a thymectomy was performed as a proported treatment for hyperthyroidism in a patient with concurrent MG. Unexpectedly, temporary postoperative improvement was noted in the patient's myasthenic symptoms as well as her thyroid dysfunction. In 1939, Blalock performed a thymectomy for removal of a thymic tumor in a 20-year-old woman with a protracted history of severe generalized MG and reported significant postoperative improvement in her myasthenia that lasted for several years. Similar results were seen in 20 additional MG patients without a preoperative diagnosis of tumor, only 2 of whom had subclinical masses on tissue examination postoperatively. These findings were published in 1944, after which thymectomy gradually gained acceptance as standard therapy for MG. Patients with a thymoma must undergo thymectomy, and all patients diagnosed with MG should have imaging of the chest (computed tomography with contrast or magnetic resonance imaging) to assess for neoplasm. All patients with thymic tumors, except those with masses spread widely throughout the mediastinum, should undergo complete resection. Ideally, the myasthenia should be controlled with appropriate immunotherapy prior to the elective scheduling of this surgery. Although preoperative imaging studies are critical, anti-striational antibody assays are also performed in a high percentage of these patients. If the histopathology suggests malignancy, postoperative radio- and chemotherapy are required and may significantly reduce tumor burden in some patients. In MG patients without a thymic mass, the indications for removal are less clear-cut, but there is general agreement that thymectomy should be used as adjunctive therapy in MG patients from early adulthood to 60 years of age. Since the thymus plays an important role in the development of the pediatric immune system, thymectomy is usually not recommended in childhood, although the limited available data suggest it may improve remission rates in the pediatric population. Patients older than 60 are generally poorer candidates for any kind of surgery, and because the thymus dramatically shrinks with age, its contribution to immune function is probably naturally reduced, making thymectomy theoretically less appealing in this group. Smaller numbers of older patients have undergone thymectomy, but some reports suggest therapeutic effects similar to those observed in younger patients. Surgery in patients with pure ocular disease and no tumor is usually not recommended.

When properly performed by experienced thoracic surgeons in conjunction with neurologists experienced in the perioperative management of MG, this surgery has a mortality rate comparable to that of general anesthesia alone. Furthermore, with careful anesthetic and critical care as well as preoperative MG stabilization, postoperative intubation and ventilation average only 1.4 days. Immediate, but transient, improvement in strength lasting several days may be noted postoperatively, with a decreased requirement for acetylcholinesterase inhibitor medication. Lasting improvement following thymectomy is usually delayed for 6–12 months and may not appear for several years in some patients. The precise contributions of thymectomy to long-term improvement and remission of the disease are difficult to quantify since virtually all patients in the modern era are also treated with immunosuppressive medication. However, up to 60–70% of patients who develop MG before age 40 and who do not have thymoma ultimately improve, with permanent remissions rates of 25–40%. The rationale for improvement following thymectomy remains a matter of debate. Antibody levels decrease slowly following thymectomy, and there is an abundance of immunologically active tissue elsewhere in the body capable of antibody production. Therefore, a decreased reservoir of antibody-producing tissue alone seems an unlikely explanation for the observed effects. More likely explanations include diminished levels of immunoactive thymic hormones and the removal of an important site for B and T lymphocyte autosensitization to the AChR.

Corticosteroids

Anterior pituitary extract was administered to two patients with MG in 1935, but steroids were not tested again until the late 1940s and early 1950s, when reports of worsening symptoms quickly following ACTH therapy discouraged further investigation for the next several years. By the mid-1960s, however, several reports suggested that this acute deterioration was transient, documenting sustained improvement and increased remission of MG if ACTH was continued beyond the initial phase. This exacerbation occurs in 50% of patients, with a more severe exacerbation in 10% of patients within 1–17 days (average onset on Day 5) after starting glucocorticoids, but it lasts an average of only 4 days. Oral prednisone therapy became extremely popular after confirmation of the immunological cause of the disease in the early 1970s and has remained a mainstay of treatment. Although glucocorticoids have a wide array of effects, those effects with more specific relevance to MG include suppression of lymphocyte reactivity to AChR and decreased AChR antibody levels in treated patients. Nonimmunological steroid effects may also play a role, as increased AChR synthesis has been documented in human muscle cell culture after the addition of dexamethasone. Unfortunately, the apparently dramatic therapeutic effect of steroids and their sudden, widespread adoption precluded any large placebo-controlled studies of their benefits and risks. However, most investigators agree that steroids are the most effective therapy for the majority patients with this condition.

There is general consensus that such therapy should begin with an intensive course, but differing induction regimens are recommended by different authorities. After high-dose steroid therapy is initiated, sustained improvement appears in most patients within 2 weeks, reaching 90% within 3 weeks. With sustained therapeutic effect, the dose is gradually tapered over many months, and maximal improvement appears within 6–9 months in most patients. During taper, many patients will reveal a threshold below which their symptoms will recur; thus, the later phases of taper should be approached cautiously. Symptomatic recurrence may lag weeks to months after a dosage change and may require a return to higher doses of steroids before control is again achieved. Some patients may require indefinite maintenance therapy with low doses, but if steroids cannot be tapered below an acceptable level, alternative immunosuppressive therapy must be considered. Steroid therapy is usually very effective, inducing remission in up to 80% of patients. However, because taper of steroids to lower dosage levels may take 1 or 2 years, the risks of long-term side effects must be considered in each patient prior to initiation of therapy.

Azathioprine

Azathioprine (AZA) is usually employed when steroid therapy fails or must be maintained at an excessive dose for effective control of symptoms. Some patients may require a combination of steroids and AZA. The major disadvantage of this medication is the long interval between initiation of therapy and its clinical effects: A response may not occur for 3–12 months. A maximal response may not occur for 1 or 2 years. This drug acts predominantly on proliferating B and T lymphocytes and reduces their numbers. Symptomatic exacerbations related to therapy, such as those seen with steroids, do not occur, but white blood cell counts and liver function tests must be monitored. These adverse effects are usually reversible with discontinuation of the drug if discovered early. An idiosyncratic flu-like reaction may also occur with fever, myalgia, generalized malaise, and vomiting and should prompt immediate discontinuation of therapy. After recovery off medication, patients may be able to tolerate another trial of therapy without recurrence of these symptoms. Mild nausea may also occur and may respond to division of the dose into thirds and administration with meals. Potential teratogenesis and mutagenesis make pregnancy relatively contraindicated, and an increased long-term risk of malignancy has been reported. Xanthine oxidase helps to metabolize this drug, so concurrent administration of allopurinol may push levels dangerously high, increasing the previously mentioned risks. Despite these concerns, most patients tolerate AZA therapy well and response rates of up to 44–71% may be achieved using this drug, although many patients require some level of simultaneous steroid therapy to achieve such results.

Cyclosporin A

Cyclosporin A decreases the production of interleukin-2 and interferon-γ by helper T cells. It has significant potential toxicity and therefore should be reserved for those cases in which steroids and/or AZA are not effective. It is one of the few agents subjected to, and proven effective in, prospective, double-blind, placebo-controlled trials. Onset of symptomatic improvement typically begins within 2 weeks, with average maximal improvement at 3 or 4 months. However, therapy must be continued indefinitely because 90% of responders will relapse with discontinuation. Side effects include significant acute nephrotoxicity (usually reversible with cessation of therapy), new-onset hypertension, mild hepatotoxicity, a slightly increased risk of malignancy, hirsutism, and gingival hyperplasia. Renal function must be monitored and increases in creatinine of 50% over baseline values or an absolute value greater than 1.5–2 mg/dl are indications for dosage reduction. Trough serum levels should also be used to guide dose adjustment. Both cyclosporin and AZA are considerably more expensive than steroids, which may be a limiting factor for some patients.

Cyclophosphamide

Due to its considerable side effects, this drug is typically reserved for the most severe and refractory cases unresponsive to other therapies. Cytoxan is an alkylating agent that interferes with DNA replication, having cytotoxic effects on lymphocytes, monocytes, and macrophages. Careful monitoring of blood counts and urine for bleeding is essential. The limited available studies of this drug report response rates of 45–75% within 1 month and a 30% remission rate, persisting only as long as the drug is continued. A number of serious side effects have been reported, including myelosuppression; hemorrhagic cystitis; malignancies of the skin, bladder, and blood; teratogenesis; alopecia; and nausea and vomiting. In addition to laboratory monitoring, patients should be well hydrated (to minimize the urinary concentration of cyclophosphamide's active and toxic metabolites in the bladder) and, if receiving intravenous therapy, might require a protective agent for the bladder. Nausea and vomiting, particularly prominent with intravenous infusions, may require antiemetic therapy.

Plasma Exchange

Plasma exchange (PEx) effectively removes a variety of macromolecules, including AChR antibodies, from the patient's blood. Evolving hematological technology enabled the clinical use of this technique during the 1960s, and its first use in MG was reported in 1976. PEx is indicated when a transient burst of relatively rapid symptomatic improvement is needed, such as in patients with a sudden progressive symptomatic deterioration. It may also have a role in reducing perioperative morbidity as pretreatment for thymectomy and to buffer steroid-induced exacerbations. Occasional patients who fail other interventions may require frequent PEx as a primary form of maintenance therapy. Improvement is usually noted within days to 4 weeks after initiation of therapy, lasts approximately 1–12 weeks, and correlates with a decrease in AChR antibody levels. In experienced centers, PEx is usually quite well tolerated, but complications can occur due to problems with vascular access (including infection, local thrombosis, and vascular perforation), removal of circulating clotting factors, dehydration (hypotension and bradycardia), and transient electrolyte disturbances. The technique is personnel and equipment intensive and expensive, but it is highly effective and the best studied temporizing measure for rapid immunotherapy in the myasthenic patient.

Intravenous Immune Globulin

High-dose intravenous immune globulin (IVIG) may work through a variety of theoretical mechanisms, including the introduction of anti-idiotypic antibodies and reduced AChR antibody production via negative feedback. Its indications are essentially those for Pex, and it has a similar time course of action in most patients. Improvement has been reported in approximately 70% of patients within 5 days of initiation of therapy, peaking at 8 or 9 days and lasting 8–12 weeks. Side effects are usually mild and can include headache, chills, fever, and nausea. Pretreatment with acetaminophen and diphenhydramine may prevent these minor reactions. Anaphylaxis may also occur, but it is much rarer than thought prior to the widespread use of this agent. In recent years, acute renal failure has also been recognized as a significant complication, occurring within days of infusion. All patients should be screened for renal insufficiency prior to infusion, but normal renal function before and during infusion, even in combination with a slow infusion rate, does not always eliminate the risk of this complication. IVIG is also a very expensive drug but may compare favorably with PEx when total costs for each therapy are tabulated.

Other Therapies

Several other immunotherapies have been reported to improve MG, including antithymocyte globulin infusions, antilymphocyte globulin infusions, splenectomy, and splenic and total body irradiation. Newer immunological agents, such as mycophenolate or CellCept (which inhibits B and T cell proliferation), may have important roles in the therapy of MG and are currently being studied. Future therapy may also include selective immunotherapy with "smart" agents designed to inhibit or eliminate the specific autoimmune responses in MG. Because T cells are integrally involved in MG autoimmunity, targeting of the CD4 surface molecule with specially engineered autoantibodies can induce immunosuppression. Oral tolerance therapy involving the oral administration of AChR antigens may also have a future role. As clinical and basic science investigation of neuromuscular junction function and disease expands further, new agents with fewer adverse effects and greater therapeutic power should follow. In future decades, with the advent of increasingly sophisticated immunomodulatory technologies, a universally effective cure for acquired myasthenia and other selective autoimmune disorders may be achievable.

—*Clifton L. Gooch*

See also–Acetylcholine; Lambert–Eaton Myasthenic Syndrome; Myasthenic Syndromes, Congenital; Oculopharyngeal Muscular Dystrophy

Further Reading

De Baets, M. H., and Oosterhuis, H. J. G. H. (Eds.) (1993). *Myasthenia Gravis.* CRC Press, Boca Raton, FL.

Drachman, D. B. (1994). Myasthenia gravis. *N. Engl. J. Med.* **330,** 1797–1810.

Gooch, C. L. (1997). Myasthenia gravis and Lambert–Eaton myasthenic syndrome. In *Neuroimmunology for the Clinician* (Y. Harati and L. A. Rolak, Eds.), pp. 263–299. Butterworth-Heinemann, Boston.

Gooch, C. L. (1998). The immunologic therapy of myasthenia gravis. In *Immunotherapy in Neuroimmunologic Diseases* (J. Zhang, D. Hafler, H. Reinhard, and M. Ariel, Eds.), pp. 75–95. Dunitz, London.

Lisak, R. P. (Ed.) (1994). *Handbook of Myasthenia Gravis and Myasthenic Syndromes.* Dekker, New York.

Oosterhuis, H. J. G. H. (1991). Myasthenia gravis. In *Clinical Neurology* (M. Seash and J. Oxbury, Eds.). Churchill Livingstone, Edinburgh, UK.

Sanders, D. B. (Ed.) (1994). Myasthenia gravis and myasthenic syndromes. *Neurol. Clin. North Am.* **12,** 305–329.

Sanders, D. B., Andrews, P. I., Barohn, R. J., *et al.* (1999). *Myasthenia Gravis*, Vol. 5. American Academy of Neurology, Minneapolis, MN.

Schonbeck, S., Chrestel, S., and Hohlfeld, R. (1990). Myasthenia gravis: Prototype of the antireceptor autoimmune diseases. *Int. Rev. Neurobiol.* **32,** 175–200.

Myasthenic Syndromes, Congenital

Encyclopedia of the Neurological Sciences
Copyright 2003, Elsevier Science (USA). All rights reserved.

ALL congenital myasthenic syndromes (CMS) stem from presynaptic, synaptic, or postsynaptic defects that compromise the safety margin of neuromuscular transmission by one or more specific mechanisms. The slow-channel CMS are transmitted by dominant inheritance; all other CMS reported to date are transmitted by recessive inheritance. In 155 CMS kinships investigated at the Mayo Clinic, the defect was presynaptic in 8%, synaptic in 16%, and postsynaptic in 75% (Table 1).

DIAGNOSIS

CMS are not uncommon but are commonly undiagnosed or diagnosed incorrectly. A generic diagnosis of a CMS can be made on clinical grounds from a history of fatigable weakness involving ocular, bulbar, and limb muscles since infancy or early childhood, a history of similarly affected relatives, a decremental electromyogram (EMG) response, and negative tests for acetylcholine receptor (AChR) antibodies. In some CMS, however, the onset is delayed, the EMG abnormalities are not present in all muscles or are present only intermittently, and the weakness has a restricted distribution. Sometimes, the following clinical or EMG clues can point to the

Table 1 CLASSIFICATION OF CMS AND INDEX PATIENTS INVESTIGATED

	No. of patients
Presynaptic defects CMS	
Choline acetyltransferase deficiency	6
Paucity of synaptic vesicles	1
Lambert–Eaton syndrome-like	1
Other presynaptic defects	4
Synaptic defect	
Endplate AChE deficiency	24
Postsynaptic defects	
Primary kinetic abnormality with/without AChR deficiency	37
Primary AChR deficiency with/without minor kinetic abnormality	67
Rapsyn deficiency	14
Myasthenic syndrome with plectin deficiency	1
No identified defect	4
Total	*155*

correct diagnosis:

1. A repetitive compound muscle action potential (CMAP) in response to a single stimulus occurs in endplate (EP) acetylcholinesterase (AChE) deficiency and in the slow-channel CMS.
2. Refractoriness to cholinesterase inhibitors and delayed pupillary light reflexes suggest EP AChE deficiency.
3. Selectively severe weakness of cervical and wrist and finger extensor muscles is found in the slow-channel CMS and in older patients with EP AChE deficiency.
4. The tendon reflexes are generally preserved but are hypoactive or absent in a CMS resembling the Lambert–Eaton syndrome, in some cases of EP AChE deficiency, and in severe cases of the slow-channel syndrome.
5. A history of recurrent apneic episodes provoked by stress suggests a defect in the resynthesis or vesicular packaging of ACh. Here, a decremental EMG is not found in rested muscle but appears after a few minutes of stimulation at 10 Hz.

DIFFERENTIAL DIAGNOSIS

In the neonatal period, infancy, and childhood, the differential diagnosis includes spinal muscular atrophy, morphologically distinct congenital myopathies, congenital muscular dystrophies, infantile myotonic dystrophy, mitochondrial myopathy, brainstem anomaly, Möbius syndrome, congenital fibrosis of the extraocular muscles, infantile botulism, and seropositive and seronegative autoimmune myasthenia gravis (MG). In older patients, the differential diagnosis includes motor neuron disease, limb–girdle or facioscapulohumeral dystrophy, mitochondrial myopathy, chronic fatigue syndrome, and seropositive and seronegative MG. Radial nerve palsy, peripheral neuropathy, and syringomyelia have been incorrectly diagnosed in some cases of the slow-channel CMS.

INVESTIGATION OF THE CMS

A deeper understanding of disease mechanisms and a precise classification of the CMS require estimation of the number of AChRs per EP, light and electron microscopic analysis of EP morphology, and electrophysiological assessment of EP function *in vitro*. Conventional microelectrode studies of EP potentials and currents readily reveal presynaptic defects in quantal release and altered postsynaptic responses to the released quanta. Patch-clamp recordings of currents flowing through single AChR channels provide precise information on the conductance and kinetic properties of the channels. If the foregoing studies indicate a defect in the candidate gene or protein, then molecular genetic analysis becomes feasible. If a mutation is discovered in the candidate gene, then expression studies with the genetically engineered mutant molecule can be performed to confirm pathogenicity and to analyze the properties of the mutant molecule. To date, the candidate gene approach has resulted in the discovery of more than 70 mutations in different subunits of the AChR and 24 mutations in the collagenic tail subunit of the EP species of AchE.

PRESYNAPTIC CMS

Paucity of Synaptic Vesicles and Reduced Quantal Release

The clinical features of this syndrome closely mimic those of autoimmune MG, but EP studies reveal no AChR deficiency. A presynaptic defect is indicated by a severe decrease (to ∼20% of normal) in the number of ACh quanta (m) released by nerve impulse. The decrease in m is due to a decrease in the number of readily releasable quanta (n), and this decrease is associated with a comparable decrease (to ∼20% of normal) in the numerical density of synaptic vesicles. The putative defect resides in the synthesis or axonal transport of vesicle precursors from the anterior horn cell to the nerve terminal or, less likely, is related to impaired recycling of the synaptic vesicles.

Abnormality in the Resynthesis or Vesicular Packaging of ACh (CMS with Episodic Apnea)

The clinical features of this disorder were recognized more than three decades ago under the rubric of familial infantile myasthenia, but it was not differentiated from MG until the autoimmune origin of MG was established and electrophysiological and morphological differences were demonstrated between MG and the congenital syndrome. Because all CMS can be familial and because most CMS present in infancy, the term familial infantile myasthenia has become a source of confusion.

The syndrome is distinguished by sudden and unexpected episodes of apnea occurring either spontaneously or precipitated by infections, fever, or excitement. In some patients the disease presents at birth with hypotonia and severe bulbar and respiratory weakness requiring ventilatory support that gradually improves but is followed by apneic attacks associated with bulbar paralysis in later life. Other patients are normal at birth and first experience the typical attacks during infancy or early childhood. Variable ptosis and fatigable weakness may persist between the attacks. The ocular movements are usually spared.

Endplate studies reveal no AChR deficiency and the postsynaptic region of the EP shows no abnormality. The miniature EP potential (MEPP) is normal in rested muscle but decreases abnormally during 10-Hz stimulation for 5 min, indicating a defect in choline reuptake by the nerve terminal, in choline acetyltransferase, or in vesicular filling with ACh. A recent study traced this syndrome in five patients to disease-associated mutations in choline acetyltransferase that reduce the expression or impair the catalytic efficiency of the enzyme. Mutations in proteins that affect choline reuptake by the nerve terminal or vesicular filling with ACh could also cause a similar syndrome but have not been identified to date.

CMS Resembling the Lambert–Eaton Syndrome

Here, EMG studies show a low-amplitude CMAP, a decremental response on low-frequency (2 Hz) stimulation, and >100% facilitation of the CMAP on high-frequency (20–40 Hz) stimulation. The defect could reside in a subunit of the presynaptic voltage-gated P/Q-type calcium channel or in a component of the synaptic vesicle release complex.

SYNAPTIC AChE DEFICIENCY

A highly disabling CMS is caused by the absence of AChE from the synaptic space. Neuromuscular transmission is compromised by smallness of the nerve terminals and their encasement by Schwann cells, which reduces the number of releasable quanta; an EP myopathy from cholinergic overactivity; and desensitization and depolarization block of AChR at physiological rates of stimulation. In the absence of AChE, the synaptic potentials are prolonged and evoke repetitive CMAPs.

The EP species of AChE is a heteromeric asymmetric enzyme composed of one to three homotetramers of globular catalytic subunits ($AChE_T$) attached to a triple-stranded collagenic tail (ColQ) that anchors the asymmetric enzyme in the synaptic basal lamina. $AChE_T$ and ColQ are encoded by $ACHE_T$ and $COLQ$, respectively. ColQ has an N-terminal proline-rich region attachment domain (PRAD), a collagenic central domain, and a C-terminal region enriched in charged residues and cystines. Each ColQ strand binds an $AChE_T$ tetramer to its PRAD. Two groups of charged residues in the collagen domain plus other residues in the C-terminal region ensure that the asymmetric enzyme is inserted into the synaptic basal lamina. The C-terminal region is also required for initiating the triple-helical assembly of the ColQ that proceeds from a C- to an N-terminal direction in a zipper-like manner. EP AChE deficiency stems from mutations in $COLQ$. The mutations either prevent attachment of $AChE_T$ to ColQ or prevent insertion of the mutated ColQ into the basal lamina.

POSTSYNAPTIC CMS

Most postsynaptic CMS identified to date stem from mutations in genes encoding subunits of AChR. Muscle AChR is a transmembrane macromolecule composed of five homologous subunits: two α, one β and one δ, and one ε in adult AChR or one γ in fetal AChR. The genes coding for α, δ, and γ are at different loci on chromosome 2q, and those coding for β and ε are at different loci on chromosome 17p. The subunits are highly homologous, have similar secondary structures, fold similarly, and are organized like barrel staves around a central cation channel. Each subunit has an N-terminal extracellular domain that comprises ~50% of the primary sequence, four putative transmembrane domains (M1–M4), and a small C-terminal extracellular domain. M2, which lines the ion channel, forms an α helix interrupted by a short stretch of β sheet. The transmembrane domains are connected by an extracellular M2/M3 linker and by intracellular M1/M2 and M3/M4 linkers. The M3/M4 linker forms a long cytoplasmic loop that likely serves as an attachment site for cytoskeletal elements and bears phosphorylatable residues that may be important for desensitization. Each AChR has two ACh-binding pockets, one at the α/ε (or α/γ) and one at the α/δ interface. Residues contributing to the binding pocket appear on three peptide loops on α and on four peptide loops on ε and γ. Recent atomic studies suggest that each ACh-binding pocket opens to the extracellular space.

Pathogenic mutations of AChR alter the kinetic properties of the receptor, reduce its expression, or both. The kinetic abnormalities of AChR either increase or decrease the synaptic response to ACh. An increased synaptic response is associated with the slow-channel syndromes, and a decreased synaptic response occurs in the fast-channel syndromes. These two syndromes are physiological opposites (Table 2).

SLOW-CHANNEL SYNDROMES

The clinical phenotypes vary. Some slow-channel CMS present in early life and cause severe disability by the end of the first decade; others present later in life and progress slowly, resulting in little disability

Table 2   KINETIC ABNORMALITIES OF ACHR

	Slow-channel syndromes	Fast-channel syndromes
Endplate currents	Slow decay	Fast decay
Channel opening events	Prolonged	Brief
Channel open state	Stabilized	Destabilized
Channel closed state	Destabilized	Stabilized
Mechanisms	Increased affinity for ACh	Decreased affinity for ACh
	Increased channel opening rate	Decreased channel opening rate
	Decreased channel closing rate	Increased channel closing rate

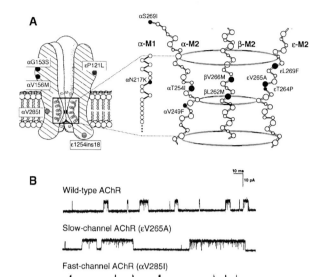

Figure 1

(A) Schematic diagram of slow-channel (solid circles) and fast-channel (shaded circles) mutations. (Left) A section through the acetylcholine receptor with two slow-channel mutations, αG153S and αV156 M, in the extracellular domain near the ACh binding site of the α subunit and three fast-channel mutations: εP121L near the ACh binding site of the ε subunit, αV156 M in the M3 domain of the α subunit, and ε1254ins18 in the long cytoplasmic loop of the ε subunit. (Right) Slow-channel mutations detected between the M2 and M3 domains of the α subunit, in the M2 domains of the α, β, and ε subunits, and in the M1 domain of the α subunit. (B) Examples of single channel currents from wild-type, slow-channel, and fast-channel AChRs expressed in HEK cells.

even in the sixth or seventh decade. Most patients show selectively severe involvement of cervical and wrist and finger extensor muscles.

The phenotypic consequences stem from prolonged opening episodes of the AChR channel in the presence of ACh (Fig. 1B). This causes cationic overloading of the junctional sarcoplasm and an EP myopathy. The EP myopathy comprises degeneration of the junctional folds with loss of AChR, widening of the synaptic space, and subsynaptic alterations consisting of degeneration of organelles, apoptosis of nuclei, and vacuolar change. The prolonged channel activation episodes prolong the EP potential so that a single nerve stimulus elicits one or more repetitive CMAPs. During physiological activity, the prolonged EP potentials undergo staircase summation, producing a depolarization block.

Solid circles in Fig. 1A show the position of 11 slow-channel mutations. The different mutations occur in different AChR subunits and in different functional domains of the subunits. Each is dominant, causing a pathological gain-of-function. Patch-clamp studies at the EP, mutation analysis, and expression studies in human embryonic kidney (HEK) cells indicate that mutations near extracellular ACh binding sites and in the N-terminal part of M1 act mainly by enhancing affinity for ACh, which promotes channel reopenings, and mutations in M2, which lines the channel pore, promote the open state by affecting gating and may or may not enhance affinity.

Quinidine is a long-lived open-channel blocker of AChR, and clinically attainable levels of the drug normalize the prolonged opening episodes of mutant slow channels expressed in HEK cells. Slow-channel patients treated with quinidine at doses producing serum levels of 0.7–2.5 µg/ml (2.1–7.7 µM/liter) are improved by clinical and EMG criteria, but a full clinical response is attained only after several months of therapy.

FAST-CHANNEL SYNDROMES

Three types of fast-channel mutations have been identified to date (Fig. 1A, shaded circles). Each fast-channel mutation operates through a different mechanism, but in each instance the channel opening events are abnormally brief (Fig. 1B) and channel opening probability in the presence of ACh is reduced. In each affected patient, the consequences of the fast-channel mutation in one allele are unmasked by a null/low expressor mutation in the second allele.

The clinical phenotypes vary from mild to severe and resemble autoimmune MG. Treatment consists of pyridostigmine, which increases the number of AChRs activated by a quantum of ACh, and 3,4-diaminopyridine, which increases the number of quanta released by nerve impulse.

Low-Affinity Fast-Channel Syndrome

This syndrome is caused by a mutation in the extracellular domain of the ε subunit εP121L. The miniature EP potentials and currents are very small, but EP AChR content and ultrastructure are normal. Expression studies indicate that the mutant AChR has a markedly decreased rate of channel opening and a reduced affinity for ACh in the open channel and desensitized states.

Fast-Channel Syndrome Due to a Gating Abnormality

This syndrome is determined by a mutation in the M3 domain of the α subunit αV285l. The primary abnormality resides in the channel gating mechanism and not in affinity for ACh. Studies of genetically engineered αV285l–AChR in HEK cells reveal that the brief channel openings are due to a slow channel opening rate constant (β), a fast channel closing rate constant (α), and a reduced probability of channel opening.

Fast-Channel Syndrome Due to Mode-Switching Kinetics

This disorder is determined by an inframe duplication in the long cytoplasmic loop of ε, ε1254ins18, which also reduces AChR expression. When expressed in HEK cells, ε1254ins18–AChR causes mode switching in the kinetics of receptor activation in which the normal high efficiency of gating is accompanied by two new modes that gait inefficiently, opening more slowly and closing more rapidly than normal. The phenotypic consequences are EP AChR deficiency and compensatory expression of fetal AChR harboring the γ instead of the ε subunit (γ-AChR), which restores electrical activity at the EP and rescues the phenotype.

PRIMARY AChR DEFICIENCY WITH OR WITHOUT MINOR KINETIC ABNORMALITY

CMS with severe EP AChR deficiency result from different types of homozygous or, more frequently, heterozygous recessive mutations in AChR subunit genes. The clinical phenotypes range from mild to very severe. Most patients respond partially to anticholinesterase drugs, and some derive additional benefit from 3,4-diaminopyridine.

Ephedrine may be of nonspecific benefit in some cases of this and other types of CMS, but its efficacy has not been rigorously documented by clinical, EMG, or experimental studies. Mutations causing severe EP AChR deficiency are concentrated in the ε subunit. There are two possible reasons for this. First, expression of the fetal-type γ subunit, although at a low level, may compensate for the absence of the ε subunit, whereas patients harboring null mutations in subunits other than ε might not survive for lack of a substituting subunit. Second, the gene encoding the ε subunit, and especially the exons coding for the long cytoplasmic loop, has a high GC content that likely predisposes to DNA rearrangements.

Morphological studies show an increased number of EP regions distributed over an increased span of the muscle fiber. The integrity of the junctional folds is preserved but AChR expression on the folds is patchy and faint. Some EP regions are simplified and small, and there is a nonspecific decrease in the number of openings between the primary and secondary synaptic clefts. The amplitude of miniature EP potentials and currents is reduced but quantal release by nerve impulse is often higher than normal. With null or low-expressor mutations in the ε subunit, single channel recordings and immunocytochemical studies reveal γ-AChR at the EP that likely rescues the phenotype.

Different types of recessive mutations causing severe EP AChR deficiency have been identified: (i) frameshifting, splice-site, or nonsense mutations causing premature termination of the translational chain; (ii) point mutations in the promoter region of a subunit gene; (iii) missense mutation in a signal peptide region; (iv) mutations involving residues essential for assembly of the pentameric receptor; and (v) missense mutations severely reducing AChR expression and also having minor kinetic effects.

CMS CAUSED BY RAPSYN DEFICIENCY

In a subset of patients with EP AChR deficiency but no mutations in AChR subunit genes, the disease-associated mutations reside in RAPSN that encodes rapsyn. Rapsyn is a 43 kDa postsynaptic protein that plays an essential role in clustering AChR at the EP. Seven tetratricopeptide repeats (TPRs) of rapsyn subserve self-association, a coiled-coil domain binds to AChR, and a RING-H2 domain associates with β-dystroglycan and links rapsyn to the subsynaptic cytoskeleton. The rapsyn mutations identified to date are recessive and impair clustering of AChR with rapsyn.

CMS ASSSOCIATED PLECTIN DEFICIENCY

Plectin is a highly conserved and ubiquitously expressed intermediate filament-linking protein concentrated at sites of mechanical stress, such as the hemidesmosomes in skin, the sarcolemma, the postsynaptic membrane, Z disks in skeletal muscle, and intercalated disks in cardiac muscle. Pathogenic mutations in plectin are associated with a simplex variety of epidermolysis bullosa (EBS), a progressive myopathy, and a myasthenic disorder.

Detailed investigation of a patient with EBS, a progressive myopathy, abnormal fatigability involving the ocular, facial, and limb muscles, a decremental EMG response, and no anti-AChR antibodies revealed that plectin expression was absent in muscle

and severely decreased in skin. Morphological studies of muscle demonstrated necrotic and regenerating fibers and a wide spectrum of ultrastructural abnormalities. Many EPs had an abnormal configuration with chains of small regions over the fiber surface, and a few EPs displayed focal degeneration of the junctional folds. The EP AChR content was normal. *In vitro* electrophysiological studies showed normal quantal release by nerve impulse, small miniature EP potentials, and fetal as well as adult AChR channels at the EP. Pyridostigmine failed to improve the patient's symptoms, but 3,4-diaminopyridine (1 mg/kg/day in divided doses) improved her strength and endurance.

—*Andrew G. Engel*

See also–Acetylcholine; Channelopathies, Genetics; Lambert–Eaton Myasthenic Syndrome; Myasthenia Gravis

Further Reading

Engel, A. G., Lambert, E. H., Mulder, D. M., et al. (1982). A newly recognized congenital myasthenic syndrome attributed to a prolonged open time of the acetylcholine-induced ion channel. *Ann. Neurol.* **11**, 553–569.

Engel, A. G., Ohno, K., Bouzat, C., et al. (1996). End-plate acetylcholine receptor deficiency due to nonsense mutations in the ε subunit. *Ann. Neurol.* **40**, 810–817.

Engel, A. G., Lambert, E. H., and Gomez, M. R. (1997). A new myasthenic syndrome with end-plate acetylcholinesterase deficiency, small nerve terminals, and reduced acetylcholine release. *Ann. Neurol.* **1**, 315–330.

Engel, A. G., Ohno, K., and Sine, S. M. (1999). Congenital myasthenic syndromes. In *Myasthenia Gravis and Myasthenic Disorders* (A. G. Engel, Ed.), pp. 251–297. Oxford Univ. Press, New York.

Harper, C. M., and Engel, A. G. (1998). Quinidine sulfate therapy for the slow-channel congenital myasthenic syndrome. *Ann. Neurol.* **43**, 480–484.

Milone, M., Wang, H.-L., Ohno, K., et al. (1977). Slow-channel syndrome caused by enhanced activation, desensitization, and agonist binding affinity due to mutation in the M2 domain of the acetylcholine receptor alpha subunit. *J. Neurosci.* **17**, 5651–5665.

Milone, M., Wang, H.-L., Ohno, K., et al. (1998). Mode switching kinetics produced by a naturally occurring mutation in the cytoplasmic loop of the human acetylcholine receptor ε subunit. *Neuron* **20**, 575–588.

Mora, M., Lambert, E. H., and Engel, A. G. (1987). Synaptic vesicle abnormality in familial infantile myasthenia. *Neurology* **37**, 206–214.

Ohno, K., Engel, A. G., Brengman, J. M., et al. (2000). The spectrum of mutations causing endplate acetylcholinesterase deficiency. *Ann. Neurol.* **47**, 162–170.

Ohno, K., Engel, A. G., Shen, X.-M., et al. (2002). Rapsyn mutations in humans cause endplate acetylcholine receptor deficiency and myasthenic syndrome. *Am. J. Hum. Genet.* **70**, 875–885.

Ohno, K., Quiram, P., Milone, M., *et al.* (1997). Congenital myasthenic syndromes due to heteroallelic nonsense/missense mutations in the acetylcholine receptor ε subunit gene: Identification and functional characterization of six new mutations. *Hum. Mol. Genet.* **6**, 753–766.

Ohno, K., Tsujino, A., Brengman, J. M., *et al.* (2001). Choline acetyltransferase mutations cause myasthenic syndrome associated with episodic apnea in humans. *Proc. Natl. Acad. Sci. USA* **98**, 2017–2022.

Ohno, K., Wang, H.-L., Milone, M., *et al.* (1996). Congenital myasthenic syndrome caused by decreased agonist binding affinity due to a mutation in the acetylcholine receptor ε subunit. *Neuron* **17**, 157–170.

Wang, H.-L., Milone, M., Ohno, K., *et al.* (1998). Acetylcholine receptor M3 domain: Stereochemical and volume contributions to channel gating. *Nat. Neurosci.* **2**, 226–233.

Myelin

Encyclopedia of the Neurological Sciences
Copyright 2003, Elsevier Science (USA). All rights reserved.

MYELIN is a multilayered membrane spiral made by Schwann cells and oligodendrocytes that surrounds large-diameter axons in both the peripheral and central nervous systems.

The rapid electrical impulse conduction by myelinated nerve fibers is made possible by the presence of the myelin sheath, which is a lipid-rich membrane wrapped around the axons of nerve cells. Myelin was first described by Virchow more than 150 years ago. Myelin is analogous to the plastic insulation surrounding electrical wires, preventing the leakage of neuronal signals to the surroundings. In fact, the characteristic appearance of white matter within the nervous system is due to the presence of myelin.

The correct formation and maintenance of myelin are key prerequisites for the normal functioning of the vertebrate nervous system. The myelin sheath has the same functions in both the central and peripheral nervous systems. The myelin sheath acts as an electrical insulator around the axon, guides the localization of axonal ion channels, and provides mechanical support. Highly regulated targeting of ion channels to specific regions is the key requirement for the very fast saltatory, "jumping" transmission of nervous impulses.

From a structural standpoint, the myelin sheath can be considered analogous to a sleeping bag rolled dozens of times very tightly around a long, round object (Fig. 1). It is clear that the outside of the myelin membrane faces the outside of the membrane in the next turn, and that the cytoplasmic sides of the membranes also interact intimately. The ultrastructure of a cross section of myelin at the electron microscopic level is characterized by alternating concentric rings, the so-called major dense lines and intraperiod lines. These lines reflect the tight packing of the membranes in myelin. The major dense lines correspond to the nearly fused cytoplasmic leaflets of opposing membranes, whereas the intraperiod line represents the extracellular side of the tightly packed membrane spiral.

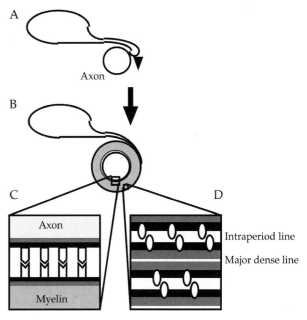

Figure 1

A schematic representation of the formation and basic structure of myelin. (A) A myelinating glial cell (Schwann cell or oligodendrocyte) contacts a large axon and starts to wrap its plasma membrane around the axon in a spiral manner. (B) In mature myelin, a thick, tightly packed membrane multilayer surrounds the axon. (C) For the normal functioning of the vertebrate nervous system, the contact between the innermost membrane of myelin and the axonal surface must be tight. This adhesion involves specific cell surface molecules from both myelin and the axon. (D) Consecutive layers of the spiral must also be in extremely intimate contact with each other. At the major dense line, the cytoplasmic faces of the myelin membrane, which also harbor myelin basic protein, are practically fused. At the intraperiod line, contacts between cell adhesion molecules, such as the homotypic interactions observed for peripheral nervous system myelin protein zero, on the extracellular face are crucial for maintaining the myelin structure. The cytoplasmic face of the myelin membrane is gray, and the extracellular face is black.

Classically, glial cells have been viewed as providers of physical and trophic support for neurons. Myelin is formed when the plasma membrane of a myelinating glial cell—an oligodendrocyte in the central and a Schwann cell in the peripheral nervous system—differentiates and wraps around the axon. It is of interest that embryologically, these two types of myelinating cells are of different origin. The two cell types also have some fundamental differences in the way in which they make myelin. Whereas a Schwann cell only makes a single segment of myelin around a single axon, an oligodendrocyte is capable of making several myelin sheaths around several central nervous system axons. For this reason, the oligodendrocyte nucleus is not found in intimate association with the outside of the myelin sheath, as is the case for the Schwann cell nucleus. Instead, it is some distance away, with the myelin sheath being formed at the end of a thin oligodendrocyte process.

Despite the differences between oligodendrocytes and Schwann cells, the structure of the myelin sheath is similar in both the central and peripheral nervous systems. It can be roughly divided into two separate domains, compact and noncompact myelin, which differ from each other structurally, functionally, and biochemically. The multilamellar structure of compact myelin is characterized by the small volume that is occupied by nonmembranous components; in other words, when the myelin sheath has compacted, nearly all water has been squeezed out. The only areas where substantial amounts of solvent remain are those adjacent to the domains of so-called noncompact myelin. In these areas, the extracellular spacing in myelin is larger than in compact myelin, and thin channels of cytoplasm are present.

Each myelin segment that is wrapped around an axon has both compact and noncompact regions; the tightly packed compact myelin constitutes most of the myelin sheath, and within the compact region and at its edges exist the more loosely packed regions of noncompact myelin. Although there is a continuous membrane surface from the cell body of the myelin-forming cell to the periaxonal membrane of myelin, in direct contact with the surface of the axon, there are many specializations within the membrane that exhibit variability in terms of structure, function, and biochemical composition. In addition to the compact myelin, these specialized domains include the surface membranes of the cell body and processes, surface and periaxonal membranes of the myelin sheath, paranodal loops, and Schmidt–Lantermann incisures. Schmidt–Lantermann incisures are a unique feature of peripheral nervous system myelin that are narrow, less tightly packed regions within compact myelin and containing some cytoplasm. The incisures allow the rapid transport of small molecules through the myelin sheath because they contain gap junctions that allow the diffusion of small molecules through the membrane.

The myelin sheath is interrupted at regular intervals along its length by indentations. These interruptions are the nodes of Ranvier, and each myelin segment located between two nodes is called an internode. The myelin sheath has an important role in guiding the localization of ion channels within the axonal plasma membrane at the nodes of Ranvier. During saltatory nerve impulse conduction, the impulse jumps from one node of Ranvier to the next; this process increases the speed of transmission of neural signals by several orders of magnitude.

Biochemically, the myelin sheath is similar to other biological membranes, but it also has some peculiarities in its biochemical composition that are likely to be of grave importance for its function in ensuring the normal conduction of nerve impulses. When inherited mutations or environmental factors affect one or more of the components that are the building blocks of myelin, the function of the nervous system is impaired, leading to neurological disease.

—*Petri Kursula*

See also–Axons; Demyelinating Disease, Pathology of; Glia; Ion Channels, Overview; Leukodystrophy; Myelin Disorders; Myelin Proteins; Nerve Injury; Nerve Roots; Oligodendrocytes; White Matter

Further Reading

Garbay, B., Heape, A. M., Sargueil, F., *et al.* (2000). Myelin synthesis in the peripheral nervous system. *Prog. Neurobiol.* **61**, 267–304.

Kandel, E. R. (1991). Nerve cells and behavior: Glial cells. In *Principles of Neural Science* (E. R. Kandel, J. H. Schwartz, and T. M. Jessell, Eds.), pp. 22–24. Elsevier, New York.

Salzer, J. L. (2002). Nodes of Ranvier come of age. *Trends Neurosci.* **25**, 2–5.

Webster, H. D. (1971). The geometry of peripheral myelin sheaths during their formation and growth in rat sciatic nerves. *J. Cell Biol.* **48**, 348–367.

Myelin Disorders

Encyclopedia of the Neurological Sciences
Copyright 2003, Elsevier Science (USA). All rights reserved.

MYELIN DISORDERS are diseases affecting either the central or the peripheral nervous system that are characterized by damage to the myelin sheath. The damage can be either due to the formation of abnormal myelin (dysmyelination) or due to the breakdown of a healthy myelin sheath (demyelination).

The myelin sheath, which is a multilayered organelle that is wrapped and compacted around large-diameter axons, has the same functions in both the central and peripheral nervous systems. When disrupted by disease or lesions, and when the myelin sheath fails to form normally because of defects in the genetic program, serious neurological symptoms result, including motor and sensory deficits. These disorders, which are usually related to the formation, structure, function, and maintenance of the myelin sheath in either the central or the peripheral nervous system, can be divided into two main groups. The first group is composed of conditions of acquired, usually immunological, origin, in which the immune system falsely directs its attack toward the patient's own tissues. An immune attack toward myelin results in the degeneration of the myelin sheath. The second group comprises those disorders caused by inherited mutations in the genes encoding the proteins of the myelin sheath or some other factors contributing to the formation of normal myelin. These disorders usually involve dysmyelination, in which abnormal myelin is formed, or hypomyelination, in which too little myelin is formed.

Both types of disease, autoimmune and inherited disorders, are encountered in both the central and peripheral nervous systems. In the central nervous system, the most common autoimmune disease is multiple sclerosis, in which faulty signals within the immune system lead to the destruction of myelin. Many of the myelin proteins, most notably myelin basic protein, are considered to be autoantigens in multiple sclerosis, but the actual factors triggering multiple sclerosis are to a large extent enigmatic. Leukodystrophies are a group of inherited diseases involving central nervous system demyelination. In the peripheral nervous system, inherited mutations in the gene encoding the predominant peripheral nerve myelin protein, protein zero, lead to Dejerine–Sottas syndrome or Charcot–Marie–Tooth disease type 1B, whereas mutations in the peripheral myelin protein

22 gene give rise to Charcot–Marie–Tooth disease type 1A. On the other hand, mutations in the gene encoding the gap junction protein connexin 32, present in noncompact regions of myelin, cause an X-linked form of Charcot–Marie–Tooth disease. In addition, changes in the gene dosage of peripheral myelin protein 22 are linked to human neuropathies. Autoantibodies directed toward the myelin-associated glycoprotein, which is present in the so-called noncompact myelin in both branches of the nervous system, are often involved in peripheral autoimmune neuropathies. Guillain–Barré syndrome is another form of peripheral neuropathy caused by an immune attack toward the myelin sheath of peripheral nerves.

Some general features are shared by the variety of myelin disorders. The condition always specifically involves either primary or secondary damage to the myelin sheath while the axons remain, at least during the initial stages of disease, relatively unaffected. Thus, the transmission of nervous impulses is slowed and dysregulated, commonly leading to sensory and motor deficits. Another common feature of myelin disorders is that there currently exists no efficient cure for them; at best, it is only possible to slow down the progression of a severely handicapping disease.

Practically all the individual myelin-specific proteins present in both the central and peripheral nervous system myelin sheaths have been linked to human disease conditions via different mechanisms. However, more detailed information on the structure and function of these proteins in the normal context of myelination is required before scientists can fully comprehend the events that take place when abnormal myelin is formed or myelin is damaged. In addition to a constantly increasing amount of information on human myelin diseases and their specific individual characteristics, an increasing number of both spontaneously occurring (e.g., the trembler mouse) and human-generated (e.g., knockout mice for most myelin protein genes) mutants for myelin-related genes in animal models have been reported in the past 10 years. These models are providing reasonable representatives of several human neurological diseases.

The treatment of myelin disorders can be envisaged to occur via two alternative mechanisms. First, approaches are being developed that would prevent demyelination. However, to be able to do so, a very intricate understanding of the events that lead to demyelination in the first place is required. Second, damaged myelin sheaths could be replaced or repaired by remyelination, and a considerable amount of research has been directed toward this possibility. However, more knowledge of the factors controlling the proliferation, migration, and differentiation of myelinating cells is required. Also complicating the situation, especially in central nervous system disorders, is the inhibitory effect of myelin and its molecular components on the ability of the axons to regenerate.

—*Petri Kursula*

See also–Leukodystrophy; Myelin; Myelin Proteins

Further Reading

Juurlink, R. H. J., Devon, R. M., Doucette, J. R., *et al.* (Eds.) (1997). *Cell Biology and Pathology of Myelin. Evolving Biological Concepts and Therapeutic Approaches.* Plenum, New York.
Steck, A. J., Schaeren-Wiemers, N., and Hartung, H. P. (1998). Demyelinating inflammatory neuropathies, including Guillain–Barré syndrome. *Curr. Opin. Neurol.* **11**, 311–318.
Steinman, L. (1996). Multiple sclerosis: A coordinated immunological attack against myelin in the central nervous system. *Cell* **85**, 299–302.
Young, P., and Suter, U. (2001). Disease mechanisms and potential therapeutic strategies in Charcot–Marie–Tooth disease. *Brain Res. Rev.* **36**, 213–221.

Myelin Proteins

Encyclopedia of the Neurological Sciences
Copyright 2003, Elsevier Science (USA). All rights reserved.

THE MYELIN SHEATH in both the central and peripheral nervous systems contains a number of proteins that are usually only expressed in myelin and have classically been studied as specific components of myelin. These proteins are called myelin proteins.

Like all other biological membranes, myelin is formed of two main components: lipids and proteins. Even though the lipid bilayer serves as a permeability barrier into which the various membrane proteins are inserted, particular lipids may modulate the biological activity of membrane-associated enzymes and other membrane proteins. Compared to other membranes, myelin has an unusually high content of lipids (70–80%). Furthermore, the lipid composition of myelin is unique, containing various gangliosides, galactocerebrosides, and up to 30% cholesterol. Some less classic functions that have been suggested for myelin lipids include signal transduction, cell adhesion, and protein transport. Although the actual amount of different proteins in myelin is lower than in the average membrane of the body, these proteins are of crucial importance to the structure and function of the myelin sheath and thus to the normal functioning of the entire nervous system.

Myelin carries a unique subset of proteins, several of which are only encountered in myelin. Furthermore, differences exist in the protein composition between central nervous system (CNS) and peripheral nervous system (PNS) myelin as well as between the domains of compact and noncompact myelin. Table 1 lists the proteins that have mostly been studied with respect to their role in the myelin sheath. Since glycoproteins are important constituents of plasma membranes in general, it is not surprising that many of the proteins in both compact and noncompact myelin are glycosylated. This addition of sugar residues is crucial for the effective adhesion between myelin and the surface of the axon as well as between consecutive turns of the glial cell plasma membrane within the myelin sheath. The intimate interactions that the myelin proteins have with the lipids of the myelin membrane, in the presence of very little solvent, are reflected in the properties of the proteins, which

Table 1   WIDELY CHARACTERIZED MYELIN PROTEINS

Protein	Abbreviation	PNS/CNS	Compartment
Protein zero	P0	PNS	Compact
Myelin basic protein	MBP	Both	Compact
Proteolipid protein	PLP	CNS	Compact
Peripheral myelin protein 22	PMP-22	PNS	Compact
Myelin-associated glycoprotein	MAG	Both	Noncompact
Myelin/oligodendrocyte glycoprotein	MOG	CNS	Noncompact
Myelin protein 2	P2	Both	Compact

often make studying these molecules in laboratory conditions unusually difficult.

At the biochemical level, important differences exist between CNS and PNS myelin. Most notably, in the CNS, certain CNS-specific proteins are present in the sheath, whereas some PNS-specific components are lacking. For example, in CNS compact myelin, the quantitatively major protein is the proteolipid protein, whereas myelin protein zero and peripheral myelin protein 22, the two most abundant PNS compact myelin proteins, are not present (Fig. 1). In noncompacted regions of the sheath, the CNS myelin-specific proteins include the putative cell adhesion molecules myelin/oligodendrocyte glycoprotein and the oligodendrocyte/myelin glycoprotein. Both CNS and PNS noncompact myelin contain substantial amounts of the myelin-associated glycoprotein, and in both branches of the nervous system the cytoplasmic face of the membranes comprising compact myelin is covered with the myelin basic protein, which is the major autoantigen in multiple sclerosis.

A diverse array of functions have been attributed to the proteins present in myelin, ranging from cell adhesion and the regulation of the cellular cytoskeleton to signal transduction and gene regulation. Myelin protein zero is an integral constituent of PNS compact myelin, and it is essential for the normal spiraling, compaction, and maintenance of PNS compact myelin. Homotypic interactions between protein zero molecules in opposing myelin membranes are most likely extremely important for the structure of compact myelin. The apparent counterpart of protein zero in the CNS myelin sheath, the

proteolipid protein, also seems to have similar functions. Myelin basic protein, which is abundant in both CNS and PNS compact myelin, is especially important for the formation of normal CNS myelin. Peripheral myelin protein 22 is involved in the initial phases of myelination, maintenance of myelin, and neuronglia interactions, whereas a role for myelin protein 2 in lipid transport has been suggested. One of the most widely studied myelin proteins, present throughout the nervous system, is the myelin-associated glycoprotein. Its two isoforms have been shown to play crucial roles in the formation and maintenance of the myelin sheath, and at the molecular level it has functions in cell adhesion, signal transduction, and the regulation of the cytoskeleton. In light of the various functions of the myelin proteins, it is not surprising that when abnormal myelin proteins are present, or when the body accidentally directs its immune system toward these proteins, severe damage to the myelin sheath and malfunctions of the nervous system occur.

—*Petri Kursula*

See also–Dystrophin and Dystrophin-Associated Proteins; G Proteins; Myelin; Myelin Disorders

Further Reading
Juurlink, R. H. J., Devon, R. M., Doucette, J. R., *et al.* (Eds.) (1997). *Cell Biology and Pathology of Myelin. Evolving Biological Concepts and Therapeutic Approaches.* Plenum, New York.
Kursula, P. (2001). The current status of structural studies on proteins of the myelin sheath. *Int. J. Mol. Med.* 8, 475–479.
Morell, P., and Quarles, R. H. (1999). Myelin formation, structure and biochemistry. In *Basic Neurochemistry: Molecular, Cellular, and Medical Aspects* (G. J. Siegel, B. W. Agranoff, R. W. Albers, S. K. Fisher, and M. D. Uhler, Eds.), 6th ed., pp. 117–144. Lippincott–Raven, New York.
Snipes, G. J., and Suter, U. (1995). Molecular anatomy and genetics of myelin proteins in the peripheral nervous system. *J. Anat.* 186, 483–494.

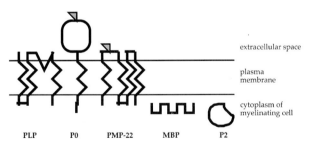

Figure 1
Schematic representation of proteins encountered in the region of compact myelin. Proteolipid protein (PLP) is specific to the central nervous system myelin, whereas myelin protein zero (P0) and peripheral myelin protein 22 (PMP-22) only reside in peripheral nervous system myelin. Myelin basic protein (MBP) and myelin protein 2 (P2), the two proteins that are not inserted into the membrane, are found throughout the nervous system. The gray triangles in P0 and PMP-22 represent carbohydrate residues attached to the extracellular domain.

Myelomeningocele

Encyclopedia of the Neurological Sciences
Copyright 2003, Elsevier Science (USA). All rights reserved.

SPINA BIFIDA literally means "spine in two parts." The term has come to encompass a wide variety of disorders, all of which share a defect in posterior midline neural, bony, or cutaneous structures. In its mildest form, spina bifida consists of the absence of the spinous process and laminar bone in one or several vertebrae, a condition that in no way affects the structural stability of the spine. In such cases, the skin over the defect is often intact; the only sign of an abnormality may be a small hair tuft over the region. More severe forms of the disorder may involve the ingrowth of subcutaneous fatty tissue through the spinal defect into the neural canal. In its most severe form, myelomeningocele, the neural elements of the spinal cord fail to close and are exposed through defects in the bone and skin to the outside world.

Meningomyeloceles are a relatively common disorder affecting approximately 3 in 10,000 births. Their incidence may be higher in northern climates than elsewhere, although no good underlying explanation exists. Equal numbers of male and female infants are affected.

Meningomyeloceles occur as a result of events during the first trimester of embryonic development. Between the third and fourth weeks of gestation, the embryo develops tissue that will become the nervous system (brain and spinal cord). Two ridges of specialized cells begin to fold over on themselves to form the neural tube (Fig. 1). The tube at the rostral (head) end of the embryo subsequently undergoes a series of convolutions that ultimately result in the formation of the brain. More caudally (tail side of the embryo), the tube elongates and its center fills in to become the spinal cord and spinal nerve roots.

Severe birth defects result if the rostral end of the tube fails to fuse. Such infants have serious brain malformations. If, however, the caudal end of the neural tube fails to fuse, a myelomeningocele develops. Proper formation of the neural tube is also essential for the surrounding tissues to develop normally. If the neural tube fails to fuse, the overlying cells destined to become bone, muscle, fat, and skin also fail to develop properly, and the spinal cord is exposed to the outside world. A myelomeningocele can occur along the entire spinal axis, but lumbar and sacral myelomeningoceles are the most common.

Many factors are associated with failure of the developing neural tube to fuse. Some theories implicate abnormal cellular adhesions, and others implicate improper cellular migrations. A deficiency of folic acid has been linked strongly to neural tube defects. Consequently, women of childbearing age are recommended to intake a daily minimum of 400 mg of folic acid.

Meningomyeloceles are usually diagnosed at birth. Typically, infants have a small reddish-brown, cystic

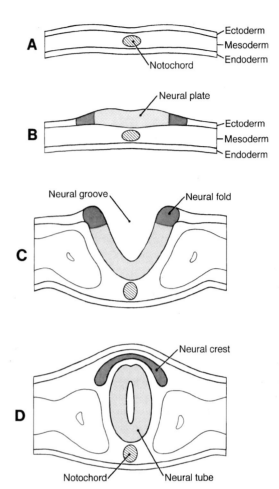

Figure 1
Development of the neural tube. In the embryo, two ridges of specialized cells elevate and fold over onto one another to create the neural tube. All elements of the developing nervous system derive from this structure [reproduced with permission from the Barrow Neurological Institute].

structure on the midline of the back (Fig. 2). The severity of the neural tube defect determines the size of the myelomeningocele. Spinal cord and nerve function inferior to the level of the meningomyelocele is usually impaired. Children with a meningomyelocele in the lumbar region usually only have control over the upper muscles of their leg (e.g., thigh and hip muscles). When meningomyeloceles are located more rostrally (e.g., neck region), the arms can also be affected. The sacral nerve roots providing control over the bladder and bowel sphincters are the caudalmost nerve roots to exit the spinal cord. They are often affected by a meningomyelocele at any level, and bowel and bladder dysfunction is commonly associated with this disorder.

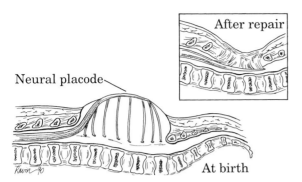

Figure 2

Thoracolumbar myelomeningocele. A newborn infant with a myelomeningocele in the midback. The cystic outpouching is composed of the neural placode (the unfused neural tube) and its attachments to surrounding tissues [reproduced with permission from the Barrow Neurological Institute].

Hydrocephalus is another common manifestation. Approximately 95% of patients with a meningomyelocele develop hydrocephalus and may require placement of a shunt. Symptoms of hydrocephalus include nausea, vomiting, eye movement problems, and headache. In more severe cases, basic bodily functions such as swallowing, breathing, and heart rate can be affected. Various brain malformations, including the so-called Chiari II malformation, are also associated with myelomeningoceles. In this disorder, the lower brainstem is abnormally kinked and descends into the cervical canal (Fig. 3). The lower brainstem, which controls basic bodily functions, can be compromised. Other malformations in the cerebral cortex can cause learning disabilities. The reason why myelomeningoceles are so closely associated with hydrocephalus and brain malformations is unclear but appears to be related to the important influences that the neural tube exerts on associated developing structures.

A meningomyelocele may be noted on an infant's first physical examination, but the evaluation for hydrocephalus and brain malformations requires further diagnostic tests. In infants whose cranial fontanelles or soft spots have not yet closed, ultrasonography can be used to determine whether large collections of cerebrospinal fluid (CSF), the hallmark of hydrocephalus, exist within the brain. Magnetic resonance imaging studies can demonstrate the same abnormalities as well as other potential brain malformations, such as the absence of the corpus callosum, the major fiber tract that connects the two cerebral hemispheres. Occasionally, fetal ultrasonography demonstrates fetal hydrocephalus or a large meningomyelocele *in utero*.

Treatment of a meningomyelocele is a multistaged process that begins with closure of the open neural tube (Fig. 4). The edges of the open neural tube are carefully excised from the surrounding skin and subcutaneous fatty tissue and reapproximated into the form of a tube. The dura, the membrane covering the spine, is then closed around the spinal cord in a water-tight fashion to prevent leakage of CSF. Subsequently, the soft tissues and skin are closed over the dural closure. Many patients with a meningomyelocele who develop hydrocephalus will likely require a shunting procedure. Depending on the severity of the meningomyelocele and the associated degree of dysfunction, patients may need additional procedures. For example, if the muscles of the lower extremity are not innervated, they can become contracted. A surgical release procedure may be needed to provide a greater range of motion. Orthopedic procedures may also be necessary to reconstruct joints that become malformed as a result of chronic muscular contraction.

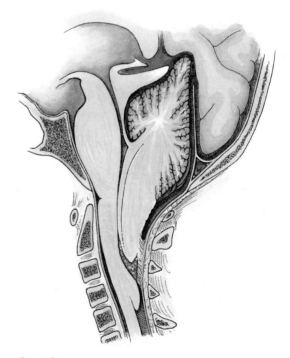

Figure 3

Chiari II malformation. Part of the brainstem, which controls basic bodily functions, is forced into the cervical canal in patients with Chiari II malformation. The cerebellum is also displaced inferiorly, worsening the crowding in the cervical canal [reproduced with permission from the Barrow Neurological Institute].

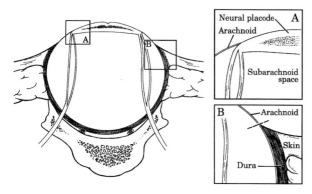

Figure 4
Myelomeningocele closure. Surgical closure of the
myelomeningocele defect involves sequential suture reconstruction
of the neural placode, the dura or spinal lining, and the overlying
muscular, fatty, and skin tissues [reproduced with permission from
Rekate, H. L. (1991). Neurosurgical management of the newborn
with spina bifida. In *Comprehensive Management of Spina Bifida*
(H. L. Rekate, Ed.). CRC Press, Boca Raton, FL].

Rehabilitative services for patients with spina
bifida are just as important as the surgical procedures. Learning disabilities may require specialized
education. Individuals with impaired bladder and
bowel function may be able to learn techniques to
achieve "social continence." Education is also needed
in the use of wheelchairs and prosthetic devices.
Overall, the treatment of a patient with a meningomyelocele requires a multidisciplinary approach.

The prognosis for individuals with a meningomyelocele depends on the severity of the disorder.
Individuals with hydrocephalus and a Chiari II brain
malformation are particularly susceptible to having
dysfunctional brainstem centers. Because these centers control basic bodily functions, patients with such
complications can die. Patients with less severe forms
of meningomyelocele, namely those in the lower
lumbar and sacral regions, may be able to live
independently to a certain degree. In fact, functional
independence often correlates with the level of the
meningomyelocele along the spinal axis.

However, patients with a meningomyelocele must
be evaluated regularly. Those with shunts for
hydrocephalus are at risk of shunt failure. Surgical
scarring at the site of meningomyelocele closure can
"tether" the spinal cord to surrounding structures. As
the child grows to adulthood, the growing spinal
cord may not tolerate this degree of traction. If
neurological deterioration is associated with such
spinal cord tethering, additional surgical maneuvers
are needed to release the spinal cord.

Advances in imaging and surgical techniques make
the *in utero* diagnosis and possible repair of
meningomyeloceles a reality. Evidence suggests that
an *in utero* surgical repair of a meningomyelocele
may lessen the severity of associated hydrocephalus
and brain malformations. Although the treatment
and prognosis for meningomyelocele have improved
during the past 50 years, further advances are
needed.

—*G. Michael Lemole, Ruth Lemole, and
Harold L. Rekate*

See also—Chiari Malformations; Hydrocephalus;
Nervous System, Neuroembryology of; Neural
Tube Defects; Sphincter Disturbances

Further Reading

McLone, D. G. (1996). Myelomeningocele. In *Neurological
Surgery* (J. R. Youmans, Ed.), 4th ed., pp. 843–860. Saunders,
Philadelphia.
Oakes, W. J. (1994). Chiari malformations and syringohydromye-
lia. In *Principles of Neurosurgery* (S. S. Rengachary and R. H.
Wilkins, Eds.), pp. 9.1–9.18. Wolfe, London.
Reigel, D. H., and Rotenstein, D. (1994). Spina bifida. In *Pediatric
Neurosurgery. Surgery of the Developing Nervous System* (W.
R. Cheek, A. E. Marlin, D. G. McLone, D. H. Reigel, and M. L.
Walker, Eds.), pp. 51–76. Saunders, Philadelphia.
Rekate, H. L. (1991). *Comprehensive Management of Spina
Bifida*. CRC Press, Boca Raton, FL.
Sutton, L. N. (1994). Spinal dysraphism. In *Principles of
Neurosurgery* (S. S. Rengachary and R. H. Wilkins, Eds.),
pp. 5.1–5.16. Wolfe, London.

Myelopathy
see Spinal Cord Diseases

Myoclonus

Encyclopedia of the Neurological Sciences
Copyright 2003, Elsevier Science (USA). All rights reserved.

MYOCLONUS is a sudden, brief, jerky, shock-like,
involuntary movement that involves extremities,
face, or trunk. It is one of the most common
involuntary movements. As with other movement
disorders, myoclonus may be classified several ways,
including phenomenologically, anatomic–physiologically, and etiologically. The etiological divisions are
physiological, essential (unknown cause), epileptic,

and symptomatic myoclonus (secondary to other underlying disorders) (Table 1). Physiological forms include benign hiccups and hypnic jerks, which are sudden movements experienced by many normal individuals upon falling asleep.

Most myoclonic jerks are caused by abrupt muscle contraction (positive myoclonus), but jerks are sometimes caused by sudden cessation of muscle contraction (negative myoclonus or asterixis). Several chemicals of the brain have been implicated in the pathophysiology of myoclonus, such as serotonin, γ-aminobutyric acid, and glycine. According to the pathophysiological mechanism underlying anatomical origin in the central nervous system, myoclonus is classified into three main categories: cortical (gray matter of the brain), subcortical (white matter of the brain), and spinal. Cortical myoclonus is most commonly encountered, is usually associated with seizures, and is commonly sensitive to stimuli such as sound or touch. Most electrophysiological studies suggest pathological hyperexcitability of the brain cortex. This is characterized on electroencephalography (EEG) studies (brain wave recording) by showing a spike preceding the myoclonus.

Subcortical myoclonus includes dystonic myoclonus, hereditary disorder well characterized by a dramatical response to alcohol, and startle syndrome, which is based on stimuli-sensitive excitability of the lower brainstem centers. Palatal myoclonus, characterized by a rhythmical vertical oscillation of the soft palate at frequencies of 100–150 per minute, is really a tremor. Various drugs have been reported to cause myoclonic jerks, including several anticonvulsants, alcohol chronically abused, methyl ethyl ketone, propofol, clozapine, bismuth subsalicylate, and serotomimetic agents that enhance serotonin activity.

Table 1 CLASSIFICATION OF CAUSES OF MYOCLONUS

Physiological myoclonus	Dementias
Sleep jerks	Creutzfeldt–Jakob disease
Anxiety induced	Alzheimer's disease
Exercise induced	Viral encephalopathies
Hiccough	Subacute sclerosing panencephalitis
Benign infantile myoclonus with feeding	Encephalitis lethargica
Essential myoclonus (no known cause)	Arbor virus encephalitis
Hereditary	Herpes simplex encephalitis
Sporadic	Postinfectious encephalitis
Epileptic myoclonus	Metabolic
Fragments of epilepsy	Hepatic failure
Isolated epileptic myoclonus	Renal failure
Photosensitivity myoclonus	Dialysis syndrome
Myoclonic absences in petit mal	Hyponatremia
Epilepsia partialis continua	Hypoglycemia
Childhood myoclonic epilepsies	Infantile myoclonic encephalopathy
Infantile spasms	Nonketotic heperglycemia
Myoclonic astatic epilepsy	Mitochondrial encephalomyopathy
Cryptogenic myoclonus epilepsy	Multiple carboxylase deficiency
Juvenile myoclonus epilepsy of Janz	Biotin deficiency
Benign familial myoclonic epilepsy	Toxic encephalopathies
Progressive myoclonus epilepsy (Unverricht–Lundborg)	Bismuth
Symptomatic myoclonus	Heavy metal poisons
Storage disease	Methyl bromide, DDT
Lafora body disease	Drugs
Lipidoses	Physical encephalopathies
Ceroid-lipofuscinosis	Posthypoxia
Sialidosis	Posttraumatic
Spinocerebellar degeneration	Heat stroke
Basal ganglia degenerations	Electric shock
Wilson's disease	Decompression injury
Torsion dystonia	Focal central nervous system damage
Halloverden–Spatz disease	Poststroke
Progressive supranuclear plasy	Postthalamotomy
Huntington's disease	Tumor
Parkinson's disease	Trauma

Most drug-induced myoclonus is dose dependent and seems to be of subcortical origin. In addition, metabolic disturbances, including sodium, calcium, and glucose disturbances secondary to liver and kidney disorders, can also produce myoclonus.

In spinal myoclonus of various forms, abnormal electrical activity spreads up and down the spinal cord through propriospinal pathways that transmit the vibratory and position sense. This disorder has been reported in association with various spinal cord diseases.

The jerks in essential myoclonus are brief (50–200 msec) and may be generalized or involve different body locations. Myoclonic jerks mainly involve the muscles of the neck or upper body and are exacerbated by action, particularly writing or out-stretching of the arms. The jerks abate during sleep and are ameliorated by alcohol. The beneficial effects of the latter are at times dramatic and nearly diagnostic; however, following the withdrawal of alcohol, there is frequently rebound worsening. Some individuals with myoclonus demonstrate associated dystonic movements, including spasmodic torticollis and blepharospasm. In spinal myoclonus, movements may be slower and spinal diseases such as multiple sclerosis may be associated with myoclonus.

The coexistence of myoclonus and epilepsy suggests a form of epileptic myoclonus that may present with either focal or generalized myoclonus. These patients have epilepsy as the dominant feature, and in most cases they have associated EEG abnormalities. Myoclonic syndromes associated with underlying diseases that cause a predominant encephalopathy (mental status changes), ataxia (wide-based gait), dementia, or other motor disorders as major features of the illness are termed symptomatic myoclonus. Symptomatic causes of myoclonus include a variety of disorders (Table 1).

The evaluation of myoclonus relies on a detailed history and neurological examination. Neuroimaging studies (head magnetic resonance imaging/computed tomography) are usually indicated for symptomatic myoclonus, such as stroke, degenerative disorders, and trauma. Electrophysiological tools, including electromyography (recording of muscle activity), EEG, and somatosensory evoked potentials (SEPs) (this test establishes the existence of sensory lesions in spinal nerve and brainstem), can be particularly valuable in distinguishing the levels of neural dysfunction in myoclonic syndromes. Blood, cerebrospinal fluid, and tissue biopsies should be utilized in appropriate clinical settings.

In most patients, myoclonus is treated purely on a symptomatic basis. The first step is to try to clarify the cause of the disorder because the treatment of the underlying cause may lead to an improvement in the myoclonus. When a toxic agent or metabolic disturbances are suspected as the cause of the myoclonus, withdrawal from the source of the poison and correction of the metabolic disturbances lead to gradual recovery. Although alcohol has been shown to alleviate the movements in a number of patients with essential myoclonus, the limitations of this pharmacological therapy are obvious. A variety of medications, several having effects on the serotoninergic system, may be used, including clonazepam, valproate, primidone, and piracetam. Postanoxic (no oxygen in the brain) myoclonus, seen after cardiac or pulmonary arrest, is particularly sensitive to 5-HTP treatment.

—*Esther Cubo and Christopher G. Goetz*

See also–Asterixis; Blepharospasm; Breath-Holding Spells; Clonus; Dyskinesias; Epilepsy, Comorbidity; Muscle Contraction, Overview

Further Reading
Papper, E. J., and Goetz, C. G. (1995). Treatment of myoclonus. In *Treatment of Movement Disorders* (R. Kurlan, Ed.), pp. 247–336. Lippincott, Philadelphia.
Shibasaki, H. (1998). Myoclonus and startle syndromes. In *Parkinson's Disease and Movement Disorders* (J. Jankovic and E. Tolosa, Eds.), pp. 453–466. Williams & Wilkins, Baltimore.

Myofascial Pain Syndrome

Editorial comment: This syndrome has received much attention in the general medical and lay press, but its definition and nature are controversial and many authors doubt its very existence. Accordingly, the editors have included two entries on this syndrome, reflecting this difference of opinion.

Myofascial Pain and Trigger Points

MUSCLE PAIN is a common medical problem in clinical practice. Pain in the muscle tissue can be caused by an acute trauma, such as direct contusion, penetration, laceration, traction, or overactivity. If the initial care is appropriate, acute muscle pain can be reduced shortly after the injury. Chronic muscle pain may or may not be caused by a direct muscle injury. Frequently, it is associated with an injury or a lesion other than that of the muscle, such as that of joints, bones, ligaments, or tendons. A common cause of chronic muscle pain is the myofascial pain syndrome (MPS), in which myofascial trigger points (MTrPs) are the cause of muscle pain. A MTrP has been defined as a highly localized painful or sensitive spot in a palpable taut band of skeletal muscle fibers. An active MTrP is one associated with spontaneous pain or pain in response to movement, whereas a latent MTrP is a sensitive spot with pain in response to compression only.

CLINICAL CHARACTERISTICS OF MYOFASCIAL TRIGGER POINTS

The clinical aspects of MTrPs, according to Travell and Simons, include the following:

1. Compression of an MTrP may elicit local pain or referred pain that is similar to a patient's usual clinical complaint (pain recognition) or may aggravate existing pain.
2. Snapping (rapid compression across the muscle fibers) may elicit a local twitch response (LTR), which is a brisk contraction of the muscle fibers in or around the taut band. Rapid insertion of a needle into the MTrP can often elicit an LTR.
3. There is a restricted range of stretch, and increased sensitivity to stretch, of muscle fibers in a taut band due to tightness of the involved muscle.
4. The muscle with an MTrP may be weak due to pain but without significant atrophy.
5. Patients with severe MTrPs may have associated autonomic phenomena, including vasoconstriction, pilomotor response, and hypersecretion.

The diagnostic criteria of an MTrP are considered to be spot tenderness (in a well-defined site), pain recognition (palpation reproduces the patient's usual pain), and a taut band (containing the MTrP). Referred pain and a local twitch response are confirmatory signs of the MTrP.

BASIC RESEARCH ON MYOFASCIAL TRIGGER POINTS

Animal Model for the Study of MTrPs

An animal model was developed by Hong and Torigoe. In rabbit skeletal muscle, taut bands similar to that in human muscle could be identified by finger palpation. When a certain sensitive site in the palpable taut band was squeezed or compressed, the rabbit would behave as if it suffered pain (e.g., screaming, kicking, or withdrawing), which was not observed when the other site was similarly irritated. When the sensitive site was stimulated mechanically with a blunt metal probe or by a needle, localized twitch responses were observed. This hyperirritable spot (MTrS) is similar to the human MTrP.

Autonomic Function and MTrPs

It has been suggested that MTrPs are a complication (or manifestation) of reflex sympathetic dystrophy (RSD) (also referred to as the complex regional pain syndrome). MTrP injection can effectively relieve muscle pain in some RSD patients. Clinically, autonomic phenomena similar to RSD may develop in extremely severe cases of MPS.

TREATMENT OF MYOFASCIAL TRIGGER POINTS

In many cases, it is difficult to find a specific cause, despite the patients' severe pain and discomfort. In such situations, pain control is the major focus of therapy.

Manual Therapy

Traditional therapy to inactivate the active MTrPs is the intermittent cold and stretch (spray and stretch) technique. The tight muscles (containing taut band and MTrP) can be stretched by intermittent cold application to the skin over that muscle. The taut band can be quickly relieved and the pain reduced after this procedure.

Deep-pressure soft tissue massage is another therapy for immediate pain relief of an MTrP. It is a localized stretch technique by manual compression on an MTrP, combined with gentle stretch of muscle fibers in an MTrP region by moving the finger following the direction of muscle fibers.

Electrotherapy

Electrical stimulation to the muscle with MTrP can provide pain relief and also relieve the tightness of the taut bands. However, therapeutic effectiveness may be only temporary. Pain relief can be obtained by stimulation of sensory nerves (TENS), but relief of muscle tightness is usually achieved by stimulating the muscle.

Thermotherapy

Application of local heat can cause direct or reflex vasodilatation to improve circulation and provide a certain degree of pain relief but may not be effective in relieving pain from MTrPs. In clinical practice, thermotherapy is a valuable adjunct to MTrP therapy in combination with other modalities such as manual therapy or electrotherapy.

Other Physical Medicine Modalities

Other physical medicine modalities, including laser therapy, exercise programs, yoga, and myofascial trigger point injection and dry needling (including acupuncture), have also been used.

—*Chang-Zern Hong*

Further Reading

Gerwin, R. D. (1992). The clinical assessment of myofascial pain. In *Handbook of Pain Assessment* (D. C. Turk and R. Melzack, Eds.), pp. 61–70. Guilford, New York.

Hong, C.-Z. (1994). Consideration and recommendation of myofascial trigger point injection. *J. Musculoskeletal Pain* 2, 29–59.

Hong, C.-Z. (1998). Algometry in evaluation of trigger points and referred pain. *J. Musculoskeletal Pain* 6, 47–59.

Hong, C.-Z. (1999). Current research on myofascial trigger points—Pathophysiological studies. *J. Musculoskeletal Pain* 7, 121–129.

Hong, C.-Z. (2000). Myofascial trigger points: Pathophysiology and correlation with acupuncture points. *Acupuncture Med.* 18, 41–47.

Hong, C.-Z., and Simons, D. G. (1998). Pathophysiologic and electrophysiologic mechanism of myofascial trigger points. *Arch. Phys. Med. Rehab.* 79, 863–872.

Mense, S. (1996). Biochemical pathogenesis of myofascial pain. *J. Musculoskeletal Pain* 4, 145–162.

Simons, D. G. (1999). Diagnostic criteria of myofascial pain due to trigger points. *J. Musculoskeletal Pain* 7, 111–120.

Simons, D. G., Travell, J. G., and Simons, L. S. (1999). *Travell & Simons's Myofascial Pain and Dysfunction: The Trigger Point Manual.* 2nd ed., Vol. 1. Williams & Wilkins, Baltimore.

Travell, J. G., and Simons, D. G. (1992). *Myofascial Pain and Dysfunction: The Trigger Point Manual*, Vol. 2. Williams & Wilkins, Baltimore.

Myofascial Pain Syndrome: A Critical Appraisal

MYOFASCIAL PAIN SYNDROME (MPS) is a controversial syndrome involving the basic unit of the muscular "trigger point" (TrP). The assessment of the TrP remains subjective, and the definition has changed in recent years as reliability studies have thrown the field into mild turmoil. The diagnosis is most popular among physiatry specialists and anesthesiologists working in pain clinics.

The revised definition of an "active" TrP now involves, at a minimum, spot tenderness in a palpable band and subject recognition of the pain. A palpable taut band is defined as a group of tense muscle fibers extending from a trigger point to the muscle attachments. Thus, some definitional circularity is involved.

The "bible" on this subject remains the two-volume work of the late internist Janet Travell and physiatrist David Simons, now in its second edition. The progenitor work and its idiosyncrasies have been reviewed elsewhere. The most significant changes in the second edition include the revamped definition of the TrP, based on reliability studies performed in the 1990s.

RELIABILITY

A major recent concern of both critics and advocates is the clinical concept of reliability; that is, can two clinicians examining the same patient be in agreement with regard to the physical findings? At least five studies have been performed with varying results and involving a gamut of parties, including physicians in various specialties, chiropractors, and physical therapists. Outcomes depend on whether "expert," trained "nonexpert," or untrained nonexpert examiners are used.

The original study is instructive and remains a landmark attempt. Until 1992, believers in MPS had never submitted their examination techniques to scientific scrutiny. However, to his credit, Dr. Simons and three other nationally recognized MPS experts agreed to test the reliability of their techniques. The four MPS experts (two physiatrists, an internist, and a neurologist) were paired with four experts on "fibromyalgia syndrome" (all rheumatologists), and examinations were performed on three groups of patients: seven patients with fibromyalgia, eight with MPS, and eight healthy controls. The following were some of the classic MPS concepts tested:

• *Taut bands*: A group of palpable, taut muscle fibers passing through an area in the muscle that is painful to palpation (i.e., a TrP).

• *Local twitch response* (LTR): A transient contraction of a group of muscle fibers in a palpable band in response to snapping palpation of the band. Much of the basic animal research has emphasized this difficult-to-find characteristic.

• *Pattern of referral/zone of reference/referred pain*: The specific region of the body at a distance from a TrP, where the phenomenon (sensory, motor, or autonomic) that it causes is observed. This has subsequently been deemphasized in the second edition of Simons' and Travell's work but traditionally has been an important factor in distinguishing the myofascial TrP from the basic building block of fibromyalgia—the tender point. The latter does not have to involve pain at a distance.

• *Active trigger point*: In 1992, this included tenderness, taut band, twitch response, and zone of reference that corresponds to the pain that is problematic to the subject.

• *Latent trigger point*: This includes tenderness, taut band, and twitch response. The latent TrP may demonstrate the zone of reference, but the zone does not correspond to pain that is problematic to a subject.

In contrast to the tender point examinations for fibromyalgia, the MPS examinations were believed to be very complicated by the noninitiated, and during the training sessions it became clear that the rheumatologists were "unable to become proficient enough in the MPS examinations." Therefore, the rheumatologists confined themselves to the part of this study dealing only with tender points and were not expected to do MPS examinations. This raised serious concerns about the reliability and variability of the MPS examination—presumably even in the hands of experienced practitioners whose specialty involves the musculoskeletal system. (This was addressed in subsequent studies by more training of both expert and nonexpert examiners.)

During the early phases of the study, not all MPS experts could examine the muscles required in the time allotted (15 min). Therefore, only restricted examinations were required—that is, eight muscles on the right side of the body. The samples of MPS patients were drawn from the practice of a well-known MPS expert, who did not participate in the study.

The results were disconcerting. Taut bands, twitch responses, and latent TrPs were found in normal controls. In fact, taut bands and twitch responses had virtually the same incidence in controls, fibromyalgia patients, and MPS patients. These false-positive results imply that even in the hands of selected and acknowledged MPS experts, the examination for these two entities has remarkably low specificity, to the point of being totally invalid. In fact, the latent

TrP does not appear to be a legitimate entity, given that normal controls were found to have these at a higher rate than either MPS or fibromyalgia patients.

In later years, after a failed attempt by a group of four expert physicians (two physiatrists and two neurologists), this group performed a second study. The physicians met for 3 hr immediately prior to the study for a training session. Definitions were studied, each clinical sign was reviewed on a live subject, and each physician examined the findings of the other three examiners. Discrepancies among the findings were evaluated and reassessed until all examiners could elicit the same signs and were in agreement about the physical findings. The amount of palpation pressure applied was varied and left up to the individual examiner. Not surprisingly, reliability scores for tenderness and taut bands were substantially improved, but LTR assessment remained less reliable.

In another experiment, four clinicians from a chiropractic college, with 54 years of experience and a total of 12 hr of training for purposes of this study alone, obtained good interexaminer agreement for a single latent trigger point in the trapezius muscle. Agreement was more than 80% for most measures, except for LTR, for which it was "very poor."

In contrast, other studies in which a "real-world" approach was taken (i.e., examiners did not have exhaustive training with each other, and experts were not used) have yielded mixed results. In a study including 12 physical therapists, a practice session of unspecified duration was used; nevertheless, the reliability results were poor, and the authors questioned the usefulness of even examining patients for TrPs. In a study performed by family practitioners, findings were found in a number of the normal controls, and palpable bands occurred without the presence of localized tenderness or pain complaints, raising doubts about the specificity of that fundamental sign.

A carefully designed study published in 2000 produced dismal results. It concluded that it is extremely difficult to obtain a gold standard for clinical palpation of myofascial TrPs. This study involved nonexpert physical medicine and chiropractic examiners compared to a single well-known expert, with prestudy practice/training levels intentionally varied. The untrained examiners received only a handout. Trained examiners had 6 hr of classroom lectures and 6 hr of hands-on training. Their findings were compared with those of the expert. The effect of training for finding taut bands was not impressive. With training, scores were still poor, compared to the nonexistent level of agreement obtained by the untrained practitioners. The findings of both groups were not different from chance for LTR assessment. Palpation of referred pain was marginally reliable among the trained examiners but not for those without training. Overall, both the trained and the untrained nonexperts failed to show acceptable reliability when compared with a single gold standard expert. There is some indication this expert may have used more force since he found that 70% of healthy subjects had taut bands.

In the nonmedical, commonsense world, this fact would raise eyebrows. The specter of nonspecificity would arise. That is, are some examiners, even known experts in the MPS community, finding false-positive results in their palpations? Not all examiners seem to possess the magic "finger of faith." However, the sincere belief of MPS advocates is that these findings are very common in the general population and have been going undiagnosed by the untrained, undereducated clinician community.

There simply does not appear to be any simple transferability of a tactile definition for TrP, and thus MPS. It remains an essentially subjective field, except in courtroom settings. In this venue, claims are commonly and confidently made that such findings are objective. Lacking a truly objective gold standard, it is understandable how difficult and central is the reliability issue. Both pathological and electrical studies have also had specificity issues—that is, "objective" findings that occur only in TrPs and not in normal tissue have not been consistently documented.

Simons and colleagues have suggested that minimum acceptable criteria for active TrPs include "the combination of spot tenderness in a palpable band and subject recognition of the pain." Appropriately, they have requested that authors of future studies on myofascial TrPs identify in the methods section specifically which TrP examinations are used as diagnostic criteria and provide detailed descriptions of how determinations are made. They note: "A consensus document that establishes official diagnostic criteria is an urgent need."

TREATMENT CONTROVERSIES

Proof of efficacy of treatment of MPS has been problematic and primarily anecdotal. A comprehensive review of 23 trials (with many others excluded due to flaws) was recently published. The authors reviewed studies in which various types of needle/injection treatments were used, and they compared (i) direct wet needling, in which an injection was aimed directly at the TrP; (ii) direct dry needling, in which a hypodermic needle or a solid needle was aimed directly at the TrP; (iii) indirect dry needling, in which the needle was placed superficially or deep into classic acupuncture points but no clear attempt was made to needle a TrP directly; and (iv) indirect wet needling, in which an injection was placed in the skin or subcutaneous tissue over a TrP.

The effect of treatment was invariably independent of the injected substance. The conclusion that wet needling is not therapeutically superior to dry needling was supported by all the high-quality trials in the review. These trials were performed during an 18-year period in many independent centers. Most important, there was no rigorous evidence that any needling therapy had an effect beyond placebo on TrP pain. MPS proponents argue that the sine qua non of spotting a TrP involves obtaining a local twitch response before needling the area, which most of these therapeutic trials did not address. However, the local twitch response is well documented to be the least reliable, most difficult to elicit property of a TrP.

To date, no controlled studies show that the various active and specific treatments for TrPs (ultrasound, injections, simple needling, vapocoolant spray, and stretching) are superior to simple massage that is not TrP oriented. The latter would be an ideal control treatment because of the known placebo effect of any hands-on therapy. Blinded assessment would be in order, with equal levels of enthusiasm shown by the various practitioners.

CONCLUSION

Currently, there is no official definition of a trigger point, and interexaminer agreement is poor even among MPS experts, unless they have spent hours with each other in a small group learning just how to agree with each other. Given the circularity involved, it is obvious that the concept of the myofascial TrP has little external validity (i.e., applicability to the majority of actual clinical situations in which informal, nonblind, nonexpert examiners believe they have found TrPs). It has been consistently shown that satisfactory agreement cannot be obtained among lesser trained persons. According to MPS advocates, this includes anyone who does not have both significant (undefined) experience and substantial hands-on training.

Logically, if there are only a handful of persons worldwide who are qualified to properly assess TrPs, then all referrals should be made exclusively to them and medical insurance payments to the thousands of practitioners who are unable to find the elusive TrP should be stopped. Moreover, there is the potential for "medicalizing" or "pathologizing" normal phenomena. Specificity is an issue when "abnormal" findings are seen consistently in normal controls without any complaints. To call them (latent) abnormalities rather than false-positive findings involves a stretch of the imagination. It takes hubris for MPS proponents to criticize the medical community at large for not acknowledging the veracity of such claims, which are not in the mainstream of medical experience.

Furthermore, there is no scientific proof of any efficacy of the varied invasive and noninvasive treatments. There are no published, properly controlled studies supporting the various treatments, but there are data showing that dry needling is equivalent to the injection of active substances. Given these issues, and the fact that no form of treatment has been shown to be superior to placebo alone, the utility and the ethics of administering and charging for such treatments can be legitimately questioned.

—*Tom Bohr*

See also–Pain, Referred

Further Reading

Bohr, T. (1995). Fibromyalgia syndrome and myofascial pain syndrome: Do they exist? *Neurol. Clin.* **13**, 365–384.
Cummings, T. M., and White, A. R. (2001). Needling therapies in the management of myofascial trigger point pain: A systematic review. *Arch. Phys. Med. Rehab.* **82**, 986–992.
Hsieh, C. Y., Hong, C. Z., Adams, A. H., *et al.* (2000). Interexaminer reliability of the palpation of trigger points in the trunk and lower limb muscles. *Arch. Phys. Med. Rehab.* **81**, 258–264.
Simons, D., Travell, J., and Simons, L. (1999). *Myofascial Pain and Dysfunction: The Trigger Point Manual.* Williams & Wilkins, Baltimore.
Travell, J., and Simons, D. (1983). *Myofascial Pain and Dysfunction: The Trigger Point Manual.* Williams & Wilkins, Baltimore.
Wolfe, F., Simons, D. G., Fricton, J., *et al.* (1992). The fibromyalgia and myofascial pain syndromes: A preliminary study of tender points and trigger points in persons with fibromyalgia, myofascial pain syndrome and no disease. *J. Rheumatol.* **19**, 944–951.

Myokymia

Encyclopedia of the Neurological Sciences

MYOKYMIA is a continuous involuntary rippling or undulating movement of muscle. It is often described as worm-like or vermicular. It is characterized electrically by grouped discharges of motor unit action potentials occurring in rhythmic or semi-rhythmic bursts of doublets, triplets, and multiplets. Intraburst firing frequency is 5–60 Hz, whereas interburst firing frequency is 2–10 Hz. The audio signal in myokymia is described as "marching."

Electrophysiological models show myokymic discharges originate from areas of axonal demyelination. The mechanism may be spontaneous generation of potentials along the demyelinated region (ectopic generation) or direct axon-to-axon transmission of nerve potentials at sites of mutual demyelination (ephaptic transmission). The myokymic firing pattern can be altered by manipulating the free or ionized calcium level of the surrounding axon. Reducing the free calcium level through hyperventilation (causing respiratory alkalosis and free calcium protein binding) or during plasma exchange enhances myokymia. Increasing free calcium levels by infusion of calcium gluconate raises the threshold for excitation and reduces myokymia.

Clinical myokymia may be broadly classified as facial myokymia and limb myokymia. Facial myokymia is more common than limb myokymia. It is observed in multiple sclerosis, Guillain–Barré syndrome, and conditions affecting the brainstem, such as pontine gliomas, cerebellar tumors, metastatic disease (tumors and meningeal carcinomatosis), and infectious mass lesions. The facial myokymia occurring in multiple sclerosis is unilateral and transient, usually lasting a few weeks but possibly lasting months. Episodes may recur and may affect the same or opposite side. Facial power is usually preserved. Facial myokymia in Guillain–Barré syndrome occurs in approximately 15% of patients. It is often bilateral. It appears early during the illness and may continue for a few weeks. Mild facial weakness is a common accompanying feature. Myokymia associated with posterior fossa tumors and metastatic disease is most often unilateral and persistent. A frequently cited but uncommonly seen cause of bilateral facial myokymia results from timber rattlesnake evenomization. It resolves after hours of receiving antivenom therapy.

Limb myokymia occurs most commonly in association with radiation injury. Radiation is frequently a treatment of choice for local tumor. Radiation plexitis (involving the brachial plexus more often than the lumbosacral plexus) with associated myokymia is reported in up to 60% of patients after radiation therapy and may occur decades after the initial exposure. Myokymia is a useful finding during electromyographic study because it may help differentiate plexitis due to radiation change from recurrent tumor. However, focal patterns of myokymia may be seen with locally invasive tumor; thus, care should be taken not to overinterpret electromyographic results. Less common causes of limb myokymia include radiculopathy and compression neuropathy (carpal tunnel syndrome and ulnar mononeuropathy). Guillain–Barré syndrome, chronic inflammatory demyelinating polyradiculopathy, cramp-fasciculation syndrome, Isaacs' syndrome (syndrome of continuous muscle fiber activity), Gold myokymia, and timber rattlesnake evenomization of the bitten extremity can cause generalized myokymia.

Treatment of myokymia is limited. Often, it is asymptomatic and requires no therapy. Symptomatic myokymia in association with inflammatory disease usually remits spontaneously. Case reports document the efficacy of antiepileptic medications in treating hyperexcitable peripheral nerve disorders: Cramp-fasciculation syndrome improves with carbamazepine therapy, and Isaacs' syndrome improves with phenytoin, carbamazepine, or plasma exchange. Gold myokymia also responds well to carbamazepine, although gold treatment must be discontinued. Treatment for myokymia in the setting of a neoplastic mass lesion should first be directed toward the underlying neoplasm, but local injection with botulinum toxin may be considered.

—*Marshall C. Freeman*

See also–Axons; Guillain-Barre Syndrome, Clinical Aspects; Isaacs' Syndrome; Multiple Sclerosis, Basic Biology; Rippling Muscle Disease; Snake Venoms

Further Reading

Gutmann, L. (1991). AAEM Minimonograph #37: Facial and limb myokymia. *Muscle Nerve* **14**, 1043–1049.
Gutmann, L. (1996). AAEM Minimonograph #46: Neurogenic muscle hypertrophy. *Muscle Nerve* **19**, 811–818.
Jamieson, P., and Katirji, B. (1994). Idiopathic generalized myokymia. *Muscle Nerve* **17**, 42–51.
Preston, C., and Shapiro, B. (1998). *Electromyography and Neuromuscular Diseases.* Butterworth-Heineman, Boston.

Myopathy, Congenital

Encyclopedia of the Neurological Sciences
Copyright 2003, Elsevier Science (USA). All rights reserved.

THE TERM CONGENITAL MYOPATHIES has been applied to a group of diverse neuromuscular disorders that typically commence in the newborn period, show little change over time with respect to weakness, and are frequently hereditary. This group of disorders may be further delineated according to specific morphological and structural characteristics of the muscle as determined by electron microscopy and histochemistry. It is now recognized that these disorders vary widely according to the severity of the presentation, the mode of inheritance (autosomal or X-linked), phenotype (physical appearance), and associated features such as skeletal abnormalities, cardiac complications, and diaphragmatic weakness. Muscle weakness may in fact be so severe as to result in premature demise, usually from respiratory failure. In addition, onset of weakness may occur at any time during childhood or even into adulthood. In some instances, the disorder may also be progressive with respect to the underlying weakness. These "exceptions to the rule" have challenged the original notion of congenital myopathies as benign, nonprogressive conditions. Furthermore, the specific structural features of muscle, such as the presence of rods in nemaline rod myopathy, may also occasionally be seen in other congenital myopathies or even in other neuromuscular conditions. Diagnosis therefore rests on a combination of history, clinical presentation, and morphological abnormalities in muscle.

Several forms of congenital myopathy, such as central core disease, nemaline rod myopathy, and centronuclear myopathy, have been well described from a clinical and morphological standpoint. Others, however, are extremely rare, and it is not clear whether the observed ultrastructural changes in the muscle are correlated with a specific phenotype and/or represent a distinct nosological entity. This group of uncertain or "questionable" disorders includes zebra body myopathy, broad A band myopathy, and trilaminar myopathy.

CLINICAL FEATURES

The congenital myopathies typically present as a "floppy infant syndrome" in the neonatal or early infantile period or with delayed motor milestones and weakness in the late-onset forms. The floppy infant is hypotonic, hyporeflexic, weak with diminished spontaneous movement, and has hyperextensibility of joints. However, these findings are not specific to neuromuscular involvement and may in fact result from any disorder of the brain, spinal cord, anterior horn cell, or peripheral nerve. The differential diagnosis is therefore vast, and accurate localization of the problem—even between the central nervous system (CNS) and peripheral nervous system (PNS)—can often be difficult. Clues to CNS involvement include associated encephalopathy, seizures, focal features on examination, hyper-reflexia, and pathological reflexes such as clonus and cross-adductor responses. Their absence suggests PNS involvement.

The severity of presentation may vary from the "classic" mild neonatal form to a severe neonatal disease often with premature demise. Associated features may suggest a specific diagnosis but are usually not sufficiently specific or reliable. Ophthalmoplegia and ptosis, for example, suggest a centronuclear/myotubular myopathy but may occur in infantile nemaline rod myopathy. The face in nemaline rod myopathy, with its narrow elongated features, facial diplegia, high arched palate, and open jaw, is typical to that disorder but nonspecific. Contractures of hands and feet may be seen in fiber type disproportion. The pattern of muscular weakness is not helpful and may be either generalized or have a proximal-to-distal Limb–Girdle distribution. Cardiac involvement may be seen in the X-linked centronuclear myopathy, late-onset nemaline rod myopathy, and, less commonly, multicore myopathy. Scoliosis is a late accompaniment of a number of the congenital myopathies.

LABORATORY DATA

Laboratory investigations are often unhelpful in diagnosis. Creatine kinase (CK) may be normal or mildly elevated. Electromyography (EMG) may show nonspecific myopathic features, namely small-amplitude, short-duration polyphasic motor unit potentials, but is normal in approximately one-third of cases. Therefore, the presence of a normal CK and EMG does not exclude a congenital myopathy, and if clinical suspicion is high, muscle biopsy is needed. Even if CK and EMG are abnormal, the findings are nonspecific; therefore, muscle biopsy is necessary for establishing the specific diagnosis. In the setting of the floppy infant, the EMG is most helpful in differentiating a neuropathy (e.g., congenital hypo-myelinating neuropathy) or anterior horn cell disease (e.g., spinal muscular atrophy) from a myopathy. The presence of an elevated CK may help to confirm clinical suspicion of a myopathy and thereby the need for a biopsy.

Many neuroimaging techniques, such as ultrasound, CAT scan, and magnetic resonance imaging, are available for assessment of structural alterations of muscle, whereas magnetic resonance spectroscopy and positron emission spectroscopy facilitate assessment of metabolic alterations. However, these are primarily research tools and unhelpful in the evaluation and management of the congenital myopathies. Rarely, they may help define diseased muscle if clinical doubt exists prior to proceeding with muscle biopsy or help define an appropriate muscle to biopsy.

The definitive diagnosis rests with muscle biopsy. Muscle may be obtained by means of either an open muscle biopsy or closed needle biopsy procedure. The muscle should be evaluated both by histochemistry and by electron microscopy.

Supplementary testing, including cardiac evaluation (electrocardiogram and echocardiogram), respiratory function testing (pulmonary function tests), polysomnogram (for sleep apnea and carbon dioxide retention from nocturnal hypoventilation), and orthopedic evaluation (for skeletal deformities and scoliosis), may be necessary. Malignant hyperthermia may be an anesthetic risk, especially with central core myopathy, nemaline rod myopathy, and minicore myopathy, but caution should be exercised in all forms.

TREATMENT

No cure exists for any form of congenital myopathy. Treatment is supportive and aimed at maximizing function and treating complications. Physical and occupational therapy are important adjuncts to any treatment regimen for monitoring and maximizing function. In some instances, late deterioration in strength may occur. Skeletal abnormalities, including hip dislocation, contractures, feet deformities, and scoliosis, are best managed with the help of an orthopedic surgeon and physical therapist. Orthotics may be necessary. Scoliosis in particular should be monitored. It may be progressive, with worsening of the curvature during puberty (due to growth spurt). Fixation and stabilization of the spine are sometimes necessary. Cardiac complications may include cardiomyopathy with heart failure and, less commonly, arrhythmias. Rarely, cardiac transplantation or cardiac pacing are required. Diaphragmatic and respiratory weakness is a common accompaniment of many of the congenital myopathies. Pulmonary functions should be monitored periodically and respiratory infections aggressively treated (antibiotics, bronchodilators, chest physical therapy, and postural drainage as necessary). Symptoms of obstructive sleep apnea (snoring) and nocturnal hypoventilation (early morning headache, fatigue, and nausea) should be monitored. When indicated, polysomnogram should be performed and early morning carbon dioxide level checked. Nasal BiPAP can provide good symptomatic relief when appropriate. Respiratory failure, especially in the neonatal period, may require tracheostomy and ventilatory support. The placement of a gastrostomy tube is often necessary for nutritional support.

SPECIFIC CONGENITAL MYOPATHIES

Central Core Myopathy

The first of the congenital myopathies to be described, central core myopathy, remains a relatively rare disorder with an elusive etiology. The histological hallmark of the disease has been the presence of centrally or eccentrically placed cores in predominantly type 1 muscle fibers that are devoid of oxidative enzyme and phosphorylase activity. There may be more than one core within a muscle fiber, and there is often a predominance of type 1 fibers. The cores may be either structured or unstructured. Myofibrillar architecture is preserved in the former, whereas in the latter the contractile apparatus has been lost. The cores show an absence of mitochondria and sarcoplasmic reticulum under electron microscopy.

Clinical Features: This myopathy usually has mild neonatal presentation with hypotonia or delayed motor milestones during infancy. The clinical course tends to be benign, with little or no progression of muscle weakness. The pattern of weakness is variable and may be proximal or generalized. Mild facial weakness may occur in the absence of ophthalmoplegia, ptosis, or bulbar weakness. Deep tendon reflexes may be normal or depressed. Congenital dislocation of the hips, contractures, and skeletal deformities may occur, including kyphoscoliosis and foot abnormalities (pes cavus, pes planus, and clubfeet). Rarely, muscle cramping following exercise has been described. Although cardiac involvement

has been reported in central core disease (mitral valve prolapse, arrhythmias, and right bundle branch block), its significance is uncertain. The association with malignant hyperthermia is well established.

Genetics: Usually inherited in an autosomal dominant pattern, the gene is linked to chromosome 19q. Some families map to the same gene locus as some autosomal dominant malignant hyperthermia families (19q13.1), suggesting that these conditions may be allelic. Mutations of the ryanodine receptor have been found in both conditions. The ryanodine receptor is an important calcium release channel in the sarcoplasmic reticulum. It is involved in calcium regulation and homeostasis during the process of muscle contraction through its intricate association with the transverse tubules. Abnormalities within this receptor and secondary problems with calcium homeostasis are thought to underlie the condition of malignant hyperthermia, a syndrome of rapid elevation of body temperature ($>42°C$), muscle rigidity, rhabdomyolysis, acidosis, and hypercarbia in response to volatile anesthetic agents (e.g., halothane, isoflurane, sevoflurane, and ether) and/or depolarizing muscle relaxants such as succinylcholine.

Nemaline Rod Myopathy

The defining histological feature is the presence of nemaline rods that typically cluster under the sarcolemma and around nuclei. These rods, from the Greek word nema meaning thread, are readily identified under light microscopy on the Gomori trichome stain. On electron microscopy, the rods are visible as dense structures with a lattice pattern of consistent periodicity in continuity with the Z lines. They are composed of predominantly α-actinin but also contain desmin, a muscle-specific intermediate filament. The abundance of rods does not relate to clinical severity. Intranuclear rods, in addition to the typical sarcoplasmic rods, may be seen in some cases of the severe neonatal presentation and appear to be unique to this form. However, rods are not unique to nemaline rod myopathy; they have been reported in other neuromuscular conditions. The muscle biopsy may also show predominance of type 1 muscle fibers.

Clinical Features: Three distinct clinical presentations are recognized: a severe, usually fatal, neonatal form; a classic neonatal or early childhood type (most common); and an adult-onset form. Hypotonia and weakness are the clinical hallmarks of this disorder. Weakness is typically more proximal than distal, although diffuse weakness may occur. The face and diaphragm are usually involved, with the diaphragmatic involvement often being prominent and disproportionate to the weakness. Extraocular muscles are rarely involved. The face has a distinctive elongated, narrow appearance, and the lower jaw is typically held open. There is facial weakness, often with limited facial expression, and a high arched palate. The voice is often nasal in quality. Swallowing difficulties and dysphagia in infancy are common and are often disproportionate to the actual weakness.

In the severe neonatal presentation, death usually results from respiratory failure and/or infection in the weeks and months following birth. Early demise is not universal, however. The infant is floppy at birth, with decreased spontaneous movement and diminished reflexes. Dysphagia and respiratory distress are prominent features. Decreased fetal movements may be noted during pregnancy, although polyhydramnios is uncommon. The classic form tends to be milder, with presentation at birth or during infancy. Occasionally, weakness and delayed motor milestones may only become evident during the first decade. The course tends to be static or slowly progressive, although, as with many muscle disorders, there may be functional deterioration at puberty coincident with a growth spurt. Hypotonia, weakness, muscle atrophy, myopathic face with distinctive phenotype, bulbar involvement (dysphagia and nasal speech), and respiratory difficulties commonly occur. Again, the diaphragmatic and respiratory involvement is disproportionate to the muscle weakness. Nocturnal hypoventilation and obstructive apnea may result in carbon dioxide retention with resultant problems of early morning headache, lethargy, and decreased appetite. Skeletal abnormalities, including arthrogryposis, clubfeet, and kyphosis, may be associated features. Intelligence is normal. Dilated cardiomyopathy has been reported but is more common in the late, adult-onset form. The late-onset or adult forms of nemaline myopathy may in fact present with isolated cardiomyopathy but more typically have mild, nonprogressive weakness.

Genetics: Sporadic, autosomal dominant and recessive patterns of inheritance have been described. Five genetic loci have been identified. These include rare mutations in the *TPM3* gene (chromosome 1q22–q23) that encodes α-tropomyosin$_{slow}$, initially described in a childhood-onset autosomal dominant family in Australia and subsequently in three other sporadic cases. More commonly, recessive mutations in the nebulin gene (*NEB*) on chromosome 2q21.2–q22, and both recessive and dominant mutations in the α-actin gene (*ACTA 1*) on chromosome 1q42.1 occur. Other rare mutations have been found in the troponin T (*TNNT1*) and β–tropomyosin (*TPM2*) genes on chromosomes 19q13 and 9p13, respectively.

Myotubular/Centronuclear Myopathy

This is an extremely rare form of congenital myopathy. The terms myotubular myopathy and centronuclear myopathy have been used synonymously to describe this condition, highlighting the unresolved debate regarding this disorder: whether the primary histological feature represents an arrest of the maturation of the muscle fiber or rather the presence of central nuclei. Favoring the former is the persistence of high levels of fetal expression of desmin, vimentin (intermediate filament proteins), and neural cell adhesion molecule (N-CAM) in the myofibers of infants with X-linked myotubular myopathy. Other histological features on muscle biopsy include smallness of muscle fibers, with occasional hypotrophy of type 1 fibers and centrally aggregated mitochondria.

Clinical Features: Two distinct clinical presentations occur: a severe X-linked form with typical early demise and a more indolent autosomal form with onset in infancy/childhood (recessive form) or late adolescence/adulthood (dominant form).

In X-linked myotubular myopathy, affected boys present in the neonatal period with severe generalized muscle weakness, hypotonia, and respiratory failure that is often fatal in the neonatal period or early infancy. Those who survive are often severely impaired and may require ongoing ventilatory support. Feeding and swallowing difficulties may be prominent. Additional features that may be present include polyhydramnios, large heads, low birth weights, arthrogryposis/contractures of hips or knees, thin ribs, and ophthalmoplegia. The main differential diagnostic concern is from congenital myotonic dystrophy, which can have similar clinical and histological features but can be excluded on the basis of DNA testing of the myotonin gene (a CTG trinucleotide repeat disorder).

In autosomal myotubular/centronuclear myopathy, onset is during infancy, childhood, adolescence, or adulthood. The recessive forms tend to occur earlier than the later onset and typically milder dominant forms. The onset of weakness and delayed motor milestones are usually present in infancy but may rarely be delayed until the second or third decade. Ocular findings including ptosis and ophthalmoplegia commonly occur and help to differentiate this form of congenital myopathy from other types. Hypotonia, hyporeflexia, and variable generalized weakness, from mild to disabling, occur. Mild facial weakness may also be present. Weakness is usually nonprogressive but may occasionally be slowly progressive. Central nervous system involvement (seizures and mental retardation) has been described. Cardiac involvement rarely occurs.

Genetics: Through linkage studies, the gene locus for X-linked myotubular myopathy was localized to the proximal Xq28 region. The gene was subsequently identified as the *MTM1* gene, which encodes a tyrosine phosphatase, myotubularin. Mutations have been identified within this gene, but there does not appear to be any correlation between the type of mutation and the severity of clinical phenotype. In an informative patient, carrier status and prenatal diagnosis may be possible, although there is a high rate of spontaneous mutation. The mechanism by which mutations result in disease is uncertain, but myotubularin appears to be involved in signal transduction during late myogenesis, and mutations resulting in a loss of function may therefore affect this process.

Minicore Myopathy

Also known as multicore myopathy, the characteristic histological features of this disorder include multifocal, circumscribed, oval-shaped cores, which have decreased or deficient ATPase and oxidative enzyme activity in type 1 and 2 muscle fibers. There is often a predominance of type 1 fibers. Ultrastructurally, there is an absence of mitochondria in the cores and a loss of sarcomere structure starting in the Z band (unstructured cores). The cores differ from those in central core myopathy, which tend to be longer, tubular in shape, and run the entire length of the fiber.

Clinical Features: Usually, there is a mild presentation with hypotonia, nonprogressive weakness, hyporeflexia, and motor developmental delay during the first year of life. The weakness may be generalized or have a proximal-to-distal gradient. The weakness tends to be mild to moderate in severity. Occasionally, a slight improvement in strength may occur with time, and rarely there may be late deterioration. Mild facial weakness, ptosis, ophthal-

moplegia, diaphragmatic involvement, cardiomyopathy, and scoliosis may be associated features. Malignant hyperthermia with anesthesia is a potential risk. Adult and late-onset presentation occurs. Although typically a benign and mild disease, severe cases and premature death have been reported.

Genetics: The gene locus has not been identified, and even the mode of inheritance remains uncertain. Although family occurrence suggests both autosomal recessive and dominant patterns of transmission, most cases appear to be sporadic.

Congenital Fiber Type Disproportion Myopathy

The defining histological feature of congenital fiber type disproportion is the predominance of type 1 muscle fibers ($\geq 80\%$), which are also smaller than type 2 fibers by more than 12%. The type 2 fibers, especially type 2b, are normal in size or may be hypertrophied. There is usually an absence of other myopathic features, such as degenerating/regenerating fibers, increased connective tissue, or central nuclei, although in a small percentage of cases these may occur. There are no ultrastructural abnormalities on electron microscopy. Although a distinctive clinical phenotype has been described, the histological features may be seen in other neuromuscular conditions. These conditions must therefore be excluded on the basis of clinical presentation and/or additional features on biopsy. Differential considerations include spinal muscular atrophy, myotonic dystrophy, congenital muscular dystrophy, nemaline rod myopathy, and centronuclear/myotubular myopathy in which fiber type disproportion may be seen. The pathogenesis of congenital fiber type disproportion is unknown, but it is thought to reflect a maturational abnormality of muscle.

Clinical Features: This myopathy is usually present as a floppy infant syndrome, with hypotonia, weakness, and hyporeflexia. Motor milestones are frequently delayed. Weakness may be of variable severity, with possible early progression of the weakness before stabilization and, in some cases, improvement in strength. Orthopedic complications include arthrogryposis, congenital dislocation of the hips, pes planus, pes cavus, and scoliosis. Torticollis and short stature may be associated features. A severe phenotype with variable ptosis, ophthalmoplegia, bulbar weakness, facial weakness, and respiratory failure with frequent early demise has also been described. Cardiac involvement is rare, although cardiomyopathy necessitating heart transplant has been reported.

Genetics: No genetic testing is available. Most cases are sporadic, although familial cases suggesting both autosomal dominant and autosomal recessive modes of transmission have been described.

Cytoplasmic Body Myopathy

This myopathy is also known as spheroid body myopathy, desmin storage myopathy, and granulofilamentous myopathy. The accumulation of cytoplasmic inclusions is the characteristic histological feature of this group of congenital myopathies. However, the cytoplasmic inclusions are nonspecific and may be seen in a number of other neuromuscular diseases. In the case of cytoplasmic body myopathy, the cytoplasmic inclusion is the principal abnormality on biopsy. The cytoplasmic body is a small, subsarcolemmal granular and filamentous structure. The filaments are 8–10 nm (intermediate filament range) and stain with desmin. The desmin gene locus has been assigned to chromosome 2q35. Desmin-staining inclusion bodies may also be seen in cardiac muscle. The clinical manifestations are heterogeneous, with a variable distribution of weakness. Adult onset may occur. Cardiac involvement is common and includes structural as well as conduction disturbances. Hypertrophic, congestive, and restrictive cardiomyopathies have all been described and may precede the skeletal myopathy by a number of years. Significant arrhythmias, including complete heart block, may also occur. Most cases are sporadic, although familial cases have suggested both autosomal dominant and recessive modes of inheritance.

Fingerprint Body Myopathy

This is an extremely rare form of congenital myopathy. The name derives from the presence of a complex arrangement of subsarcolemmal lamellae inclusions that appear as a fingerprint pattern under electron microscopy. Light microscopy may be normal or show type 1 fiber predominance. Fingerprint bodies have also been reported in other neuromuscular disorders. Reported cases suggest an autosomal dominant pattern of inheritance.

Hyaline Body Myopathy

Hyaline bodies are subsarcolemmal, moderately dense, disorganized filaments that are not limited by a surrounding membrane. Visible under light microscopy, they appear to have a predilection for type 1 fibers and are pale under H&E staining. Under electron microscopy, they appear to be in continuity with thick myosin filaments.

Other Extremely Rare Congenital Myopathies

A number of other extremely rare structural myopathies with distinctive histological features have been described, often in only one or two case reports. These include reducing body myopathy, zebra body myopathy, sarcotubular myopathy, tubular aggregate myopathy, trilaminar myopathy, and broad A band myopathy.

—Neil Friedman

***See also*—**Muscle Biopsy; Myopathy, Endocrine; Myopathy, Metabolic; Myopathy, Overview; Myopathy, Toxic

Further Reading

Bodensteiner, J. B. (1994). Congenital myopathies. *Muscle Nerve* **17**, 131–134.
Dubowitz, V. (1995). *Muscle Disorders in Childhood*, 2nd ed. Saunders, London.
Engel, A. G., and Franzini-Armstrong, C. (Eds.) (1994). *Myology*, 2nd ed. McGraw-Hill, New York.
Goebel, H. H. (1996). Congenital myopathies. *Semin. Pediatr. Neurol.* **3**, 152–161.
Goebel, H. H. (1999). Congenital myopathies: The current status. *J. Child Neurol.* **14**, 30–31.
Kaplan, J.-C., and Fontaine, B. (2000). Neuromuscular disorders: Gene location. *Neuromuscular Dis.* **10**, I–XV.
Sarnat, H. B. (1994). New insights into the pathogenesis of congenital myopathies. *J. Child Neurol.* **9**, 193–201.

Myopathy, Endocrine

Encyclopedia of the Neurological Sciences
Copyright 2003, Elsevier Science (USA). All rights reserved.

MYOPATHIES are associated with a number of different endocrinopathies related to thyroid, parathyroid, adrenal, and pituitary dysfunction (Table 1). These "endocrine myopathies" are typically characterized by the insidious onset of proximal muscle weakness, and recovery generally occurs with treatment of the underlying hormonal abnormality. In most instances, the myopathy associated with endocrine disease is a minor component of the clinical disorder; however, occasionally, as in patients with a thyrotoxic myopathy, the neuromuscular manifestations may be the presenting feature of the endocrinopathy.

Table 1   ENDOCRINE MYOPATHIES

	Clinical features	Laboratory features	Histopathology	Prognosis following treatment
Hyperthyroid myopathy	Proximal weakness (predominantly shoulder girdle) Prominent muscle atrophy Occasional bulbar, ocular, or respiratory weakness Fasciculations, myokymia (uncommon) Muscle cramps, pain (uncommon) Hyperactive reflexes	CK level: normal or low EMG: myopathic; occasional fasciculations, fibrillations	Normal or non-specific myopathic features	Resolution of symptoms within several months once euthyroid state is achieved
Hypothyroid myopathy	Muscle pain, cramps, stiffness, fatigue Slight proximal weakness Muscle hypertrophy (rare atrophy) Myoedema Hypoactive reflexes with delayed relaxation	CK level; elevated 10–100× normal EMG: usually normal; occasionally myopathic; rare positive sharp waves, fibrillation potentials, or complex repetitive discharges	Normal or nonspecific myopathic features	Resolution of symptoms within 1 year; some patients may have permanent residual weakness
Hyperparathyroid myopathy	Proximal weakness (predominately legs) Muscle atrophy Muscle cramps Paresthesias Occasional bulbar or respiratory weakness Hyperactive reflexes	CK level: normal or elevated EMG: usually normal; occasionally myopathic; rare positive sharp waves, fibrillation potentials, and fasciculations	Nonspecific myopathic features; prominent type 2 atrophy	Improvement of strength within days to months
Hypoparathyroid myopathy	Parethesias Muscle pain Tetany Mild proximal weakness Hypoactive or absent reflexes	CK level: normal or elevated EMG: doublets or multiplets occasional fasciculations	Nonspecific myopathic features Decreased glycogen phosphorylase	Resolution of symptoms
Steroid myopathy	Proximal weakness (predominantly legs) Muscle atrophy Muscle tenderness Normal reflexes	CK level: normal Elevated urinary creative levels EMG: Normal except myopathic motor units may be seen in severely affected muscles	Preferential atrophy of type 2 fibers Lipid droplets/glycogen accumulation in type 1 fibers	Recovery within 1–4 months of steroid withdrawal or removal of tumor
Addison's disease	Mild proximal weakness Muscle fatigue	CK level: normal EMG: usually normal; occasionally myopathic	Normal	Resolution of symptoms
Acromegaly	Proximal weakness Muscle fatigue Occasional muscle hypertrophy	CK level: normal or mildly elevated EMG: usually normal; occasionally myopathic	Normal Muscle fiber hypertrophy/atrophy and/or necrotic fibers may be seen	Improvement in 50% within 1 year

THYROID DISORDERS

Hyperthyroid Myopathy

Clinical Features: The majority of patients with hyperthyroidism will demonstrate evidence of weakness and/or muscle atrophy on clinical examination. In 5% of cases, muscle weakness is the presenting complaint and precedes, by several months, other clinical symptoms of hyperthyroidism. Although hyperthyroidism occurs more commonly in women, the myopathy secondary to this endocrinopathy occurs equally in men and women. The severity of the weakness correlates with the duration of the thyrotoxic state rather than the degree of chemical dysthyroidism.

Thyrotoxic myopathy is characterized by proximal muscle weakness and atrophy. The proximal upper extremities can be more prominently affected in some cases, resulting in severe shoulder girdle atrophy with scapular winging. Distal extremity weakness occurs in approximately 20% of patients and can be an isolated manifestation. Fasciculations and myokymia are occasionally seen, which probably reflects thyrotoxicosis-induced irritability of the anterior horn cells or peripheral nerves. Muscle cramps and pain may also occur, but these are relatively uncommon symptoms. Muscle stretch reflexes are preserved and often brisk due to shortened relaxation times. Dysphagia, dysphonia, aspiration pneumonia, and respiratory insufficiency may also occur in approximately 15% of patients due to weakness of the bulbar, esophageal, and respiratory muscles. Rarely, rhabdomyolysis with myoglobinuria can occur in severe thyrotoxicosis. Exophthalmos and extraocular muscle dysfunction as well as a clinical syndrome similar to hypokalemic periodic paralysis may also occur in some hyperthyroid patients.

Laboratory Features: Primary hyperthyroidism is diagnosed on the basis of elevated thyroxine (T4) levels and occasionally only on elevated triiodothyronine (T3) levels, whereas the thyroid-stimulating hormone (TSH) level is low. Serum creatine kinase (CK) levels are often low in thyrotoxic myopathy, probably related to increased clearance of the enzyme from the blood.

Routine motor and sensory nerve conduction studies are normal. Abnormalities on needle electromyography (EMG) examination are seen in approximately 90% of patients. In proximal muscles, there is usually evidence of brief-duration, polyphasic motor unit potentials. Fasciculations, fibrillations, and positive sharp waves are unusual but may be found in distal muscles. Complex repetitive discharges and focal or generalized myokymia rarely occur. These electrodiagnostic abnormalities correlate with the degree of muscle atrophy and weakness but not the severity of thyrotoxicosis and resolve once a euthyroid state is achieved.

Histopathology: Routine muscle biopsies usually do not reveal any significant abnormalities in patients with clinical features of thyrotoxic myopathy. Nonspecific findings occur in approximately one-fourth of patients and include slight fatty infiltration, muscle fiber atrophy of all types, connective tissue proliferation, variability in fiber size, scattered necrotic fibers, decreased glycogen, and increased central nuclei.

Treatment: Successful treatment of the hyperthyroid state will result in resolution of the myopathy generally over a period of several months. Improvement in strength usually precedes the reversal of muscle atrophy. Propanolol can be effective in treating the systemic symptoms of thyrotoxicosis as well as improve proximal and bulbar muscle strength.

Hypothyroid Myopathy

Clinical Features: Neuromuscular symptoms commonly occur in patients with hypothyroidism and include proximal weakness, fatigue, myoedema, cramps, muscle stiffness, and myalgias. Muscle pain is probably the most common feature, occurring in up to half of patients with hypothyroidism. Proximal weakness tends to develop insidiously over months and occurs in approximately 25% of patients. Weakness is accompanied by either muscle hypertrophy or, rarely, muscle atrophy. Myoedema, sometimes referred to as the mounding phenomenon, is seen in 30–60% of hypothyroid patients and consists of a local knot of contraction induced in a muscle by percussion. Typically, the mound lasts for 30–60 sec and is electrically silent. Although characteristic, this phenomenon is not specific for hypothyroid myopathy and can occur in various states of malnutrition, aging, and in some normal subjects. The ankle reflex may demonstrate a delayed relaxation phase in approximately two-thirds of patients, a finding best demonstrated by having the patient kneel on a chair while the clinician strikes the Achilles tendon.

Laboratory Features: The CK levels are typically elevated 10–100 times normal, which may lead to an erroneous diagnosis of polymyositis. The serum myoglobin levels may also be increased. The diagnosis can be established based on low circulating thyroxine levels. TSH levels are elevated in primary hypothyroidism and depressed in hypothalamic-pituitary failure.

Nerve conduction studies are usually normal, slow motor or sensory studies suggesting a concomitant peripheral neuropathy. Patients with hypothyroidism are also more susceptible to the development of entrapment neuropathies such as carpal tunnel syndrome. Insertional activity on needle EMG studies is usually normal, although rarely positive sharp waves, fibrillation potentials, and/or complex repetitive discharges may be demonstrated. Motor unit potentials may be normal or occasionally be of short duration, low amplitude, and polyphasic, particularly in severely affected muscles.

Histopathology: Muscle biopsy findings are typically nonspecific and tend to correlate with the duration and severity of the myopathy. Abnormalities may include variability in fiber size, atrophy of type 2 fibers (occasionally type 1 fibers), increased central nuclei, glycogen accumulation, vacuoles, ring fibers, and increased connective tissue. Scattered hypertrophic, necrotic, and/or regenerating fibers have also been reported.

Treatment: Treatment with thyroid hormone usually induces remission of the myopathy; however, it may take a year or more before full doses can be used and the patient's symptoms resolve. Unfortunately, in some cases permanent residual weakness may result despite return to a euthyroid state.

PARATHYROID DISORDERS

Hyperparathyroid Myopathy

Clinical Features: Proximal muscle weakness and atrophy is very common in patients with osteomalacia but relatively infrequent in primary hyperparathyroidism or in hypercalcemia from other causes. The weakness is usually insidious in onset, preferentially involving the lower extremities, and can be progressive over a period of months or years. Cramps, paresthesias, hoarseness, dysphagia, respiratory insufficiency, and cognitive changes have also been reported in association with hyperparathyroidism. Muscle stretch reflexes are typically

brisk with flexor plantar responses, although there have been rare reports of extensor plantar responses associated with a spastic paraparesis.

Laboratory Features: Serum CK levels are usually normal or only slightly elevated in all forms of hyperparathyroidism. In primary hyperparathyroidism, serum calcium, parathyroid hormone, and 1,25-dihydroxy vitamin D levels are usually elevated and serum phosphate levels are low. In secondary hyperparathyroidism due to renal failure, 1,25-dihydroxy vitamin D levels are low. Noninvasive imaging techniques, such as thallium/technetium scintigraphs and magnetic resonance imaging, may be useful in identifying abnormal parathyroid glands. In osteomalacia, serum calcium, phosphate, and 1,25-dihydroxy vitamin D levels are low, whereas serum alkaline phosphatase levels are elevated in 80–90% of cases.

Nerve conduction studies can be expected to be normal; however, a concomitant peripheral neuropathy may be present in patients with associated renal failure or nutritional deficits. Needle EMG examination is typically normal, but occasionally positive sharp waves, fibrillation potentials, or fasciculations may be identified, especially in the anterior tibialis muscle. There is a mixture of normal and short-duration, polyphasic motor unit action potentials. Occasionally, in longstanding disease, long-duration, large-amplitude motor unit action potentials may also be observed.

Histopathology: Muscle biopsies usually demonstrate nonspecific myopathic features. Atrophy of predominantly type 2 fibers is the most common abnormality.

Treatment: In symptomatic patients, medical or surgical treatment usually results in improvement of muscle strength within days to months. Patients with amyotrophic lateral sclerosis with concomitant elevations in parathyroid hormone due to parathyroid adenomas do not improve following parathyroidectomy.

Hypoparathyroid Myopathy

Clinical Features: Patients with hypocalcemia related to hypoparathyroidism may present with symptoms of paresthesias, muscle pain, and/or tetany. Mild proximal weakness has been rarely reported. On examination, patients may be hypo- or areflexic. In addition, they may demonstrate a Chvostek's sign (ipsilateral facial contraction upon tapping the facial nerve at the external auditory meatus) or a Trousseau's sign (interphalangeal joint extension, metacarpophalangeal joint flexion, and thumb adduction elicited by occluding venous return from an arm).

Laboratory Features: The CK level may be elevated, even in the absence of objective weakness. The diagnosis can be made on the basis of low serum calcium and parathyroid hormone levels and elevated serum phosphate levels.

Nerve conduction studies are normal. Needle EMG examination reveals normal insertional activity, although fasciculation potentials can be observed in some patients. The most striking abnormality is the spontaneous occurrence of motor unit action potentials that fire rapidly in succession, creating so-called doublets or multiplets. Otherwise, motor unit action potential morphology and recruitment are normal.

Histopathology: Muscle biopsies may reveal nonspecific myopathic features resulting from muscle damage induced by episodes of tetany. Decreased glycogen phosphorylase activity has also been reported.

Treatment: Neuromuscular symptoms associated with hypoparathyroidism improve following correction of the hyperphosphatemia and hypocalcemia with vitamin D and calcium administration.

ADRENAL DISORDERS

Cushing's Syndrome and Steroid Myopathy

Clinical Features: Corticosteroid-induced myopathy is the most common endocrine-related muscle disease. An excess of either endogenous corticosteroids (Cushing's syndrome) or exogenous corticosteroids (related to steroid therapy) can result in muscle weakness and atrophy. The occurrence of an associated myopathy in patients with Cushing's syndrome is approximately 50–80%. The incidence of exogenous corticosteroid myopathy is unknown, but it occurs almost twice as often in women. Prednisone doses of 30 mg/day or more have been associated with an increased risk of myopathy, although the incidence of corticosteroid-induced weakness does not necessarily correlate with the duration of treatment or dosage. Alternate-day dosing appears to reduce the risk, as does the use of nonfluorinated synthetic glucocorticoids. Muscle weakness may begin within several weeks of initiation of steroid therapy but typically develops after chronic administration of high doses of oral steroids. An acute myopathy resulting in prolonged paralysis and respiratory failure can occur in patients receiving high doses of intravenous corticosteroids with or without the concomitant administration of neuromuscular blocking agents (acute quadriplegic myopathy).

On examination, patients demonstrate proximal muscle atrophy and weakness, which is typically most severe in the lower extremities. Muscle tenderness may be elicited by palpation. Facial, ocular, bulbar, and distal extremity muscles tend to be spared. Muscle stretch reflexes initially remain intact.

Laboratory Features: The serum CK is invariably normal but may approach the upper limit of normal. The serum potassium level may be low as a result of glucocorticoid excess. Elevated urinary creatine levels may be the best indicator of a steroid myopathy. Nerve conduction studies should be normal since glucocorticoids do not appreciably affect the function of the peripheral nerves. Needle EMG studies typically show no evidence of abnormal insertional or spontaneous activity. Motor unit potential morphology is also normal, except in patients with severe atrophy, in which case myopathic features may be demonstrated.

Histopathology: The main abnormality on muscle biopsy is preferential atrophy of type 2 fibers, especially type 2B fibers. A distinct absence of significant necrosis or regeneration is observed. Lipid droplets and glycogen accumulations are prominent features, usually in type 1 fibers.

Treatment: Treatment of neuromuscular symptoms related to exogenous steroids includes cessation or reduction of steroid dosage, switching to an alternate-day regimen or a nonfluorinated compound, and initiation of an exercise program to minimize disuse atrophy. Recovery in Cushing's syndrome, following removal of the glucocorticoid excreting tumor, typically occurs within 1–4 months.

Adrenal Insufficiency (Addison's Disease)

Clinical Features: Adrenal insufficiency commonly results in symptoms of muscle fatigability and cramping, although mild objective weakness may occur. Muscle weakness is more commonly seen in patients with associated electrolyte disturbances or concurrent endocrinopathies.

Laboratory Features/Histopathology: Serum CK levels are normal. Electrodiagnostic studies are typically unremarkable, although short-duration motor unit potentials without polyphasia or abnormal spontaneous activity have been reported in several cases. Muscle biopsies are essentially normal.

Treatment: Symptoms improve following proper replacement of adrenal hormones and correction of any underlying electrolyte abnormalities.

PITUITARY DISORDERS

Acromegaly

Clinical Features: The duration of acromegaly rather than serum growth hormone levels correlates with the incidence of myopathy. Proximal muscle weakness and fatigue typically develop insidiously and represent a late clinical manifestation of acromegaly. Muscle weakness is usually mild and not associated with muscle atrophy; rather, muscle hypertrophy may be seen.

Laboratory Features: Serum CK levels may be normal or mildly elevated. Nerve conduction studies are frequently abnormal due to associated entrapment neuropathies. Short-duration, low-amplitude motor unit potentials may be detected in proximal muscles in the absence of associated positive sharp waves or fibrillation potentials.

Histopathology: The muscle biopsy may be normal or show evidence of fiber size variability with hypertrophy and atrophy of both type 1 and type 2 muscle fibers. A small number of necrotic muscle fibers may also be seen.

Treatment: Muscle strength typically shows little improvement in the first few weeks after pituitary surgery. However, approximately 50% of patients will show some clinical improvement within 1 year. Improvement has not been shown to be related to normalization of growth hormone levels.

—*Carlayne E. Jackson*

See also–Addison's Disease; Cushing Syndrome; Myopathy, Congenital; Myopathy, Metabolic; Myopathy, Overview; Myopathy, Toxic; Thyroid and Thyroid Disorders

Further Reading

Engel, A. G. (1981). Metabolic and endocrine myopathies. In *Disorders of Voluntary Muscle* (J. N. Walton, Ed.), 4th ed., pp. 664–711. Churchill Livingstone, Edinburgh, UK.
Kissel, J. T., and Mendell, J. R. (1992). The endocrine myopathies. *Handb. Clin. Neurol.* **18**, 527–551.
Layzer, R. B. (1985). Endocrine disorders. In *Neuromuscular Manifestations of Systemic Disease* (R. B. Layzer, Ed.), pp. 79–137. Davis, Philadelphia.

Myopathy, Metabolic

Encyclopedia of the Neurological Sciences

METABOLIC myopathies comprise a broad group of disorders caused by defects in the biochemical pathways producing adenosine triphosphate (ATP), the energy currency of the cell. Skeletal muscle is particularly vulnerable to impoverishment of ATP because this tissue consumes large amounts of energy. Therefore, impaired ATP production can cause progressive skeletal muscle weakness. Alternatively, metabolic myopathies can present as exercise intolerance with recurrent, acute, and reversible episodes of muscle dysfunction that manifest as muscle cramps and breakdown of muscle (rhabdomyolysis), which in turn allows creatine kinase (CK) and myoglobin to spill into the patient's serum. When there is massive muscle breakdown, myoglobin passes through the kidneys and is visible as dark urine (pigmenturia myoglobinuria). In some metabolic myopathies, both progressive weakness and episodic muscle dysfunction coexist.

Numerous causes of metabolic myopathies exist due to the many biochemical reactions required to produce cellular energy. Skeletal muscle uses three major sources of ATP: fatty acids, glycogen, and high-energy phosphate compounds such as phosphocreatine. The type and duration of muscle activity dictate the relative proportions of energy derived from these three sources. At rest, fatty acid oxidation accounts for the bulk of ATP production. During the first several minutes of moderate exercise, high-energy phosphate compounds regenerate ATP from adenosine diphosphate (ADP). After 5–10 min of exercise, glycogen becomes the major energy source, and after longer periods of exertion fatty acids are the predominant sources of ATP. As a consequence, defects of glycogen breakdown such as myophosphorylase deficiency (McArdle's disease), are evident after relatively short intervals of moderate to intense exercise, such as walking uphill or sprinting short distances. In contrast, disorders of fatty acid metabolism, such as carnitine palmitoyltransferase

(CPT) II deficiency, are more likely to produce symptoms after prolonged periods of exercise. In this entry, the main clinical and biochemical features of several metabolic myopathies are described according to etiologies.

BASIC PRINCIPLES OF MUSCLE ENERGY METABOLISM

To describe the numerous metabolic steps involved in the breakdown of fatty acid and glycogen to form ATP is beyond the scope of this entry and readers may refer to other sources for further details. Nevertheless, a brief overview of the major biochemical pathways may be helpful to place the various metabolic myopathies into a broader perspective. These processes include lipid metabolism, glycogen metabolism, the Krebs or tricarboxylic acid cycle (TCA), and oxidative phosphorylation (Fig. 1).

Most of the body's lipids are stored in adipocytes, which release free fatty acids that are then incorporated into muscle and other cells. Short 4-carbon and medium 8-carbon chain fatty acids freely cross the mitochondrial membranes, whereas long-chain and very long-chain 14- to 24-carbon chain fatty acids must be transported into mitochondria. Within the mitochondrial matrix, fatty acids undergo β-oxidation to form acetyl coenzyme A (acetyl-CoA), which in turn is processed by the Krebs or tricarboxylic acid cycle (Fig. 2). Therefore, metabolic disorders of lipid metabolism can be caused by defects of fatty acid transport or β-oxidation.

In contrast to lipids, most of the body's glycogen is contained in liver and muscle. Liver stores of glycogen are mainly responsible for maintaining blood glucose levels, whereas muscle glycogen is mainly used for internal consumption to produce ATP. Glucose is osmotically active; therefore, high concentrations of glucose cannot be stored. However, large amounts of the relatively insoluble glycogen can be sequestered in cells. Glycogen constitutes approximately 1% of the total muscle mass and is maintained within a narrow range of concentrations by a balance between glycogen synthesis and degradation. Defects in either process can cause clinical disorders. Glycogen synthesis involves several enzymes and is controlled mainly by glycogen synthetase, which adds glucosyl residues from UDP-glucose to the end of glycogen molecules. Every 8–12 residues, branches of glycogen are added to the stems to produce highly branched glycogen molecules. Breakdown of glycogen is primarily regulated by phosphorylase, which liberates glucose-1-phosphate from glycogen (Fig. 2). Glucose is degraded by a series of reactions called glycolysis to form pyruvate, which can be converted by pyruvate dehydrogenase complex to acetyl-CoA.

In the mitochondrial matrix, acetyl-CoA, derived from both glycolysis and β-oxidation, enters the Krebs cycle to produce reduced nicotinamide adenine dinucleotide and reduced flavin adenine dinucleotide, which transfer reducing equivalents (electrons) to the mitochondrial respiratory chain that leads to ATP through oxidative phosphorylation (Fig. 1). The transfer of electrons through complexes I–IV of the respiratory chain induces protons pumping from the mitochondrial matrix into the intermembrane space, resulting in an electrochemical gradient across the inner mitochondrial membrane. This proton gradient is utilized by complex V of the respiratory chain to produce ATP. Because many reactions are involved in energy metabolism, there are numerous biochemical defects that cause metabolic myopathies.

DEFECTS OF GLYCOGEN METABOLISM

During moderate- to high-intensity exercise [70–80% of maximum aerobic capacity (VO_2 max)], glycogen is the major source of stored energy for ATP production. When glycogen metabolism is defective, the supply of substrate for energy production cannot meet the demands of intense exercise. The resulting symptoms include exercise intolerance, muscle cramps, and myoglobinuria. Other organ systems depend on glycogen metabolism; therefore, liver, kidney, heart, and brain can also be affected. Fasting hypoglycemia is another manifestation.

Of the 12 different glycogenoses, 10 have been associated with neuromuscular syndromes (Fig. 1). The two forms without neuromuscular involvement are type I, due to glucose-6-phosphatase deficiency that causes liver and kidney dysfunction, and type VI, due to hepatic phosphorylase deficiency that affects liver and erythrocytes. Four types of glycogen storage disease present with skeletal muscle symptoms: type V, muscle phosphorylase deficiency; type VII, phosphofructokinase (PFK) deficiency; type X, muscle phosphoglycerate mutase (PGAM-M); and type XI, muscle lactate dehydrogenase (LDH-M). Type II, acid maltase deficiency (AMD), and type VIII, phosphorylase b kinase (PBK) deficiency, have multiple clinical phenotypes and can present with a myopathy or with multiorgan disease. The other

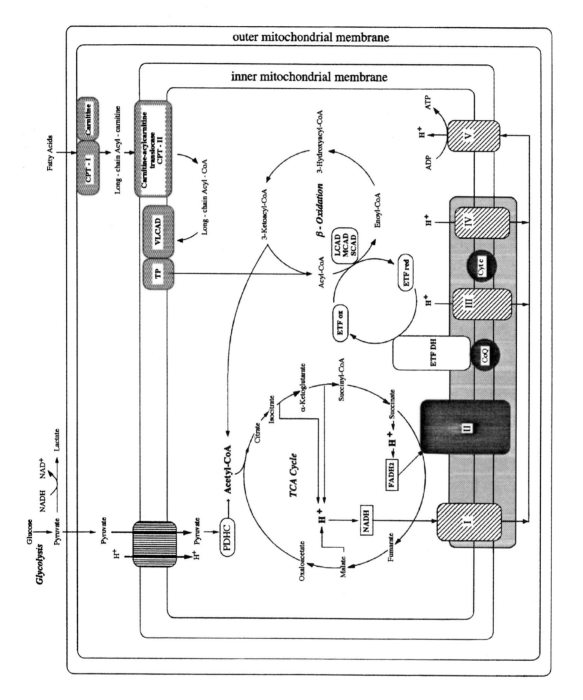

Figure 1

Schematic representation of mitochondrial metabolism. CPT, carnitine palmitoyltransferase; VLCAD, very long-chain acyl-CoA dehydrogenase; TP, trifunctional enzyme; PDHC, pyruvate dehydrogenase complex; CoA, coenzyme A; TCA, tricarboxylic acid; LCAD, long-chain acyl-CoA dehydrogenase; MCAD, medium-chain acyl-CoA dehydrogenase; SCAD, short-chain acyl-CoA dehydrogenase; ETF, electron transfer flavoprotein; CoQ, coenzyme Q; Cyt c, cytochrome c. Roman numerals refer to mitochondrial respiratory chain enzymes.

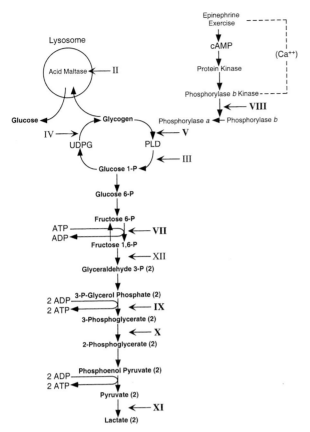

Figure 2
Scheme of glycogen metabolism and glycolysis. Roman numerals denote muscle glycogenoses due to defects in the following enzymes: II, acid maltase; III, debrancher; IV, brancher; V, myophosphorylase; VII, phosphofructokinase; VIII, phosphorylase b kinase; IX, phosphoglycerate kinase; X, phosphoglycerate mutase; XI, lactate dehydrogenase; and XII, aldolase. Bold numerals designate glycogenoses associated with exercise intolerance, cramps, and myoglobinuria. Nonbold numerals correspond to glycogenoses causing weakness.

glycogen storage diseases are generalized disorders with multiple tissue involvement.

Generalized Glycogen Storage Diseases

Glycogen storage disease type II, AMD, is distinct from the other forms of glycogen metabolism defects in that the enzyme is located in lysosomes rather than in the cytosol. Clinically, three forms have been defined by ages at onset: infantile, childhood, and adult AMD. Infantile AMD (Pompe's disease) presents in the first weeks or months of life with diffuse hypotonia and weakness, including respiratory muscles; macroglossia is common. There is marked cardiomegaly and mild hepatomegaly. The disease is invariably fatal before age 2 due to pulmonary and

cardiac failure. Childhood and adult AMD are primarily disorders of skeletal muscle manifesting as slowly progressive weakness. The childhood form can resemble Duchenne's muscular dystrophy. Respiratory muscle weakness out of proportion to limb weakness can be a clinical clue to the diagnosis.

Debrancher deficiency (type III) is clinically characterized by childhood-onset liver dysfunction with hepatomegaly, growth failure, fasting hypoglycemia, and, occasionally, hypoglycemic seizures. Patients tend to spontaneously resolve at puberty and lead normal adult lives; however, cirrhosis and hepatic failure may develop later. Type IIIa affects both muscle and liver, whereas type IIIb spares muscle. The myopathy primarily affects distal leg and intrinsic hand muscles and is slowly progressive and rarely incapacitating. After muscle phosphorylase has shortened the peripheral chains of glycogen to approximately four glucosyl units, producing a partially digested polysaccharide called phosphorylase-limit-dextran, the debrancher enzyme removes the residual oligosaccharide "twigs."

Branching enzyme deficiency (Andersen's disease, type IV) is typically a severe, rapidly progressive disease of infancy that is clinically dominated by liver dysfunction with hepatosplenomegaly, cirrhosis, and death by age 4 due to hepatic failure or gastrointestinal bleeding. Muscle wasting, hypotonia, and contractures are prominent. In Askenazi, Jewish patients with adult polyglucosan body disease (APBD), brancher enzyme deficiency has been identified in leukocytes. Although urinary disturbances are often an early and important manifestation, APBD is characterized by late-onset (fifth or sixth decade) progressive upper and lower motor neuron degeneration, sensory neuropathy, bladder and bowel incontinence, and, in some patients, dementia. Branching enzyme catalyzes the final step of glycogen synthesis by adding short glucosyl chains (approximately seven glucosyl units) to linear peripheral chains of glycogen.

PBK deficiency (type VIII) has been associated with four distinct phenotypes based on the mode of inheritance and tissue involvement: (i) liver disease, typically a benign condition of infancy or childhood with hepatomegaly, growth retardation, delayed motor development, and fasting hypoglycemia and usually inherited as an X-linked trait; (ii) liver and muscle disease with a static myopathy inherited as an autosomal recessive trait; (iii) myopathy alone, also inherited in an autosomal recessive pattern; and (iv) fatal infantile myopathy. In patients with myopathy, serum CK is variably increased. PBK is composed of four subunits (α, β, γ, and δ) and acts on two enzymes—glycogen synthetase and phosphorylase. Specifically, PBK converts phosphorylase from the less active b form to the more active a form while converting glycogen synthetase from a more active dephosphorylated form to a less active phosphorylated form.

Aldolase deficiency (type XII) was identified in a 4-year-old boy with exercise intolerance, mild weakness, developmental delay, hemolysis, and repeated episodes of rhabdomyolysis during febrile illnesses. The muscle biopsy did not reveal excess glycogen by histochemistry; however, it showed an isolated severe defect in aldolase activity by biochemical analysis (4% of normal). A homozygous point mutation was identified.

Glycogen Storage Diseases Primarily Affecting Skeletal Muscle

Myophosphorylase deficiency (McArdle's disease, type V), muscle phosphofructokinase (PFK, type VII) deficiency (Tarui's disease), phosphoglycerate kinase (PGK) deficiency (type IX), and lactate dehydrogenase (LDH) A deficiency (type XI) present with similar myopathic features: exercise intolerance with premature fatigue, myalgia, and cramps in exercising muscles that are relieved by rest. Symptoms are more likely to occur during intense isometric exercise (lifting heavy weights) or during less intense but sustained dynamic exercise, such as walking up stairs. Most patient experience a "second wind" phenomenon: If they slow down or rest briefly at the onset of symptoms, they can resume exercising at the original pace. Patients often experience acute muscle necrosis and myoglobinuria after exercise that, if severe, can cause acute renal failure. Some patients develop fixed weakness, which is more common in older patients. PFK deficiency can also cause a hemolytic anemia, jaundice, and gouty arthritis, which can be helpful in making the diagnosis. PGK deficiency can be clinically asymptomatic or may manifest as hemolytic anemia, seizures, and mental retardation with or without myopathy. Isolated myopathy with intolerance of vigorous exercise, cramps, and myoglobinuria has been reported in a few patients with PGK deficiency. Mutations in the genes encoding the enzymes have been identified in all four of these disorders.

DEFECTS OF LIPID METABOLISM

Lipids are the most important and efficient fuel source in the body. Fatty acids are particularly vital during periods of fasting because liver glycogen stores are depleted within a few hours of a meal. The fatty acids serve three major functions: Partial oxidation of fatty acids in the liver produces ketones, which are an important auxillary fuel for almost all tissues and especially the brain; fatty acids constitute a major energy source in cardiac and skeletal muscle, particularly during rest and during prolonged exercise; and ATP produced from fatty acid oxidation provides energy for gluconeogenesis and ureagenesis.

Carnitine Deficiency

L-Carnitine is a vital molecule for the transport of LCFA into mitochondria. Other physiological functions of L-carnitine include buffering of acyl-CoA/CoASH ratio, scavenging of potentially toxic acyl-CoA, and oxidation of branched-chain amino acids. Approximately 75% of L-carnitine is derived from dietary sources, whereas the rest is synthesized in liver and kidney. In contrast, 95% of the total body carnitine is stored in muscle.

Primary deficiencies of L-carnitine manifest in three phenotypic forms: dilated cardiomyopathy, myopathic with lipid storage, and hypoketoic hypoglycemia with recurrent encephalopathy. Patients frequently show overlapping phenotypes. The age at onset of symptoms ranges from 1 month to 7 years, with a mean of approximately 2 years. The dilated cardiomyopathy is progressive and ultimately fatal unless treated with L-carnitine supplementation. The myopathic form is the least common phenotype and is usually associated with a cardiomyopathy, encephalopathy, or both. The myopathy presents with motor delay, hypotonia, or slowly progressive proximal limb weakness. Acute metabolic encephalopathy is associated with hypoketotic hypoglycemia usually in younger infants. Typically, the episodes are triggered by intercurrent illnesses and stress complicated by recurrent vomiting and decreased oral intake. Persistent central nervous system signs can develop due to severe hypoglycemic encephalopathy and cardiac or respiratory arrest.

Laboratory studies can reveal low serum carnitine concentrations (usually less than 10% of normal) while the acyl-carnitine ester fraction is proportionally decreased. The diagnosis can be confirmed by documenting decreased carnitine uptake in cultured skin fibroblasts. Primary carnitine deficiency responds dramatically to oral L-carnitine therapy (daily doses of 100–200 mg/kg of body weight in divided doses). Although primary carnitine deficiencies are important to identify, secondary carnitine deficiencies are more common and are due to a variety of underlying defects. Causes of secondary carnitine deficiencies include defects of β-oxidation, malnutrition states, excessive carnitine loss (i.e., renal Fanconi syndrome), and valproic acid therapy that causes iatrogenic carnitine excretion.

Carnitine Palmitoyltransferase Deficiency

Mitochondria contain two CPTs that are vital in the transport of long-chain fatty acids into mitochondria. CPT I is located in the inner aspect of the outer mitochondrial membrane, and CPT II is bound to the inner mitochondrial membrane.

CPT I deficiency presents in infancy as attacks of fasting-induced, life-threatening hypoketotic hypoglycemia. The hypoglycemic episodes manifest as lethargy, coma, and seizures and may cause death. They may cause psychomotor developmental delay, hemiplegia, or generalized epilepsy. Myopathy is not a typical manifestation but has been reported. The diagnosis is confirmed by demonstrating decreased CPT I activity in cultured fibroblasts, leukocytes, or hepatocytes. However, CPT I activity is normal in skeletal muscle, accounting for the absence of clinical myopathy. Two tissue-specific isoforms of CPT I exist: liver and muscle. Mutations in the liver isoform have been reported.

CPT II deficiency, in contrast to CPT I deficiency, has variable clinical manifestations. Three forms of CPT II deficiency have been described: infantile, late infantile, and adult. The early infantile phenotype is rare and presents at birth with severe hypoketotic hypoglycemia and generalized steatosis, and it usually causes death within a few days. Multiple organ malformations are often present. The late-infantile hepatomuscular form is clinically similar to CPT I deficiency, with acute episodic fasting hypoglycemia and hypoketosis, lethargy, coma, and death. Seizures, hepatomegaly, cardiomegaly, arrhythmias, and pancreatitis have been described. In both infantile forms, CPT II activity is less than 10% of normal.

The adult form of CPT II deficiency is a common cause of exercise-induced myoglobinuria. The disorder typically presents in young adulthood with complaints of muscle pain and pigmenturia after prolonged exercise. Severe bouts of rhabomyolysis with myoglobinuria can cause acute renal failure. Some infants have presented with acute muscle breakdown induced by fever. Adult patients may also have acute rhabomyolysis precipitated by fever or other stress. Lipid storage cardiomyopathy has also been reported. CPT activity is less than 30% of normal. Mutations in the CPT II gene have been identified.

β-Oxidation Defects

The breakdown of fatty acids in the mitochondria requires two distinct but linked systems: the inner mitochondrial membrane portion, which metabolizes long-chain acyl-CoA, and the matrix β-oxidation spiral, which acts on medium- and short-chain acyl-CoA.

β-Oxidation Defects of the Inner Mitochondrial Membrane System: Very long-chain acyl-CoA dehydrogenase (VLCAD) deficiency presents in infancy with hypoketotic hypoglycemia, hepatic steatosis, cardiomyopathy, and elevated plasma levels of long-chain acylcarnitines. Metabolic acidosis, dicarboxylic aciduria, and increased serum CK with myoglobinuria have also been noted. Mutations in the VLCAD gene have been identified.

Trifunctional protein (TP) is a multienzyme complex with three functions, as the name implies: long-chain 3-hydroxy-acyl-CoA dehydrogenase (LCHAD), enoyl-CoA hydratase, and 3-ketoacyl-CoA thiolase. Most patients with TP defects have isolate LCHAD deficiency, whereas a small number of individuals have a combined defect of all three enzymes. The clinical features of LCHAD deficiency include infantile onset; Reye's-like episodes; hypoketotic hypoglycemia with hepatic dysfunction; progressive myopathy, recurrent myoglobinuria, or both; cardiomyopathy; and sudden infant death syndrome.

Treatment of patients with inner mitochondrial membrane defects of fatty acid metabolism includes dietary therapy. Specifically, patients should avoid long periods of fasting and long-chain fatty acids. They should be treated with intravenous glucose during acute intercurrent illnesses.

β-Oxidation Defects of the Mitochondrial Matrix System: The mitochondrial β-oxidation matrix system shortens the fatty acid backbone of acyl-CoA by two carbon fragments during each turn of the β-oxidation spiral. In this process, acetyl-CoA is produced and is a substrate for the Krebs cycle. In addition, electron transfer flavoprotein (ETF) is reduced. The reduced ETF provides reducing equivalents to the oxidative phosphorylation pathway. Human diseases can be caused by defects in several steps in these mitochondrial matrix proteins.

Defects of long-chain, medium-chain, and short-chain acyl-CoA dehydrogenases present in infancy.

Medium-chain acyl-CoA dehydrogenase (MCAD) is the most frequent defect of β-oxidation. MCAD typically begins in the first 2 years of life with fasting intolerance, nausea, vomiting, hypoketotic hypoglycemia, lethargy, and coma; however, clinical expression is variable and some patients are asymptomatic. MCAD activity in most tissues (fibroblasts, lymphocytes, and liver) is low (2–20% of normal). Early diagnosis and treatment can lead to good long-term outcome. Dietary therapy is aimed at avoidance of fasting and adequate caloric intake. LCAD deficiency and short-chain acyl-CoA dehydrogenase (SCAD) deficiency have been documented in only a few patients.

Multiple acyl-CoA dehydrogenase deficiency (MAD) or glutaric aciduria type II is a clinical syndrome characterized by metabolic acidosis, hypoketotic hypoglycemia, strong, sweaty feet odor, and early death. There are three distinct clinical presentations of MAD deficiency: a severe neonatal form with congenital abnormalities; a severe neonatal form without congenital abnormalities; and a mild, late-onset form. The biochemical abnormality is decreased activities of various acyl-CoA dehydrogenases with urinary excretion of large amounts of numerous organic acids. The three defects that lead to MAD deficiency are ETF deficiency, ETF–coenzyme Q oxidoreductase deficiency, and riboflavin (B$_2$) responsive MAD.

MITOCHONDRIAL RESPIRATORY CHAIN DEFECTS

Mitochondria are unique mammalian organelles because they possess their own genetic material, mitochondrial DNA (mtDNA), which is a small (16.5 kilobases), circular molecule. Each mtDNA encodes 22 transfer RNAs (tRNA), 13 polypeptides, and two ribosomal RNAs. The mtDNA-encoded polypeptides are functionally important because they are subunits of the respiratory or electron transport chain. However, the vast majority of the mitochondrial proteins are encoded in the nuclear DNA (nDNA). Thus, mitochondria are the products of two genomes. Defects in either genome can cause mitochondrial dysfunction. To date, most of the respiratory chain defects that have been characterized at the molecular genetic level are due to mtDNA mutations; however, the number of identified nDNA mutations is growing rapidly.

An important principle of mtDNA genetics is heteroplasmy. Each mitochondrion contains 2–10 copies of mtDNA; in turn, each cell contains multiple mitochondria. Therefore, there are numerous copies of mtDNA in each cell. Alterations of mtDNA may be present in some of the mtDNA molecules (heteroplasmy) or in all of the molecules (homoplasmy). As a consequence of heteroplasmy, the proportion of a deleterious mtDNA mutation can vary widely. An individual who harbors a large proportion of mutant mtDNA will be more severely afflicted by the mitochondrial dysfunction than a person with a low percentage of the same mutation; therefore, there is a spectrum of clinical severity among patients with a given mitochondrial mutation.

A second factor that can influence the expression of a mtDNA mutation in a person is the tissue distribution of the mutation. The best example of tissue distribution variation is large-scale mtDNA deletions. Infants with a high proportion of deleted mtDNA in blood can develop Pearson's syndrome of sideroblastic anemia often accompanied by exocrine pancreatic dysfunction. Presumably, these infants have a high proportion of deleted mtDNA in the bone marrow stem cells. Some children survive the anemia with blood transfusions and subsequently recover because the stem cells with a high proportion of deleted mtDNA are under a negative selection bias. Later in life, however, these children may develop the multisystem mitochondrial disorder Kearns–Sayre syndrome (KSS), characterized by ophthalmoplegia, pigmentary retinopathy, and cardiac conduction block. Thus, variable tissue distribution broadens the clinical spectrum of pathogenic mtDNA mutations.

The third factor that determines clinical manifestations of a mtDNA mutation is tissue threshold effect. Cells with high metabolic activities are severely and adversely affected by mtDNA mutations; therefore, these disorders tend to disproportionately affect brain and muscle (encephalomyopathies).

A fourth unusual characteristic of mtDNA is maternal inheritance. During the formation of the zygote, the mtDNA is derived exclusively from the oocyte. Thus, mtDNA is transmitted vertically in a non-Mendelian fashion from the mother to both male and female progeny. This inheritance pattern is important to recognize in determining whether a family is likely to harbor a mtDNA mutation. A caveat to this principle is the fact that maternal relatives who have a lower percentage of a mtDNA mutation may have fewer symptoms (oligosymptomatic) than the proband or they may even be asymptomatic. Therefore, in taking the family history, it is important to ask about the presence of subtle symptoms or signs in maternally related family members who might be oligosymptomatic.

These peculiar features of "mitochondrial genetics" contribute to the clinical complexity of human mitochondrial disorders. Variable heteroplasmy of mtDNA mutations produces an extensive range of disease severity, whereas tissue distribution and tissue threshold of mtDNA mutations explain the frequent but variable involvement of multiple organ systems. In addition to mtDNA mutations, nDNA defects can also cause mitochondrial dysfunction. In fact, nDNA encodes most of the electron transport chain components, and recently the first nDNA mutation associated with a defect in oxidative phosphorylation was identified. Finally, a third group of genetic mitochondrial disorders includes defects of intergenomic communication due to mutations of nDNA genes regulating replication and expression of the mitochondrial genome.

Mitochondrial DNA Mutations

The mitochondrial encephalomyopathies comprise a heterogeneous group of multisystem disorders. The discovery of distinct mtDNA mutations demonstrated that, in general, clinical phenotypes have specific genotypes; however, some patients do not fit the description of any clinical syndrome or have an atypical presentation for a particular mtDNA mutation. Clinicians often encounter patients who are suspected of having a mitochondrial encephalomyopathy; therefore, clinical classification of the mitochondrial disorders is of pragmatic significance in guiding the diagnostic evaluation and in directing the therapy.

Rowland and colleagues defined KSS by the obligate triad of ophthalmoplegia, pigmentary retinopathy, and onset before age 20, with at least one of the following features: cardiac conduction block, ataxia, and cerebrospinal fluid protein >100. Approximately 90% of KSS patients have single large-scale rearrangements of the mtDNA—deletions, duplications, or both. Typically, KSS patients are sporadic because the mtDNA rearrangements seem to originate in oogenesis or early zygote formation.

In contrast to KSS, myoclonus epilepsy ragged-red fibers (MERRF) syndrome is maternally inherited. The disease is clinically defined by seizures, myoclonus, ataxia, and ragged-red fibers in the muscle biopsy. Other common clinical manifestations associated with MERRF are hearing loss, dementia,

peripheral neuropathy, short stature, exercise intolerance, lipomas, and lactic acidosis. Although the majority of MERRF patients have a history of affected maternally related family members, not all have the full syndrome. An A-to-G transition mutation at nucleotide 8344 (A8344G) of the mtDNA tRNA^{Lys} gene has been found in approximately 90% of MERRF patients tested. Within families with an MERRF proband, oligosymptomatic and asymptomatic members harbor the same mtDNA mutation, but the phenotype is presumably attenuated by heteroplasmy and tissue distribution of the mtDNA mutation.

Mitochondrial encephalomyopathy, lactic acidosis, and stroke-like episodes (MELAS) syndrome is another maternally inherited disorder whose defining clinical features include stroke-like episodes at a young age (typically before age 40); encephalopathy manifest as seizures, dementia, or both; and mitochondrial dysfunction with lactic acidosis, ragged-red fibers, or both. In addition, to secure the diagnosis, at least two of the following clinical features should be present: normal early development, recurrent headaches, or recurrent vomiting. Other commonly encountered manifestations include myopathic weakness, exercise intolerance, myoclonus, ataxia, short stature, and hearing loss. It is uncommon for more than one family member to have the full MELAS syndrome; in most pedigrees, there is only one MELAS patient with oligosymptomatic or asymptomatic relatives in the maternal lineage. A mutation in the tRNA$^{Leu(UUR)}$ gene (A3243G) has been identified in approximately 80% of MELAS patients.

In addition to these three phenotypes, many other clinical syndromes are associated with oxidative phosphorylation defects. Despite the complexity and the heterogeneity of mitochondrial disorders, there are several clinical themes common to all. First, the disorders tend to affect children and young adults. Second, the syndromes are often multisystemic. Third, maternal inheritance is pathognomonic of mtDNA point mutations, whereas patients with single large-scale rearrangements tend to be sporadic. Fourth, there is great variability of phenotypic expression in families with mtDNA point mutations.

Nuclear DNA Mutations

The first nDNA causing a mitochondrial respiratory chain defect was described in 1994 and 1995 in a pair of siblings with Leigh syndrome who were found to have compound heterozygous mutations in the flavoprotein subunit of complex II. Since then, additional mutations encoding subunits of complexes I and II have been identified in a small number of patients mainly with Leigh syndrome. Curiously, sequencing of genes encoding complex IV (COX) subunits have not revealed mutations. However, defects have been identified in three different genes involved in COX assembly: *SURF1*, *SCO2*, and *COX10*. *SURF1* mutations have been associated with Leigh syndrome, whereas patients with *SCO2* mutations had Leigh-like features with a severe hypertrophic cardiomyopathy. The patient with a homozygous mutations in the *COX10* gene had a multisystem disorder characterized by encephalopathy, myopathy, and renal tubulopathy. These mutations are likely the tip of the iceberg of nuclear mutations causing mitochondrial myopathies.

Intergenomic Communication

A growing number of autosomal diseases have been associated with mtDNA depletion and multiple deletions. These disorders are thought to disrupt the normal cross-talk that regulated the integrity and quantity of mtDNA. Autosomal dominant progressive external ophthalmoplegia with multiple mtDNA deletions was the first of these disorders to be identified. MtDNA depletion syndrome was originally reported in infants with severe hepatopathy or myopathy. Mitochondrial neurogastrointestinal encephalomyopathy was the first disease of intergenomic communication to be molecularly defined. This autosomal recessive disorder is associated with depletion and multiple deletions of mtDNA and is due to mutations in the gene encoding thymidine phosphorylase, a cytosolic enzyme that is thought to contribute to the regulation of nucleotide pools in the mitochondria. The identification of additional genetic causes of intergenomic communication defects will likely provide insight into the normal dialogue between the two genomes.

CONCLUSION

Metabolic myopathies comprise a diverse group of disorders that are related to energy metabolism. Many of these diseases have been well characterized at the biochemical level, and molecular genetics studies are rapidly revealing the specific etiologies. Our expanding knowledge in this field will enhance our scientific understanding and, it is hoped, will translate into therapies for patients with these devastating diseases.

—*Michio Hirano*

See also—Carnitine Deficiency; Glycogen Storage Diseases; Mitochondrial Encephalomyopathies, Overview; Mitochondrial Encephalopathy, Lactic Acidosis and Stroke (MELAS); Myopathy, Congenital; Myopathy, Endocrine; Myopathy, Overview; Myopathy, Toxic; Respiratory Chain Disorders

Further Reading

Di Donato, S. (1997). Diseases associated with defects of beta oxidation. In *The Molecular and Genetic Basis of Neurological Disease* (R. N. Rosenberg, S. B. Prusiner, S. DiMauro, and R. L. Barchi, Eds.), 2nd ed., pp. 939–956. Butterworth-Heinemann, Boston.

DiMauro, S., and Andreu, A. (2000). Mutations in mtDNA: Are we scraping the bottom of the barrel? *Brain Pathol.* 10, 431–441.

DiMauro, S., and Bonilla, E. (1997). Mitochondrial encephalomyopathies. In *The Molecular and Genetic Basis of Neurological Disease* (R. N. Rosenberg, S. B. Prusiner, S. DiMauro, and R. L. Barchi, Eds.), 2nd ed., pp. 201–235. Butterworth-Heinemann, Boston.

DiMauro, S., Servidei, S., and Tsujino, S. (1997). Disorders of carbohydrate metabolism: Glycogen storage diseases. In *The Molecular and Genetic Basis of Neurological Disease* (R. N. Rosenberg, S. B. Prusiner, S. DiMauro, and R. L. Barchi, Eds.), 2nd ed., pp. 1067–1097. Butterworth-Heinemann, Boston.

Hirano, M., and Vu, T. H. (2000). Defects of intergenomic communication: Where do we stand? *Brain Pathol.* 10, 451–461.

Sue, C. M., and Schon, E. A. (2000). Mutations in nuclear DNA: A promising start. *Brain Pathol.* 10, 442–450.

Myopathy, Overview

Encyclopedia of the Neurological Sciences
Copyright 2003, Elsevier Science (USA). All rights reserved.

MYOPATHIES are diseases of skeletal muscle in which there is a primary structural or functional impairment of muscle. Myopathies can be differentiated from other disorders of the motor unit by characteristic clinical and laboratory findings. In addition, the disorders of muscles can be categorized and subdivided so that it is generally possible to characterize a particular myopathy based on its distinctive features. Myopathies can be broadly classified into hereditary and acquired disorders (Table 1).

CLINICAL ASSESSMENT

The most important aspect of evaluating a patient with a myopathy is the information obtained from the history. After taking the history, the physician

Table 1   CLASSIFICATION OF MYOPATHIES

Hereditary
   Muscular dystrophies
   Myotonias and channelopathies
   Congenital myopathies
   Metabolic myopathies
   Mitochondrial myopathies
Acquired
   Inflammatory myopathies
   Endocrine myopathies
   Myopathies associated with other systemic illness
   Drug-induced/toxic myopathies

should have a reasonable preliminary diagnosis that places the patient into one of the categories in Table 2. The findings on the physical examination, particularly the pattern of weakness, help to further determine the diagnosis. The results of the laboratory studies (blood tests, electromyogram, muscle biopsy, and molecular studies) serve to confirm the preliminary diagnosis arrived at from the history and physical examination.

History

Symptoms of muscle disease can be classified as negative, due to loss of function, and positive, due to new additional function complaints.

Negative Symptoms: Weakness, a loss of muscle strength, is the most common symptom of a patient with muscle disease. If the weakness is in the legs, patients will complain of difficulty climbing stairs, rising from a low chair or toilet, or rising from the floor. When the arms are involved, patients notice trouble lifting objects (especially over their heads) and washing or brushing their hair. These symptoms in the arms and legs indicate proximal muscle weakness, which is probably the most common site of weakness in a myopathic disorder. Rarely, patients with myopathies may complain of poor handgrip (difficulty opening jar tops and turning doorknobs) or tripping due to ankle weakness from distal muscle weakness. Some myopathies involve "proximal" cranial muscles and patients complain of a change in speech (dysarthria) or swallowing (dysphagia) and droopy eyelids (ptosis).

It is important to determine the tempo of the weakness. Patients should be asked if the weakness is present all of the time or if it is intermittent. Myopathies can present with either constant weakness (muscular dystrophies and inflammatory myopathies) or episodic periods of weakness with normal

strength interictally (periodic paralysis due to channelopathies or metabolic myopathies due to certain glycolytic pathway disorders). Muscle disorders can have acute (less than 4 weeks), subacute (4–8 weeks), or chronic (more than 8 weeks) periods over which time the weakness evolves. The episodic disorders have acute weakness that can return to normal strength within hours or days. The tempo of the disorders with constant weakness can vary from (i) acute or subacute in some inflammatory myopathies (dermatomyositis and polymyositis) to (ii) chronic slow progression over years (most muscular dystrophies) or (iii) fixed weakness with little change over decades (congenital myopathies). Finally, both constant and episodic myopathic disorders can have symptoms that may be monophasic or relapsing. For example, a myositis can occasionally have an acute monophasic course and return to normal strength within weeks or months. Patients with channelopathies or metabolic myopathies can have recurrent attacks of weakness over many years, whereas a patient with acute rhabdomyolysis due to a toxin such as cocaine may have a single episode.

Although weakness may be the most reliable negative symptom of a patient with a myopathy, many patients who complain of diffuse global "weakness" or fatigue (lack of stamina) do not have a disorder of muscle, particularly if the neurological examination is normal. Fatigue is a nonspecific symptom. On the other hand, abnormal fatigability after exercise can result from certain metabolic and mitochondrial myopathies and it is important to define the duration and intensity of exercise that provokes it.

Positive Symptoms: Muscle pain (myalgia) is another nonspecific symptom of some myopathies. Myalgias may be episodic (metabolic myopathies) or

Table 2   CLUES FROM THE PHYSICAL EXAMINATION TO DIAGNOSIS OF MYOPATHIES

Distribution of weakness
   Proximal—limb–girdle
   Proximal arms/distal legs—scapuloperoneal
   Proximal (quadriceps) legs/distal (finger and wrist flexors) arms—inclusion body myositis
   Distal—distal myopathy
   Ocular and/or pharyngeal
   Neck extensors
Atrophy or enlargement
Myotonia or stiffness

nearly constant (inflammatory muscle disorders). However, muscle pain is usually not common in most muscle diseases and pain is more likely to be due to bone or joint disorders. It is rare for a muscle disease to be responsible for vague aches and discomfort in muscle regions in the presence of a normal neurological examination and laboratory studies.

A specific category of pain is the involuntary muscle cramp. Cramps are usually localized to a particular muscle region and last from seconds to minutes. They are usually benign, occurring in normal individuals, and do not reflect an underlying disease process and, in particular, are seldom a feature of a primary myopathy. Cramps can occur with dehydration, hyponatremia, azotemia, myxedema, and in disorders of the motor neuron (especially amyotrophic lateral sclerosis) or nerve.

Muscle contractures are uncommon but can superficially resemble a cramp. They usually last longer than cramps and are provoked by exercise in patients with glycolytic enzyme defects. They can be distinguished from cramps with needle electromyography: Contractures are electrically silent, whereas cramps are associated with rapid-firing motor unit discharges.

Myotonia is the phenomenon of impaired relaxation of muscle after forceful voluntary contraction. Patients can complain of muscle stiffness or persistent contraction in almost any muscle group, particularly involving the hands and eyelids. They will note difficulty releasing their handgrip after a handshake, unscrewing a bottle top, or turning a doorknob. They have difficulty opening their eyelids if they shut their eyes forcefully. The myotonia improves with repeated exercise, the so-called warm-up phenomenon. Paramyotonia is the paradoxical occurrence of exercise making the myotonia worse. Myotonia is due to repetitive depolarization of the muscle membrane. Exposure to cold makes myotonia and paramyotonia worse.

If a patient complains of exercise-induced weakness and myalgias, they should be asked if their urine has ever turned dark or red during or after these episodes, indicating myoglobinuria. Myoglobinuria follows excessive release of myoglobin from muscle during periods of rapid muscle destruction (rhabdomyolysis).

Other crucial points in the history concern the age at onset of symptoms. Did the weakness (or other symptoms) first manifest at birth or was onset in the first, second, third, etc., decade? Identifying the age at which symptoms began can provide important clues to the diagnosis. For example, of the muscular dystrophies, symptoms in Duchenne's dystrophy usually are noted by age 3, whereas most facioscapaulohumeral and limb–girdle dystrophies begin in adolescence or later. Disorders such as myotonic dystrophy and oculopharyngeal dystrophy may not become symptomatic until middle age or later. Of the inflammatory myopathies, dermatomyositis occurs in children and adults, polymyositis rarely occurs in children but in any decade in the adult years, and inclusion body myositis is a myositis of the elderly.

The family history is obviously of great importance in correctly diagnosing the hereditary myopathies. A detailed family tree should be completed to search for autosomal dominant, recessive, and X-linked patterns of transmission. Identifying a particular hereditary pattern can not only help in correctly diagnosing the disorder but also is of importance regarding genetic counseling.

Finally, precipitating factors should be explored in the history. Is the patient taking legal or illegal drugs or exposed to toxins that can produce a myopathy? Does exercise provoke attacks of weakness, pain, or urine discoloration, raising the possibility of a glycolytic pathway defect? Do episodes of weakness precede or occur in association with a fever, a feature of carnitine palmitoyltransferase deficiency? Does the ingestion of a carbohydrate meal precede an attack of weakness, suggesting a periodic paralysis? Does cold exposure precipitate muscle stiffness, a characteristic finding in myotonic myopathies?

Signs on Neurological Examination

In order to determine if a particular muscle group is weak, it is important to know what muscles to test and how to grade the power at the bedside. In examining the upper limbs, it is necessary to assess shoulder abduction, adduction, and external and internal rotation; elbow flexion and extension; wrist flexion and extension; and finger and thumb extension, flexion, and abduction. Muscle groups that should be tested in the lower extremities include hip flexion, extension, abduction, and adduction; knee flexion and extension; ankle dorsiflexion, plantar flexion, inversion, and eversion; and toe extension and flexion. Neck flexors should be assessed in the supine and neck extensors in the prone positions. Finally, cranial nerve muscles such as eye lids, extraocular muscles controlling eye movements, upper and lower facial muscles of expression, tongue, and palate should be examined. All muscle groups should be tested bilaterally, preferably against gravity. Knee extension and hip flexion should be tested in the seated position, knee flexion should be tested prone, and abduction should be tested in the lateral decubitus position. If testing against gravity is not done, the presence of significant muscle weakness can escape recognition.

Assessment of muscle strength is usually based on the Medical Research Council of Great Britain (MRC) grading scale of 0 to 5:

- 5—normal power
- 4—active movement against gravity and resistance
- 3—active movement against gravity
- 2—active movement only with gravity eliminated
- 1—trace contraction
- 0—no contraction

In addition to manual muscle testing, muscles should be inspected for atrophy or hypertrophy. Atrophy of proximal limb muscles is common in long-standing myopathies. However, certain myopathies have atrophy in specific groups that correspond to severe weakness in those muscles and can be a clue to the diagnosis. Atrophy around the periscapular muscles may be associated with scapular winging. Selective atrophy of the quadriceps muscles and forearm flexor muscles is highly suggestive of inclusion body myositis. Distal myopathies may have profound atrophy in anterior or posterior lower leg compartments. Muscles can become diffusely hypertrophic in some myotonic conditions such as myotonia congenita. Muscle hypertrophy can also occur in disorders such as amyloidosis and sarcoidosis and hypothyroid myopathy. In Duchenne's and Becker's dystrophy, the calves can become enlarged, but this usually reflects pseudohypertrophy of the muscle due to replacement with connective tissue and fat. Focal muscle enlargement can be due to a neoplastic or inflammatory process, ectopic ossification, or tendon rupture. Rarely, partial denervation of various causes can produce focal muscle hypertrophy.

Musculoskeletal contractures can occur in many myopathies of a long-standing duration. However, contractures developing early in the course of the disease, especially at the elbows, can be a clue to Emery–Dreifuss dystrophy and Bethlem myopathy.

Muscle twitches or fasciculations can be noted on inspection. However, fasciculations are generally not a manifestation of a muscle disease but occur in the setting of denervation or as a benign process.

It is important to observe the patient performing functional activities. Watch the patient walking to look for a wide-based waddling gait with hyperlordosis, which is a sign of pelvic muscle weakness; rising from a chair, from a squat, or from a seated position on the floor (Gower's sign); or climbing stairs, noting whether there is a need to use the arms, another sign of proximal weakness in the lower extremities. The inability to walk on the heels or toes can indicate weakness in the anterior and posterior distal leg muscles, respectively. Observe the patient talk and smile to determine if there is facial weakness. Is there the so-called "horizontal smile" indicating lower facial muscle weakness? Is the patient unable to close his or her eyes completely when asked to do so, indicating upper facial muscle weakness? Are the upper eyelids drooping so that they touch the pupil, indicating ptosis? Is the speech hypernasal, indicating pharyngeal muscle involvement?

Finally, if the patient complains of muscle stiffness, the physician should attempt to elicit myotonia. This can be done by asking the patient to squeeze the examiner's finger and then observe for the patient's inability to relax the handgrip. Additionally, the muscles can be directly percussed with a reflex hammer. Observe for a slow, persistent contraction and delayed relaxation. The muscles that can be most easily percussed to search for myotonia are the thenar and wrist/finger extensor muscle groups. Facial myotonia can also be observed after forceful voluntary eye closure. The patient will be unable to easily open their eyes after this maneuver.

Other aspects of the neurological examination need to be assessed in all potential myopathy patients to ensure that they are not involved. The sensory examination should be normal in muscle disease. Reflexes are usually preserved early in the disease process. Once the myopathy is advanced and the muscles are extremely weak, reflexes can become hypoactive or unelicitable.

Patterns of Weakness

Once the muscles have been inspected, tested for power, and functional activity has been observed, an attempt should be made to place the patient in one of the patterns of muscle weakness that can occur in myopathic disorders. The various patterns of muscle weakness can be divided into six broad groups:

1. The most common pattern of muscle disease is weakness that is exclusively or predominantly in proximal muscles of the legs and arms, or the

so-called limb–girdle distribution. Neck flexor and extensor muscles can also be affected. This pattern of weakness can be seen in many hereditary and acquired myopathies and therefore is the least specific in arriving at a particular diagnosis. It is not known why most myopathic disorders selectively involve proximal muscles.

2. *The pattern of distal weakness in the upper extremities or lower extremities (anterior or posterior compartment muscle groups) (Table 3):* Selective weakness and atrophy in distal extremity muscles is more often a feature of neuropathies but is uncommonly due to a primary muscle disease. When this pattern of weakness is determined to be due to a myopathic rather than a neuropathic disorder, a diagnosis of distal myopathy is appropriate.

3. *The pattern of proximal upper extremity weakness of the periscapular muscles and distal lower extremity weakness of the anterior compartment—the scapuloperoneal pattern (Table 3):* The scapular muscle weakness is

Table 3   MYOPATHIES THAT CAN HAVE PROMINENT DISTAL WEAKNESS

Late adult-onset distal myopathy type 1 (Welander)
Late adult-onset distal myopathy type 2 (Markesbery/Udd)
Early adult-onset distal myopathy type 1 (Nonaka)
Early adult-onset distal myopathy type 2 (Miyoshi)
Early adult-onset distal myopathy type 3 (Laing)
Desmin myopathy
Childhood-onset distal myopathy
Infantile onset (before age 2)
Juvenile onset (before age 15)
Myotonic dystrophy
Facioscapulohumeral dystrophy[a]
Scapuloperoneal myopathy[a]
Oculopharyngeal dystrophy
Emery–Dreifuss humeroperonal dystrophy[a]
Inflammatory myopathies
  Inclusion body myositis
  Polymyositis
Metabolic myopathy
  Debrancher deficiency
  Acid-maltase deficiency[a]
Congenital myopathy
  Nemaline myopathy[a]
  Central core myopathy[a]
  Centronuclear myopathy
Nephropathic cystinosis

[a] Scapuloperoneal pattern can occur.

Table 4   MYOPATHIES WITH PTOSIS OR OPHTHALMOPLEGIA

Ptosis usually without ophthalmoplegia
  Myotonic dystrophy
  Congenital myopathies
    Centronuclear myopathy
    Nemaline myopathy
    Central core myopathy
  Desmin storage myopathy
Ptosis with ophthalmoplegia
  Oculopharyngeal muscular dystrophy
  Oculopharyngodistal myopathy
  Chronic progressive external ophthalmoplegia (mitochondrial myopathy)

usually accompanied by scapular winging. When this pattern is associated with facial weakness, it is highly suggestive of facioscapulohmeral dystrophy. Other hereditary myopathies can be associated with a scapuloperoneal syndrome—for example, scapuloperoneal dystrophy, Emery–Dreifuss dystrophy, congenital myopathies, and acid maltase deficiency.

4. *The pattern of distal upper extremity weakness in the distal forearm muscles (wrist and finger flexors) and proximal lower extremity weakness involving the knee extensors (quadriceps):* This pattern is essentially pathognomonic for inclusion body myositis. In addition, the weakness is often asymmetric between the two sides, which is uncommon in most myopathies.

5. *Predominant involvement of ocular or pharyngeal muscles (Table 4):* The combination of ptosis, ophthalmoplegia without diplopia, and pharyngeal weakness should suggest the diagnosis of oculopharyngeal dystrophy, especially if the onset is in middle age or later. Ptosis and ophthalmoplegia without prominent pharyngeal involvement is a hallmark of many of the mitochondrial myopathies. Ptosis and facial weakness without ophthalmoplegia or pharyngeal weakness is a common feature of myotonic dystrophy and facioscapulohumeral dystrophy. Patients with ocular or pharyngeal involvement can also have the typical pattern of limb–girdle weakness.

6. *Prominent neck extensor weakness:* Some myopathic conditions have a dramatic degree of weakness of the neck extensor muscles. The term dropped head syndrome has been used in this situation (Table 5). The neck flexors may or may not be weak. Significant neck extensor weakness occurs in the setting of a myopathy

Table 5 MYOPATHIES AND OTHER NEUROMUSCULAR CONDITIONS WITH PROMINENT NECK EXTENSOR WEAKNESS

Myopathies
Isolated neck extensor myopathy
   Polymyositis
   Dermatomyositis
   Inclusion body myositis
   Carnitine deficiency
   Facioscapulomumeral dystrophy
   Myotonic dystrophy
   Congenital myopathy
   Hyperparathyroidism
Other neuromuscular disorders
   Myasthenia gravis
   Amyotrophic lateral sclerosis

that also has one of the previously outlined phenotypic patterns. For example, a patient with a limb–girdle pattern of weakness may also have significant neck extensor involvement. However, occasionally isolated neck extensor myopathy may occur as a distinct muscle disorder. Prominent neck extensor weakness is common in two other neuromuscular diseases—amyotrophic lateral sclerosis and myasthenia gravis.

Although these six patterns of myopathy have limitations, they are useful in narrowing the differential diagnosis. Other neuromuscular diseases can also present with one of these weakness patterns. For example, although proximal more than distal weakness is most often seen in a myopathy, patients with acquired demyelinating neuropathies (Guillain–Barré syndrome and chronic inflammatory demyelinating polyneuropathy) often have proximal as well as distal muscle involvement. Demyelinating neuropathies will have sensory and reflex loss. Ocular, pharyngeal, and proximal limb weakness is a frequent feature of neuromuscular junction transmission disorders such as myasthenia gravis. However, these patients will also have diplopia, weakness that fluctuates, and additional laboratory features that will lead to the correct diagnosis.

Associated Organ Involvement or Systemic Illness

Involvement of organs or tissues other than muscle can provide additional diagnostic clues. Cardiac disease can be associated with myotonic dystrophy, a dystrophinopathy, Emery–Dreifuss dystrophy, and certain types of periodic paralysis. Hepatomegaly can occur in sarcoidosis and in the myopathies associated with deficiencies of acid maltase, debranching enzyme, and carnitine. Intrinsic pulmonary involvement can be seen in some of the inflammatory myopathies and sarcoidosis. Evidence of a diffuse systemic disorder can indicate a collagen–vascular disease, amyloidosis, sarcoidosis, endocrine myopathies, or mitochondrial disorders.

LABORATORY STUDIES FOR THE EVALUATION OF MYOPATHY

Serum Enzymes of Muscle Origin

Creatine kinase (CK) occurs in high concentration in the sarcoplasm of skeletal and cardiac muscle. The MM isoenzyme of CK predominates in skeletal muscle, MB occurs primarily in cardiac muscle, and BB is mainly in brain. When skeletal muscle is injured, CK can leak into the blood. Therefore, an elevated serum CK occurs in many muscle diseases. However, the absence of an elevated serum CK does not rule out a myopathy. In addition, the elevation of serum CK does not necessarily imply a primary myopathic disorder. CK is often elevated in normal individuals for days after strenuous voluntary exercise. Involuntary prolonged muscle contraction from a motor seizure can elevate CK. Serum CK is above the normal range in some African individuals, in individuals with large muscles, and after minor muscle trauma [e.g., electromyogaphy (EMG)]. Finally, other neuromuscular disorders such as motor neuron disease can produce a moderate increases in CK (usually less than 1000 IU/liter). Serum CK is normal in peripheral neuropathies and neuromuscular junction disorders.

Other enzymes that can be released from injured skeletal muscle include aspartate aminotransferase (AST), alanine aminotransferase (ALT), and lactate dehydrogenase. Serum CK is the most sensitive for muscle disease and it is rarely necessary to measure for these other enzymes in the evaluation of a myopathy. Enzymes such as AST and ALT are elevated in hepatic disease. Since AST and ALT are often measured in large screening chemistry panels, their elevation should prompt CK measurement to determine if the source is muscle or liver. If a patient with an inflammatory myopathy is treated with a drug that may have hepatotoxicity as a side effect, it is not sufficient measure ALT and AST; the liver-specific enzyme γ-glutamic transferase should be followed.

In general, CK isoenzymes are not helpful in evaluating myopathies. CK-MM elevations are typical of muscle disease, but CK-MB is also elevated in myopathies and does not indicate that cardiac disease is present.

Needle EMG

Abnormal Needle EMG Activity at Rest: In a normal individual, there is no recorded electrical activity from a muscle when it is at rest. Electrical activity at rest is abnormal. Spontaneous rhythmic discharges of a single muscle fiber called fibrillation or positive sharp waves occur when there has been a disconnection between the nerve and the muscle it innervates. Fibrillations are seen most often in nerve diseases but can occur in active myopathies. For example, if a muscle fiber becomes injured due to an inflammatory myopathy, it can lose its connection with the nerve terminal and fibrillate. The finding of fibrillation potentials at rest in a patient suspected of a myopathy usually indicates active, ongoing muscle fiber degeneration. Since a fibrillation represents the discharge of a single muscle fiber, it cannot be detected on clinical examination but can only be observed on needle EMG.

Myotonia is another abnormal spontaneous discharge of muscle that occurs in the same myopathies, such as myotonic dystrophy, myotonia congenita, periodic paralysis, and acid maltase deficiency. On EMG, myotonia consists of high-frequency repetitive discharges that spontaneously increase and decrease in amplitude and frequency, and it has the sound of a dive-bomber or motorcycle. It represents repeated muscle fiber depolarization due to an irritable muscle membrane. Myotonic discharges can accompany clinical myotonia or can be subclinical. Myotonia almost always indicates a myopathy but is rarely present in neuropathic disorders. A third spontaneous electrical phenomenon, the complex repetitive discharge, is usually the result of nerve disease but occasionally is observed in myopathies. The complex repetitive discharge differs from myotonia in that it starts and stops abruptly and does not wax and wane in frequency and amplitude. It sounds like a jackhammer.

Fasciculations are to be distinguished from fibrillations and myotonia. A fasciculation represents a spontaneous discharge of a motor unit, which is a group of muscle fibers of the same histochemical type under the control of a single anterior horn cell and thus innervated by the same axon. These can be observed clinically as a small muscle twitch or movement. Electrically, a fasciculation is a large-amplitude potential that consists of the simultaneous involuntary depolarization of a group of muscle fibers. Although they do not necessarily imply neuromuscular disease and occur in many normal patients, fasciculations can occur in diseases of the motor neuron or nerve. Neither clinical nor electrical fasciculations are a feature of muscle disorders.

Activity with Movement: When the patient voluntarily contracts the muscle, individual motor unit action potentials are assessed. Motor units are normally triphasic potentials, and a normal motor unit recorded with the EMG needle consists of approximately 10 or more muscle fibers innervated by the same axon that are simultaneously depolarizing. Myopathic motor unit potentials are small, brief polyphasic potentials (<4 msec). In a myopathy, multiple small motor units are recruited with only minimal voluntary effort. This myopathic pattern occurs because the number of motor units is normal, but there are fewer functioning muscle fibers within each unit; therefore, more units are required to generate a degree of force.

The EMG can be normal in a patient with a myopathy. However, if the needle EMG examination shows evidence of myopathic motor units, this is further evidence that the patient may indeed have a myopathy. In addition, multiple muscles can be sampled with needle EMG. Needle EMG can be useful in confirming the clinical phenotype of muscle involvement established on the neurological examination. EMG can also provide a clue as to which muscles have had recent or ongoing muscle injury and can be a guide as to which muscle to biopsy.

Muscle Biopsy

A muscle specimen can be obtained through either an open or a closed (needle or punch) biopsy procedure. The open biopsy technique is a minor surgical procedure that is done under local anesthesia. Most centers perform primarily open muscle biopsies, but this is in large part determined by the expertise of the histology laboratory in which the tissue is processed. Not all laboratories are able to process the tissue adequately for all of the necessary studies from a small punch biopsy specimen. On the other hand, the advantage of a punch biopsy is that it is minimally invasive and multiple specimens can be obtained. Whether an open or punch biopsy procedure is performed, the tissue must be processed in a laboratory that has researchers who are skilled in the evaluation of muscle tissue.

Muscles that are moderately weak should be biopsied. Biopsies should generally not be taken from severely weak muscles (MRC grade 2 or less). Muscles that have recently been studied by needle EMG may have artifacts from the needle insertion; therefore, these muscles should not be biopsied. Occasionally, the muscle to biopsy can be guided by abnormalities on a imaging procedure, such as muscle ultrasound, computed tomography, or magnetic resonance imaging.

Biopsy specimens are analyzed using light microscopic, electron microscopic, biochemical, and molecular genetic studies. In most instances, light microscopic observations are sufficient to make a pathological diagnosis. Muscle tissue examined under light microscopy is primarily performed using frozen specimens. The tissue is examined for muscle fiber size, shape, fiber type distribution, and the presence of fiber degeneration (necrosis) or regeneration. Structural changes such as central nuclei, disorganization of myofibrils and sarcoplasm (e.g., target fibers, ring fibers, and central cores), and vacuoles can be observed with light microscopy. Connective tissue and blood vessels are examined for inflammation and whether there is increased collagen and fat. In addition to standard stains such as hemotoxylin and eosin and Gomori trichrome, various enzymatic reactions are performed. The myosin ATPase stains at alkaline (pH 9.4) and acidic (pH 4.3 and 4.6) distinguish the type 1 and type 2 fibers. Type 1 fibers (slow-twitch, fatigue-resistant, oxidative metabolism) stain lightly at alkaline and darkly at acidic pHs. Type 2 fibers (fast-twitch, fatigue-prone, glycolytic metabolism) stain darkly at alkaline and lightly at acidic pHs. Normally, there is a random distribution of the two histochemical fiber types and there are generally twice as many type 2 as type 1 fibers. Oxidative enzyme stains (NADH dehydrogenase, succinate dehydrogenase, and cytochrome *c* oxidase) are useful for identifying myofibrillar and mitochondrial abnormalities. Stains for glycogen (periodic acid–Schiff) and fat (oil red O) can suggest excess accumulations of these substances. Qualitative biochemical enzyme stains can be performed for phosphorylase and phosphofructokinase. Amyloid deposition can be assayed with Congo red or crystal violet staining. Acid and alkaline phosphatase reactions can highlight necrotic and regenerating fibers, respectively. Finally,

immunological techniques can stain for muscle proteins that are deficient in some muscular dystrophies (e.g., dystrophin in Duchenne's and Becker's dystrophy) or for products that are increased in certain inflammatory myopathies (e.g., membrane attack complex in dermatomyositis).

The muscle biopsy can be useful to establish if there is evidence of either a neuropathic or a myopathic disorder. A neuropathy can produce denervation atrophy with small angular fibers, groups of atrophic fibers, and, as a result of reinnervation, groups of fibers of the same histochemical type and target fibers. These features should not be present in a myopathy. Typical myopathic abnormalities include central nuclei, both small and large hypertrophic round fibers, split fibers, and degenerating and regenerating fibers. Inflammatory myopathies produce mononuclear inflammatory cells in the endomysial and perimysial connective tissue between fibers and occasionally around blood vessels. The atrophy of fibers located on the periphery of a muscle fascicle, perifascicular atrophy, is a common finding in a particular inflammatory myopathy, dermatomyositis. Any long-standing chronic myopathy can produce an increase in connective tissue and fat. Mitochondrial disorders can be suspected by identifying ragged-red fibers on the Gomori trichrome stain and various abnormal staining patterns on the oxidative stains. The enzymatic stains can demonstrate a nonspecific type 1 fiber predominance in a number of myopathies.

Electron microscopy (EM) evaluates ultrastructural components of muscle fibers. In most myopathic disorders, EM is not required to make a pathological diagnosis. However, EM is important in the study of certain disease states with abnormal light microscopic, especially congenital myopathies (ex nemaline rod and central core) and mitochondrial disorders. Findings detected only by EM are seldom of importance.

In the evaluation of metabolic and mitochondrial myopathies, a portion of the muscle tissue can be processed for biochemical analysis to determine the specific enzyme defect. Western blot determinations from muscle tissue can be performed for certain muscle proteins. Currently, this analysis is usually limited to the dystrophin assays in potential dystrophinopathies when the light microscopic immune stains and the molecular genetic studies are inconclusive in establishing Duchenne's or Becker's dystrophy.

Molecular Genetic Studies

Specific molecular genetic defects are known for an increasing number of myopathies. Usually, the presence of a mutation can be determined by blood DNA analysis without relying on direct muscle DNA analysis. Molecular genetic testing can help in both diagnosis and carrier detection.

Other Tests

Blood Studies: The importance of serum enzymes was previously outlined. Other blood tests that are important include electrolyte determinations for potassium (particularly for the periodic paralysis), sodium, calcium, phosphate, and, rarely, magnesium. Endocrine myopathies are usually evaluated through blood assays for establishing thyroid, parathyroid, or adrenal gland dysfunction. Serological determinations for systemic lupus erythematosis, rheumatoid arthritis, and other immunological markers (e.g., Jo-1 antibodies) can occasionally be useful in a patient with an inflammatory myopathy.

Forearm exercise testing in patients with a suspected metabolic myopathy is often performed to determine if there is a defect in the glycolytic enzyme pathway. Following vigorous exercise, serum lactate is measured. In disorders such as phosphorylase deficiency (McArdles disease), the characteristic elevation of serum lactate after exercise is absent. Forearm testing is normal in all disorders of fat metabolism and mitochondrial and also in some glycolytic disorders with fixed muscle weakness such as acid maltase deficiency. On the other hand, acid maltase deficiency is a rare metabolic myopathy in which a decrease in the deficient enzyme, α-glucosidase, can be directly measured in white blood cell assays from blood.

Urine Studies: Urine analysis can detect the presence of myoglobinuria. This should be suspected if the urine tests positive for blood but no red blood cells are seen.

Quantitation of urinary creatinine excretion is useful to determine if there is a decrease in muscle mass but requires that the patient be on a meat-free diet and must be done over a period of 72 hr or more.

Imaging and Spectroscopy Studies: Techniques to image muscle include computed tomography, magnetic resonance imaging, and ultrasound. Muscle imaging is seldom useful to diagnose a myopathy. However, in selective patients undergoing muscle biopsy in whom it is unclear from the neurological examination and needle EMG which muscle to biopsy, an imaging procedure may be helpful. Muscle imaging has been of interest as a research technique in unusual myopathies to provide information regarding the extent and distribution of the disease. In addition, magnetic resonance spectroscopy is a useful research tool in the study of various metabolic myopathies.

—*Richard J. Barohn*

See also—Electromyography (EMG); Muscle Biopsy; Muscle Strength, Assessment of; Muscle Tone; Ophthalmoplegia; Ptosis

Further Reading

Carpenter, S., and Karpati, G. (2001). *Pathology of Skeletal Muscle*, 2nd ed. Oxford Univ. Press, New York.

Dumitru, D., Amato, A. A., and Zwarts, M. (2002). *Electrodiagnostic Medicine*, 2nd ed. Hanley & Belfus Inc., Philadelphia.

Engel, A. G., and Franzini-Armstrong, C. (Eds.) (1994). *Myology*, 2nd ed. McGraw-Hill, New York.

Griggs, R. C., Mendell, J. R., and Miller, R. G. (1995). *Evaluation and Treatment of Myopathies*. Davis, Philadelphia.

Karpati, G., Hilton-Jones, D., and Griggs, R. C. (2001). *Disorders of Voluntary Muscle*, 7th ed. Cambridge Univ. Press, Cambridge.

Katirji, B., Kaminski, H. J., Preston, D. C., *et al.* (2002). *Neuromuscular Disorders in Clinical Practice*. Butterworth-Heinemann, Boston.

Medical Research Council (2000). *Aids to the Examination of the Peripheral Nervous System*. Balliére Tindall, London.

Pourmand, R. (2001). *Neuromuscular Diseases: Expert Clinicians' Views*. Butterworth-Heinemann, Boston.

Preston, D. C., and Shapiro, B. E. (1998). *Electromyography and Neuromuscular Disorders: Clinical-Electrophysiologic Correlations*. Butterworth-Heinemann, Boston.

Myopathy, Toxic

Encyclopedia of the Neurological Sciences
Copyright 2003, Elsevier Science (USA). All rights reserved.

A NUMBER of medications and abused substances cause myopathy, a disturbance in muscle structure, function, or both. The overall incidence is uncertain, but this occurrence is relatively common. Therefore, all patients who present with symptoms of myopathy should have their drug list carefully scrutinized, and they should be asked about potential exposures to illicit drugs and alcohol.

Since toxins can also cause neuropathy and sometimes neuromuscular junction dysfunction either with or without myopathy, it is important to distinguish these disorders. Myopathies typically present with shoulder and hip girdle weakness in conjunction with preserved tendon reflexes (at least early in the course) and normal sensation. Neuromuscular junction (NMJ) disorders may include these features, but ocular and bulbar involvement are more common than in myopathies. In addition, NMJ disorders, especially myasthenia gravis, usually have a substantial diurnal variation in symptoms. Peripheral neuropathies tend to involve distal muscles predominantly and usually lead to loss of tendon reflexes early in conjunction with paresthesias.

Toxic myopathies can present acutely, subacutely, or chronically. The acute myopathies tend to be characterized by symmetric and proximal-predominant or generalized limb weakness. Acute myopathies usually occur due to rhabdomyolysis or less fulminant muscle necrosis, and they are sometimes accompanied by muscle pain, especially when rhabdomyolysis is present. Sometimes, compartment syndromes occur. The serum creatine kinase (CK) may be highly elevated, and rhabdomyolysis may precipitate renal failure in up to one-third of patients with myoglobinuria. The serum CK tends to peak between 1 and 3 days and can decline by 3–5 days. Electrolyte imbalances including hypophosphatemia, hyperkalemia, hypokalemia, and hypocalcemia may occur. Electrodiagnostic studies usually reveal normal nerve conductions, and needle electrode examinations reveal fibrillation potentials with or without so-called "myopathic" changes, namely low-amplitude, short-duration, and polyphasic motor unit potentials (MUPs). The pathological features are muscle necrosis, myophagocytosis, and eventually regeneration.

The subacute to chronic myopathies tend to present with proximal limb and neck flexor weakness with or without associated pain. The serum CK levels are variable, and electromyography findings are usually myopathic with fibrillation potentials if there is muscle necrosis, inflammation, or muscle membrane irritability. Occasionally, the pathological changes are characteristic if not pathognomonic. The remainder of this entry discusses the better characterized toxic myopathies.

ACUTE MYOPATHIES

Rhabdomyolysis

Rhabdomyolysis may occur from the toxic illicit drugs and pharmacological agents listed in Table 1.

Table 1 TOXIC CAUSES OF ACUTE MYOPATHY

Rhabdomyolysis
  Substance of abuse
    Alcohol
    Amphetamines
    Barbiturates
    Cocaine
    Ectasy
    LSD
    Opiates
  Prescribed drugs
    Anesthetics (malignant hyperthermia)
    Antibiotics including amphoterecin
    Cholesterol-lowering agents
    Cimetidine
    ε-Aminocaproic acid
    Lithium
    Neuroleptics (neuroleptic malignant syndrome)
    Propofol
    Retinoids
    Serotonin reuptake inhibitors (serotonin syndrome)
    Theophyllines
  Organic chemicals
    Toluene
  Miscellaneous
    Hypokalemia (including drug-and licorice-induced)
  Critical illness myopathy
    Intravenous corticosteroids
    Neuromuscular junction blocking agents

In some instances, a causal relationship is unproven. For example, infections can cause rhabdomyolysis; therefore, antibiotic-associated rhabdomyolysis may sometimes be questioned. In addition, environmental toxins such as snake venom can cause myoglobinuria. Significant hypokalemia from numerous medical conditions and drugs, such as diuretics, and chronic licorice ingestion can cause rhabdomyolysis. Rhabdomyolysis can also occur in the setting of hypermetabolic syndromes, such as malignant hyperthermia, serotonin syndrome, and neuroleptic malignant syndrome.

Usually, the mechanism of rhabdomyolysis is uncertain, but ultimately cellular injury appears to occur from an increase in free sarcoplasmic or mitochondrial calcium with activation of proteolytic enzymes. The process is reversible when the causative agent is discontinued. Treatment consists of analgesics and crystalloid intravenous hydration with urine alkalinization to prevent renal failure.

Critical Illness Myopathy

Critical illness myopathy (CIM) is a common cause of acute myopathy in intensive care unit patients. CIM is recognized either during or after treatment with high-dose intravenous corticosteroids given with or without neuromuscular junction blocking agents. Rarely, patients have not had exposures to these pharmacological agents but have only multi-organ dysfunction or the systemic inflammatory response syndrome.

Patients present with failure to wean from mechanical ventilation (diaphragm weakness), generalized limb weakness, or both. Sometimes, facial, bulbar, and, less often, extraocular muscles are affected; tendon reflexes are reduced or normal.

The serum CK is often elevated, but as many as 50% of patients may have normal serum CKs, probably because the serum CK is assessed after the presumed period of peak elevation. Electrophysiological studies usually show normal sensory responses with low or sometimes normal motor amplitudes. Needle electrode examination often reveals diffuse fibrillation potentials with myopathic MUPs. Fibrillation potentials can occur as early as 7 days after exposure to intravenous corticosteroids. Histological findings range from atrophy of type 2 more than type 1 fibers to muscle necrosis, but the most common feature is loss of myosin thick filaments. Myosin loss should be suspected when there is patchy or absent staining of nonnecrotic fibers on myosin-ATPase-reacted sections. In the appropriate setting, such a finding is almost pathognomonic of critical illness myopathy. If necessary, myosin loss could be confirmed either by ultrastructural studies or by immunohistochemistry.

The cause of CIM is uncertain, but there is likely a disassembly of myosin monomers, overexpression of calpain (a calcium protease), and possibly an increase in proteosomes. Although CIM patients have considerable morbidity due to prolonged ventilator requirement and weakness that usually results in difficulty ambulating for approximately 8 weeks, they usually have a full recovery.

SUBACUTE TO CHRONIC MYOPATHIES

A subacute to chronic myopathy occurs in approximately 10% of patients treated with corticosteroids (CS) (Table 2). Perhaps cancer patients have a higher incidence. The weakness tends to be painless. It affects proximal lower more than upper extremity muscles. It tends to occur after months but sometimes after only 2 weeks of therapy. Rarely, there may be respiratory muscle weakness. Usually, dose

Table 2   TYPICAL LABORATORY FEATURES OF SUBACUTE–CHRONIC TOXIC MYOPATHIES[a]

Drug	Serum creatine kinase level	Nerve conductions/ electromyogram	Muscle pathology	Other
Corticosteroids	Normal	Myopathic or normal MUPs, no fibrillations	Type 2 fiber atrophy	
Colchicine	Increased	Myopathic MUPs with FP, myotonia, axonal PN	Autophagic vacuoles; myopathic and neurogenic changes	
Chloroquine/ hydroxychloroquine	Increased	Axonal PN, myopathic MUPs with FP	Autophagic vacuoles curvilinear inclusions on EM	Cardiomyopathy
Amiodarone	Increased	Demyelinating or axonal PN, myopathic MUPs, no fibrillations	Mild vacuolar myopathy	Lipid inclusions in nerve
Cholesterol-lowering agents	Increased	Myopathic MUPs with FP, may have myotonic discharges	Necrosis, regeneration, ± inflammation	
Zidovudine	Increased	Myopathic MUPs with FP	Ragged red fibres	
D-Penicillamine	Increased	Myopathic MUPs with FP	Inflammatory mypothy	Possible cardiac involvement
Alcohol	Normal	Myopathic MUPs, no fibrillations, axonal PN in some	Type 2 fiber atrophy, mild myopathy	
Ipecac	Increased	Myopathic MUPs, may have FP	Cytoplasmic body myopathy	

[a] Abbreviations used: MUPs, motor unit potentials; PN, polyneuropathy; FP, fibrillation potentials; EM, electron microscopy.

equivalents of at least 10 mg or more of prednisone per day are necessary to cause myopathy. Treatment consists of reducing the CS dose as much as possible and perhaps switching to an alternate-day regimen or a nonfluorinated compound.

Vacuolar myopathies can occur from agents that block mitosis, such as colchicine and vincristine, and from amphiphilic compounds that alter cell membranes, such as chloroquine, hydroxychloroquine, amiodarone, and perhexilene. These drugs also cause peripheral neuropathy. The neuropathy from vincristine usually overshadows the myopathy. The mitosis blockers can also affect cardiac muscle, and amiodarone can affect the optic nerve. Usually, the drugs have been taken for months before symptoms occur.

Colchicine neuromyopathy tends to present in patients with renal insufficiency and in patients who are also receiving cyclosporine and lipid-lowering agents. Hydroxychloroquine myopathy is similar to but milder than chloroquine myopathy. The treatment for all these disorders is discontinuation of the offending agent.

Most cholesterol-lowering agents can cause a subacute to chronic, often painful necrotizing myopathy and sometimes overt rhabdomyolysis possibly due to disruption of sarcolemmal membranes. Clofibrate, gemfibrozil, and the "statin" drugs, especially lovastatin, have all been associated with a necrotizing myopathy. Up to 0.5% of lovastatin-treated patients develop myopathy. Cyclosporine can potentiate the myopathy. The myopathy improves gradually when the drugs are discontinued.

A mitochondrial myopathy can be induced by zidovudine, which inhibits human immunodeficiency virus reverse transcriptase. Affected patients have proximal muscle weakness with or without myalgias. The myopathy usually improves weeks after discontinuation of zidovudine. It may be difficult or impossible to differentiate zidovudine myopathy from HIV-related noninflammatory myopathy unless the myopathy improves upon discontinuation of the drug. HIV can also cause an inflammatory myopathy that can be differentiated from noninflammatory zidovudine myoathy by muscle biopsy. Suramin can also induce a mitochondrial myopathy.

Inflammatory myopathy can rarely be caused by D-penicillamine. The myopathy is not necessarily dose related and can occur at any time during the course of treatment with the drug. Patients have the typical pattern of proximal weakness but sometimes with dysphagia and myalgias. Cardiac muscle can also be affected. Patients may recover when the drug is withdrawn, but corticosteroids have also been used to induce remission. Penicillamine can also induce myasthenia gravis (MG), sometimes in conjunction with an inflammatory myopathy. These patients harbor acetylcholine receptor binding antibodies and usually have a decremental response with repetitive nerve stimulation. The clinical features are indistinguishable from nonpenicillamine-related MG.

Alcohol, in addition to causing rhabdomyolysis, can commonly cause a chronic painless myopathy with muscle atrophy. Cardiomyopathy may be present, and affected patients may also have an alcoholic peripheral neuropathy. The pathogenesis is uncertain; alcohol may cause defective skeletal muscle protein synthesis.

Ipecac, the antiemetic agent that contains emetine, can cause a subacute myopathy in patients such as bulimics who abuse ipecac. Patients can develop proximal or diffuse weakness with myalgias and cardiac involvement. The myopathy may occur from an effect on actin and other myofibrillar proteins.

ε-Aminocaproic acid, which is rarely used as an antifibrinolytic agent, can rarely cause a necrotizing, painful myopathy after prolonged use.

In the past, toxic myopathies occurred due to environmental toxins (e.g., toxic oil syndrome) as well as from adulterated pharmacological compounds (e.g., eosinophilia myalgia syndrome from L-tryptophan).

—*David Lacomis*

***See also*–Myasthenia Gravis; Myopathy, Congenital; Myopathy, Endocrine; Myopathy, Metabolic; Myopathy, Overview; Neuropathy, Toxic; Substance Abuse**

Further Reading

Dalakas, M. C. (1992). Inflammatory and toxic myopathies. *Curr. Opin. Neurosurg.* **5**, 645–654.

Douglass, J. A., Tuxen, D. V., Horne, M., et al. (1992). Myopathy in severe asthma. *Am. Rev. Respir. Dis.* **146**, 517–519.

Estes, M. L., Ewing-Wilson, D., Chou, S. M., et al. (1987). Chloroquine neuromyotoxicity. Clinical and pathological perspective. *Am. J. Med.* **82**, 447–455.

George, K. K., and Pourmand, R. (1997). Toxic myopathies. *Neurol. Clin.* **15**, 711–730.

Knochel, J. P. (1993). Mechanisms of rhabdomyolysis. *Curr. Opin. Rheumatol.* **5**, 725–731.

Lacomis, D., Giuliani, M. J., Van Cott, A., et al. (1996). Acute myopathy of intensive care: Clinical, EMG, and pathologic aspects. *Ann. Neurol.* **40**, 645–654.

London, S. F., Gross, K. F., and Ringel, S. P. (1991). Cholesterol-lowering agent myopathy (CLAM). *Neurology* **41**, 1159–1160.

Pascuzzi, R. M. (1998). Drugs and toxins associated with myopathies. *Curr. Opin. Rheumatol.* **10**, 511–520.

Poels, P. J. E., and Gabreels, F. J. M. (1993). Rhabdomyolysis: a review of the literature. *Clin. Neurol. Neurosurg.* **95**, 175–192.

Preedy, V. R., Salisbury, J. R., and Peters, T. J. (1994). Alcoholic muscle disease: Features and mechanisms. *J. Pathol.* **173**, 309–315.

Rago, R. P., Mile, J. M., Sufit, R. L., Spriggs, D. R., and Wilding, G. (1994). Suramen-induced weakness from hypophosphatemia and mitochondrial myopathy. *Cancer* **73**, 1954–1959.

Rana, S. S., Giuliani, M. J., Oddis, C. V., *et al.* (1997). Acute onset of colchicine myoneuropathy in cardiac transplant recipients: Case studies of three patients. *Clin. Neurol. Neurosurg.* **99**, 266–270.

Road, J., Mackie, G., Jiang, T., *et al.* (1997). Reversible paralysis with status asthmaticus, steroids, and pancuronium: Clinical electrophysiological correlates. *Muscle Nerve* **20**, 1587–1590.

Showalter, C. J., and Engel, A. G. (1997). Acute quadriplegic myopathy: Analysis of myosin isoforms and evidence for calpain-mediated proteolysis. *Muscle Nerve* **20**, 316–322.

Slater, M. S., and Mullins, R. J. (1998). Rhabdomyolysis and myoglobinuric renal failure in trauma and surgical patients: A review. *J. Am. Coll. Surg.* **186**, 693–716.

Myophosphorylase Deficiency
see Glycogen Storage Diseases

Myositis, Inflammatory

Encyclopedia of the Neurological Sciences

THE INFLAMMATORY MYOPATHIES comprise three major and distinct subsets: polymyositis (PM), dermatomyositis (DM), and inclusion body myositis (IBM). The diseases are clinically important because they represent the largest group of acquired and potentially treatable myopathies both in children and in adults. The cause of PM, DM, and IBM is unknown, but an autoimmune pathogenesis is strongly implicated. In this entry, the distinct clinical, immunopathological, and histological criteria of these disorders are discussed and the currently available therapies are presented.

CLINICAL SIGNS

General Clinical Features

The incidence of PM, DM, and IBM is approximately 1 in 100,000. DM affects both children and adults, and it affects females more often than males. PM is the most uncommon of the three subsets and presents after the second decade of life. IBM is more common in white men (men:women ratio 3:1).

All three forms have in common a myopathy characterized by proximal and often symmetric muscle weakness that develops relatively subacutely (weeks to months) or slowly (over years), as in IBM. Patients report increasing difficulty with everyday tasks predominantly requiring the use of proximal muscles, such as getting up from a chair, climbing steps, stepping onto a curb, lifting objects, or combing their hair. Fine motor movements that depend on the strength of distal muscles, such as buttoning a shirt, sewing, knitting, or writing, are affected only late in the course of DM and PM but early in IBM. Falling is common among patients with IBM because of early involvement of the quadriceps muscle and buckling of the knees. Ocular muscles remain normal but mild facial muscle weakness can be seen in up to 60% of IBM patients. The pharyngeal and neck extensor muscles are often involved, causing dysphagia or fatigue and, occasionally, difficulty in holding up the head. In advanced cases, and rarely in rapidly evolving cases, respiratory muscles may also be affected. Sensation remains normal.

Dermatomyositis

DM is a distinct clinical entity identified by a characteristic rash accompanying or, more often, preceding the muscle weakness. The skin manifestations include a heliotrope rash (blue-purple discoloration) on the upper eyelids with edema, a flat red rash on the face and upper truck, and erythema of the knuckles with a raised violaceous scaly eruption (Gottron rash) that later results in scaling of the skin. The erythematous rash can also occur on other body surfaces, including the knees, elbows, malleoli, neck and anterior chest (often in a V sign), or back and shoulders (shawl sign), and it may be exacerbated after exposure to the sun. In some patients, the rash is pruritic, especially in the scalp, chest, and back. Dilated capillary loops at the base of the fingernails are also characteristic of DM. The cuticles may be irregular, thickened, and distorted, and the lateral and palmar areas of the fingers may become rough and cracked, with irregular, "dirty" horizontal lines resembling mechanic's hands. The degree of weakness can be mild, moderate, or severe leading to quadraparesis. Occasionally, muscle strength appears normal; hence the term dermatomyositis sine myositis. When muscle biopsy is performed in such cases, however, significant perivascular and perimysial inflammation is seen. In children, DM resembles the adult disease, except there are more frequent extramuscular manifestations. A common early abnormality in children is "misery," defined as an irritable child that feels uncomfortable, has a red flush on the face, is fatigued, does not feel well enough to socialize, and has a varying degree of proximal muscle weakness. A tiptoe gait due to flexion contracture of the ankles is also common.

DM usually occurs alone, but it may occur simultaneously with systemic sclerosis and mixed connective tissue disease.

Polymyositis

Unlike in DM, in which the rash secures early recognition, the actual onset of PM cannot be easily determined. Patients present with subacute onset of proximal muscle weakness and myalgia that may exist for several months before they seek medical advise. The diagnosis of PM is one of exclusion. It is best diagnosed and defined as an inflammatory myopathy that develops subacutely, usually over weeks to months; progresses steadily; and occurs in adults who do not have a rash, involvement of the extraocular and facial muscles, family history of a neuromuscular disease, history of exposure to myotoxic drugs or toxins, endocrinopathy, neurogenic disease, dystrophy, biochemical muscle disorder, or IBM as determined by muscle enzyme histochemistry and biochemistry.

PM is rare. It is a syndrome of diverse causes that may occur separately or in association with systemic autoimmune or connective tissue diseases and certain known viral or bacterial infections. In addition to D-penicillamine and zidovudine, in which the myopathy has endomysial inflammation, myotoxic drugs such as emetine, chloroquine, steroids, cimetidine, ipecac, and lovostatin do not cause PM but instead elicit a toxic noninflammatory myopathy.

Inclusion Body Myositis

IBM is the most common acquired myopathy in men older than 50 years. Although it is often suspected when a patient with presumed PM does not respond to therapy, involvement of distal muscles, especially foot extensors and deep finger flexors, in almost all cases may be a clue to early clinical diagnosis. Some patients present with falls because their knees collapse due to early weakness of the quadriceps muscles. Others present with weakness in the small muscles of the hands, especially finger flexors, and complain of inability to hold certain objects such as golf clubs, play the guitar, turn keys, or tie knots. The

weakness and the accompanied atrophy can be asymmetric, with selective involvement of the quadriceps, iliopsoas, triceps, biceps, and finger flexors in the forearm. Dysphagia is common, occurring in up to 60% of patients, especially late in the disease. Because of the distal and, occasionally, asymmetric weakness and atrophy and the early loss of the patellar reflex owing to severe weakness of the quadriceps muscle, a lower motor neuron disease is often suspected, especially when serum creatine kinase (CK) is not elevated. Sensory examination is generally normal. Contrary to early suggestions, the distal weakness does not represent neurogenic involvement but rather is part of the distal myopathic process, as confirmed with macro electromyography (EMG). IBM is associated with systemic autoimmune or connective tissue diseases in at least 20% of cases and with $DR\beta_10301$ and $DQ\beta_10201$ alleles in the DR and DQ phenotypes in up to 75% of patients.

A subset of patients with familial IBM, occurring in members of the same generation with the typical clinical, histological, and immunopathological phenotype of the sporadic form, are designated as having familial inflammatory IBM. These cases are different from those with the hereditary form of IBM, which comprises a group of various ill-defined, vacuolar, distal > proximal myopathies of recessive or dominant inheritance with a clinical profile different from that of the sporadic disease. A distinct subset of patients with hereditary IBM present with characteristic sparing of the quadriceps muscle. This disease, originally described in Iranian Jews but later in many ethnic groups, is a distinct genetic, noninflammatory, vacuolar myopathy caused by mutations in the gene encoding the VDP-N-acetylglucosamime 2-epimerase/N-acetylmannosamine kinase on chromosome 9p1.

Progression of IBM is slow but steady. After a number of years, patients may require a cane or support for ambulation. Some patients with symptoms for 10 years or more may require the use of wheelchairs. Progression is faster, leading to a need for assistive devices earlier when the disease begins later in life, presumably because of lesser muscle reserves.

Extramuscular Manifestations

In addition to the primary disturbance of the skeletal muscles, extramuscular manifestations may also be prominent and include (i) dysphagia due to involvement of the oropharyngeal striated muscles and distal esophagus; (ii) cardiac abnormalities consisting of atrioventricular conduction defects, tachyarrythmias, low ejection fraction, and dilated cardiomyopathy;

(iii) pulmonary involvement as the result of primary weakness of the thoracic muscles, drug-induced pneumonitis (e.g., from methotrexate), or interstitial lung disease (which develops in up to 10% of patients with anti-Jo-1 antibodies); (iv) subcutaneous calcifications in patients with DM, which sometimes extrude onto the skin, causing ulcerations and infections; (v) gastrointestinal ulcerations, seen rarely in childhood DM due to vasculitis and infections; (vi) contractures of the joints, especially in childhood DM; (vii) general systemic disturbances, such as fever, malaise, weight loss, arthralgia, and Raynaud's phenomenon, when the inflammatory myopathy is associated with a connective tissue disorder; and (viii) an increased incidence of malignancies in patients with DM but not PM or IBM. Because tumors are usually discovered not by a radiological blind search but by abnormal findings on medical history and physical examination, it is our practice to recommend a complete annual physical examination with breast, pelvic, and rectal examinations, urinalysis, complete blood cell count, blood chemistry tests, and a chest x-ray film.

DIAGNOSIS

The clinically suspected diagnosis of PM, DM, or IBM is established or confirmed by several methods.

Muscle-Derived Serum Enzyme Levels

The most sensitive enzyme is CK, which in the presence of active disease can be elevated as much as 50 times higher than the normal level. Although CK usually parallels disease activity, it can be normal in active DM and in some patients with PM or DM associated with a connective tissue disease, reflecting the restriction of the pathological process to the intramuscular vessels and perimysium. In IBM, CK is not usually elevated more than 10-fold, and in some cases it may be normal, even at the beginning of the illness. Along with CK, serum SGOT, SGPT, LDH, and aldolase may be elevated.

Electromyography

Needle EMG shows non-disease-specific myopathic motor unit potentials characterized by short-duration, low-amplitude polyphasic units on voluntary activation and increased spontaneous activity with fibrillations, complex repetitive discharges, and positive sharp waves. Mixed myopathic and neurogenic potentials (polyphasic units of short and long duration) are more often seen in IBM, but they can be seen in both PM and DM as a consequence of muscle fiber regeneration and chronicity of the disease. Contrary to previous reports, macro-EMG studies have failed to show a neurogenic pattern of involvement in IBM patients.

Muscle Biopsy

Muscle biopsy shows characteristic features for each subtype of disease. In DM, the hallmark histological findings consist of perivascular and interstitial inflammation, necrosis, phagocytosis and degeneration of muscle fibers around the fascicle or within a muscle fasciculus in a wedge-like shape due to microinfarcts within the muscle, and perifascicular atrophy that can be seen even without inflammation. In PM, the muscle biopsy shows endomysial infiltrates, scattered in several foci, consisting of lymphocytes invading healthy muscle fibers and phagocytosis of necrotic fibers. In IBM, the following are histological hallmarks: (i) basophilic granular inclusions distributed around the edge of slit-like vacuoles (rimmed vacuoles); (ii) angulated or round fibers scattered or in small groups; (iii) eosinophilic cytoplasmic inclusions; (iv) endomysial inflammation with T cells invading healthy muscle fibers in a pattern identical to that for PM; (v) tiny deposits of Congo red or crystal violet-positive amyloid within or next to some vacuoles. The amyloid, seen in approximately 80% of our patients, immunoreacts with β-amyloid protein, which is the type of amyloid sequenced from the amyloid fibrils of blood vessels of patients with Alzheimer's disease; (vi) characteristic filamentous inclusions seen by electron microscopy in the cytoplasm or myonuclei, prominent in the vicinity of the rimmed vacuoles, which immunoreact among others for tau, ubiquitin, chymotrypsin, and prion. Although demonstration of the filaments by electron microscopy was deemed essential for the diagnosis of IBM, this is no longer necessary if all the characteristic light microscopic features including the amyloid deposits are present. Furthermore, such filaments are not unique to IBM; and (vii) abnormal mitochondria, seen as ragged-red fibers, which are often negative with cytochrome oxidase and contain mitochondrial DNA deletions.

PATHOGENESIS

Immunopathology of DM

The primary antigenic targets in DM are components of the vascular endothelium of the endomysial blood vessels and the capillaries. The earliest pathological alterations are changes in the endothelial cells consisting of pale and swollen cytoplasm with microvacuoles and undulating tubules in the smooth endoplasmic reticulum followed by obliteration, vascular necrosis, and thrombosis. Such alterations occur early in the disease by the C5b-9 membranolytic attack complex (MAC), the lytic component of the complement pathway that is deposited on the capillaries before the onset of inflammatory or structural changes in the muscle fibers. MAC and the active fragments of the early complement components C3b and C4b are increased in patients' serum. The activation of complement, perhaps by putative anti-endothelial cell antibodies, is believed to be responsible for the induction of cytokines, which in turn upregulate the expression of VCAM-I and ICAM-I on the endothelial cells and facilitate the exit of activated lymphoid cells to the perivascular, perimysial, and endomysial spaces. The majority of these cells are B cells and CD4$^+$ cells.

Sequentially, the disease begins with activation or complement, formation, and deposition of MAC on the endomysial microvasculature, osmotic lysis of the endothelial cells, necrosis of the capillaries, perivascular inflammation, ischemia, and muscle fiber destruction, often resembling microinfarcts. The perifascicular atrophy often seen in more chronic stages is a reflection of the endofascicular hypoperfusion that is prominent distally. Finally, there is a marked reduction in the number of capillaries per each muscle fiber, with dilatation of the remaining capillaries in an effort to compensate for the impaired perfusion.

Immunopathology of Polymyositis and Inclusion Body Myositis

Cytotoxic T Cells and T Cell Receptor Rearrangement: In PM and IBM, there is evidence for an antigen-directed cytotoxicity mediated by cytotoxic T cells, as supported by the presence of CD8$^+$ cells that surround major histocompatibility (MHC)-1-expressing, non-necrotic muscle fibers that eventually invade and destroy. These CD8$^+$ T cells are activated, exert cytotoxicity to their autologous myotubes *in vitro*, send spike-like processes that traverse the basal lamina, and contain perforin and granzyme granules that are directed toward the surface of the fibers and upon release induce necrosis of the myofibers (Fig. 1). The Fas-dependent (apoptotic) pathway is not involved in myocytic cell death

or in the death of the autoinvasive T cells, despite the expression of Fas antigen on the muscle fibers and Fas-L on the autoinvasive CD8$^+$ cells. This may be related to coexpression by the muscle fibers of various antiapoptotic molecules, including the death suppressor molecule Bcl-2; the FLICE (Fas-associated death domain-like IL-1-converting enzyme)-inhibitory protein (FLIP), which inhibits Fas death receptor signaling; and the human IAP-like protein (hILP), which inhibits the executioner caspases (Fig. 1).

The T cells recognize an antigen by the T cell receptor (TCR), a heterodimer of two α and β chains encoded by multiple gene families in the V (variable), D (diversity), J (joining), and C (constant) regions of the TCR. The part of the TCR that recognizes an antigen is the CDR3 region, which is encoded by genes in the V–J and V–D–J segments of the TCR gene. If the endomysial T cells are selectively recruited by a muscle-specific autoantigen, use of the V and J genes of the TCR should be restricted and the amino acid sequence in their CDR3 region should be conserved. In patients with PM and IBM, but not DM, only certain T cells of specific TCR-α and TCR-β families are recruited to the muscle from the circulation. Cloning and sequencing of the amplified endomysial or autoinvasive TCR gene families have demonstrated a restricted use of the Jβ gene with a conserved amino acid sequence in the CDR3 region suggesting that CD8$^+$ cells are specifically selected and clonally expanded *in situ* by muscle-specific autoantigens. Sequential muscle biopsy specimens obtained during a 2-year period have shown persistent clonal restriction and amino acid sequence homology in the CDR3 determining region.

MHC Expression for Antigen Presentation: Muscle fibers normally do not express a detectable amount of MHC class I or II antigens. In PM and IBM, however, widespread overexpression of MHC occurs early, even in areas remote from the inflammation, probably upregulated by cytokines such as interferon-γ (IFN-γ) and tumor necrosis factor-α (TNF-α). Another MHC molecule of interest is HLA-G, which is also upregulated on the muscle fibers in a pattern similar to MHC-I. The exact role of HLA-G in PM and IBM is unclear.

Costimulatory Molecules: For antigen presentation, the MHC-I-expressing muscle fibers should coexpress the B7 family of costimulatory molecules (B7-1, B7-2, or BB1), whereas the autoinvasive CD8$^+$ T cells express the counter-receptors CD28 and CTLA-4. It has been shown that the BB1 (CD80)

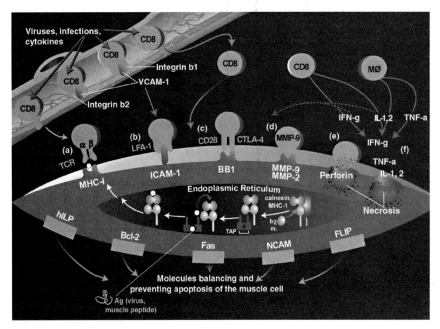

Figure 1

Molecules, receptors, and their ligands involved in exiting of the T cells through the endothelial cell wall and recognizing muscle antigens on the surface of muscle fibers. Sequentially, the LFA-I/ICAM-I binding anchors the cytoskeletal molecules in the nascent immunological synapse. This allows the interaction of TCR/MHC with the sampling of MHC–peptides complex and the engagement of BB1 and CD40 costimulatory molecules with their ligands CD28, CTLA, and CD40L—the prerequisites for antigen recognition. Metalloproteinases facilitate the attachment of T cells to the muscle surface. Muscle fiber necrosis occurs via the perforin granules released by the autoinvasive T cells. A direct myocytotoxic effect exerted by the released IFN-γ, IL-1 or TNF-α may also occur. Muscle fiber cell death is mediated through necrosis and not apoptosis, presumably because of the counterbalancing effect or protection by the antiapoptotic molecules Bcl-2, hILP, and FLIP, which are upregulated in PM and IBM muscles. Fas is also expressed in the muscle, but it does not mediate apoptosis. The upregulated NCAM on degenerating muscle fibers may enhance regeneration. (See color plate section.)

is expressed on MHC-I-positive muscle fibers and makes cell-to-cell contact with their CD28 or CTLA-4 ligand on the autoinvasive CD8$^+$ T cells (Fig. 1).

Cytokines, Cytokine Signaling, Chemokines, and Metalloproteinases: Overexpression of signal transduction and activation of transducers type I (STAT-1), indicative of cytokine upregulation, occurs early in the muscle fibers of PM and IBM. Polymerase chain reaction studies have confirmed a varying degree of amplification of mRNA of the various cytokines, including interleukin1 (IL-1), IL-2, TNF-α, IFN-γ, transforming growth factor-β (TGF-β), granulocyte macrophage colony-stimulating factor, IL-6, and IL-10. Some of these cytokines, such as IFN-γ, IL-1b, and TNF-α, may also exert a direct cytotoxic effect to the muscle fibers (Fig. 1). Others, such as TGF-β, may promote chronic tissue inflammation and fibrosis.

Chemokines, a class of small cytokines, are molecules known to participate in leukocyte recruitment and activation at the sites of inflammation. Chemokines such as IL-8, RANTES, or MCP-I are constitutively expressed on myoblasts or after proper induction by IFN-γ. In the muscles of PM, DM, and IBM, MCP-I and MIP-1a are also expressed in the endomysial inflammatory cells and the neighboring extracellular matrix and may play a role in trafficking of the activated T cells to the muscle or in promoting tissue fibrosis.

Another group of molecules facilitating T cell adhesion to matrices and endothelial cells or the transmigration of lymphocytes is the metalloproteinases (MMPs), a family of calcium-dependent zinc endopeptidases. MMPs, which are also involved in the remodeling of the extracellular matrix and amyloid, are upregulated on the non-necrotic and MHC-I-expressing muscle fibers of patients with PM and IBM. Furthermore, MMP-2 immunostains the autoinvasive CD8$^+$ T cells that make cell-to-cell contact with muscle fibers (Fig. 1), thereby facilitating T cell adhesion or enhancing T cell-mediated cytotoxicity by degrading extracellular matrix proteins.

Association with Viral Infections

Several viruses, including coxsackieviruses, influenza, paramyxoviruses, cytomegalovirus, hepatitis C, and Epstein–Barr virus, have been indirectly associated with chronic and acute myositis. A possible molecular mimicry phenomenon has been proposed for the coxsakieviruses because of structural homology between Jo-1, a histidyl transfer RNA synthetase, and the genomic RNA of an animal picornavirus, the encephalomyocarditis virus. However, very sensitive polymerase chain reaction studies have repeatedly failed to confirm the presence of such viruses in these patients' muscle biopsies.

Retroviruses provide the best evidence of a viral connection. They have been associated with inflammatory myopathy in monkeys infected with the simian immunodeficiency virus and in humans infected with HIV and HTLV-I. In HIV- or HTLV-1-positive patients, PM or IBM can occur as an isolated clinical phenomenon, as the first clinical indication of HIV infection, or concurrently with other manifestations of AIDS and HTLV-1. Viral antigens are not detected or amplified within the muscle fibers; they are detected only in rare endomysial macrophages, indicating the absent of persistent infection or viral replication within the muscle. Because the immunopathology of HIV or HTLV-1 PM and IBM is identical to that described earlier for the retroviral-negative PM and IBM, a T cell-mediated and MHC-I-restricted cytotoxic process appears to be a common pathogenetic mechanism in both retroviral-negative and retroviral-positive PM and IBM.

The Presence of Autoantibodies

Various autoantibodies against nuclear (anti-nuclear antibodies) and cytoplasmic antigens, directed against cytoplasmic ribonucleoproteins involved in translation and protein synthesis, are found in up to 20% of patients with inflammatory myopathies. They include antibodies against various synthetases, translation factors, and proteins of the signal-recognition particles. The antibody directed against the histidyl transfer RNA synthetase, called anti-Jo-1, accounts for 75% of all anti-synthetases, and it is clinically useful because up to 80% of patients with anti-Jo-1 antibodies have interstitial lung disease. In general, these antibodies may be non-muscle-specific because they are directed against ubiquitous targets; they may represent epiphenomena since they have no proven pathogenic significance; they occur in all three subtypes (PM, DM, and, rarely, IBM), despite their clinical and immunopathological differences; they occur in less than one-fifth of patients, most of whom have or develop interstitial lung disease; and they are also seen in patients who do not have active myositis but only lung disease.

The Role of Nonimmune Factors in s-IBM

In IBM, the presence of amyloid deposits within some of the vacuolated muscle fibers, the finding of abnormal mitochondria, and the resistance of the disease to immunotherapies have generated reasonable concerns that in addition to the autoimmune components mentioned earlier, there is also a degenerative process. Of interest, the amyloid is accompanied by all the other proteins seen in the β-amyloid of Alzheimer's disease, including β-APP, chymotrypsin, ApoE, and phosphorylated tau. Whether these deposits are secondary, related to the chronicity of the disease, or generated *de novo* and contribute to disease pathogenesis is unclear. Mitochondrial abnormalities associated with mitochondrial DNA deletions are common in IBM but appear to be secondary and do not impair muscle oxidative metabolism. The vacuolated muscle fibers express mitogen-activated protein kinases (MAPKs), specifically the active P42 MAPK, indicating abnormal intracellular protein phosphorylation. The chaperone, αB crystalline stress protein, is also upregulated in the apparently healthy, nonvacuolated muscle fibers in IBM. Whether this is a sign of a stressor effect before vacuolar formation or whether it serves as a putative autoantigen remains to be determined.

TREATMENT

Because the specific target antigens in DM, PM, and IBM are unknown, the current immunosuppressive therapies are nonselective and most are empirical. The goal of therapy in inflammatory myopathies is to improve strength and to enable patients to perform activities of daily living. Although when strength improves, serum CK declines concurrently, the reverse is not always true because most of the immunosuppressive therapies can result in a decrease in serum muscle enzymes without necessarily improving muscle strength. Several agents are used in the treatment of PM and DM.

Corticosteroids

Prednisone is the first-line drug of this empirical treatment. After 3 or 4 weeks of high-dose prednisone (80–100 mg per day), the drug is tapered over a 10-week period to an 80- to 100-mg single dose every other day by gradually reducing an alternate "off day" dose by 10 mg per week or faster if necessitated by side effects. Although almost all patients with PM or DM respond to steroids to some degree and for some period of time, a number of them fail to respond or become steroid resistant.

Immunosuppressive Drugs

The decision to start an immunosuppressive drug in PM or DM patients is based on the following factors: need for its "steroid-sparing" effect, when despite steroid responsiveness the patient has developed significant complications; attempts to lower a high steroid dosage have repeatedly resulted in a new relapse; an adequate dose of prednisone for at least a 2- or 3-month period has been ineffective; and a rapidly progressive disease with evolving severe weakness and respiratory failure. The preference for selecting the next immunosuppressive therapy is empirical. The choice is usually based on the clinician's prejudices, personal experience with each drug, and his or her assessment of the relative efficacy and safety ratio. The following immunosuppressive agents are used:

- *Azathioprine*: This is a derivative of 6-mercaptopurine and it is given orally. Although lower doses (1.5–2 mg/kg) are commonly used, we prefer higher doses (up to 3 mg/kg) for effective immunosuppression.
- *Methotrexate*: This is an antagonist of folate metabolism. It has a faster action than azathioprine. It is given orally starting at 7.5 mg weekly for the first 3 weeks and increasing gradually by 2.5 mg per week to a total of 25 mg weekly. A relevant side effect is methotrexate pneumonitis, which can be difficult to distinguish from interstitial lung disease of the primary myopathy, often associated with Jo-1 antibodies.
- *Cyclophosphamide*: Our preference for this alkylating agent is to give it intravenously up to 1 g/m^2/month. Cyclophosphamide has not been effective in our hands, despite occasional promising results reported by others.
- *Chlorambucil*: It is an antimetabolite that has been tried in some patients with variable results.
- *Cyclosporine*: Although the toxicity of the drug can be monitored by measuring optimal trough serum levels, its effectiveness in PM and DM is uncertain. A report indicating that low doses of cyclosporine may be of benefit in children with DM needs confirmation. The advantage of cyclosporine is that it acts faster than azathioprine or methotrexate.
- *Mycophenolate mofetil*: This is emerging as an interesting, promising, and well-tolerated drug at doses up to 2 g per day.
- *Plasmapheresis*: This was not helpful in a double-blind, placebo-controlled study that we conducted.
- *Total lymphoid irradiation*: It has been helpful in rare patients with PM or IBM, but it has been ineffective in IBM. The long-term toxicity of this treatment precludes its use.
- *Intravenous immunoglobulin*: Based on a double-blind study, intravenous immunoglobulin (IVIg) is effective in DM patients with refractory disease. Not only does strength improve but also the underlying immunopathology resolves. The benefit is short-lived (not more than 8 weeks), requiring repeated infusions every 6–8 weeks to maintain improvement. The drug has also been effective in most PM patients, but no controlled studies have been performed. The mechanism of action of IVIg in DM may be inhibition of the deposition of activated complement fragment on the capillaries or suppression of cytokines and activated T cells. IVIg also exerted some benefit, although not statistically significant, in up to 30% of patients with IBM in a controlled, double-blind study. Although the improvement was not dramatic, it positively affected patients for a period of time. A second controlled study showed similar effects. A third controlled study that investigated whether IVIg in combination with prednisone is better than prednisone alone showed no benefit of IVIg.

—*Marinos C. Dalakas*

***See also*-Inclusion Bodies**

Further Reading

Amemiya, K., Granger, R. P., and Dalakas, M. C. (2000). Clonal restriction of T-ceptor expression by infiltrating lymphocytes in inclusion body myositis persists over time: Studies in repeated muscle biopsies. *Brain* 123, 2030–2039.

Askanas, V., and Engel, W. K. (1988). Sporadic inclusion body myositis and hereditary inclusion body myopathies. *Arch. Neurol.* 55, 915–920.

Askanas, V., Serdaroglu, P., Engel, W. K., *et al.* (1992). Immunocytochemical localization of ubiquitin in inclusion body myositis allows its light-microscopic distinction from polymyositis. *Neurology* 42, 460–461.

Cupler, E. J., Leon-Monzon, M., Miller, J., et al. (1996). Inclusion body myositis in HIV-I and HTLV-I infected patients. *Brain* **119**, 1887–1893.

Dalakas, M. C. (1991). Polymyositis, dermatomyositis and inclusion-body myositis. *N. Engl. J. Med.* **325**, 1487–1498.

Dalakas, M. C. (1995). Immunopathogenesis of inflammatory myopathies. *Ann. Neurol.* **37**, S74–S86.

Dalakas, M. C. (1998). Controlled studies with high-dose intravenous immunoglobulin in the treatment of dermatomyositis, inclusion body myositis and polymyositis. *Neurology* **51**, 537–545.

Dalakas, M. C. (1998). Molecular immunology and genetics of inflammatory muscle diseases. *Arch. Neurol.* **55**, 1509–1512.

Dalakas, M. C. (2001). The molecular and cellular pathology of inflammatory muscle diseases. *Curr. Opin. Pharmacol.* **1**, 300–306.

Dalakas, M. C., and Karpati, G. (2001). The inflammatory myopathies. In *Disorders of Voluntary Muscle* (G. Karpati, Hilton-Jones, and R. C. Griggs, Eds.), 7th ed., pp. 636–659. Cambridge Univ. Press, Cambridge, UK.

Eisenberg, I., Avidan, N., Potikha, T., et al. (2001). The UDP-N-acetyglucosamine 2-epimerase/N-acetylmannosamine kinase gene is mutated in recessive hereditary inclusion body myopathy. *Nat. Genet.* **29**, 83–87.

Emslie-Smith, A. M., and Engel, A. G. (1990). Microvascular changes in early and advanced dermatomyositis: A quantitative study. *Ann. Neurol.* **27**, 343–356.

Engel, A. G., Hohfeld, R., and Banker, B. Q. (1994). The polymyositis and dermatomyositis syndromes. In *Myology* (A. G. Engel and C. Franzini-Armstrong, Eds.), 2nd ed., pp. 1335–1383. McGraw-Hill, New York.

Griggs, R. C., Askanas, V., Di Mauro, S., et al. (1995). Inclusion body myositis and myopathies. *Ann. Neurol.* **38**, 705–713.

Hohlfeld, R., and Engel, A. G. (1994). The immunobiology of muscle. *Immunol. Today* **15**, 269–274.

Kissel, J. T., Mendell, J. R., and Rammohan, K. W. (1986). Microvascular deposition of complement membrane attack complex in dermatomyositis. *N. Engl. J. Med.* **314**, 329–334.

Mendell, J. R., Sahenk, Z., Gales, T., et al. (1991). Amyloid filaments in inclusion body myositis. *Arch. Neurol.* **48**, 1229–1234.

Sivakumar, K., and Dalakas, M. C. (1996). The spectrum of familial inclusion body myopathies in 13 families and description of a quadriceps sparing phenotype in non-Iranian Jews. *Neurology* **47**, 977–984.

Myotonia

Encyclopedia of the Neurological Sciences
Copyright 2003, Elsevier Science (USA). All rights reserved.

MYOTONIA refers to the delayed relaxation of muscle after voluntary contraction or percussion. This delayed relaxation may be accompanied by electrical silence or by various types of electrical discharge, including so-called myotonic discharges. Myotonic discharges are the repetitive discharges of single muscle fibers, with waxing and waning in frequency and amplitude that produce a sound that has been likened to that of a dive bomber.

—*Michael J. Aminoff*

See also–Electromyography (EMG); Myotonic Disorders; Rippling Muscle Disease

Myotonic Disorders

Encyclopedia of the Neurological Sciences
Copyright 2003, Elsevier Science (USA). All rights reserved.

CHLORIDE CHANNEL MYOTONIAS: MYOTONIA CONGENITAS

THE MYOTONIA CONGENITAS are nondystrophic disorders that may be autosomal dominant (Thomsen's disease) or, more commonly, recessive (Becker's myotonia) (Table 1). Onset of myotonic stiffness, the predominant symptom, occurs between infancy and the teen years. The myotonia is generalized, painless, and may follow sudden physical exertion after a period of rest. However, subsequent repetitive muscle contractions result in resolution of the stiffness associated with myotonia. This "warm-up" phenomenon distinguishes myotonia congenita from disorders associated with sodium channel mutations, in which repetitive muscle contractions lead to increased muscle stiffness. Muscle hypertrophy is common, especially in the lower limbs, and is more pronounced in Becker's myotonia than in the dominant form. Furthermore, in Becker's myotonia there is transient weakness in addition to the stiffness at the initiation of movements following a period of prolonged inactivity, but muscle strength normalizes following several contractions.

Serum creatine kinase (CK) is normal or slightly elevated in both forms of myotonia congenitas, and electromyography (EMG) shows myotonic discharges but no myopathic features. Muscle biopsy is usually normal, although nonspecific abnormalities, such as increased variability in fiber size, increased number of fibers with central nuclei, and lack of type IIB fibers, may be present in some patients. The myotonia may respond to procainamide, quinine, phenytoin, dantrolene, tocainide, and mexiletine.

Myotonia congenitas are due to mutations of the gene coding for the skeletal muscle voltage-sensitive chloride channel (CLCN1) on chromosome 7q35.

Table 1 CHARACTERISTICS OF MYOTONIC DISORDERS AND CHANNELOPATHIES[a]

Syndrome	Molecular defect	Inheritance	Age of onset	Muscle involvement	Characteristics of myotonia	Provocative stimuli	Periodic paralysis
Myotonia congenita of Thomsen	Chloride channel, CLCN1 gene, Chromosome 7q35	Autosomal dominant	Infancy/early childhood	Hypertrophy; rarely weakness	Occurs with sudden exertion after rest; prominent with eye closure; warm-up phenomenon	Myotonia: prolonged rest or maintenance of same posture	No
Generalized myotonia (Becker)	Chloride channel, CLCN1 gene, Chromosome 7q35	Autosomal recessive	Late childhood/teens	Hypertrophy in legs; rarely wasting and weakness late in course; transient weakness after complete rest	Occurs with sudden exertion after rest and with eye closure; warm-up phenomenon	Myotonia: prolonged rest or maintenance of same posture	No
Paramyotonia congenita	Sodium channel, SCN4A gene, Chromosome 17q23–q25	Autosomal dominant	Birth	No permanent myopathy	Paradoxic (face, tongue, neck, grips)	Paralysis: exposure to cold, rest following exercise Myotonia: exercise	Yes (focal)
Hyperkalemic periodic paralysis	Sodium channel, SCN4A gene, Chromosome 17q23–q25	Autosomal dominant	First/second decades	Late myopathy	Paradoxic (eyelids, grips)	Paralysis: potassium; rest after exercise; fasting; cold exposure followed by exercise	Yes
Potassium-aggravated myotonias	Sodium channel, SCN4A gene, Chromosome 17q23–q25	Autosomal dominant	First decade	Very rarely late myopathy; hypertrophy	Face, paraspinal muscles; paradoxic in eyelids, grip, limbs; pain with myotonia	Myotonia: rest after exercise; cold; potassium	Rare
Hypokalemic periodic paralysis	Calcium channel, CACNL1A3 gene, Chromosome 1q31–q32	Autosomal dominant	Second decade	Late myopathy	No myotonia	Not applicable for myotonia Paralysis: carbohydrate intake; cold; rest after intense exercise	Yes

[a] Modified from Moxley (1997).

Several missense and splice mutations have been reported in the autosomal dominant form. Similarly, a (T to G) mutation leading to a substitution of cysteine for phenylalanine in the transmembrane D8 domain of the channel protein has been identified in 15% of recessive cases. The identified mutations putatively lead to decreased chloride conductance across the transverse tubules, resulting in muscle membrane hyperexcitability. As a consequence, afterdepolarization and repetitive firing occur, manifesting clinically as myotonia.

SODIUM CHANNEL MYOTONIAS

Paramyotonia Congenita

The clinical hallmarks of this disorder, which was originally described by Eulenberg in 1886, are the temperature-sensitive nature of the myotonia and episodic paralysis. Myotonia worsens with repetitive activity, especially in a cold environment (hence, paramyotonia). The paramyotonia is present at birth, persists throughout life, and affects predominantly the face, tongue, neck, and hands. Episodic paralysis precipitated by cold, rest following exercise, and potassium intake affects some individuals beginning in the second decade. The weakness is presumably a result of prolonged inactivation of sodium channels and associated membrane inexcitability. Unlike other conditions discussed in this entry, patients with paramyotonia congenita do not develop muscle atrophy or permanent weakness. Transmission is autosomal dominant, with complete penetrance. The disorder is due to numerous mutations in the gene coding the voltage-sensitive sodium channel of skeletal muscle (SCN4A, chromosome 17q23–q25), particularly in the voltage-sensing region of domain IV. There is considerable phenotypic variation between families with the same mutation. On the other hand, there is also considerable overlap in symptoms among patients with different mutations. Laboratory findings are essentially normal, except for high CK in some patients. Muscle biopsy shows no specific pathological features. Acetazolamide is effective in preventing attacks of periodic paralysis and in controlling myotonia. Mexiletine is also an effective symptomatic treatment in these patients.

Hyperkalemic Periodic Paralysis

Hyperkalemic periodic paralysis is transmitted as an autosomal dominant trait. Similar to paramyotonia congenita and potassium-aggravated myotonia, this disorder is due to mutations in the α subunit of the voltage-sensitive sodium channel (SCN4A). These mutations presumably alter the gating properties of the channel. The onset is usually in late childhood or adolescence. Attacks of periodic weakness are shorter than in the hypokalemic disorder (lasting minutes to hours) and may be precipitated by rest after heavy exercise, by cold, or by fasting. Unlike hypokalemic periodic paralysis, only a brief rest following exercise may elicit the symptoms. Sustained, low-level exercise may abort an attack or reduce its severity. Clinical or electrical evidence of myotonia is present in most affected families and may be subtle. Weakness, not myotonia, is the main clinical complaint and may be permanent in later stages of the disease. Serum potassium concentrations are variably increased during the attacks, and attacks may be induced by administration of potassium. Rarely, the increase in serum potassium may be high enough to cause electrocardiograph (ECG) changes (high-amplitude T waves). The attack presumably ends when excess potassium is excreted in the urine. At the end of an attack, mild weakness, myalgias, elevated CK level, and diuresis may be present. The most frequent findings in muscle biopsies are vacuoles and tubular aggregates, which have features identical to those observed in the hypokalemic form, but they are usually less numerous. Treatment is similar to that of paramyotonia congenita and may include preventive and abortive measures. Preventive treatment includes medications to reduce serum potassium (acetazolamide and thiazide diuretics), diet modifications (frequent high-carbohydrate, low-potassium meals with avoidance of fasting), and cold exposure avoidance. Abortive measures include carbohydrate ingestion or a low level of exercise at the beginning of an attack and inhalation of a β-adrenergic agent (metaproterenol, albuterol). The β-adrenergic agents are believed to exert their therapeutic effect by stimulating the sodium–potassium pump.

Potassium-Aggravated Myotonia

This entity encompasses the conditions previously known as myotonia fluctuans, myotonia permanens, chronic myotonia, and acetazolamide-responsive myotonia. They are inherited as an autosomal dominant trait and, like paramyotonia congenita and hyperkalemic periodic paralysis, are associated with mutations in the α subunit of the sodium channel. Potassium ingestion, cold exposure, and rest after exercise provoke symptoms (muscle stiffness, muscle spasms, and cramps) in patients with these diseases. Unlike paramyotonia congenita and hyperkalemic periodic paralysis, they are rarely associated with periodic weakness. The myotonia in these patients is relieved by acetazolamide and mexiletine.

The mutations associated with the sodium channel myotonias result in an abnormal gain of channel function and lead to an impairment of fast inactivation of the channel. As a result, there is a persistent influx of sodium into the muscle cell. Sequential depolarization of the cell occurs, resulting in sustained contraction (myotonia). Periodic paralysis occurs if the mutation results in a more profound sodium ion influx, causing the muscle cell to enter a partially depolarized, inexcitable state.

CALCIUM CHANNEL DISEASE: HYPOKALEMIC PERIODIC PARALYSIS

Although not associated with myotonia, this condition is included here because it, like other conditions discussed, is associated with a defect in an ion channel (i.e., a channelopathy). It is the most common form of periodic paralysis and has an estimated prevalence of 1 per 100,000. This condition is characterized by attacks of flaccid paralysis involving trunk and limb muscles, typically sparing respiratory, facial, and ocular muscles. Attacks typically begin in the second decade, may last hours to days, and may be precipitated by carbohydrates intake, cold, or rest after intense exercise. Typically, the patient wakes up with severe weakness on the morning following a day of vigorous exercise and ingestion of a large high-carbohydrate meal. Patients usually have a full recovery after the attacks, but they may develop fixed mild to moderate weakness over time. This weakness is most prominent in proximal leg muscles. In some patients, the course is benign, and resolution of symptoms occurs in the fifth or sixth decade. Transmission is autosomal dominant, with variable penetrance (reduced in females and complete in males). The disorder is due to mutations in the voltage-dependent calcium channel of the muscle fibers (CACNL1A3, chromosome 1q31–q32). During attacks, muscle is depolarized and unexcitable, and EMG shows electrical silence or a markedly decreased number of motor unit action potentials. Nerve conduction studies may show no or small compound motor action potential (CMAP). Serum potassium concentrations are characteristically decreased from baseline levels (but may still be in the normal range in some cases), probably due to a shift of potassium into the muscle. If the potassium level is low enough, there may be ECG changes, such as sinus bradycardia and T wave abnormalities. Phosphorus level may also decrease during attacks. CK may be elevated between attacks and more so after an attack. Muscle biopsies taken during and between attacks show tubular aggregates and numerous vacuoles, which may be empty or contain granular or hyaline material. Provocative testing with oral glucose load followed by insulin injection should be done judiciously and with close ECG monitoring. Preventive treatments include acetazolamide and avoidance of large carbohydrate-rich meals. Oral potassium during attacks may help alleviate symptoms.

—*Tuan Vu*

See also–Channelopathies, Clinical Manifestations; Myotonia; Myotonic Dystrophy

Further Reading

Barchi, R. L. (1996). Molecular pathology of the period paralysis. In *The Molecular and Genetic Basis of Neurological Disease* (R. N. Rosenberg, S. B. Prusiner, S. DiMauro, and R. L. Barchi, Eds.), pp. 723–731. Butterworth-Heinemann, Boston.

Brown, R. H. (1993). Ion channel mutations in periodic paralysis and related myotonic diseases. *Ann. N. Y. Acad. Sci.* 707, 305–316.

Davies, N. P., and Hanna, M. G. (1999). Neurological channelopathies: Diagnosis and therapy in the new millennium. *Ann. Med.* 31, 406–420.

Gutmann, L. (2000). Periodic paralyses. *Neurol. Clin.* 18, 195–202.

Jentsch, T. J. (1996). Myotonia congenita. In *The Molecular and Genetic Basis of Neurological Disease* (R. N. Rosenberg, S. B. Prusiner, S. DiMauro, and R. L. Barchi, Eds.), pp. 715–721. Butterworth-Heinemann, Boston.

Moxley, R. T., III (1997). Myotonic disorders in childhood: Diagnosis and treatment. *J. Child Neurol.* 12, 116–129.

Surtees, R. (2000). Inherited ion channel disorders. *Eur. J. Pediatr.* 159, S199–S203.

Myotonic Dystrophy

Encyclopedia of the Neurological Sciences
Copyright 2003, Elsevier Science (USA). All rights reserved.

ALTHOUGH CLASSIFIED as a muscular dystrophy, myotonic dystrophy (DM: OMIM 160900, also known as dystrophia myotonica, myotonia atrophica, and Steinert's disease) is a multisystem disease inherited as an autosomal dominant trait. It is the most common form of muscular dystrophy and has a prevalence of approximately 5/100,000, affecting approximately 300,000 people worldwide at any given time.

CLINICAL FEATURES

The clinical features of the disease are highly variable, and DM is compatible with long life in some individuals. In its classic form, the disease begins between adolescence and 50 years of age with muscle weakness and stiffness. In the limbs, the weakness is most prominent distally, affecting the finger flexor and foot extensor muscles initially; proximal weakness appears later in the course and causes difficulty with walking. Involvement of cranial and facial muscles results in ptosis, ophthalmoparesis, dysarthria, and dysphagia. In addition, the temporalis and sternocleidomastoid muscles are small and weak. Because of cranial and facial muscle involvement and frontal baldness, patients with DM have a distinctive long, lean facial appearance (Fig. 1). Diaphragmatic involvement may occur early or late and may lead to hypoventilation and hypersomnia. Coexisting with the weakness is myotonia, which can be induced by action or percussion. Myotonia is a phenomenon of impaired relaxation, which may be clinically elicited by asking the patient to grasp forcefully or to close the eyes tightly. Following the contraction, a patient with DM cannot release the grip or open the eyes quickly. As a result, certain activities of daily living, such as opening doors and buttoning, are impaired. Electrophysiologically, myotonia is characterized by afterdischarge of varying frequencies and waxing and waning amplitudes; this activity continues after relaxation begins. Myotonia is due to an abnormality of the muscle membrane, but the molecular basis is unknown.

In keeping with the multisystemic nature of the disease, ocular involvements including cataracts, low intraocular pressure, retinal degeneration, corneal keratopathy, sluggish pupillary reactions, slow and hypometric saccades, and decreased smooth pursuit performance have been described. Characteristic lens findings include iridescent/polychromatic opacities and subcapsular plaque opacities. These findings are readily detectable by slit-lamp examination and are a sensitive marker because they are seen in patients with minimal additional signs of the disease. However, they are not specific to DM and may be seen very rarely in normal individuals.

Cardiac manifestations include conduction defects (progressive prolongation of the PR and QRS

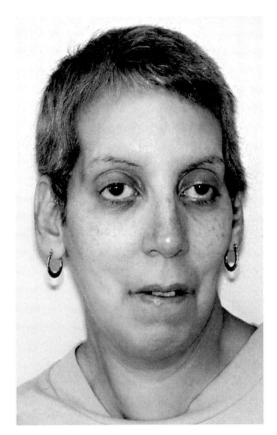

Figure 1
A 49-year-old woman with myotonic dystrophy. Involvement of cranial and facial muscles results in ptosis, ophthalmoparesis, and facial diplegia. Also apparent in this patient are temporalis wasting and receding frontal hairline. These features result in a distinctive facial appearance.

intervals), arrhythmias (atrial and ventricular), and mitral valve prolapse. Sudden death from cardiac arrhythmias is the second most common cause of death after respiratory insufficiency. Contractile function of the heart is usually preserved. There is a general correlation between the likelihood of cardiac involvement and severity of limb weakness and size of the trinucleotide repeat.

Gastrointestinal symptoms and signs include dysphagia, aspiration, bowel dysmotility, megacolon, abdominal pain, gallstones, anal sphincter laxity, and fecal incontinence. Two-thirds of DM patients have elevated liver enzyme levels, most commonly γ-glutamyltransferase. However, the reason for the elevation in liver enzymes is unknown since it is not accompanied by hepatomegaly, cirrhosis, or portal hypertension. Furthermore, liver function test results do not correlate with size of the CTG repeat expansion, severity of weakness, disease duration, and serum levels of creatine kinase (CK), glucose, or lipids.

Balding is common, and hair follicle tumor (pilomatricoma) may also occur. Endocrinological manifestations include parathyroid adenoma, insulin resistance, and testicular atrophy. Dysregulation of the hypothalamic–pituitary–adrenal axis is commonly seen, leading to decreased levels of testosterone, dehydroepiandrosterone sulfate (DHEAS), DHEA, androstenedione, and 17-α-hydroxyprogesterone and abnormal secretion of growth hormone. Fertility in both men and women with DM is not significantly diminished, so the disease is propagated.

Neurobehavioral manifestations are common and have an adverse impact on the quality of life. Obsessive–compulsive, passive–aggressive, avoidant, and schizotypic traits, along with apathy and depression, in some individuals with DM contribute to their social isolation and employability. Mental retardation disables those who survive the neonatal complications of congenital DM. Many individuals with the classic form also have mild cognitive impairment, particularly in recent memory and spatial orientation. The cognitive impairment and personality traits appear to be independent of the muscular involvement and sociocultural environments and may be related to the genetic defect affecting the central nervous system. Indeed, white matter abnormalities on magnetic resonance imaging (MRI) are common, and histopathological findings in the brain, including rod-like intracytoplasmic neuronal inclusions, neuronal loss, ventriculomegaly, abundant Alzheimer's neurofibrillary tangles (NTFs), disturbed cortical architecture, cortical heterotopia, and severe loss and disordered arrangement of myelin sheaths and axons, have been reported. The disturbed cortical architecture and heterotopia suggest that there is interference with nerve cell migration during early embryonic development. The distribution of NTFs and the characteristics of the associated tau proteins in DM are not identical to those of Alzheimer's disease, suggesting that these findings are not due to comorbidity.

Other manifestations include cranial hyperostosis, talipes, and decreased serum immunoglobulins. Polyneuropathy may coexist with the myopathy. Hypersomnia is extremely common (up to 40% of patients in one series) and may be related to nocturnal hypoventilation, obstructive sleep apnea, or central mechanisms.

Women with DM have an increased incidence of obstetric complications, including increased rate of spontaneous abortion, polyhydramnios, prolonged and ineffective labor, retained placenta, placenta previa, and anesthetic and surgical complications. In addition, muscle weakness and respiratory compromise may worsen during pregnancy.

In terms of life expectancy, the mean age at death in various series was between 43.5 and 54.3 years, with a median survival of 60 years for males and 59 years for females. CTG repeat length and earlier death were weakly correlated. The most frequent causes of death are pneumonia and cardiac arrhythmias, each accounting for approximately 30%. In addition, approximately half of patients are wheelchair dependent shortly before death.

GENETICS

The penetrance of the gene is almost 100%. The disease is caused by an unstable cytosine–thymine–guanine repeat (CTGn) expansion both in the 3'-untranslated region of a gene encoding a serine/threonine, cAMP-dependent, protein kinase (DMPK) and in the promoter region of the immediately adjacent homeodomain gene SIX5 on chromosome 19q13.3. In general, the size of the expansion appears to be proportional to the severity and correlates to earlier onset of the disease, especially at the extreme ends of the spectrum. However, there is significant clinical overlap associated with the number of repeats, and prediction of prognosis based on expansion size may be inaccurate. Healthy individuals have alleles between 5 and 35 repeats, and alleles ranging from 35 to 49 repeats are considered "premutation." As a general rule, mildly affected individuals have between 50 and 150 repeats, patients with DM have between 100 and 1000 repeats, and children with the congenital form often have more than 1000 repeats. In any individual, there is a high level of somatic mosaicism (different allele or repeat size in different tissues). Alleles in muscle cells are consistently larger than those in circulating lymphocytes; therefore, blood test may not accurately reflect the size of the repeat in muscle or other tissues (i.e., it is theoretically possible that the repeat expansion may be borderline in blood but significant in other tissues). In addition, there is an increase in repeat size and repeat size heterogeneity over the life of most patients, with bias toward further expansion. This expansion in repeat size over time may explain the clinical progression of the disease. No cases of DM have been identified with point mutation, deletion, or duplication of the *DMPK* gene.

It is unclear why the repeats cause DM; their location suggests that they could not directly affect the structure of the protein translated from the gene. In fact, *DMPK* knockout mice do not have myotonia and other DM symptoms. Multiple mechanisms have been proposed, including alteration of the DNA in the chromatin due to the expansion, alteration of expression of RNA-binding proteins resulting in alterations of RNA metabolism, and reduction of *DMPK* resulting in interference with the signal transduction pathway.

The expanded repeats in DM result in several interesting genetic phenomena, including anticipation (increasing severity and decreasing age at onset of an inherited disease in successive generations). Anticipation is due to the accumulation of larger expansion repeats in the progenies and is more frequent in maternal than paternal transmission. However, after a few generations of increasingly larger repeats and progressively more severe disease, the offspring may no longer be reproductively fit. It is possible that segregation distortion maintains the disease in a population. Normal individuals may carry a small normal allele on chromosome 19 and a large normal allele on the other allele; for unknown reasons, the larger allele is transmitted to the offspring. Occasionally, a mutation may cause the large normal allele to become a small expanded repeat (transition mutation). This small expansion may be transmitted through several generations with minor changes; however, at some point, significant intergenerational enlargement occurs, causing symptoms. The opposite situation, contraction of the expanded repeat from one generation to the next, may also occur. In one series, contraction of the repeat size in leukocyte DNA was found in 6.4% of DM offspring; nevertheless, anticipation occurs in approximately half of offspring, especially when DM is maternally transmitted. It is unknown why anticipation occurs despite a reduction in repeat size; however, ascertainment biases, somatic mosaicism, and unknown maternal factors may play a role.

DIAGNOSIS

As mentioned previously, the appearance of DM patients is distinctive, and the diagnosis is often apparent by visual inspection. Distal more than proximal weakness and myotonia are usually evident on clinical examination and electromyography (EMG). Diaphragmatic weakness may be apparent clinically or on pulmonary function tests. In addition, involvement of other systems (e.g., cataracts and hypogonadism) should be identified. Cardiac conduction defects may be detected by electrocardiogram (ECG) or by 24-hr monitoring. CK is normal or mildly increased, and hepatic enzymes may be elevated. Examination of relatives is often useful, especially when the disorder is suspected in a neonate or child. Although morphological features are not specific, the muscle of DM patients shows increased internal nuclei, muscle fiber atrophy, ring fibers, and sarcoplasmic masses (Fig. 2). DNA testing for expanded CTG repeat is useful to confirm the diagnosis, to clarify an uncertain diagnosis, and to determine the carrier status. Obviously, pretest genetic counseling and maintenance of confidentiality are required. Prenatal testing using cultured amniocytes or chorionic villus samples is accurate in identifying DM in the fetus. Diagnosis of DM should be confirmed in at least one other family member to exclude other entities. Differential diagnoses include disorders of chloride and calcium channel mutations, especially when myotonia is the presenting symptom. Foot drop may be the presenting symptom and may raise the possibility of Charcot–Marie–Tooth disease.

TREATMENT

Although no treatment has been shown to reverse the effects of DM, palliative measures may maintain function and prevent sudden death. Cataract removal can improve vision, and orthoses can improve gait abnormality due to foot drop. Antiepileptic agents, such as phenytoin and quinine, may decrease the

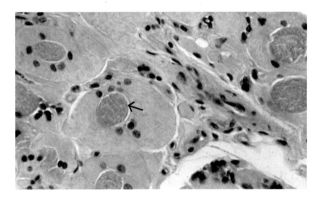

Figure 2
Muscle biopsy of a patient with myotonic dystrophy. Muscle section shows increased internal nuclei, muscle fiber atrophy, and sarcoplasmic masses (arrow) (courtesy of Dr. Arthur P. Hays).

myotonia; however, patients with DM seldom consider myotonia a bothersome symptom. Troglitazone, which is used in the treatment of insulin resistance, has also been anecdotally reported to reduce myotonia. Periodic ECG or Holter monitor identify conduction defects, and cardiac pacemaker is indicated for third-degree heart blocks. However, heart block and rhythm abnormalities may occur in patients with normal ECG; therefore, patients must be advised to report any suggestive symptoms. Bilevel positive airway pressure is useful in patients with nocturnal hypoventilation.

Because of a reduction of hormonal levels in patients with DM, treatments with hormones have been tried. Most studies have been small, and confirmation of their results using a larger population is lacking. In a pilot study, DHEAS (200 mg/day) was reported to improve activities of daily living, increase muscular strength, decrease myotonia, and decrease arrhythmia. The mechanism by which DHEAS exerts its effect is unknown. Testosterone and recombinant human growth hormone increased muscle mass but did not improve muscle function or strength. Similarly, because insulin resistance was observed in patients with DM, recombinant human-like growth factor I (IGF-1) was also tested and found to have modest effects on the insulin sensitivity index, insulin action, glucose disposal, protein synthesis, body weight, lean body mass, manual muscle strength, and neuromuscular function.

Surgery Risks

Perioperative complications are more frequent in individuals with DM, affecting 8–43% of those undergoing surgical procedures. The most common complications are pulmonary in nature (acute ventilatory failure, atelectasis, and pneumonia). These complications are more frequent in patients undergoing upper abdominal surgeries and in those with more severe proximal weakness. The likelihood of pulmonary complications was not associated with any particular anesthetic drug. Patients with DM may also develop tachyarrhythmias and heart block perioperatively.

Proximal Myotonic Myopathy

Soon after the identification of the genetic defect in DM, it became apparent that at least 2% of patients do not have the expansion of the CTG repeats or point mutations in the *DMPK* gene. In the past decade, several clinical variations on the theme of myotonia, predominantly proximal weakness, and

the absence of trinucleotide repeat in the *DMPK* gene have been described (Table 1).

Thornton *et al.* reported three patients from two families who had the characteristic features of DM (frontal balding, cataracts, cardiac conduction abnormalities, testicular atrophy, myotonia, muscle weakness, hypersomnia, and psychiatric symptoms) but without expanded CTG repeat in the *DMPK* gene. In addition, the authors noted three features that were atypical for DM: the lack of anticipation, the proximal distribution of weakness, and hypertrophied (rather than atrophic) limb muscles. Some have proposed that this entity be called Thornton–Griggs–Moxley disease.

Ricker and colleagues reported 17 German families without expanded CTG repeats in the *DMPK* gene and called the disorder proximal myotonic myopathy (PROMM). In Germany, PROMM prevalence may be comparable to that of DM, and it has also been described in families from other countries. Initial symptoms occurred between 20 and 60 years of age. These patients have proximal without distal leg weakness, electromyographic and intermittent clinical myotonias, elevated CK, cataracts, and myalgias. Unlike DM patients, who do not usually complain about myotonia, patients with PROMM often complain about myotonia and stiffness. The myotonia is not clinically present in all individuals and may be intermittent, induced by vigorous muscle contraction, and asymmetric. The quality of relaxation is different, being jerky and stepwise. Most patients developed slowly progressive, proximal leg weakness. Some patients also had weakness in neck flexion, arm abduction, and elbow extension, but none had weakness of the hands, feet, or face. None had significant muscle atrophy, and some had calf hypertrophy, which may be asymmetrical. A few patients also had fluctuations in weakness, and in some exercise transiently improved motor strength. Some patients with PROMM experience a peculiar, annoying pain. The pain may be burning, tearing, or jabbing. It is most pronounced at rest, variable in intensity, and refractory to treatment. Some complain of increased sensitivity to pain, with significant local pain that persists for up to 30 min following being stuck in their muscles. Cataracts, with the typical features of the type seen in DM, were present in many patients before age 50. Cardiac arrhythmias and mental retardation were rare features. Many patients also had elevated γ-glutamyltransferase, unexplained by alcohol abuse or other liver diseases. The overall level of disability is less than that of DM,

Table 1 COMPARISON OF FEATURES OF MYOTONIC DYSTROPHY, PROXIMAL MYOTONIC MYOPATHY, AND PROXIMAL MYOTONIC DYSTROPHY[a]

Characteristics	DM	PROMM	PDM	DM2
Age of onset (years)	10–50	20–60	27–35	8–50
First symptoms	Weakness	Stiffness, myalgia, weakness, cataracts	Weakness	Weakness
Myotonia				
Clinical	+	±	−	+
EDX	+	+	+	+
Weakness distribution	Distal > Proximal	Proximal	Proximal > Distal	Proximal and Distal
Face/jaw	+	−	+	+
Fluctuation	−	+	−	
Ptosis	+	−	−	
Atrophy	+	±	+	+
Myalgia	−	+	−	+
Laboratory findings				
↑ CK	+	+	+	+
↑ γ-Glutamyltransferase	+	+	−	+
Anticipation	+	?	?	?
Congenital form	+	−	?	−
Cardiac disease				
Conduction defect	+	+	−	+
Myocardial defect	±		+	+
Liver involvement	+	+		
Cognitive dysfunction	+	−	?	−
Hypersomnia	+	+[b]	−	+
Peripheral neuropathy	±	−	−	−
Hearing loss	+	+[c]	+	+
Hypogonadism	+	+	+	+
Diabetes	+	−	+	±
Cataract	+	+	+	+

[a] Abbreviations used: DM, myotonic dystrophy; PROMM, proximal myotonic myopathy; PDM, proximal myotonic dystrophy; DM2, myotonic dystrophy type 2; +, commonly present; −, absent; ±, present in some individuals; ?, unknown or undetermined.
[b] In a Norwegian family (Sun et al., 1999).
[c] Phillips et al. (1998).

and patients in Ricker et al.'s study did not develop late-onset mental deterioration, hypersomnia, dysarthria, dysphagia, and respiratory complications. However, later accounts noted that cognitive deficits and cerebral white matter abnormalities on MRI were not uncommon. Endocrine abnormalities, including insulin resistance, thyroid dysfunction, and hypogonadism, have also been reported. Perioperative complications are rare: Only 1 of 35 patients in a series had dark urine, muscle pain, and transient renal insufficiency after minor surgery. This patient had a higher CK level than the usual mild elevation. Therefore, preoperative measurement may be useful in identifying those at risk. In approximately two-thirds of the parent–child pairs, the child had earlier onset and more severe disease, suggesting anticipation. A congenital form has not been clearly

identified. Linkage of PROMM to the gene loci responsible for paramyotonia (skeletal muscle sodium channel, chromosome 17) and myotonia congenita (skeletal muscle chloride channel, chromosome 7) has been excluded.

Phillips et al. reported on a family in which three generations were affected with an autosomal dominant disorder resembling PROMM. These patients had proximal myopathy, subclinical EMG myotonia, cataracts, and no abnormal expansion of the CTG repeat in the DMPK gene. The distinguishing feature of this family was severe deafness, which was not described in Ricker et al.'s families. Sun et al. described another Norwegian family with PROMM but with myalgia as a prominent symptom, along with ptosis, dysphagia, frontal balding, and hypersomnia.

Proximal Myotonic Dystrophy

Udd *et al.* described a Finnish family with PROMM-like features that they called proximal myotonic dystrophy (PDM). Like PROMM, individuals from this family had an autosomal dominant disorder with proximal weakness, cataracts, and electrophysiological myotonia. However, unlike in other PROMM patients, the myopathy was more severe, and these patients did not have myalgias, symptomatic myotonia, or muscle stiffness. Instead, they had significant dystrophic–atrophic changes in proximal muscles, late-onset progressive deafness, atherosclerotic cardiovascular disease, and hypogonadism.

Myotonic Dystrophy Type 2

Day and colleagues reported on a family from Minnesota with a novel form of DM that they called myotonic dystrophy type 2 (DM2). The clinical features of this family were similar to those of DM: autosomal dominant transmission, myotonia, weakness, frontal balding, polychromatic cataracts, infertility, and arrhythmias. Elevated CK (up to 7.5 times normal) was seen in 12 of 15 individuals. Muscle biopsies showed fiber size variability, centrally located nuclei, severely atrophic fibers, swirled sarcomere organization, necrotic fibers, and significant endo- and perimysial fibrosis. Anticipation is possible but could not be definitely demonstrated due to sample size and large variation in the age at onset. However, these patients also did not have the CTG expansion, and the gene locus was not linked to chromosome 19. The authors distinguished this disease from PROMM because the pattern of weakness in their patients was not purely proximal (of the 18 individuals with weakness, the pattern was both proximal and distal in 11, purely distal in 5, and proximal in only 2).

Ranum *et al.* (1998) reported that is linked to the long arm of chromosome 3. In eight of nine German families with PROMM, the disease locus was also linked to the same region as that of DM2 on chromosome 3. PDM also mapped to this region, raising the possibility that these diseases are allelic or caused by mutations in closely linked and functionally related genes. Recently, DM2 was reported to be associated with a CCTG expansion (mean, ~5000 repeats) in intron 1 of the zinc finger protein 9 on chromosome 3. However, in some PROMM kindred, the disease locus is on neither chromosome 3 nor 19, suggesting that at least one other locus is responsible for this phenotype.

Congenital Myotonic Dystrophy

Congenital myotonic dystrophy is almost exclusively maternally transmitted. The condition may be suspected prenatally by polyhydramnios and decreased fetal movement. Affected infants have severe hypotonia, facial weakness, difficulty in sucking and feeding, and respiratory distress. There is also an increase in frequency of germinal matrix hemorrhage. The absence of clinical and often electrical myotonia in these infants is an important negative finding; therefore, it is often diagnostically useful to examine the mother. The most significant pathological abnormality in the muscle biopsy is immaturity of muscle fibers. The fibers are small and have the histological features of myotubes, with basophilic cytoplasm and centrally located nuclei. There is also a high incidence of cardiac disease (conduction system defect and, very rarely, myocardial abnormalities), gastrointestinal dysfunction, and hearing loss. In a small series, the mortality rate was 25% before 18 months of age, and only approximately half survived to the mid-30 s. For those who survived past infancy, cognitive impairment, attention deficit, anxiety disorders, and speech dysfunction were common, and three-fourths needed special education.

—Tuan Vu

***See also*–Muscle Contraction, Overview; Muscular Dystrophy: Emery–Dreifuss, Facioscapulohumeral, Scapuloperoneal, and Bethlem Myopathy; Muscular Dystrophy: Limb–Girdle, Becker, and Duchenne; Myotonic Disorders; Trinucleotide Repeat Disorders**

Further Reading

Day, J. W., Roelofs, R., Leroy, B., *et al.* (1999). Clinical and genetic characteristics of a five-generation family with a novel form of myotonic dystrophy (DM2). *Neuromuscular Dis.* 9, 19–27.

International Myotonic Dystrophy Consortium (2000). New nomenclature and DNA testing guidelines for myotonic dystrophy type 1 (DM1). *Neurology* 54, 1218–1221.

Moxley, R. T., III (1996). Proximal myotonic myopathy: Mini-review of a recently delineated clinical disorder. *Neuromuscular Dis.* 6, 87–93.

Moxley, R. T., III (1997). Myotonic disorders in childhood: Diagnosis and treatment. *J. Child Neurol.* 12, 116–129.

Phillips, M. F., Rogers, M. T., Barnetson, R., *et al.* (1998). PROMM: The expanding phenotype. A family with proximal, myotonia, and deafness. *Neuromuscular Dis.* **8**, 439–446.

Ranum, L. P. W., Rasmussen, P. F., Benzow, K. A., *et al.* (1998). Genetic mapping of a second myotonic dystrophy locus. *Nat. Genet.* **19**, 196–198.

Ricker, K., Koch, M. C., Lehmann-Horn, F., *et al.* (1995). Proximal myotonic myopathy—Clinical features of a multisystem disorder similar to myotonic dystrophy. *Arch. Neurol.* **52**, 25–31.

Sun, C., Henriksen, O. A., and Tranebjærg, L. (1999). Proximal myotonic myopathy: Clinical and molecular investigation of a Norwegian family with PROMM. *Clin. Genet.* **56**, 457–461.

Thornton, C. (1999). The myotonic dystrophies. *Semin. Neurol.* **19**, 25–33.

Udd, B., Krahe, R., Wallgren-Pettersson, C., *et al.* (1997). Proximal myotonic dystrophy—A family with autosomal dominant muscular dystrophy, cataracts, hearing loss and hypogonadism: Heterogeneity of proximal myotonic syndromes? *Neuromuscular Dis.* **7**, 217–228.

Myxedema
see Thyroid and Thyroid Disorders

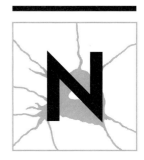

Narcolepsy

Encyclopedia of the Neurological Sciences
Copyright 2003, Elsevier Science (USA). All rights reserved.

NARCOLEPSY is a neurological disorder characterized by excessive daytime sleepiness that is typically associated with cataplexy, sleep paralysis, and hypnagogic hallucinations. For more than a century, narcolepsy was a disorder of unknown etiology. It is now thought that the disorder is due, in part, to a dysfunction of hypocretin activity in the hypothalamus.

Historically, the word narcolepsy was first coined by Gélineau in 1880 to designate a pathological condition characterized by irresistible episodes of sleep of short duration recurring at close intervals. In the same article, he wrote that attacks were sometimes accompanied by falls or "astasias." In the 1930s, Daniels emphasized the association of cataplexy, hypnagogic hallucinations, sleep paralysis, and excessive daytime sleepiness. Yoss and Daly called these symptoms the "tetrad" of narcolepsy, and Vogel described sleep-onset rapid eye movement (REM) in narcoleptic patients. Narcolepsy is a neurological syndrome that is characterized by abnormal sleep, including excessive daytime sleepiness with often disturbed nocturnal sleep and pathological manifestations related to rapid REM.

Narcolepsy is not a rare condition. The prevalence of narcolepsy has been calculated to be approximately 0.02–0.05% of the general population. Age at onset varies from childhood to the fifth decade, with a peak in the second decade. The first symptoms often develop at approximately the time of puberty. The peak age at which reported symptoms occur is between 15 and 25 years, but narcolepsy and other symptoms have been noted at 5 or 6 years; a second, smaller peak of onset has been noted between 35 and 45 years. Special circumstances, such as an abrupt change of sleep–wake schedule, head trauma, or a severe psychological stress (e.g., death of a relative or divorce), may precede the occurrence of the first symptom.

CLINICAL PRESENTATION

Narcolepsy can be thought of as a chronic neurological disorder in which the boundaries between the awake, sleeping, and dreaming brain are blurred. The awake narcoleptic will feel sleepy. The sleeping narcoleptic will have disturbed sleep due to arousals. REM-like activity such as cataplexy and dream imagery will interrupt the awake state. Narcolepsy is characterized by a set of clinical symptoms including abnormal sleep features, overwhelming episodes of sleep, excessive daytime somnolence (EDS), hypnagogic hallucinations, disturbed nocturnal sleep, and manifestations of paroxysmal muscular weakness, cataplexy, and sleep paralysis.

Unwanted episodes of sleep recur several times a day, not only in favorable circumstances, such as monotonous sedentary activity or after a meal, but also in situations in which the subject is fully involved in a task. The duration of the episode may vary from a few minutes, if the subject is in an uncomfortable position, to more than 1 hr if the subject is reclining. Narcoleptics characteristically wake up refreshed, and there is a variable length refractory period before the next episode occurs.

Apart from sleep episodes, patients may feel abnormally drowsy. They may have an unpleasant level of low alertness that is responsible for poor performance at work, memory lapses, and even gestural or speech automatisms. This low alertness may persist despite the use of maximum dosage of stimulant medication.

Cataplexy is an abrupt and reversible decrease or loss of muscle tone, most frequently elicited by emotions such as laughter or anger, surprise, or abrupt strain. It may involve certain muscles or the entire voluntary musculature. Typically, the jaw sags, the head falls forward, the arms drop to the side, and the knees unlock. The severity and extent of cataplectic attacks can vary from a state of absolute powerlessness, which seems to involve the entire voluntary musculature, to a limited involvement of certain muscle groups or to no more than a fleeting sensation of weakness extending more or less throughout the body. The patient may complain of blurred vision. Complete paralysis of extraocular muscles has never been reported, however, but the palpebral muscle may be affected. Speech may be impaired, and respiration may become irregular during an attack, which may be related to weakness of the abdominal muscles. Long diaphragmatic pauses have never been recorded, but short diaphragmatic pauses similar to those seen during nocturnal REM sleep can be noted. Complete loss of muscle tone, which results in a total collapse with risk of serious injuries, including skull and other bone fractures, may be noted during a cataplectic attack. The attacks are commonly not this dramatic, however, and may go unnoticed by nearby individuals. An attack may consist only of a slight buckling of the knees. Patients may perceive this abrupt and short-lasting weakness and may simply stop or stand against a wall. The condition may be slightly more obvious when there is a combination of sagging jaw and inclined head. The duration of each cataplectic attack (partial or total) is highly variable and usually ranges from a few seconds to 2 min but may rarely last up to 30 min. Attacks can be elicited by emotion, stress, fatigue, or heavy meals. Laughter and anger seem to be the most common triggers, but the attacks can also be induced by a feeling of elation. Cataplexy may be induced merely by remembering a happy or funny situation, and it may also occur without clear precipitating acts or emotions. Cataplexy is associated with an inhibition of monosynaptic H reflexes and tendon reflexes. H reflex activity is fully suppressed physiologically only during REM sleep, emphasizing the relationship between the motor inhibition of REM sleep and the sudden atonia and areflexia seen during a cataplectic attack.

Sleep paralysis is a terrifying experience that occurs in the narcoleptic on falling asleep or on awakening. Patients find themselves suddenly unable to move the limbs, to speak, or even to breathe deeply. This state is frequently accompanied by hallucinations. During an episode of sleep paralysis, the patient is powerless to move the extremities, speak, or open the eyes even though they are fully aware of the condition and able to recall it completely afterward. In many episodes of sleep paralysis, but especially the first occurrence, the patient may be prey to extreme anxiety associated with the fear of dying. This anxiety is often greatly intensified by the terrifying hallucinations that may accompany the sleep paralysis. With more experience of the phenomenon, however, the patient usually learns that episodes are brief and benign, rarely lasting longer than 10 min and always ending spontaneously.

Hypnagogic hallucinations occur at sleep onset and often involve visual images; manifestations usually consist of simple forms (colored circles, parts of objects, and so forth) that are constant or changing in size. The images may present abruptly in black and white but more often in color. Auditory hallucinations are also common, although other senses are seldom involved. The auditory hallucinations can range from a collection of sounds to an elaborate melody. The hallucinations may also occur upon awakening. The term hypnopompic hallucination is used when this phenomenon occurs upon awakening. When these hallucinations occur along with sleep paralysis, the experience can be particularly frightening. Sleep paralysis with hypnagogic and hypnopompic hallucinations has been singled out as a particularly likely source of beliefs concerning supernatural phenomenon. Patients may report feeling a "presence" that can be perceived as threatening or evil. An intense sense of dread and terror is very common.

Initial Symptoms

EDS and irresistible sleep episodes usually occur as the first symptoms, either independently or associated with one or more other symptoms. They are enhanced by high environmental temperature, indoor activity, and idleness. Symptoms may abate with time but never resolve completely. Attacks of cataplexy generally appear in conjunction with abnormal episodes of sleep but may occur as much as 20 years later. They occasionally occur before the abnormal sleep episodes, in which case they are a major source of difficulty in diagnosis. They can vary in frequency from a few episodes during the subject's entire lifetime to one or several episodes per day.

Hypnagogic hallucinations and sleep paralysis do not affect all subjects and are often transitory. Disturbed nocturnal sleep seldom occurs in the first stages, and its occurrence generally increases with age. Narcolepsy leads to a variety of complications, such as driving- or machine-related accidents; difficulties at work, resulting in disability, forced retirement, or job dismissal; impotence; and depression.

DIAGNOSTIC CRITERIA

The most widely accepted diagnostic criteria are published in the *International Classification of Sleep Disorders Diagnostic and Coding Manual*. Undoubtedly, the presence of cataplexy is pathognomonic of narcolepsy, but it may be difficult to rely on this criterion alone, particularly when cataplexy is partial (i.e., limited to the head and neck or neck and upper arms). To help confirm the diagnosis, nocturnal polysomnogram and the Multiple Sleep Latency Test (MSLT) are performed. The nocturnal polysomnogram recording includes electroencephalography (EEG) (C3/A2, C4/A1, O1/A2, and O2/A1 of the international 10–20 electrode placement system), chin electromyography (EMG), right and left electrooculogram, electrocardiogram, anterior tibialis EMG, and breathing measurements. The breathing measurement techniques always include nasal–oral airflow, thoracic and abdominal effort, and non-invasive measurement of oxygen saturation or transcutaneous PO_2. Intercostal EMG and esophageal pressure measurements may be performed if there is concern of subtle sleep-disordered breathing causing excessive daytime sleepiness. The polysomnogram is scored using the standard international recommendations of Rechtschaffen and Kales. This recording is always performed on subjects free of any medication for at least 15 days.

The MSLT was designed by Carskadon and Dement to measure physiological sleep tendencies in the absence of alerting factors. It consists of four or five scheduled 20-min naps, during which the subject is polygraphically monitored. The latency between lights-out time and sleep onset is calculated for each nap. The type of sleep, REM or non-REM, is also noted. The MSLT records the latency for each nap, the mean sleep latency, and the presence or absence of REM sleep in any of the naps. On the basis of polygraphic recording, REM sleep that occurs within 15 min of sleep onset is considered a sleep-onset REM period. Mean MSLT scores less than 5 min are generally considered to be in the pathological range; those more than 10 min are considered normal. The range between 5 and 10 min represents a gray zone. Narcoleptics typically have scores of less than 5 min and at least two sleep-onset REM episodes. The MSLT may sometimes need to be repeated before the diagnosis of narcolepsy is established. The MSLT requires the patient's motivation and cooperation in order to obtain valid results.

PATHOPHYSIOLOGY

The investigation of the pathophysiology of narcolepsy was greatly advanced when it was reported that 100% of Japanese narcoleptic patients studied presented a class 2 antigen of the major histocompatibility complex known at the time as DR2. British, French, Canadian, and U.S. investigators confirmed that the vast majority of studied Caucasian narcoleptics were also DR15 DQw6 DW2-positive. Progress in the typology of class 2 antigens led to the creation of a new nomenclature in 1990, and the term DR15 replaced DR2. However, it was demonstrated in 1989 that DR2 DQwl was neither sufficient nor necessary for the development of narcolepsy in independent and familial cases. The link between the HLA marker and narcolepsy is stronger than that of any other known HLA marker to a disease. This has led to speculation that narcolepsy may have an autoimmune component. To date, no such mechanism has been identified. Narcolepsy patients do not have the expected serological markers of an autoimmune disease.

A better understanding of the genetics and pathophysiology of narcolepsy has been possible due to the discovery of the disease in animals such as dogs and horses. This has allowed for the development of an animal model for research. A Doberman model of the disease has led to the discovery of a narcolepsy gene. The canine narcolepsy is caused by a defective receptor to hypocretin. Hypocretin, also known as orexin, is a neurotransmitter located in the lateral hypothalamus with wide projections throughout the brain. Different subtypes of hypocretin were identified. Subsequently, it has been found that many narcoleptics are deficient in hypocretin 2. Many narcoleptics have decreased levels of hypocretin in the cerebral spinal fluid.

DIFFERENTIAL DIAGNOSIS OF HYPERSOMNOLENCE

There are several entities that need to be well differentiated in patients with EDS. Narcolepsy is a common differential diagnostic consideration, but it is not the most difficult. The requirement of an association of EDS, a positive history of cataplexy, and the presence of two or more sleep-onset REM periods during up to 4 days of repeated MSLT should allow appropriate differentiation. However, the narcolepsy syndrome may initially present as isolated EDS, and the positive diagnosis may be in doubt for months or even years. Neither HLA typing nor sleep-onset REM periods are pathognomonic.

Cataplectic attacks may be confused with seizures. In particular, atonic seizures or drop attacks may be diagnosed instead of cataplexy. This results in inappropriate therapy. The main distinguishing feature is the retention of consciousness in an attack of cataplexy. The patient should not be amnesic during brief episodes of cataplexy.

The complaint of sleepiness and positive MSLT findings may also be similar in patients with significant daytime sleepiness as a sequela of severe head trauma. Past medical history, which often includes an initial coma after head trauma, is enlightening in these cases.

The daytime somnolence seen in association with communicating hydrocephalus of unknown etiology also does not differ clinically from central nervous system (CNS) hypersomnia. Imaging of the brain, which confirms the hydrocephalus, distinguishes this syndrome from idiopathic CNS hypersomnia. A careful history will differentiate these patients from those with chronic insufficient nocturnal sleep who have daytime sleepiness.

Obstructive sleep apnea syndrome may also be misdiagnosed as narcolepsy. The term narcolepsy has been in use in medicine for many more years than has the term obstructive sleep apnea. The term narcolepsy was often used to describe any form of unexplained hypersomnolence. Thus, patients with obstructive sleep apnea may report having older relatives diagnosed with narcolepsy. Both are chronic conditions with decreased alertness. Patients with narcolepsy report that brief naps are refreshing, whereas patients with obstructive sleep apnea may feel worse or more tired. Cataplexy is only found in narcoleptics. The clinician must keep in mind that obstructive sleep apnea is more common with advancing age. Therefore, an older narcoleptic patient could have worsening daytime alertness due to developing obstructive sleep apnea. Typically, the degree of excessive daytime sleepiness is not progressive with aging in narcolepsy. For unknown reasons, the comorbidity of narcolepsy and obstructive sleep apnea is higher than predicted by their prevalence.

TREATMENT

The goal of all therapeutic approaches in narcolepsy is to control the narcoleptic symptoms and to allow the patient to continue full participation in familial and professional daily activities. However, drug prescriptions must take into account possible side effects, with the consideration that narcolepsy is a lifelong illness and patients must take medication for years. Tolerance or addiction may be seen with some compounds. Treatment of narcolepsy must thus balance avoidance of secondary side effects, avoidance of tolerance, and maintenance of all activities.

There may be a major difference in which side effects are acceptable to the physicians and which side effects are acceptable to the patients. On the one hand, some patients will not accept even mild tremor, even though they may be much more alert with even small doses of stimulants, whereas other patients readily accept tremor, fidgety behavior, irritability, and nocturnal insomnia as the price they pay to maintain alertness all day.

Historically, the drugs most widely used to treat EDS are the CNS stimulants (Table 1). Amphetamines were first proposed in 1935. The alerting effect of a single oral dose of amphetamine is maximal 2–4 hr after administration, and many patients require a single daily or twice-daily dose. However, a number of side effects, including irritability, tachycardia,

Table 1   MEDICATIONS FOR NARCOLEPSY

Medication	Dosage
Stimulants/alerting agents	
Modafinil	200–400 mg
Dextroamphetamine	20–60 mg/day
Methamphetamine	20–60 mg/day
Methylphenidate	10–60 mg/day
Pemoline	150 mg/day
Cataplexy antagonist	
γ-Hydroxybutyrate	2–3 g at bedtime
Protriptyline	10–40 mg/day
Clomipramine	25–200 mg/day
Fluoxetine	20–60 mg/day

nocturnal sleep disturbances, and sometimes tolerance and drug dependence, may occur. The use of methylphenidate was later encouraged because of faster action and lower frequency of side effects. Pemoline, an oxazolidine derivative with a longer half-life and a slower onset of action, is used less frequently. In rare cases, it is associated with severe hepatotoxicity. If pemoline is used, periodic liver function test monitoring is required.

Use of modafinil, a newer medication, may also result in substantial improvement. Modafinil's mechanism of action is not entirely clear, but modafinil does have important advantages over traditional stimulants. It has a safer cardiovascular profile and a lower risk of substance abuse. The longer half-life allows for once-a-day dosing, and it does not interfere with nocturnal sleep. Modafinil is currently the preferred medication for newly diagnosed narcoleptics. Modafinil's most common side effect is transient headaches, particularly with high starting dosages. This may be avoided by starting with a lower dosage.

The management of cataplexy is ideally part of a comprehensive narcolepsy treatment plan. Successful treatment typically must combine both behavioral and pharmacological treatments. The situation is analogous to other chronic conditions, such as juvenile diabetes mellitus, in which a combination of diet with medication can control the disease. Patients with narcolepsy–cataplexy will benefit from the healthy sleep habits referred to as sleep hygiene. Some patients with narcolepsy with relatively mild cataplexy may prefer not to take medication for their cataplexy, in part to avoid medication side effects. Also, some patients learn to anticipate the attacks. Finally, cataplexy does not typically progress in severity over time and sometimes may improve slightly during the course of the disease.

Cataplexy does not usually respond to the stimulant medications used to treat the sleepiness of narcolepsy. Narcoleptics typically take a medication to improve alertness and a different medication to avoid cataplexy attacks. Pharmacological treatment options for cataplexy may change due to the recent discovery of a gene responsible for narcolepsy. Cataplexy seems to respond best to medications with noradrenergic reuptake blocking properties. Medications used effectively include tricyclic antidepressants, such as clomipramine, protriptyline, and imipramine. Selective serotonin reuptake inhibitors, such as fluoxetine and venlafaxine, are effective and have fewer undesirable side effects than the tricyclic

antidepressants. Some patients have benefited from monoamine oxidase inhibitors (MAOIs), such as phenelzine. If an MAOI is used, stimulant drugs or tricyclics cannot be used. The interactions of MAOIs with modafinil have not been studied and caution should be used when concomitantly administering MAOIs with modafinil. Two of these medications, clomipramine and fluoxetine, have been more commonly used. Both of these drugs have active noradrenergic reuptake blocking metabolites (desmethylclomipramine and norfluoxetine), through which the therapeutic effect may be mediated.

The novel agent γ-hydroxybutyrate (GHB) is very effective and well tolerated in the treatment of cataplexy among narcoleptics. This is a precursor to γ-aminobutyric acid. This medication usually does not improve daytime sleepiness. The medication does increase slow-wave sleep without changing the amount of REM sleep. The dosage is usually approximately 2 or 3 g given at bedtime. In the United States, GHB is a very controversial compound. It has become a popular drug of abuse among some segments of society and has been given the notorious nickname of the date rape drug. The medication has strong sedating properties when mixed with alcohol. Attempts to classify GHB in the same category as heroin, cocaine, and other street drugs have been made. It has been shown to have medical benefit in cataplexy, but it should be used with caution in patients with a known history of substance abuse. To date, GHB has not been approved by the Food and Drug Administration. It is being used in the United States as part of ongoing research trials. GHB is effective in controlling cataplexy but not the other symptoms of narcolepsy.

Nocturnal sleep disturbances seem to be better controlled by GHB than by the benzodiazepines. The advantage of improving nocturnal sleep is significant not only for daytime sleepiness but also for cataplexy. However, stimulant medications are often necessary with GHB. Patients who present with all the clinical symptoms of narcolepsy frequently need a combination of drugs, particularly stimulants and tricyclics; GHB or a hypnotic may be needed at night.

Two other therapeutic approaches must be emphasized: short daytime naps and support groups. A 15- to 20-min nap taken three times daily will help maintain a satisfactory level of vigilance. Naps may have to be repeated throughout the day because the "refractory" sleep period after naps oscillates between 90 and 120 min. Undoubtedly, narcolepsy is a disabling disorder leading in many instances to loss of gainful employment because of daytime sleepiness and automatic behavior. It is also a disorder often poorly understood by patients, family members, and peers that can result in rejection from families and other social entities, divorce, loss of self-esteem, and depressive reactions. For these reasons, and in consideration of age of onset, it is important to put narcoleptic patients in contact with support groups and to help with the creation of regional narcolepsy associations and patient groups.

The aim of narcolepsy treatment is maintenance of the patient's wakefulness and alertness throughout the day. However, the medications currently available often have significant side effects. Treatment plans must therefore be tailored to individual preference and tolerance, with good communication between the physician and the patient.

—*Rafael Pelayo and Kin Yuen*

See also–Cataplexy; Drowsiness; Excessive Daytime Sleepiness; Insomnia; Multiple Sleep Latency Test (MSLT); REM (Rapid Eye Movement) Sleep; REM Sleep Behavior Disorder; Sleep Disorders; Sleep Paralysis; Sleep–Wake Cycle

Further Reading

Carskadon, M. A., Dement, W. C., Mitler, M., *et al.* (1986). Guidelines for the Multiple Sleep Latency Test (MSLT): A standard measure of sleepiness. *Sleep* **9**, 519–524.

Diagnostic Classification Steering Committee (M. J. Thorpy, Chairman) (1997). *International Classification of Sleep Disorders Diagnostic and Coding Manual.* American Association of Sleep Disorders, Rochester, MN.

Melberg, A., Ripley, B., Lin, L., *et al.* (2001). Hypocretin deficiency in familial symptomatic narcolepsy. *Ann. Neurol.* **49**, 136–137.

Nishino, S., Arrigoni, J., Shelton, J., *et al.* (1993). Desmethyl metabolites of serotonergic uptake inhibitors are more potent for suppressing canine cataplexy than their parent compounds. *Sleep* **16**, 706–712.

Rechtschaffen, A., and Kales, A. (Eds.) (1968). *A Manual of Standardized Terminology: Techniques and Scoring Systems for Sleep Stages of Human Subjects.* UCLA Brain Information Service/Brain Research Institute, Los Angeles.

Scharf, M. B., Lai, A. A., Branigan, B., *et al.* (1998). Pharmacokinetics of gammahydroxybutyrate (GHB) in narcoleptic patients. *Sleep* **21**, 507–514.

Vogel, G. (1960). Studies in psychophysiology of dreams. III. The dream of narcolepsy. *Arch. Gen. Psychiatry* **3**, 421–428.

Wing, Y. K., Lee, S. T., and Chen, C. N. (1994). Sleep paralysis in Chinese: Ghost oppression phenomenon in Hong Kong. *Sleep* **17**, 609–613.

Yoss, R. E., and Daly, D. D. (1968). On the treatment of narcolepsy. *Med. Clin. North Am.* **52**, 781–787.

Neck and Arm Pain

Encyclopedia of the Neurological Sciences
Copyright 2003, Elsevier Science (USA). All rights reserved.

PHYSIOLOGICALLY, pain can arise in any of three fundamental ways. Nociceptive pain arises when diseases or injuries of viscera or somatic tissues (bone, joints, ligaments, and muscles) stimulate the peripheral receptors of peripheral nerves. Neurogenic pain arises when the axons in the trunk of a peripheral nerve are stimulated somewhere along their course by inflammation, mechanical irritation, or injury. Each of these processes generates ectopic impulses in the affected axons at the site of disease or injury. Although the impulses are generated in the axon, they are perceived as having arisen in the territory subtended by the affected nerve. A subset of neurogenic pain is radicular pain, in which the axons are irritated or damaged in a dorsal root or at the dorsal root ganglion. Central pain arises when neurons in the dorsal horn or thalamus become spontaneously active as a result of being disinhibited or deafferentated. Central pain can occur as a result of ischemic injury to the central nervous system or as a result of disruption of peripheral nerves or central tracts. In either case, the neurons to which the injured nerves or tracts previously relayed cease to maintain receptors, their membranes become unstable, and they become spontaneously active.

All three pain mechanisms can affect the neck and upper limb. Each gives rise to a different constellation of symptoms and signs. Each invites a different approach to investigation and treatment.

NOCICEPTIVE NECK PAIN

Sources and Mechanism

Experiments in normal volunteers have demonstrated that neck pain can be produced by noxious stimulation of the posterior neck muscles and the synovial joints of the cervical spine. This pain is referred to characteristic, segmental locations (Fig. 1). If severe enough, the pain may radiate into the head, the upper limb, or the anterior chest wall. When referred to the head, somatic referred pain is perceived as, and may present as, headache. In the anterior chest wall it may mimic angina. In the upper limb, somatic referred pain may be mistaken for radicular pain.

The segmental patterns of somatic referred pain do not follow dermatomes but reflect the pattern of

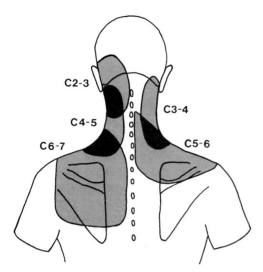

Figure 1
Map of the distribution of somatic referred pain from the zygapophysial joints at the segments indicated, produced by experimental noxious stimulation of the joint in normal volunteers (based on Dwyer *et al.*, 1990).

segmental innervation of the deep tissues of the neck and upper limb. Therefore, the location of pain does not implicate a particular structure as the source but reflects its segmental innervation. Consonant with this rule, observations in patients undergoing provocation discography reveal that the patterns of pain arising from the cervical intervertebral disks are essentially identical to those of the ipsisegmental zygapophysial joints. The mechanism of somatic referred pain is convergence. When afferents from a spinal structure converge on the same dorsal horn neurons that receive afferents from the head, upper limb, or chest wall, the cerebral cortex has no means of determining the exact origin of the stimulus and ascribes it to anywhere or everywhere within the regions subtended by those dorsal horn neurons.

Nociceptive pain has a deep, aching quality or may feel like an internal pressure expanding into and across the region in which it is perceived. Importantly, nociceptive pain is not associated with neurological signs. Its associated features are protean and simple. They are restriction of movement and muscle guarding, either or both of which may result in an abnormal posture or attitude of the neck.

Epidemiology: Neck pain is common. The annual incidence rate of acute neck pain is approximately 10%, and the prevalence of chronic neck pain is approximately 14%. It is more common among manual workers, office workers, secretaries, and

sewing machine operators. The risk factors for neck pain are occupation, physical stress at work, mental stress at work, previous injury, and working with machines. Psychological and personality factors have been refuted as risk factors for neck pain; they account for only 2% of the variance in symptoms of neck pain. Significant, however, are occupational psychosocial factors such as poor cooperation and camaraderie among employees, inability to influence one's work, and too great work demands.

The natural history of neck pain is relatively benign. Approximately 43% of patients recover fully within 10 years; 25% have only fleeting or minor symptoms, but 25% of patients still have moderate symptoms and approximately 7% remain or become severely disabled. Neck pain after whiplash has a good prognosis. Within 12 months, approximately 75% are asymptomatic, with the percentage increasing to 82% by 2 years. Approximately 20% of patients remain with symptoms, but only 4% are severely disabled. In the general community, the frequency of chronic neck pain due to whiplash is only approximately 1% or less; thus, whiplash represents only a fraction of the causes of chronic neck pain.

Etiology

There are many possible causes of neck pain. Some are uncommon and nonthreatening (in an immediate sense), such as rheumatoid arthritis, ankylosing spondylitis, Reiter's syndrome, psoriatic arthritis, and crystal arthropathies. Some are uncommon but serious because of the immediate threats they pose to life or well-being. These include fractures, tumors, infections, and metabolic disorders of the cervical spine; dissecting aneurysms of the vertebral or carotid arteries; and spinal hematomas.

In most cases of acute neck pain, however, the cause and source of pain are unknown. This deficit in knowledge arises because no population studies have pursued the causes of pain in patients with acute neck pain. Nor should they, given the self-limiting nature of most episodes. With respect to chronic neck pain, once tumors, infections, and other rare causes have been excluded, the known causes are few. The best available data implicate injuries to the cervical zygapophysial joints as the cause of pain in at least 50% of patients with chronic neck pain after whiplash. Outside the context of whiplash, the prevalence of cervical zygapophysial joint pain is not known. Some authorities maintain that disorders of the cervical intervertebral disks can cause neck pain; others believe in myofascial disorders. However, no epidemiological data indicate how commonly either of these conditions are the basis for neck pain.

Cervical spondylosis is not a cause of neck pain. It is a normal age change that correlates poorly, if at all, with the presence of neck pain. It is equally prevalent in individuals who do not have neck pain. Indeed, osteoarthrosis of the synovial joints of the cervical spine is slightly more common in individuals who do not have neck pain.

Although feared as a cause of neck pain (for medicolegal reasons), fractures of the neck are actually not common. In accident and emergency settings, only approximately 3% of patients suspected of having a fracture prove to have fractures upon cervical radiography.

History

In patients presenting simply with neck pain, no aspect of history allows a diagnosis to be pinpointed in the majority of cases. Typically, the patient presents with pain and limited movement but no other features. However, history is critical in screening for serious and rare conditions. These should be suspected if the patient has a past history of cancer, risk factors for infection (such as body penetration or sepsis elsewhere in the body), unusually severe and unremitting pain, or pain that is not relieved by rest or sleep. Neurological symptoms suggest a neurological disorder. Cerebrovascular features suggest vertebral or carotid vascular disease. Fractures should be suspected in light of external trauma to the head or neck, such as in a fall or a blow. Inertial injury, as occurs in whiplash, is very unlikely to cause a significant fracture.

Physical Examination

Conventional clinical examination does not provide a diagnosis of neck pain. Various techniques lack reliability, validity, or both. At best, clinical examination can detect tenderness and restricted range of movement, and it allows the physician to describe the patient's presentation. However, none of these features allow a specific, pathoanatomical diagnosis to be rendered. Otherwise, physical examination principally serves to rule out features of a neurological, systemic, or other serious disorder.

Investigations

For acute neck pain, pain alone is not an indication for investigations. Investigations are indicated by associated features, such as neurological or cerebrovascular symptoms and signs, a history of cancer, risk factors for infection, or a genuine suspicion of a metabolic disorder. If these are absent, investigations for screening purposes are not justified. Large population studies showed that in no case did plain radiography of the neck reveal a diagnosis that was not already suspected from the history, and in no instance would a serious disease have been missed had the radiographs not been obtained. In the vast majority of patients with neck pain, plain radiography reveals nothing that correlates with pain, nor does computed tomography (CT) or magnetic resonance imaging (MRI). Physicians need legitimate medical reasons to request these investigations. Neck pain is not one of them.

In due course, a reasonable indication for medical imaging is persistence of pain and failure to respond to treatment. In this case, imaging might be undertaken to rule out rare or occult disorders. For this purpose, MRI has the greatest sensitivity and specificity. Its role, however, is to rule out tumors, infections, and metabolic disorders. Not even MRI will establish the cause of chronic neck pain in the majority of cases. However, in litigious societies such as the United States, physicians often obtain these studies defensively.

If a definitive diagnosis of the source of chronic neck pain is required or desired, invasive procedures will need to be employed. The best validated procedures are diagnostic blocks of the cervical zygapophysial joints. These joints can be anesthetized under fluoroscopic control using intraarticular injections of local anesthetic or by blocking the nerves that innervate them—the medial branches of the cervical dorsal rami. Medial branch blocks are the more expedient test and easier to perform. When performed under double-blind conditions, these blocks serve to pinpoint one of the zygapophysial joints as the source of the patient's pain. The use of controlled blocks is essential to reduce the risk of false-positive responses, which is high if only single diagnostic blocks are used.

Cervical provocation discography is designed to test if an intervertebral disks is the source of pain. It involves stressing the target disk with an injection of contrast medium into the nucleus pulposus. Provocation discography, however, needs to be carefully undertaken and interpreted. It carries a high false-positive rate, and it is uncommon for a single disk to be painful; most often, two or more disks appear to be symptomatic.

Treatment

Many options are available for the treatment of neck pain. However, despite their popularity, few interventions have been validated by randomized, double-blind, controlled trials. Moreover, many interventions have been studied, but the abundant literature refutes more treatments than it vindicates.

For the treatment of acute neck pain, the use of collars, transcutaneous electrical nerve stimulation (TENS), neck school, spray and stretch, laser therapy, and traction have been found to confer no benefit greater than that of placebo or even no treatment. For acute neck pain after whiplash, multimodal therapy, tailored physiotherapy, and manual therapy are each more effective than rest and analgesia in that they hasten recovery during the first 4 weeks after onset of pain. However, by 12 weeks, the results are not better. The only conservative intervention that has been shown to achieve significant long-term gains is home exercises. In the treatment of whiplash, a 1-week course of NSAIDs followed by encouragement and insistence to resume normal activities has been found to be as efficacious as any other intervention.

For the conservative therapy of chronic neck pain, there are no data on the efficacy of short-wave diathermy, collars, traction, TENS, laser therapy, neck school, spray and stretch, or trigger point therapy. Magnetic necklaces have only a placebo effect. Acupuncture is no more effective than sham TENS or sham acupuncture. Physiotherapy is no better than acupuncture. Manual therapy is better than massage and traction but is not better than using salicylates while on a waiting list. Intensive exercises are no more effective than less intensive exercises; both achieve only modest improvements (25%) in pain and disability. Intraarticular injections of corticosteroids for cervical zygapophysial joint pain offer no long-term and little short-term benefit. One uncontrolled study attests to the efficacy of a 4-week, multimodal treatment program involving graded return to activity, abolishing pain behavior, and restoring muscle strength and endurance. At 6-month follow-up, pain was reduced to "healthy" levels in 46% of patients, disabilities were reduced to normal levels in 38%, cognitive and behavioral complaints were eliminated in approximately 90%, 65% of patients returned to work, 58% ceased to use drugs, and 81% ceased to pursue medical care.

Surgical treatment, in the form of anterior cervical fusion, is performed in some centers for persistent neck pain. Studies of this therapy claim success, but outcome measures are few and lacking in rigor. Some studies report disappointing results, particularly for surgical therapy of neck pain after whiplash.

Much stronger evidence obtains for cervical radiofrequency neurotomy. In this procedure, the medial branches of the cervical dorsal rami are coagulated in order to denervate painful cervical zygapophysial joints. A randomized, double-blind, controlled trial established that this procedure is not a placebo. Moreover, it is the only treatment for neck pain that has been shown to be able to consistently achieve complete abolition of pain and concomitant restoration of activities of daily living. Complete relief of pain persists for approximately 9 months and more than 1 year in some cases. Although the pain returns once the nerves recover, the procedure can be successfully repeated to reinstate relief. The indication for this treatment is complete relief of pain upon anesthetizing the cervical zygapophysial joints under double-blind conditions.

An Algorithm

Based on the best available evidence, an appropriate algorithm for the management of neck pain is the following:

• Obtain a careful history. If there has been significant trauma, obtain radiographs to screen for fractures, and manage accordingly. If there are reasons to suspect tumor, infection, vascular disease, or a systemic disorder, investigate and manage accordingly.

• Perform a physical examination to confirm that there is no basis to suspect a serious disorder.

• Implement conservative management but review the patient and remain vigilant for the late onset of associated features that might implicate a serious disorder.

• Provide an explanation of the patient's problem. Be reassuring that there is no serious cause for the pain and no need for concern. Provide simple analgesia, if required. Implement a course of home exercises. Encourage and assist with resumption of normal activities, in a graded fashion if required.

• Monitor the patient's progress. Remain vigilant for the onset of associated features that might implicate a serious disorder.

• If the patient is not improving, entertain the possibility of manual therapy to expedite recovery.

• Consider if recovery is being impeded by psychosocial factors, such as the work environment, legal issues, fears, or inappropriate and counter-productive beliefs. Deal with these issues, or engage specialist services if required.

• If the patient's pain persists, undertake MRI to screen for occult disorders.

• If the patient's pain threatens to become chronic or has become chronic, undertake controlled, zyga-pophysial joint blocks; if these are positive, under-take radiofrequency neurotomy. Consider if discography and anterior fusion might be an option; undertake these judiciously.

• Consider referral to a competent multidisci-plinary pain program that might deal with the patient's pain beliefs and undertake graded return to activity.

CERVICAL RADICULOPATHY

Cervical radicular pain and cervical radiculopathy usually, if not typically, occur concomitantly. Although they are different phenomena, they are often mistakenly regarded as one and the same thing. The features of one are often confused with those of the other. As a result, it is difficult to disentangle the features of radicular pain from the composite picture. However, the features of radicu-lopathy are easier to retrieve, describe, and explain. Accordingly, those features are described here as a prelude to the more exacting issue of cervical radicular pain.

Definition and Mechanism

Radiculopathy is a condition in which conduction is blocked in the axons of a spinal nerve by a disorder that affects the roots of that nerve. When the dorsal root is affected, the clinical feature of conduction block is numbness in a dermatomal distribution. When the ventral root is affected, weakness occurs in a myotomal distribution. Depression or loss of reflexes can occur as a result of the afferent arc being interrupted in the dorsal root, the efferent arc being interrupted in the ventral, or both. In contrast to conduction block, paraesthesiae are ectopic impulses generated from a peripheral nerve as a result of ischemia of that nerve. They are a prominent feature of radiculopathy and suggest that the affected root is being rendered ischemic. If paraesthesiae occur before or in the absence of numbness, this suggests a disorder that is sufficient to compromise the blood supply of the nerve root but that has not yet compromised the conduction in the axons of the affected root.

Clinical Features

The clinical features of radiculopathy are paraesthe-siae, numbness, weakness, and loss of reflexes. These can occur in various combinations, depending on the extent to which the nerve roots are affected by the causative pathology. In the surgical literature, para-esthesiae and hyporeflexia are the most common features expressed by patients diagnosed as having cervical radiculopathy, followed by numbness and weakness. The critical and distinguishing feature of any of these symptoms and signs is their segmental distribution.

Etiology

By way of mechanism, the causes of cervical radiculopathy can be summarized as any lesion that encroaches on a cervical nerve root or compromises its blood supply. Rare causes include tumors and cysts of the nerve roots or their meninges, angioma and arteritis of the cervical radicular arteries, and tumors and other disorders of the vertebral bodies or zygapophysial joints that impinge upon a cervical nerve root. More common causes are cervical disk protrusion and foraminal stenosis caused by osteo-phytes of the vertebral body or of the zygapophysial joint related to the affected nerve root. Trauma is the alleged precipitant in fewer than 20% of cases.

Epidemiology

The prevalence of cervical radiculopathy has not been measured. Its incidence, however, is either 5.5 or 38.4 cases per 100,000 population per year. The cardinal risk factors are diving, coughing, and heavy lifting. There are no explicit data on the natural history of cervical radiculopathy, but anecdotal reports and inferences drawn from controlled trials of treatment suggest a good prognosis. Approximately 70% of patients improve with time, with all symptoms resolving in 20%. In the long term, perhaps only 10% of patients remain severely disabled.

Differential Diagnosis

A diagnosis of cervical radiculopathy should be self-evident when a patient complains of numbness, weakness, or paraesthesiae in a segmental distribu-tion. Few conditions resemble radiculopathy. The classic differential diagnosis includes myelopathy and spinal cord lesions, but the cardinal features of these conditions are long-tract signs and involvement of the lower limbs. Similarly, multiple sclerosis lacks a clear segmental pattern. Peripheral neuropathy may share some of the clinical features of radiculopathy, but the distinction lies in the different patterns of distribution of a segmental nerve and a peripheral nerve. Clinically, the features of a C8 radiculopathy may be indistinguishable from those of an ulnar nerve lesion at the wrist, but if there is no evidence of a lesion at the wrist, nerve conduction studies can resolve the difficulty.

Physical Examination

Testing for numbness and weakness is a reliable procedure. Agreement between observers in detecting these features is moderate to good, with kappa scores of 0.4 to more than 0.6. (In this regard, the kappa score measures agreement between observers, with a score of 1.0 indicating perfect agreement and a score of 0 indicating no agreement beyond chance alone.) It is also reasonably valid in determining which segment is affected.

Clinical examination is also a valid procedure for cervical radiculopathy. Hyporeflexia is the most valid sign, followed by numbness and weakness. The presence of these features predicts quite well the presence of radiculopathy, as confirmed by surgery. However, they do not necessarily indicate which segment is affected. For that purpose, a dermatomal distribution of paraesthesiae is the most accurate feature.

Neurological symptoms and signs are usually enough to establish an accurate diagnosis of cervical radiculopathy. Accessory tests contribute little to improving confidence in diagnosis. These tests include the compression test, in which the patient's neck is flexed laterally to the side of pain in an effort to close the intervertebral foramen and aggravate nerve root compression; the traction test, in which the patient's head is lifted by the examiner in an effort to decompress the affected nerves; and the abduction test, in which abduction of the arm is supposed to aggravate compression of the affect nerve roots. A positive compression test increases the specificity of physical assessment but decreases its sensitivity. As a result, confidence in the diagnosis is increased but fewer patients are diagnosed as positive overall. Manual traction is infrequently positive in patients with radiculopathy and lends little to diagnostic confidence, nor does the abduction test for the same reason.

Investigations

Special investigations are not indicated in the diagnosis of cervical radiculopathy. The diagnosis can be made confidently upon history and physical examination alone. Investigations may be required to establish the exact cause of radiculopathy, but these may not be required unless and until symptoms persist. In that event, plain radiographs are of little value because, of the conditions relevant to cervical radiculopathy, they can show only osteophytes or advanced tumors or metabolic bone disease. The preferred investigation is MRI, coupled with a plain film if required to identify osteophytes that are poorly resolved by MRI. Although CT and CT myelography have been used in the past, these investigations lack sensitivity and specificity for rarer and unusual causes of radiculopathy and offer no advantage if MRI is available.

Electrodiagnostic studies serve little purpose in the investigation of cervical radiculopathy. They are superfluous if a diagnosis can already be made confidently on the basis of history and physical examination. Their role is limited to the assessment of patients with peripheral neuropathy that genuinely might resemble radiculopathy. For the determination of the segmental level affected, electrodiagnostic studies have poor accuracy. Their role in this regard is superfluous if imaging is undertaken. However, other authors believe they have an important role in determining the functional relevance of any imaging abnormalities and in detecting radiculopathies not related to mechanical factors.

Treatment

Conspicuously, there are no data from controlled studies on the efficacy of conservative therapy for radiculopathy. Ironically, although the features of radiculopathy are used as the basis for diagnosing radicular pain, it seems that treatment is undertaken exclusively for pain; treatment is not directed at relieving numbness, weakness, or paraesthesiae. It would also not be logical to undertake conservative therapy for radiculopathy. No form of manual therapy, and no amount of manual therapy or exercise, has any prospect of relieving a nerve root compression, nor does any form of drug therapy. Traction causes a trivial displacement of cervical vertebrae, and any increase in the diameter of an intervertebral foramen is lost within minutes of releasing the traction.

Surgery is the only treatment for cervical radiculopathy that has a logical biological basis. In this regard, cervical nerve roots can be decompressed anteriorly by discectomy with or without subsequent interbody fusion or posteriorly by foraminotomy.

However, even the surgical literature does not report the success rate of relieving features of radiculopathy. It, too, is preoccupied with the relief of pain.

CERVICAL RADICULAR PAIN

Definition and Mechanisms

By definition, cervical radicular pain is pain that is caused by irritation or a disorder of a cervical nerve root. For this reason, in descriptions and studies, cervical radicular pain has been confused with cervical radiculopathy. However, the mechanisms of the two conditions must be different. The neurological signs of radiculopathy are caused by conduction block. Radicular pain is not caused by conduction block. It requires the ectopic generation of nociceptive impulses. This requires either inflammation of the nerve root or compression of the dorsal root ganglion. Experiments in laboratory animals have demonstrated that compression of a normal nerve root does not generate activity in nociceptive afferents.

Clinical Features

There are few explicit data on the clinical features of cervical radicular pain. Although it may be regarded that radicular pain often accompanies radiculopathy, the features of the radiculopathy are not the features of pain. Whereas the paraesthesiae and numbness of cervical radiculopathy follow a dermatomal distribution, cervical radicular pain does not. The common claim that radicular pain follows a dermatomal distribution is patently wrong and probably stems from inattention to the actual distribution of pain or confusion of the distribution of paraesthesiae with the distribution of pain.

Experiments involving the artificial stimulation of cervical nerve roots reveal that radicular pain has a widespread distribution that differs markedly between individuals. Significantly for clinical purposes, radicular pain is perceived extensively around the shoulder girdle (i.e., proximally), where it bears no relationship to the corresponding dermatome. Even when it extends distally into the upper limb, cervical radicular pain bears no more than a superficial and inaccurate resemblance to dermatomes (Fig. 2). This is understandable because radicular pain has no obligation to be exclusively cutaneous. If a cervical nerve root is irritated, the afferents from deep somatic tissues it transmits will be affected. Consequently, cervical radicular pain will largely be felt deeply in the tissues subtended by the affected nerve root.

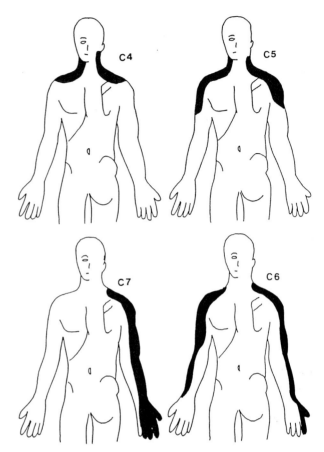

Figure 2
Maps of the most consistent patterns of distribution of cervical radicular pain produced in normal volunteers by mechanical stimulation of the spinal nerves (based on Slipman *et al.*, 1998).

Of particular difficulty is the distinction between cervical radicular pain and somatic referred pain. Either can be perceived in the shoulder girdle, and when limited to that distribution they cannot be distinguished on the basis of distribution or quality. A distinction can be made, however, if the pain radiates further distally into the upper limb. No clinical studies have reported somatic referred pain extending beyond the upper arm, whereas cervical radicular pain commonly does so. Consequently, pain extending beyond the elbow and into the hand is unlikely to be somatic referred pain and is most likely to be radicular pain. Confidence in the diagnosis is enhanced if such a distal referral of pain is accompanied by features of radiculopathy.

However, if the pain is felt only proximally, one cannot be confident that it is radicular pain, or only radicular pain, even in the presence of radiculopathy. The proximal pain may be somatic referred pain, wholly or in part. Indeed, surgeons warn that whereas arm pain is usually the result of nerve compression, pain in the neck, shoulder girdle, and anterior chest is probably referred pain from the disk (which is responsible for the nerve root compression). Failure to appreciate this distinction can lead to inappropriate, incomplete, or inadequate treatment. Although nerve root decompression may successfully relieve arm pain, it will not relieve more proximal pain if that is referred from a structure and disorder that is not addressed by the decompression.

Investigations

No imaging studies or electrodiagnostic studies are indicated for cervical radicular pain. Neither type of study can show pain. Nor can they show the mechanism or cause of pain. If radicular pain is associated with radiculopathy, imaging studies are justified to define the cause of the radiculopathy. In that event, the cause of radicular pain can be inferred as the same as the cause of the radiculopathy. However, in the absence of radiculopathy, one has no legitimate grounds for invoking nerve root irritation as the basis for pain and no grounds for not considering the pain to be somatic referred pain and investigating it accordingly.

Treatment

Data are available on the effectiveness of conservative therapy for cervical radicular pain. They are not complimentary. Although often referred to in the surgical literature, conservative therapy for cervical radicular pain has never been defined. It involves various combinations of drugs, physical therapy, traction, collars, bed rest, exercise, and TENS. There are no explicit data on the efficacy of drug therapy for cervical radicular pain, but most of the other elements of conservative therapy have been tested, either individually or in combinations.

Traction offers no benefit greater than that of sham traction. Nor are traction or collars more efficacious than placebo heat or placebo tablets. When assessed by self-report, and when compared to patients treated with isometric exercises or with traction, a greater proportion of patients who received no treatment failed to improve. However, when assessed by a physician the three groups of patients did not differ statistically with respect to outcome. Physiotherapy confers no greater benefit than that of simply wearing a rigid collar for three months.

In all studies of the efficacy of conservative therapy for cervical radicular pain, recovery cannot be distinguished from the effects of natural history or the nonspecific effects of attention and "something being done." Moreover, virtually all studies report patients who failed treatment and had to undergo surgery.

Surgery is the mainstay for intractable cervical radicular pain. Most of the literature attests to good results, regardless of the technique used. However, within this literature better results are reported in smaller studies and in those from the United States. Larger studies from Europe claim more modest results. The only randomized, controlled study found no difference in outcome between patients treated surgically and those treated with physiotherapy or with a collar. However, the results from surgery in that study were far worse than those claimed in uncontrolled studies. One long-term study warns that although surgery for radicular pain is largely successful, in only approximately 64% of patients is the relief obtained permanent, approximately 16% develop recurrent neck pain, and a further 16% develop recurrent radicular pain.

CENTRAL PAIN

Brachial plexus avulsion is the most vivid example of central pain affecting the cervical region. The diagnosis is obvious given a history of injury causing downward thrust to the shoulder girdle and the presence of a denervated upper limb. Pain rarely if ever occurs in patients in whom the roots of the brachial plexus are disrupted distal to the dorsal root ganglion. Avulsion of the roots proximal to the ganglion is a prerequisite for the production of pain, which suggests that lack of trophic influence from the dorsal root ganglion, in addition to the absence of afferent input, is necessary for the production of pain. The pain is typically burning in quality, which is characteristic of central pain.

Although the diagnosis is obvious from the presenting clinical features, investigations might be undertaken to demonstrate which roots have been avulsed. These can involve MRI, myelography, and somatosensory evoked potentials.

The pain is virtually resistant to conservative therapy. Medications, even opioids, have a poor reputation of efficacy. This correlates with the pathophysiology of deafferentation pain that involves dorsal horn neurons ceasing to maintain receptors, particularly the inhibitory receptors that are required for opioids and tricyclic antidepressants to exert an analgesic effect. Resumption of normal activities, and the distraction that doing so entails, is the most effective conservative measure. The one treatment that can abolish the pain is dorsal root entry zone lesioning. This entails coagulating with a radio frequency electrode the dorsal horn neurons at the segments from which the nerve roots have been avulsed.

Syringomyelia is another condition that technically constitutes a possible cause of central pain affecting the cervical region. It differs from brachial plexus avulsion in that peripheral afferents remain intact. Instead, the syrinx may interrupt the axons of second-order nociceptive neurons, whereupon the deafferentated neurons are located in the thalamus and brainstem. The diagnosis is provided by the presence of a suspended sensory segment. The differential diagnosis includes spinal cord injury and intramedullary tumors. MRI is the quintessential method of demonstrating the causative lesion.

Like all central pains, the pain of syringomyelia is difficult to treat because of the extensive disruption to patterns of neural activity. Drainage of the syrinx may prevent progression of the neurological defect but offers little prospect of relief of pain. The most recent textbook of pain medicine offers no therapeutic alternative for this condition.

—*Nikolai Bogduk*

See also–Facial Pain; Nerve Injury; Neuropathic Pain Syndromes; Neuropathy, Axillary; Pain, Assessment of; Pain, Overview; Radiculopathy; Radiculopathy, Cervical, Surgery

Further Reading

Aker, P. D., Gross, A. R., Goldsmith, C. H., *et al.* (1996). Conservative management of mechanical neck pain: Systematic overview and meta-analysis. *Br. Med. J.* **313**, 1291–1296.

Bogduk, N. (1994). Innervation and pain patterns of the cervical spine. In *Physical Therapy of the Cervical and Thoracic Spine* (R. Grant, Ed.), 2nd ed., pp. 65–76. Churchill-Livingstone, New York.

Bogduk, N. (1998). Treatment of whiplash injuries. In *Cervical Flexion–Extension/Whiplash Injuries. Spine: State of the Art Reviews.* (G. A. Malanga, Ed.), Vol. 12, pp. 469–483. Hanley & Belfus, Philadelphia.

Bogduk, N. (1999). *Medical Management of Acute Cervical Radicular Pain. An Evidence-Based Approach.* Newcastle Bone and Joint Institute, Newcastle, Australia.

Bogduk, N. (1999). The neck. *Bailliere's Clin. Rheumatol.* **13**, 261–285.

Borchgrevink, G. E., Kaasa, A., McDonagh, D., *et al.* (1998). Acute treatment of whiplash neck sprain injuries: A randomized trial of treatment during the first 14 days after a car accident. *Spine* **23**, 25–31.

Dwyer, A., Aprill, C., and Bogduk, N. (1990). Cervical zygapophyseal joint pain patterns I: A study in normal volunteers. *Spine* **15**, 453–457.

Loeser, J. D. (Ed.) (2001). *Bonica's Management of Pain*, 3rd ed. Lippincott Williams & Wilkins, Philadelphia.

Lord, S. M., McDonald, G. J., and Bogduk, N. (1998). Percutaneous radiofrequency neurotomy of the cervical medial branches: A validated treatment for cervical zygapophysial joint pain. *Neurosurg. Q.* **8**, 288–308.

Slipman, C. W., Plastaras, C. T., Palmitier, R. A., *et al.* (1998). Symptom provocation of fluoroscopically guided cervical nerve root stimulation: Are dynatomal maps identical to dermatomal maps? *Spine* **23**, 2235–2242.

Vendrig, A. A., van Akkerveeken, F., and McWhorter, K. R. (2000). Results of a multimodal treatment program for patients with chronic symptoms after a whiplash injury of the neck. *Spine* **25**, 238–244.

Wynn-Parry, C. B. (1980). Pain in avulsion lesions of the brachial plexus. *Pain* **9**, 41–53.

Necrosis
see Cell Death

Necrotizing Encephalopathy
see Subacute Necrotizing Encephalomyelopathy

Neglect Disorders

Encyclopedia of the Neurological Sciences
Copyright 2003, Elsevier Science (USA). All rights reserved.

NEGLECT is the failure to report, respond to, or orient to meaningful or novel stimuli. These failures are primarily for stimuli or actions that occur on the side contralateral to a hemispheric lesion; however, these deficits may also be ipsilateral. If these deficits can be accounted for by either elemental sensory deficits, such as a hemianopsia, or motor defects, such as a hemiparesis, then these failures are not considered to be neglect. Neglect and related disorders are severely disabling and patients with neglect are less likely to be able to live independently than even patients with global aphasia.

SUBTYPES OF NEGLECT

Many different behavioral abnormalities or subtypes of neglect have been reported. The subtypes are distinguished by several different factors, including the following:

- *Domain:* Spatial neglect, personal neglect, and representational or imagery neglect
- *Input or output demands:* Inattention or sensory neglect versus intentional or motor neglect
- *Means of eliciting:* Unilateral stimuli (inattention) or actions (motor neglect) versus bilateral stimuli (extinction to simultaneous stimuli) or actions (motor extinction)
- *Spatial distribution:* Horizontal, vertical, and radial
- *Reference frames:* Viewer centered, environmentally centered, and object centered. Other neurobehavioral disorders, such as anosognosia, are often associated with neglect; however, they will not be discussed here.

CLINICAL SIGNS AND SYMPTOMS

Sensory Neglect or Inattention

Sensory neglect or inattention is a form of selective unawareness. Sensory neglect may be defined by its modality (e.g., tactile, visual, and auditory). Sensory neglect may be associated with an ipsilesional attentional bias and an inability to disengage from stimuli in ipsilesional space.

To test for inattention, the patient is presented with stimuli (visual, tactile, and auditory modalities) or no stimuli to either the ipsilesional or contralesional sides of the body in random order. Each time a stimulus or nonstimulus is presented, the examiner says "now." If the patient makes more contralesional than ipsilesional errors, they have evidence of inattention. If a patient consistently fails to detect any contralesional stimulus, it may be difficult to determine if the patient's problem is inattention or an elemental sensory defect. There are several means by which these deficits can be differentiated. In the auditory modality, because hemispheric lesions do not cause contralesional deafness, if a patient fails to detect auditory stimuli that come from the contralateral portion of space, they have inattention. In the visual modality, inattention may be body or head hemispatial, such that the patient is unaware of visual stimuli that come from the contralateral side of space or the side of the body or head, rather than

being hemiretinal. Therefore, patients who cannot detect contralesional stimuli may be able to detect these stimuli if their heads or eyes are deviated to the ipsilesional side (such that the contralesional retinal field now falls in ipsilesional hemispace). When a patient cannot detect stimuli that fall on one side of the retina or one side of the body, they may either be inattentive or have a primary sensory defect. Techniques such as caloric stimulation, in which cold water is injected into the ear on the same side as the inattention, may allow the person to detect contralateral visual and tactile stimuli and thereby help discriminate between inattention and deafferentation. Optokinetic nystagmus and vibration of neck muscles have also been used for similar purposes. Psychophysiological techniques such as evoked potentials or galvanic skin responses may also help demonstrate that a defect is inattention rather than deafferentation.

Extinction to Simultaneous Stimulation

Many patients who are first unaware of stimuli may recover and be able to detect isolated stimuli that are presented to the contralesional side of the body or hemispace. However, when presented with two or more simultaneous stimuli they may demonstrate unawareness of the contralesional stimulus(extinction). Like inattention, extinction may also be defined by the modality of stimulation (tactile, visual, and auditory).

Extinction is tested in a manner similar to that used to test for inattention. To test for extinction, the patient is presented with stimuli (visual, tactile, and auditory modalities) or no stimuli to the ipsilesional side, the contralesional side, or both sides of the body or hemispace in random order. Each time a stimulus or nonstimulus is presented, the examiner says "now" and the patient responds by saying "right," "left," "both," or "neither." If a patient is able to detect contralesional stimuli when presented alone but with bilateral simultaneous stimulation only detects the ipsilesional stimuli, the patient exhibits extinction.

Intentional or Motor Neglect

Patients with neglect may fail to normally respond to stimuli in contralateral hemispace or on the contralesional side of the body. However, this failure to respond may be related not to unawareness of the stimulus but rather an inability to initiate a movement.

There are several forms of intentional neglect. Patients who appear to be hemiplegic may not have damage to the corticospinal system as determined by imaging or magnetic stimulation. This pseudohemiplegia is termed limb akinesia or motor neglect. Other subjects may be unable to move a limb in contralesional hemispace but may be able to move it in ipsilesional hemispace. This disorder has been termed hemispatial akinesia. Similarly, patients may be impaired in moving the head, eyes (e.g., gaze paresis), or even arm in a contralesional direction (directional akinesia). Some patients who can move the contralesional limb alone have difficulty initiating movement of this limb at the same time as they are starting to move the ipsilesional limb (motor extinction).

Hypokinesia is a milder form of intentional neglect in which there is a delay in initiating a movement. Movements of reduced amplitude (hypometria) may also occur in the limbs, eyes, or head. Movement may also be directional or hemispatial. Motor impersistence is the inability to sustain a movement or posture. In general, when one tests for impersistence the examiner asks the patient to maintain a posture for a given period of time. Motor impersistence may also be seen in the limbs, eyes, or head. It may also be hemispatial or directional.

Patients with limb akinesia or motor neglect may appear to have a hemiparesis. However, unlike patient with weakness, many patients with limb akinesia can be encouraged to move the extremity and then may show normal strength. Unlike patients with a hemiparesis, who show signs of effort or even shoulder movement, patients with limb akinesia may fail to show these signs. Transcranial magnetic stimulation may be used to demonstrate an intact corticospinal tract in those patients who cannot be encouraged to move.

One of the best means for testing for hypokinesia is by performing reaction times. These can be performed for the limbs (limb hypokinesia), head, or eyes in a hemispace (hemispatial akinesia) and in a direction (directional hypokinesia).

To test for hypometria, one directs the patient to move a certain distance and then ascertains if the subject undershot their mark. However, one must use a testing procedure that enables one to dissociate inattention (to the target) from hypometria. For example, before having a patient saccade to a target, the patient should be able to see the target. If the patient then makes multiple small saccades until they reach the target, the patient has a directional hypometria of their eyes. To test for hemispatial or directional impersistence, one usually asks a patient to maintain a posture (e.g., "look leftward and keep looking leftward until I tell you to stop") for 15 sec.

Hemispatial Neglect

Patients with hemispatial neglect fail to act on environmental stimuli that are contralateral to their hemispheric lesion. For example, when eating food from a tray, they may just eat the food that is ipsilateral to their hemispheric lesion.

Hemispatial neglect may occur in all three dimensions of space: horizontal (right and left), vertical (up and down), and radial (near and far). Therefore, tests that assess spatial neglect should evaluate all three dimensions. There are three bedside tests used to test for spatial neglect: line bisection, target cancellation, and drawing. Each of these tests may assess different functions. When performing the line bisection task, a patient is presented with a line and asked to find the middle of the line. Longer lines are more likely to detect neglect than are shorter lines. With very short lines, a patient with neglect may err by placing a mark in the portion of the line that is in contralesional hemispace. By placing the entire line in contralesional hemispace, neglect is more likely to be detected than by placing the line in ipsilateral hemispace. Putting cues on the ipsilateral side of the line may also increase neglect, and having cues on the contralesional side may reduce neglect.

When performing the cancellation test, a sheet of paper with targets is placed before the patient and the patient is asked to mark out or cancel all the targets. Increasing the number of targets, placing them randomly on the sheet, and using foils that are difficult to discriminate from the targets are methods that can be used to increase the sensitivity of the task. While the patient is performing the cancellation task, it is important to see the means by which they explore the sheet (i.e., from left to right versus right to left). Most normal people explore from left to right. Patients with left side neglect often start from the right and explore right to left.

Drawing should be tested by both having the patient copy the examiner's drawing and having the patient draw spontaneously. Copying asymmetrical nonsense figures is usually a more sensitive test for neglect than copying symmetrical familiar figures. The more detailed the drawing, the more sensitive the task. If a patient has difficulty copying one side of a figure, they may have an attentional or an intentional deficit. If the subject does not draw one side spontaneously, they may have an intentional or representational deficit (i.e., the memory of one side of the object is no longer present because it was destroyed by the lesion).

To dissociate attentional from intentional hemispatial neglect, one can use different forms of the crossed response task, in which the subject acts in ipsilateral space when presented contralesional stimuli and acts in contralesional space when present with ipsilesional stimuli. This can be performed using a variety of techniques, including video cameras with monitors, strings and pulleys, and mirrors.

When a patient has hemispatial neglect, they may be neglecting the contralesional part of space that is opposite the eyes, head, or body (viewer-centered frame of reference). Alternatively, they may be using an environmental frame of reference. One can dissociate viewer-centered from environmentally centered neglect by having the patient bisect lines in the upright position and then having the patient bisect lines when lying down on their right or left side. If the patient's performance does not change with a change of positions, their neglect is viewer centered; if the patient's neglect changes, it is environmentally centered.

Personal Neglect

Patients with personal neglect may be unaware of the side of their body that is contralateral to a hemispheric lesion. Other patients are not even aware that portions of their contralateral body belong to them. This is called asomatognosia.

Patients with personal neglect may fail to groom or even dress one side of their body. They may complain that someone is in bed with them. To more formally test for personal neglect, one can ask the subject to show or point to different portions of the right or left side of their body. One can perform a cancellation-type task in which one puts small pieces of sticky paper on different areas of the patient's body and asks them to take them all off. Last, one can perform a bisection task in which a horizontal line is placed before the subject, who is asked to show, by pointing, the position on the line that is directly across from the middle of their chest (e.g., midsagittal plane).

Representational Imagery Neglect

Representational imagery neglect may be spatial or personal. When patients are asked to image an object, scene, or body part, they may report only those items that are ipsilateral to their lesion.

Patients should be asked to recall details of a familiar scene from a particular perspective; for example, "When you walk into your living room, what do you see?"

PATHOPHYSIOLOGY

Pathology

Neglect and related disorders can be induced by a wide variety of diseases, including stroke, degenerative diseases, and tumors, and trauma. In humans, neglect is most commonly associated with lesions that involve the right parietal lobe. However, there are other areas in which lesions in humans have been reported to induce neglect, including the dorsolateral frontal lobes, the mesial frontal lobes including the cingulate gyrus, the thalamus and mesencephalic reticular formation, and the basal ganglia.

Attention

The brain has a limited capacity to process incoming information. Attention is the process by which the brain triages incoming stimuli according to their significance. Lesions and functional imaging studies suggest that attention is mediated by a corticolimbic reticular network. One attends to stimuli that have biological significance and ignores stimuli that are irrelevant. In order to attend to a stimulus, one must know what the stimulus is and where it is located. The ventral portion of the visual system (e.g., ventral temporal lobe) is important for determining the type of stimuli (What?), and the dorsal portion codes the spatial location (Where?). The somatosensory and auditory systems may also be categorized into "what" and "where" subsystems. These what and where systems converge and integrate in man's parietal lobe. In addition to knowing what and where, one has to determine significance. The parietal lobe also receives input from both the cingulate gyrus and the dorsolateral frontal lobes. The dorsolateral frontal lobes are important in mediating goal-oriented behaviors and may provide this system with information about long-term goals. The cingulate gyrus is part of the limbic system and may provide this system information about biological needs and drives. Because the parietal lobe receives input from the perceptual–cognitive systems and receives conative and motivational information, it may be an ideal place to make attentional computations. The parietal lobe not only has reciprocal relations with the cortical areas from which it receives information but also appears able to modulate the activity of the reticular activating system (cortical control of arousal). Therefore, lesions of the parietal and frontal lobes, as well as the cingulate gyrus, impair a person's ability to make attentional computations.

Intention

The brain not only has a limited capacity to process incoming information but also has a limited ability to prepare for action and to act. The process by which the brain triages and prepares for action is called intention. Lesion studies and functional imaging suggest that the frontal lobes play a critical role in intention. The intentional and attentional systems have to be interactive. Therefore, not only do the frontal lobes have to influence the parietal lobes but also the parietal lobes must influence the frontal lobes. The parietal lobe has strong reciprocal projections with the arcuate and periarcuate regions of the dorsal lateral frontal lobe. The arcuate region or frontal eye field is important for the initiation of purposeful saccades, and the periarcuate region is important for the initiation of voluntary arm movements. It has been demonstrated that lesions of this region as well as this region's projections to the basal ganglia, cingulate gyrus, and thalamus are part of a motor-intentional system that when injured may be associated with motor-intentional neglect.

Right–Left Asymmetries

Neglect can be seen with either right or left hemisphere lesions. However, in humans neglect is more common and severe with right hemisphere lesions than with left hemisphere lesions. These asymmetries of neglect appear to be related to asymmetrical attentional representations of the body and space. Electrophysiological and functional imaging studies suggest that whereas the left hemisphere attends primarily to the right side or in a rightward direction, the right hemisphere can attend to both sides or in both directions. Similarly, although the left hemisphere prepares the right side for action (or prepares for rightward actions), the right hemisphere can prepare both sides for action (or prepare for action in either direction). Lastly, the right hemisphere appears to have more control of the reticular activating system than does the left, and right parietal lesions are associated with a greater reduction of an arousal response than are left hemisphere lesions.

—Kenneth M. Heilman, Edward Valenstein, and Robert T. Watson

See also–Anosognosia; Cognitive Impairment; Parietal Lobe; Perception and Perceptual Disorders; Perceptual-Motor Integration; Sensory Receptors, Overview

Further Reading

Halligan, P. W., and Marshall, J. C. (1994). *Spatial Neglect.* Erlbaum, Hillsdale, NJ.

Heilman, K. M., Watson, R. T., and Valenstein, E. (1993). Neglect and related disorders. In *Clinical Neuropsychology* (K. M. Heilman and E. Valenstein, Eds.), pp. 279–336. Oxford Univ. Press, New York.

Rafal, R. (1997). Hemispatial neglect. In *Behavioral Neurology and Neuropsychology* (T. E. Feinberg and M. J. Farah McGraw, Eds.), pp. 319–336. McGraw-Hill, New York.

Neonatal Seizures

Encyclopedia of the Neurological Sciences
Copyright 2003, Elsevier Science (USA). All rights reserved.

A NEONATAL SEIZURE is a sudden paroxysmal event characterized by stereotypic, repetitive abnormal movements. They are most often generated by an epileptic process in the brain (abnormal, hypersynchronous neuronal discharges), although other pathophysiological mechanisms may also be involved. Seizures that occur in newborn infants are often considered as a group of distinct entities because, when compared to those of older children and adults, their clinical manifestations are unusual, their treatment may differ, and they may have distinct impact later.

Although some neonatal seizures may be considered of epileptic origin, they usually are not considered epilepsy per se since the seizures are typically self-limited, thought to be primarily reactive to acute brain injury, and rarely extend beyond this period. Although occasionally seizures persist and evolve into epilepsy, this is infrequent.

Specific terms define the neonatal period—the age of the infant and, secondarily, the stage of physiological and neurological development. Stage of development in turn will influence the clinical manifestations of seizures, important etiological factors, therapeutic strategies, and long-term outcome following seizures. The neonatal period is defined as the first 28 days of life when the infant is born at term (40 weeks of gestation). The number of days following birth is referred to as the chronological age. The gestational age (GA) is defined in weeks as the duration of pregnancy prior to birth based on historical data, fetal head ultrasound, or neonatal examination. In clinical settings, the conceptional age (CA) of the infant is most often calculated as the sum of the GA and the chronological age calculated to the greatest completed week. Thus, for any infant, regardless of GA, the neonatal period will end at 44 weeks CA. Estimates of CA relate directly to a variety of issues concerning neonatal seizures since the CA indicates the stage of brain development. In clinical practice, neonates are encountered between 26 and 44 weeks CA, spanning a period of rapid brain growth and development.

THE CLINICAL PROBLEM

Seizures that occur in the newborn period represent unique and difficult challenges with regard to seizure recognition, accurate classification, and determination of pathophysiology. In addition, there is a diversity of etiologic and risk factors associated with seizures, limited therapeutic options, and uncertain determinants of prognosis. It has long been suggested that the immature brain is more resistant to seizure-induced injury than the mature brain. However, recent animal investigations suggest a less benign effect.

Seizure occurrence ranges from 1.8 to 3.5/1000 live births. Occurrence rates vary according to several risks factors, most notably the related factors of birth weight, CA, and associated age-dependent etiologies. Thus, a greater frequency of seizures has been reported in premature or low-birth-weight infants compared with full-term and normal-weight infants.

Seizures occur more often in the neonatal period than at any other time of life. Most neonatal seizures occur within the first week of life, and the majority of these occur within the first few days of life. Timing of onset may be related to an age-dependent enhanced epileptogenesis of the developing brain, a period of rapid brain growth and development in the perinatal period, and a hazardous environment into which the neonate is born. Since most neonatal seizures are reactive to an acute central nervous system (CNS) disorder, their timing and clinical manifestations are most likely due to the presence and impact of specific etiologic or risk factors during specific periods of brain development.

CLINICAL AND ELECTROENCEPHALOGRAPHIC CHARACTERIZATION AND CLASSIFICATION

Motor and Nonmotor Phenomena

The clinical seizures that occur in the neonate have unique features compared to those of older children and adults. There is a rich history of clinical investigations of neonatal seizures initiated by pioneering descriptions of clinical and electroencephalographic (EEG) seizures in the mid-1950s, most notably by a group of French investigators. They recognized generalized tonic seizures, unifocal and multifocal clonic seizures, bilateral but asynchronous clonic seizures, and myoclonic seizures, and they emphasized features that are relatively unique to neonates: multifocality, asynchrony of clonic activity on the two sides of the body, non-Jacksonian patterns of migration, and the lack of generalized tonic–clonic seizures. They also developed the concept of so-called "anarchic" seizures in neonates, referring to clinical events not previously classified in older children or adults: paroxysmal oral–buccal–lingual movements, limb movements of progression (bicycling, pedaling, and stepping), and ocular signs. These events were eventually referred to as "subtle" seizures, and this description, in association with the consolidation of the understanding of clinical features of neonatal seizures, evolved to a more widespread appreciation of and general interest in neonatal seizures as events with unique clinical qualities.

Nonmotor phenomena manifestations have also been described, such as vasomotor changes, apnea, pallor, changes in respiration, changes in heart rate, excessive salivation, and elevation in blood pressure. It has recently been suggested that these phenomena do not occur in isolation as the sole manifestation of a seizure but rather occur most often in association with motor phenomena.

As in the investigation of other seizure types, EEG video monitoring in neonates has provided the basis for the most verifiable classification system. A current description of seizure types is given in Table 1 and a working classification system is given in Table 2, both of which are based on time-synchronized, EEG video monitoring.

EEG Manifestations

The age at which the developing brain can consistently initiate and sustain electrical activity has not been firmly established, although it is believed that electrical seizure activity in the neonate is rare before 34 or 35 C.A. The definition of an EEG seizure is relatively arbitrary: paroxysmal rhythmic activity of at least 10 sec in duration with seizure discharges tending to be longer with increasing CA. Electrographic seizures are also characterized by region of onset and focality, waveform morphology, and, if present, migration. They most frequently appear in

Table 1   CLINICAL CHARACTERISTICS, CLASSIFICATION, AND PRESUMED PATHOPHYSIOLOGY OF NEONATAL SEIZURES

Classification	Characterization	Presumed pathophysiology
Focal clonic	Repetitive, rhythmic contracts of muscle groups of the limbs, face, or trunk	Epileptic
	May be unifocal or multifocal	
	May occur synchronously or asynchronously in muscle groups on one side of the body	
	May occur simultaneously but asynchronously on both sides	
	Cannot be suppressed by restraint	
Focal tonic	Sustained posturing of single limbs	Epileptic
	Sustained asymmetrical posturing of the trunk	
	Sustained eye deviation	
	Cannot be provoked by stimulation or suppressed by restraint	
Generalized tonic	Sustained symmetrical posturing of limbs, trunk, and neck	Nonepileptic
	May be flexor, extensor, or mixed extensor/flexor	
	May be provoked or intensified by stimulation	
	May be suppressed by restraint or repositioning	
Myoclonic	Random, single, rapid contractions of muscle groups of the limbs, face, or trunk	Epileptic or nonepileptic
	Typically not repetitive or may recur at a slow rate	
	May be generalized, focal, or fragmentary	
	May be provoked by stimulation	
Spasms	May be flexor, extensor, or mixed extensor/flexor	Epileptic
	May occur in clusters	
	Cannot be provoked by stimulation or suppressed by restraint	
Motor automatisms		
Ocular signs	Random and roving eye movements or nystagmus (distinct from tonic eye deviation)	Nonepileptic
	May be provoked or intensified by tactile stimulation	
Oral–buccal–lingual movements	Sucking, chewing, tongue protrusions	Nonepileptic
	May be provoked or intensified by stimulation	
Progression movements	Rowing or swimming movements	Nonepileptic
	Pedaling or bicycling movements of the legs	
	May be provoked or intensified by stimulation	
	May be suppressed by restraint or repositioning	
Complex purposeless movements	Sudden arousal with transient increased random activity of limbs	Nonepileptic
	May be provoked or intensified by stimulation	

the central or temporal regions, although other regions may generate seizures. The discharges are most often unifocal but may be multifocal. When multifocal, the seizures may occur simultaneously in different brain regions, but they often occur asynchronously. Waveform frequency, voltage, and morphology may vary considerably. The seizures may differ from one to the next within the same infant or be very consistent in appearance. The appearance of the seizure may change within a single seizure or it may remain relatively monomorphic. A single discharge may be confined to one well-circumscribed brain region or it may spread to other brain regions by a gradual widening of the field of the focus, an

abrupt change from region to region, or a migration of the electrical seizure from one area to another.

Most EEG seizures occur in association with clinical events, although some seizures are characterized only by electrical seizure activity. These include seizure discharges of the depressed brain, alpha seizure discharges, EEG seizures that occur in pharmacologically paralyzed infants, and those that occur in infants treated with antiepileptic drugs (AEDs). Seizure discharges of the depressed brain are low in amplitude, long in duration, and highly localized. They are associated with background EEG activity that is depressed and undifferentiated. An alpha seizure discharge is characterized by the sudden appearance of sustained rhythmic 8- to 12-Hz activity in the temporal or central region. Neither of these electrical events is associated with clinical seizures; both occur in infants with diffuse encephalopathy and the occurrence of either type of discharge suggests a poor prognosis.

Use of medications may also result in circumstances in which EEG seizures occur in the absence of clinical events. The most obvious situation is when a neonate is pharmacologically paralyzed for respiratory care. A less obvious circumstance is when neonates with EEG and clinical seizures are treated with AEDs. The initial response may be the control of the clinical events while the electrical events continue; this is referred to as "decoupling" of the clinical from electrical events.

Methods of Classification

A number of methods are applied to the classification of neonatal seizures. If clinical and EEG data are available, seizures may be classified in the broadest terms according to clinical and electrical temporal relationships as electroclinical (clinical seizures overlap temporally with EEG seizure activity), electrical only (no clinical events overlapping with EEG seizure activity), or clinical only (clinical events with no overlapping electrical events) (Table 2). Clinical seizures may also be described in relation to accompanying electrical seizure activity recorded on EEG: When closely associated, the events are designated electroclinical in nature. Seizures may also be classified according to predominant clinical type or according to the sequence of clinical components. In most clinical settings, classification according to predominant clinical type is appropriate. In addition, neonatal seizures may be classified according to pathophysiology, either epileptic or nonepileptic in origin. Less frequently used but equally as important is a classification system based on etiology—symptomatic or cryptogenic (idiopathic). Over time, there may be a trend to classify neonatal seizure according to electroclinical relationships, predominant clinical type, sequence of clinical events, pathophysiology, and etiologic grouping. This detail of classification may lead to more focused methods of treatment and more accurate determination of prognosis.

Neonatal Seizure Syndromes

Some neonatal seizures may be classified according to syndrome. In most cases, neonatal seizures do not

Table 2 CLASSIFICATION OF NEONATAL SEIZURES BASED ON ELECTROCLINICAL FINDINGS

Clinical seizures with a consistent electrocortical signature (pathophysiology: epileptic)
  Focal clonic
    Unifocal
    Multifocal
    Hemiconvulsive
    Axial
  Focal tonic
    Asymmetrical truncal posturing
    Limb posturing
    Sustained eye deviation
  Myoclonic
    Generalized
    Focal
  Spasms
    Flexor
    Extensor
    Mixed extensor/flexor
Clinical seizures without a consistent electrocortical signature (pathophysiology: presumed nonepileptic)
  Myoclonic
    Generalized
    Focal
    Fragmentary
  Generalized tonic
    Flexor
    Extensor
    Mixed extensor/flexor
  Motor automatisms
    Oral–buccal–lingual movements
    Ocular signs
    Progression movements
    Complex purposeless movements
Electrical seizures without clinical seizure activity

herald a chronic, postneonatal, convulsive disorder and can be classified as situation related. Thus, the term epilepsy is rarely applied to this age group. However, some seizures do occur in the neonatal period that persist, evolve into a chronic disorder, and are best characterized as true neonatal epilepsies. These include benign neonatal convulsions, benign neonatal familial convulsions (two syndromes with relatively good long-term outcomes), and early myoclonic encephalopathy (EME) and early infantile epileptic encephalopathy (EIEE) (both associated with a poor outcome and often considered catastrophic) (Table 3). These so-called catastrophic neonatal seizure syndromes may evolve over time to become other epileptic syndromes in surviving older infants and children. The concept of age-dependent epileptic encephalopathy was first applied to EIEE evolving to West syndrome and then

Table 3 COMPARISON OF EARLY MYOCLONIC ENCEPHALOPATHY (EME) AND EARLY INFANTILE EPILEPTIC ENCEPHALOPATHY (EIEE)[a]

	EME	EIEE
Age of onset	Neonatal period	Within first 3 months
Neurological status at onset	Abnormal at birth or at seizure onset	Always abnormal, even prior to seizure onset
Characteristic seizure type	Erratic or fragmentary myoclonus	Tonic spasm
Additional seizure types	Massive myoclonus	Focal motor seizures
	Simple partial seizures	Hemiconvulsions
	Infantile spasms (tonic)	Generalized seizures
Background EEG	Suppression burst	Suppression burst
Etiology	Inborn errors of metabolism	Cerebral dysgenesis
	Familial	Anoxia
	Cryptogenic	Cryptogenic
Natural course	Progressive impairment	Static impairment
Incidence of death	Very high, occurring in infancy	High, occurring in infancy, childhood, or adolescence
Status of survivors	Vegetative state	Severe mental retardation
		Quadriplegia, and bedridden
Long-term seizure evolution	Infantile spasms	West syndrome Lennox–Gastaut Syndrome

[a]Based on data from Aicardi (1997) and Ohtahara *et al.* (1992).

Lennox–Gastaut syndrome, with the epileptic expression of the encephalopathy in a given infant dependent on the stage of brain maturation. Watanabe and colleagues recently described this evolution, in addition to EIEE, in infants with EME, holoprosencephaly, tuberous sclerosis, other symptomatic epilepsies, and some cryptogenic etiologies.

PATHOPHYSIOLOGY OF SEIZURE TYPES

Epileptic Events

Initially, all neonatal seizures were thought to be of epileptic origin, but recent data suggest that some types of clinical seizures may be generated by a nonepileptic mechanism. Focal clonic, focal tonic, and some types of myoclonic events are generated by an epileptic mechanism (i.e., initiated and maintained by abnormal, paroxysmal, and hypersynchronous electrical discharges of cortical neurons) and occur in close association with EEG seizure activity. These types of clinical events are referred to as epileptic neonatal seizures.

Nonepileptic Events

Generalized tonic seizures and so-called subtle seizures (or motor automatisms) are generated by a nonepileptic mechanism, such as an exaggerated reflex response. When they occur spontaneously, these clinical events have the appearance and responsive features of reflex behaviors. They can also be provoked by tactile stimulation of the infant. Increased levels of stimulation of the infant (spatial and temporal) result in increased intensity of the response, and both provoked and spontaneous events can be suppressed by restraint of the infant. Although these clinical events may occur in the absence of EEG seizure activity, their designation as nonepileptic in origin is based on their clinical similarities to reflex behaviors and not the absence of EEG seizure activity associated with clinical seizure activity. Because tonic posturing and motor automatisms occur in infants with forebrain depression due to diffuse brain injury, and because they manifest characteristics of movements generated or mediated at the brainstem level, these types of clinical events have been referred to as brainstem release phenomena and are considered nonepileptic neonatal seizures.

ETIOLOGY

Regardless of seizure type, at onset, thorough evaluation is conducted for each infant to determine seizure etiology since there may be etiologic-specific therapies and because etiology may be the overriding determinant of long-term outcome. Table 4 lists the most frequently identified etiologies in order of frequency of occurrence. From a clinical perspective, the major categories of etiologic factors initially

Table 4 MOST FREQUENTLY OCCURRING ETIOLOGIES OF NEONATAL SEIZURES[a]

Hypoxia–ischemia
Intracranial hemorrhage
   Intraventricular
   Intracerebral
   Subdural
   Subarachnoid
Infection, CNS
   Meningitis
   Encephalitis
   Intrauterine
Infarction
Metabolic
   Hypoglycemia
   Hypocalcemia
   Hypomagnesemia
Chromosomal anomalies
Congenital abnormalities of the brain
Neurodegenerative disorders
Inborn errors of metabolism
Benign neonatal convulsions
Benign familial neonatal convulsions
Drug withdrawal or intoxication

[a] Listed in relative order of frequency. Not listed is unknown etiology, which is encountered in approximately 10% of cases (although some cases in this category may be benign neonatal convulsions) (from Mizrahi and Kellaway, 1998).

considered are hypoxia–ischemia, metabolic disturbances (e.g., hypoglycemia, hypomagnesium, and hypocalcemia), infection (e.g., CNS, systemic, or intrauterine), structural brain lesions (e.g., hemorrhage, infarction, and malformations), familial disorders, and inborn errors of metabolisms (e.g., amino acidurias, urea cycle defects, organic acidurias, mitochondrial disorders, paroxysmal disorders, and metabolic substrate deficiencies). Typically, the assessment for etiology is individualized and based on specific clinical, historical, and laboratory data obtained for each affected infant. This is done with the understanding that in clinical practice there may be more than one factor that may contribute to seizure onset in a single infant.

For some categories of etiology, there are specific diagnostic criteria that are universally accepted, but for others there continues to be debate, particularly regarding the diagnosis of hypoxic–ischemic encephalopathy. The definitions of this disorder may vary among practitioners, investigators, or clinical centers. In general, the diagnosis is based on a number of factors, including perinatal history, serial Apgar scores, umbilical blood gas determinations, acid–base balance, the presence of multisystem impairment, and the neurological examination. Even utilizing strict criteria, it is not clear whether they accurately predict outcome, including the eventual development of cerebral palsy.

There are also risk factors that may have an indirect impact on seizure occurrence, such as relatively young gestational age, low birth weight, extremes of maternal age or the presence of maternal fever, and some circumstances of labor and delivery. Any may coexist with other specific etiologic factors.

THERAPY

General Considerations

The factors to be considered that form the basis of therapy are accurate seizure diagnosis, precise characterization and classification of seizure type, appropriate interpretation of the EEG findings, identification of etiology, and determination of the pathophysiology of seizures and the severity of the epileptic neonatal seizures. The duration of epileptic seizures, their rate of recurrence, and the potential for spontaneous resolve may determine whether AEDs are given since some epileptic seizures may be too brief, infrequent, or self-limiting to justify such therapy.

Initial Medical Management

Supportive measures are initially undertaken based on principles of general medical management, cardiovascular stabilization, and respiratory support. Although all neonates with seizures may not require these measures, others do, particularly when seizures occur in critically ill neonates, when seizures are frequent or prolonged, or when seizures are associated with clinically significant changes in respiration, heart rate, or blood pressure as a consequence of the seizures themselves or vigorous AED therapy.

Etiology-Specific Therapy

In neonates with symptomatic seizures, etiology-specific therapy is directed to limit further CNS injury and to contribute to the control of seizures. In some cases, etiology-specific therapy may be the only treatment needed, such as in the correction of some metabolic disturbances, whereas in other circumstances in which brain injury has already occurred, both etiology-specific and AED therapy may be needed to control seizures. In other circumstances, some seizures may not be responsive to AED therapy unless the underlying causes are successfully treated.

Acute AED Therapy

The most frequently utilized AEDs in the acute treatment of neonatal seizures are phenobarbital, phenytoin, and a benzodiazepine (diazepam or lorazepam) given intravenously: 20 mg/kg of phenobarbital is given as a loading dose, followed by increments of 10 mg/kg as may be required to achieve serum levels between 20 and 40 µg/ml; 20 mg/kg of phenytoin is given as a loading dose to achieve serum levels between 15 and 20 µg/ml; 0.1–0.3 mg/kg diazepam is given in repeated dosages; and 0.05 mg/kg lorazepam is given in repeated dosages. Phenobarbital is almost universally accepted as the first-line AED and phenytoin as the second-line AED. Typically, a benzodiazepine (diazepam or lorazepam) is given if these fail. However, because of perceived enhanced efficacy, the use of initial benzodiazepine treatment prior to administration of first-line, longer acting AEDs has recently been given greater consideration.

The relative efficacy of both phenobarbital and phenytoin has recently been called into question. Painter and colleagues found no significant difference in seizure control in terminating acute electrographically confirmed clinical neonatal seizures; approximately 60% of the two treatment groups responded completely to drug treatment, suggesting that neither proved as efficacious as is generally believed. There are few other controlled studies on the relative efficacy of various AEDs in the initial treatment of neonatal seizure.

Recent investigations of fosphenytoin in neonates (not yet approved by the U.S. Food and Drug Administration for use in neonates) indicate that pharmacological properties in this age group are similar to those reported for older infants. The conversion half-life of fosphenytoin and resultant plasma total and free (unbound) phenytoin concentration–time profiles following intravenous administration in neonates are similar to those of older children and adults, although the range of values is greater in neonates. The absence of a potentially irritative solute as found in phenytoin is thought to substantially reduce the potential for irritation of blood vessels and skin at the site of infusion. In addition, fosphenytoin may be administered intramuscularly. Both of these features make this AED an attractive alternative to phenytoin in neonates.

A number of other medications have been tried with varying success to control neonatal seizures that have not been controlled by the first- or second-line AEDs. Adjuvant and alternative AEDs reported to be useful in neonatal seizure therapy are summarized in detail elsewhere. Those given intravenously include clonazepam, lidocaine, midazolam, and paraldehyde. Those given orally include carbamazepine, primidone, valproate, vigabatrin, and lamotragine. None have been proven efficacious.

End Point of Acute Therapy

The determination of the appropriate end point of acute therapy may not be straightforward. In untreated infants with electroclinical seizures, clinical epileptic seizures occur in a time-locked relationship to EEG seizure activity. An initial response to acute AED administration is the cessation of clinical seizures, although EEG seizure activity may persist (decoupling). The response of the electrical seizures to either increasing dosages of an AED or the addition of other AEDs is variable. Even as AED dosage and number increase, these electrical discharges may be difficult to eliminate. Attempts to further control the electrical seizure activity may result in high-dosage AED therapy and/or polypharmacy and may produce CNS depression, systemic hypotension, and respiratory depression. Thus, the potential risks of aggressive AED treatment must be weighed against any potential benefits of therapy.

Relative Risks and Benefits of Acute Therapy

There is no clear consensus as to what, if any, sequelae may be associated with the occurrence of epileptic seizures in the developing brain. It has been suggested that although the immature brain may be more susceptible to the generation of epileptic seizures in response to injury compared to the brains of older children and adults, the neonatal brain is also more resistant to seizure-induced injury compared to the mature brain. Some animal studies indicate that there are transient changes with perhaps limited significance in the CNS at a cellular or molecular level or in brain circuitry, although these issues have not been comprehensively addressed in human newborns. However, recent data raise the possibility that seizures in the immature animal may not cause immediate CNS injury but may increase the likelihood of seizure-induced injury if additional seizures occur later in life. Data also indicate that animals that experience seizures in the neonatal period may be more emotional labile later in life or have impaired memory compared to animals that do not.

The relative risks of AEDs have also not been well determined. Experimental data suggest some alterations in cell growth and energy substrate utilization with AEDs, although the applicability of these findings to human neonates has been questioned and the relative risks are considered small compared to the overall potential gain. There are few studies of the adverse systemic effects of acute AED therapy, although acute and aggressive treatment may result in CNS depression, hypotension, bradycardia, cardiac arrhythmia, and respiratory depression.

Balanced Regimen of Acute AED Therapy

The previously discussed considerations have led to the development of a proposed balanced AED regimen for acute treatment that may minimize perceived risks and maximize therapeutic effectiveness. Acute therapy is initiated with the goal of eliminating clinical seizures with phenobarbital. If clinical or EEG seizures persist, phenobarbital dosage is increased; then, if necessary, phenytoin is added and later, if required, a benzodiazepine is also added. If clinical seizures are controlled but electrical seizures persist, phenobarbital and then phenytoin dosages are increased to obtain high therapeutic serum levels. After seizure control is attained or reaches acceptable levels based on trials of initial therapy, maintenance therapy is established. The AEDs listed previously as adjuvant therapies are typically not utilized.

Chronic AED Therapy and Its Eventual Discontinuation

When a therapeutic effect is obtained acutely, infants are typically placed on maintenance doses of the successful AED (phenobarbital or phenytoin). However, the chronic levels of these AEDs may be difficult to stabilize over time for the following reasons: Drug metabolism may be conceptionally age dependent or altered by underlying systemic disease, phenobarbital elimination may be slowed in asphyxiated infants who may have concomitant hepatic or renal dysfunction, and maintenance dosing requirements are relatively lower early in the course of therapy but increase later. There may also be problems with maintenance of therapeutic levels of phenytoin because of its nonlinear kinetics and the rapid decrease in elimination rates during the first weeks of life. Thus, careful monitoring of AEDs early in the

course of chronic therapy is necessary to prevent adverse effects associated with drug buildup and, perhaps, seizure breakthrough as AED metabolism increases and levels decline.

There are no well-defined practice guidelines for the discontinuation of chronic therapy, although reports of maintenance schedules range from 1 week to 12 months after the last seizure. Recently, short-term AED therapy has been advocated, with AED withdrawal 2 weeks following the infant's last clinical seizure and in the absence of electrical seizure activity on EEG.

PROGNOSIS

Outcome of neonatal seizures is measured in terms of survival, neurological disability, developmental delay, and the presence of postneonatal epilepsy. Most clinical studies describe an increased frequency of these measures in subjects who experience seizures as newborns. The objectives of rapid diagnosis, accurate identification of etiology, and successful AED treatment of neonatal seizures are to prevent such adverse sequelae and to improve long-term outcomes of affected neonates, although few investigations have conclusively linked cessation of seizures and prognosis. Overall, it appears that the primary factor that predicts outcome is the underlying cause of the seizures rather than specific characteristics of the epileptic events. However, Volpe emphasized the impact of gestational age, in addition to etiology, on prognosis. Mortality increases with the greater degree of prematurity, although sequelae in survivors in Volpe's analysis is similar for various birth-weight groups.

In a representative study, Ortibus and colleagues reported that 28% of those with neonatal seizures died, 22% of survivors were neurologically normal at an average age of 17 months, 14% had mild abnormalities, and 36% had severe abnormalities. Methods of multivariant analyses have been proposed to predict the ultimate outcome of neonates who experience neonatal seizures. Factors that have been considered include features of the interictal EEG from one or serial recordings, the ictal EEG, the neurological examination at the time of seizures, the character or duration of the seizures, etiology, findings on neuroimaging, conceptional age, and birth weight. Use of multiple rather than single factors appears to provide the most accurate prediction of outcome. For example, outcome is less reliable when based solely on EEG variables from a single recording obtained at seizure onset than when based on a combination of imaging findings and clinical and EEG data. However, all variables relate to a single factor—the degree of brain injury at the time of seizure occurrence; this, in turn, relates to etiology.

Of special interest is the relationship of postneonatal epilepsy and neonatal seizures, which is reported to occur in up to 28% of survivors with variable types of neonatal seizures. Watanabe and colleagues considered in detail a select population of infants with neonatal seizures that persisted and could be classified as epilepsy of neonatal onset. In most of these infants, the initial epileptic syndrome evolved into West syndrome, and it evolved into symptomatic localization-related epilepsy in fewer cases.

—Eli M. Mizrahi

See also–Epilepsy, Epidemiology; Epilepsy, Risk Factors; Epilepsy Treatment Strategies; Epileptic Seizures; Febrile Seizures

Acknowledgment

Research in the Section of Neurophysiology, Department of Neurology, Baylor College of Medicine is supported in part by the Peter Kellaway, PhD, Endowment for Research.

Further Reading

Aicardi, J. (1997). Overview: Neonatal syndromes. In *Epilepsy: A Comprehensive Textbook* (J. Engel, Jr., and T. A. Pedley, Eds.), pp. 2243–2245. Lippincott–Raven, Philadelphia.

Camfield, P. R. (1997). Recurrent seizures in the developing brain are not harmful. *Epilepsia* 38, 735–737.

Dreyfus-Brisac, C., and Monod, N. (1964). Electroclinical studies of status epilepticus and convulsions in the newborn. In *Neurological and Electroencephalographic Correlative Studies in Infancy* (P. Kellaway and I. Petersén, Eds.), pp. 250–272. Grune & Stratton, New York.

Fenichel, G. M. (1997). Paroxysmal disorders. *Clinical Pediatric Neurology*, 3rd ed., pp. 1–43. Saunders, Philadelphia.

Holmes, G. L., and Ben-Ari, Y. (2001). The neurobiology and consequences of epilepsy in the developing brain. *Pediatr. Res.* 49, 320–325.

Lanska, M. J., Lanska, D. J., Baumann, R. J., et al. (1995). A population-based study of neonatal seizures in Fayette County, Kentucky. *Neurology* 45, 724–732.

Leppert, M., Anderson, V. E., Quattlebaum, T. G., et al. (1989). Benign familial neonatal convulsions linked to genetic markers on chromosome 20. *Nature* 337, 647–648.

Mizrahi, E. M., and Kellaway, P. (1987). Characterization and classification of neonatal seizures. *Neurology* 37, 1837–1844.

Mizrahi, E. M., and Kellaway, P. (1998). *Diagnosis and Management of Neonatal Seizures*. Lippincott–Raven, New York.

Nelson, K. B., and Emery, E. S. (1993). Birth asphyxia and the neonatal brain: What do we know and when do we know it? *Clin. Perinatol.* 20, 327–344.

Ohtahara, S., Ohtsuka, Y., Yamatogi, Y., et al. (1992). Early-infantile epileptic encephalopathy with suppression-bursts. In *Epileptic Syndromes in Infancy, Childhood and Adolescence* (J. Roger, M. Bureau, Ch. Dravet, F. E. Dreifuss, A. Perret, and P. Wolf, Eds.), 2nd ed., pp. 25–34. Libbey.

Ortibus, E., Sum, J., and Hahn, J. (1996). Predictive value of EEG for outcome and epilepsy following neonatal seizures. *Electroencephalogr. Clin. Neurophysiol.* 98, 175–185.

Painter, M. J., Scher, M. S., Stein, A. D., et al. (1999). Phenobarbital compared with phenytoin for the treatment neonatal seizures. *N. Engl. J. Med.* 341, 485–489.

Scher, M. S., Aso, K., Beggarly, M., et al. (1993). Electrographic seizures in preterm and full-term neonates: Clinical correlates, associated brain lesions, and risk for neurologic sequelae. *Pediatrics* 91, 128–134.

Volpe, J. J. (1995). *Neurology of the Newborn*, pp. 172–207. Sanders, Philadelphia.

Watanabe, K., Miura, K., Natsume, J., et al. (1999). Epilepsies of neonatal onset: Seizure type and evolution. *Dev. Med. Child Neurol.* 41, 318–322.

Nerve Conduction Studies

Encyclopedia of the Neurological Sciences
Copyright 2003, Elsevier Science (USA). All rights reserved.

NERVE CONDUCTION STUDIES (NCS) are neurophysiological techniques that record the responses of motor and sensory fibers to electrical stimulation. NCS are a central part of the electromyographic (EMG) examination and are generally used in conjunction with late responses (F responses and H reflex) and needle electromyography.

The EMG examination is an extension of the clinical examination. It is primarily designed by a physician to answer clinical questions and is always preceded by history taking and a physical examination. The pattern of findings, if abnormal, results in diagnostic insights into the pathology of disorders of peripheral spinal cord, spinal roots, limb plexuses, peripheral nerves, neuromuscular junctions, and muscles.

ANATOMICAL AND PHYSIOLOGICAL CONSIDERATIONS

The peripheral nerves are composed of a large number of fibers varying in diameter from 1 to 20 μm. The largest fibers are myelinated, conduct impulses at high speed, and include proprioceptive, cutaneous sensory (touch and pressure modalities), and motor fibers. They are outnumbered by un-myelinated fibers (UFs) by a ratio of 4–6 to 1. The large myelinated fibers (MFs) have the lowest excitation threshold to electrical stimulation and are therefore tested only by conventional NCS. Thus, the NCS may be strictly normal in disorders affecting UFs and small MFs.

The myelin sheath is an insulator that is periodically interrupted by the nodes of Ranvier. Transmembrane ion exchange occurs in the nodes of Ranvier during the depolarization generating an action potential. In MFs, the conduction proceeds from node to node and is therefore termed saltatory, in contrast to continuous conduction in UFs. The distance between consecutive nodes of Ranvier or internodal length is constant in a normal MF. It varies in a direct relationship to the outer diameter of the fiber, the myelin thickness, the axon diameter, and the conduction velocity (CV).

Each subset of MFs tested in a given conduction study comprises fibers of different diameters and CVs. These fibers are synchronously excited by electrical stimulation, and a compound response is recorded from a muscle [compound motor action potential (CMAP)] or a nerve trunk [nerve action potential (NAP)]. The onset latency of the evoked response is one of the essential parameters used in electrodiagnosis and corresponds to the CV of the fastest fiber among those excited by the stimulus. Therefore, the calculated CV is the maximum CV of this subset of fibers.

PATHOLOGICAL PROCESSES AFFECTING PERIPHERAL NERVE FIBERS

Two processes may affect MFs—axonal degeneration and demyelination. The best known type of axonal degeneration is Wallerian degeneration that follows the loss of continuity of a fiber. In this type of degeneration, the axon and its myelin sheath degenerate in the segment no longer connected to the cell body. This occurs after a delay of up to 10 days, depending on the length of peripheral axon isolated. During this period, conduction persists in the anatomically isolated segment for several days, although function is interrupted, and ultimately fails as the axon degenerates. Axonal degeneration also occurs in axonal neuropathies, in which it is presumably caused by failure of neuronal mechanisms that maintain peripheral processes. In this situation, the largest and longest axons tend to be affected first leading to a length- and size-dependent

neuropathy, with symmetrical deficits in the distal lower extremities initially and centripetal progression. Repair of axonal degeneration occurs in favorable situations via sprouting of immature axons from the axonal stump. These sprouts may find their way to the original targets of degenerated fibers, although this process is generally incomplete. In the initial stage of successful regeneration of motor fibers, the safety factor of conduction and neuromuscular transmission is reduced and occasional failure may occur at either level. As the regenerated fibers mature, the safety factor increases, probably due to thickening of the myelin sheath and strengthening of the neuromuscular junction. Regardless of the diameter of the parent axon, the sprouts exhibit uniformly short internodes, resulting in the persistence of slow CV after full maturation. This is seen, for instance, in motor nerves after transection followed by successful surgical repair. In partial denervation, the deficits may be compensated by collateral reinnervation, whereby sprouts originating from intact axons reinnervate the denervated targets. This process has been extensively studied in motor fibers and results in a several- to many-fold enlargement of functional motor units. The reinnervated motor units are characterized by an increase in size and fiber density. These form the pathological basis for the generation of reinnervated motor unit potentials (MUPs), characterized by increased duration, polyphasia, and high amplitude. In parallel with the conduction abnormalities seen in immature axons, reinnervated MUPs may exhibit instability of some of their components, causing the "jiggle" phenomenon, and/or satellite potentials that are initially unstable and mature to become stable, strictly time-locked components of the MUP. Some late components of the CMAP in denervation-reinnervation, sometimes termed axon reflexes, exhibit the same features.

Primary demyelination occurs in immune-mediated polyneuropathies, such as the typical demyelinating variant of Guillain–Barré syndrome (GBS) and chronic inflammatory demyelinating polyradiculoneuropathies (CIDPs). Pathologically, the change is focal and consists of segmental lysis of the myelin sheath, leaving the axon naked (segmental demyelination). This causes focal failure of conduction or conduction block (CB), the pathophysiological basis for the neurological deficits in these disorders. Repair of these demyelinated foci occurs with a faster temporal course than axonal regeneration and may be hastened by therapy. The newly formed myelin sheath is also characterized by uniformly short internodes, resulting in residual focal slowing of conduction. The new internodes are initially thinly myelinated, causing a reduction in the safety factor of conduction that subsequently improves as the myelin sheath thickens. Primary demyelination also occurs in chronic and acute compression of nerves. The resulting conduction abnormalities, focal slowing, or CB are useful for the neurophysiological diagnosis of these conditions. In both compressive and demyelinating immune-mediated neuropathies, the demyelinating lesions are rarely pure; some axons undergo degeneration as well. This combination of lesions may complicate the recognition of the primary pathological process.

A third type of primary myelin disorder is appropriately termed dysmyelinating. This is seen in genetically determined polyneuropathies classically known as the Charcot–Marie–Tooth syndrome, demyelinating variant. This is a heterogeneous clinical entity in which several molecular defects have been identified and likely alter the normal development of myelin. Short internodes and markedly reduced CVs are hallmarks of these disorders, in which secondary axonal degeneration also occurs through unknown mechanisms, causing the distal muscle atrophy typical of the clinical syndrome.

TECHNICAL CONSIDERATIONS

The NCS are routinely performed noninvasively using percutaneous electrical stimulation and surface recordings. Stimulation is applied in incremental steps until the evoked response reaches a maximal amplitude. It is recommended to exceed this supramaximal level of stimulation by 10–20% to account for variability in stimulus efficiency due to minute changes in electrode position relative to the stimulated nerve.

In motor conduction studies, the recording electrodes are affixed over the target muscle using a tendon–belly montage: The active electrode is positioned over the motor point and the reference electrode over the distal tendon, which is an electrically inactive structure. The position of the active electrode may require optimization to obtain a sharp negative onset and a maximal amplitude of the recorded CMAP. The nerve trunk is generally stimulated at different points. The most distal stimulation generates a CMAP whose latency is termed distal motor latency (DML). The DML

represents conduction along heterogeneous segments, including motor axons, their terminal branches, and the neuromuscular junction. Therefore, it is expressed in milliseconds because a CV would be meaningless. On more proximal stimulation, the CMAP has a longer latency, with its amplitude being equal or slightly decreased relative to the distal response (Fig. 1). The DML is subtracted from the proximal latency and divided into the distance separating the distal and proximal stimulation points, resulting in the maximum CV between these points expressed in meters per second.

Sensory conduction studies may be performed orthodromically or antidromically. The recorded sensory NAP is smaller than the CMAP by a 10^3 order of magnitude. The sensory NAP is measured in microvolts, compared to millivolts for the CMAP. As a result, the signal-to-noise ratio should be maximized. To do so, signal averaging is frequently required, particularly when the NAP amplitude is pathologically low. The latency of the NAP is generally measured to the onset of the negative deflection (Fig. 2), in which case it reflects the

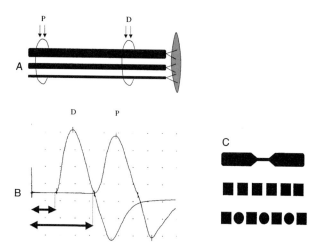

Figure 1

(A) Schematic representation of the population of motor fibers connected to their target muscle: large-, intermediate-, and small-diameter fibers are shown. D and P indicate the sites of distal and proximal stimulation in a routine conduction study. (B) CMAPs elicited by distal (D) and proximal (P) stimulations in a normal median nerve. Note that the corresponding waveforms are similar in configuration with a slight decrease in amplitude and slightly longer duration of the proximal one, corresponding to the physiological dispersion expected from the spectrum of conduction velocities of motor fibers. The short double arrow indicates the DML and the longer double arrow the latency of the response on proximal stimulation. Calibration: 2 msec and 5 mV. (C) Symbols used in the following figures depicting (top to bottom) segmental demyelination, remyelination, and axonal degeneration.

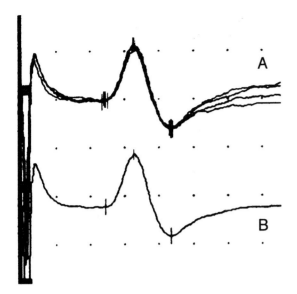

Figure 2
Sensory nerve action potential recorded antidromically in the wrist to digit 2 segment in a normal median nerve. (A) Superimposition of unaveraged responses (note the baseline noise and the slight variation of onset latency determined automatically by the EMG machine). (B) Average of eight responses revealing a noiseless baseline and clear takeoff of the negative phase. Calibration: 2 msec and 10 μV.

maximum CV of the fibers stimulated. In rare instances, the latency is measured to the peak of the negative deflection. The normal values differ in both instances, and for appropriate retrospective evaluation of a study, the technique used and the corresponding normal values should be mentioned in the report.

COMPLEMENTARY TECHNIQUES

Nerve conduction studies routinely assess the distal and intermediate part of the peripheral nervous system. They readily document abnormalities in the segments of nerve accessible to percutaneous stimulation. In the lower extremities, the segments of nerves distal to the popliteal fossa are accessible for investigation. In the upper extremities, the most proximal stimulation site is Erb's point. Conventional bipolar stimulation in the supraclavicular regions has intrinsic limitations that in our experience can be overcome with an alternative method of stimulation.

Motor conduction in the proximal segments of the peripheral nervous system can also be indirectly assessed by the recording of F responses, elicited by the antidromic depolarization of a subset of the

alpha motor neurons. F responses are elicited by supramaximal stimulation of motor nerves at the most distal stimulation site available. At least 10 stimulations should be used, and the sweep duration and gain should be appropriately adjusted (sweep of 50 msec in the upper extremities and 100 msec in the lower extremities and gain of 200–500 μV per division). The responses are much smaller than the CMAP and represent the backfiring of a subpopulation (5–10%) of the fastest conducting alpha motor neuron in response to antidromic depolarization. F responses vary in onset latency and configuration from stimulation to stimulation. The parameters used clinically always include the minimal latency and generally the maximal latency as well. Some authors use the mean latency of at least 10 F responses. F responses do not require any distance measurement, and normal values are expressed as a function of height. Because F responses explore a long conduction distance (approximately twice the length of the limb examined), they are very sensitive to mild conduction slowing and are frequently abnormal in mild polyneuropathies with normal values of routine CVs. They are also useful in the detection of proximal conduction slowing or block. We believe that recording of F responses should be systematically included in every motor conduction study.

Spinal root stimulation can also be performed at the cervical level with minimally invasive techniques. The stimulation is most reliably effected using a monopolar needle electrode inserted parasagittally through the cervical paraspinal muscles to reach the vertebral lamina. This electrode is used as the cathode, with the anode being a surface electrode placed more caudally on the midline. This technique is not nerve selective; selectivity is obtained through selection of the target muscle(s). Anatomical overlaps such as in the thenar eminence can be overcome by use of collision studies. This method is useful for detecting proximal CB or slowing and enhances the sensitivity of the neurodiagnostic approach to multifocal demyelinating neuropathies.

Finally, the sensory conduction studies reflect function in the distal segment of the peripheral sensory system. In selected cases, they are usefully supplemented by somatosensory evoked potentials, which assess sensory conduction along the whole peripheral and central sensory pathway, and may reveal proximal conduction abnormalities that cannot be documented with conventional sensory conduction studies.

NORMAL VALUES

Ideally, each laboratory should develop its own normal values, and the techniques should be consistent with those used to generate the normative data. In practice, many clinical neurophysiologists use literature data or the data generated in the laboratory at which they trained. Care should be taken to ensure that data are comparable. For instance, some electromyographers use fixed distances for DML determination, whereas others use variable distances fitting the anatomy of individual patients. In the first case, a single number expresses the cutoff between normal and abnormal findings, whereas in the second case the DML must be related to a normogram factoring in the conduction distance to determine whether the DML is normal or abnormal. The techniques used for surface measurement of conduction distances should also be consistent with those used to collect reference data.

NONPHYSIOLOGICAL FACTORS AFFECTING THE RESULTS

Conduction velocity is temperature dependent. In our experience, inadequate temperature control is the most common source of spurious slowing of nerve conduction. Assessment of conduction in the distal parts of the extremities (DMLs and sensory conduction latencies) is most vulnerable to temperature-related slowing. Therefore, it is essential to monitor the skin temperature throughout the recording session and to maintain temperature higher than 34°C in the hand and higher than 32°C in the foot.

Other common pitfalls stem from undetected spread of stimulating current to neighboring peripheral nerves, common in areas in which several nerves lie in close proximity, such as median and ulnar nerves at the wrist (particularly if the wrist is small) or the peroneal and the posterior tibial nerve in the popliteal fossa. Frequently, this results from use of excessive stimulation intensity. Such technical errors are easily avoided by systematically monitoring the twitch elicited by the supramaximal stimulus, in addition to the waveform.

ANOMALOUS INNERVATION

The patterns of anomalous innervation that may affect the results of conduction studies are described elsewhere in this encyclopedia. The electromyographer and technicians should be thoroughly familiar with the effects of the Martin–Gruber anastomosis on median and ulnar conduction studies as well as those of an accessory peroneal branch. Occasionally, complex situations require multiple simultaneous stimulations and collision studies to clarify the anomalous anatomical pattern underlying aberrant results.

PATHOLOGICAL FINDINGS

Motor Conduction Studies

Distal Motor Latency: In pathological situations, prolongation of the DML should be interpreted in light of the amplitude and configuration of the distal CMAP. In severe neuropathy when the CMAP amplitude is very low, a prolonged DML may be difficult to interpret. It may stem from survival of the smallest slow-conducting motor axons, regeneration of the distal portion of the motor axons, or primary pathology of the myelin sheath (Fig. 3). A mildly prolonged DML is common in distal axonopathies, which are particularly distal in the lower extremities when the CMAP is of low amplitude. A markedly prolonged DML, especially when the CMAP amplitude is normal or near normal, is suggestive of primary demyelinating lesions as seen in carpal tunnel syndrome, the demyelinating variant of GBS, or CIDP. Marked prolongation of the DML in excess to that expected from more proximal conduction slowing (as documented by the terminal latency index) is noted in generalized demyelinating polyneuropathies with distal predominance, such as that associated with anti-MAG antibodies.

Dispersion of the Distal CMAP: This finding often reflects the increase in range of CVs of the motor fibers in the segment considered. This may be seen in primary demyelinating lesions affecting some but not all motor fibers (demyelinating GBS and CIDP) (Fig. 4). It can also be seen in advanced axonal neuropathies in which only few reinnervated motor units survive and summate asynchronously, resulting in a multipeaked and prolonged waveform due to cancellation of positive and negative phases of individual MUPs.

Slowing of Conduction Velocity: Conduction velocities are calculated by recording CMAPs obtained on stimulation of the same nerve at two locations separated by a known distance. Mild conduction slowing is generally defined as slowing within 30% of the lower limit of normal. It reflects either loss of

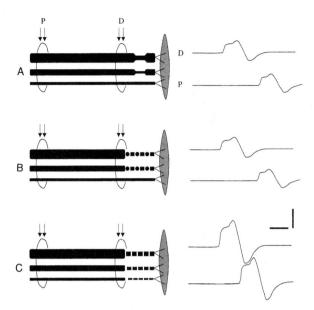

Figure 3
Pathophysiological mechanisms leading to a prolonged DML. (Right) Diagrammatic representation of distal (top) and proximal (bottom) waveforms. (A) Distal conduction block of the large and intermediate MFs. Distal conduction relies on the slower conduction small MFs, hence the prolonged DML and low-amplitude CMAP. The corresponding CV is moderately slow in the forearm because the conduction along the larger fibers does not contribute to the CMAP. This is the mechanism of conduction slowing in the forearm noted in some cases of carpal tunnel syndrome. (B) Distal degeneration of the large and intermediate MFs as seen in a dying back neuropathy. As in A, the large and intermediate MFs are not functionally active, hence the prolonged DML, low-amplitude CMAP, and moderately slow CV in the forearm. (C) Remyelinating changes in the distal segment of all motor fibers causing a prolonged DML with a normal CMAP amplitude and a normal CV in the forearm. Calibration: 5 msec and 5 mV.

function or slowing of conduction in the fastest conducting motor fibers. It is commonly noted in "dying-back" axonal neuropathies, in which the largest motor fibers are disconnected from their target muscle by a process of axonal degeneration (Fig. 5B). When mild, this slowing may not be apparent because of the broad range of normal values. It is easier to document mild slowing over long conduction distances, which is the reason why F response latencies are the most sensitive in the detection of mild motor axonal dysfunction. Another possible cause of mild conduction slowing is metabolic changes affecting the peripheral nerves. An example in the clinical realm is the conduction slowing occasionally noted in newly diagnosed type I diabetics, which is subsequently corrected by adjustment of insulin therapy and normalization of glucose

levels. It should be noted that mild slowing may also be due to demyelinating lesions affecting the largest motor fibers; of course, this finding is not specific for demyelination (Fig. 5). Slowing is also occasionally seen in the forearm segment of the median nerve, upstream from a compressive lesion at the carpal tunnel. This slowing is due to a distal conduction block of the largest motor fibers, which are functionally disconnected from their target but conduct normally in the forearm, and whose conduction is not reflected in the measure of CV in the forearm (Fig. 5C). The CB at the wrist can be document by step stimulation (inching studies) across the wrist. The same mechanism can be invoked in the genesis of mild, focal conduction slowing in

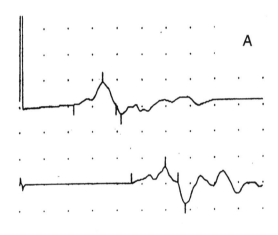

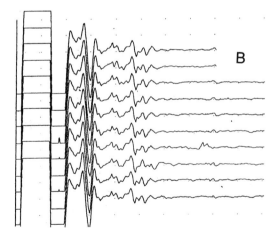

Figure 4
Dispersion of the CMAP. (A) CIDP: distal (top) and proximal (bottom). Note the desynchronization of the CMAP that changes in configuration from proximal to distal due to phase cancellation. Calibration: 2 msec and 2 mV. (B) Demyelinating GBS. Dispersion of the CMAP on high gain recordings, recurrent stimulations. Note the multiple late, time-locked components. Calibration: 10 msec and 500 µV.

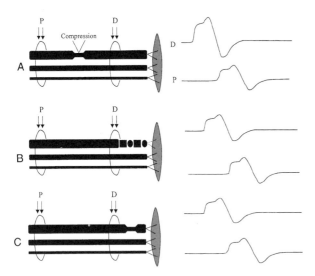

Figure 5

Pathophysiological mechanism leading to moderate slowing of motor conduction velocity. In all situations, there is no contribution of the fastest conducting fibers to the CMAP elicited on proximal stimulation. This occurs through CB in the intermediate segment (A), distal CB (C), or distal axonal degeneration (B) of the largest motor fibers.

compression neuropathies (ulnar nerve at the elbow or peroneal nerve at the fibular head) (Fig. 5A). Also in chronic compressive neuropathies, focal demyelination–remyelination is an alternative explanation to focal conduction slowing.

Severe conduction slowing is defined as a reduction in CV exceeding 30% of the lower limit of normal. Figure 6 exemplifies the mechanisms of severe conduction slowing in common pathophysiological situations. It should be emphasized that this 30% cutoff was determined empirically by experts whose aim was to define criteria specific for primary demyelination. Therefore, one should keep in mind that patients who do not reach this degree of slowing may nonetheless have primary demyelinating lesions. In such patients, the yield of neurophysiological studies is significantly augmented by sampling of multiple nerves, study of F response latencies, spinal root stimulation, attention to the values of the DMLs, and the presence of partial CB.

Motor CB is defined as a marked decrease in CMAP amplitude from a given stimulation site relative to a more distal one. It is the consequence of conduction failure in a subset of motor fibers between these two points. Recognition of CB is easy if both the distal and the proximal responses compared are well synchronized. A difference in CMAP amplitude exceeding 50% is generally considered

diagnostic. A more complex situation is that in which the proximal response is desynchronized, posing the problem of a pseudo-CB. In both instances, CB and pseudo-CB, the underlying pathology is almost always primary demyelinative. Conduction block may also occur in the very distal segments of motor fibers or in proximal segments such as the spinal roots. In these cases, the neurophysiological documentation of CB relies on indirect methods (F response abnormalities), spinal root stimulation techniques, needle EMG data (decreased recruitment of normal MUPs in a muscle with normal CMAP amplitude), or comparison of subsequent studies. Figure 7 indicates conduction abnormalities noted in different localizations of focal CB.

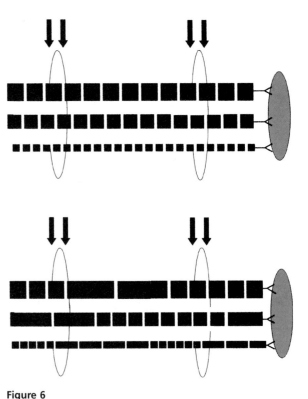

Figure 6

Pathophysiological mechanism leading to severe slowing of motor conduction velocity. Widespread demyelination–remyelination is noted in both cases. (Top) Normal internodes are interposed between short, remyelinated internodes, with the lesions being scattered throughout the entire length of MFs, as in CIDP or demyelinating GBS. (Bottom) Universally short internodes throughout, as in some common variants of Charcot–Marie–Tooth type 1. In the latter situation, synchronous CMAPs are frequently recorded because all CVs are slowed to the same extent. In the former, the range of conduction velocities is increased and desynchronization of the CMAP and phase cancellation are likely to occur.

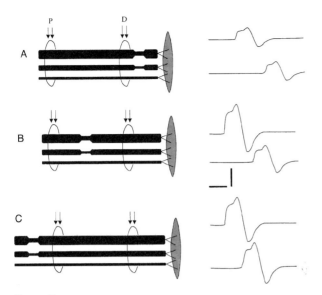

Figure 7
Effect of focal demyelination in different locations on DML, CV, and CMAP amplitude. (A) Distal demyelination causing prolonged DML and low-amplitude CMAP (see Fig. 3A). Demyelination in the intermediate segment causing CB and CV slowing. (C) Proximal conduction block. All routine conduction parameters are normal. The CB may be revealed indirectly by prolonged F response latencies, reflecting conduction along the intact small MFs, or directly by proximal stimulation techniques. Calibration: 5 msec and 5 mV.

Sensory Conduction Studies

The surface sensory NAP is generated by fibers 7 μm in diameter or more, with the bulk of the amplitude of the NAP due to action potentials in fibers >9 μm. Therefore, loss of these large fibers through axonal degeneration quickly leads to a decrease in amplitude and then loss of the surface NAP, leaving only a very small window of opportunity to detect mild slowing. Near-nerve recording techniques would be more sensitive in the detection of NAP slowing but are no longer routinely used.

Slowing of NAP conduction, however, is seen in situations in which demyelination–remyelination affect a large subset of the large MFs, such as mild, chronic compression neuropathies. Indeed, slowing of sensory or mixed (palm to wrist) conduction is the mainstay of the neurodiagnosis of early carpal tunnel syndrome. Slow sensory CVs are also often noted in the dysmyelinating neuropathies causing Charcot–Marie–Tooth syndrome type 1. Because the nerve fibers are universally affected to the same extent, the sensory NAP remains synchronized and sensory slowing can be demonstrated with routine techniques. It should be noted that some cases of

dysmyelinating neuropathies do not show the uniform slowing described previously and may therefore mimic acquired demyelinating neuropathies.

In acquired demyelinating neuropathies (demyelinating variant of GBS and CIDP), the nerve fibers are unevenly affected, which may lead to dispersion and loss of the NAP via phase cancellation, without correlative sensory deficits. It should be kept in mind that in all preceding instances, pathology may also involve secondary axonal degeneration, providing an alternative explanation for an absent NAP.

CONCLUSION

Nerve conduction studies are powerful tools for the diagnosis of peripheral nerve disorders. They are generally complemented by F response studies and needle electromyography. They are essential for the assessment of focal neuropathy and their localization and severity. In generalized neuropathy, emphasis is placed on the distinction between primary demyelinating and primary axonal neuropathies. In this regard, some findings are unequivocally diagnostic of primary demyelination, including marked prolongation of DMLs with normal or near-normal CMAP amplitudes and severe slowing of CVs and CB. Other findings are ambiguous because they may reflect either primary demyelination or axonal degeneration. These include moderate slowing of CVs, low-amplitude CMAPs (which may be caused by either motor unit loss or distal CB), and absent sensory potentials. In difficult cases, multiple nerve studies, F responses, and proximal conduction studies may be very helpful in obtaining an accurate diagnosis.

—Didier Cros and Peter Siao

***See also*–Conduction Block; Denervation; Electromyography (EMG); Impulse Conduction; Neuropathies, Entrapment; Sensation, Assessment of**

Further Reading

American Association for Electrodiagnostic Medicine. AAEM guidelines in electrodiagnostic medicine. *Muscle Nerve* **199**, S1–S30.

Buchtal, F., Rosenfalk, A., and Behse, F. (1975). Sensory potentials of normal and diseased nerves. In *Peripheral Neuropathies* (P. J. Dyck, P. K. Thomas, and E. H. Lambert, Eds.), pp. 442–464. Saunders, Philadelphia.

Cros, D., Chiappa, K. H., Gominak, S., *et al.* (1990). Cervical magnetic stimulation. *Neurology* **40**, 1751–1756.

Cros, D., Gominak, S., Shahani, B. T., *et al.* (1992). Comparison of electrical and magnetic stimulation in the supraclavicular region. *Muscle Nerve* **15**, 587–590.

Gominak, S. C., and Cros, D. (1993). A 66-year-old woman with a 19-year history of progressive weakness of all extremities. *N. Engl. J. Med.* **329**, 1182–1190.

Hall, S. M., Hughes, R. A., Atkinson, P. E., *et al.* (1992). Motor nerve biopsy in severe Guillain–Barre syndrome. *Ann. Neurol.* **31**, 441–444.

Kaku, D. A., England, J. D., and Sumner, A. J. (1994). Distal accentuation of conduction slowing in polyneuropathy associated with antibodies to myelin-associated glycoprotein and sulphated glucuronyl paragloboside. *Brain* **117**, 941–947.

Kimura, J. (1979). The carpal tunnel syndrome: Localization of conduction abnormalities within the distal segment of the median nerve. *Brain* **102**, 619–635.

Lachman, T., Shahani, B. T., and Young, R. R. (1980). Late responses as aids to diagnosis in peripheral neuropathy. *J. Neurol. Neurosurg. Psychiatry* **43**, 156–162.

Lewis, R. A., Sumner, A. J., and Shy, M. E. (2000). Electrodiagnostic features of inherited demyelinating neuropathies: A reappraisal in the era of molecular diagnosis. *Muscle Nerve* **23**, 1472–1487.

Menkes, D. L., Hood, D. C., Ballesteros, R. A., *et al.* (1998). Root stimulation improves the detection of acquired demyelinating polyneuropathies. *Muscle Nerve* **21**, 298–308.

Rosenbaum, R. B., and Ochoa, J. L. (1993). Acute and chronic mechanical nerve injuries: Pathologic, physiologic and clinical correlations. In *Carpal Tunnel Syndrome and Other Disorders of the Median Nerve*, pp. 197–232. Butterworth-Heinemann, Boston.

Roth, G., and Magistris, M. R. (1987). Detection of conduction block by monopolar percutaneous stimulation of the brachial plexus. *Electromyogr. Clin. Neurophysiol.* **27**, 45–53.

Triggs, W. J., Cros, D., Gominak, S. C., *et al.* (1992). Motor nerve inexcitability in Guillain–Barre syndrome. The spectrum of distal conduction block and axonal degeneration. *Brain* **115**, 1201–1302.

Nerve Fibers
see Axons

Nerve Injury

Encyclopedia of the Neurological Sciences
Copyright 2003, Elsevier Science (USA). All rights reserved.

INJURY can occur at any point along the length of a peripheral nerve as it courses from the root through the plexus and then to the target organ (Fig. 1). There are a number of mechanisms whereby peripheral nerves may be directly traumatized,

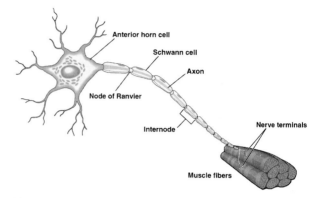

Figure 1

Innervation of a muscle by a myelinated motor nerve. An internode represents a segment of axon surrounded by a myelin sheath. Each one is separated from its neighbor by a node of Ranvier.

including compression, traction, drug injection, and laceration. Furthermore, damage may also occur from toxins, ischemia, infection, and physical agents such as freezing, electrical current, and radiation exposure.

In order to understand the pathophysiology of peripheral nerve injury, it is important to be familiar with the anatomical components of a peripheral nerve and its supporting tissues (Fig. 2). One of the principal sites of peripheral nerve injury is the axon, which is composed largely of neurofilaments and microtubules that ferry substances (e.g., organelles) between the nerve cell body and the axon terminal. Injury may also affect specialized neuronal sheath cells called Schwann cells, which are intimately associated with all peripheral nerve axons. In larger (myelinated) nerves, these cells generate concentric layers of myelin around the axon to form a sheath, whereas in smaller (unmyelinated) nerves a single Schwann cell associates with several axons via a single layer of myelin. Trauma can also affect the connective tissue that invests individual axons (endoneurium), nerve fascicles (perineurium), and entire nerve trunks (epineurium), one of the principal functions of which is to protect the underlying nerve from injury by mechanical deformation. A layer of loose areolar tissue, the mesoneurium, extends from the epineurium to surrounding tissue structures and may serve as an endoneurial cushion as well as allowing a degree of mobility in the longitudinal plane. Finally, injury can lead to peripheral nerve ischemia by compromising blood flow through the extensive network of blood vessels that course throughout the connective tissue sheath and the nerve.

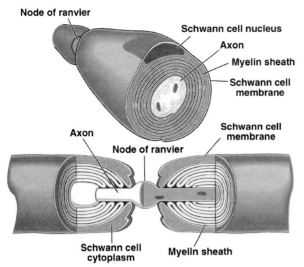

Figure 2

Histological components of a myelinated nerve. The central axon is surrounded by concentric layers of myelin that have been laid down by the Schwann cell.

PATHOGENESIS

Irrespective of cause, there is a limited range of responses to peripheral nerve injury, namely segmental demyelination, Wallerian degeneration, or axonal degeneration. These may occur alone or in combination.

Segmental Demyelination

Since the Schwann cell and myelin sheath lie outside the axon, they are relatively more vulnerable to injury from external compression. However, myelin degeneration can also occur secondary to axonal injury. In either case, myelin erosion occurs at the site of injury, thus exposing a localized segment of the underlying axon. This process is called segmental demyelination, the functional consequence of which is a slowing in nerve conduction across the injury site through a reduction in the efficiency of action potential propagation. Severe degrees of demyelination completely prevent the passage of impulses across the site of injury, acting like a roadblock to the flow of traffic on either side. This is called conduction block and clinically manifests as numbness and/or weakness. Segmental demyelination is not restricted to traumatic nerve injury; it is also encountered in a number of peripheral neuropathies, such as Guillain–Barré syndrome and multifocal motor neuropathy with conduction block.

Wallerian Degeneration

Wallerian degeneration (Fig. 3) occurs when axonal continuity is compromised by axotomy (e.g.,

transection from a sharp blade or severe crush). Communication is lost between the cell body and the segment of nerve distal to the site of injury. As a consequence, the distal segment and its myelin sheath degenerate into spheroid-shaped segments called ellipsoids during a 3- to 5-day period. In addition, a limited degree of degeneration occurs proximal to the injury site until a node of Ranvier is encountered or, if very proximal, degeneration includes the cell body. The separation of an axon segment from its cell body (and the trophic factors that it generates) is not the sole instigator of Wallerian degeneration. Indeed, post-traumatic axonal degeneration appears to be an active rather than a passive process involving a complex series of molecular interactions between traumatized nerves and surrounding tissues. The details of the initiating events remain to be fully elucidated, but evidence indicates that a key event is an increase in intraaxonal calcium that activates proteases, which then degrade the axon cytoskeleton.

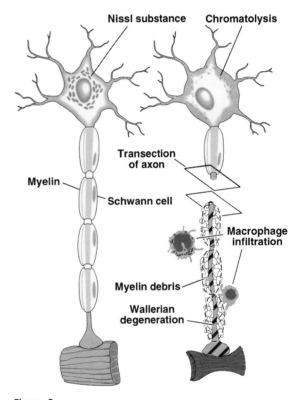

Figure 3

Wallerian degeneration: Loss of axonal continuity due to an axotomy lesion causes breakdown of the distal axon over a period of 3–5 days. The myelin surrounding the distal stump also degenerates, and during chromatolysis the cell body becomes swollen with accumulating proteins that will be needed to begin the process of regeneration. The nucleus moves to an eccentric position and the Nissl substance becomes fragmented.

Since the maintenance of healthy myelin requires contact with the axon, Wallerian degeneration is also associated with breakdown of the myelin sheath by myelin-derived lipases and proteinases. Schwann cells (and later macrophages) assist in further myelin breakdown. Schwann cells also proliferate and undergo morphological changes and are induced to generate molecules that will be required for the regenerative phase that is soon to follow.

Within 2 or 3 days of injury, chemical signals (possibly chemokines and interleukin-10) attract cells of the monocyte/macrophage system that sweep into the region. These cells then clear away debris, leaving connective tissue fibroblast cells and rows of Schwann cells in their wake.

Proximal to the injury site, the nerve cell body is deprived of essential trophic factors and consequently either undergoes programmed cell death (apoptosis) or a potentially reversible process called chromatolysis. In the latter situation, axotomy causes the cell body to swell with accumulating proteins. This is not simply due to a traffic jam caused by disruption of the normal flow of substances to and from the cell body; rather, it reflects increased production of proteins that will be required in the regenerative phase that is soon to follow. This switch in function of the cell body is evident through the granular appearance of the endoplasmic reticulum and the eccentric position adopted by the nucleus to accommodate the buildup of new proteins.

Post-traumatic degeneration affects not only the damaged nerve but also those tissues that are intimately associated with it. In a process called synaptic stripping, microglial cells in the central nervous system replace the myriad of synaptic terminals that were present on the nerve cell body. At the other end of the nerve, degeneration begins to take effect in the target tissue. When one considers this in the context of a motor nerve, axotomy interrupts the supply of trophic factors that are important in muscle fiber maintenance and growth. Within weeks of being deprived of this important material, the target muscle begins to degenerate. Indeed, if significant reinnervation fails to take place subsequently, the muscle becomes completely replaced by fibrotic material.

Axonal Degeneration

Toxic and metabolic derangements (e.g., hexacarbon toxicity) may precipitate a process akin to Wallerian degeneration called axonal degeneration. The most distal part of the axon and its myelin sheath degenerate first; the process then proceeds proximally toward the nerve cell body at a rate of 2 or 3 mm/day. This "dying back" neuropathy may ultimately extend to involve related tracts of the central nervous system. Such neuropathies are often described as being length dependent; those regions of the nerve that are most distant from the nerve cell body (and its trophic factors) are most vulnerable. Spencer and Schaumburg refer to these disorders as central and peripheral distal axonopathies to emphasize that changes also occur in the largest axons of the spinal cord.

CLASSIFICATION

Based on his extensive wartime experience, Seddon introduced a three-tiered classification system for traumatic nerve injury in 1943. The first type, neurapraxia, is a block in conduction along a segment of the axon without loss of axonal continuity. In this situation, action potentials can propagate above and below the injured segment but not at the site of injury. This functional deficit results from segmental demyelination, which allows current to leak away from the internodal membrane and thus reduces the efficiency of action potential propagation along the nerve. This kind of injury is commonly encountered in compression and entrapment neuropathies, and the prognosis for recovery is generally excellent. In both the upper and lower extremities, the most common sites for compressive nerve injury are those at which a peripheral nerve crosses over a relatively exposed joint or bony protuberance. A good example is the wrist drop that occurs when a person under the influence of alcohol falls asleep with one arm draped over the back of a chair (Saturday night palsy), thus compressing the radial nerve in the upper arm against the spiral groove of the humerus. Significant segmental demyelination occurs at the compression site causing conduction block, and the unfortunate patient awakens unable to elevate the wrist or straighten the fingers. However, one usually sees a very satisfactory recovery during the ensuing 10–12 weeks as the conduction block resolves. Other relatively common sites for nerve compression include the elbow (ulnar nerve), fibular head (common peroneal nerve), and wrist (median nerve; carpal tunnel syndrome).

Seddon's second type of injury, axonotmesis, occurs when the axon has been damaged (with a degree of loss of continuity) in the setting of an intact connective tissue sheath. Wallerian degeneration of

Table 1   SEDDON'S AND SUNDERLAND'S CLASSIFICATION OF NERVE TRAUMA

Injured nerve component	Process	Classification	
		Seddon	Sunderland
Myelin	Conduction block	Neurapraxia	Grade 1
Axon	Loss of axonal continuity with intact endoneurium	Axonotmesis	Grade 2
Endoneurium	Loss of axonal and endoneurial continuity	Neurotmesis	Grade 3
Perineurium	Loss of axonal, endoneurial, and perineurial continuity	Neurotmesis	Grade 4
Epineurium	Loss of axonal, endoneurial, perineurial, and epineurial continuity	Neurotmesis	Grade 5
Combination	Combination of other levels	Combination of other levels	Grade 6

the axon occurs distal to the site of injury. This type of injury has many causes, including more severe compression/entrapment, and also occurs as a result of traction and laceration injuries. An example of such a lesion is a more severe case of longstanding carpal tunnel syndrome, a chronic nerve entrapment disorder caused by compression of the median nerve at or just beyond the wrist. Demyelination is the principal component of the disorder in its earlier stages. However, as the condition progresses, a degree of axon loss also occurs that, if left unattended, may lead to wasting of median-innervated hand muscles.

The third and most severe type of nerve injury, neurotmesis, involves loss of axonal continuity and disruption of the connective tissue sheath. Severe traction, crush, and laceration injuries often lead to neurotmesis, and the prognosis for satisfactory recovery is generally poor.

In 1947, Sunderland introduced a modified form of the previously mentioned classification (Table 1), including five as opposed to three degrees of injury. First- and second-degree injuries correspond to Seddon's neurapraxia and axonotmesis, respectively. Third-degree nerve injury involves loss of both axonal and endoneurial continuity with intact perineurium and epineurium. Fourth-degree injury involves loss of continuity of all components of the nerve trunk except the epineurium, whereas fifth-degree injury involves complete transection of the entire nerve trunk. At the time of his original writing, Sunderland recognized that many instances of nerve trauma do not fit neatly into this classification. In 1989, it was proposed that a sixth degree of nerve injury be added to Sunderland's classification encompassing mixed-pattern injuries to different fascicles within the same nerve. These injuries are particularly challenging to diagnose and treat, and the pattern of recovery may be difficult to predict. For example, gunshot wounds to the brachial plexus below the level of the clavicle may cause severe sixth-degree injuries encompassing regions of neurapraxia and axonotmesis involving multiple cords and terminal nerves. Some nerves may recover fairly quickly, indicating that they were affected by neurapraxia. However, the patient may never gain useful function in muscles innervated by more severely affected nerves.

—*Brian Eamon Murray*

See also–Axons; Electrical and Lightning Injuries; Myelin; Nerve Regeneration; Nerve Repair; Neuropathies, Entrapment; Neuropathies, Overview; Nodes of Ranvier

Further Reading

Birch, R., Bonney, G., Payan, J., *et al.* (1986). Peripheral nerve injuries. *J. Bone Jt. Surg.* **68B**, 2–21.

Flores, A., Lavernia, C. J., and Owens, P. W. (2000). Anatomy and physiology of peripheral nerve injury and repair. *Am. J. Orthop.* **29**, 167–173.

Hughes, P. M., and Perry, V. H. (2000). The role of macrophages in degeneration and regeneration in the peripheral nervous system. In *Degeneration and Regeneration in the Nervous System* (N. R. Saunders and K. M. Dziegielewska, Eds.), pp. 263–283. Harwood Academic, Amsterdam.

Sanes, J. R., and Jessell, T. M. (2000). The formation and regeneration of synapses. In *Principles of Neural Science* (E. R. Kandel, J. H. Schwartz, and T. M. Jessell, Eds.), 4th ed., pp. 1108–1110. McGraw-Hill, New York.

Seddon, H. J., Medawar, P. B., and Smiths, H. (1943). Rate of regeneration of peripheral nerves in man. *J. Physiol. (London)* **102**, 191–201.

Spencer, P. S., and Schaumburg, H. H. (1984). Experimental models of primary axonal disease induced by toxic chemicals. In *Peripheral Neuropathy* (P. J. Dyck, P. K. Thomas, and E. H. Lambert, *et al.*, Eds.), 2nd ed., pp. 636–649. Saunders, Philadelphia.

Sunderland, S. (1947). Rate of regeneration of I: Sensory nerve fibres and II: Motor fibres. *Arch. Neurol. Psychiatry* **58**, 1–14.

Nerve Regeneration

Encyclopedia of the Neurological Sciences

THE PERIPHERAL NERVOUS SYSTEM has a significantly greater regenerative capacity than the mature central nervous system. This relates not only to intrinsic differences in the content between peripheral and central neurons but also to the properties of their support tissues. Robust regeneration in the peripheral nervous system occurs in lesions that remain in continuity largely because connective tissue elements are spared. During Wallerian degeneration, there is extensive molecular cross talk between many tissues and cell populations that stimulate connective tissue fibroblasts and Schwann cells to proliferate. Chains of Schwann cells surrounded by basement membrane tubes, called bands of Büngner, form at the gap between the nerve stumps, whereas others migrate into the distal stump. The cell body reacts to axotomy by increasing production of proteins that will be required to repair the damage. Thus, coincident with the process of Wallerian degeneration, the stage is being set for a subsequent phase of regeneration during which new axons, fresh myelin, and new target connections are made. There are three principal mechanisms that facilitate and regulate peripheral nerve regeneration.

First, chemotropic factors released by Schwann cells attract axonal sprouts to the distal stump. Immediately following axotomy, Schwann cells release stored ciliary neurotrophic factor, an injury factor that stimulates and mobilizes inflammatory cells and scavenger cells. The basal laminae of Schwann cells also express increased levels of such molecules as cadherins, immunoglobulin superfamily factors, and laminin, which promote sprouting of new axons. In addition, they increase production of other neurotrophic factors, including nerve growth factor (NGF), insulin-like growth factor, and brain-derived neurotrophic factor (BDNF), and they send out processes that make contact with the growing axon and help guide it to the distal stump.

Second, a network of adhesion molecules, such as the recently discovered protein ninjurin, is present on the distal stump. These molecules provide a finely tuned contact guidance system promoting axon growth along the correct tissue planes. In addition, the stump produces neurotrophic factors such as BDNF and NGF that promote the growth of axons.

Third, inhibitory factors, including members of the semaphorin family, are released from the surrounding perineurium. They prevent misdirected growth of axonal sprouts.

The tip of a growing axon is called the growth cone, which is a motile structure that is able to navigate toward the correct target under guidance from surrounding signals (Fig. 1). The growth cone emerges from a nontraumatized site just proximal to the actual injury. It consists of three components, the first of which is a central core rich in mitochondria and microtubules. The other structures, filopodia and lammellipodia, are motile elements rich in actin, myosin, and microtubules that can physically move the growth cone in any desired direction. The finger-like filopodia, extending from the tips of the growth cone, bear an array of surface receptor molecules that respond to a myriad of signals in the local microenvironment. These are passed into the interior of the growth cone, causing a structural rearrangement of the actin cytoskeleton and the microtubular network. The net effect of this activity is a change in the shape of the tip of the growth cone and movement toward the desired target (Fig. 2).

The average rate of nerve regeneration after axon injury is 1–1.5 mm/day (1 in. per month). However, this may vary depending on the caliber of the affected nerve and the nature of the injury. For example, axon sprouts may arise from the proximal stump within hours of a clean transection from a sharp blade, whereas axotomy caused by crush from a blunt object may be followed by retrograde degeneration for approximately 1 cm before anterograde regeneration begins. This "dying back" process takes approximately 1 week, during which time the axon sprouts must bypass damaged tissue before

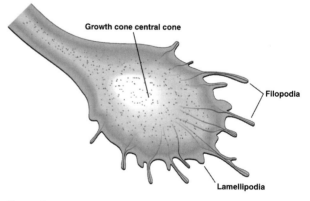

Figure 1
The growth cone.

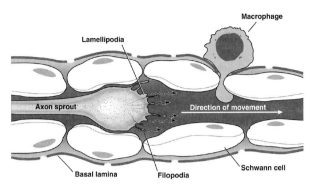

Figure 2

Illustration of an axon sprout migrating through a Band of Büngner. The axon sprout moves towards its distal target under the influence of a host of signals from the microenvironment. The Schwann cells in the Band of Büngner are vital in producing these chemical signals.

traversing the gap between nerve stumps. In some instances, debris and scar tissue may be present in the gap and significantly impede adequate contact of the axon sprout with the distal stump. A complication that may arise from this is the formation of an irregular, multicompartmentalized mass of tissue containing fibroblasts, axon sprouts, Schwann cells, and capillaries formed by disorganized regrowth of the new axon. This irregular mass lesion, called a neuroma, frequently develops when traumatic injury has breached the endoneurium (Sunderland grade 3 and higher). Although a neuroma may be readily appreciated at the proximal stump of a completely transected nerve, it may not be visible to the naked eye upon visual inspection of lesions in continuity. In the latter situation, one may suspect a neuroma when clinical recovery is less satisfactory than expected, with persistent neurological deficit and/or persistent pain. The latter is due to abnormal electrical hyperexcitability of the mass tissue, whereas the former represents failed target reinnervation.

In addition to axon regrowth, the process of nerve regeneration also involves the formation of a new myelin sheath. Schwann cells that have proliferated at the injury site begin to elaborate fresh myelin along the section of new axonal material; newly made internodes tend to be somewhat thinner and generally shorter (and more variable) in length than their predecessors. This process is relatively rapid so that after pure demyelinating lesions, it is not unusual to witness a full clinical recovery within a few weeks. Successful nerve regeneration must be functional as well as anatomical. Autonomic axons must effectively innervate blood vessels and vice versa, sensory fibers must reestablish communication

between the cell body and sensory organs, and terminal segments of newly grown motor nerve axons must develop into specialized neuromuscular junctions. It is interesting that motor axons make their contacts at the precise sites at which previous synapses were present on the target muscle. Research shows that the basal lamina of the target muscle membrane releases substances that guide the new axon terminals to these highly specific locations.

In axonotmesis lesions, the endoneurial sheath remains in continuity, whereas the axon has lost continuity. Consequently, it is highly likely that motor axonal sprouts will migrate along the endoneurial sheath of denervated motor fibers. However, if there is more significant distortion of the original architecture, such as a Sunderland third-degree injury in which the stumps are very closely apposed, it is quite possible for motor fibers to travel into the endoneurial sheaths of the wrong target muscle or even into former sensory tracts. For example, inappropriate reinnervation can be seen after injury to the facial nerve. Aberrant regrowth of facial nerve visceromotor fibers intended for the salivary glands into nerve sheaths destined for innervation of the lacrimal apparatus results in crocodile tears during mealtimes (i.e., saliva production is associated with the anomalous production of tears). Similarly, misdirected regrowth of some facial motor fibers into the wrong muscle can result in synkinesis; aberrant reinnervation of the orbicularus oris muscle by fibers that are intended for the orbicularis oculi muscle results in the phenomenon of involuntary retraction of the angle of the mouth when the eyelid is voluntarily closed.

Even in healthy individuals, nerve regeneration is rarely 100% efficient, and patients often report residual deficits, such as subtle loss of fine motor function in hand muscles that are otherwise functioning normally. It is likely that many factors contribute to this clinical picture, including a failure of new motor axons to distinguish between fast-twitch and slow-twitch fibers and less efficient conduction through segments wrapped in freshly made, albeit thinner, myelin. Furthermore, in long-standing nerve injuries, degeneration of intramuscular nerve sheaths and scar formation in the muscle militate against successful reinnervation.

Nerve regeneration is also hampered in many disease states. For example, in diabetic peripheral polyneuropathy the rate of regeneration fails to keep pace with degeneration. Recent research on gene regulation of the peripheral nerve cell body responses in injured diabetic nerve indicates that there is a delay in activating certain immediate early genes that are important in initiating the process of regeneration. Many of these genes code for neurotrophic factors, and a delay in their production may underlie the pathogenesis of a variety of peripheral neuropathies. Indeed, there is experimental evidence that recombinant human nerve growth factor (rhNGF), a member of the neurotrophic factor family, may be effective as a therapeutic agent in small-fiber sensory polyneuropathy. Peripheral sensory neurons are less well protected by the blood–nerve barrier than motor neurons, and thus circulating therapeutic substances have better access to sensory neuron cell bodies. Furthermore, NGF is naturally trophic for small-caliber sensory and autonomic fibers. Human clinical trials of subcutaneously administered rhNGF have been carried out in patients with sensory neuropathy associated with human immunodeficiency virus (HIV) and in patients with diabetic polyneuropathy. To date, however, no clear benefit has been noted in terms of nerve fiber regrowth (although pain symptoms were noted to improve significantly in the HIV neuropathy study).

In general, successful clinical recovery from a nerve injury depends on many factors, the most important of which is the principal underlying pathophysiology. It is unusual for a neurapractic injury to cause a persistent deficit for more than 6 weeks; if so, it is likely that a degree of axonotmesis has also occurred. The clinical recovery rate for axonotmesis and neuronotmesis lesions is far less predictable. The process of Wallerian degeneration and regeneration is slow (approximately 1 in./month), and many muscles will completely degenerate if they do not gain reinnervation within 24–36 months. Thus, one of the key issues is the distance of the injury from the nearest target organ (e.g., a muscle). For example, if there is an 18-in. distance between a severe axon loss injury and the target muscle (e.g., an injury to the lower cord of the brachial plexus), it is quite likely that there will be only a limited functional reinnervation of the target muscle (e.g., small intrinsic hand muscle). When loss of continuity occurs, there is a further delay in clinical recovery because of the necessary process of retrograde degeneration, axon sprouting, regrowth across the gap to the distal stump, and maturation of the distal connections. Thus, the recovery rate of unrecognized or untreated neurotmesis lesions tends to be worse than that of axonotmesis lesions.

—*Brian Eamon Murray*

See also–Axons; Myelin; Nerve Injury; Nerve Repair; Neurolysis

Further Reading

Apfel, S. C. (1999). Neurotrophic factors in the therapy of diabetic neuropathy. *Am. J. Med.* **107**, 34S–42S.

Bisby, M. A. (2000). Regeneration in the peripheral nervous system. In *Degeneration and Regeneration in the Nervous System* (N. R. Saunders and K. M. Dziegielewska, Eds.), pp. 239–262. Harwood Academic, Amsterdam.

Fawcett, J. W., and Keynes, R. J. (1990). Peripheral nerve regeneration. *Annu. Rev. Neurosci.* **13**, 43–60.

Sanes, J. R., and Jessell, T. M. (2000). The guidance of axons to their targets. In *Principles of Neural Science* (E. R. Kandel, J. H. Schwartz, and T. M. Jessell, Eds.), 4th ed., pp. 1069–1086. McGraw-Hill, New York.

Sanes, J. R., and Jessell, T. M. (2000). The formation and regeneration of synapses. In *Principles of Neural Science* (E. R. Kandel, J. H. Schwartz, and T. M. Jessell, Eds.), 4th ed., pp. 1108–1114. McGraw-Hill, New York.

Nerve Repair

Encyclopedia of the Neurological Sciences

A TRAUMATIC INJURY may cause damage to one or several components of a peripheral nerve. A compressive injury may cause a functional deficit in the myelin sheath surrounding the axon of the peripheral nerve but spare the axon and associated connective tissue elements (Seddon's neurapraxia or Sunderland's grade 1). This may cause a block in electrical conductivity across the site of injury and thus manifest as either weakness or numbness depending on the primary function of the affected nerve. Alternatively, a traumatic event may wholly or partly sever the axon across its width but spare the endoneurium and other connective tissue elements, thus leaving the nerve in continuity (axonotmesis or grade 2). Finally, certain injuries may actually disrupt myelin, axon, and connective tissue elements, which in the most severe cases completely transect a nerve trunk leaving a gap interposed between the proximal and distal nerve stumps (neurotmesis or grades 3–5).

The correct classification of nerve injury is of great prognostic importance. Neurapractic injuries generally recover extremely well during a period of less than 6 weeks, but the prognosis for axonotmesis and neurotmesis lesions is far less certain since axons do not have the same kind of regenerative capabilities as myelin. As such, surgical intervention is sometimes required to repair axonotmesis and neurotmesis lesions.

EVALUATION OF THE INJURY

When called on to evaluate a traumatic peripheral nerve injury, it is paramount to consider the likelihood of success or failure of functional end organ reinnervation. This process is dependent on many factors, including the nature of the injury, the presence of infection and/or debris in the injury site, vascular supply, distance between the stumps, and the distance of the injury from the target organ. Thus, a careful history and a detailed clinical examination are the key initial elements in the evaluation process. One can often diagnose a neurapractic injury based on a history of a compressive event and a clinical scenario of rapid clinical recovery. Similarly, it is relatively easy to diagnose a neurotmesis lesion in an open wound caused by laceration from a sharp blade since the severed nerve may be clearly visible to the naked eye. However, it is sometimes difficult to distinguish a mild from severe injury based on this initial evaluation. Crush, stretch, and contusive injuries may be complex: Multiple plexus elements and nerves may be involved, and there may be coexisting regions of neurapraxia, axonotmesis, and neurotmesis all manifesting with the same symptoms (weakness and/or sensory disturbance). Furthermore, 70% of lesions remain in continuity and not all may be clearly identified by visual inspection or palpation.

As a consequence, a number of ancillary testing techniques have been developed to aid in the correct classification and subsequent management of nerve injuries. The electrodiagnostic examination (EDX) is the most useful and most frequently employed technique. It consists of two components—the nerve conduction study (NCS) and the needle electrode examination (NEE). The NCS assesses the amplitude and latencies of compound muscle action potentials (CMAPs) and sensory nerve action potentials (SNAPs), whereas the NEE evaluates muscle recruitment and whether there is evidence of active muscle degeneration due to axon loss. The EDX is used to provide a more precise localization of the site of injury and differentiate an axon loss lesion from one that is primarily due to demyelinating conduction block (neurapraxia). It can also more objectively measure the severity of the lesion and monitor the rate and extent of recovery over time. The first complete EDX should be performed no earlier than 3

weeks after the original insult to allow time for any potential axon loss to appear in the form of loss of CMAP and SNAP amplitudes, reduced muscle recruitment, and evidence of active axon loss (fibrillation potentials and positive sharp waves). Serially performed EDX examinations are particularly valuable in discriminating between grade 2–4 lesions, all of which may be clinically similar in the earlier stages. Early reinnervation of target muscle may be identified electrically in the form of small, polyphasic, and unstable nascent muscle potentials. The presence of such potentials may predate any clinical evidence of muscle activity and suggests a milder injury and a better functional outcome.

Other techniques may also be used to assist in the evaluation of nerve injury. Somatosensory evoked potentials (SSEPs) have been used to identify very proximal sites of nerve injury that cannot be adequately assessed by EDX. As such, SSEPs are mainly used in the evaluation of nerve root avulsion injuries, although they are limited by their inability to yield information about the anterior nerve rootlets as they exit the spinal cord.

Magnetic resonance imaging (MRI) is also useful in the evaluation of traumatic nerve injury. A novel technique, called MR neurography, can identify discontinuity (neurotmesis) lesions very early after injury, although hemorrhage at the trauma site may limit accurate assessment. Using this technique, one may detect high signal and swelling in individual nerve fascicles caused by crush and compression injuries and also identify meningoceles caused by nerve root avulsion. Furthermore, MR neurography can be used to assess the integrity of suture sites after nerve grafting has been performed and even reveal the presence of neuromas in continuity. Moreover, T2-weighted MRI sequences can show high signal in denervated muscle and thus may be useful in the evaluation of very proximal muscles that cannot be easily assessed by EDX. Unfortunately, many of these novel MRI techniques are not widely available, and expertise in interpretation of images is limited to a few centers.

Approximately 70% of injuries leave the nerve in continuity. The injury site may appear quite normal to the naked eye and feel normal when palpated. Thus, it is often necessary to carry out intraoperative electrophysiological nerve studies to evaluate the precise nature and extent of the injury. The technique entails the placement of stimulating and recording needle electrodes onto the nerve above and below the injury site and recording nerve action potentials

(NAPs). If the latter are unattainable across a segment of nerve, this indicates the presence of a significant nerve injury at that site, and the surgeon may classify the injury, identify its precise location(s), and localize healthy nerve or fascicle stumps.

SURGICAL REPAIR

Since the mid-1970s, modern microsurgical techniques have been developed to repair many kinds of injury and achieve satisfactory functional outcome. Peripheral nerve repair is delicate by nature, with a good result depending on the skill of the surgeon and careful patient selection.

One of the most common and important surgical procedures is external neurolysis, which entails isolation of the nerve by careful dissection above and below the site of injury and mobilization of vascular, connective tissue and related neural elements. Indeed, external neurolysis is often the only intervention required in the surgical management of nerve lesions that are in continuity with recordable NAPs. Occasionally, a patient may suffer a pain syndrome caused by an incomplete nerve lesion, which may be effectively relieved by internal neurolysis; this entails dissecting out healthy fascicles from injured ones and then removing excess scar tissue.

Primary neurorrhaphy is the term applied to direct end-to-end suturing of the nerve stumps above (proximal) and below (distal) the site of injury and is the procedure of choice whenever possible. Two basic techniques are used for end-to-end coaption and suturing of nerve stumps—epineurial repair and fascicular repair. In the former (Fig. 1), sutures are placed through the epineurial connective tissue

sheath using local landmarks to approximate the correct alignment of proximal and distal nerve stumps. Under the influence of neurotophic factors, the proximal nerve end grows toward the distal stump. Epineurial repair is the preferred technique when dealing with smaller nerves, such as those in the hand and lower forearm.

In fascicular repair (Fig. 1), the surgeon places sutures through the perineurium surrounding individual proximal and distal nerve fascicles. Nerve fascicles, particularly in the proximal portions of the nerve, do not lie longitudinally side by side but intertwine in an arrangement called fasciculation (not to be confused with the term applied to the spontaneous contraction of part of a muscle belly). Thus, it is important to correctly identify the particular pattern of each nerve so as to line up the correct proximal and distal nerve fascicle stumps. A number of techniques have been developed to assist in proper alignment of fascicles, including histochemical staining of nerve ends, aligning landmark blood vessels, and intraoperative electrophysiological studies. Fascicular repair is the preferred technique when dealing with larger, more proximal nerve segments, such as those in the upper arm and the brachial plexus.

Primary neurorrhaphy is not the preferred method for certain kinds of nerve injury. A significant gap may preclude direct end-to-end anastomosis because excessive tension is placed on the repaired nerve. Experimental work has shown that if a nerve is stretched to a length 8% more than the original, there is a 46% decrease in effective blood flow within the nerve. Thus, an end-to-end anastomosis under tension may expose the nerve to the risk of ischemic injury. Furthermore, there may be excessive deformation of the nerve as it crosses joints and bony structures, causing scar formation and adhesions in the operative region.

NERVE GRAFTS

A nerve graft is used when the gap between the stumps of a transected nerve cannot be brought together without exerting excessive tension. The gold standard in nerve grafting is the use of autogenous donor grafts, which are harvested (with prior consent) from other parts of the patient's body. These are typically small-caliber sensory nerves, such as the lateral antebrachial cutaneous nerve, sural nerve, and sensory branch of the posterior interosseous nerve, the loss of which is not significantly

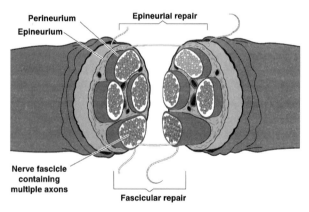

Figure 1
Epineurial repair (top) and fascicular repair (bottom).

disabling to the patient. The donor graft is sutured in place between the nerve stumps in the trauma site.

Nerve regeneration across nerve grafts may not be quite as effective as that seen with a direct end-to-end anastomosis because axonal sprouts must cross two suture lines and the entire length of the interposed graft. In addition, graft material does not produce as much biochemical support in the form of tropic and trophic factors to assist the regenerative process. The anatomical alignment of donor and recipient nerve tissue may be quite dissimilar, which may make it difficult to align similar fascicular patterns between nerve stumps. Finally, survival of the graft very much depends on its ability to be vascularized by the local blood supply. In cases in which the vascular bed is poor, a section of nerve with its own blood supply, a vascularized nerve graft, may be indicated.

It is not always desirable to use autogenous nerve grafts, especially when the distance between stumps is great or when there are multiple nerve injuries. Research is ongoing regarding the potential use of human cadaver grafts, which would be in plentiful supply and also obviate the need to sacrifice healthy donor nerves in the patient. However, insertion of this "foreign" material stimulates a robust immune response in the recipient, which currently necessitates the administration of potent immunosuppressant drugs to prevent graft rejection. Another experimental approach is to bridge the gap with nonnerve tubular material, which serves as a conduit across which regenerating axonal sprouts pass. A number of different entubulation materials are under investigation, including collagen, mesothelium, muscle, vein, and artery. In addition, fully synthetic (e.g., glycolide trimethylene carbonate, silicone, and polyglycolic acid) and semisynthetic entubulation materials are also being developed. Future use may also be made of reservoir devices or matrices that release neurotrophic factors such as ciliary neurotrophic factor into the regenerating graft site.

A variation on nerve grafting called neurotization is used to improve the functional outcome of brachial plexus avulsion injuries when no proximal stump is available. The general principal is to substitute the injured nerve that is unlikely to recover with an axon donor that is functioning normally. For example, the surgeon may transfer an intercostal nerve (the axon donor) to the distal stump of the musculocutaneous nerve or transfer the spinal accessory nerve to the distal stump of the suprascapular nerve.

Neurotization can also be used when no distal stump is available. The surgeon first splits the nerve into fascicles and then directly inserts them into the end plate region of the muscle belly. It is also possible to carry out muscle transfers that are subsequently neurotized and vascularized; for example, one could replace a nonfunctional biceps muscle in the arm with the gracilis muscle from the lower extremity.

TIMING OF SURGERY

Open Injuries

The timing of nerve repair is important to ensure the best possible outcome. A prime consideration in this regard is the nature of the injury. After a clean transection (e.g., from a razor blade), it is relatively easy to locate the wound and carry out a neurological examination. Many surgeons operate within the first 72 hr, surgically exploring the wound and carrying out an end-to-end suture repair.

The course of action is less clear-cut with neurotmesis lesions in open wounds caused by blunt trauma or jagged edges (e.g., from a chainsaw blade). These not only deform the nerve stumps but also damage soft tissue and blood vessels in the trauma site. Furthermore, axonotmesis lesions may flank an obvious transection for a long distance. Early exploration of the wound enables the surgeon to evaluate the damage and clean up the debris. However, the decision to proceed to a direct end-to-end repair is often very difficult: If the nerve stumps are immediately sutured together, there is an increased risk of fibrosis, which may impede subsequent nerve regeneration across the repair site. In light of this possibility, many surgeons tack the nerve ends to adjacent soft tissue and close the wound for a few weeks until an early secondary repair can be performed, at which time it is relatively easy to visually identify fibrosis at the nerve endings. It is common practice to also perform intraoperative NAP recordings to both classify and define the extent of the lesions.

Neurotmesis lesions in open wounds are by no means the only indication for early surgical exploration. Other reasons include the presence of pain or swelling, acute compression from an expanding blood clot or blood vessel, or progressively worsening clinical signs.

Closed Injuries

Most injuries to peripheral nerve are from blunt trauma and lack an open wound. The lesions are usually in continuity and are typically caused by traction or compression. Unless there is a pressing need for early intervention (e.g., compression from an expanding pseudoaneurysm), it is common practice to avoid early surgery in these patients. Instead, they are evaluated both clinically and electrophysiologically every 2–5 months to assess whether or not there is good functional recovery. If the patient fails to improve or begins to deteriorate, surgical intervention is usually indicated. When performing these delayed procedures it is important to perform intraoperative NAPs to detect the presence of neuromas lying beneath the surface of an apparently healthy nerve.

OUTCOME OF NERVE REPAIR

Overall, the results of surgery depend on many factors, including the nature of the injury, the time to referral to a specialist center, and the expertise of the surgical team. At Louisiana State University Medical Center, a major specialist center with a 35-year experience in the surgical management of nerve injury, it has been reported that good functional outcome is seen in approximately 90% of cases when a recordable NAP is obtained. In addition, approximately 70% of direct end-to-end anastomoses and 50% of graft repairs are associated with good outcome.

In general, pure motor and pure sensory nerves fare better than mixed nerves after surgical repair. Superior results are more frequently seen in children, patients who are operated on earlier, and when shorter nerve grafts (<3 in.) are used.

Protective sensory recovery is possible even years after the original nerve injury, but long delays in repair of motor nerves may prove ineffective because muscle fibers degenerate and are replaced by scar tissue within 24–36 months of significant nerve injury.

In the postoperative phase, it is important for the patient to receive physical therapy in order to maximize limb function while simultaneously protecting the integrity of the repair site. Adequate outpatient follow-up is also an important part of the surgical management of nerve repair, allowing the doctor and patient to accurately assess the rate and extent of recovery and determine if further intervention is necessary.

—*Brian Murray*

See also–Axons; Microneurosurgery; Nerve Injury; Nerve Regeneration

Further Reading

Flores, A. J., Lavernia, C. J., and Owens, P. W. (2000). Anatomy and physiology of peripheral nerve injury and repair. *Am. J. Orthop.* **29**, 167–173.

Kline, D. G. (2000). Nerve surgery as it is now and as it may be. *Neurosurgery* **46**, 1285–1293.

Millesi, H. (1998). Nerve grafts: Indications, techniques, and prognoses. In *Management of Peripheral Nerve Problems* (G. E. Omer, A. Van Beek, and M. Spinner, Eds.), pp. 280–289. Saunders, Philadelphia.

Spinner, R. J., and Kline, D. G. (2000). Surgery for peripheral nerve and brachial plexus injuries or other nerve lesions. *Muscle Nerve* **23**, 680–695.

Nerve Roots

Encyclopedia of the Neurological Sciences
Copyright 2003, Elsevier Science (USA). All rights reserved.

NERVE ROOTS connect the spinal cord to the peripheral nerve. At each spinal segment there are two pairs of roots on each side of the cord—the anterior roots and the posterior roots (Fig. 1). The two converge and perforate the arachnoid and dura close to each other. The anterior roots carry large motor axons of cells whose cell bodies are in the anterior gray matter of the spinal cord. The anterior roots from the first thoracic segment to the first lumbar segment also carry small myelinated axons from neurons in the intermediolateral column of the gray matter. These axons leave the motor root just outside the dura to enter the paravertebral autonomic chain and the sympathetic ganglia. The posterior roots carry sensory fibers of various

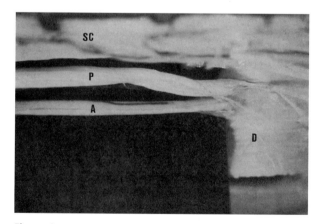

Figure 1
Anterior (A) and posterior (P) roots and the location at which they run through the dura. A piece of black paper was placed behind the roots and the spinal cord (SC) but in front of the dura (D).

diameters from the posterior root ganglia into the spinal cord. These ganglia lie at the gap between vertebrae where the nerve roots pass after running through the dura. The posterior roots enter the capsule of the ganglia, where their axons are connected to the ganglion cells by thin processes. Just beyond the ganglia, the anterior and posterior roots join and merge. At this point, the roots are considered to end and the peripheral nerve begins.

The main components of nerve roots are thus axons, with their concomitant myelin sheaths. Axons larger than 2 μm in diameter are covered with myelin. For a distance of up to approximately 100 μm, the part of a root immediately adjacent to the spinal cord contains oligodendroglial cells, and the axons are covered by the myelin that they make—the so-called central myelin. Beyond 100 μm, oligodendroglial cells are replaced by Schwann cells and the peripheral myelin that they produce.

Where the roots travel through the subarachnoid space, they are bathed in cerebrospinal fluid. The roots are covered by a single layer of arachnoid cells until near the point at which they leave the subarachnoid space, and the arachnoid cells are replaced by layered perineurial cells. A few vessels run in roots. Some of the larger arteries furnish blood to the spinal cord, whereas the smaller ones only supply the roots.

—Stirling Carpenter

See also–Axons; Dorsal Root Ganglion; Myelin; Spinal Cord Anatomy; Spinal Roots

Nerve Sheath Tumors

Encyclopedia of the Neurological Sciences
Copyright 2003, Elsevier Science (USA). All rights reserved.

NERVE SHEATH tumors arise from cranial nerves, spinal nerve roots, or peripheral nerves. Because these structures are anatomically part of the peripheral nervous system (PNS), nerve sheath tumors arise outside of the central nervous system (CNS) but through expansion and subsequent compression may cause CNS dysfunction.

ETIOLOGY

Nerve sheath tumors are derived from neoplasia of the Schwann cell, the PNS counterpart of the oligodendrocyte in the CNS and the manufacturer of PNS myelin. The two distinct categories of nerve sheath tumors are neurofibromas, a mixture of proliferating Schwann cells and fibroblasts interdigitated between nerve fibers, and schwannomas, which are neoplastic Schwann cells. The term schwannoma is now used interchangeably with neurinoma, neurilemmoma, and, in some cases, neuroma. The vast majority of nerve sheath tumors display benign biological behavior, but malignant degeneration of neurofibromas occurs in a small percentage of cases.

Two autosomal dominant neurocutaneous syndromes, neurofibromatosis I (mutation on chromosome 17) and neurofibromatosis II (mutation on chromosome 22), involve a preponderance of nerve sheath tumors. Neurofibromatosis I (peripheral or von Recklinghausen's neurofibromatosis) consists of peripheral and subcutaneous neurofibromas in addition to other clinical features. The hallmark of neurofibromatosis II (central neurofibromatosis) is bilateral acoustic neuromas (vestibular schwannomas).

CLINICAL FEATURES

Acoustic neuromas represent approximately 5–10% of all intracranial tumors and are the most common cranial nerve schwannoma. These tumors arise from the vestibular division of the eighth cranial nerve and exhibit a female preponderance. Trigeminal schwannomas arise from cranial nerve 5, account for only 0.07–0.36% of all intracranial tumors, and are the second most common cranial nerve sheath tumor. On cranial magnetic resonance imaging (MRI), trigeminal schwannomas are often dumbbell-shaped, extending from the posterior fossa into Meckel's cave (a space or dural sac beneath the dura mater containing the fifth cranial nerve ganglion) of the middle fossa (Fig. 1). Cranial nerve schwannomas and neurofibromas of the facial, glossopharyngeal or vagal (jugular foramen schwannomas), and hypoglossal nerves are quite rare and may be identified as solitary tumors but are more likely to be a manifestation of neurofibromatosis.

Spinal nerve root schwannomas and neurofibromas are rare and most commonly arise from sensory roots. These lesions often grow through spinal neural foramina, forming a dumbbell-shaped lesion on MRI (Fig. 2). Spinal nerve root sheath tumors are commonly multiple as part of neurofibromatosis.

Peripheral nerve sheath tumors most commonly involve cutaneous nerves and represent neurofibromas

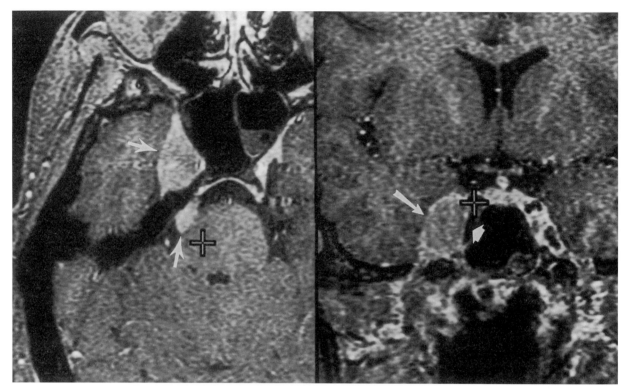

Figure 1
Contrast-enhanced axial (left) and coronal (right) magnetic resonance images of a trigeminal schwannoma in a patient with trigeminal neuralgia. Arrows on the axial image indicate the separate posterior fossa and middle fossa components. The narrow arrow on the coronal image indicates the Meckel's cave/cavernous sinus middle fossa component, and the arrowhead shows the location of the carotid artery traversing the cavernous sinus.

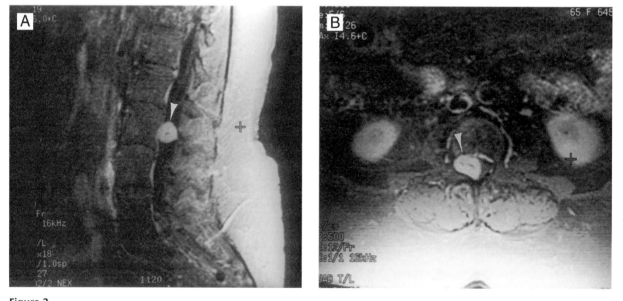

Figure 2
Contrast-enhanced sagittal (A) and axial (B) magnetic resonance images of a lumbar spinal nerve root sheath tumor (arrows) in a patient with an L3 radiculopathy. Note the dumbbell-shaped appearance on the axial image where the tumor traverses the neural foremen.

secondary to neurofibromatosis. These lesions may be plexiform neurofibromas, tortuous collections of enlarged cutaneous nerves, or nodular. Peripheral nerve sheath tumors are often palpable, tender masses that become symptomatic secondary to pain.

Nerve sheath tumors most commonly present due to symptoms and signs related to dysfunction of the nerve of origin. However, as these lesions enlarge they may cause dysfunction of adjacent CNS structures. In the case of acoustic neuromas, the three most common presenting symptoms are hearing loss, tinnitus, and dysequilibrium. With larger lesions, facial pain or numbness (trigeminal nerve dysfunction), facial weakness (facial nerve dysfunction), or symptomatic hydrocephalus (fourth ventricular compression) may be observed. Trigeminal schwannomas typically present with facial pain (trigeminal neuralgia) and numbness.

Spinal nerve root sheath tumors most commonly present with pain and/or motor dysfunction relative to the root of origin. Spinal cord compression with resultant myelopathy occurs as lesions expand.

TREATMENT OPTIONS

Spinal and peripheral nerve sheath tumors are generally treated by surgical excision when symptomatic. Spinal nerve root tumors may have intradural and extradural components; therefore, a combined intradural and extradural approach to excision is often necessary.

Treatment of cranial nerve sheath tumors is more controversial. Options include observation with serial imaging over time in patients with no or minor symptoms, stereotactic image-guided radiosurgery, fractionated radiotherapy, and conventional microsurgical skull base approaches to resection. With large lesions >3 cm in diameter causing symptomatic compression of surrounding brain structures, most authors agree that a microsurgical approach alone or followed by radiosurgery is warranted. With smaller lesions symptomatic of the cranial nerve of origin, radiosurgery versus microsurgery is debated. Patient factors such as age and general medical condition influence decisions regarding the best treatment option.

—*Timothy F. Witham and Douglas Kondziolka*

See also–Acoustic Neuroma; Brain Tumors, Biology; Brain Tumors, Genetics; Central

Nervous System Tumors, Epidemiology; Childhood Brain Tumors; Glial Tumors; Metastases, Brain; Oligodendrocytes; Pituitary Tumors; Primary Central Nervous System Lymphoma and Germ Cell Tumors; Spinal Cord Tumors, Biology of; Spinal Cord Tumors, Treatment of

Further Reading

Muthukumar, N., Kondziolka, D., and Lunsford, L. D. (1998). Stereotactic radiosurgery for other skull base lesions. In *Gamma Knife Brain Surgery* (L. D. Lunsford, D. Kondziolka, and J. C. Flickinger, Eds.), pp. 128–144. Karger, New York.

Okazaki, H. (1989). *Fundamentals of Neuropathology, Morphologic Basis of Neurologic Disorders*. Igaku-Shoin, New York.

Nervous System, Neuroembryology of

Encyclopedia of the Neurological Sciences
Copyright 2003, Elsevier Science (USA). All rights reserved.

THE ESSENCE of classic embryology is descriptive morphogenesis; that is, detailed observations of gross and microscopic changes in organs and tissues in the developing embryo and fetus. This aspect is timeless and will never become obsolete. The new neuroembryology integrates classic embryology with insight provided by recent data on the molecular genetic programming of neural development. Interactions of genes or their transcription products specify differentiation; developmental genes may be expressed only transiently in the embryo or may continue throughout life. After development is completed, these same genes may continue to be expressed in order to conserve the identity of individual cellular types even in the adult. They may also provide clues to hereditary degenerative processes that begin after the nervous system is mature.

Malformations are aberrations in neural development resulting from genetic mutations or lesions acquired in fetal life. These dysgeneses are traditionally taught as a series of sequential and overlapping developmental processes: proliferation of neuroepithelial cells, apoptosis, cell migration, differentiation and maturation of neuroblasts and glioblasts, axonal growth toward target cells, dendritic sprouting, synaptogenesis, and myelination cycles. These categories provided a basis for classifying malformations as hypoplasias of midline structures, disorders of neuroblast migration, aberrant axonal projections, disturbances of synaptogenesis, and others. These older concepts of developmental processes remain valid, but we also must consider the defective expression or coexpression of transcription products of various developmental genes. Genes determine and coordinate every aspect of neuroembryonic development, from gastrulation and the creation of a neuroepithelium to the last detail of postnatal synaptogenesis and myelination. The new neuroembryology encompasses traditional and emerging concepts of how the nervous system forms, matures, and functions at every developmental stage. Each concept is fragmentary without the complement of the other.

The term development may occasionally be confusing because it is used in two different ways, which in the end are in harmony. As used here, development refers to morphogenesis and the molecular genetic basis for it. Clinical neurologists and pediatricians also use the term development to identify the progressive functional changes of maturation: the acquisition of motor, cognitive, linguistic, and intellectual skills at particular ages, along with emotional and psychological maturation. Both uses of the term are equally valid within their distinct contexts. Ultimately, the important issue is not to memorize when a child can take the first unaided steps but to understand why they do not walk before 1 year of age.

GASTRULATION

Gastrulation is the birth of the nervous system. In simple chordates, such as amphioxus and amphibians, gastrulation is the invagination of a spherical blastula. In birds and mammals, the blastula is collapsed as a flattened, bilayered disk, and gastrulation appears not as an invagination but as a groove between two ridges on one surface of this disk, the primitive streak on the epiblast. The primitive streak establishes in each embryo the basic body plan of all vertebrates: a midline axis, bilateral symmetry, rostral and caudal ends, and dorsal and ventral surfaces. As the primitive streak extends forward, an aggregate of cells at one end is designated the primitive node or Hensen's node. Hensen's node defines the rostral end. Cells of the epiblast on either side move toward the primitive streak, stream through it, and emerge beneath it to pass into the narrow cavity between the two sheets of cells—the epiblast above and the hypoblast below; these migratory cells give rise to the mesoderm and endoderm internally, and some then replace the hypoblast.

After extending approximately halfway across the blastoderm (epiblast), the primitive streak with Hensen's node reverses the direction of its growth to retreat, moving posteriorly as the head fold and neural plate form anterior to Henson's node. As the node regresses, a notochordal process develops in the area rostral to it, and somites begin to form on either side of the notochord, with the more caudal somites differentiating first, and successive ones differentiating anterior to somites already formed. The notochord induces epiblast cells to form neuroectoderm.

INDUCTION

Induction is a term denoting the influence of one embryonic tissue on another so that the inducer and the induced differentiate as discrete mature tissues. In the case of the nervous system, the creation and subsequent development of the neural tube may be defined in terms of gradients of inductive influences. Induction usually occurs between germ layers, as with the notochord (mesoderm) inducing the floor plate of the neural tube (ectoderm). The visceral endoderm mediates ectodermal forebrain development by suppressing posteriorizing signals in the formation of the head. Induction may also occur within a single germ layer. An example is the optic cup (neuroectoderm) inducing the formation of a lens and cornea from the overlying epithelium (surface ectoderm) that otherwise would have differentiated simply as more epidermis. Neural induction is the differentiation or maturation of structures of the nervous system from undifferentiated ectodermal cells due to the influence of surrounding embryonic tissues.

Induction was discovered in 1924 by Hans Spemann and Hilde Mangold, who demonstrated that the dorsal lip of the newt gastrula was capable of inducing the formation of an ectopic second nervous system when transplanted to another site in a host embryo, in another individual of the same species, or in a ventral site of the same embryo. This dorsal lip of the amphibian gastrula, also known as the Spemann organizer, is homologous with Hensen's node of embryonic birds and mammals. Transplantation of the primitive node in a manner similar to that in the Spemann and Mangold experiments in amphibians yields similar results. The first gene isolated from the Spemann organizer was *goosecoid* (*gsc*), which encoded a homeodomain protein (defined later) able to recapitulate the transplantation of the dorsal lip tissue. When injected into an ectopic site, *gsc* also normally induces the prechordal mesoderm and contributes to prosencephalic differentiation. Another gene, *Wnt8C*, expressed in Hensen's node and before the primitive streak is fully formed, is also essential for the regulation of axis formation and later for hindbrain patterning in the region of the future rhombomere 4 (r4). The regulatory gene *Cnot*, with major domains in the primitive node, notochord, and prenodal and postnodal neural plate, is another important molecular factor responsible for the induction of prechordal mesoderm and for the formation of the notochord in particular. The *gooseberry* (*Gox*) gene (transcription factor) is unique in being the only identified gene to be expressed in the primitive streak that loses expression at the onset of notochord formation. The *Gox* gene probably regulates the primitive streak positively by promoting its elongation or negatively by suppressing formation of the notochordal process. Another possible function is to promote a mesodermal lineage of epiblast cells as they ingress through the primitive streak. Several other genes essential in creating the fundamental architecture of the embryo and its nervous system are already expressed in the primitive node, and many reappear later to influence more advanced stages of ontogenesis.

The specificity of induction is not the inductive molecule but, rather, the receptor in the induced cell. This distinction is important because foreign molecules similar in structure to that of the natural inductor molecule may sometimes be erroneously recognized by the receptor as identical; such foreign molecules may behave as teratogens if the embryo is exposed to such a toxin. Induction occurs during a precise temporal window; the time of responsiveness of the induced cell is designated its competence, and it is incapable of responding before or after the precise time. Induction receptors are not necessarily in or on the plasma membrane of the cell, but they may be in the cytoplasm or the nucleoplasm. Retinoic acid is an example of a nuclear inducer. In some cases, the stimulus acts exclusively at the plasma membrane of target cells and does not require actual penetration of the cell. The receptors that represent the specificity of induction are also genetically programmed; the gene *Notch* is particularly important in regulating the competence of a cell to respond to inductive cues from within the neural tube and in surrounding embryonic tissues.

Some mesodermal tissues, such as smooth muscle of the fetal gut, can act as mitogens on the neuroepithelium by increasing the rate of cellular proliferation, but this phenomenon is not true neural induction because the proliferating cells do not differentiate or mature. Some organizer and regulatory genes of the nervous system, such as *Wnt1*, also exhibit mitogenic effects, and insulin-like growth factor and basic fibroblast growth factor also act as mitogens.

The early formation of the neural plate is not accomplished exclusively by mitotic proliferation of neuroepithelial cells; it is also accomplished by a conversion of surrounding cells to a neural fate. In amphibians, a gene known as *Achaete-scute* (*XASH3*) is expressed very early in the dorsal part of the embryo from the time of gastrulation and acts as a molecular switch to change the fate of undifferentiated cells to become neuroepithelium rather than surface ectodermal or mesodermal tissues. Some cells differentiate as specific types because they are actively inhibited from differentiating as others; all ectodermal cells are preprogrammed to form neuroepithelium, and neuroepithelial cells are preprogrammed to become neurons if not inhibited by genes that direct their differentiation along a different lineage, such as epidermal, glial, or ependymal.

SEGMENTATION

More than a century ago, the concept of segmentation was already a highly debated issue by biologists who were intrigued by the repeating units along the rostrocaudal axis of many worms and insects and by the somites of embryonic vertebrates. Segmentation of the neural tube creates intrinsic compartments that restrict the movement of cells by physical and chemical boundaries between adjacent compartments. These embryonic compartments are known as neuromeres.

The spinal cord has the appearance of a highly segmented structure but is not intrinsically segmented in the embryo, fetus, or the adult; instead, it corresponds in its entirety to the caudalmost of the eight neuromeres that create the hindbrain. The apparent segmentation of the spinal cord results from clustering of nerve roots imposed by the true segmentation of surrounding tissues derived from mesoderm—tissues that form the neural arches of the vertebrae, the somites, and associated structures. Neuromeres of the hindbrain are designated rhombomeres. Nearly the entire cerebellar cortex—the vermis, flocculonodular lobe, and lateral hemispheres—develops from r1, but the mesencephalic neuromere contributes to the formation of part of the rostral cerebellum. The dentate and other deep cerebellar nuclei are formed in r2. The rostral end of the neural tube forms a mesencephalic neuromere and four (possibly six) forebrain neuromeres, segregated as two diencephalic and four telencephalic prosomeres. Segmentation of the human embryonic brain into neuromeres is summarized in Table 1.

The segments of the embryonic neural tube are distinguished by physical barriers formed by processes of early specializing cells that resemble the radial glial cells that appear later in development and also by chemical barriers from secreted molecules that repel migratory cells. Cell adhesion is increased in the boundary zones between rhombomeres, which also contributes to the creation of barriers against cellular migration in the longitudinal axis. Limited mitotic proliferation of the neuroepithelium occurs in the boundary zones between rhombomeres. Although cells still divide in this zone, their nuclei remain near the ventricle during the mitotic cycle and do not move as far centrifugally within the elongated

cell cytoplasm during the interkinetic gap phases as they generally move. The rhombomeres of the brainstem may also be visualized as a series of transverse ridges and grooves on the dorsal surface, the future floor of the fourth ventricle; these ridges are gross morphological markers of the hindbrain compartments.

The first evidence of segmentation is a boundary that separates the future mesencephalic neuromere from r1 of the hindbrain. More genes play a role in this initial segmentation of the neural tube than in any boundaries that subsequently form to separate other neuromeres. The mesencephalic–metencephalic region appears to develop early as a single independent unit or "organizer" for other neuromeres rostral and caudal to that zone.

PATTERNING OF THE NEURAL TUBE

Basic characteristics of the body plan are called patterning. They are the anatomical expression of the genetic code within the nuclear DNA of every cell, but they also may result from signals from neighboring cells, carried by molecules that are secretory translation products of various families of organizer genes, each in a highly precise and predictable temporal and spatial distribution.

The early development of the central nervous system (CNS) of all vertebrates, even before the closure of the neural placode or plate to form the neural tube, requires establishment of a fundamental body plan of bilateral symmetry, cephalization (or the identity of head and tail ends), and dorsal and ventral surfaces. These axes of the body and of the CNS require the expression of genes that impose gradients of differentiation and growth. Genes that determine polarity and gradients of the anatomic axes are called organizer genes. Many are expressed not only in the CNS but also in other organs and tissues. The bilateral symmetry of many organs and programmed asymmetries, probably including such neural structures as the different targets of the left and right vagal nerves and left–right asymmetries in the cerebral cortex, is determined in part by genes of symmetry expressed as early as in the primitive node, such as *Zic3*, *Pitx2*, and *Lefty 1* and *2*.

The RNA that represents a transcript of the DNA translates a peptide, a glycoprotein, or some other molecule that acts to induce or occasionally serve as a growth factor. Some genes also stimulate or inhibit the expression of others, or there is an antagonism or equilibrium between certain families of genes,

Table 1   SEGMENTATION OF THE NEURAL TUBE[a]

Neuromere	Derived structures in mature CNS
Rhombomere 8	Entire spinal cord; caudal medulla oblongata; cranial nerves (CNs) XI, XII
Rhombomere 7	Medulla oblongata, CN IX, X; neural crest
Rhombomere 6	Medulla oblongata; CN VIII, IX
Rhombomere 5	Medulla oblongata; CN VI, VII; no neural crest
Rhombomere 4	Medulla oblongata; CN VI, VII; neural crest
Rhombomere 3	Caudal pons, CN V; no neural crest
Rhombomere 2	Caudal pons, CN IV, V; cerebellar nuclei
Rhombomere 1	Rostral pons, cerebellar cortex
Mesencephalic neuromere	Midbrain, CN III, neural crest; rostral cerebellum
Diencephalic prosomere 2	Dorsal diencephalon
Diencephalic prosomere 1	Ventral diencephalon
Prosencephalic prosomere 2	Telencephalic nuclei, olfactory bulb
Prosencephalic prosomere 1	Cerebral cortex; hippocampus; corpus callosum

[a]Rhombomere 3 is associated with the first branchial arch, r4 and r5 are associated with the second branchial arch, and r7 is associated with the third branchial arch.

exemplified by those that exert a dorsoventral gradient and those that cause a ventrodorsal gradient.

Organizer and Regulator Genes

The difference between an organizer gene and a regulator gene is the function of the gene, and the same gene often serves both roles at different stages of development. Organizer genes are expressed earlier and are responsible for the gradients of the neural axes, symmetry, and differentiation of fundamental tissues, such as neuroectoderm and neural crest. Regulator genes are expressed later and determine cellular lineage and the differentiation of specific types of cells. The term structural gene is avoided because it may be ambiguous: To some, it refers to molecular structure, and to others it refers to anatomical structure.

Evolutionary Conservation of Genes

The sequences of DNA nucleotides are so primordial to animal life that identical or nearly identical base pairs exist in all vertebrates and all invertebrates, from the simplest worms to the most complex primates. The evolutionary biologists of the 19th century, such as Charles Darwin and Thomas Huxley, were constantly searching for "missing links" between mammals and other vertebrates, between man and other primates, and especially between invertebrates and vertebrates because comparative anatomy did not provide a satisfying answer. They never found the missing links because the technology of their day could not elucidate this profound question. The missing link sought by the 19th-century evolutionary biologists is the identical sequence of nucleic acid residues that forms the same organizer genes in all animals, from the simplest worms to humans.

Despite evolutionary conservation of genes, there may be some variability between species in the compartmental site within the embryonic neural tube of structures programmed by these genes. For example, the abducens motor nucleus forms in r6 in elasmobranchs (sharks) but in r5 in mammals; the trigeminal–facial boundary shifts from r4 in lampreys to r3 in birds and mammals.

Not all genes are conserved in evolution, however, and some appear for the first time in primates or even only in humans. An example is the *SMN* gene at the human 5p13 locus, mutations of which are responsible for autosomal recessive spinal muscular atrophies (Werdnig–Hoffmann and Kugelberg–Welander diseases).

Transcription Factors and Homeoboxes

The genes that program the development of the nervous system are specific series of DNA base pairs linked to small proteins called transcription factors. These transcription factors are essential for the functional expression of the gene. A common transcription factor is the basic helix–loop–helix structure. It is so fundamental to the evolution of life that it appears for the first time in certain bacteria, even before a cell nucleus, to concentrate the DNA evolved.

The zinc finger is another DNA-binding, gene-specific transcription factor structure. It consists of 28 amino acid repeats with pairs of cysteine and histidine residues and with each sequence folded around a zinc ion. *Krox20* (this gene name is applied to the mouse; it is redesignated *EGR2* in humans) is a zinc finger gene expressed in alternating rhombomeres, especially r3 and r5; neural crest tissue does not differentiate from these two rhombomeres, although it does in adjacent segments, including r4. *Krox20* also serves an additional function in the peripheral nervous system (PNS), in which it regulates myelination by Schwann cells. *Krox20* regulates the expression of some other genes, most notably those of the *Hox* family. Examples of other zinc fingers include *Zic*, *TFIIIA*, *cSnR* (*snail-related*), and *PLZF* (*human promyelocytic leukemia zinc finger*).

Growth factors, which are also molecules encoded by DNA sequences, influence the establishment of the plan of the neural tube by behaving biologically as transcription factors. Basic fibroblast growth factor behaves as an auxiliary inductor of the longitudinal axis with a rostrocaudal gradient during the formation of the neural tube.

Some transcription factors include homeoboxes, which are restricted DNA sequences of 183 base pairs of nucleotides that encode a class of proteins sharing a common or very similar 60-amino acid motif called the homeodomain. Homeodomains contain sequence-specific DNA-binding activities and are integral parts of the larger regulatory proteins, the transcription factors. Homeoboxes or homeotic genes are classified into various families with a common molecular structure and similar general expression in ontogenesis. Homeoboxes are especially associated with genes that program segmentation and rostrocaudal gradients of the neural tube. Some of the important families of homeobox genes in the development of the vertebrate nervous system are *Gsc*, *Hox*, *En*, *Wnt*, *Shh*, *Nkx*, *LIM*, and *Otx*.

FAMILIES OF DEVELOPMENTAL GENES OF THE CENTRAL NERVOUS SYSTEM

The genes that program the axes and gradients of the neural tube may be classified as families by their similar nuclei acid sequences and by their similar general functions, although important differences occur within a family in the site or neuromere in which each gene is expressed and the anatomical structures they form. A dorsalizing gene has a dorsal territory of expression and causes the ventral parts of the neural tube to differentiate as dorsal structures if influences from ventralizing genes do not antagonize them with sufficient strength and vice versa. An example is the development of the somite. The sclerotome (which forms cartilage and bone of the vertebral body) is normally ventral to the myotome (which forms muscle cells) and the dermatome. Ectopic cells of the floor plate or the notochord implanted next to the somite of the chick embryo cause a ventralization of the somite; excess cartilage and bone are formed, and there is a deficiency of muscle and dermis. The floor plate, or notochord in this instance, is the ventralizing inductor of the mesodermal somite, and the genetic factor responsible is the transcription product of the gene *Sonic hedgehog* (*Shh*), which also serves as a strong ventralizing gradient force in the neural tube. If a section of notochord is implanted ectopically dorsal or lateral to the neural tube, a second floor plate forms opposite the notochord and motor neurons differentiate on either side of it, despite the presence of a normal floor plate and motor neurons in the normal position. *Shh*, a strong gene of the ventrodorsal gradient that becomes expressed as early as in the primitive node, induces the ventralization of a dorsal region of the neural tube or duplicates the neural tube. Such an influence in the human fetus, the so-called split notochord, could explain the rare cases of diplomyelia or diastematomyelia. Excessive *Shh*, particularly its N-terminal cleavage product, upregulates floor plate differentiation at the expense of motor neuron formation and may induce duplication of the neuraxis. *Shh* also exerts a strong influence in the differentiation of ventral and medial structures of the prosencephalon, and defective expression due to the mutation of this gene is thought to be the molecular basis of the human malformation holoprosencephaly.

To establish an equilibrium with genes with a ventralizing influence, other families of genes exercise a dorsalizing influence, causing the differentiation of dorsal structures of the neural tube; the *Pax* family is an example. The *Wnt* family is also dorsalizing in the hindbrain; *in situ* hybridization shows its transcription products expressed diffusely only in the early neuroepithelium and restricted to dorsal regions as the neural tube develops. The zinc finger gene *Zic2* has a dorsalizing gradient in the forebrain. The rostrocaudal axis of the neural tube and segmentation, or formation of neuromeres, is directed in large part by a family of 38 genes, classified into four groups, called *Hox* genes. Each of the *Hox* genes is expressed in certain rhombomeres and not in others. In addition to their functions in establishing the compartments or rhombomeres of the brainstem and effecting differentiation of certain anatomical structures, *Hox* genes also serve as guides of growth cones that form the long descending and ascending pathways between the brain and spinal cord.

Many genes exert influences on the expression of others, and some serve redundant functions with others. The gene *En1* has a strong domain in the mesencephalic neuromere and also in r1, the rhombomere that forms the rostral half of the pons and the cerebellar cortex. This same territory corresponds to the neuromeric expressions of *Wnt1* and *Wnt3*, and one of these *Wnt* genes is necessary to augment the expression of *En1*; if there is a loss of *Wnt1* or *Wnt3* by mutation, the other *Wnt* gene is able to compensate and no malformation of the brain is observed in homozygotes. The overlapping and redundant expression of these two *Wnt* genes provides a kind of plasticity at the molecular level for the developing nervous system. If *Wnt1* expression is lost, however, the expression of *Wnt3* is insufficient to compensate in the rostral regions of the future brainstem, and the result is a defective midbrain and pons and cerebellar hypoplasia. The genes *En1* and *En2* have similar functions, with differences in some details, and are demonstrated in the human fetus and the mouse.

Many regulatory genes change their territories of expression in different stages of development, increasing to include more rhombomeres or broader expression early in development and decreasing to more restricted domains later. The expression of a gene in the wrong neuromere, called ectopic expression, sometimes interferes with normal development.

Retinoic Acid

Retinoic acid, the alcohol of which is vitamin A, is a hydrophobic molecule secreted by the notochord and by ependymal floor plate cells. Retinoid-binding proteins and receptors are already strongly expressed in mesenchymal cells of the primitive streak and in the preoptic region of the early developing hindbrain. Ependymal cells other than those of the floor plate and neuroepithelial cells have retinoic acid receptors but do not secrete this compound. Retinoic acid diffuses across the plasma membrane without requiring active transport and binds to intracellular receptors. It enters the cell nucleus, where it binds to a specific nuclear receptor protein, changing the structural configuration of that protein and enabling it to attach to a specific receptor on a target gene, where the complex formed by retinoic acid and its receptor then functions as a transcription factor for neural induction. Other transcription factors of developmental genes already mentioned are the basic helix–loop–helix and zinc fingers.

Retinoic acid functions as a polarity molecule for determining the anterior and posterior surfaces of limb buds and, in the nervous system, is important in segmentation polarity and is a strong rostrocaudal polarity gradient. Excessive retinoic acid acts on the neural tube of amphibian tadpoles to transform anterior neural tissue to a posterior morphogenesis, resulting in extreme microcephaly and suppression of optic cup formation. Failure of optic cup formation may result from retinoic acid suppression by genes of the *LIM* family, such as *Islet3* and *Lim1*. Retinoic acid upregulates homeobox genes, those of the *Hox* family and *Krox20* in particular, and causes ectopic expression of these genes in rhombomeres in which they are not normally expressed. An excess of retinoic acid, whether endogenous or exogenous, such as in mothers who take an excess of vitamin A during early gestation, results in severe malformations of the hindbrain and spinal cord. A single dose of retinoic acid administered intraperitoneally to maternal hamsters on Embryonic Day 9.5 results in the Chiari type II malformation and often causes meningomyelocele in the fetuses. In cell cultures of cloned CNS stem cells from the mouse, retinoic acid enhances neuronal proliferation and astroglial differentiation.

PRINCIPLES OF GENETIC PROGRAMMING

The molecular genetic regulation of neural tube development may be summarized as a series of principles of genetic programming:

1. Developmental genes are reused repeatedly. Nature recognizes useful genes and uses them repeatedly during embryonic development, but de-

velopmental genes play different roles at different stages. An organizer gene of the neural axis or of segmentation may later serve as a regulator gene for the differentiation and maintenance of specific cells of the CNS. Genes of growth factors are also reused at different stages; the fibroblast growth factor gene *EGF8* is active during gastrulation but later contributes to cardiac, craniofacial, midbrain, cerebellar, and forebrain development. The classification of a gene as an organizer or regulator therefore depends on the specific embryonic stage and its function at that stage of development.

2. Domains of organizer genes change in successive stages. The domains, or territories of expression, of organizer genes are usually diffuse initially and become more localized or confined to certain neuromeres as the neural tube develops.

3. Relative gene domains may differ in various neuromeres. The domain of one gene may be dorsal to another in rostral neuromeres and ventral to it in caudal neuromeres at any given stage of development. Examples are *Nkx2.2* and *Nkx6.1*, both of which are coexpressed throughout most of the length of the neural tube. The domain of *Nkx2.2* is dorsal to that of *Nkx6.1* in the diencephalic and mesencephalic neuromeres, but it shifts to a position ventral to that of *Nkx6.1* in the hindbrain and spinal cord.

4. Some genes activate, regulate, or suppress the expression of others. Some organizer genes act sequentially; an already expressed gene initiates the expression of another that follows or that becomes coexpressed. Failure of the first gene may result in a lack of expression of others, producing a more extensive developmental defect than might be anticipated from loss of the first gene alone. An example is the normal cascade of *Pax2* activating *Wnt1* at the mesencephalic–metencephalic boundary at the beginning of neuromere formation; *Wnt1* then activates *En1* and *En2*. Another example is the activation by *Shh* of *Nkx2.1* in the rostral neural plate and *Nkx6.1* in the caudal neural plate. Some genes act by inhibiting or antagonizing the genetic programs of others. *Notch* and *Achaete-scute* change the fate of undifferentiated cells to form neuroepithelium and signal the formation of the neural plate; *Numb* and *Delta* antagonize these genes and inhibit neural differentiation. *Bone morphogenic protein-4* (*BMP4*), expressed in Hensen's node, inhibits ectodermal germ cells from forming neural tissue and promotes epidermal differentiation, but *Noggin* inhibits *BMP4*, allowing neural plate formation to proceed. The formation of dorsal structures,

including the neural plate in the early embryo, depends on the lack of *BMP4* expression. *Wnt1* and *Wnt3* cause neural crest cells to form melanocytes instead of proceeding with neuronal fates. All neuroepithelial cells are preprogrammed to form neurons; glial and ependymal cells can form only when this program is inhibited. An example of gene inhibition by another gene during a more advanced stage of development is the suppression of *Mash1* in hippocampal neurons by the coexpression of *Hes1*. *Mash1* increases neurite outgrowth, but *Hes1* represses the activation of *Mash1* transcription.

5. Defective homeoboxes usually have reduced domains or result in deletions of entire neuromeres. A defective homeobox gene, especially one of segmentation, usually is expressed in fewer neuromeres than normal, representing a reduction in its domain. It may even lose all of its expression. These changes occur in the homozygous and not the heterozygous state of genetic animal models.

6. Some genes may compensate for the loss of others if their domains overlap (redundancy and synergy). Some genes coexpressed in the same neuromeres may compensate, in part or in full, for the loss of expression of one of the pair such that anatomical development, maturation, and function of the nervous system proceed normally. An example is the coexpression of *Wnt1* and *Wnt3* in the myelencephalic rhombomeres. If *Wnt1* is defective in r4–r9 of the mouse but *Wnt3* continues to be normally expressed, the hindbrain develops normally. This principle is known as redundancy. In the continued expression in adult life of some regulator genes to conserve cell identity, oculomotor, trochlear, and abducens neurons, but not hypoglossal or spinal motor neurons, are conserved by *Wnt1* and *LIM* family genes, and these may compensate for loss of expression of other genes in all motor neurons to preserve normal extraocular muscle innervation in spinal muscular atrophy. A variation of the principle of redundancy is synergy, a cooperation of two or more genes to produce effects that none is capable of achieving alone. An example is the synergy between *Pax2* and *Pax5* in midbrain and cerebellar development. If one of this pair is lost, partial but not total compensation may occur.

7. An organizer gene may be upregulated to be expressed in ectopic domains. Certain molecules may act as teratogens in the developing nervous system if the embryo is exposed to an excess, whether the excess is exogenous or endogenous in origin. The inductive mechanism is the upregulation of organizer

genes to become expressed in ectopic domains such as in neuromeres, in which they do not normally play a role in development. An example is retinoic acid, which induces ectopic expression of *Hox* genes. Upregulation of some genes may suppress the expression of others, contributing to dysgenesis. Overexpression of LIM proteins containing only *Islet3*-encoded homeodomains in the zebrafish causes early termination of expression of *Wnt1*, *En2*, and *Pax2* in the midbrain neuromere and r1. This results in severe mesencephalic and metencephalic defects and prevents formation of optic vesicles; these defects can be rescued by the simultaneous overexpression of *Islet3*.

8. Developmental genes regulate cell proliferation to conserve constant ratios of synaptically related neurons. An example is the fixed ratio maintained between Purkinje cells and granule cells in the cerebellar cortex. This ratio is lower in less complex mammals than in humans. The ratio was 1:778 in mice and 1:2991 in humans in one study and 1:449 in rats and 1:3300 in humans in another. In regulating granule cell proliferation, *Shh* and its receptor *patched* (*ptc*) are important genes. The Ptc protein is localized to granule cells and *Shh* to Purkinje cells, providing a molecular substrate for signaling between these synaptically related neurons to establish the needed amount of granule cell production. *Shh* in Purkinje cells acts as a mitogen on external granule cells. To make the system even more complex, *ptc* also interacts through activation of another gene, *smoothened*. A hemizygous deletion of *ptc* in mice results in uncontrolled, excessive proliferation of granule cells and often leads to neoplastic transformation to medulloblastoma. Mutation in the human *ptc* gene is associated with sporadic basal cell carcinomas of the skin and primitive neuroectodermal tumors of the cerebellum; this gene is involved in at least a subset of human medulloblastomas. Theoretically, the focal loss of *ptc* expression may also be a basis for dysplastic gangliocytoma of the cerebellum, also known as Lhermitte–Duclos disease, a focal hamartoma rather than a neoplasm.

9. Overexpression of genes programming the ventrodorsal or dorsoventral gradients manifests as hyperplasia or duplication of paramedian structures of the neuraxis.

10. Underexpression of genes programming the ventrodorsal or dorsoventral gradients manifests as aplasia, hypoplasia, or noncleavage ("fusion") of paramedian structures of the neuraxis.

11. Minor genetic mutations may change cell lineage within or between traditional germ layers. Small mutations in some genes may cause them to behave as other genes that are closely related in molecular structure but that encode programs for other cells or tissues, not even necessarily within the same embryonic germ layer of ectoderm, mesoderm, or endoderm. These arbitrary germ layers, to which all embryonic tissues were previously assigned, may be an artificial separation.

12. Organizer and regulator genes are conserved in phylogenetic evolution but may expand into a larger number of distinct varieties with distinctive functions in more evolved species. Although most fundamental genes are highly conserved in evolution and may be demonstrated in the simplest invertebrates as well as in all vertebrates including humans, a few genes appear for the first time in mammals and a few make an initial appearance in humans without any animal counterpart. An example is the *SMN* gene, mutations of which are responsible for spinal muscular atrophy.

NEURULATION

Bending of the neural placode to form the neural tube requires extrinsic and intrinsic mechanical forces in addition to the dorsalizing and ventralizing genetic effects discussed earlier (Table 2). These forces arise in part from the growth of the surrounding mesodermal tissues on either side of

Table 2 FACTORS INVOLVED IN CLOSURE OF NEUROEPITHELIUM TO FORM THE NEURAL TUBE

Extrinsic mechanical forces
Surrounding mesodermal tissues
Surface epithelium
Intrinsic mechanical forces
Wedge shape of floor plate cells
Differential growth in dorsal and ventral zones
Adhesion molecules
Orientation of mitotic spindles of neuroepithelium
Large fetal central canal
Molecular genetic programming
Induction of floor plate by Sonic hedgehog
Ventralizing gene transcription products
Dorsalizing gene transcription products
Genetic transcription products that regulate axonal guidance (attraction and repulsion) across midline and in longitudinal axis
Separation of neural crest

the neural tube—the future somites. After surgical removal of mesoderm and endoderm from one side of the neuroepithelium in experimental animals, the neural tube still closes, but it is rotated and becomes asymmetrical. The mesoderm appears to be important for orientation but not for closure of the neural tube. Expansion of the surface epithelium of the embryo is the principal extrinsic force for the folding of the neuroepithelium to form the neural tube. Cells of the neural placode are mobile and migrate beneath the surface ectoderm, raising the lateral margins of the placode toward the dorsal midline. The growth of the whole embryo does not appear to be an important factor because neurulation proceeds equally well in anamniotes (e.g., amphibians) that do not grow during this period and in amniotes (e.g., mammals) that grow rapidly at this time.

Among the intrinsic forces of the neuroepithelium, the cells of the floor plate have a wedge shape, narrow at the apex and broad at the base, that facilitates bending. Although the width of the floor plate is small, its site in the ventral midline is crucial and sufficient to allow a significant influence. It represents another aspect of floor plate induction by the notochord, apart from its influence on the differentiation of neural cells. Ependymal cells that form the floor plate are the first neural cells to differentiate, and they induce growth of the parenchyma of the ventral zone more than in the dorsal regions; this mechanical effect may also facilitate curving of the neural placode. The direction of proliferation of new cells in the mitotic cycle, determined in part by the orientation of the mitotic spindle, is another mechanical force shaping the neural tube. Adhesion molecules are probably also important mechanical factors for neurulation. In later stages, the ependymal cell-lined central canal, which is much larger in the fetus than in the newborn, may have a role in exerting a centrifugal force for the tubular shape, although in early spinal cord development the central canal is a tall, narrow, midline slit, and only later in fetal life does it assume a rounded contour as seen in transverse sections.

Neuroepithelial cells of the neural placode or plate downregulate the polarity of their plasma membrane so that apical and basilar surfaces are not as distinct before neural tube closure; cell differentiation generally involves such changes in cell polarity. The rostrocaudal orientation of most mitotic spindles of the neuroepithelium and the direction in which they push by the mass of daughter cells they form also influence the shape of the neural tube.

The neural tube closes in the dorsal midline first in the cervical region, and closure then extends rostrally and caudally. The anterior neuropore of the human embryo closes at 24 days and the posterior neuropore closes at 28 days because the distances from the cervical region are not equal. The traditional view of a continuous zipper-like closure is an oversimplification. In the mouse embryo, the neural tube closes in the cranial region at four distinct sites, with the closure proceeding bidirectionally or unidirectionally and in general synchrony with somite formation. An intermittent pattern of anterior neural tube closure involving multiple sites has also been described in human embryos. In this closure, the principal rostral neuropore closes bidirectionally to form the lamina terminalis, an essential primordium of the forebrain.

Bending of the neural plate to form the neural tube is primary neurulation. The term secondary neurulation refers only to the most caudal part of the spinal cord (i.e., conus medullaris) that develops from the neuroepithelium caudal to the site of posterior neuropore closure. This part of the spinal cord forms as a solid cord of neural cells in which ependymal cells differentiate in its core and "canalize" the cord, often giving rise to minor aberrations. It was previously believed that this is the manner in which the entire spinal cord of fishes is formed, but dorsal folding of the neural plate occurs as in other vertebrates.

A rare anomaly of a human tail may occur. A true vestigial tail is the most distal remnant of the embryonic tail and contains adipose and connective tissue, central bundles of striated muscle, blood vessels, and nerves. It is covered by skin, but bone, cartilage, and spinal cord are lacking. Pseudotails are usually an anomalous elongation of the coccygeal vertebrae, but they may contain lipomas, gliomas, teratomas, or even a thin, elongated parasitic fetus. Pseudotails often cause tethering of the spinal cord or may be associated with spinal dysraphism. Pseudotail malformations may be the site of neoplasia, such as subependymoma. Upregulation of a ventralizing gene such as *SHH* at the caudalmost level of the neural tube may be the pathogenesis.

EXPRESSION OF REGULATOR GENES AFTER THE FETAL PERIOD: CONSERVATION OF CELL IDENTITY

Many developmental genes continue to be expressed after the period of ontogenesis and into adult life. In particular, those that direct the differentiation of particular types of cells may preserve the unique identity of these distinct cells in the mature state. In the cerebellar cortex, *Wnt3* preserves the identity of Purkinje cells; *Pax3* is responsible for the preservation of the Bergmann glia; and granule cells are supported by several genes, the most important being *Pax6*, *Zic1*, and *Math*. If one of these genes fails to be expressed, there may be compensation because of the principle of redundancy. However, if this phenomenon is incomplete or fails to occur, the motor neurons may never differentiate or may later die by apoptosis and disappear. Theoretically, such a mechanism could explain human cases of granuloprival cerebellar hypoplasia, in which there are sparse or no granule cells despite a normal complement of Purkinje cells and other cellular elements of the cerebellar cortex. However, the preservation of *Wnt3* expression in Purkinje cells also depends in part on its relations with granule cells; thus, synaptic contacts probably also impart genetic information between mature neurons.

Genetic expression to preserve cell identity also occurs in motor neurons. The earliest stimulus of motor neuron differentiation is *Shh*, induced by the notochord and floor plate. However, *Shh* also has a symbiotic relationship with *Nkx2.2*, which helps select neuronal identity by interpreting graded *Shh* signals and allowing them to become expressed at appropriate concentration gradients. Despite their similar morphological appearance and function in ocular and spinal motor neurons, differences exist in the genes that program their development and maintenance. *Wnt1* knockout mice fail to develop oculomotor and trochlear nuclei and their extraocular muscles are altered or deficient, but spinal and hypoglossal motor neurons are not altered. Even among the three pairs of motor nuclei subserving the various extraocular muscles, abducens motor neurons may be selectively involved or spared in relation to motor neurons of the trochlear and oculomotor nuclei. Members of the large *LIM* gene family, particularly *Lim1*, *Lim2*, *Islet1*, and *Islet2*, are also expressed in motor neurons, and each gene in this family defines a subclass of motor neurons for the topographical projection of axonal projections. Insulin-like growth factor has also been identified as a regulator of apoptosis of developing motor neurons and may express a differential effect. These differences in genetic programming of motor neurons in various neuromeres perhaps explain oculomotor sparing with progressive degeneration of spinal and hypoglossal motor neurons in spinal muscular atrophy (i.e., Werdnig–Hoffmann disease).

ANATOMICAL AND PHYSIOLOGICAL PROCESSES OF CENTRAL NERVOUS SYSTEM DEVELOPMENT

Traditional embryology recognizes a series of developmental processes that are not entirely sequential because of much temporal overlap as the various processes proceed simultaneously.

Redundancy

One of the most important principles of neuroembryology is that of redundancy. The redundancy of some genes with overlapping domains and their ability to compensate for a lack of expression of the other has been mentioned. Another form of redundancy occurs in the production of neuroblasts. Neuroblasts are overproduced by 30–50% in all regions of the nervous system, depending on the number of symmetric mitotic cycles, followed by apoptosis of the surplus cells that are not needed for matching to targets. Immature axonal projections are redundant because many collaterals form diffuse projections, followed during maturation by retraction of many, resulting in fewer but more specific connections. Synapses are also overly produced, followed by synaptic pruning to provide greater precision. Acetylcholine receptors are initially diffusely distributed along the myotube, but with maturation as a myofiber they decrease and become confined to the innervation site.

Embryological Zones of the Neural Tube

After neurulation, the closed neural tube has an architecture of two concentric rings as viewed in transverse section. The inner ring is the ventricular zone, consisting of the proliferative, pseudostratified columnar neuroepithelium; the outer ring is the marginal zone, a cell-sparse region of fibers and extracellular matrix proteins. Details of the mitotic patterns in the ventricular zone are discussed later.

With further development, four concentric zones appear. A subventricular zone outside the proliferative ventricular zone is composed of postmitotic, premigratory neuroblasts and glioblasts and radial glial cells. After radial migration of neuroblasts begins, an intermediate zone is formed by the radial glial processes and the migratory neuroblasts adherent to them; this intermediate zone eventually becomes the deep subcortical white matter of the cerebral hemispheres. In the cerebrum, migratory neuroblasts destined to form the cerebral cortex begin to form an unlaminated cortical plate within the marginal zone, dividing the zone. The outermost, cell-sparse region is thereafter known as the molecular layer (eventually layer 1 of the mature cerebral cortex), and the innermost portion of the marginal zone isolated by the intervening cortical plate is known as the subplate zone. This region contains many neurons that form transitory pioneer axons to establish the corticospinal and other long projection pathways, but eventually the subplate zone becomes incorporated into layer 6 of the maturing cortex and disappears as a distinct anatomical region.

The two, and later four, concentric zones clearly identified in the cerebrum are similar, although in modified form in the brainstem and spinal cord, but they become even further altered in the cerebellum by means of an apparent inversion, with the granule cells migrating from the surface inward rather than from the periventricular region outward. An ependymal epithelium eventually forms at the ventricular surface of the ventricular zone, creating an additional, innermost zone not present in the embryo except for the floor plate in the ventral midline.

Separation and Migration of the Neural Crest

Neural crest cells arise from the dorsal midline of the neural tube at the time of closure or soon thereafter and migrate extensively along prescribed routes through the embryo to differentiate as the PNS, including dorsal root and sympathetic ganglia, chromaffin cells such as those of the adrenal medulla and carotid body, melanocytes or pigment cells, and a few other cell types of ectodermal and mesodermal origin. The facial skeleton, including the orbits, connective tissue of the eye, ciliary ganglion, part of the trigeminal ganglia, and Schwann cells of nerves, is also formed by neural crest. The vertebrate gene *Slug*, a homolog of the *Snail* gene of insects, is expressed in early neural crest before its migrations begin and probably is important in its differentiation.

The most rostral origin of neural crest cells from the neural tube is from the midbrain neuromere. These cells migrate as a uniform sheet, whereas those migrating from hindbrain and spinal cord rhombomeres do so segmentally. Rhombomeres 3 and 5 do not appear to generate neural crest cells; alternative hypotheses are that these cells undergo accelerated apoptosis or deviate rostrally and caudally to migrate with cells of adjacent rhombomeres. Migratory pathways of neural crest cells outside the neural tube are created in large part by attractant and repulsive molecules secreted by surrounding tissues, such as the otic capsule, the somites, and the vertebral neural arches. Neural crest cells possess integrin receptors for interacting with extracellular matrix molecules. Changes in the distribution of extracellular matrix components impose migratory guidance limits as well.

The origin of neural crest cells is incompletely understood because they represent diverse mature populations that include elements of mesodermal and ectodermal primitive germ layers. Why neural crest precursors are so heterogeneous, why neural crest stem cells with multiple potentials exist, and even whether stem cells arising from the neural tube are joined by surrounding cells from the mesoderm are not as well understood as the pathways they follow within the body of the embryo. As with other parts of the neural tube, neural crest tissue follows a rostrocaudal gradient of differentiation. The fate of neural crest cells is influenced by whether they migrate early or late and by neurotrophic factors; for example, neurotrophin-3 (NT-3) is essential for survival of sympathetic neuroblasts and the innervation of specific organs.

Neuroepithelial Cell Proliferation

Early cleavages in the fertilized ovum to form the blastula and the blastomere (gastrula) involve a simple proliferation of cells cycling between the mitotic (M phase) and resting (S phase) states, a process similar to DNA replication in bacteria. As the neuroectoderm forms in the epiblast at post-ovulatory Week 3 in the human embryo, it becomes organized as a pseudostratified columnar epithelium, a sheet of bipolar cells all oriented so that one cytoplasmic process extends to the dorsal (future ventricular) surface and the other process extends to the ventral (future pial) surface. The nucleus of each of these spindle-shaped cells moves to and fro within its own cytoplasmic extensions. M phase occurs at or near the ventricular surface, and S phase occurs at the other end. Transitional periods between these two states are known as gap phases: G_1 when the nucleus moves distally toward the surface and G_2 when the nucleus approaches the ventricular surface. The introduction of gap phases in the mitotic cycle

allows for adjustments to be made in the replication of DNA during G_1, and the sequence ensures that G_2 cells do not undergo an extra round of S phase, which could lead to a change in ploidy as the chromosomes segregate in the dividing cell. In this way, errors may be corrected before the next mitosis, allowing more plasticity than the all-or-none principle of simple cell division.

Mitoses continue to occur at the ventricular surface as the neural plate folds and becomes a neural tube. The differentiation of an ependyma at the ventricular surface signals the termination of mitotic activity and the ventricular zone because the remaining cells in the periventricular region are all postmitotic premigratory neuroblasts and glioblasts—hence, they belong to the subventricular zone.

Because mitoses increase cell populations exponentially, a finite number of mitotic cycles are needed to produce the requisite number of neurons needed in a given part of the nervous system. In the cerebrum of the rat, 10 mitotic cycles in the ventricular zone generate all the neurons of the cerebral cortex; in the human, 33 mitotic cycles generate a much larger number of neurons than simply three times the number in the rat cortex. Eight symmetrical mitotic cycles are required to produce the minimum essential number of motor neuroblasts in the spinal cord of the chick (Table 3). Many organizer genes are also mitogens.

The orientation of the mitotic spindle at the ventricular surface is important to the fate of the daughter cells after each mitosis because certain gene products are distributed asymmetrically within the mother cell and because with some orientations both daughter cells cannot retain an attachment to the

Table 3   GENERATION OF MOTOR NEURONS IN THE LUMBAR SPINAL CORD OF THE CHICK EMBRYO[a]

	No. of cells
Progenitor stem cells	60
Motor neuroblasts generated	24,000
Mature motor neurons required	12,000
Motor neurons generated in seven symmetrical mitotic cycles	7,680
Motor neurons generated in eight symmetrical mitotic cycles	15,360

[a] Adapted from Bursk, M. J., and Oppenheim, R. W. (1996). Programmed cell death in the developing nervous system. *Brain Pathol.* **6**, 427–446.

ventricular wall. *Notch* and *Numb* are genes with antagonistic functions situated at opposite poles of the neuroepithelial cell. If the cleavage plane of the mitotic spindle is perpendicular to the ventricular surface, each of the daughter cells retains an attachment to that surface and inherits equal amounts of *Notch* and *Numb*. This situation is called symmetrical cleavage, and both daughter cells reenter the mitotic cycle in the same manner as their common precursor cell. If, however, the mitotic spindle is parallel to the ventricular surface, the two daughter cells are unequal because only one can retain an attachment to the ventricle, and one inherits most of the *Notch* while the other inherits most of the *Numb* gene product. This situation is called asymmetrical cleavage. Only the cell at the ventricular surface reenters the mitotic cycle, and the other, more distal cell completes its final mitosis and rapidly moves away from its sister to begin differentiation as a neuroblast and to prepare for radial migration from the subventricular zone.

Neuronal Polarity

Neuronal polarity establishes from which side of the cell the axon will sprout and from which cell surfaces the dendrites will form, and it is determined in part at the time of the final mitosis. Microtubule arrays are the most fundamental components of the mitotic spindle, forming during prophase as the centrosome replicates. The "minus" ends of the microtubules remain associated with the centrosome, whereas the "plus" ends emanate outward, with the duplicated centrosomes driven to opposite poles of the cell as a direct result of microtubule organization. The mitotic spindle consists of regions in which microtubules are uniformly oriented in tandem and in parallel and other regions in which the microtubules are more haphazardly oriented; the former become the axonal end of the cell, and the latter become the opposite pole, or the dendritic end. Mitochondrial DNA also plays a role in polarizing the nerve cell, possibly by modulating calcium homeostasis.

Although sparse, mitotic activity of neuronal precursors continues to be seen in the postnatal human infant in the outer half of the external granule cell layer of the cerebellum. External granule cells do not complete migration until after 1 year; hence, the potential for regeneration after prenatal and even postnatal loss of some of these cells exists. Another well-documented region of continued neuronal turn-

over in the human nervous system is the primary olfactory neurons.

A few neuroblasts appear to undergo division even during migration, providing exceptions to the general rule. A population of quiescent neuroepithelial stem cells in the subventricular zone of the mammalian forebrain retains a proliferative potential even in the adult. Much research is directed at mobilizing this population of progenitor cells to increase in number so as to provide a source of neuronal replacement in neurodegenerative diseases and acquired brain and spinal cord damage.

Apoptosis

In every region of the nervous system, 30–70% more neuroblasts are generated than are required at maturity. Surplus cells survive for a period of days or weeks and then spontaneously undergo a cascade of degenerative changes and disappear without inflammatory responses to cell death or the proliferation of glial "scars." This physiological process of programmed cell death, or apoptosis, was discovered in 1949 by Hamburger and Levi-Montalcini, who demonstrated its occurrence in the spinal dorsal root ganglion of the chick embryo. The phenomenon has subsequently been confirmed by numerous other independent investigators. It is a general principle of development in all animals, from the simplest worms to humans, and involves all organ systems, not just the nervous system. Examples of apoptosis that continues throughout life are found in any tissue that has a constant turnover of cells, such as the 120-day half-life of erythrocytes and the continuous replacement of intestinal mucosal epithelial cells (of mesodermal origin) and of epidermal cells of the skin (of ectodermal origin). Without programmed cell death, final cell numbers of neurons and glia could not be controlled and precision of synaptic circuitry would be impossible to achieve.

Apoptosis differs from cell death by necrosis (e.g., from ischemia, hypoxia, toxins, and infections) in several important morphological details, in addition to the absence of tissue reaction to the loss, except for the removal of the cellular debris by phagocytic microglial cells (i.e., modified macrophages). In neural cell apoptosis, the sequence begins with shrinkage of the nucleus, condensation of chromatin, and increased electron opacity of the cell and is followed by the disappearance of the Golgi apparatus, loss of endoplasmic reticulum, and disaggregation of polyribosomes. The final events are formation of ribosomal crystals and breakdown of the nuclear membrane. Mitochondria are preserved until the late stages of apoptosis, whereas they swell and disintegrate early in cellular necrosis.

Apoptosis is genetically patterned, as are other events in nervous system development. The process is programmed into every cell, but its expression is blocked by the inhibitory influence of certain genes, such as *bcl-2* and the immediate early protooncogene *c-fos*. Mitochondrial DNA is a regulatory factor in the expression of *bcl-2*, here of apoptosis. This genetic regulation is also modulated by trophic factors of other cells in the vicinity that preserve metabolic integrity. For example, nerve growth factor and basic fibroblast growth factor block cell death and preserve the identity of various cell lineages in the nervous system. The apoptotic process may be accelerated or retarded by metabolic factors such as plasma concentrations of thyroid hormone, serum ammonia, local neurotoxins (including excitatory amino acids such as aspartate), lactic acidosis, and imbalances of calcium and electrolytes.

Synaptic relations constitute another environmental factor within the brain that affects apoptosis. An inverse relationship exists between the rate of apoptosis of spinal motor neurons and synaptogenesis. On the afferent side, neurons degenerate if they fail to be innervated or lose their entire afferent supply because of the loss of presynaptic neurons. This phenomenon is called trans-synaptic degeneration and is exemplified in the lateral genicular body after optic nerve lesions and in the inferior olivary nucleus after destruction of the central tegmental tract. On the efferent side, motor neurons degenerate if they fail to match with target muscle fibers or their muscle targets are removed, such as after amputation of a limb bud of an embryo or amputation of an extremity in the adult.

Proteins programmed from exons 7 and 8 of the *survival motor neuron* (*SMN*) gene at the 5q11–q13 locus are defective in spinal muscular atrophy (Werdnig–Hoffmann and Kugelberg–Welander diseases). *SMN* is an example of a gene that normally arrests apoptosis in spinal motor neurons after all muscular targets are matched. This degenerative disease occurs because a physiological process in the early fetus becomes pathological in late fetal life and the postnatal period due to its failure to stop, with continued progressive death of motor neurons. The protein of a second gene, also at the 5q11–q13 locus, is called neuronal apoptosis inhibitory protein.

Apoptosis occurs in two phases. The first is the programmed death of incompletely differentiated cells and represents the numerically most important phase of this process. Even completely undifferentiated neuroepithelial cells undergo apoptosis, but the factors that select these short life cycles are poorly understood. The second phase is the cell death of mature, well-differentiated neurons. This process continues in the early postnatal period in the rat cervical spinal cord.

Neuroblast Migration

Almost no neurons occupy sites in the mature human brain where these cells underwent terminal mitosis and began differentiation. In some simple vertebrates, such as the salamander, mature neurons are often situated in the periventricular zone where they originated, but in humans such periventricular maturation is regarded as heterotopical and pathological. Neuroblasts migrate to sites often distant from their birthplace to establish the needed synaptic relations with similar and different types of neurons and to send axonal projections grouped with similar fibers to form tracts or fascicles to distant sites along the neuraxis. The synaptic architecture of the cerebral or cerebellar cortices would not be possible without such neuroblast migration.

Several mechanisms subserve neuroblast migration. The most important from the standpoint of transporting most neuroblasts, whether into cortical or nuclear structures, is the use of radial glial fiber guides. In the cerebrum, each glial cell of the subventricular zone develops a long, slender process that spans the entire cerebral mantle to terminate as an end foot on the pial membrane at the surface of the brain. These specialized radial glial cells are transitory, and after all migration is complete they retract the radial process and mature to become fibrillary astrocytes of the subcortical white matter. Glial growth factor, or neuroregulin, is an inducer of the radial glial cell and acts by initiating the expression of the brain lipid-binding protein (BLBP), a fundamental protein of the radial glial cell and an important marker of the migratory phase. Neuroepithelial cells destined to become neurons induce the extension of the radial glial process, as shown in cultures of purified radial glial cells.

The radial glial process of these cells serves the unique function during fetal life of guiding migratory cells, neuroblasts, and glioblasts from the subventricular zone, or germinal matrix, to their destination in the cerebral cortex or in other forebrain structures. They perform this function as a "monorail," with migratory cells gliding along their surface. Fetal ependymal cells also have basal processes that extend into the germinal matrix, but they do not reach as far as the cortex or even into the deep white matter, they differ morphologically, and they serve entirely different functions that do not include the guidance of migratory cells. In the cerebellum, the specialized Bergmann glial cells, which occupy the Purkinje cell layer and have radiating processes that extend to the surface of the cerebellar cortex, provide a similar function for the migration inward of granule cells from the fetal external granular layer to the mature internal site within the folia. Bergmann cells and their processes persist into adult life, unlike the change that occurs before birth in the radial glial cells of the cerebrum. BLBP is expressed in Bergmann cells along with the radial glial cells of the cerebrum.

The transport of migratory neuroepithelial cells along the radial glial fiber requires a number of adhesion molecules to prevent the cell from detaching too early, to lubricate its path of travel, and perhaps to provide nutrition to the cell as it moves and continuously changes position in relation to capillaries within the white matter parenchyma. These molecules are secreted by the migratory neuroblast or the radial glial cell, or others are already present in the extracellular matrix. Astrotactin is a protein molecule produced by the neuroblast during migration that helps adhere the cell to the radial glial fiber and is essential in establishing the laminar architecture of the neocortex, the hippocampus, the olfactory bulb, and the cerebellar cortex. The gene that encodes astrotactin is also related to the synthesis of epidermal growth factor and fibronectin. Examples of molecules synthesized by the radial glial cell for purposes of neuroblast adhesion are S-100β protein and L1 neural cell adhesion molecule (NCAM); the defective expression of the gene that regulates the L1-CAM protein results in polymicrogyria, pachygyria, and X-linked recessive fetal hydrocephalus. Other molecules synthesized by the radial glial cell have also been identified.

Some molecules contributing to cell adhesion, such as fibronectin, laminins, and collagen type IV (necessary for the formation of basement membranes), are found in the extracellular matrix. In addition to providing a substrate for normal neuroblast and glioblast migration, the motility and infiltration of brain parenchyma by neoplastic cells

of neural origin depend largely on extracellular matrix proteins.

Reelin (Reln) is a gene and glycoprotein transcription product secreted by Cajal–Retzius neurons in the cerebrum and by external granule cells in the cerebellum that is essential to terminal migration and the laminal architecture of cortices. The reeler mouse is a model that lacks expression of the *Reln* gene and exhibits severe disruption of laminated structures of the brain. Another gene and its protein Disabled-1 (*Dab1*) act downstream of *Reln* in a signaling pathway of laminar organization and function in phosphorylation-dependent intracellular signal transduction.

Not all cells migrating within the developing brain use radial glial fibers. Some migrations proceed along the axons of previously established cells in the brainstem, olfactory bulb, and cerebellum using the axons in the same manner as radial glial fibers. Tangential migrations perpendicular to the radial glial fibers also occur in the cerebral cortex and contribute to a mixture of clones in any given region so that all neurons are not from the same neuroepithelial stem cells originating in the same zone of the germinal matrix. The site of origin of these cells migrating tangentially is not well documented, but they probably originate outside the proliferative ventricular zone. They may even represent the persistent stem cells that have only recently been recognized in the adult brain and are of great interest because of their potential value in regeneration of the damaged nervous system if they can be stimulated and mobilized. How these tangential migrations occur, skipping from one radial glial fiber to another or traveling between radial glia, has not been resolved.

At the surface of the cerebrum, the migratory neuroblasts reverse direction so that the earlier migrations are displaced into deeper layers of the cortical plate by the recent arrivals. Layer 6 therefore represents the earliest wave of radial neuroblast migration from the subventricular zone, and layer 2 consists of the last neurons to migrate.

Cajal–Retzius neurons of the molecular zone are the first neurons to mature in the early telencephalon. They are present in the marginal zone before the first wave of radial migrations from the subventricular zone occurs and are important to the architectural integrity of the developing cortex. They appear to influence cell placement within the cortical plate, even before distinct lamination occurs. They form a preplate plexus and innervate pyramidal cells in the cortical plate of the future layer 6, later synapsing with pyramidal cells in all layers. They thus create the first intrinsic synaptic circuits of the cerebral cortex. Cajal–Retzius neurons synthesize γ-aminobutyric acid (GABA), acetylcholine, several neuropeptides (e.g., neuropeptide Y, somatostatin, and cholecystokinin), and calcium-mediating proteins that include calretinin, calmodulin, and parvalbumin. They express two genes important in neuroblast migration, *Reln* and *LIS*. Cajal–Retzius neurons probably originate in either the mesencephalic neuromere or the ganglionic eminence. They were previously thought to be transitory neurons of the fetal brain, but it has been demonstrated that they persist in the molecular layer after maturity, although they are very sparse. In addition to the principal functions of Cajal–Retzius neurons in mediating neuroblast migration and cortical organization and in forming the first cortical synaptic circuits, they may have roles in maintaining the integrity of radial glial cells, cortical repair during development, and modulating neurogenesis in the neuroepithelium by their influence on GABA$_A$ receptors.

The pial membrane and the subpial granular layer of Brun (which in the human fetal cerebrum is a transitory layer of glial cells, unlike the cerebellar cortex, in which the external granule cell layer is neuroblasts) are important in reversing the direction of migration as cells arrive at the surface. Deficiency of these components in malformations such as holoprosencephaly results in extensive overmigration, with neuronal ectopia in the leptomeninges.

Several genes are defective in disorders of neuroblast migration in humans. The *LIS1* gene at the 17p13.3 locus is responsible for lissencephaly type 1 in Miller–Dieker syndrome and in isolated lissencephaly. The gene that encodes the gene product or signaling protein called *doublecortin* is defective or unexpressed in X-linked dominant subcortical laminar heterotopia, also known as band heterotopia or double cortex. Bilateral periventricular heterotopia, another X-linked dominant trait, is associated with deficiency of expression of *FILAMIN-1*. The neural cell adhesion molecule L1-CAM is implicated in hemimegalencephaly, X-linked recessive hydrocephalus with pachygyria, and aqueductal stenosis; *Reln* is probably defective in these cases as well.

Genetically programmed disturbances in neuroblast migration may be categorized anatomically into three phases. Early migratory disturbances, such as periventricular nodular heterotopia, illustrate total failure of subventricular neuroblasts to migrate; these cells simply mature in their embryonic site but cannot establish the intended synaptic relations. The middle phase of migration is represented by disorders in which neuroblasts begin to migrate but their journey is arrested before they reach the cortical plate (e.g., subcortical laminar heterotopia). The late phase of migration produces abnormal positioning of neurons in the cortical plate and abnormal lamination of the cortex, often associated with abnormal gyration at the macroscopic level, such as the lissencephalies and pachygyria.

Axonal Pathfinding

The outgrowth of a single axon precedes the formation of the multiple dendrites and is one of the first morphological events marking the maturation of a neuroblast in becoming a neuron. It sometimes occurs during the course of migration before the cell has arrived at its final destination, and in some cases (e.g., the external granule cells of the cerebellum) it occurs before migration starts. The tip of the growing axon, called the growth cone by Ramón y Cajal, is neither pointed nor blunt; it is a constantly changing complex of cytoplasmic fingers or extensions, the filopodia, enclosed by a membrane that extends between filopodia to form veils or webs. The cytoplasm of the filopodia is filled with microtubules, filaments, and mitochondria. Filopodia extend and retract with amoeboid movements.

To develop polarity, by which an axon emerges at one site and not at others, neuroblasts share membrane protein-sorting mechanisms with epithelial cells, the other important polarized cells. The axonal cell surface is analogous to the apical plasma membrane of epithelial cells, such as ependymal cells or intestinal mucosal cells, and the somatodendritic plasma membrane is analogous to the basolateral epithelial surface. A complex interaction of sorting signals from glycolipid proteins within the plasma membrane and soluble attachment protein receptors that promote the docking of vesicles with target membranes results in intracellular membrane fusions that differ in various parts of the neuroblast plasma membrane and are required for membrane assembly during axonal growth. Neuronal polarity is determined by mitochondrial and somatic nuclear DNA.

Three fundamental mechanisms guide axons to their destination, which may be a great distance from the cell body. A fourth mechanism, proposed a century ago, has again been resurrected as plausible.

• *Cell–cell interactions*: Molecular signals generated by the target cell induce the growth cone to form a synapse. This mechanism is effective only as the axon approaches within 1 or 2 mm of the target.

• *Cell–substrate interactions*: Molecules known as integrins bind the cell to an extracellular protein matrix, such as fibronectin or laminin. Such substrates serve as adhesive surfaces for growth cones, allowing them to pull themselves forward, and may provide directional cues as attractants or repellents.

• *Chemotactic interactions*: Secretory molecules may release powerful attractants or repellents to keep the axon aligned along an intended course in its intermediate trajectory. Growth cones are exquisitely sensitive to certain chemicals and grow toward or away from these molecules.

• *Electrical or electromagnetic fields*: It was once thought that electrical or electromagnetic fields were important influences in orienting the growing axon; this discarded theory is being reconsidered in a more modern context, although it is still poorly substantiated. Local electrical fields may change the course of growing axons by altering the receptive properties of their membranes to neurotransmitters and attractant and repellent molecules.

The family of glycosaminoglycans and proteoglycan molecules are important examples of growth cone repellents in the developing CNS. An example is keratan sulfate (unrelated biochemically to the epidermal protein keratin). This compound is secreted in many tissues of the fetal body at sites where nerves are not needed or desired: the epiphysial plates of growing bones, the epidermis (to prevent nerves from growing through the skin), the notochordal sheath, and the developing neural arches of the vertebrae (to segment and guide nerve roots from the spinal cord between rather than through the somites). The highly segmented somites are important early guides of neural crest cellular migration and of axonal projections peripherally. Within the CNS, fetal ependymal cells synthesize keratan sulfate, in part to prevent axons from growing into the ventricles of the brain and in part to prevent aberrant decussation of developing long tracts and wandering of axons toward wrong targets. The dorsal median raphe that separates the dorsal columns of the two sides of the spinal cord in the dorsal midline, probably programmed by dorsalizing genes such as those of the *Pax* family, is composed of ependymal roof plate processes that secrete keratan sulfate when the axons of the

dorsal columns are growing rostrally. The raphe serves to repel growth cones that might otherwise decussate prematurely, before reaching the gracile and cuneate nuclei of the medulla oblongata. The effects of such repellent molecules are selective, however; keratan sulfate secreted by the floor plate and the dorsal median septum of the midbrain collicular plate does not prevent the passage of commissural fibers at those sites, although it repulses axons of descending and ascending long tracts. Perhaps the passage of commissural fibers is mediated by attractants of such fibers as netrin that overcome a negative influence of keratan sulfate. The floor plate also repulses axons of developing motor neurons, such that they extend into the spinal roots only on the side of their soma.

Another family of proteins, the semaphorins (formerly called collapsins), act mainly as growth cone repellents in neural tissue, including the floor plate, and throughout the body in nonneural tissues. The midline septa, composed of floor plate and roof plate basal processes, act as chemical barriers to some axons but are not physical barriers despite their appearance in histological stained sections because commissural axons easily pass through them. Other examples of growth cone attractants are nerve growth factor and S-100β protein. Another secretory protein that repels axonal growth cones at the midline is the product of the gene *Slit*.

The decision regarding attraction or repulsion of an axonal growth cone results not only from secreted molecules but also from the axonal response. Axons of the longitudinal pathways are attracted to the floor plate for decussation, but after a single crossing the axonal growth cone no longer recognizes the attractant molecule and, in fact, becomes repelled by it so that aberrant second decussations to the original side do not occur. The axonal response to an external signal depends on the internal state of the axon.

The cytoskeleton plays a central role in axonal guidance. The internal organization of actin filaments and microtubules changes rapidly within the growth cone before large-scale changes in growth cone shape occur. These changes are evoked by local environmental molecules that stabilize local changes of cytoskeletal polymers in the growth cone. Although microtubule assembly in the growing axon is required for the axon to extend along its pathway, drugs that disrupt microtubule assembly do not impede assembly and growth at the axonal tip. Growth cone collapse is a part of the normal process of axonal growth and may become pathological if excessive; it is induced by a platelet-activation factor.

Homeobox-containing genes are involved in the regulation of axonal growth. A gene expressed early in neuronal differentiation, *TOAD64* ("turned on after division," with an identical nucleotide sequence to *unc33* in nematodes), is strongly expressed by its protein transcription product in growth cones and is downregulated after axonal projection is complete. Mutations in this gene result in aberrations in axonal outgrowth in the mouse. The overexpression of *Hox2* reverses axonal pathways from r3. Boundary regions between adjacent domains of regulatory gene expression influence where the first axons extend. Initial tract formation is associated with the selective expression of certain cell adhesion molecules and their regulatory gene transcripts.

Some long tracts are preceded by pioneer axons formed by transitory neurons, which appear to serve as guides for the growth cones of permanent axons and without which the permanent axons detour to heterotopical sites. An example is the pioneer axons from subplate neurons as the cortical plate is beginning to form. These pioneer axons establish the internal capsule and precede the passage of axons from pyramidal cells of future layers 5 and 6 of the cortex and also provide pioneer callosal axons of the hippocampus. Subplate neurons originate with the Cajal–Retzius neurons before the formation of the cortical plate. After the pyramidal cell axons are guided into the internal capsule, the pioneer axons and their cells of origin either disappear by apoptosis or become incorporated into the deep layers of the maturing cortex so that the subplate zone is no longer recognized histologically.

Dendritic Proliferation and Synaptogenesis

Dendrites sprout only after the axon begins its projection from the same neuron. The branching pattern of dendrites and the formation of spines on these dendritic arborizations, on which synapses form, are varied and characteristic for each type of neuron. In the cerebral cortex, synaptogenesis occurs after migration of the neuron to its mature site is complete. In the cerebellar cortex, however, external granule cells project bipolar axons as parallel fibers in the molecular zone and form synapses with Purkinje cell dendrites before migrating to their mature site in the interior of the folium.

An excessive number of synapses usually form, and many are later deleted, with retraction of redundant collateral axons. Transitory neurons, such as the Cajal–Retzius neurons of the fetal cerebral cortex, form temporary synapses. As with other aspects of neural development, there is a critical period of synapse elimination. Class I major histocompatibility complex glycoproteins may be involved in synaptic remodeling during fetal development and infancy. In the optic system, considerable amounts of these surface-expressed proteins are demonstrated on neurons of the lateral geniculate body in the late fetal and early postnatal periods, when synaptogenesis and especially synaptic retraction are most active. Most of the dendritic arborizations and synapatogenesis in the cerebral cortex occur during late gestation and early infancy, a circumstance that renders this developmental process particularly vulnerable to toxic, hypoxic, ischemic, and metabolic insults in the postnatal period, especially in neonates born prematurely. When an axonal terminal reaches a dendritic spine and cell–cell contact is achieved, a chemical synapse usually forms rapidly. Some "promiscuous" neurons may even secrete transmitter before contacting their targets, inducing an overabundance of synapses that then undergo additional electrical activity-dependent refinement. Dendritic spines determine the dynamics of intracellular second-messenger ions such as calcium and probably provide for synaptic plasticity by establishing compartmentalization of afferent input based on biochemical rather than electrical signals.

Neurotrophins play an important role in the modulation of synaptogenesis as selective retrograde messengers. Trans-synaptic signaling by neurotrophins and neurotransmitters may also influence neuronal architecture, such as neurite sprouting and dendritic pruning. The effects of neurotrophic factors may even be lamina specific within the cortex and have opposite effects in different layers. Brain-derived neurotrophic factor (BDNF) stimulates dendritic growth in layer 4 neurons, whereas NT-3 inhibits this growth. In contrast, BDNF is inhibitory and NT-3 is stimulatory for neuroblasts in layer 6. Prostaglandins and their inducible synthetase enzymes (e.g., cyclooxygenase-2) are expressed by excitatory neurons at postsynaptic sites in the cerebral cortex and hippocampus. They modulate N-methyl-D-aspartate-dependent responses such as long-term potentiation and show a spatial and temporal sequence of expression that may be demonstrated in the fetal brain by immunocytochemistry. This expression is highly localized to dendritic spines and reflects functional rather than structural features of synapse formation. Prostaglandin signaling of cortical development and synaptogenesis in particular are mediated through dendrites; this is also likely the case for neurotrophin signaling.

Glial cells are important in promoting dendritic development. In addition to axodendritic and axosomatic synapses, a few specialized sites in the developing brain show dendrodendritic contacts. An example is the spines of olfactory granule cells.

The electroencephalogram (EEG) is the most reliable and accessible noninvasive clinical measure of functional synaptogenesis in the cerebral cortex of the preterm infant. The maturation of EEG patterns involves a precise and predictable temporal progression of changes with conceptional age, including the development of sleep–wake cycles.

Neuronal and Glial Cell Maturation

Neuronal and epithelial cells are the most polarized cells of the body. Epithelial cells must have apical and basal surfaces, and neurons must form an axon at one end and dendrites at other cell surfaces. The development of cell polarity is one of the first events in neuronogenesis. The structural and molecular differences that distinguish the axonal and dendritic domains play an integral role in every aspect of neuronal function.

Two other features distinguish neurons from all other cells in the body: an electrically polarizing and excitable plasma membrane and secretory function. Muscle cells have excitable membranes but do not secrete; endocrine and exocrine cells are secretory but do not have polarized membranes. Only neurons have both.

The development of electrical polarity of the cell membrane is an important maturational feature that denotes when a neuroblast becomes a neuron. This process depends on the development of ion channels and on a means of delivering continuous energy production necessary to maintain a resting membrane potential. This membrane potential is mediated by voltage-gated ion channels and does not require other energy-generating mechanisms, such as the adenosine triphosphatase pumps mediated by Na^+/K^+, Ca^{2+}, or Mg^{2+}. The importance of glial cells for ion transport in this regard may be greater than once believed, and astrocytes play an important role in regulating the cerebral microenvironment in addition to their nutritive functions and their contribution to the blood–brain barrier.

The onset of synthesis of neurotransmitter substances, their transport down the axon, and the formation of terminal axonal storage vesicles for these compounds denote the transition from neuroblast to neuron. Transmitter biosynthesis may begin before neuroblast migration is completed, although the secretion of these substances is delayed until synapses are formed with target cells. Some substances that later serve as neurotransmitters, including most of the neuropeptides, acetylcholine, and GABA, may be synthesized early in embryonic or fetal life, before they could possibly function as transmitters, and they may serve a neurotrophic function.

A number of proteins are produced by mature neurons and not by immature nerve cells. Antibodies against such proteins may be employed to demonstrate the maturation of neuroblasts in the human fetal brain (at autopsy) by immunocytochemistry. One such example is neuronal nuclear antigen. By coupling such studies with immunocytochemical markers of axonal maturation, such as the use of antibodies against synaptic vesicle proteins, it is possible to demonstrate the temporal relation of terminal axonal maturation and the maturation of their target neuron. This sequence may be altered in some cerebral malformations and may explain why some infants with severe malformations such as holoprosencephaly have intractable epilepsy, whereas others with similar anatomical lesions identified by imaging or histopathological examination have few or no seizures.

Some genes appear to be essential for the regulation of trophic factors or differentiation and growth of the individual neural cell. *TSC1* and *TSC2* are genes that produce protein products called hamartin and tuberin, respectively, which are defective in neural and nonneural tissues in patients with tuberous sclerosis. *TSC1* is localized on chromosome 9q34 but accounts for only a minority of patients with this autosomal dominant disease. *TSC2* is located at the 16p13.3 locus.

Myelination

As with other aspects of nervous system development, myelination cycles (i.e., the time between onset and termination of myelination in a given pathway) are specific for each tract and precisely time linked. Some pathways myelinate in a rostrocaudal progression. At birth, the human corticospinal tract is myelinated in the corona radiata, the internal capsule, the middle third of the cerebral peduncle, and the upper pons. It is very lightly myelinated in the pyramids, and it is unmyelinated in the spinal cord. Other pathways myelinate in their proximal and distal portions simultaneously. Some pathways myelinate early and others late, but no axons myelinate during the growth of the axonal growth cone before it reaches its target. The medial longitudinal fasciculus acquires myelin at 24 weeks of gestation and is fully myelinated within 2 weeks. The corticospinal tract begins myelinating at approximately 38 weeks of gestation and is not complete until 2 years of age. The corpus callosum begins myelination at approximately 4 months postnatally and is not complete until late adolescence. The last tract to complete myelination is the ipsilateral association bundle that interconnects the anterior frontal and the temporal lobes: It is not complete until 32 years of age.

Myelination cycles as determined by special myelin stains of sections of fetal and postnatal CNS tissue at autopsy are summarized in Table 4. The traditional stain is Luxol fast blue, but newer methods using gallocyanin stain and immunocytochemical demonstration of myelin basic protein provide earlier detection of myelin formation at the light microscopic level. Electron microscopy is the most sensitive morphological method for documenting the onset of myelination in brain tissue. The sequences of proteins and lipids incorporated into myelin may also be studied biochemically at autopsy in immature brains.

Myelination may be determined in living patients by magnetic resonance imaging (MRI). T1-weighted MRIs are more sensitive than T2-weighted sequences early during myelination, and T2-weighted images are more sensitive as myelination advances with maturation. However, the current generation of imaging does not show the earliest onset of myelination that can be demonstrated histologically. This difference in sensitivity accounts for the slightly different myelination data used by neuroradiologists and neuropathologists (Table 5).

Myelination depends on the normal differentiation and integrity of oligodendrocytes in the CNS and Schwann cells in the PNS. As with other developmental processes in the nervous system, the programming of differentiation of these myelin-producing cells and myelin formation is under genetic regulation. The *Krox20* mouse gene (*ERG2* in humans), previously discussed as a zinc finger homeobox gene expressed in r3 and r5, also plays an important role in myelination by Schwann

Table 4   MYELINATION CYCLES IN THE HUMAN CENTRAL NERVOUS SYSTEM BASED ON MYELIN TISSUE STAINS[a]

Pathway	Cycle Begins	Cycle Completed
Spinal motor roots	16 weeks	42 weeks
Spinal sensory roots	20 weeks	5 months
Cranial motor nerves III–VI	20 weeks	28 weeks
Ventral commissure, spinal cord	24 weeks	4 months
Dorsal columns, spinal cord	28 weeks	36 weeks
Medial longitudinal fasciculus	24 weeks	28 weeks
Habenulopeduncular tract	28 weeks	34 weeks
Acoustic nerve	24 weeks	36 weeks
Trapezoid body and lateral lemniscus	25 weeks	36 weeks
Acoustic radiations (thalamocortical)	40 weeks	3 years
Inferior cerebellar peduncle (inner part)	26 weeks	36 weeks
Inferior cerebellar peduncle (outer part)	32 weeks	4 months
Middle cerebellar peduncle (pontocerebellar)	42 weeks	3 years
Superior cerebellar peduncle	28 weeks	6 months
Medial lemniscus	32 weeks	12 months
Optic nerve	38 weeks	6 months
Optic radiations (geniculocalcarine)	40 weeks	6 months
Ansa reticularis	28 weeks	8 months
Fornix	2 months	2 years
Mammillothalamic tract	8 months	6 years
Thalamocortical radiations	2 months	7 years
Corticospinal (pyramidal) tract	38 weeks	2 years
Corpus callosum	2 months	14 years
Ipsilateral intracortical association fibers, frontotemporal and frontoparietal	3 months	32 years

[a]Myelination was determined by light microscopy using Luxol fast blue and other myelin stains; composite is from various authors. Gestational age is stated in weeks; postnatal age is stated in months and years. From Sarnat (1992).

cells. It is ironic that *Krox20/ERG2* is expressed only in r3 and r5, rhombomeres that do not form neural crest tissue, but adjacent and intervening rhombomeres do form this tissue and Schwann cells are derived from neural crest. The *PMP22* gene, which is defective in several hereditary motor–sensory neuropathies, programs proteolipid protein by encoding an axonally regulated Schwann cell protein incorporated into peripheral myelin;

Table 5 FIRST APPEARANCE OF MYELINATION IN THE HUMAN BRAIN BASED ON MAGNETIC RESONANCE IMAGING[a]

Anatomical region	T1-weighted	T2-weighted
Middle cerebellar peduncle	Birth	Birth to 2 months
Cerebral white matter	Birth to 4 months	3–5 months
Internal capsule, posterior limb		
Anterior portion	Birth	4–7 months
Posterior portion	Birth	Birth to 2 months
Internal capsule, anterior limb	2–3 months	7–11 months
Corpus callosum, genu	4–6 months	5–8 months
Corpus callosum, splenium	3–4 months	4–6 months
Occipital white matter		
Central	3–5 months	9–14 months
Peripheral	4–7 months	11–15 months
Frontal white matter		
Central	3–6 months	11–16 months
Peripheral	7–11 months	14–18 months
Centrum semiovale	2–6 months	7–11 months

[a] Modified from Barkovich, A. J. (1995). *Pediatric Neroimaging*, 2nd ed. Raven Press, New York.

however, whether it serves a function in the CNS is uncertain. The oligodendrocytes, which ensheathe and myelinate axons in the CNS, develop from primitive O4 cells in response to ventralizing influences in the neural tube, such as *Shh*, and are inhibited from differentiating by dorsalizing gradients.

In addition to their role in generating myelin sheaths around some axons, oligodendrocytes express nerve growth factor and may secrete other molecules that stimulate the growth of axons. Insulin-like growth factor may also play a role in central myelination and conserving axonal integrity. Gangliosides are complex lipids that form part of the myelinating membranes of oligodendrocytes and Schwann cells, and their composition is important in the development of myelin.

Oligodendrocytes may ensheathe several axons in the CNS, but in the PNS each Schwann cell myelinates only a single axon, although some Schwann cells may enclose 1–4 unmyelinated axons. At midgestation, a single Schwann cell may enclose as many as 25 axons, but this number becomes smaller with progressive maturation.

Myelination is an important parameter of the maturation of the brain in a clinically measurable index. Delayed myelination occurs in many metabolic diseases involving the nervous system, in fetal and postnatal malnutrition if the lipids and proteins are not available to be incorporated, and sometimes as a nonspecific feature of global developmental delay.

ROLE OF FETAL EPENDYMA

The ependyma of the mature brain is little more than a decorative lining of the ventricular system, serving minor functions in the transport of ions and small molecules between the ventricles and the cerebral parenchyma and perhaps having a small immunoprotective role. The fetal ependyma, however, is an essential and dynamic structure that contributes to a number of developmental processes. The floor plate is the first region of the neuroepithelium to differentiate as specific cells, and it forms the ventral midline of the ependyma in the spinal cord and brainstem as far rostrally as the midbrain. However, a floor plate is not recognized in the prosencephalon, in diencephalic neuromeres perhaps because of the infundibulum in the ventral midline, or in the telencephalon. The floor plate has active expression of *Shh* and contributes to the differentiation of motor neurons and other parts of the ependyma. It also secretes retinoic acid, unlike other ependymal cells that merely have retinoid receptors.

The ependyma develops in a precise temporal and spatial pattern. The last surfaces of the ventricular system to be completely covered by ependyma are in the lateral ventricles at 22 weeks of gestation. In some areas of the neuraxis, it is advantageous for ependymal differentiation to be delayed as long as possible to permit the requisite number of neuroblasts to be produced in the ventricular zone because after the ependyma forms in a particular region, all mitotic activity ceases at the ventricular surface. One function of the fetal ependyma is to regulate the arrest of mitotic proliferation of neuroepithelial cells. Mature human ependymal cells *in vivo* have minimal or no mitotic potential for regeneration, but rat ependymal cells *in vitro* may be induced to proliferate by epidermal growth factor and fibroblast growth factor-2.

The fetal ependyma is structurally different from that of the adult. Rather than the simple cuboidal epithelium in the adult, it is a pseudostratified columnar epithelium, with each cell having at least a slender cytoplasmic process contacting the ventricular surface, although its nucleus may be at some distance. This arrangement is required because ependymal cells do not divide after differentiation, and a provision is needed for enough cells to cover the entire ventricular surface; the "extra" layers of ependymal cells become thinned as the ependyma spreads to cover the expanding ventricular surface during growth of the fetus. At the basal surface of fetal ependymal cells is a process that radiates into the parenchyma. This process may reach the pial surface of the spinal cord and brainstem, but it never spans the entire cerebral hemisphere and extends only into the subventricular zone (i.e., the germinal matrix) and into the deeper portions of the intermediate zone. The fetal ependyma also differs from that in the adult in expressing certain intermediate filament proteins, such as vimentin, glial fibrillary acidic protein, and other molecules such as the S-100β protein. As in the adult, the fetal ependyma is ciliated at its apical (ventricular) surface.

Ependymal cells are important elements in guiding the intermediate trajectories of axonal growth cones. In some places, the basal processes of fetal ependymal cells form mechanical tunnels to guide axonal growth in developing long tracts. Ependymal cells and their processes also secrete molecules that attract or repel axons and that may be specific for some but not other axons. Floor plate ependymal cells synthesize netrin, a diffusible neurotropic factor, permitting the passage of commissural axons but repelling fibers of longitudinal tracts (185–187). Netrin may be bifunctional, acting as an attractant of decussating axons at some sites (e.g., the floor plate in the spinal cord) but as a repellent at other sites (e.g., trochlear axons). In the developing dorsal columns of the spinal cord, the dorsal median raphe formed by ependymal cells of the roof plate prevents wandering of rostrally growing axons to the wrong side of the spinal cord by secreting a proteoglycan, keratan sulfate, that strongly repels axonal growth cones. Ependymal processes do not guide migratory neuroblasts, despite their resemblance to radial glial fibers.

The loss of S-100β protein from ependymal cells of the lateral ventricles appears to coincide with the end of cell migration from the subventricular zone and the beginning conversion of radial glial cells into mature astrocytes. Whether the ependyma induces this conversion is uncertain, but circumstantial evidence suggests such a function.

—*Harvey B. Sarnat*

See also–Axons; Brain Development, Normal Postnatal; Cell Death; Central Nervous System, Overview; Dendrites; Ependyma; Glia; Myelin; Neural Tube Defects; Neurogenetics, Overview; Neurons, Overview; Vertebrate Nervous System, Development of

Further Reading

Bass, P. W. (1999). Microtubules and neuronal polarity: Lessons from mitosis. *Neuron* **22**, 23–31.

Bovolentá, P., and Dodd, J. (1990). Guidance of commissural growth cones at the floor plate in embryonic rat spinal cord. *Development* **109**, 435–447.

Bronner-Fraser, M. (1995). Origins and developmental potential of the neural crest. *Exp. Cell Res.* **218**, 405–417.

des Portes, V., Pinard, J. M., Billuart, P., *et al.* (1998). A novel CNS gene required for neuronal migration and involved in X-linked subcortical laminar heterotopia and lissencephaly syndrome. *Cell* **92**, 51–61.

Dodd, J., and Schuchardt, A. (1995). Axon guidance: A compelling case for repelling growth cones. *Cell* **81**, 471–474.

Dorsky, R. I., Moon, R. T., and Raible, D. W. (1998). Control of neural crest cell fate by the *Wnt* signalling pathway. *Nature* **396**, 370–373.

Eksioglu, Y. Z., Scheffer, I. E., Cardena, P., *et al.* (1996). Periventricular heterotopia: An X-linked dominant epilepsy locus causing aberrant cerebral cortical development. *Neuron* **16**, 77–87.

Guthrie, S. (1996). Patterning the hindbrain. *Curr. Opin. Neurobiol.* **6**, 41–48.

Higgins, D., Burack, M., Lein, P., *et al.* (1997). Mechanisms of neuronal polarity. *Curr. Opin. Neurobiol.* **7**, 599–604.

Marín-Padilla, M. (1998). Cajal–Retzius cells and the development of the neocortex. *Trends Neurosci.* **21**, 64–71.

Qiu, M., Shimamuira, K., Sussel, L., *et al.* (1998). Control of anteroposterior and dorsoventral domains of Nkx-6.1 gene expression relative to other *Nkx* genes during vertebrate cns development. *Mech. Dev.* **72**, 77–88.

Rakic, P. (1995). Radial versus tangential migration of neuronal clones in the developing cerebral cortex. *Proc. Natl. Acad. Sci. USA* **92**, 11323–11327.

Roy, N., Mahadevan, M. S., McLean, M., *et al.* (1995). The gene for neuronal apoptosis inhibitory protein is partially deleted in individuals with spinal muscular atrophy. *Cell* **80**, 167–178.

Sarnat, H. B. (1992). Regional differentiation of the human fetal ependyma: Immunocytochemical markers. *J. Neuropathol. Exp. Neurol.* **51**, 58–75.

Sarnat, H. B. (1992). *Cerebral Dysgenesis: Embryology and Clinical Expression*. Oxford Univ. Press, New York.

Sarnat, H. B., and Flores-Sarnat, L. (2002). Cajal–Retzius and subplate neurons and their role in cortical development. *Eur. J. Paediatr. Neurol.* **6**, 91–97.

Sarnat, H. B., and Menkes, J. H. (2000). How to construct a neural tube. *J. Child Neurol.* **21**, 109–124.

Smith, J. L., and Schoenwolf, G. C. (1997). Neurulation: Coming to closure. *Trends Neurosci.* **20**, 510–517.

Tabin, C. J., and McMahon, A. P. (1997). Recent advances in hedgehog signalling. *Trends Cell. Biol.* **7**, 442–446.

Yakovlev, P. I., and Lecours, A.-R. (1967). The myelination cycles of regional maturation of the brain. In *Regional Development of the Brain in Early Life* (A. Minkowsky, Ed.), pp. 3–70. Davis, Philadelphia.

Nervous Tissue, Non-Neural Components of

NERVOUS TISSUE is composed of nerve cells and their processes along with a number of other cell types, most of which are classified as glia and seem to be essential for normal function.

The most plentiful type of cell in the central nervous system is the oligodendroglial cell. Myelin sheaths are formed from the membranes of these cells. The white matter of the brain is filled with axons connecting one brain area to another, and most of these axons are ensheathed in myelin. It is the myelin that makes the white matter appear white. The gray matter contains neuronal cell bodies along with numerous dendritic processes and less numerous axons. Myelin in the cortical gray matter is generally limited to large axons entering from the white matter or projecting to other areas. Each segment of a myelin sheath is connected to an oligodendroglial cell body by a slender process, but the entire trajectory from sheath to cell body can rarely be visualized. A single oligodendroglial cell may support 2–20 segments of myelin, all on different axons. The cell bodies of the myelin-forming oligodendroglia tend to occur in rows between the axons (Fig. 1). Oligodendroglia also occur as perineuronal satellites, especially around the large neurons of the sixth (deepest) cortical layer. The function of these satellites is obscure. Predecessors of oligodendroglial cells exist in the brain but are few and their identification is difficult.

Astrocytes are a second type of glia and are found in all brain regions. Like oligodendroglia, they may be placed as perineuronal satellites. They are usually star shaped, as their name implies, with several processes extending from a small cell body (Fig. 2). The ends of the processes form broad feet that encircle vessels. Molecules entering the brain from the vasculature must either pass through the exiguous extracellular space or transit the astrocytic cytoplasm. Astrocytic processes also broaden out at

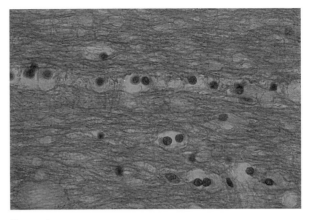

Figure 1
A hematoxylin and eosin-stained section of cerebral white matter showing interfascicular oligodendroglia, of which little more than the nucleus is visible.

the pial boundary of the brain, where they are probably responsible for formation of the basal lamina. Astrocytic processes tend to envelop synapses, especially complex synaptic glomeruli, and to lie next to nodes of Ranvier. These localizations suggest some metabolic role. Astrocytes are coupled to one another by gap junctions, which allow passage of small molecules from the cytoplasm of one to another. These junctions are permeable to calcium, for example. The type of intermediate filament that astrocytes make is called glial fibrillary acidic protein (GFAP). The astrocytes in the cerebral cortex and the putamen and caudate nucleus normally differ from those in other regions of the brain by having very few GFAP filaments in their processes. This led early investigators to call them protoplasmic astrocytes, in contrast to the fibrous astrocytes in the white matter and elsewhere. When these protoplasmic astrocytes respond to almost any pathological stimulus, they begin making GFAP and become fibrous astrocytes. Astrocytes react to almost any injury to the nervous system. They may divide, and they may put forth extra processes, increasing the amount of GFAP within the processes. Their paranuclear cytoplasm may increase its volume. The result of these changes is called gliosis. The functions of astrocytes are not well understood. They probably have a role in promoting the mechanical stability of the brain. They also probably have a role in maintaining the homeostasis of the extracellular milieu of the central nervous system, especially with regard to levels of extracellular potassium. They contain the enzyme glutamine

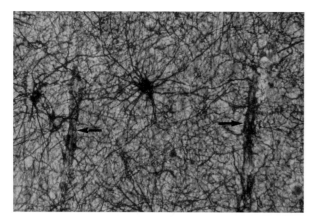

Figure 2
Cajal gold sulfate stain showing a large astrocyte with many processes, two of which are directed to nearby capillaries (arrows). The terminal processes that ensheathe the capillaries are not well shown on this kind of section.

synthase, which they may use to metabolize glutamate and γ-aminobutyric acid, both important neurotransmitters.

Ependymal cells are the third type of glial cells. Their extent is much more limited since they line the ventricular system and the central canal of the spinal cord. They are more or less cuboidal in shape, with cilia and microvillae on their ventricular surface. They are linked to one another by desmosomes and gap junctions. A tracer substance introduced experimentally into the ventricle of an animal will move easily into the tissue past the ependyma, except in the lower part of the third ventricle. In this region, modified ependymal cells called tanycytes are joined by tight junctions, and they have stout processes that end on vessels inside the hypothalamus.

Microglial cells are sometimes classified as glia, although they are probably derived from blood monocytes. They are resting cells with a phagocytic potential, evenly spaced in the gray and white matter. Special stains show that they have at least two short branching processes. When the nervous system is injured, they can enlarge and divide and probably become macrophages, in which case they may be impossible to distinguish from blood-borne macrophages, which may arrive in much greater numbers.

The tissue of the nervous system contains vessels that supply oxygen and substrates and remove carbon dioxide and wastes. These vessels are unusual in having numerous mitochondria, tight junctions between their endothelial cells, and no fenestrations.

These features are consistent with the selective uptake of molecules into the brain through the loosely termed blood–brain barrier. The arteries and veins are surrounded by a space whose outer limit is formed by a basal lamina covering astrocytic processes.

The composition of the peripheral nervous system differs from that of the central nervous system. Astrocytes, oligodendroglia, and ependymal cells are absent, but there is an element known as Schwann cells. These cells wrap axons like oligodendroglia do, but they differ in several ways. Each Schwann cell forms only one segment of myelin on one axon, and the Schwann cell cytoplasm and nucleus remain in contact with the sheath. Schwann cells also wrap very small axons without making myelin. The proteins of the myelin in nerves are slightly different from those in the brain. Sensory neurons of the peripheral nervous system are found in autonomic and dorsal root ganglia. Satellite cells, which are modified Schwann cells, line the surface of these neurons. Of course, the somatic motor neuron cell bodies are within the spinal cord or brainstem.

—*Stirling Carpenter*

See also—Ependyma; Glia; Microglia; Myelin; Neurons, Overview; Oligodendrocytes

Further Reading

Berry, M., and Butt, A. M. (1997). Structure and function of glia in the central nervous system. In *Greenfield's Neuropathology* (D. I. Graham and P. L. Lantos, Eds.), 6th ed., pp. 63–83. Arnold, London.

Neuralgias, Cranial

Encyclopedia of the Neurological Sciences
Copyright 2003, Elsevier Science (USA). All rights reserved.

TRIGEMINAL NERVE

THE TRIGEMINAL or fifth cranial nerve (CN V) supplies sensory and some motor innervation to the head and scalp. It innervates the muscles of mastication (masseter and temporalis) and supplies sensory fibers to the face, conjunctiva, cornea, and mucous membranes of the mouth, nose, and paranasal sinuses. The dura of the middle and anterior cranial fossae is also innervated by CN V. The trigeminal is the largest cranial nerve and includes the large sensory trigeminal ganglion, called the semilunar or gasserian ganglion, located in Meckel's cave, a dural reflection in the medial temporal fossa. The postganglionic sensory fibers aggregate into three divisions: the ophthalmic supplying the eye and forehead to the midcrown, the mandibular supplying the face below the eye and above the mouth, and the maxillary supplying the face below the mouth. The preganglionic sensory fibers enter the brainstem in the midpons and pursue separate and complicated courses. The small pain and temperature afferents descend and synapse with second-order neurons in the descending trigeminal tract, which stretches from the midpons to C2. The stretch receptors, which subserve the jaw jerk reflex afferent arc, synapse with second-order afferents in the principal sensory nucleus of CN V in the mid- to upper pons. The light touch-pressure afferents ascend and synapse in the mesencephalic nucleus of CN V. In all cases, they then cross over and ascend to the thalamus via the trigeminothalamic tract and synapse again in the posteromedial nucleus before third-order afferents pass to the sensory cortex behind the motor strip.

Several disorders may affect the peripheral branches of the trigeminal nerve, the gasserian ganglion, and the sensory and motor roots.

Trigeminal Neuralgia (Tic Douloureux)

This entity was originally described by Arateus in the first century AD, by John Locke in 1677, and by John Fothergill in 1776.

Clinical Symptoms: Trigeminal neuralgia (TN) is paroxysmal and extremely painful. The overall incidence for both sexes is 4.3 per 100,000 persons per year and is higher for women (ration of 3:2) and the elderly. The typical age of onset is 52–58 years for the idiopathic form and 30–35 years for the symptomatic or secondary form.

The pain is usually felt unilaterally within the distribution of one or more divisions of the CN V but typically involves the second and third divisions. Involvement of the first division can occur but always indicates a possible secondary cause. The pain is frequently triggered by a sensory stimulus to the mucosa, skin, or teeth—the "trigger point"—in the distribution of the affected trigeminal division. The quality of the pain is described as electric shock-like, shooting, or lancinating. Each attack lasts only a few seconds, but the pain may be repetitive at short intervals.

The tongue is uncommonly affected, even though it is innervated by the mandibular division. The pain rarely lasts more than a few seconds or a minute or two, but it may be so intense that the patient involuntarily winces. The paroxysms of pain recur frequently, both day and night, but nocturnal pain during sleep is rare. Some patients suffering from TN complain of discomfort, itching, and sensitivity of the face. Patients refuse to apply makeup on the affected side of the face, avoid brushing their teeth or shaving on that side, and often eat or talk out of the other side of the mouth. Sometimes, the wind is enough to trigger an attack. These patients frequently experience remissions of months to 1 year or more. This is an important historical feature since it effectively eliminates a secondary cause such as an infiltrating carcinoma, which is often difficult to diagnose early.

Physical Findings: In primary TN, there is no evidence of sensory or motor impairment. As mentioned previously, personal hygiene may be neglected on the affected side of the face. Examination of the face may be difficult because the patient is reluctant to let the examiner touch the skin for fear of triggering an attack. Secondary TN may be associated with signs of sensory loss in an affected division along with weakness and atrophy of the muscles of mastication and involvement of neighboring cranial nerves. Bilaterality is highly suggestive of multiple sclerosis or other intrinsic brainstem lesions such as an arteriovenous malformation (AVM) or tumor.

Pathology: There are degenerative changes within the gasserian ganglion in patients with TN. Demyelination of the axons in the main sensory root may be associated with vascular compression of the nerve.

Pathogenesis: Trigeminal neuralgia is one of the most thoroughly investigated pain syndromes. Its cause is multifactorial. Considered idiopathic in the past, the etiology is now attributed in most cases, with some dissenters, to vascular compression of the preganglionic trigeminal nerve fibers in the posterior fossa producing partial demyelination of nerve fibers. Progressive arteriosclerotic changes of the vertebrobasilar system, accelerated by aging and hypertension, cause ectasia of vessels with deviation of their course resulting in trigeminal nerve root compression. This is thought to result in abnormal transmission and processing of impulses. Multiple sclerosis, schwannomas, cerebellopontine angle tumors, AVMs, and other local lesions account for a small proportion of cases.

Treatment and Management: Management of TN can be either medical or surgical. The drug of choice is carbamazepine, which is effective in 75% of patients. Carbamazepine must be initiated with small doses of 100 mg and increased slowly as tolerated. The therapeutic range of 4–12 µg/ml generally can be achieved with doses ranging from 600 to 1200 mg per day. During the first few months of therapy, regular blood counts are mandatory to monitor for development of agranulocytosis, a rare but serious complication.

Second-line options include phenytoin, baclofen, valproic acid, gabapentin, clonazepam, and lamotrigine. These are thought to be less effective than carbamazepine but can be tried alone or in combination when there is evidence of failure or intolerance to carbamazepine. An acute attack can sometimes be aborted by administering 250 mg of phosphenytoin. Other options include alcohol block of the peripheral nerve as it leaves the foramen or the use of three different techniques to perform percutaneous destruction of the ganglion: balloon microcompression, radio frequency lesioning, and glycerol injection.

Microvascular decompression of the nerve as it leaves the brainstem, developed by Jannetta and colleagues at the University of Pittsburgh, is the preferred open surgical approach in refractory patients. This requires a posterior fossa craniectomy but is safe in experienced hands and generally provides long-lasting benefit. It is also applicable to vascular compression syndromes associated with TN, hemifacial spasm, and glossopharyngeal neuralgia.

Trigeminal Neuropathy

This disorder is quite rare. Generally, the pain is more chronic and not as frequently lancinating as in TN. In addition, there is usually objective sensory loss in one or more divisions. The pain and numbness may cross several divisions of CN V and are often bilateral, although one side may be affected before the other for a long period of time. In some cases, the motor branches are also affected. In all cases, vigorous attempts should be made to exclude a secondary process, especially squamous cell carcinoma. This can be difficult to diagnose early since it infiltrates into foramina and often does not present with a discrete mass. Careful radiography of the skull base with high-resolution computed tomography and high-

quality magnetic resonance imaging (MRI) with contrast enhancement should be performed and interpreted by skilled radiologists to detect these early malignancies. ENT consultation should be obtained. The idiopathic cases are often associated with collagen vascular diseases, such as Sjogren's syndrome and mixed connective disease. Although the pathology is not conclusive, a vasculitis affecting the nerve is the prevalent theory. Treatment is symptomatic with medications for neuropathic pain. These patients generally do not respond to the same treatments as those for primary TN and generally require a comprehensive pain management approach.

Secondary or "Symptomatic" Trigeminal Neuropathy

These patients may present with progressive numbness interspersed with pain or may present with symptoms similar to those of idiopathic TN. Clues to the possibility of a secondary cause include young age of onset, bilaterality, associated sensory loss or motor dysfunction, initial involvement of the ophthalmic division, spread of pain from one segment to another, and involvement of other cranial nerves. For patients presenting with typical TN-type pain, intrinsic brainstem lesions such as multiple sclerosis, tumors, and AVMs need to be excluded with appropriate tests, usually MRI. These patients generally respond to typical TN drugs but not as well as in primary TN. For patients with atypical TN pain, more extensive imaging studies and ENT evaluation are required, as discussed previously. These patients usually harbor an underlying disorder or malignancy and have to be followed carefully. Even a negative initial workup does not exclude an underlying disorder, and retesting, especially if symptoms worsen or spread, should be considered. These patients respond poorly or not at all to typical TN drugs and often require a comprehensive pain management approach.

Atypical Facial Pain

These patients have a chronic pain syndrome affecting the face without objective findings on exam or testing. The pain is often burning or aching. It also involves the face in a nondermatomal fashion, either involving parts of adjacent trigeminal nerve divisions or spreading in the occipital or cervical nerve territory. The symptoms tend to be chronic and unrelenting. Patients are often depressed and functionally impaired. The clinician must first rule out a secondary problem, as discussed previously.

Treatment usually consists of pain management, often with psychiatric treatment for depression.

GLOSSOPHARYNGEAL NERVE

The glossopharyngeal or ninth cranial nerve (CN IX) mediates taste, salivation, and (with CNs X and XII) swallowing. It mediates input from the carotid body, which contains chemoreceptors that monitor the carbon dioxide and oxygen concentration of the blood. It contains general somatic afferent, general visceral afferent, special visceral afferent, special visceral efferent, and general visceral efferent components. It is predominately a sensory nerve that exits the brainstem from the postolivary sulcus with CNs X and XI. It exits the skull via the jugular foramen with CNs X and XI.

Glossopharyngeal Neuralgia

Glossopharyngeal neuralgia is a rare disorder similar in quality and periodicity to that of TN. The pain is described as sharp, stabbing, shooting, burning, cutting, shock-like, and paroxysmal, and it is distributed in the glossopharyngeal nerve and the upper fibers of the vagus nerve. Patients complain of unilateral pain in the throat, posterior third of the tongue, tonsillar region, larynx, nasopharynx, and pinna of the ear. The painful attack may be triggered by chewing, speaking, swallowing, coughing, and laughing. Generally, patients are older than 40 years. The paroxysm of pain can cause syncope or bradycardia.

Glossopharyngeal neuralgia is idiopathic or associated with oropharyngeal malignancies, peritonsillar infections, vascular compression of the nerve, or Eagle's syndrome, which consists of dysphagia and unilateral pharyngeal pain radiating to the ear, worsened by swallowing, possibly due to compression of the neurovascular structure by an elongated styloid process.

Treatment with carbamazepine and phenytoin has had mixed success. Posterior fossa craniectomy with microvascular decompression, similar to the procedure in TN, is often successful in typical cases. Microvascular decompression of the ninth cranial nerve root entry zone can also relieve the pain.

—*Omar Figueroa and John J. Kelly, Jr.*

See also–Facial Pain; Glossopharyngeal Nerve (Cranial Nerve IX); Trigeminal Nerve (Cranial Nerve V)

Neural Tube Defects

Encyclopedia of the Neurological Sciences
Copyright 2003, Elsevier Science (USA). All rights reserved.

DURING early embryological development, certain tissues notably influence the development of adjacent tissues; this process is known as induction. It involves the inducing tissues, the inductor, and the induced tissue and characterizes the early development of the human central nervous system. It is hallmarked by the formation of a primitive neural tube by a process known as neurulation. This critical step occurs during the third and fourth weeks of gestation and is the result of progressive inductive events on the dorsal aspect of the embryo. At approximately 18 days of gestation, a neural plate is formed. Under continued inductive influences, invagination of the lateral margins of the neural plate occurs to form a neural grove followed by dorsal midline fusion (Fig. 1). Closure begins at the level of the low brainstem and appears to proceed in both a rostral and caudal direction by multisite closure, eventually forming a tube with open apertures at both ends. The sites of closure are most likely controlled by specific genes. The cephalic end of the neural tube, the anterior neuropore, closes at approximately 24–26 days of gestation, whereas the caudal end, the posterior neuropore, closes at approximately 27–29 days of gestation.

Disturbances of this process result in defects in neural tube formation and are associated with abnormalities in the development of the cranium, axial skeleton, nervous system, and corresponding meningovascular and dermal coverings (Table 1). The most severe form of neural tube disruption is craniorachischisis with a complete failure of neurulation. Most of these cases are aborted in early pregnancy. Disruption of anterior (rostral) neural tube closure results in anencephaly and cranium bifidum, whereas disruption of the posterior (caudal) neural tube results in spinal dysraphism. The term spinal dysraphism refers to all spinal anomalies that have incomplete embryonic closure of any combination of midline mesenchymal, osseous, and nervous tissue structures.

A variety of environmental influences including teratogenic exposures during early pregnancy in both experimental animals and humans have been associated with an increased incidence of neural tube defects. These also include radiation, maternal hyperthermia, gestational diabetes, vitamin A

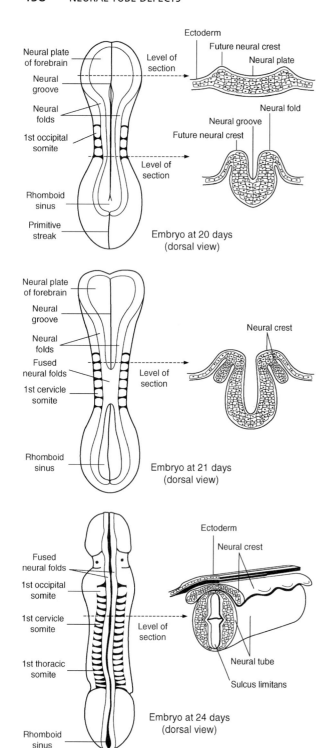

Figure 1

Illustrations demonstrating the process of neurulation with the transformation of the neural plate to a closed neural tube. [Reproduced with permission from Brass, A. (Ed.) (1986). *The CIBA Collection of Medical Illustrations. Vol. 1, Nervous System, Part 1, Anatomy and Physiology* (F. H. Netter, Illustrator). CIBA, West Caldwell, NJ.]

deficiency, administration of valproic acid or carbamazepine, and folic acid deficiency. Daily oral supplementation with 400 µg of folic acid during early pregnancy is now recognized as an important factor in decreasing the incidence of neural tube defects by as much as 50%.

SPINA BIFIDA

The term spina bifida refers to a developmental abnormality with incomplete closure of the bony lamina and the spinous processes of the spine. Spina bifida occulta is the failure of fusion of the posterior vertebral arches unaccompanied by any herniation of spinal contents or defect of the overlying skin. Spina bifida cystica (aperta) refers to an associated protrusion of all or part of the contents of the spinal canal through the bony defect and includes meningoceles, myeloceles, and myelomeningoceles.

Spina bifida is not an uncommon phenomenon; it is estimated to occur in at least 5% of the general pediatric population. Spina bifida occulta is the most common type and is clinically asymptomatic; the diagnosis is usually made by incidental radiographs of the spine obtained for some other reason. Although there is a bony defect in the vertebral arch establishing the diagnosis, the overlying skin is intact and there is no neurological involvement. However, there can be associated overlying cutaneous findings, such as hyperpigmentation over the spine, a patch of hair, a dermal sinus tract, or a subcutaneous mass secondary to an associated lipoma. Spina bifida occulta is most commonly seen in the lower lumbar region involving the lamina of L_5 and S_1. No surgical intervention is necessary.

OCCULT SPINAL DYSRAPHISM

When a spina bifida occulta is associated with neurological abnormalities, the condition is referred to as an occult spinal dysraphism. This results from a distortion of the spinal cord or roots by associated fibrous bands or masses beneath the intact dermis and epidermis. This category includes the tethered cord syndrome, spinal lipomas, diastematomyelia, and diplomyelia. Of these, the tethered cord syndrome (tight filum terminale syndrome) is the most common. Early clinical features suggestive of a potential occult spinal dysraphism include overlying cutaneous abnormalities that include a hair tuft, subcutaneous mass, pigmentary abnormalities, and dimples or tracts (Table 2). In a recent study

Table 1 NEURAL TUBE DEFECTS

Total neurulation failure
  Craniorachischisis
Anterior (rostral) neural tube closure defects
  Anencephaly
  Cranium bifidum
Posterior (caudal) neural tube closure defects (spinal dysraphism)
  Spina bifida occulta
  Occult spinal dysraphism
    Tethered cord syndrome
      Thick filum terminale syndrome
      Spinal lipoma
    Split cord malformations
      Diastematomyelia (SCM I)
      Diplomyelia (SCM II)
  Spina bifida cystica
    Meningocele
    Myelocele
    Myelomeningocele

evaluating infants with high-risk cutaneous stigmata, no infant (0 of 160) with a "simple dimple" (defined as midline, measuring <5 mm, and within 2.5 cm of the anus) had an occult spinal dysraphism.

In the tethered cord syndrome, the spinal cord is fixed to the surrounding spine and usually results from a thickened filum terminale appearing to anchor the conus medullaris to the base of the vertebrae (tight filum terminale syndrome). Radiographically, this is characterized by a short, thick filum (>2 mm) and a low position of the conus medullaris. A conus below the L2–L3 disk space is always abnormal. Tethering can also be associated with a spinal lipoma, dermal sinus, or diastematomyelia and diplomyelia. Clinically, the tethered cord syndrome usually presents with slowly progressive lower extremity weakness, foot or leg length abnormalities, scoliosis, gait abnormalities, urological dysfunction, and/or changes of the myotatic reflexes. Occasionally, clinical symptoms can present abruptly. Although the pathophysiology of the symptoms and signs remains obscure, it appears that with growth there is stretching of nerve fibers and possibly vascular compromise resulting in decreased oxidative metabolism. The sudden onset of symptoms and signs may be related to sudden vascular insufficiency.

Early diagnosis and management of these lesions have been greatly aided by the use of ultrasonography in infants and/or magnetic resonance imaging (MRI). Computed tomography (CT) may be helpful for visualizing anomalous bony structures and diastematomyelia spurs. Routine radiographic stu-

dies of the spine in patients younger than 1 year of age are usually insufficient to document a bony defect due to the poor ossification of the posterior elements of the spine. Even in older children, 10% or more may have normal spine films.

Surgical intervention should be undertaken to release spinal cord tethering before there is significant clinical deterioration. Although surgical intervention will halt further neurological progression, it may not restore lost function, especially in patients who have an abrupt onset of symptoms. Following surgery for a spinal lipoma, only 25% of patients will have any improvement in their preexisting neurological status, and only 50% with a thickened filum terminale may improve. Prophylactic surgical intervention in asymptomatic children has become standard treatment to lessen the possibility of poor recovery from preexisting neurological deficits. However, the timing of surgery in the asymptomatic infant is controversial.

Diastematomyelia is a split spinal cord usually separated by a fibrous or bony septum anchoring the spinal cord to the vertebrae. Recently, the term split cord malformation (SCM) has been applied to diastematomyelia (SCM I) and diplomyelia (SCM II). The distinction between these two malformations is based on the integrity of the dural coverings and the presence or absence of intervening mesenchymal tissue. With SCM I, there are two dural sacs and a bony or fibrous spur. With SCM II, there is a single dural sac and intradural fibrous band. In either condition, there is usually progressive neurological, urological, and orthopedic deterioration. Clinical findings on examination can include scoliosis, kyphosis, leg length discrepancy, foot deformities, bladder disturbances, and a myelopathy. Infants may present with congenital scoliosis, frequently with overlying cutaneous abnormalities. Most lesions occur in the lumbosacral region and are somewhat more common in females. Detection can

Table 2 CUTANEOUS ABNORMALITIES ASSOCIATED WITH AN OCCULT SPINAL DYSRAPHISM

Hair tuft/patch
Subcutaneous mass
Hemangioma
Skin tag
Cutis aplasia (congenitial dermal atrophy)
Pigmented macule
Dimples and tracts

be accomplished by ultrasonography, even prenatally. MRI of the spine is the preferred neuroimaging technique. Surgical resection of the spur usually does not result in clinical improvement, although it can halt progression of neurological deterioration. The role of surgery before clinical deterioration occurs is controversial.

Occult malformations along the spinal canal and neuraxis can present with episodes of recurrent meningitis due to external contamination of the cerebrospinal fluid. Malformations include dermal sinuses, neurenteric fistulas, temporal bone fistulas, and basal encephaloceles or meningoceles.

MENINGOCELE

The meningocele is a protrusion of a spinal fluid-filled sac of meninges through a bony defect in the posterior elements of the spine without associated neural tissue herniation. This is the mildest form of spina bifida cystica. It is not associated with a neurological deficit. These fluid-filled protrusions over the midline spine are covered by normal skin or a membrane (Fig. 2). Membranous lesions more commonly occur rostrally, whereas skin-covered lesions occur anywhere along the spine. Membranous meningoceles and meningoceles in the high cervical region may be associated with aqueductal stenosis, hydromyelia, or Chiari malformation. Meningoceles that contain adipose tissue are called lipomeningoceles. Infants with meningoceles should undergo evaluation for an occult dysraphic anomaly, such as a tethered cord or split-cord malformation. Rarely, meningoceles may be anterior, presenting as an intraabdominal or pelvic mass. With a small meningocele and integrity of the overlying skin,

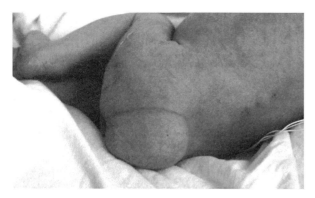

Figure 2
Newborn infant with intact covering of a lumbosacral meningocele. Lower extremity function is normal.

surgical intervention is not necessarily required. Meningoceles account for approximately 5% of patients with spina bifida cystica.

MYELOCELE AND MYELOMENINGOCELE

A localized lack of closure of the posterior neural tube is the essential defect accounting for myelocele and myelomeningocele. As a result, there is a defect in the corresponding neural, mesenchymal, osseous, and other ectodermal tissue. The myelocele is defined as having a midline plaque of neural tissue lying exposed, flush with the surface of the skin. With the more common myelomeningocele, there is elevation of the neural plaque above the skin surface by expansion of the subarachnoid space ventral to the plaque (Fig. 3). In the United States, the incidence of these defects was estimated to be 0.2–0.4 per 1000 live births in 1989. Lumbar (thoracolumbar, lumbar, and lumbosacral) involvement is most common, accounting for approximately 80% of all myelomeningoceles. Neurological, urological, and orthopedic impairment varies depending on the location and extent of the spinal lesion (Table 3). All spinal levels will have some sphincter and bladder disturbances. Sensory disturbances below the level of the lesion are usually profound. Most children with spinal levels below S1 are able to walk unaided, whereas those with levels above L2 are often dependent on a wheelchair for much of their physical activities. Scoliosis is a significant problem for children with levels above L2, whereas it is unusual in children with levels below S1.

Hydrocephalus secondary to an associated Chiari malformation type 2 with or without aqueductal stenosis frequently presents at birth or soon thereafter. It occurs in approximately 90% of children with thoracolumbar, lumbar, or lumbosacral levels, and it is present in approximately 60% of children with nonlumbar levels. Early identification using sonography or CT scanning is warranted. MRI is preferable to better delineate the extent of brainstem involvement in the infant presenting with brainstem signs, including stridor, apnea, cyanotic spells, and dysphagia. Earlier surgical treatment of the hydrocephalus with ventriculoperitoneal shunt placement has been shown to improve the cognitive outcome of infants with myelomeningoceles. Medical management with diuretics and osmotic agents is only a temporizing measure for infants who are too small or medically unstable to undergo surgery.

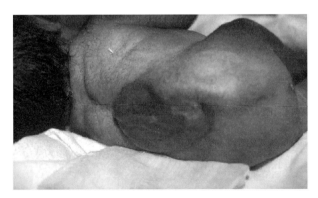

Myelomeningocele may be inherited as an autosomal recessive or dominant trait. The recurrence risk of a neural tube defect after the birth of an affected child is estimated to be approximately 4–8%, increasing to at least 10% after the birth of two affected children. The risk in children with an affected parent is approximately 3%. Neural tube defects have been reported in children with trisomies 13 or 18 and triploidy. Antenatal diagnosis can be made by obtaining an elevated α-fetoprotein (AFP) level in the amniotic fluid at 14–16 weeks of gestation. AFP is a component of the fetal nervous system, and it is believed to leak into the amniotic fluid from an open tube defect. Closed lesions are not associated with an elevated AFP level. Maternal serum AFP screening between 16 and 18 weeks of gestation can also be used and has a serum sensitivity of approximately 89% and a specificity of 98%. Maternal serum acetylcholinesterase (AchE) levels have also been reported to be elevated with open tube defects. AChE sensitivity appears to be approximately 100% and ultimately may be a better diagnostic test than the serum AFP. Ultrasonography is an imaging technique of high sensitivity—approximately 100% in high-risk pregnancies referred for confirmation—and in many centers it is used to further evaluate women with elevated serum levels of AFP.

The optimal management of the child with a myelomeningocele should begin before birth. Although further confirmation is necessary, there are early reports of endoscopic fetal surgery at 24 and 30 weeks of gestation attempting to cover the open spinal lesion with a maternal skin graft. These reports suggest a decreased need for postnatal ventriculoperitoneal shunt placement. Delivery by

Table 3 NEUROLOGICAL DEFICITS WITH MYELOMENINGOCELES[a]

Lesion level	Disability
Above L3	Paraplegia, complete
	Nonambulatory
	Bladder and rectal dysfunction
L4 and below	Intact hip flexion and adduction
	Ambulatory with aids, braces
	Bladder and rectal dysfunction
S1 and below	Intact foot dorsiflexors, partial hip flexors and knee extensors
	Ambulatory with aids
	Bladder and rectal dysfunction
S3 and below	Normal lower extremity motor function
	Saddle anesthesia
	Variable bladder and rectal dysfunction

[a] Adapted from Menkes, J. H., and Sarnat, H. B. (2000). *Child Neurology*, 6th ed. Lippincott Williams & Wilkins. Philadelphia.

elective cesarean section prior to the onset of labor is believed to minimize mechanical pressure and trauma to the spinal cord and to minimize neurological deficits. In a pivotal study of 160 infants with myelomeningoceles, those delivered by elective cesarean section prior to the onset of labor showed better motor function than those delivered by cesarean section after the onset of labor or those delivered vaginally.

After birth, the management of a child with a myelomeningocele requires early and aggressive intervention and a multidisciplinary approach. In the neonatal period, closure of the open defect is usually performed within 24–48 hr. Hydrocephalus needs to be identified and surgically treated early. Bladder dysfunction and urinary incontinence may be a significant problem, and the prevention of genitourinary tract infections frequently requires regular intermittent catheterization and prophylactic antibacterial drugs. Congenital orthopedic defects may be significant, requiring early intervention. After the neonatal period, coordinated multidisciplinary clinics for children with spinal defects provide optimal outpatient care for a chronic disorder that requires the attention of multiple medical and surgical specialists. The long-term outcome of children born with myelomeningocele has improved greatly. In one study, 53% were community ambulators and 58% attended normal school and were grade appropriate.

—*Thomas K. Koch*

Figure 3
Newborn infant with a large thoracolumbar myelomeningocele. Note the neural plate-like structure in the midline of the lesion.

See also–Anencephaly; Brain Development, Normal Postnatal; Central Nervous System Malformations; Diastematomyelia; Myelomeningocele; Nervous System, Neuroembryology of; Vertebrate Nervous System, Development of

Further Reading

Bruner, J. P., Tulipan, N., and Paschall, R. L. (1999). Fetal surgery for myelomeningocele and the incidence of shunt-dependent hydrocephalus. *J. Am. Med. Assoc.* **282,** 1819–1825.

Canadian Task Force on the Periodic Health Examination (1994). Periodic health examination, 1994 update 3. Primary and secondary prevention of neural tube defects. *Can. Med. Assoc. J.* **151,** 159.

Dias, M. S., and Pang, D. (1995). Split cord malformations. *Neurosurg. Clin. North Am.* **6,** 339–358.

DiPietro, M. A. (1993). The conus medullaris: Normal US findings throughout childhood. *Radiology* **188,** 149–153.

Hammock, M. K., Milhorat, T. H., and Baron, I. S. (1976). Normal pressure hydrocephalus in patients with myelomeningocele. *Dev. Med. Child Neurol. Suppl.* **37,** 55–68.

Hemphill, M., Freeman, J. M., and Martinez, C. R. (1982). A new, treatable source of recurrent meningitis: Basioccipital meningocele. *Pediatrics* **70,** 941–943.

Herman, J. M., McLone, D. G., and Storrs, B. B. (1993). Analysis of 153 patients with myelomeningocele or spinal lipoma reoperated upon for a tethered cord. Presentation, management and outcome. *Pediatr. Neurosurg.* **19,** 243–249.

Holmes, L. B. (1994). Spina bifida: Anticonvulsants and other maternal influences. *CIBA Foundation Symp.* **181,** 232–238.

Kriss, V. M., and Desai, N. S. (1998). Occult spinal dysraphism in neonates: Assessment of high-risk cutaneous stigmata on sonography. *Am. J. Roentgenol.* **171,** 1687–1692.

Loft, A. G., Hogdall, E., Larsen, S. O., *et al.* (1993). A comparison of amniotic fluid alpha-fetoprotein and acetylcholinesterase in the prenatal diagnosis of open neural tube defects and anterior abdominal wall defects. *Prenatal Diagn.* **13,** 93–109.

Lorber, J. (1961). Systematic ventriculographic studies in infants born with meningomyelocele and encephalocele. *Arch. Dis. Child* **36,** 381.

Luthy, D. A., Wardinsky, T., and Shurtleff, D. B. (1991). Cesarean section before the onset of labor and subsequent motor function in infants with meningomyelocele diagnosed antenatally. *N. Engl. J. Med.* **324,** 662–666.

McKusick, V. A. (1994). *Mendelian Inheritance in Man: A Catalog of Human Genes and Genetic Disorders,* 11th ed. Johns Hopkins Univ. Press, Baltimore.

McLone, D. G., and La Marca, F. (1997). The tethered cord syndrome: Diagnosis, significance, and management. *Semin. Pediatr. Neurol.* **14,** 192–208.

Miller, A., Guille, J. T., and Bowen, J. R. (1993). Evaluation and treatment of diastematomyelia. *J. Bone Jt. Surg. Am.* **75,** 1308–1317.

Naidich, T. P., McLone, D. G., and Harwood-Nash, D. C. (1983). Spinal dysraphism. In *Modern Neuroradiology: Computed Tomography of the Spine and Spinal Cord* (T. H. Newton and G. Potts, Eds.), pp. 299–353. Clavedel, San Anselmo, CA.

Steinbok, P., Irvine, B., and Cochrane, D. D. (1992). Long-term outcome and complications of children born with meningomyelocele. *Childs Nervous Syst.* **8,** 92–96.

Van Allen, M. I., Kalousek, D. K., and Chernoff, G. F. (1993). Evidence for multi-site closure of the neural tube in humans. *Am. J. Med. Genet.* **47,** 723–743.

Yen, I. H., Khoury, M. J., and Erickson, J. D. (1991). The changing epidemiology of neural tube defects—United States, 1968–1989. *Am. J. Dis. Child* **146,** 857–861.

Neuroacanthocytosis

Encyclopedia of the Neurological Sciences
Copyright 2003, Elsevier Science (USA). All rights reserved.

NEUROACANTHOCYTOSIS is a rare hereditary disorder with both neurological and hematological (blood cell) abnormalities. This combination of a blood–brain disorder suggests that a general cell membrane defect underlies all elements of the condition. Acanthocytes are abnormal red blood cells that have a spiny appearance under the microscope. Neuroacanthocytosis is a familial condition with autosomal dominant, recessive, or even X-linked inheritance. Cases have been genetically linked to abnormalities in chromosome 9q21. The condition causes a variety of involuntary movements, including chorea, tics, dystonia, and parkinsonism. Patients can also develop self-mutilatory behavior in which they bite themselves and cause body injury. Weakness, termed amyotrophy, and loss of deep tendon reflexes also occur. One of the most distinguishing features of neuroacanthocytosis is eating dystonia due to facial and tongue contortions that expel food from the mouth by involuntary tongue protrusion. Involuntary vocalizations such as grunts, sniffs, and guttural sounds also occur, and patients have altered walking. Although the mechanism of acanthocyte formation in the red blood cells is unknown, abnormal protein:fatty acid ratios and, in some cases, abnormal red blood cell surface antigens have been found in this condition.

Neuroacanthocytosis has been suggested to represent a biochemical disorder of calcium-based or other cellular membrane channels similar to several other unusual neurological disorders, including the periodic ataxias and some of the paroxysmal dyskinesias. Acanthocytes are seen on a fresh blood smear in most patients, but the red blood cells may require special incubation techniques to show the acanthocyte pattern. Neuroimaging studies, including computerized tomography or magnetic resonance imaging, of the brain may demonstrate atrophy or shrinkage of the cerebral cortex or the deeper brain region known as the caudate nucleus. Positron emission tomography studies suggest that the neuro-chemical system involving dopamine is altered, and reduced brain activity and receptor protein density in the caudate and the other basal gangliar nucleus known as the putamen have been documented. There is no known treatment for the underlying disorder, but the symptoms of chorea and other hyperkinesias usually involve the use of dopamine-blocking agents in the form of neuroleptics (haloperidol and fluphe-nazine) or dopamine-depleting drugs (reserpine or tetrabenazine). With disease progression, most care is supportive, and a dementia with memory deficits and impulsive, poor judgment predominates. Although progression is variable, death usually occurs within 15 years of diagnosis.

—*Christopher G. Goetz*

See also–Movement Disorders, Overview

Further Reading

Kartsounis, L. D., and Hardie, R. J. (1996). The pattern of cognitive impairment in neuroacanthocytosis. *Arch. Neurol.* **53,** 77–80.

Kutcher, J. S., Kahn, M. J., Andersson, H. C., *et al.* (1999). Neuroacanthocytosis masquerading as Huntington's disease. *J. Neuroimaging* **9,** 187–189.

Rubio, U. P., Danek, A., and Stone, C. (1997). Chorea-acanthocytosis: Genetic link to chromosome 9q21. *Am. J. Hum. Genet.* **61,** 899–908.

Stacy, M., and Jankovic, J. (1995). Rare movement disorders associated with metabolic and neurodegenerative diseases. In *Movement and Allied Disorders of Childhood* (M. M. Robertson and V. Eapen, Eds.), pp. 177–198. Wiley, Chichester, UK.

Neurobehavioral Disorders

see individual entries; e.g., Attention Deficit Disorder; Autism; Hyperactivity

Neurocardiogenic Syncope

Encyclopedia of the Neurological Sciences
Copyright 2003, Elsevier Science (USA). All rights reserved.

THE TERM neurocardiogenic syncope (also referred to as vasovagal or neurally mediated syncope) refers to episodes of a transient centrally mediated hypotension and bradycardia that can ultimately lead to loss of consciousness. The medical term for fainting, "syncope" is derived from the Greek term *synkoptein*, which is usually translated as "to cut short."

Neurocardiogenic syncope can have a fairly diverse presentation ranging from a "common faint" to quite sudden dramatic loss of consciousness similar to Stokes–Adams attacks or aborted sudden death. Frequently, affected individuals demonstrate no observable underlying structural heart disease or alterations in the cardiac conducting system.

Until relatively recently, patients suffering from recurrent unexplained syncope were subjected to a long series of tedious, expensive, and all too often unrewarding evaluations that were routinely ordered in an attempt to disclose a potential etiology. Often, this would include ambulatory electrocardiography, electroencephalography, exercise tolerance testing, glucose tolerance testing, as well as computed axial tomography and/or magnetic resonance scans of the brain. Not infrequently, cardiac catheterization and electrophysiological testing were also performed. However, historically, despite this extensive series of examinations (often costing up to $16,000 per patient), a probable cause of syncope was elaborated in less than 40% of cases. This represents a cost of approximately $800 million per year spent on the diagnosis of syncope in the United States alone. A study by Linzer *et al.* found that the degree of functional impairment experienced by patients with recurrent unexplained syncope is not dissimilar to that seen with chronic debilitating diseases such as rheumatoid arthritis. Recurrent syncope places the patient at risk for bodily trauma from falls, whereas syncope during driving can imperil the life of the patient and others as well. A single syncopal episode in an elderly patient can produce injury profound enough to require nursing home placement at a tremendous cost to the patient, the family, and society in general.

In the past, many investigators believed that many syncopal events might be due to transient episodes of altered autonomic tone producing profound hypo-tension and bradycardia. However, it was not until relatively recently that there existed an effective modality for reproducing the syncopal event and confirming the diagnosis. At the same time, much of the pathophysiology of these disorders remained an enigma due to the relative inability to observe and make recordings during spontaneous events.

By the mid-1980s, a team of investigators in London postulated that an individual's predisposition to episodes of neurocardiogenic hypotension could be uncovered by the use of a strong orthostatic stimulus such as the effects of gravity produced by strong prolonged upright posture. Since the landmark study by Kenny *et al.* in 1986, numerous centers throughout the world have found that head-upright tilt table testing (HUTT) is a safe and effective means of revealing a patient's predisposition to neurocardiogenic syncope. At the same time, the ability to provoke these episodes in the controlled laboratory setting has provided a tremendous opportunity to directly observe the events that occur during syncope, thereby greatly enhancing our knowledge of these disorders.

This entry discusses the current understanding of the pathophysiology of neurocardiogenic syncope, its clinical characteristics, the use of tilt table testing in diagnosis, and potential therapeutic options that can be employed.

PATHOPHYSIOLOGY

Fainting is one of the oldest of medical maladies and has been the subject of medical inquiry for centuries. Reports on fainting appear in the works of Hippocrates, Galen, and Maimonides. In the late 1700s, the British physician John Hunter observed that some patients would faint quite easily during phlebotomy and speculated that excessive vasodilation may be the cause. A century later, Foster reported that fainting was often accompanied by profound bradycardia. Sir Thomas Lewis reported in 1932 that although the administration of atropine could prevent bradycardia during syncope, hypotension and loss of consciousness would nonetheless occur, and he used the term "vasovagal" to describe the event.

By the 1940s, there was a growing interest in the body's responses to sudden changes in position, focusing on the body's responses to the stresses produced by air flight and the effects of the microgravity environment experienced during space travel. It was during this period that HUTT was first used to provide a controlled method by which the body's responses to incremental changes in position could be carefully measured. These observations revealed that in the normal person approximately 25–30% of the circulating blood volume is in the thorax. The assumption of upright posture produces a gravity-mediated downward displacement of approximately 300–800 cc of blood (approximately 6–8 ml/kg) to the abdomen and the lower extremities. This relatively rapid decline in central blood volume results in a decrease in venous return to the heart. This produces less stretch on the cardiac mechanoreceptors (or C fibers) located in the basilar portions of the right and left ventricles, decreasing their frequency of afferent impulse formation because of less stretch on the receptors. These mechanoreceptors communicate directly to the dorsal vagal nucleus of the brainstem, and as the afferent output decreases a reflex increase in sympathetic output occurs, with a resultant increase in chronotrophy and peripheral vascular resistance. At the same time, there is input from mechanically sensitive afferents from the aorta (vagus nerve) and the carotid sinus (glossopharyngeal nerve), which are stimulated when stretched by increases in blood pressure. The increased afferent activity that occurs with an increase in blood pressure inhibits sympathetic outflow and slows heart rate, with the reverse happening when the pressure decreases. Therefore, the normal response to upright posture is an increase in heart rate and diastolic pressure and no change or only a slight decrease in systolic blood pressure.

Although the exact sequence of events that occurs in syncope is incompletely understood, a basic understanding of the process is emerging. One hypothesis holds that in predisposed individuals, there is a failure of the peripheral vasculature to contract properly during upright posture. Peripheral venous pooling is excessive, resulting in a relatively sudden decline in central venous return to the heart. The reason for the failure of peripheral vascular tone to increase has yet to be elucidated. The abrupt decline in ventricular filling causes an exceptionally vigorous ventricular contraction that is so forceful that it results in the activation of a large number of mechanoreceptors that would normally respond only to mechanical stretch. The resultant influx of neural traffic to the brainstem (particularly to the nucleus tractus solitarii) seems to mimic the information it would receive during hypertension. This then causes a rapid decrease in sympathetic output with an apparently "paradoxical" reflex decrease in both heart rate and peripheral vascular resistance. Echocardiographic observations have been forwarded to support this view.

Several investigators have expressed doubts at the aforementioned theories. Classic episodes of neurocardiogenic syncope have been provoked during HUTT in patients who have undergone cardiac transplantation, a condition in which the heart is supposedly denervated. Other researchers have pointed out that mechanoreceptors are also present in the atria as well as the pulmonary arteries and have suggested that sudden C-fiber activation in any area may provoke neurocardiogenic hypotension in predisposed individuals.

Sir Thomas Lewis is credited with first using the term "vasovagal syncope" to describe this sequence of events. However, it is now believed that although parasympathetically mediated bradycardia can occur, the most important action is that of peripheral vasodilation leading to hypotension. Most investigators now believe that this occurs as a result of sympathetic withdrawal from skeletal muscle, along with a possible increase in beta-receptor responsiveness or a decrease in alpha-receptor responsiveness.

Recently, the central nervous system's (CNS) role in the pathogenesis of syncope has been explored. These investigations have mainly employed hemorrhagic shock as an animal model because a relatively small but sudden loss of volume during acute hemorrhage can cause an abrupt, paradoxical sympathoinhibition with resultant profound hypotension and bradycardia. At the time of this "paradoxical" hypotension and bradycardia, these animal studies have shown an increase in adrenal nerve activity as well as a decrease in renal sympathetic nerve activity.

A series of insightful animal studies have demonstrated that sudden alterations in the CNS levels of serotonin (5-hydroxytryptamine) appear to trigger sympathetic withdrawal. It has also been shown that the sequence can be effectively blocked by the central serotonin-blocking agent methysergide. Abboud reported that the brainstem administration of serotonin results in inhibition of renal sympathetic nerve activity, excitation of adrenal sympathetic nerve activity, and hypotension. These observations support the concept that a precipitous surge in central serotonin levels contributes to the mechanism of sympathetic withdrawal seen during neurocardiogenic syncope. This idea has been supported by preliminary observations from clinical trials using serotonin reuptake inhibitors in the treatment of patients with refractory neurocardiogenic syncope. The principle action of the serotonin reuptake inhibitors is to block the presynaptic reuptake of serotonin, thereby leading to a progressive increase in intrasynaptic serotonin concentrations. This progressive buildup in intrasynaptic serotonin results in a postsynaptic downregulation in receptor density. It has been postulated that this downregulation in postsynaptic receptor density could have the same

results as could be achieved by directly blocking receptor sites (as with methysergide), namely blunting the responses to sudden fluctuations in serotonin levels. To date, clinical trials with fluoxetine hydrochloride, sertraline hydrochloride, and paroxetine in patients with otherwise refractory neurocardiogenic syncope have demonstrated a response rate of approximately 60%.

It is thought that there are at least seven major groups of serotonin receptors, each of which contains a number of subreceptors. These various receptors and subreceptors exert control over a number of activities in different areas of the brain, with some receptor subtypes having direct antagonistic effects on others (an organizational system similar to that seen with prostaglandins). Current studies are attempting to better determine the actual serotonin receptor subtypes associated with the events surrounding neurocardiogenic syncope and to develop pharmacological agents directed specifically toward these receptors.

A second group of central mediating substances that has been investigated is the endogenous opiates. In studies using the aforementioned hemorrhagic shock model, it has been observed that inhibition of renal sympathetic activity occurs when opiate receptor antagonists are administered. Other studies have demonstrated that the intracisternal injection of the opiate receptor antagonist nafoxone counteracts the vasodilation produced with acute hemorrhagic shock. Ferguson reported that the intravenous administration of nafoxone in humans augments the cardiopulmonary baroreflex excitation of sympathetic activity, whereas Perna *et al.* found that plasma ß endorphin levels increase in patients with tilt-induced syncope. However, these findings have been tempered by the fact that opiate antagonists have not proven to be successful in preventing neurocardiogenic syncope brought on by lower body negative pressure.

A number of recent investigations have examined the potential role of the cerebral vasculature in the production of syncope. It had been thought that autoregulation of cerebral blood flow occurred solely at the local level in response to arterial blood pressure changes. Arteriolar vasodilation would occur in response to a decrease in systemic blood pressure and vasoconstriction would take place as the systemic pressure increased, with both processes acting to maintain cerebral blood flow at a constant level. However, by using transcranial Doppler ultrasonography (TCD), a number of investigators have demonstrated that cerebral vasoconstriction, instead of the predicted vasodilation, occurs during head-upright, tilt-induced syncope in the presence of profound hypotension. These apparently paradoxical alterations in cerebral vascular resistance (i.e., arteriolar vasoconstriction) could potentially play a role in the pathogenesis of neurocardiogenic syncope. Indeed, several reports suggest that syncope may occur because of cerebral vasoconstriction alone in the absence of systemic hypotension.

CLINICAL ASPECTS

Neurocardiogenic syncope may have a wide and variant number of presentations. There appear to be a number of potential triggers that all may lead to neurocardiogenically mediated hypotension and bradycardia. Upright posture, the postprandial state, sodium restriction, diuretic use, vigorous exercise in warm environments, or extremely stressful situations are but a few of the possible triggers to consider. Drugs such as alcohol can easily increase a person's predisposition to these episodes. It also appears that rapid change in time zone during air travel (jet lag) may also facilitate these tendencies.

There appear to be three distinct phases to a syncopal event: the presyncopal event or aura, the actual loss of consciousness, and the postsyncopal period. Patients with typical vasovagal syncope will usually report a long history of recurrent events extending from adolescence. The situations that cause syncope in these patients are those that provoke fear, anxiety, and emotional distress (activities that result in increased sympathetic stimulation). Interestingly, this appears similar to the responses seen in some animal species that are placed in a situation in which neither fight or flight are possible. Animals presented with these conditions experience sudden loss of sympathetic tone, leading to bradycardia, vasodilation, and cessation of motion, often referred to as "playing dead."

The aura phase is characterized by warning phenomena that can include diaphoresis, weakness, dizziness, vertigo, epigastric discomfort, palpitations, visual blurring, headache, nausea, and vomiting. The aura may last between one second and several minutes, a period that will give a perceptive patient the opportunity to lie down and abort (or at least diminish the severity of) a syncopal event. Studies categorizing the frequency of various presyncopal symptoms in patients have reported that the most common are dizziness (44%), sweating (33%), blurred vision (33%), nausea (29%), and abdominal discomfort (11%).

The patient often does not remember the actual loss of consciousness. People who witness an event will usually say that the patient looked ashen or pale in color, with diaphoresis, cold skin, and dilated pupils. On rare occasions there may be urinary or even fecal incontinence. Occasionally, patients may demonstrate tonic and/or clonic movements. When convulsions occur during syncope, this means that the cerebral anoxic threshold has been reached, thereby allowing an acute "decortication" to occur. The convulsive movements usually (but not always) begin after the loss of consciousness with tonic contractions of extended legs, arms extended in adduction, and a backward elevated throw of the head (opisthotonos). These differ from the decreasing frequency and increasing amplitude sequence that is usually characteristic of epileptic grand mal seizures. The loss of consciousness is often short, with quick recovery and minimal, if any, postictal confusion. While awake immediately following syncope the patient may experience nausea, headache, nervousness, or dizziness.

It is important to realize, however, that although the preceding description applies to the majority of patients with neurocardiogenic syncope, a substantial minority may have atypical presentations. Many older patients seem not to sense the decrease in blood pressure and thus give no history of any prodrome at all. These elderly patients describe "drop attacks" similar to those seen with atrioventricular heart block. This lack of warning of impending syncope can lead to serious injury due to trauma suffered during a fall (a particular problem in older patients, for whom falls are a leading cause of morbidity and mortality). Although in most patients the loss of consciousness during syncope is brief, there are occasional patients in whom unconsciousness may be prolonged (up to 15 min). In some patients the convulsive movements seen during neurocardiogenic syncope may be surprisingly similar to those seen during a typical epileptic seizure, and rare patients may experience urinary or rectal incontinence as well as a significant postictal period.

It should be kept in mind that many patients suffering from neurocardiogenic syncope can experience a decrease in blood pressure that although not sufficient to produce a full loss of consciousness, will nonetheless be sufficient to cause symptoms of cerebral hypoperfusion. These hypotensive events will be experienced as lightheadedness, vertigo, dizziness, and a sense of disequilibrium. In some elderly patients, episodes of neurocardiogenic hypotension may produce focal neurological deficits that can appear remarkably similar to transient ischemic attacks manifested by disorientation, dysarthria, and even visual field cuts.

There appears to be very rare cases in which severe neurocardiogenic syncope may be lethal. Periods of asystole during neurocardiogenic syncope have been documented to be 73 sec in duration and there are two reports of polymorphic ventricular tachycardia induced during tilt table testing. Episodes of near fatal cardiac asystole have been reported during tilt table testing. Engle and other investigators have proposed that periods of prolonged asystole can degenerate into asystole and death, particularly if this occurs in the setting of preexisting coronary artery disease, myocardial dysfunction, or aortic stenosis.

Some investigators have reported an increased incidence of neuropsychiatric disturbances in patients suffering from documented recurrent neurocardiogenic syncope. These disorders include somatization disorder, major depression, and panic disorders. In addition, patients with neurocardiogenic syncope have a high incidence of chronic vascular and migraine headaches.

The ability to clinically reproduce the syncopal or near syncopal event is often important in establishing a diagnosis and, occasionally, assessing the responses to therapy. In the past, a number of various maneuvers were used to trigger neurocardiogenic responses, including carotid sinus massage, Valsalva maneuver, hyperventilation, and ocular compression. However, these were mostly discarded for use in neurocardiogenic syncope because of relatively low sensitivities and poor correlation with clinical events.

HUTT

As alluded to previously, physiologists had employed tilt table testing for a number of years as a method of applying a controlled orthostatic stress whereby the body's responses to changes in posture could be studied. In the course of these investigations, some researchers incidentally noted that occasional subjects suddenly became hypotensive and faint. However, it was not until the report of Kenny *et al.* in 1986 that HUTT was first employed as a diagnostic modality for provoking hypotension and bradycardia in patients with unexplained syncope.

Several factors have added support to the concept that a head-upright, tilt-induced syncope closely parallels its occurrence spontaneously. First, both tilt-induced and spontaneous syncopal episodes are accompanied by similar prodromal sensations, including lightheadedness, pallor, diaphoresis, nausea, and loss of postural tone. Second, the sequences of observed changes in heart rate and blood pressure seen in both spontaneous and tilt-induced syncope are quite similar. Lastly, the changes in serum catecholamines and other hormones are essentially the same during spontaneous and tilt-induced episodes. Indeed, in regard to the last observation, the finding that catecholamine levels increase sharply before the onset of syncope has led a number of investigators to use a concomitant isoproterenol infusion in conjunction with head-upright tilt as a method for increasing the sensitivity of the test. At the same time, concerns have been expressed that injudicious use of isoproterenol may achieve higher levels of sensitivity at the expense of specificity. Recently, the use of a number of other potential provocative agents has been explored, including edrophonium, nitroglycerin, and adenosine triphosphate.

When HUTT is employed alone (in the absence of provocative stimuli outside of gravity), it is able to distinguish between symptomatic patients and asymptomatic control subjects with a level of accuracy that is comparable to other clinically useful testing procedures. The bulk of the published literature has reported that HUTT without pharmacological provocation at angles between 60 and 80° has a specificity of approximately 90%. When tilt table testing is used in conjunction with low-dose isoproterenol infusions, most of the available literature has shown a specificity of between 80 and 90%.

The exact sensitivity of HUTT is difficult to assess because there is no real gold standard against which it can be compared. In considering sensitivity, one must bear in mind that the aforementioned physiological alterations that culminate in syncope could potentially occur in most people if a sufficient orthostatic stress was continued over a long enough period. Thus, tilt table testing does not identify a fixed "pathology"; rather, it is employed to illustrate an enhanced susceptibility to what is an otherwise normal response. In many aspects, this is used in much the same way that electrophysiological testing is employed in the evaluation of syncopal patients with known structural heart disease. Some authors have suggested that the actual sensitivity of tilt table testing may be underestimated in that otherwise normal controls who have a false-positive test may in reality have an enhanced susceptibility to clinical syncopal events. Recent reports have given validity to this concept because false-positive controls have later experienced spontaneous syncopal events.

By the very nature of the processes that it seeks to evaluate, it is obvious that tilt table testing is not perfect. It is difficult to duplicate the exact clinical and environmental factors that may culminate in syncope in every patient. One must also remember that orthostatic stress is only one of a number of stimuli known to provoke autonomic decompensation and syncope in predisposed individuals. These limitations notwithstanding, tilt table testing can be used to confirm the physician's clinical suspicions and serves as an aid in establishing a diagnosis in a patient whose history and physical findings have not yielded a cause for recurrent syncope. As alluded to previously, use of tilt table testing is similar in respect to the way electrophysiological testing is used, namely to determine whether a particular substrate is present. When employed in the evaluation of syncope, the results of either test are not taken alone but rather they are assessed in the context of the history, physical findings, and any other relevant data to arrive at a reasonable diagnosis and treatment plan. It is wise to remember that unless one is lucky enough to record the physiological alterations that occur during a spontaneous episode, the diagnosis of syncope is virtually always a "leap of faith" in regard to extrapolation of any test to the patient's actual condition. These patients frequently will serve as a reminder that medicine is an interface of both art and science. Recently, the American College of Cardiology released an expert consensus statement on the use of tilt table testing in assessing syncope, which is recommended for further information.

USES AND RESPONSES TO UPRIGHT TILT TABLE TESTING

In the course of investigations into recurrent syncope and other autonomic disorders using tilt table testing, a variety of different response patterns have been noted. At the same time, it has become clear that there are a number of possible uses for tilt table testing other than evaluation of recurrent syncope.

In respect to the various response patterns seen, we have found it useful to define five broad groups (Fig. 1). One must remember that any attempt to clarify natural phenomena is, by its very nature,

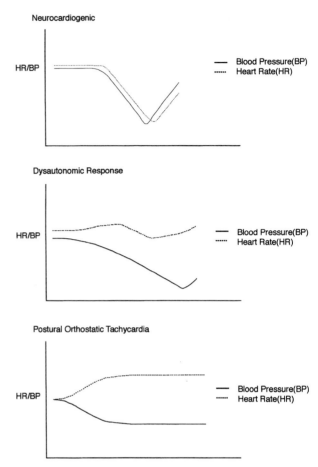

Figure 1
Classic neurocardiogenic (vasovagal) response. Blood pressure (BP) and heart rate (HR) patterns observed in abnormal response to tilt table testing. POTS, postural orthostatic tachycardia syndrome.

arbitrary and that these categories are still in a state of evaluation.

The first response pattern is that of the neurocardiogenic (or vasovagal) episode. This is characterized by an abrupt decrease in systemic pressure that is usually followed by a decrease in heart rate. Clinically, in between episodes, these patients are for the most part normal with few other complaints. They tend to be younger, often in the adolescent age group, although we have occasionally seen elderly patients with this pattern. In small children, episodes of breath holding may induce neurocardiogenic episodes. Although many patients are adolescents, we have seen a number of preadolescent patients as well. These patients have a somewhat "hypersensitive" autonomic system and syncope can be provoked by a number of different vagal stimuli, such as carotid sinus stimulation, mechanical stimulation of the esophagus and rectum, micturition, and cough. Occasionally, these patients will exhibit long episodes of asystole both clinically and during tilt table testing. These patients have been referred to as having "malignant" neurocardiogenic syncope that may mimic or lead to sudden death. Periodically, these patients will have profound asystole and hypotension provoked during tilt table testing that requires prolonged resuscitative efforts to terminate.

The second response pattern is termed dysautonomic. Here, one sees a gradual parallel decline in both systolic and diastolic blood pressure that culminates in loss of consciousness. Heart rate either remains unchanged or increases slightly. These patients tend to be older adults, although we have seen the pattern in young people and even in children. In contrast to the pure neurocardiogenic group, syncope is but one of a number of complaints and the patients rarely feel well. They often demonstrate other signs of autonomic dysfunction, such as abnormal sweating and thermoregulatory control. Dysautonomic patients can demonstrate a pattern of supine hypertension in conjunction with upright hypotension and syncope.

Ours and other centers have recently elaborated on a third important subgroup that is referred to as the postural orthostatic tachycardia syndrome (POTS). Patients in this subgroup demonstrate an increase of at least 30 beats per minute (or a maximum rate of 120 beats per minute) within the first 10 min of upright tilt, usually without profound hypotension. It is currently postulated that these individuals suffer from a milder form of autonomic dysfunction in which the major defect is the inability to regulate peripheral vascular resistance appropriately, which is then offset by an excessive increase in heart rate. Occasionally, these patients have been diagnosed with "inappropriate" sinus tachycardia. Following radio frequency catheter modification of the sinoatrial node, these patients have experienced a resolution of their tachycardia but have been left with a profound degree of orthostatic hypotension. The most common complaints of the patient with POTS (other than palpitations) are extreme fatigue and exercise intolerance. There is an emerging body of evidence showing that there may be a considerable degree of overlap between POTS and chronic fatigue syndrome.

The response of the cerebrovasculature to neurocardiogenic syncope has been investigated using TCD. A number of studies have demonstrated that during tilt-induced neurocardiogenic syncope, cerebral arteriolar constriction occurs concomitant with, or occasionally preceded by, the onset of hypotension and loss of consciousness. Recently, several investigators have reported cases of tilt-induced syncope due to cerebral vasoconstriction alone (as observed using TCD) in the absence of systemic hypotension. This pattern is called cerebral syncope.

The final response pattern is referred to as the psychogenic or psychosomatic response. In these patients, head-upright tilt induces a syncopal episode that occurs in the absence of any demonstrable change in heart rate, blood pressure, encephalographic tracing, or transcranial blood flow pattern. These individuals frequently suffer from severe underlying psychiatric disorders that can range from conversion reactions to anxiety disorders and major depression. It is important to remember that patients suffering from conversion reactions are not conceivably aware of their actions. Studies of patients with psychogenic syncope have shown that a significant number are young people, especially young women, who are frequently the victims of sexual abuse. Psychogenic syncope in an abused child or adolescent may be a "cry for help" that needs to be recognized. These cries should not be uttered in vain.

THERAPY OF NEUROCARDIOGENIC SYNCOPE

A detailed discussion of all the potential treatment options that can be employed in patients with neurocardiogenic syncope is beyond the scope of this entry. However, some basic principles will be outlined. The therapeutic approach to the patient with neurocardiogenic syncope needs to be individualized to meet the requirements of each patient because the severity of the condition varies markedly. In many cases, syncope is infrequent and occurs only under unusual conditions. Therefore, first and foremost, the physician needs to educate the patient and their family as to the nature of the problem and to avoid any identifiable precipitating factors, such as extreme heat, dehydration, and alcohol consumption. In addition, one must determine if the hypotensive event is primary in nature or due to some potentially reversible cause, such as pharmacological agents, anemia, or other disease processes (Table 1). Patients who experience prodromal symptoms should be advised to lie down at their onset. In many younger patients, simply increasing salt and fluid intake may be sufficient to prevent further syncopal episodes. Biofeedback has been

Table 1 PHARMACOLOGICAL AGENTS THAT MAY CAUSE OR WORSEN ORTHOSTATIC INTOLERANCE

Angiotensin-converting enzyme inhibitors
Alpha receptor blockers
Calcium channel blockers
Beta blockers
Phenothiazines
Tricyclic antidepressants
Bromocriptine
Ethanol
Opiates
Diuretics
Hydralazine
Ganglionic blocking agents
Nitrates
Sildenafil citrate
Monoamine oxidase inhibitors

quite helpful in some patients, particularly in those whose neurocardiogenic syncope has well-defined psychological triggers. Moderate exercise is often useful in maintaining venous return by strengthening the skeletal muscle pump. Some have advocated "tilt training" with prolonged periods of standing to desensitize people to the neurocardiogenic reflex. Sleeping with the head of the bed propped up may reduce the excessive loss of sodium water during recumbency at night in patients with dysautonomic syndromes.

Despite these efforts, there will still be patients in whom sudden unpredictable syncopal episodes continue to occur with little or no warning. In these individuals, particularly those who have suffered injury due to trauma suffered as a consequence of syncope, some form of prophylactic therapy is usually required.

A variety of pharmacotherapies have been used to prevent neurocardiogenic syncope (Table 2). Perhaps the most widely used are the ß1-adrenergic blocking agents. It has been postulated that these agents act in their negative inotropic actions, which retard the aforementioned increase in inotropy and result in rapid mechanoreceptor activation. Although there are numerous reports of efficacy of these agents in preventing syncope, there are also reports that these agents may actually exacerbate syncope (prosyncope). Some investigators have found that beta-blocker therapy tends to be more effective in patients who required isoproterenol provocation during upright tilt than in patients whose syncope was provoked during passive tilt alone. Transdermal

scopolamine was reported to be effective; however, it is poorly tolerated. Disopyramide has also been reported to be effective, possibly via its negative inotropic, anticholinergic, and direct vasoconstrictive effects. However, Morillo et al. questioned the usefulness of the agent.

The agent that we employ frequently in the therapy of these patients is hydrofludrocortisone. A mineral corticoid, it promotes sodium retention and volume expansion. However, its more important action seems to be a peripheral vasoconstrictive effect that occurs because of increased alpha-receptor sensitivity to endogenous catecholamines. The agent seems to be particularly effective in young people and in patients with dysautonomic response on tilt table testing (who do not have a concomitant supine hypertension).

Because the major problem with these disorders is often a failure of the peripheral vasculature to respond properly, it seems logical to use a peripheral vasoconstrictor in therapy. A number of different agents have been employed with varying degrees of success. The methylated xanthine theophylline causes peripheral adenosine receptor blockade, thereby increasing the peripheral vascular tone. However, tolerance of the dosages required to be effective is often poor. Pseudoephedrine has been used with success in treating children, although in our experience there is a significant problem with tachyphylaxis. Oral dextroamphetamine was found to be effective in the treatment of severely refractory patients with neurocardiogenic syncope. The agent methylphenidate is a safe, effective, and well-tolerated agent in treating otherwise refractory individuals. However, concerns about abuse and dependency have limited its use.

These problems have recently been addressed by the release of the alpha-stimulant agent midodrine hydrochloride. Similar to methylphenidate, it does not cross the blood–brain barrier and thus is free of central nervous system stimulant effects. It has a relatively short half-life and must be given three times a day. It works particularly well if given in combination with fludrocortisone. A recent double-blind study by Ward et al. demonstrated midodrine's effectiveness in treating neurocardiogenic syncope.

Following initial anecdotal observations, we explored the use of the serotonin reuptake inhibitors for the treatment of patients unresponsive to or intolerant of other forms of therapy. In separate studies, both fluoxetine hydrochloride and sertraline hydrochloride produced a beneficial response in 50%

Table 2 TREATMENT OPTIONS[a]

Therapy	Method or dose	Common problems
Head-up tilt of bed	45° head-up tilt of bed (often will need footboard)	Hypotension; sliding off bed; leg cramps
Elastic support hose	Require at least 30–40 mmHg ankle counter pressure; work best if waist high	Uncomfortable; hot; difficult to get on
Diet	Fluid intake of 2–2.5 liters/day; Na$^+$ intake of 150–250 mEq/day	Supine hypertension; peripheral edema
Exercise	Aerobic exercise (mild) may aid venous return; water exercise particularly helpful	May lower blood pressure if done too vigorously
Fludrocortisone	Begin at 0.1–0.2 mg/day; may work up to doses not exceeding 1.0 mg/day	Hypokalemia; hypomagnesemia; peripheral edema; weight gain; congestive heart failure
Methylphenidate	5–10 mg po tid given with meals; give last dose before 6 pm	Agitation; tremor; insomnia; supine hypertension
Midodrine	2.5–10 mg every 2–4 hr; may use up to 40 mg/day	Nausea; supine hypertension
Clonidine	0.1–0.3 mg po bid or patches placed 1/week	Dry mouth; bradycardia hypotension
Yohimbine	8 mg po bid tid	Diarrhea; anxiety; nervousness
Ephedrine sulfate	12.5–25 mg po tid	Tachycardia; tremor; supine hypertension
Fluoxetine	10–20 mg po qd (requires 4–6 weeks of therapy)	Nausea; anorexia; diarrhea
Erythropoietin	4000 IU^2 twice a week	Requires injections; burning at site; increase hematocrit; CVA
Pindolol	2.5–5.0 mg po bid to tid	Hypotension; congestive heart failure; bradycardia
Desmopressin	An analog of vasopressin used as a nasal spray	Hyponatremia

[a] Abbreviations used: Bid, twice daily; po, by mouth; tid, three times a day; qd, every day.

of otherwise untreatable patients. Later, the more selective agent, nefazodone hydrochloride, was reported to have a 60% response rate. It is thought that these agents, by preventing rapid shifts in central serotonin levels, blunt the cerebral triggers for sympathetic withdrawal, thereby reducing the susceptibility to neurocardiogenic events.

This concept was recently confirmed when Girolamo et al. reported the results of a randomized, double-blind, placebo-controlled trial of paroxetine in neurocardiogenic syncope. During a 25-month follow-up period, the recurrence rate of syncope was 18% in the paroxetine group versus 53% in the placebo group ($p < 0.0001$). Coincidentally, recently observations have suggested that the β-adrenergic blocking agents may have significant effects on cerebral serotonergic activity, an action that may contribute to their therapeutic actions.

Perhaps no aspect of therapy has generated more controversy than the role of permanent cardiac pacing in the management of patients with refractory neurocardiogenic syncope whose episodes are associated with significant bradycardia or asystole. It is estimated that at least 25% of patients with neurocardiogenic syncope have only modest bradycardia and would not be candidates for pacing.

The initial investigations of the use of permanent cardiac pacing in the treatment of recurrent neuro-cardiogenic syncope found that VVI pacing is not only ineffective but also can actually worsen the syncope because of retrograde ventriculoatrial conduction. In the original article by Kenny et al. on the use of tilt table testing in neurocardiogenic syncope, they also reported that dual-chamber cardiac pacing could be an effective therapy. Fitzpatrick et al. explored the use of tilt table testing together with temporary dual-chamber pacing, finding that DVI pacing with hysteresis could stop 85% of tilt-induced syncopes. Samoil et al. later independently confirmed these findings. However, Sra et al. reported on the effects of temporary pacing in 22 patients: twenty with sinus rhythm during atrioventricular sequential pacing and two with atrial fibrillation who had ventricular pacing only. Each of these patients had an initial positive baseline tilt table test and then underwent a repeat test with pacing (at a rate 20% above the resting supine heart rate). One patient remained asymptomatic, one had dizziness without hypotension, and 15 had presyncope instead of full syncope, whereas only five patients had full syncope. Later, each patient underwent repeat tilt table testing while receiving pharmacological therapy. Metoprolol was effective in 10 of 22 patients, theophylline in three of 13 patients, and disopyramide in six of nine patients. The investigators then concluded that pacing was of little benefit. Interestingly, other investigators have concluded that the same data support the idea that pacing could offer a clear benefit in some patients.

Petersen *et al.* presented data on the long-term effects of permanent cardiac pacing in patients with severe recurrent syncope as well as reproducible tilt-induced neurocardiogenic syncope (with a significant bradycardic component). Thirty-seven patients who underwent permanent dual-chamber pacemaker implantation were followed for 50 ± 24 months. Approximately 85% displayed a marked reduction in symptoms, whereas 27% had complete elimination of symptoms. The overall frequency of syncopal episodes decreased from 137 to 11 per year. Of interest was the observation that the clinical factors that predicted a good outcome with pacing included a younger age (56 years as opposed to 76 years) and the absence of a recognizable prodrome before spontaneous events.

The American Vasovagal Pacemaker Study was the first randomized trial to test whether permanent pacing with rate-drop responsiveness would reduce the likelihood of syncope in patients with frequent vasovagal syncope. Fifty-four patients were randomized to pacemaker placement or medical therapy. Ultimately, six of 27 paced patients had syncope compared to 19 of 27 patients treated medically. This corresponds to a 91% reduction in risk of developing syncope in the paced group. Additional trials evaluating the role of pacing in syncope are under way.

In any discussion of pacing, it should be kept in mind that in neurocardiogenic syncope, the decrease in blood pressure usually precedes the decrease in heart rate, and syncope could be well under way before bradycardia becomes manifest. Therefore, pacing onset as determined by rate criteria alone may represent "too little, too late." The development of a pacemaker sensor technology that allows for either a direct or indirect measurement of blood pressure could potentially allow for the onset of pacing at a point much earlier in the syncopal process. In regard to current devices, the units that we favor are those that incorporate a surge hysteresis function, such that the device is triggered by the development of a low heart rate and then reacts by pacing at a rate sufficient to prevent (or at least retard) the development of hypotension.

We do not consider pacing as first-line therapy because many patients respond to medical therapy. However, in patients with a significant bradycardic component and who have proven drug refractory, permanent pacing may greatly prolong the time from the onset of symptoms to syncope and may sometimes prevent loss of consciousness altogether. Especially in those individuals who experience little or no warning prior to syncope (i.e., drop attacks), cardiac pacing may elicit a more gradual decline in pressure that can be perceived by the patient as a prodrome and may allow him or her to take evasive actions, such as lying down, at its onset.

An assessment of the efficacy of any form of therapy can be made by observing a reduction or elimination of the patient's clinical episodes or by noting the response on repeat tilt table testing. Although several studies have reported that the absence of syncope during repeat upright tilt table testing after the initiation of therapy (in those with an initial positive response) appears to predict the absence of clinical responses over the long term, others have questioned the usefulness of follow-up testing.

The wide range of possible therapeutic options available can easily leave the practitioner confused as to how to start a rational treatment process. In many ways, treatment is currently more an art than a science. Initially, the physician must take into account any associated diseases or conditions that exist in the patient to ensure the compatibility of therapy. Next, the patient's response during upright tilt table testing must be examined.

In young people who display either a classic neurocardiogenic or dysautonomic response, we tend to start with fludrocortisone and continue it for at least 2 or 3 weeks. If there is no response or insufficient response, we will usually add a second agent. Although beta blockers are often useful in those individuals with a classic neurocardiogenic or POTS response, they tend to be less useful or even counterproductive in patients with a dysautonomic pattern. In many patients, we use the serotonin reuptake inhibitors as second-tier therapy. In severe refractory patients, we add a third agent, most often a vasoconstrictor such as methylphenidate or midodrine; these two agents are often quite useful in dysautonomic or POTS patients. We have observed that a low-dose combination of several agents that work by different mechanisms is often more effective and better tolerated than are large doses of a single agent. The practitioner should also be mindful of the fact that the body is a dynamic substrate that can change over time, and therapies may also have to be modified over time to keep abreast of these changes.

Many adolescents with neurocardiogenic syncope will "grow out of it" after several years. In these groups, the major thrust should be to get them through the symptomatic period and then to discontinue therapy. For this reason, we are most reluctant to employ permanent cardiac pacing in young people and do so only if we believe the patient's life is at risk. Therapy can be safely stopped in 80% of adolescents with neurocardiogenic syncope after two years. This is not true of older patients, whose therapy may have to be continued indefinitely.

SUMMARY

The disorder that is currently known as neurocardiogenic syncope is a complex disturbance in autonomic nervous system function with a wide variety of clinical manifestations. Tilt table testing has emerged as a valuable tool for inducing periods of neurocardiogenic syncope, not only allowing for confirmation of the diagnosis but also permitting more detailed observations of the pathophysiology of the condition. More detailed studies are necessary to better understand this common malady and to establish better diagnostic and therapeutic modalities.

—*Blair Grubb, Yousuf Kanjwal, and Daniel J. Kosinski*

See also—Falls and Drops; Syncope; Vertigo and Dizziness

Further Reading

Abboud, F. M. (1993). Neurocardiogenic syncope. *N. Engl. J. Med.* **328**, 1117–1119.

Benarroch, E. (1993). The central autonomic network: Functional organization, dysfunction, and perspective. *Mayo Clinic Proc.* **68**, 988–1001.

Benditt, D., Ferguson, D., Grubb, B. P., *et al.* (1996). Tilt-table testing for assessing syncope. *J. Am. Coll. Cardiol.* **28**, 263–275.

Calkins, H. (1999). Pharmacologic approaches to therapy for vasovagal syncope. *Am. J. Cardiol.* **84**, 200–250.

DiGirolamo, E., DiIorio, C., Satabtini, P., *et al.* (1994). Effects of paroxetine hydrochloride, a selective serotonin reuptake inhibitor, on refractory vasovagal syncope: A randomized, double blind, placebo controlled study. *J. Am. Coll. Cardiol.* **24**, 490–494.

Engle, G. L. (1978). Psychologic stress, vasodepressor (vasovagal) syncope, and sudden death. *Ann. Intern. Med.* **89**, 403–412.

Grubb, B. P. (1998). Neurocardiogenic syncope. In *Syncope: Mechanisms and Management* (B. P. Grubb and B. Olshansky, Eds.), pp. 78–106. Futura, Armonk, NY.

Grubb, B. P. (1998). Dysautonomic syncope. In *Syncope: Mechanisms and Management* (B. P. Grubb and B. Olshansky, Eds.). Futura, Armonk, NY.

Grubb, B. P., and Karas, B. J. (1998). The potential role of serotonin in the pathogenesis of neurocardiogenic syncope and related autonomic disturbances. *J. Intervent. Cardiac Electrophysiol.* **2**, 325–332.

Grubb, B. P., and Kosinski, D. (1997). Tilt table testing: Concepts and limitations. *PACE* **20**, 781–787.

Grubb, B. P., Gerard, G., Roush, K., *et al.* (1991). Differentiation of convulsive syncope and epilepsy with head up tilt table testing. *Ann. Intern. Med.* **115**, 871–876.

Grubb, B. P., Wolfe, D., Gerard, G., *et al.* (1992). Syncope and seizures of psychogenic origin: Identification with upright tilt-table testing. *Clin. Cardiol.* **15**, 839–842.

Grubb, B. P., Gerard, G., Roush, K., *et al.* (1992). Cerebral vasoconstriction during head upright tilt-induced vasovagal syncope: A paradoxic and unexpected response. *Circulation* **84**, 1157–1164.

Grubb, B. P., Kosinski, D., Temesy-Armos, P., *et al.* (1997). Responses of normal subjects during upright tilt-table testing with and without low dose isoproterenol infusion. *PACE.*

Grubb, B. P., Samoil, D., Kosinski, D., *et al.* (1998). Cerebral syncope: Loss of consciousness associated with cerebral vasoconstriction in the absence of systemic hypotension. *PACE* **21**, 652–658.

Kosinski, D., Grubb, B. P., and Temesy-Armos, P. (1995). Pathophysiologic aspects of neurocardiogenic syncope. *PACE* **18**, 716–721.

Lurie, K., and Benditt, D. (1996). Syncope and the autonomic nervous system. *J. Cardiovasc. Electrophysiol.* **7**, 760–776.

Mahanondal, N., Bhuripanya, K., Kangkagate, C., *et al.* (1995). Randomized placebo controlled trial of oral atenolol in patients with unexplained syncope and positive upright tilt-table test results. *Am. Heart J.* **130**, 1250–1253.

McGrady, A., and Bernal, G. (1986). Relaxation-based treatment of stress induced syncope. *J. Behav. Ther. Exp. Psychiatry* **17**, 23–27.

Morillo, C. A., Leitch, J. W., Yee, R., *et al.* (1993). A placebo controlled trial of disopyramide for neurally mediated syncope induced by head up tilt. *J. Am. Coll. Cardiol.* **22**, 1843–1848.

Perna, G. P., Ficola, U., Salvatori, P., *et al.* (1990). Increase of plasma beta-endorphins in vasodepressor syncope. *Am. J. Cardiol.* **65**, 929–930.

Rea, R., and Thomas, M. (1993). Neural control mechanisms and vasovagal syncope. *J. Cardiovasc. Electrophysiol.* **4**, 587–595.

Sheldon, R. (1999). Role of pacing in the treatment of vasovagal syncope. *Am. J. Cardiol.* **84**, 26Q–32Q.

Wallin, B. G., and Sundlaff, G. (1982). Sympathetic outflow to the muscles during vasovagal syncope. *J. Autonomous Nervous Syst.* **6**, 284–291.

Ward, C. R., Gray, J. C., Gilroy, J. J., *et al.* (1998). Midodrine: A role in the management of neurocardiogenic syncope. *Heart* **79**, 45–49.

Wayne, H. H. (1961). Syncope: Physiologic considerations and an analysis of the clinical characteristics in 510 patients. *Am. J. Med.* **30**, 418–438.

Wieling, W., and Lieshout, T. (1993). Maintenance of postural normotension in humans. In *Clinical Autonomic Disorders* (P. Low, Ed.), pp. 63–67. Little, Brown, Boston.

Neurocysticercosis

Encyclopedia of the Neurological Sciences
Copyright 2003, Elsevier Science (USA). All rights reserved.

HUMAN cysticercosis is invasion of tissue by the larval stage (a cysticercus) of the pork tapeworm *Taenia solium.* Cysticerci of the central nervous system (CNS) are the most common of neurological parasitic infections in the world, rendering cysticercosis one of the most frequent neurological disorders. Cysticercosis is endemic to Latin America, Asia, and Africa, but it is also commonly seen in eastern and southern Europe and in countries with high rates of immigration from endemic areas, such as the United States. In many neurological centers in Latin America, for instance, cysticercosis is the most frequent cause of late-onset epilepsy, adult hydrocephalus, and chronic meningitis. Cysticercosis is far more common in areas with domestic breeding of pork and poor human waste sanitation.

TRANSMISSION

Cysticercus is the embryo of the intestinal cestode *T. solium.* Both humans and pigs may act as intermediate hosts for cysticercus, but humans are the only host of the adult intestinal cestode and are required to complete the life cycle. Intestinal tapeworms are acquired by eating undercooked pork containing cysticerci, whereas human cysticercosis is a fecal–oral infection caused by ingestion of eggs excreted in the feces of a human tapeworm carrier. Eggs ingested by either humans or swine lose their coat in the gastrointestinal tract, pass into the blood circulation, and are carried to the brain, muscles, or eye, where the cysticerci will evolve. Should humans eat insufficiently cooked pork meat infected with cysticerci, the embryo evaginates from the cyst within the initial portion of the small intestine and firmly attaches to the intestinal wall. In a few weeks, this embryo, initially measuring 1 or 2 mm, will grow to a very large worm 2 or 3 m long. The adult tapeworm will produce, on a daily basis, mature, fertile proglottides, thus closing the life cycle of the parasite. A single carrier of *T. solium* can become an asymptomatic, continuous, and extensive source of cysticercosis for the community. Taenia eggs are infective even after long exposures in the environment.

PATHOGENESIS AND CLINICAL FEATURES

Onset of symptoms may be from 1 to 35 years after exposure. Symptoms result from migration or arrest of larval forms in host tissues, particularly the CNS. In approximately 35% of neurocysticercosis cases, a single parasite occurs in brain parenchyma. In these patients, the infection may go unnoticed or the patient may experience occasional seizures. In another 35% of cases, various parasites infect the brain parenchyma producing, in addition to epilepsy, a protean mixture of neurological and psychiatric manifestations related to the topography of lesions. The number of parasites may vary from few to countless, and the clinical picture may include a discrete symptom, such as headache or dizziness, or a life-threatening disorder such as cysticercotic encephalitis. Lesions may be scattered throughout the brain parenchyma, or cysts may grow in clusters, producing a clinical picture similar to that of a brain tumor. The stage of the infection can also vary from live cysticerci to quiescent infections with calcified granulomas, in which the parasites degenerated and the active cyst was replaced by a remnant granuloma. In other patients (approximately 30% of cases), cysticerci lodge in the meninges, producing chronic arachnoiditis whose clinical manifestations are due to widespread inflammation, vasculitis, hydrocephalus, and multiple small brain infarctions. This is the most severe form of neurocysticercosis. The inflammatory process is distributed throughout the nervous system by cerebrospinal fluid (CSF) circulation, and the meningitis may outlast effective destruction of the parasites. The prognosis in these cases is closely related with the intensity of the inflammatory process in the subarachnoid space. Sustained results on periodic CSF analysis of more than 100 mg/dl of protein and more than 50 cells/mm^3 may produce hydrocephalus secondary to inflammatory and fibrotic obstruction to CSF absorption. Ventricular or eye cysticercosis is rare ($<1\%$ of cases).

DIAGNOSIS

Diagnosis is by neuroimaging studies—computed tomography or magnetic resonance. Immunodiagnostic tests in serum are unreliable, mostly due to a high percentage of false positives (approximately 30%) among healthy subjects from endemic areas and also to a high percentage of false negatives (approximately 30%) in serum from neurocysticercosis (NCC) patients with radiological evidence of few parasites. Serological tests are negative in subjects with brain granuloma as permanent sequelae of a previous cysticercus, and they are frequently negative in patients with solitary CNS lesions.

TREATMENT

Treatment and prognosis of NCC largely depend on the location of parasites. Parenchymal cysticercosis is usually cured with cysticidal drugs, whereas meningeal cysticercosis frequently requires additional measures: shunting for hydrocephalus and chronic antiinflammatory treatment. Two cysticidal drugs, albendazole and praziquantel, are highly effective for the elimination of parasites. Effectiveness (i.e., elimination of parenchymal cysticerci as seen by imaging studies) is approximately 80% for albendazole, 70% for praziquantel, and more than 90% with the sequential use of both drugs. Two drugs are used in succession in cases of partial results with a single drug. Albendazole is given in doses of 15 mg/kg/day twice daily for 1 week. Oral prednisone (50 mg) given each morning during the first 4 days of treatment prevents most reactions to the sudden destruction of the parasites, such as headache and vomiting. Praziquantel is given in a single-day schedule with a total dose of 75 mg/kg divided in three doses of 25 mg administered at 2-hr intervals (e.g., at 7, 9, and 11 AM) accompanied by a normal breakfast (which increases the plasma levels of praziquantel). Prednisone (50 mg) is also administered 3 hr after the last dose and again each morning for the next 3 days. Therapeutic efficacy is evaluated by neuroimaging study 1 or 2 months after treatment. In cases of partial results with one drug, the other cysticidal drug can be administered. In cases of chronic meningitis, the inflammatory process is the therapeutic priority. A useful scheme is 50 mg of prednisone three times a week (e.g., Monday, Wednesday, and Friday). Therapeutic response is evaluated by periodic analysis of CSF. In refractory cases, steroid treatment should be continued for several years.

PREVENTION

Cysticercosis is an eradicable disease. Proper sanitary implementation, adequate disposal of human feces, compulsory search and treatment of *T. solium* carriers, and community education about the life cycle of the parasite are highly effective preventive measures.

—*Julio Sotelo*

See also–Parasites and Neurological Diseases, Overview; Tropical Neurology

Further Reading

Martinez, H. R., Rangel-Guerra, R., Arredondo-Estrada, J. H., et al. (1995). Medical and surgical treatment in neurocysticercosis: A magnetic resonance study of 161 cases. *J. Neurol. Sci.* **130**, 25–34.
Pitella, J. E. H. (1997). Neurocysticercosis. *Brain Pathol.* 7, 681–693.
Salgado, P., Rojas, R., and Sotelo, J. (1997). Cysticercosis: Clinical classification based on imaging studies. *Arch. Intern. Med.* **157**, 1991–1997.
Sotelo, J. (1997). Treatment of brain cysticercosis. *Surg. Neurol.* 48, 110–112.
Sotelo, J., and Jung, H. (1998). Pharmacokinetic optimisation of the treatment of neurocysticercosis. *Clin. Pharmacokinetics* 34(6), 503–515.

Neuroepidemiology, Overview

Encyclopedia of the Neurological Sciences
Copyright 2003, Elsevier Science (USA). All rights reserved.

A USEFUL definition of epidemiology is "the science of the natural history of diseases." This concept is based on the original roots of the word: *logos*, from *legein*, to study; *epi*, (what is) on; and *demos*, the people. In epidemiology, the unit of study is a person affected with the disorder in view. Therefore, diagnosis is the essential prerequisite. Thus, the neurologist must be an essential part of any inquiry into neuroepidemiology, the epidemiology of neurological diseases. The content and uses of epidemiology are described in Fig. 1.

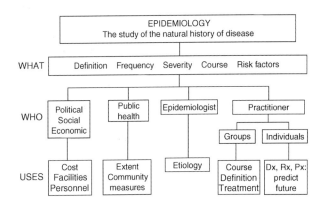

Figure 1
Epidemiology: content and uses. Dx, diagnosis; Rx, treatment; Px, prognosis (adapted with permission from Kurtzke, 1977).

After diagnosis, the most important question is the frequency of a disorder. Much of this type of information has been based on case series from clinic and hospital databases. However, whether taken as numerator alone (case series) or compared with all admissions (relative frequency), the difficulty with such data is that one has little assurance that what has been included is representative of the total population. Such case material needs to be referenced to its proper denominator, its true source: the finite population at risk.

POPULATION-BASED RATES

Ratios of cases to population, together with the period to which they refer, make up population-based rates. Those commonly measured are the incidence rate, mortality rate, and the so-called prevalence rate. They are ordinarily expressed in unit-population values. For example, 10 cases among a community of 20,000 represents a rate of 50 per 100,000 population or 0.5 per 1000.

The incidence or attack rate is the number of new cases of a disease beginning in a unit of time in a population. This is usually given as an annual incidence rate in cases per 100,000 population per year. The date of onset of clinical symptoms ordinarily is the time of accession, although occasionally the date of first diagnosis is used.

The mortality or death rate is the number of deaths in a population in a period with a particular disease as the underlying cause, such as an annual death rate per 100,000 population. The case:fatality ratio is the proportion of those affected who die from the disease.

The (point) prevalence rate is more properly called a ratio, but it refers to the number of those affected at one time within the community, again expressed per unit of population. If there is no change in case:fatality ratios over time and no change in annual incidence rates (and no migration), then the average annual incidence rate multiplied by the average duration of illness in years equals the prevalence rate.

When the numerator and denominator for a rate refer to an entire community, their quotient is a crude rate for all ages. When both terms of the ratio are delimited by age or sex, these are age-specific or sex-specific rates. Such rates for consecutive age groups, from birth to the oldest group of each sex, provide the best description of a disease within a community.

In comparing rates between two communities for an age-related disorder (such as stroke or epilepsy),

there may be differences in crude rates solely because of differences in the age distributions of the denominator populations. This can be avoided by comparing only the individual age-specific rates between the two, but this rapidly becomes unwieldy. Methods exist for adjusting the crude rates for all ages to permit such comparisons. One such method involves taking for each community each age-specific rate and multiplying it by the proportion of a "standard" population that the same age group represents. The sum of all such products provides an age-adjusted (to a standard) rate, or a rate for all ages adjusted to a standard population. One common standard in the United States is its population for a given census year.

The major focus of this entry is morbidity rates (i.e., incidence and prevalence). Space precludes attention to survey methods, risk factors, treatment comparisons, and statistical methods, which are all intrinsic aspects of epidemiology. Regarding neuroepidemiology per se, the material presented here is but a sketch of some highlights for a few major diseases chosen to represent the field.

CEREBROVASCULAR DISEASE

Stroke is the third leading cause of death in the United States, with an estimated 731,000 strokes occurring annually. Cerebrovascular disease has been variably classified, particularly in mortality data. The general usage in morbidity studies has been to subdivide into subarachnoid hemorrhage (SAH), intracerebral hemorrhage, thrombotic acute brain infarct or cerebral thrombosis, cerebral embolism, and ill-defined acute cerebrovascular accident. Cerebral arteriosclerosis and transient ischemic attacks are generally not included within the corpus of acute cerebrovascular disease or stroke.

Mortality Rates

International death rates from stroke have varied notably. In Europe, rates in Finland and Scotland have been considerably higher than those of neighboring countries. Overall, there has been a modest male excess. Average annual age-adjusted death rates in the 1950s were near 100 per 100,000 population, and in many countries rates decreased to approximately 70 per 100,000 in the 1980s.

In the United States, the annual age-adjusted death rates decreased dramatically during the past century, and the decline continues. The adjusted rate for 1991 was 27 per 100,000. The decline in adjusted rates was regular during this entire period for white males and females. The much higher rates for nonwhites, approximately 90% of whom are black, followed a similar but steeper time course for women, but nonwhite males seemed to start their decline only in the 1950s. The rates by sex and race seemed to be converging by the mid-1980s.

There were similar decreasing rates for other countries between 1950 and 1990, including Australia, New Zealand, Canada, and all of western Europe. There was an even more dramatic decrease in Japan. Reported rates actually increased for Czechoslovakia, Yugoslavia, Bulgaria, Poland, and Hungary.

Morbidity Rates

Like the temporal trends in stroke death rates, stroke incidence has decreased over time. In Rochester, Minnesota, the age-adjusted average annual incidence rate declined from 200 per 100,000 population during 1945–1954 to 107 per 100,000 during 1975–1979. The decrease was for both sexes, for essentially all ages, and for both cerebral hemorrhage and thrombosis; it was not found for SAH, however. An extension of the Rochester data through 1989 showed a 13% increase in total stroke incidence rates for 1985–1989 versus 1975–1979. The most prominent increases were in those 85 years or older.

Average annual age-adjusted incidence rates by sex show a modest, but possibly increasing, male excess. In recent years, the annual incidence rate in Europe and North America has been approximately 120–150 per 100,000 population, and in Asia the rate may now be similar. The age-adjusted rate for Taiwan from 1986 to 1990 was 145 per 100,000. In Hiroshima–Nagasaki, Japan, the age-adjusted incidence rate for cerebral infarction declined from 490 per 100,000 in 1972 to 120 per 100,000 in 1988. Equivalent rates for cerebral hemorrhage approximated 100 and 20 per 100,000, respectively. Rates in the United States for blacks remain higher than those for whites. Incidence rates increase sharply with age, but not quite as steeply as death rates increase. Including undefined acute cerebrovascular disease, approximately 80–90% of all strokes in whites are thromboembolic cerebral infarcts, with 10–15% being cerebral hemorrhage and 4–8% SAH. In Asia, the incidence of cerebral hemorrhage is approximately twice as high as in the West, but there has never been any definite excess of SAH in the Orient.

The World Health Organization's Multinational Monitoring of Trends and Determinants in Cardiovascular Disease project is an ongoing study to compare incidence and mortality of stroke across multinational populations adjusted to a "world standard population." The highest incidence rates of 18 countries were in men in Kuopio, Finland, and Novosibirsk, Russia (adjusted incidence rates >300 per 100,000). In women, the highest rates were in Novosibirsk. The highest rates for both sexes were more than three times higher than those in Friuli, Italy. In half the populations, the stroke incidence rates were twice as high in men as in women.

Prevalence rates in the early 1980s were approximately 600 per 100,0000 in the West and 900 per 100,000 in Asia. Reports from Rochester, Minnesota, have shown an increase in the average point-prevalence rate with time.

PRIMARY NEOPLASMS

In clinical experience, approximately 85% of primary CNS tumors are intracranial and 15% are intraspinal. For the brain, the major groupings are the gliomas (40–50%, of which approximately half are glioblastoma multiforme) and the meningiomas (15–20%). Pituitary adenomas plus neurilemmomas, especially acoustic, comprise another 15–20%. The most common spinal cord tumors are neurofibroma and meningioma, followed by ependymoma and angioma.

Morbidity Rates

Average annual incidence rates for primary brain tumors in the more complete surveys have ranges mostly between 10 and 15 per 100,000 population, including pituitary tumor rates at 1 or 2 per 100,000. Primary tumors of the spinal cord are recorded at approximately 1 per 100,000, and in one survey peripheral nerve tumors had a rate of 1.5 per 100,000.

From the late 1960s to the late 1980s, the incidence of primary brain neoplasms at least doubled in the United States. The Connecticut Tumor Registry showed a dramatic increase in incidence for age groups 65–84 years, with relatively stable rates for younger cohorts. For the 65- to 69-year-old age group, the incidence rate increased from 18.4 per 100,000 in 1965–1969 to 28.3 per 100,000 in 1985–1988. Similar increases were seen in older age groups. There was a trend of increasing incidence for the 1890 and 1900 birth cohorts, implying a cohort effect. Whether these cohort trends are due to environmental effects or improved diagnostic capabilities is not clear. Using a retrospective analysis, Desmeules and colleagues argued in 1992 that only 20% of the recent increased incidence in brain tumor cases can be accounted for by improved diagnostic capabilities of computed tomography and magnetic resonance imaging scans.

In all but the Rochester, Minnesota, studies, age-specific incidence rates for glioblastoma multiforme have shown a sharp peak at approximately age 60. In the Rochester study, the rate continued to rise with increasing age, especially when tumors first diagnosed at postmortem were included. The male preponderance inferred from death data is seen for the entire glioma group, particularly for glioblastoma. There is also evidence suggesting an increased incidence of glioblastoma in recent years. There was a similar trend in malignant brain tumor death rates over time.

In meningioma, the age-specific rates continue to increase with age to the oldest group, and there is a female preponderance. The suspected excess in blacks was borne out in a survey in the Los Angeles County Cancer Surveillance program. Age-adjusted average annual incidence rates were 1.8 per 100,000 male and 2.7 per 100,000 female. Respective non-Hispanic white rates were 1.8 and 2.5 per 100,000; for blacks, they were 2.5 and 3.6 per 100,000.

CONVULSIVE DISORDERS

Classification of convulsive disorders or the epilepsies has varied considerably. For epidemiological purposes, they have been classified as epilepsy, isolated (single) seizures, febrile convulsions, and acute symptomatic seizures. Patients categorized as having epilepsy are usually subdivided into idiopathic (or primary) and secondary. Secondary epilepsy has a presumed cause, with recurrent seizures after recovery from the acute insult. All partial-focal or focal-onset seizures are by definition secondary. Absence seizures are almost always primary or idiopathic, as are many grand mal seizures.

Morbidity Rates

Average annual incidence rates as of 1980 were approximately 20–70 per 100,000 population per year. There was a slight male excess, which averaged approximately 1.2 to 1.0, and almost a 2 to 1 black:white ratio. Later surveys showed annual rates

of 24 per 100,000 for Kuopio, Finland; 34 per 100,000 for Västerbotten, Sweden; and 52 per 100,000 for Rochester, Minnesota. There seems to be support for a high incidence of epilepsy in Central and South America, as suggested by their death and prevalence rates. Elsewhere in the West, an expected range of annual incidence is 30–60 per 100,000 with a reasonable general estimate of 50 per 100,000. With concomitant prevalence rates, an average duration of active seizure disorder could then be calculated to be approximately 13 years.

Age-specific incidence rates vary by type of seizure. Myoclonic seizures were the major type diagnosed during the first year of life; they were also the most common in the 1- to 4-year-old age group but rarely occurred after 5 years of age. Absence (petit mal) seizures peaked in the 1- to 4-year-old age group and did not begin in patients older than 20. Complex partial (psychomotor) and generalized tonic–clonic (grand mal) seizures both had fairly consistent incidence rates of 5–15 per 100,000 in patients aged 5–60 after low maxima at ages 1–4; for patients 70 years old and older, the rates of both were sharply higher.

Point prevalence rates for epilepsy are available from a number of community surveys. Rates from industrialized countries range between 300 and 900 per 100,000 population. An overall estimate of the point prevalence of active epilepsy may be taken as approximately 600–700 per 100,000 population. Prevalence rates from developing countries have tended to be more variable, with a range between 300 and 5700 per 100,000. Differing methodological approaches and definitions of epilepsy help to explain some of this variation. Temporally, prevalence rates have tended to increase in recent years in several surveys. Males and blacks have higher rates than females and whites.

DEMENTIA

Dementia is an acquired decline in memory and other cognitive functions sufficient to affect daily life in an alert patient. Alzheimer's disease (DAT) is the most common cause of dementia, representing approximately 70% of cases. Current U.S. estimates show that the disorder affects approximately 3–4 million U.S. citizens with an annual cost of $67.3 billion. Vascular dementia is the next most common cause, accounting for 10–15% of cases. A small proportion of dementias are reversible and include intoxications, metabolic derangements, infections, deficiency states, and cardiopulmonary disorders. Because DAT is the most common form of dementia and the focus of most epidemiological studies on dementia, we focus on DAT here.

Morbidity Rates

Utilizing incidence rates from eight recent Occidental surveys, an unweighted average rate for each age group was age adjusted to the 1960 U.S. population. The overall adjusted rate for DAT was 102 per 100,000, all ages. If this figure represents 70% of all dementias, then other dementias would provide an incidence of approximately 45 per 100,000. Unlike the marked increased data for prevalence since the 1980s, the incidence data for dementia appear to be fairly constant.

Predicting the lifetime risk for dementia is difficult due to the steep increase in incidence of dementia with increasing age and the competing risk of death due to other causes. Cumulative incidence estimates for dementia overestimate the risk when the likelihood of an alternative cause of mortality is high. Seshandri *et al.* used the Framingham cohort to estimate the lifetime risk of all-cause dementia and DAT. At age 65, the remaining lifetime risk for developing DAT for men was 6.3%, and it was 12% for women. This doubling of risk for women is due to the fact that women live longer and experience a longer period of risk. Other studies have reported cumulative incidence rates ranging between 21 and 49.6%.

Breteler *et al.* summarized the prevalence rates for DAT from five European studies and four U.S. studies, yielding an unweighted average adjusted rate of 338 per 100,000 population, all ages. If this comprises 70% of all prevalent cases of dementia, then one could estimate a rate of 145 per 100,000 for non-Alzheimer's dementia. Rounding these figures gives 350 for DAT plus 150 for other dementias, or a total of 500 per 100,000. With a rounded incidence of 150 per 100,000, this would provide an estimated duration of life of slightly more than 3 years after onset.

Jorm *et al.* performed a meta-analysis of the prevalence studies of dementia from 1945 to 1985. For moderate and severe dementia, the estimated rates in the analysis were 2800 per 100,000 for the 70- to 74-year-old group and 5600 for the 75- to 79-year-old age group. Rates for dementia doubled every 5.1 years of age. Furthermore, age-specific rates were not different between men and women.

PARKINSON'S DISEASE

Parkinsonism is a clinical syndrome characterized by tremor, bradykinesia, rigidity, and abnormal gait and posture. This syndrome has several causes, including drugs, toxins, and head trauma, but the most common variety is Parkinson's disease. The etiology of Parkinson's disease (PD) is unknown but believed to be related to multiple environmental and genetic influences.

Morbidity Rates

Few studies have evaluated the incidence of parkinsonism. A recent study described the incidence of parkinsonism and its specific types among residents of Rochester, Minnesota, between 1976 and 1990. The average annual incidence of parkinsonism was 26 per 100,000 population, all ages, or 139 per 100,000 person-years in the age group 65–99 years. The incidence increased steeply with age and PD was the most common type of parkinsonism (42%). Men had a higher incidence than women (all ages) for all types of parkinsonism except drug-induced.

Community-based surveys during the past 20 years have reported prevalence rates of PD ranging from 31 per 100,000 in Benghazi, Libya, to 244 per 100,000 in Alberta, Canada. Incidence rates for the same period have been between 5 and 20 per 100,000.

OVERVIEW OF NEUROLOGICAL DISORDERS

Morbidity and mortality rates for neurological disorders provide us with data regarding their numerical impact on the community. Tables 1 and 2 represent the best estimates for incidence and prevalence available. All rates have been rounded and, unless otherwise specified, refer to the population of all ages, even though the disorder favors one gender or age group. Furthermore, in view of the limited sources of data, the information is largely applicable to sites of economically developed countries, predominantly those of Europe and North America. Therefore, these rates should be regarded as a general guide only; they may vary considerably in different populations. The rates are cited as cases per 100,000 population. For cases in a given community or country, these rates are multiplied by the appropriate population factor. For example, in a population of 200 million with a rate of 10 per 100,000, there would be 20,000 cases.

Regarding morbidity, for the 63 disorders in Table 1, the combined average annual incidence rates equal more than 2600 per 100,000 population or 2.6%.

Table 1   APPROXIMATE AVERAGE ANNUAL INCIDENCE RATES (PER 100,000 POPULATION), ALL AGES[a]

Disorder	Rate	Disorder	Rate
Herpes zoster	400	Cerebral palsy	9.0
Migraine	250	Congenital malformations of central nervous system	7.0
Brain trauma	200	Mental retardation, severe	6.0
Other severe headache	200[b]	Mental retardation, other	6.0[b]
Acute cerebrovascular disease	150	Malignant primary brain tumor	5.0
Other head injury	150[b]	Metastatic cord tumor	5.0
Transient postconcussive syndrome	150	Tic douloureux	4.0
Lumbosacral herniated nucleus pulposus	150	Multiple sclerosis	3.0[d]
Lumbosacral pain syndrome	150[b]	Optic neuritis	3.0[d]
Dementia	150	Dorsolateral sclerosis	3.0
Neurological symptoms (with no defined disease)	75	Functional psychosis	3.0[b]
Epilepsy	50	Spinal cord injury	3.0
Febrile fits	50	Motor neuron disease	2.0
Méniére's disease	50	Down's syndrome	2.0
Mononeuropathies	40	Gullian–Barré syndrome	2.0
Polyneuropathy	40	Intracranial abscess	1.0
Transient ischemic attacks	30	Benign cord tumor	1.0
Bell's palsy	25	Cranial nerve trauma	1.0
Single seizures	20	Acute transverse myelopathy	0.8
Parkinsonism	20	All muscular dystrophies	0.7
Cervical pain syndrome	20[b]	Chronic progressive myelopathy	0.5
Persistent postconcussive syndrome	20	Polymyositis	0.5
Alcoholism	20[b]	Syringomyelia	0.4
Meningitides	15	Hereditary ataxias	0.4
Encephalitides	15	Huntington's disease	0.4
Sleep disorders[c]	15	Myasthenia gravis	0.4
Subarachnoid hermorrhage	15	Acute disseminated encephalomyelitis	0.2
Cervical herniated nucleus pulposus	15	Charcot–Marie–Tooth disease	0.2
Metastatic brain tumor	15	Spinal muscular atrophy	0.2
Peripheral nerve trauma	15	Familial spastic paraplegia	0.1
Blindness	15	Wilson's disease	0.1
Benign brain tumor	10	Malignant primary cord tumor	0.1
Deafness	10[b]	Vascular disease cord	0.1

[a] Modified and updated from Kurtzke (1982) and Kurtzke and Wallin (2000).
[b] Rate for those who should be seen by a physician competent in neurology (10% of total).
[c] Narcolepsies and hypersomnias (with sleep apnea).
[d] Rate for high-risk areas.

This includes eight disorders for which only one-tenth of the incident cases were thought to require attention by a physician competent in clinical neurology: the two vertebrogenic pain syndromes, nonmigrainous headache, nonbrain head injury, alcoholism, psychosis, nonsevere mental retardation, and deafness. Total blindness data were taken as an estimate for the proportion of all the visually impaired that should see a neurologist. Overall incidence rates are easily calculated, but here we are aiming at data likely relevant to readers. Even if we exclude all headaches, trauma, vertebrogenic pain, vision loss, deafness, and psychosis, there are still more than 1200 new cases of neurological disease each year in every 100,000 of the population—well over 1 case for every 100 people.

For the 61 disorders listed in Table 2, the point prevalence rates in like manner contain only 10% of the nonmigrainous headache, vertebrogenic pain, alcoholism, and nonbrain head injury and 20% of

Table 2   APPROXIMATE AVERAGE ANNUAL POINT PREVALENCE RATES (PER 100,000 POPULATION), ALL AGES[a]

Disorder	Rate	Disorder	Rate
Migraine	2000[b]	Dorsolateral sclerosis	30
Other severe headache	1500[b]	Peripheral nerve trauma	30
Brain trauma	800	Other head injury	30
Epilepsy	650	Acute transverse myelopathy	15
Acute cerebrovascular disease	600	Metastatic brain tumor	15
Lumbosacral pain syndrome	500[b]	Chronic progressive myelopathy	10
Alcoholism	500[b]	Optic neuritis	10
Dementia	500	Encephalitides	10
Sleep disorders[c]	300	Vascular disease spinal cord	9
Méniére's disease	300	Hereditary ataxias	8
Lumbosacral herniated nucleus pulposus	300	Syringomyelia	7
Cerebral palsy	250	Motor neuron disease	6
Parkinsonism	200	Polymyositis	6
Transient ischemic attacks	150	Progressive muscular dystrophy	6
Febrile fits	100	Malignant primary brain tumor	5
Persistent postconcussive syndrome	80	Metastatic cord tumor	5
Herpes zoster	80	Meningitides	5
Congenital malformations of central nervous system	70	Bell's palsy	5
Single seizures	60	Huntington's disease	5
Multiple sclerosis	60[d]	Charcot–Marie–Tooth disease	5
Benign brain tumor	60	Myasthenia gravis	4
Cervical pain syndrome	60[b]	Familial spastic paraplegia	3
Down's syndrome	50	Intracranial abscess	2
Subarachnoid hemorrhage	50	Cranial nerve trauma	2
Cervical herniated nucleus pulposus	50	Myotonic dystrophy	2
Transient postconcussive syndrome	50	Spinal muscular atrophy	2
Spinal cord injury	50	Guillain–Barré syndrome	1
Tic douloureux	40	Wilson's disease	1
Neurological symptoms without defined disease	40	Acute disseminated encephalomyelitis	0.6
Mononeuropathies	40	Dystonia musculorum deformans	0.3
Polyneuropathies	40		

[a] Modified and updated from Kurtzke (1982) and Kurtzke and Wallin (2000).
[b] Rate for those who should be seen by a physician competent in neurology (20% of migraine, 10% of all others).
[c] Narcolepsies and hypersomnias (with sleep apnea).
[d] Rate for high-risk areas.

migraine, but they exclude completely all mental retardation, psychosis, deafness, and blindness. The total exceeds 9700 per 100,000 population. Again, if we exclude entirely all the disorders previously mentioned, there is still a prevalence rate of approximately 3800 per 100,000 population, or 3.8% of the people who at any one time require the care of a physician competent in clinical neurology. In a U.S. population of 274.6 million (Department of Health and Human Services 2000 projected population), this means 10.4 million people are affected.

Not all neurological disorders are referred to neurologists, even in the most socioeconomically advanced countries; in many countries, the neurologist is primarily a consultant rather than the physician who manages these disorders, and in others there is an admixture. Of course, there are countries not limited to the Third World in which there is a dearth of neurologists and other specialists. However, regardless of the type of practice a given country deems appropriate for a neurologist, the patients will still exist. Therefore, the data in Tables 1 and 2 could well serve as a basis for at least a rational allocation of available resources in any country for the teaching, research, and patient care of neurological disorders.

—*Mitchell T. Wallin and John F. Kurtzke*

See also–Alzheimer's Disease, Epidemiology; Brain Injury, Traumatic: Epidemiological Issues; Central Nervous System Tumors, Epidemiology; Epidemiology, Overview; Epilepsy, Epidemiology; Multiple Sclerosis, Epidemiology; Parkinson's Disease, Epidemiology; Stroke, Epidemiology

Further Reading

Bower, J. H., Maraganore, D. M., McDonnell, S. K., *et al.* (1999). Incidence and distribution of parkinsonism in Olmsted County, Minnesota, 1976–1990. *Neurology* **52**, 1214–1220.

Breteler, M. M., Claus, J. J., van Duijn, C. M., *et al.* (1992). Epidemiology of Alzheimer's disease. *Epidemiol. Rev.* **14**, 59–82.

Brown, R. D., Whisnant, J. P., Sicks, J. D., *et al.* (1996). Stroke incidence, prevalence, and survival: Secular trends in Rochester, Minnesota, through 1989. *Stroke* **27**, 373–380.

Desmeules, M., Mikkelsen, T., and Mao, Y. (1992). Increasing incidence of primary malignant brain tumors: Influence of diagnostic methods. *J. Natl. Cancer Inst.* **84**, 442–445.

Ernst, R. L., and Hay, J. W. (1994). The US economic and social costs of Alzheimer's disease revisited. *Am. J. Public Health* **84**, 1261–1264.

Jorm, A. F., Korten, A. E., and Henderson, A. S. (1987). The prevalence of dementia: A quantitative integration of the literature. *Acta Psychiatr. Scand.* **76**, 465–479.

Klein, R. J., and Schoenborn, C. A. (2001, January). Age adjustment using the 2000 projected US population. Healthy People Statistical Notes No. 20. National Center for Health Statistics, Hyattsville, MD.

Kurtzke, J. F. (1977). Multiple sclerosis from an epidemiological viewpoint. In *Multiple Sclerosis: A Critical Conspectus* (E. J. Field, Ed.), pp. 83–142. University Park Press, Baltimore.

Kurtzke, J. F. (1982). The current neurologic burden of illness and injury in the United States. *Neurology* **32**, 1207–1214.

Kurtzke, J. F., and Wallin, M. T. (2000). Neuroepidemiology. In: Bradley, W. G., Daroff, R. B., Fenichel, G. M., and Marsden, C. D. (Eds.), *Neurology in Clinical Practice*. 3rd ed., Vol. 1, Butterworth-Heinemann, Boston, pp. 759–776.

Seshadri, S., Wolf, P. A., Beiser, A., *et al.* (1997). Lifetime risk of dementia and Alzheimer's disease. The impact of mortality on risk estimates in the Framingham Study. *Neurology* **49**, 1498–1504.

Stegmayr, B., Asplund, K., Kuulasmaa, K., *et al.* (1997). Stroke incidence and mortality correlated to stroke risk factors in the WHO MONICA Project. An ecological study of 18 populations. *Stroke* **28**, 1367–1374.

Neurofibromas
see Nerve Sheath Tumors

Neurofibromatosis

Encyclopedia of the Neurological Sciences
Copyright 2003, Elsevier Science (USA). All rights reserved.

DIAGNOSTIC criteria for both neurofibromatosis 1 (NF1) and neurofibromatosis 2 (NF2) have been proposed by the National Institutes of Health (NIH) (Table 1). Revisions of these criteria have been proposed, but use of revised criteria should be made with caution because they are not clinically or molecularly validated. When the NIH criteria are applied strictly, it is rare to find an overlap between NF1 and NF2 in a single patient. Other forms of neurofibromatosis include mosaic disease and schwannomatosis.

CLINICAL FEATURES

The major clinical manifestations of NF1 are cafe au lait macules, cutaneous neurofibromas, freckling of the axillae and groin, and Lisch nodules (Fig. 1). Other common findings are deep-seated neurofibromas, learning disabilities, scoliosis, hypertension, migraine, and disorders of growth and development (short stature and precocious or delayed puberty). Rare but potentially serious complications include malignant peripheral nerve sheath tumors (previously known as malignant schwannoma),

Table 1   DIAGNOSTIC CRITERIA FOR NF1 AND NF2[a]

The diagnostic criteria for NF1 are met in an individual if **two** or more of the following are found:
  1. Six or more cafe au lait macules of significant size
  2. Two or more neurofibromas
  3. Freckling in the axillary or inguinal regions
  4. Optic glioma
  5. Two or more Lisch nodules
  6. A distinctive osseous lesion
  7. A first-degree relative with NF1

The diagnostic criteria for NF2 are met by an individual with the following:
  1. Bilateral vestibular schwannoma
  or
  2. A first-degree relative with NF2 and either
   a. Unilateral vestibular schwannoma
   or
   b. Two of the following:
    Meningioma
    Glioma
    Schwannoma
    Characteristic cataract

[a] Adapted from Gutmann *et al.* (1997).

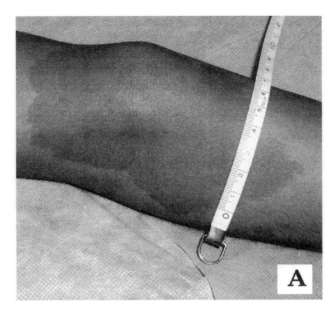

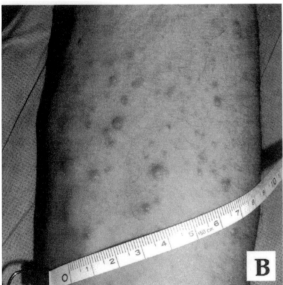

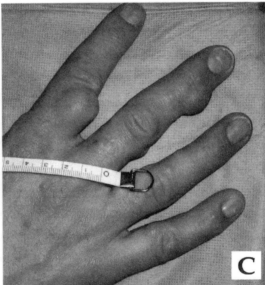

Figure 1
Typical skin findings in NF1 include (A) cafe au lait macules, (B) cutaneous neurofibromas, and (C) subcutaneous neurofibromas.

pseudoarthrosis, and pheochromocytoma. T2-weighted changes on magnetic resonance imaging scan are a common finding but alone are of little clinical significance (Fig. 2).

The defining clinical feature of NF2 is bilateral vestibular schwannoma, which is pathognomonic for the disease (Fig. 3). Initial symptoms include tinnitus, hearing, loss and balance dysfunction. Approximately half of individuals with NF2 develop meningiomas. Most such tumors are intracranial, although spinal meningioma is not uncommon. Other spinal cord tumors include nerve root schwannomas, ependymomas, and, rarely, astrocytomas. Schwannomas may develop along other cranial nerves, in the brachial and lumbar plexuses, and along peripheral nerves. The only nontumorous manifestations of NF2 are ocular, including posterior subcapsular lens opacity progressing to cataract, retinal hamartoma, and epiretinal membrane.

The clinical course of NF1 and NF2 varies widely. Most NF1 patients have multiple cafe au lait macules by the first birthday, and nearly all meet clinical

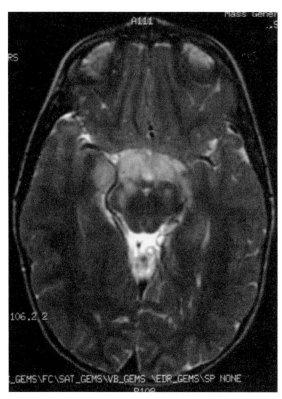

Figure 2
T2-weighted changes in the optic tracks and chiasm are common in NF1 patients. Less than 10% of children with such changes will develop progressive or symptomatic disease.

criteria by age 5. Many major manifestations, such as severe mental disability, seizure disorder, and plexiform tumors, are also obvious in early childhood. Manifestations of NF1 are clearly age dependent, with cutaneous tumors usually appearing at approximately the time of puberty. Malignancy is rarely encountered before the third decade. The average age of onset of symptoms among NF2 patients is 18–22 years. Younger diagnosis can be achieved with greater clinical suspicion of the at-risk individual and careful attention to subtle features, such as asymptomatic skin tumors and cataract. Most NF2 patients have a relentless course with progressive deafness, balance dysfunction, and death. Newer and more aggressive treatment strategies may have a positive impact on the natural history of NF2 in the near future.

Both NF1 and NF2 are autosomal dominant disorders with full penetrance. Approximately half of all cases are due to new mutations with clinically unaffected parents. There appears to be a relatively high rate of mosaicism among founders that can mitigate the phenotype. NF1 shows great intrafamilial heterogeneity, with affected relatives having widely different clinical courses. NF2 shows much greater homogeneity within families, especially with regard to age of onset and total tumor load.

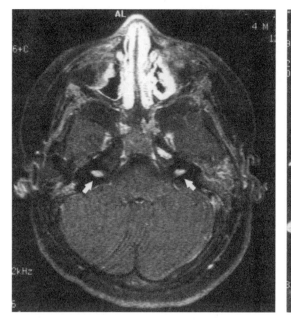
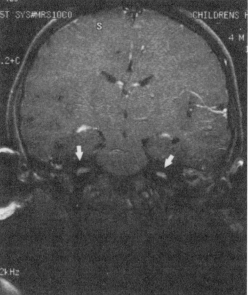

Figure 3
Bilateral vestibular schwannomas (BVSs; arrows) originate within the internal auditory canal at the point where the eighth cranial nerve acquires a Schwann cell sheath. Small BVSs are best visualized on contrast-enhanced MRI scan obtained at 3-mm slice thickness through the skull base.

MANAGEMENT

Management of NF includes anticipatory guidance for families at all stages of disease. Patients with NF1 should undergo a complete neurological evaluation and blood pressure evaluation annually. Children should also have a developmental assessment and annual ocular examination. Imaging can be reserved for those with unexplained or progressive symptoms. In an adult, unexplained pain should always be considered a sign of malignancy until proven otherwise. Management of patients with NF2 is often deferred to a specialized center. All NF2 patients should undergo annual cranial imaging, hearing evaluation, and ocular examination. Many also require more frequent imaging and spinal cord imaging. Two excellent patient support groups exist, providing educational brochures, patient-to-patient contact, and lay and professional conferences [the National Neurofibromatosis Foundation (http://www.nf.org) and NF, Inc. (http://www.nfinc.org)].

MOLECULAR BIOLOGY

The *NF1* gene was cloned from human chromosome 17 in 1990. It encodes a large and complex transcript with an open reading frame of 8454 base pairs. This has made molecular analysis of *NF1* mutations cumbersome, and little rationale currently exists for molecular genetic analysis in clinical practice. Approximately 15% of the NF1 protein product is a GTPase activating protein for the protooncogene RAS, which may play a role in the tumor suppressor gene activity of this molecule. The function of the remaining 85% of the protein remains unknown.

The *NF2* gene was cloned from human chromosome 22 in 1993. Its protein product is a member of the protein 4.1 family of cytoskeletal-associated proteins that link the spectrin actin cytoskeleton to the membrane. Mutational analysis of *NF2* has proceeded at a much more rapid pace because of its smaller size, and many studies have proven that it functions as a true tumor suppressor gene in NF2-related tumor types. Presymptomatic and prenatal diagnosis based on molecular genetic identification of mutations in *NF2* and/or linkage analysis is a powerful tool for identification of affected offspring at a young age.

—*Mia MacCollin*

See also–Canavan Disease; **Childhood Brain Tumors; Glial Tumors; Meningiomas; Spinal Cord Tumors, Treatment of**

Further Reading

American Academy of Pediatrics Committee on Genetics (1995). Health supervision for children with neurofibromatosis. *Pediatrics* **96**, 368–372.

Evans, D. G., Wallace, A. J., Wu, C. L., *et al.* (1998). Somatic mosaicism: A common cause of classic disease in tumor-prone syndromes? Lessons from type 2 neurofibromatosis. *Am. J. Hum. Genet.* **63**, 727–736.

Gusella, J. F., Ramesh, V., MacCollin, M., *et al.* (1999). The neurofibromatosis 2 tumor suppressor. *Biochim. Biophys. Acta* **1423**, M29–M36.

Gutmann, D. H. (1998). Recent insights into neurofibromatosis type 1: Clear genetic progress. *Arch. Neurol.* **55**, 778–780.

Gutmann, D. H., Aylsworth, A., Carey, J. C., *et al.* (1997). The diagnostic evaluation and multidisciplinary management of neurofibromatosis 1 and neurofibromatosis 2. *J. Am. Med. Assoc.* **278**, 51–57.

MacCollin, M., Woodfin, W., Kronn, D., *et al.* (1996). Schwannomatosis: A clinical and pathologic study. *Neurology* **46**, 1072–1079.

Neurogenesis
see **Central Nervous System, Overview**

Neurogenetics, Overview

Encyclopedia of the Neurological Sciences
Copyright 2003, Elsevier Science (USA). All rights reserved.

NEUROGENETICS applies the study of inherited traits to the nervous system and the behaviors and diseases that are the consequence of normal or abnormal functioning. Gregor Mendel, an Austrian monk, is generally credited with performing the first controlled genetic experiments. By observing the inheritance of specific traits in garden peas, he formulated the fundamental rules of genetics. In contrast to previous animal and plant breeders, Mendel did not stop at the descriptive level; by analyzing the ratios of observed traits in the offspring he was able to conclude that there must be dominant and recessive traits.

Mendelian or unifactorial inheritance refers to a pattern of inheritance that can be explained on the basis of mutation in a single gene. Thus, the presence or absence of a genetic character depends on the genotype at a single locus. Mendelian disorders can be autosomal dominant, autosomal recessive, and

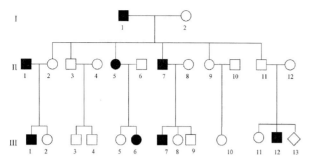

Figure 1
Pedigree segregating a dominant disease-causing allele (e.g., Huntington disease). Affected individuals are indicated by black symbols. The mutant allele is dominant to the wild-type alleles, and the disease phenotype is seen in heterozygotes. Offspring have a 50% risk of inheriting the disease. Offspring who inherit the normal allele will not develop the disease or pass it on to their offspring. The disease appears over multiple generations, which appears as vertical transmission in the pedigree notation. Males and females are evenly affected, and the disease is passed on from affected fathers or mothers to male and female offspring with equal probabilities. Note that the individual II-11 is nonpenetrant. He has an affected child but is apparently normal himself.

X-linked, and they are caused by mutations in a single gene. A trait is dominant if it is manifest in the heterozygote. Dominant alleles exert their phenotypic effect despite the presence of a normal (wild-type) allele on the second homologous chromosome. Thus, if the phenotypes associated with genotypes AA and AB are identical but are different from the BB phenotype, the A allele is dominant to allele B (Fig. 1). Conversely, the B allele is recessive to allele A.

Recessive mutations lead to phenotypic consequences only when both alleles contain mutations (Fig. 2). If the mutations on both alleles are different, this is referred to as compound heterozygosity. An example is a patient with Friedreich's ataxia whose mutation is an expansion of the intronic GAA repeat on one allele, whereas the other allele carries a missense mutation. X-linked disorders usually affect only males (Fig. 3). The mutation resides on the X chromosome. Females normally do not show a

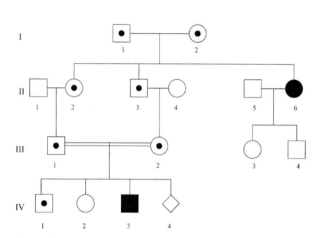

Figure 2
Pedigree segregating recessive disease alleles such as Friedreich ataxia. Only individuals homozygous for the disease gene will develop the disease; heterozygous individuals (indicated by a symbol with a center dot) are clinically normal because they carry one normal copy and one mutated copy of the gene. Since heterozygotes may pass on an abnormal gene to their offspring, they are called carriers. Parents of affected individuals are usually carriers of the disease gene, and each parent contributes one abnormal copy to the offspring. Disease risk to siblings is 25%, 50% of siblings will be carriers, and 25% will have two normal copies of the gene. In contrast to autosomal dominant inheritance, in which vertical transmission is observed, horizontal aggregation is typical for recessive disorders, in which multiple individuals in one generation are affected. Consanguinity may be present in pedigrees with autosomal recessive inheritance and is indicated by a double vertical line connecting the consanguineous parents.

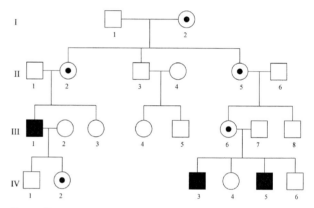

Figure 3
Pedigree segregating an X-linked disorder such as Duchenne's muscular dystrophy. In these disorders, the mutation lies on the X chromosome. Since females have two X chromosomes, they are usually clinically normal in X-linked recessive disorders. Sons of carrier females are at 50% risk to inherit the mutation and to develop clinical signs. Affected males carry one copy of the mutated allele but no normal allele. Daughters of affected males are carriers with 100% risk because all paternal X chromosomes carry the mutated allele. Since sons receive their X chromosome from the mother, they cannot pass the disease on when they have a normal phenotype. Thus, X-linked recessive disorders show only affected males, but transmission of the disease occurs through unaffected mothers. Male-to-male transmission excludes X-linked inheritance. Although carrier females are usually clinically normal, occasional carrier females are mildly symptomatic or show biochemical signs of the disease. X-linked dominant diseases are rare. When a trait is X-linked dominant, females are also affected. However, the disease is usually more severe in the hemizygous males. Rett syndrome only occurs in females and may be an example of an X-linked dominant disease that leads to the death of male embryos *in utero*.

phenotype but can be carriers of the disease-causing mutation. When mutations occur in mitochondrial DNA, the disease is passed on solely through the mother (Fig. 4).

In contrast to monogenic disorders, complex genetic traits cannot be explained on the basis of mutations in a single gene, and a phenotype is only observed when mutations in several genes have occurred. Examples of complex genetic traits are multiple sclerosis and stroke.

Neurogenetics was initially focused on childhood metabolic diseases, and then it branched out to chromosomal mapping of inherited disease due to defects in unknown proteins. This was made possible by the advent of a large number of genetic markers that could be used for genetic linkage analysis, which is a powerful tool to detect the chromosomal location of disease genes. It is based on the observation that genes that reside physically close on a chromosome remain linked during meiosis.

For most neurological diseases for which the underlying biochemical defect was not known, the identification of the chromosomal location of the disease gene was the first step in its eventual isolation. In this manner, genes have been isolated from all types of neurological diseases, including neurodegenerative diseases such as Alzheimer's, Parkinson's, or ataxias; diseases of ion channels leading to periodic paralysis or hemiplegic migraine; and tumor syndromes such as neurofibromatosis 1 and 2.

When a chromosomal location for a disease phenotype has been established, genetic linkage analysis determines whether the disease phenotype is caused only by mutation in a single gene or whether mutations in other genes can give rise to an identical or similar phenotype. Often, it is found that similar phenotypes can be caused by mutations in very different genes. For example, the autosomal dominant spinocerebellar ataxias are caused by mutations in different genes but have very similar phenotypes.

In addition to providing novel, genotype-based classifications of neurological diseases, genetic linkage analysis can aid in diagnosis. However, in contrast to direct mutational analysis, such as detection of an expanded CAG repeat in the Huntington gene, diagnosis using flanking markers requires the analysis of several family members.

—Stefan M. Pulst

See also–Friedreich's Ataxia; Huntington's Disease; Nervous System, Neuroembryology of (see also specific entries in the Neurogenetics section; e.g., Down's Syndrome)

Further Reading

McKusick, V. A. (1996). History of medical genetics. In *Emory and Rimoin's Principles and Practice of Medical Genetics* (D. L. Rimoin, J. M. Connor, and R. E. Pyeritz, Eds.), 3rd ed. Churchill Livingstone, New York.
Pulst, S. M. (1999). Genetic linkage analysis and neurologic disease. *Arch. Neurol.* **56,** 667–672.
Pulst, S. M. (2000). Introduction to medical genetics. In *Neurogenetics* (S. M. Pulst, Ed.), pp. 1–264. Oxford Univ. Press, New York.

Neuroimaging, Overview

Encyclopedia of the Neurological Sciences
Copyright 2003, Elsevier Science (USA). All rights reserved.

THE FIRST imaging tool applied to the nervous system was the x-ray. X-rays of the skull and spine (which primarily only allowed the distinction of bone and calcified structures) were soon augmented by techniques to increase the contrast between different soft tissues. X-ray techniques still in current use include angiography (injection of an x-ray dense material into the blood to define the walls of blood vessels) and myelography (injection of an x-ray dense material into the cerebrospinal fluid to define the spinal cord and nerve roots). The past 30 years have witnessed an explosion in the field of both clinical

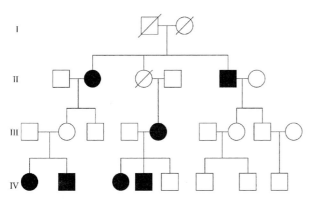

Figure 4
Pedigree showing maternal inheritance. This pattern is seen with mitochondrial mutations because all mitochondrial DNA in a fetus is contributed by the oocyte. The mitochondrial genome is distinct from the nuclear genome. However, the number of mutant mitochondria in each offspring may vary, resulting in extremely variable phenotypes. All children are at risk to inherit at least some mutated mitochondria.

and research neuroimaging, beginning with the development of x-ray computed tomography (CT) in the early 1970s, followed by positron emission tomography (PET) in the late 1970s and magnetic resonance imaging (MRI) in the 1980s. The ability of x-ray CT to provide highly accurate cross-sectional images of the brain, spine, and their coverings completely changed the practice of clinical neurology and neurosurgery in less than a decade. PET uses the principles of CT together with internally administered radioactive molecules to obtain measurements of physiological processes in the brain. The capability of MRI to provide accurate structural images of the spinal cord and even higher resolution brain images has led to increasing reliance on this techniques for neurological diagnosis.

Neuroimaging refers to the use of radiological and other techniques to create images of the living human nervous system. The field of neuroradiology can be broadly defined as the clinical application of neuroimaging tools for either the diagnosis (diagnostic neuroradiology) or treatment (therapeutic neuroradiology) of diseases affecting the nervous system.

Neuroimages may be structural or physiological. Structural neuroimaging provides information about the macroscopically visible structure of bone, neural, and vascular tissues as a substitute for direct visualization at surgery or autopsy. Because of the close correspondence of these images to visible changes in diseased tissue, structural neuroimaging is the cornerstone of clinical neuroradiology. Angiography, x-ray CT, proton MRI, and ultrasound are all structural neuroimaging techniques. Physiological neuroimaging is concerned with measuring biological processes in the nervous system and their alteration in disease states. A similar term, functional neuroimaging, is often used interchangeably. In physiological neuroimaging, an understanding of the physical or chemical basis for the image is essential since the goal is to use this signal to measure a physiological or biological process. Doppler ultrasound, PET, single photon emission tomography (SPECT), MRI, and magnetic resonance spectroscopy all provide physiological neuroimaging data (Fig. 1).

PET has led the way in the research field of physiological brain imaging, providing new insights

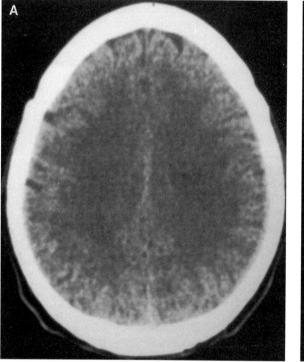
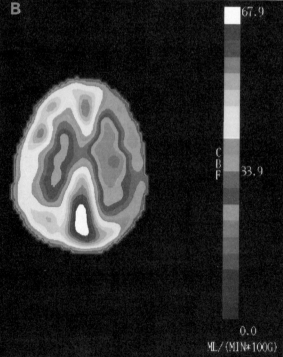

Figure 1

Structural and functional neuroimages from a man with right carotid occlusion and transient ischemic attacks manifested by left arm and leg weakness. (A) The structural x-ray CT image shows normal gray and white matter in both hemispheres with no evidence of any structural abnormality. (B) The physiological PET cerebral blood flow image shows reduced cerebral blood flow in the part of the brain supplied by the occluded carotid artery. (See color plate section.)

into the biology of both normal and diseased human brain. PET methods for measuring cerebral blood flow, cerebral metabolism, and neuroreceptors are widely used for research applications. MRI techniques to measure cerebral blood flow and for measuring cerebral metabolism based on the use of proton MRI signals sensitive to venous blood oxygen levels are being developed. Both PET and MRI can be used to investigate the regional localization of normal human brain function by detecting changes in regional cerebral blood flow.

Diagnostic neuroradiology primarily relies on structural imaging techniques for the definition of anatomy and structural lesions, such as tumors, infections, and aneurysms. Clinical applications of physiological imaging that can be considered to be classified in the category of diagnostic neuroimaging include Doppler ultrasound for the evaluation of arterial and venous pathology and SPECT and PET for the identification of epileptic foci.

The field of therapeutic neuroradiology, also referred to as interventional neuroradiology or endovascular neurosurgery, uses imaging techniques to guide catheters or needles introduced through small skin punctures for the treatment of diseases affecting the nervous system. Common interventional neuroradiological procedures include angioplasty of stenoses of the vessels of the head and neck, endovascular obliteration of saccular intracranial aneurysms, embolization (blockage of the arterial supply using a variety of different materials) of vascular tumors or vascular malformations, and direct thrombolysis for acute ischemic stroke. Dramatic improvements in imaging systems, catheters and guidewires, and intravascular devices (such as platinum coils for aneurysms and small, flexible angioplasty balloons) are responsible for the rapid growth of this field. These procedures are currently performed in dedicated angiographic suites. Interventional MR scanners are being developed and evaluated for some of these procedures. Nonvascular interventions include biopsies, spinal nerve root injections and epidural injections for the treatment of pain, and vertebroplasty for pathological stress fractures of the spine.

—*William J. Powers and Colin P. Derdeyn*

See also–Computerized Axial Tomography (CAT); Magnetic Resonance Imaging (MRI); Physiological Brain Imaging; Positron Emission Tomography (PET); Single-Photon Emission Computed Tomography (SPECT)

Further Reading

Connors, J. J., 3rd, and Wojak, J. C. (1998). *Interventional Neuroradiology: Strategies and Practical Techniques.* Saunders, Philadelphia.
Grossman, R. I., and Yousem, D. M. (1994). *Neuroradiology: The Requisites.* Mosby-Year Book, St. Louis.
Osborn, A. G. (1994). *Diagnostic Neuroradiology.* Mosby-Year Book, St. Louis.
Wagner, H. N., Jr., Szabo, Z., and Buchanan, J. W. (1995). *Principles of Nuclear Medicine.* Saunders, Philadelphia.
Zimmerman, R. A., Gibby, W. A., and Carmody, R. F. (2000). *Neuroimaging: Clinical and Physical Principles.* Springer-Verlag, New York.

Neuroimmunology, Overview

Encyclopedia of the Neurological Sciences
Copyright 2003, Elsevier Science (USA). All rights reserved.

THE NERVOUS SYSTEM has long been considered an immunologically privileged site. This concept was based on the premise that (i) there is a more or less strict anatomical separation between the systemic immune compartment (blood) and the neural tissue, (ii) major histocompatibility complex (MHC) molecules required for antigen presentation are absent in normal circumstances, (iii) there is no lymphatic drainage, and (iv) immune surveillance by T cells is lacking. It is now obvious that most of these assumptions are not tenable. The blood–brain and the blood–nerve barrier restrict access of immune cells and soluble mediators to a certain degree, but this restriction is not complete, neither anatomically (e.g., the blood–nerve barrier is absent or relatively deficient at the roots, in the ganglia, and the motor terminals) nor functionally. Activated T lymphocytes can penetrate intact barriers irrespective of their antigen specificity and, in certain circumstances, release cytokines that upregulate the expression of MHC class II molecules. Moreover, the nervous system contains intrinsic cellular populations that have the potential to act as antigen presenters.

ANTIGEN PRESENTATION IN THE NERVOUS SYSTEM

In the central nervous system (CNS), cells participating in the formation of the blood–brain barrier, specifically perivascular microglia or pericytes but also endothelial cells, can serve as competent antigen presenting cells by upregulation of class II MHC molecules. Microglia are the dominant parenchymal antigen presenters, whereas the relevance of astrocytes in unclear. Interestingly, MHC class II inducibility in microglia cells appears to be regulated by neurotrophins released by electrically active neurons, assigning an immune regulating function to neuronal cells within the CNS.

In the peripheral nervous system (PNS), Schwann cells, in addition to forming the myelin sheath, can express MHC class II antigens and have been shown *in vitro* to present antigen to autoreactive T cells. They also exhibit MHC class I antigens, which mark them as targets for T cell-mediated cellular cytotoxicity. Schwann cells can generate toxic and immunosuppressive mediators, such as leukotrienes, prostanoids, and nitric oxide. This raises the possibility that these cells act as antigen presenters as well as immunoregulators within the PNS.

PATHOGENESIS OF NEUROIMMUNOLOGICAL DISEASES

For most neurological autoimmune disorders, the ultimate cause has not been established. The breakdown of self-tolerance is crucial. Peripheral activation of potentially self-reactive T lymphocytes in the normal repertoire by infectious agents represents another mechanism. In autoimmune diseases such as multiple sclerosis (MS) or Guillain–Barré syndrome (GBS), several lines of evidence implicate infection as a potential trigger of disease. Alternatively, the release of sequestered autoantigens due to tissue damage could provoke or perpetuate ongoing immune reactions. Another possible role in the genesis of autoimmunity has been attributed to a group of peptides derived from viral and bacterial pathogens called superantigens. They have a distinct mode of binding to MHC molecules that enables them to activate large numbers of T or B cells. Bystander activation implicating the "accidental" activation of effector immune cells may also play an important role in the pathogenesis of immune-mediated disorders of the nervous system.

Alternatively, structural similarities between microbial and self-antigens could activate autoreactive T cells—a mechanism termed molecular mimicry. T lymphocytes can recognize microbial as well as self-peptides with similar amino acid sequence. On the other hand, a single T cell receptor can recognize several peptides with various degrees of sequence homology. The first human autoimmune disorder proposed to result from such misguided T cell cross-reactivity was rheumatic fever and its associated CNS disorder, Sydenham's chorea, after infection

with hemolytic streptococci. The principle of molecular mimicry has also been invoked in the pathogenesis of GBS following infection with *Campylobacter jejuni* or certain viruses.

The precise pathomechanisms are much better understood in antibody-mediated disorders, such as myasthenia gravis (MG) and Lambert–Eaton myasthenic syndrome (LEMS). In both disorders, autoantibodies target specific receptors along the neuromuscular junction, inducing a dysfunction of neuromuscular transmission.

SELF-LIMITATION OF THE IMMUNE RESPONSE

Several neurological disorders provide evidence that autoimmunity caused by autoreactive T cells can be self-limited. Examples are monophasic diseases such as acute disseminated encephalomyelitis and GBS. Other forms of autoimmune diseases are episodic but persistent (e.g., relapsing–remitting forms of MS) or chronic and progressive (e.g., primary or late stages of MS or chronic inflammatory demyelinating polyradiculoneuropathy [CIDP]). It is unclear which mechanisms determine the duration and extent of the autoimmune response, but apoptosis of autoaggressive T cells or restoration of a disturbed Th1/Th2 balance have been proposed as underlying mechanisms.

THE ROLE OF GENES

It has long been established that autoimmunity is under genetic control. Clinical evidence points to hereditary susceptibility factors linked to MHC haplotype, immunoglobulin genes, and others. Genetic susceptibility was traditionally studied in animal models such as experimental autoimmune encephalomyelitis or neuritis, in which resistant and highly susceptible strains exist. In the resistant strains, experimental tools were developed to break tolerance and set off a fulminant autoimmune reaction.

EFFECTOR MECHANISMS OF TISSUE DAMAGE

Within the nervous system, various effector mechanisms utilized by the immune system can induce tissue damage:

1. *Autoreactive CD4$^+$ T cell-driven mechanisms:* Through the release of proinflammatory cytokines, T$_H$1 lymphocytes activate macrophages

to enhance phagocytosis and release of noxious molecules, such as reactive oxygen and nitrogen oxide metabolites, complement, and proteases. This mechanism is critically involved in the pathogenesis of demyelinating diseases such MS and GBS.

2. *CD8+ T lymphocytes:* These are instrumental in launching cytotoxic attacks on MHC class I displaying targets. These T cells destroy targets primarily by the release of cytotoxic granules, perforin, and granzymes. Neurons or oligodendrocytes represent such MHC class I-expressing target cells in certain neuroimmunological diseases.

3. *Antibody-dependent cellular cytotoxicity:* This toxic program is activated by antibodies binding via Fc receptors to mononuclear phagocytes. It results in an antigen-specific attack by an effector cell through the cellular release of cytoplasmic granules containing granzymes or perforins or induces phagocytosis by macrophages. Such mechanisms are critically involved in GBS.

4. *Antibodies exhibit various effector mechanisms:* They can block functionally relevant epitopes, such as certain receptors relevant for neurotransmission or nerve conduction in MG, LEMS, or GBS. On the other hand, antibodies can modulate the expression of functionally relevant epitopes. For example, in MG, antibodies are able to cross-link the acetylcholine receptors (AchRs) on the membrane surface,

Table 1 IMMUNE-MEDIATED DISORDERS OF THE NERVOUS SYSTEM[a]

Disorder	Target autoantigens (candidates)	Histopathology/Pathomechanisms
CNS		
Multiple sclerosis	Myelin/oligodendrocyte proteins (e.g., MBP, MOG, MAG, PLP, αB cristallin)	Heterogeneous: multifocal inflammation, demyelination, axonal loss, loss of oligodendrocytes, colocalization of IgG and complement in the lesion
Stiff-person syndrome	Glutamic acid decarboxylase-containing GABAergic neurons	No significant observations
Rassmussen's encephalitis	Glu receptor-3 on neurons	Inflammation and neuronal loss
Neuromuscular junction		
Myasthenia gravis	Postsynaptic AChRs MuSK in some cases	Reduced folding and AchR density; deposition of IgG and complement
Lambert–Eaton myasthenic syndrome	Presynaptic voltage-gated calcium channels	Loss of calcium channels at the motor nerve terminal
Neuromyotonia (acquired)	Voltage-gated potassium channels	Heterogeneous
PNS		
Guillain–Barré syndrome	Gangliosides such as GM1 (especially axonal form), GQ1b (Miller–Fisher variant), and related glycolipids	Macrophage-mediated multifocal demyelination, axonal loss, IgG and complement deposition
CIDP	P_0, glycolipids	Same as for Guillain–Barré syndrome
Multifocal motor neuropathy	Ganglioside GM1	Focal demyelination, deposition of IgM at the nodes of Ranvier
Monoclonal gammopathy-associated neuropathies	MAG, unknown targets	Segmental demyelination without inflammatory infiltration, IgM and complement deposition on the myelin sheath
CNS/PNS		
Paraneoplastic syndromes	Various (e.g., Hu, Ri, Yo)	Neuronal loss, gliosis, perivascular inflammatory infiltration
Muscle		
Dermatomyositis	Unknown	Complement-mediated vasculopathy, perimysial and perivascular infiltration with CD4+ T cells and B cells
Polymyositis	Unknown	Endomysial infiltrates consisting of CD8+ cells

[a] Abbreviations used: AChR, acetylcholine receptor; CIDP, chronic inflammatory demyelinating polyradiculoneuropathy; CNS, central nervous system; Glu, glutamat; MAG, myelin-associated glycoprotein; MBP, myelin basic protein; MOG, myelin oligodendrocyte glycoprotein; MuSK, muscle-specific kinase; PLP, proteolipid protein; PNS, peripheral nervous system.

resulting in their accelerated internalization and degradation (a process termed antigenic modulation). Finally, antibodies can activate the complement system by the classic pathway, yielding proinflammatory mediators and the lytic C5b–9 terminal complex. In demyelinating diseases of the CNS and the PNS, complement activation results in myelin breakdown and axonal damage. In MG, antibodies targeting the AChRs on the postsynaptic membrane induce complement-mediated lysis. Similarly, in dermatomyositis and vasculitic disorders activation of the complement cascade results in severe tissue damage.

CONCLUSION

Table 1 lists neurological diseases considered to be autoimmune in nature or immune mediated and summarizes candidate antigens and potentially operating pathogenic mechanisms. Detailed aspects on clinical presentation and treatment can be found in the individual entries assigned to these diseases.

—*Hans-Peter Hartung and Bernd C. Kieseier*

See also–Immune System, Overview; Neurogenetics, Overview (see also specific entries in the Neuroimmunology section)

Further Reading

Aloisi, F., Ria, F., and Adorini, L. (2000). Regulation of T-cell responses by CNS antigen-presenting cells: Different roles for microglia and astrocytes. *Immunol. Today* **21**, 141–147.

Antel, J. P., and Owens, T. (1999). Immune regulation and CNS autoimmune disease. *J. Neuroimmunol.* **100**, 181–189.

Antel, J., Birnbaum, G., and Hartung, H.-P. (Eds.) (1998). *Clinical Neuroimmunology*. Blackwell, Malden, MA.

Archelos, J. J., and Hartung, H.-P. (2000). Pathogenetic roles of autoantibodies in neurological diseases. *Trends Neurosci.* **23**, 317–327.

Davidson, A., and Diamond, B. (2001). Autoimmune diseases. *N. Engl. J. Med.* **345**, 340–350.

Gold, R., Archelos, J. J., and Hartung, H.-P. (1999). Mechanisms of immune regulation in the peripheral nervous system. *Brain Pathol.* **9**, 343–360.

Hartung, H.-P., Toyka, K. V., and Kieseier, B. C. (2002). Immune mechanisms in neurological disease. In *Diseases of the Nervous System: Clinical Neuroscience and Therapeutic Principles* (A. K. Asbury, G. M. McKhann, W. I. McDonald, P. J. Goadsby, and J. McArthur, Eds.). Cambridge Univ. Press, Cambridge, UK.

Hohlfeld, R. (1997). Biotechnological agents for the immunotherapy of multiple sclerosis. Principles, problems and perspectives. *Brain* **120**, 865–916.

Neuroleptic Malignant Syndrome
see Malignant Hyperthermia

Neurolysis

Encyclopedia of the Neurological Sciences
Copyright 2003, Elsevier Science (USA). All rights reserved.

SPINAL NERVE TRUNKS are wrapped in sheaths of connective tissue. If these enveloping layers of connective tissue are dissected away, the nerve can be separated into individual bundles or fascicles. The connective tissue components of peripheral nerves are the endoneurium, perineurium, and epineurium (Fig. 1).

The endoneurium specifies the delicate collagenous sheath that envelops individual myelinated or unmyelinated nerve fibers. A bundle of nerve fibers is called a fasciculus or funiculus and is surrounded by a circular arrangement of connective tissue called perineurium. The connective tissue that surrounds the perineurium and binds fascicles into a single nerve trunk is the epineurium. The epineurium is further divided into a dense outer layer, called the superficial epineurium, and the interfascicular epineurium. The latter is the layer of loose connective tissue that extends between fasciculi (Fig. 1). Depending on the extent and severity of injury, the scarring that follows injury and damage to peripheral nerves involves these different components of the nerve trunk.

The procedure of neurolysis involves releasing the nerve trunk from scar tissue and constrictive adhesions. The extent and invasiveness of neurolysis depend on the pattern and extent of injury. External neurolysis is defined as freeing the nerve trunk from external scar tissue or releasing any compression extrinsic to the nerve. Internal neurolysis involves freeing and separating individual fasciculi from each other as well as from interfascicular scar tissue.

External neurolysis is based on the assumption that the internal architecture of the nerve is intact but that the superficial epineurium may be intimately scarred to the surrounding tissue, and it may be impossible to free the nerve from the scar tissue without excising the scarred superficial epineurium. Therefore, the terms epineurotomy and epineurectomy have been applied to describe the extent of

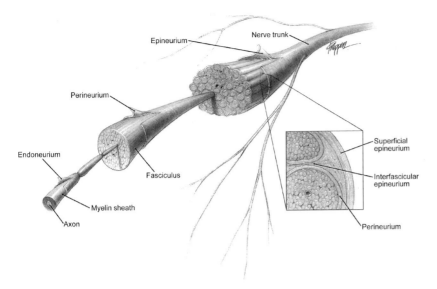

Figure 1
The various layers of a nerve trunk are outlined. The epineurium consists of connective tissue surrounding the nerve trunk, which is subdivided in the superficial epineurium, which wraps around the nerve trunk, and the interfascicular epineurium. The latter also extends between nerve fascicles, which are covered by perineurium. The endoneurium serves as a mantle for individual nerves (reprinted with permission from the Barrow Neurological Institute).

neurolysis with appropriate descriptive terms. In epineurotomy, a longitudinal incision is made through the superficial epineurium, along the area of compression, to expose the underlying fascicles and interfascicular connective tissue.

Epineurectomy involves the excision and partial or total removal of the scarred or thickened superficial epineurium. The injection of warm saline within a nerve trunk is called saline neurolysis. This procedure is used to help define the extent of interfascicular scarring and does not dissolve the scar.

TECHNIQUE

In external neurolysis, the entire nerve trunk is identified and carefully isolated proximal and distal to the site of involvement. The nerve should never be approached directly through the scar tissue. An electric nerve stimulator is used to identify and preserve functioning portions of the nerve. Initially, the neurolysis is confined to those portions of the nerve that are unattached to the vessel. Total epineurectomy can decrease the vascular supply to the nerve by removing the blood vessels attached to the nerve in this layer. Neurolysis should be terminated if the nerve and vessel are so firmly attached to each other that attempts to decompress or free the nerve completely would sever the vessel. A total epineurectomy should be performed when scar

tissue has already compromised the microcirculation. All bleeding and oozing should be controlled to prevent scar tissue from reforming and to avoid new inflammation and deformation. At a minimum, loupe magnification is recommended for this procedure.

Technically, internal neurolysis is a more difficult and invasive procedure. The nerve is exposed as in external neurolysis. The superficial epineurium is incised longitudinally (i.e., an epineurotomy is performed), and the underlying individual fasciculi are identified and dissected away from the perifascicular scar tissue under magnification. The nerve bundles or fascicles are then separated within the nerve trunk. The fine interfascicular communications, blood vessels, and perineurium are damaged as a result. An internal saline injection can help identify interfascicular communications, but this procedure is controversial. The injection of saline into a nerve trunk causes fibrosis and is thought to disorganize the architecture. The nerve becomes edematous, thereby disturbing visualization of the surgical field and regeneration of the nerve. Saline should never be injected into the fasciculi, and the perineurium should only be opened if leprosy bacillus is involved.

ADVERSE EFFECTS

Improved microsurgical techniques have greatly reduced the risks of neurolysis; thus, it is now a useful procedure. Most of the adverse effects of neurolysis are related to intra- and epineural fibrosis occurring in response to the procedure. In animal studies, the injection of saline (saline neurolysis) causes inflammation and increases the amount of fibrosis.

Intra- and epineural fibrosis adversely affects the nerve trunk mostly by increasing and aggravating the size of scar tissue and by constricting the fascicles. This constriction interferes with the axon transport system and compresses nutrient vessels, thereby impairing circulation, nutrition, and regeneration of the recovering nerve. Furthermore, the interfascicular connections, fascicles, or trunk could be destroyed and cause paralysis.

Although the microsurgical technique has reduced the damage associated with neurolysis, it remains a potentially dangerous procedure. Therefore, this procedure is only justified when scarring and fibrosis are preoperatively evaluated to be more severe than the fibrosis that might follow the surgical procedure. Neurolysis is undertaken with the intent of restoring the environment to facilitate the regeneration of injured nerve fibers.

INDICATIONS

Neurolysis has been performed to treat many different peripheral nerve lesions, with more or less good outcomes. The appropriate surgical management of radial, ulnar, and median nerve lesions has been associated with excellent functional recovery. However, treating carpal tunnel syndrome with neurolysis remains controversial.

Overall, neurolysis is performed mostly to evaluate and treat neural lesions in intact nerves. This group of injuries includes mechanical, thermal, and injection injuries as well as acute and chronic compression syndromes. However, neurolysis can be used to treat injuries when neural continuity is lost, such as lacerations, fracture-associated injuries, and gunshot injuries. For these lesions, neurolysis is performed circumferentially above and below the site of injury. Epineural scarring is resected and the entire injured segment is exposed. Furthermore, nerve action potentials are measured to identify functioning fibers. Split or partial graft repairs may then be performed when fascicles are lacerated, neural continuity is lost, or fascicles of the injured segment do not transmit action potentials. Furthermore, nerves are explored and neurolysis is performed to relieve pain associated with leprous neuritis by

removing compressive scar tissue and adhesions, to assist regeneration, and to follow patients with an unsatisfactory or arrested recovery.

—*Sam Safavi-Abbasi, Iman Feiz-Erfan, and Andrew G. Shetter*

See also—Fasciculation; Microneurosurgery; Nerve Injury; Nerve Regeneration

Further Reading
Dellon, A. L. (1989). Review of treatment results for ulnar nerve entrapment at the elbow. *J. Hand Surg.* **14A**, 688–700.
Frykman, G. K., Adams, J., and Bowen, W. W. (1981). Neurolysis. *Orthop. Clin. North Am.* **12**, 325–342.
Kim, D. H., Kam, A. C., Chandika, P., *et al.* (2001). Surgical management and outcomes in patients with median nerve lesions. *J. Neurosurg.* **95**, 584–594.
Kim, D. H., Kam, A. C., Chandika, P., *et al.* (2001). Surgical management and outcomes in patients with radial nerve lesions. *J. Neurosurg.* **95**, 573–583.
Spinner, M. (1980). Management of nerve compression lesions of the upper extremity. In *Management of Peripheral Nerve Problems* (G. E. Omer, Jr., and M. Spinner, Eds.), pp. 569–592. Saunders, Philadelphia.

Neuromuscular Disorders, Overview

Encyclopedia of the Neurological Sciences
Copyright 2003, Elsevier Science (USA). All rights reserved.

THE NEUROMUSCULAR disorders comprise a variety of disease states that affect the lower motor and sensory neurons, the spinal (motor and sensory) roots, peripheral nerves, neuromuscular junctions, and muscles. Figure 1 shows an overview of the general organization of the peripheral nervous system. Figure 2 depicts the major cell types of the peripheral nervous system—the lower motor neuron (anterior horn cell) and sensory neuron (dorsal root ganglion cell). We describe the clinical manifestations associated with disorders affecting these elements of the peripheral nervous system and comment on their underlying causes.

DISORDERS OF THE MOTOR NEURONS

Clinical Picture

As further anatomical background, Fig. 3 expands on Fig. 2 and shows that a group of muscle fibers is normally supplied by a single lower motor neuron

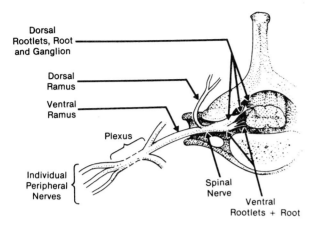

Figure 1

General organization of the peripheral nervous system to show the formation of the nerve roots (formed from "rootlets"), spinal nerves, plexuses, and individual nerve trunks [reproduced with permission from Stewart, J. D. (1993). *Focal Peripheral Neuropathies*. Raven Press, New York].

and that we designate this cell, its axon, and the muscle fibers it innervates as the motor unit. When a disease process leads to the loss of lower motor neurons (a condition also known as denervation), the result is muscle weakness, fasciculations (or muscle twitches), and atrophy (or reduction in muscle mass) in muscles previously innervated by the affected motor neurons. These clinical features are referred to as lower motor neuron signs.

Weakness is characterized by loss of strength and may be described as mild, moderate, or severe. Alternatively, it may be measured by the Medical Research Council scale in which strength is rated from 5 (normal) to 0 (no movement at all). The scale is outlined as follows: 5, normal; 4, movement against resistance; 3, movement against gravity; 2, movement with gravity eliminated; 1, flicker of movement; 0, no movement.

Fasciculations are spontaneous visible twitches in a muscle resulting from the contractions of many of the individual muscle fibers belonging to an electrically excitable motor unit. Atrophy is the visible, gross loss of muscle bulk or mass over time that reflects at the microscopic level the denervation atrophy of many individual muscle fibers belonging to an affected motor unit (Fig. 4).

Lower motor neurons are distributed throughout the brainstem and spinal cord; thus, lower motor neuron signs may appear in muscles innervated by both cranial and spinal nerves. For example, degeneration and loss of motor neurons in the right hypoglossal nucleus in the medulla of the brainstem

would be expected to cause weakness, atrophy, and fasciculations of the right side of the tongue. A similar process affecting motor neurons in the right cervical spinal cord would cause lower motor neuron signs in the right hand.

In some clinical settings, degeneration of lower motor neurons is accompanied by loss of cortical motor neurons. These latter cells are also called Betz

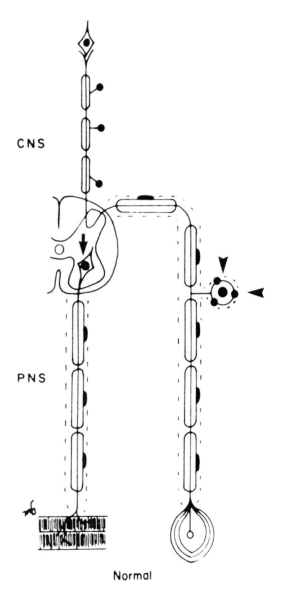

Normal

Figure 2

Diagram of the lower motor neuron (anterior horn cell; arrow) and its axon innervating muscle and also a sensory neuron (dorsal root ganglion cell; arrowheads) with its axon supplying a touch receptor [reproduced with permission from Schaumburg, H. H., Berger, A. R., and Thomas, P. K. (1992). *Disorders of Peripheral Nerves*. Davis, Philadelphia].

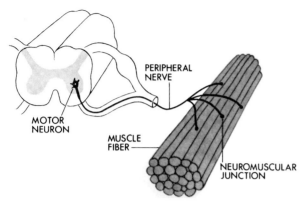

Figure 3
The motor unit. Note the motor neuron, its axon, and the many muscle fibers that are innervated by it [reproduced with permission from Layzer, R. (1975). *Primary Care* **2**, 235].

cells, and they project heavily myelinated fibers to connect with lower motor neurons of the brainstem and spinal cord. The fibers projecting to the brainstem lower motor neurons are collected in a pathway called the corticobulbar tract, and the fibers projecting to the lower motor neurons in the spinal cord are found in the corticospinal tract (Fig. 5). When Betz cells are lost, a group of clinical findings emerge that are referred to as upper motor neuron signs. These comprise increased muscle tone or spasticity, increased reflex activity or hyper-reflexia, and pathological reflexes, such as the Babinski sign.

Causes of Motor Neuron Disorders

There are two major categories of motor neuron disorders: genetically determined and acquired. For example, the spinal muscular atrophies—purely lower motor neuronal in character—are autosomal recessive in nature and may present in infancy, childhood, or adult life. Amyotrophic lateral sclerosis (ALS), on the other hand, is the most commonly occurring acquired disease (except for 5–10% of cases that are inherited) of mid- to later adult life. ALS affects both lower and upper motor neurons (Fig. 5) and is characterized by a combination of muscle weakness, atrophy, fascicu- lations, and spasticity with hyper-reflexia, often in the same limb. This disease usually begins in one body region (e.g., the right hand) and then spreads to other regions over the course of 3–5 years, ultimately affecting all muscles under voluntary control, with a few exceptions (ocular and sphincter muscles).

DISORDERS OF THE SENSORY NEURONS

Clinical Picture

To provide further anatomical background, Fig. 6 depicts the various sensory neurons and their respective axons as they project to the peripheral nerves. Also shown is the peripheral component of the sympathetic nervous system that projects to the skin via peripheral nerves and is important for supplying blood vessels, sweat glands, and other skin components. Degeneration or loss of peripheral sensory neurons located in the spinal sensory ganglia lead to some combination of the following signs and symptoms: sensory impairment, disap- pearance of tendon reflexes, impaired coordination due to defective proprioception, and pain and paresthesias. Disorders that affect these sensory neurons exclusively are known as sensory neurono- pathies, and the resulting clinical picture is purely sensory (sensory symptoms and signs with preserved motor function).

Causes of Sensory Neuron Disorders

As noted for the motor neuron disorders, there are also two major categories of sensory neuron dis- orders: genetically determined and acquired. In the latter category are the sensory neuronopathies associated with Sjogren's syndrome, small cell lung carcinoma (a paraneoplastic syndrome), and neuro- toxic drugs. A typical presentation for an acquired sensory neuronopathy might comprise the subacute

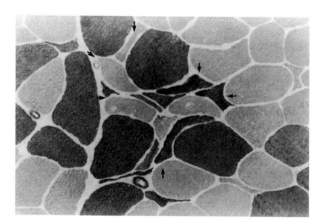

Figure 4
Muscle biopsy showing early denervation. There are small groups of angulated atrophic fibers (arrows) that have lost their innervation. Compare to the adjacent, still innervated muscle fibers of normal size [reproduced with permission from Mitsumoto, H., Chad, D. A., and Pioro, E. P. (1998). *Amyotrophic Lateral Sclerosis*. Davis, Philadelphia].

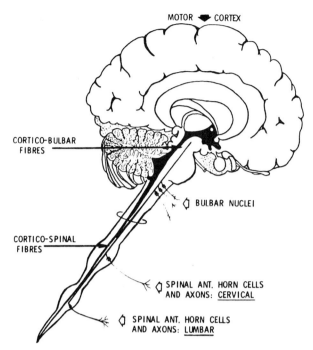

Figure 5
Diagram showing the involvement of motor nerves in the cortex, brainstem, and spinal cord in amyotrophic lateral sclerosis [reproduced with permission from Pryce-Phillips, W., and Murray, J. J. (1992). *Essential Clinical Neurology*, 4th ed., p. 660. Elsevier, New York].

to chronic evolution (over months) of tingling paresthesias and pain in the feet, poor balance with frequent falls, and clumsiness in upper extremity movements.

DISORDERS OF THE NERVE ROOTS

Clinical Picture

Damage to a nerve root or roots leads to a set of symptoms and signs referable to the injured root (radiculopathy) or roots (polyradiculopathy). In clinical practice, the nerve roots that are most commonly compromised are those in the cervical (C5–C8) and the lumbosacral (L4–S1) regions. The symptoms are numbness, pain, and weakness in either the arm or leg, and the signs comprise loss of sensation in the dermatome (the sensory territory of the affected root), reduction or loss of reflex activity subserved by the nerve root and its respective reflex arc in question, and weakness in the myotome (the motor territory innervated by the root in question). When the disease process affects thoracic roots, the major manifestation is pain and numbness in the dermatomes of the affected nerve roots.

Causes of Nerve Root Disorders

The most common causes of radiculopathy are nerve root compression by a herniated nucleus pulposus or by osteophytes complicating spondylotic arthropathy. Figure 7 shows the anatomy of different types of disk herniation in the lumbosacral region. Other causes of radiculopathy or polyradiculopathy are diabetes, Lyme disease, and carcinomatous meningitis (metastases to nerve roots).

DISORDERS OF PERIPHERAL NERVE

Clinical Picture

There are three major clinical presentations of peripheral nerve disease: focal, multifocal, and diffuse. The focal category comprises mononeuropathy, characterized by numbness, sensory loss, pain, and weakness in the territory of an affected nerve. Multifocal peripheral nerve disease is characterized by multiple mononeuropathies wherein symptoms and signs occur in the distribution of two or more nerves. The diffuse disorder, polyneuropathy, is usually characterized by symptoms and signs referable to dysfunction of both sensory and motor fibers, with findings widely and symmetrically distributed, affecting the lower and the upper extremities. In some instances, the disorders causing polyneuropathy target sensory, autonomic, or motor fibers selectively.

The clinical manifestations of polyneuropathy comprise symptoms of numbness and tingling as well as weakness. Typically, distal portions of the extremities are affected before the more proximal, and the legs before the arms. Accordingly, in the early stages of the disease process, the physical

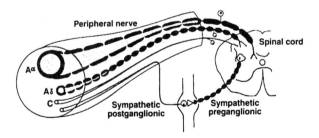

Figure 6
Peripheral nerve showing sensory and sympathetic fibers. Note the unipolar neurons of the sensory fibers: The Aα are heavily myelinated and rapidly conducting; the Aδ are thinly myelinated; and the C are unmyelinated, derived from both the unipolar sensory neurons and the postganglionic sympathetic neurons [reproduced with permission from Fields, H. L. (1987). *Pain*. Figure 2.1, p. 14. McGraw Hill, New York].

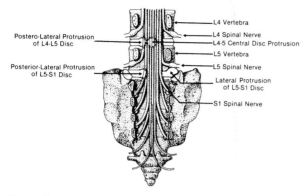

Postero-Lateral Protrusion of L4-L5 Disc

Posterior-Lateral Protrusion of L5-S1 Disc

L4 Vertebra
L4 Spinal Nerve
L4-5 Central Disc Protrusion
L5 Vertebra
L5 Spinal Nerve
Lateral Protrusion of L5-S1 Disc
S1 Spinal Nerve

Figure 7
Dorsal view of the lower lumbar spine and sacrum showing the different types of herniations and the way in which different roots and the cauda equina can be compressed [reproduced with permission from Stewart, J. D. (1993). *Focal Peripheral Neuropathies.* Raven Press, New York].

examination findings are loss of sensation in the toes and attenuated tendon reflexes at the ankles. At this early stage, motor findings may be minimal or limited to mild atrophy and weakness of intrinsic foot muscles. With continued activity of the disease process, sensory loss may spread more proximally to the feet and ankles and possibly to more rostral levels. Loss or reduction of tendon reflexes also may progress to higher levels (the knees); weakness may spread from the feet per se to the legs where the foot dorsi- and plantar flexor muscles may be affected. At a later stage of the disease, the hands may also become involved with sensory loss and weakness of hand intrinsic muscles (those that comprise the thenar [base of the thumb] and hypothenar [base of the little finger] eminences). A less common clinical scenario for the presentation of a polyneuropathy is the early onset of proximally predominant symptoms and signs.

Causes of Peripheral Nerve Disorders

The mononeuropathies are most often caused by compression or entrapment, with median mononeuropathy at the wrist or peroneal mononeuropathy at the fibular head being common examples. Figure 8 shows the clinical features of severe long-standing compression of the median nerves, with evidence for loss of both sensory and motor fibers. The multiple mononeuropathies have several potential causes, including ischemia from vasculitis or diabetic vasculopathy, immune-mediated multifocal demyelination, and genetically determined myelinopathy with predisposition to nerve palsy from compression. The causes of polyneuropathy are numerous, including

genetic, diabetic, and other endocrine, immunological, infectious, toxic, and paraneoplastic causes. The time course of polyneuropathy may be acute, subacute, or chronic; the underlying pathology may be primarily axon loss or demyelinating; and the major fiber types affected may be a combination of sensory, motor, and autonomic.

DISORDERS OF THE NEUROMUSCULAR JUNCTION

Clinical Picture and Causes

There are two forms of neuromuscular junction disorder: one that stems from abnormalities of the postsynaptic component and another caused by disturbances of presynaptic structure and function. The most common postsynaptic disorder, myasthenia gravis, presents with weakness affecting all skeletal muscles, especially those that are cranial nerve innervated, particularly ocular muscles. Figure 9 shows both healthy and myasthenic neuromuscular junctions visualized by electron microscope. Typically, early symptoms include lid droop and double vision followed in some patients by difficulty chewing, swallowing, and speaking and possibly generalized limb weakness. In a small percentage of patients, respiratory muscle weakness may develop. The clinical findings are purely motor and comprise ptosis, diplopia, jaw weakness, dysarthria, dysphagia, and limb muscle weakness. A characteristic of the weakness found in myasthenia gravis is fatigability, a term that denotes the increasing weakness a

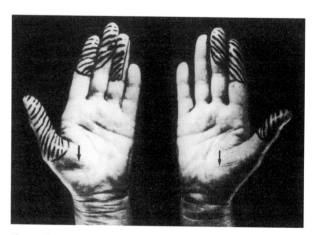

Figure 8
Severe bilateral median mononeuropathies at the wrists (carpal tunnel syndrome). Note the cross-hatching representing areas with sensory loss and also observe the marked muscle atrophy (arrows), especially for the left hand.

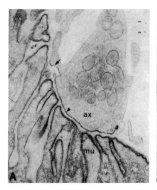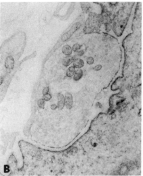

Figure 9
Electron microscopic images showing the neuromuscular junctions from an experimental animal (rabbit) model with experimental autoimmune myasthenia gravis. ax, the axonal presynaptic portion; mu, the muscle postsynaptic region. (A) Normal neuromuscular junction. Note the normally abundant folds of the postsynaptic membrane (arrowheads). (B) Myasthenic neuromuscular junction. Note the extremely simplified postsynaptic membrane.

muscle will demonstrate after it has been repeatedly activated.

The two postsynaptic disorders encountered in clinical practice are Lambert–Eaton myasthenic syndrome (LEMS), an immune-mediated disorder, and botulism, a toxic disorder. In both, generalized weakness is the major symptom and sign. In LEMS, the clinical course is usually subacute to chronic, whereas botulism is typically acute in its presentation. In both, there is an increase in muscle strength after repeated contraction of a weak muscle—a phenomenon referred to as postactivation facilitation.

DISORDERS OF MUSCLE

Clinical Picture

Disorders of muscle are known as myopathies, and their main manifestation is skeletal muscle weakness. Although any skeletal muscle may be affected, most diseases of muscle target limb–girdle and proximal muscle groups, with variable and often less pronounced involvement of distal muscles. Thus, the examination of a patient with myopathy will usually disclose weakness of the following groups: neck flexors and extensor muscles, the shoulder and pelvic girdle muscles, and the humeral and femoral muscles. Figure 10 depicts a patient with a myopathy having difficulty standing from the seated position because of weakness in the region of the hips. In long-standing myopathies, loss of muscle bulk may occur. In some patients with muscular dystrophy, severe muscle wasting associated with joint contractures

and spine abnormalities such as kyphoscoliosis may develop. For myopathies in general, the sensory and tendon reflex examinations are normal. With notable exceptions, in most myopathies the cranial nerve-innervated muscles are normal. For example, ocular muscles are typically targeted in certain myopathies with abnormal mitochondria, facial muscles may be weakened in at least one form of muscular dystrophy (facioscapulohumeral dystrophy), and pharyngeal muscles may be weakened in some of the muscular dystrophies (myotonic dystrophy) and in about 30% of patients with inflammatory myopathy.

Causes of Muscle Disorders

Muscle diseases may be grouped into one of two main categories: genetically determined and acquired. The muscular dystrophies are a group of muscle diseases that are genetically determined and progressive (also known as dystrophic myopathies).

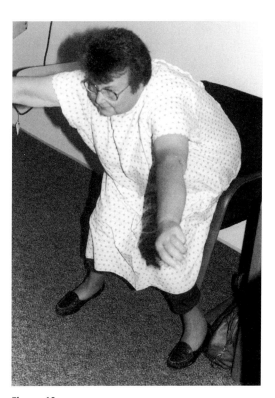

Figure 10
This patient has a severe myopathy secondary to an excess of corticosteroid hormone caused by Cushing's syndrome. Because of marked weakness in the muscles of the pelvis and thighs, she has a wide stance as she attempts to rise from a chair and her movements are labored and effortful [reproduced with permission from Lacomis, D., and Chad, D. A. (1996). Myopathic disorders. In *Practical Neurology of the Elderly* (J. L. Sage and M. H. Mark, Eds.). Dekker, New York].

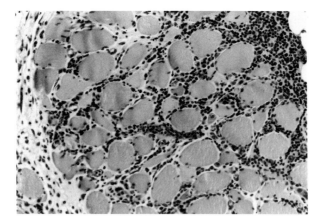

Figure 11
Light microscopic cross-section image of a muscle biopsy specimen from a patient with polymyositis. Note the inflammatory cells surrounding muscle fibers.

They are genetically heterogeneous, and for many the molecular genetic aspects are well understood. These include the X-linked dystrophinopathies (Duchenne, which is the severe form, and the more mild and variable Becker form) and the trinucleotide repeat autosomal dominant disorder myotonic muscular dystrophy. Other genetically determined disorders include the congenital myopathies, which are slowly progressive and relatively benign, and the metabolic myopathies, comprising disorders of glycogen and lipid metabolism and the mitochondrial myopathies. Included in the acquired group of muscle disorders are endocrine, metabolic, inflammatory (polymyositis, dermatomyositis, and inclusion body myositis), and toxic myopathies. Figure 11 shows a light microscopic image of a muscle biopsy specimen from a patient with polymyositis.

—*David A. Chad*

See also–Muscle Contraction, Overview; Nerve Roots; Neuromuscular Transmission Disorders; Neurons, Overview (see also specific entries in the Neuromuscular Disorders section)

Neuromuscular Disorders, Sleep and

Encyclopedia of the Neurological Sciences
Copyright 2003, Elsevier Science (USA). All rights reserved.

COMPROMISE of the ventilatory mechanism is the principal consequence of a neuromuscular dysfunc- tion in the individual who is asleep. Here, I include alterations of the lower motor neuron, the neuro- muscular junction, and muscle. Physiological reduc- tion of general muscle tone in non-rapid eye movement (REM) sleep and loss of muscle tone and activity of intercostal muscles with preservation of diaphragmatic drive in REM sleep determine a unique series of circumstances that bring about the patterns of involvement in patients with neuromus- cular disorders.

During sleep, there are powerful mechanisms that control ventilation and ultimately awaken the person should an obstruction occur. The control of breath- ing is different in non-REM and REM sleep. Signals from a medullary respiratory center drive the respiratory muscle groups that include the dia- phragm, intercostal muscles, and pharyngeal dilator muscles. Both hypoxia and hypercapnia stimulate arousals independently, but when combined, hypoxia increases the sensitivity to arousals caused by PCO_2. Cough is suppressed during sleep and can only occur after an arousal. Laryngeal stimulation during sleep causes reflex apnea.

In non-REM sleep, electromyographic activity increases in intercostal muscles as the ventilatory rate decreases, suggesting increased upper airway resistance that reflects a partial impediment to air flow. Detailed studies of pharyngeal electromyo- graphic (EMG) activity during non-REM sleep have shown a decrease in activity in dilator muscles that likely contributes to the relative upper airway resistance encountered in this stage.

In REM sleep, muscle atonia reduces significantly the activity of intercostal muscles without affecting diaphragmatic muscle tone that may even be increased to compensate for the intercostal loss. Upper airway resistance is also higher during REM sleep, contributing to a decreased efficiency of the ventilatory effort that results in mild hypoxemia.

NEUROMUSCULAR FACTORS CAUSING SLEEP-RELATED RESPIRATORY DYSFUNCTION

Determinant Factors

Diaphragmatic weakness is the major determinant of the pattern of ventilatory compromise in patients with neuromuscular disease. The diaphragm may be weak in isolation or as part of a generalized muscle involvement. Diaphragmatic muscle weakness be- comes specifically manifest during REM sleep when the diaphragm is the only effective muscle pump (Fig. 1). Patients with diaphragmatic paralysis cannot breathe while supine, even in the awake state. Lesser forms of diaphragmatic muscle weakness become apparent during REM sleep, particularly if the patient lies supine. Individuals with neuromuscular disease and diaphragmatic involvement exhibit the greatest oxygen desaturations in REM sleep so that this stage becomes a test of diaphragmatic muscle function.

Phrenic nerve damage resulting in diaphragmatic paralysis may be part of the spectrum of involvement in some diffuse neuropathies and in motor neuron disease. Unilateral paralysis is asymptomatic, but bilateral paralysis is invariably symptomatic and may be life threatening; paresis with partial diaphrag-

matic dysfunction may cause manifestations of sleep-related ventilatory insufficiency. Bilateral paralysis causes orthopnea with difficulty on inspiration out of proportion to the cardiopulmonary status. In the supine posture, patients complain of profound difficulty breathing that is the result of a reduction in lung volume and increased inspiratory effort as the abdominal contents rise into the thorax. In severe or acute cases, patients present with nocturnal orthopnea, cyanosis, and fragmented sleep followed by morning headaches, vomiting, and daytime lethargy.

The severity of hypoventilation and the depth of oxygen desaturation in non-REM sleep are determined by the degree of involvement of chest wall and accessory respiratory muscles. Undiagnosed bilateral diaphragmatic paralysis of any cause may lead to

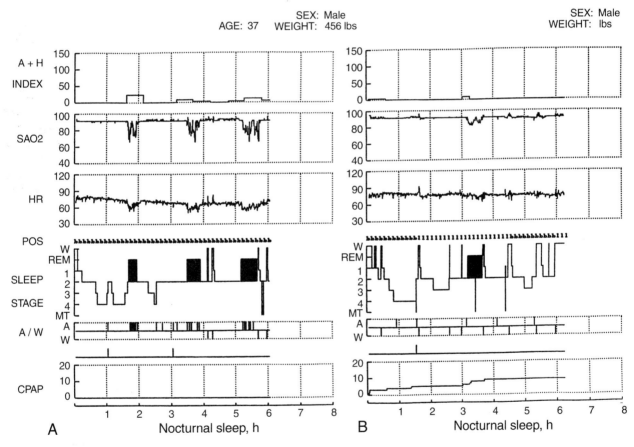

Figure 1
(A) Hypnogram of 37-year-old obese man showing diaphragmatic insufficiency manifested in REM sleep (sleep stage) by clusters of oxygen desaturation events (SAO$_2$) that correlate with a higher respiratory disturbance index (A + H index), heart instability (HR), and arousals (A/W). (B) CPAP application at 10 cm H$_2$O reduces respiratory disturbance events (A + H index), depth of desaturation events (SAO$_2$), heart instability (HR), and arousals (A/W) during REM sleep. Nocturnal sleep progresses hourly from "lights out" at 0 to final awakening at 6. Hypnogram constructed from overnight polysomnogram. SAO$_2$, saturation of oxygen measured with finger oximetry; HR, heart rate measured by ECG; POS, body position in sleep; sleep stage, architecture of sleep; A/W, arousals and awakenings; jerks, leg jerks; CPAP, continuous positive airway pressure.

acute cardiopulmonary failure and death. Some reports describe unexplained failure to wean from respirator as the presenting manifestation of diaphragmatic paralysis in patients with undiagnosed motor neuron disease or myopathies.

Phrenic nerve paralysis has been reported in patients with Charcot–Marie–Tooth disease (hereditary motor and sensory neuropathy) complicated with diabetes mellitus and in spinal cord injury, poliomyelitis, Guillain–Barré syndrome, diabetes, diphtheric neuropathy, beri-beri, alcoholic neuropathy, brachial plexus neuropathy, lead neuropathy, trauma, amyotrophic lateral sclerosis (ALS), myotonic dystrophy, Duchenne's muscular dystrophy, paraneoplastic syndrome, and idiopathic conditions.

Contributing Factors

Restrictive lung disorder contributes to the ventilatory disturbance in patients with neuromuscular disease. This may be the consequence of chest wall muscle weakness, scoliosis, and pulmonary microatelectases that result from chronic hypoventilation, repeated episodes of aspiration, and retained secretions. These changes may lead to perfusion of nonventilated lung parenchyma, aggravating hypoxemia.

Weakness of pharyngeal muscle dilators increases inspiratory upper airway resistance and may precipitate obstructive sleep apnea in patients with neuromuscular disorders. Weakness of pharyngeal muscle dilators facilitates the reduction of the pharyngeal lumen during negative intrathoracic pressures and tends to collapse the pharyngeal wall, increasing resistance to the flow of air in the upper airway.

Structural anomalies, such as craniofacial dysmorphias and micrognathia, reduce the oropharyngeal lumen. Patients with congenital myopathies and muscular dystrophies commonly have poor development of facial bones and mandible.

Anatomical alterations of the oropharyngeal area, including tonsillar hypertrophy and macroglossia, are nonspecific disorders that may also be present in patients with neuromuscular disease.

Scoliosis is a common occurrence in these patients. Postural alteration of the spine causes a disadvantage of intercostal muscle and diaphragmatic function that is translated in a less efficient inspiratory mechanism.

Sedentariness, which is very common in weak patients, promotes obesity, another factor that burdens ventilatory efficiency during sleep. Obese patients exhibit reduction of intercostal muscle

function, and subjects with abdominal obesity have limitation of diaphragmatic function that is particularly evident during REM sleep. Accumulation of fat in oropharyngeal soft tissues contributes to restriction of the oropharyngeal lumen.

Associated Factors

In some forms of congenital myopathy, there is evidence of impairment of respiratory chemosensitivity that may be familial in nature. The combination of ventilatory muscle dysfunction and reduced central ventilatory drive is particularly dangerous.

Neuromuscular disorders with associated central neurological disease may show other patterns of involvement. Although ventilatory dysfunction is the prime sleep-related abnormality in most patients with a neuromuscular disorder, some sleep/wake alterations cannot be explained solely on the basis of a peripheral respiratory disorder. Patients with myotonic dystrophy may have hypersomnia that is not corrected with ventilatory assistance or that appears in excess of, or in the absence of, a ventilatory impediment. These patients have an intrinsic form of hypersomnia that is poorly understood but may be related to neuronal damage in the dorsomedial nucleus of the thalamus. In some forms of congenital myopathy, there is impairment of respiratory chemosensitivity with reduced sleep-related ventilatory drive independent of hypoxemia and hypercapnia, suggesting a central dysfunction and not a mere blunting of chemosensitivity.

CONSEQUENCES OF SLEEP-RELATED VENTILATORY DYSFUNCTION

Sleep-related ventilatory deficit in patients with neuromuscular disease may cause nocturnal hypoxemia or episodes of oxygen desaturation that precipitate restlessness, arousals, and sleep fragmentation. Depending on the severity of the ventilatory deficit, patients may have continuous alveolar hypoventilation, even in the awake state, that in the most advanced circumstances becomes complicated with CO_2 retention. Patients with sleep-related ventilatory deficit usually exhibit secondary daytime excessive somnolence, a development that should prompt testing with polysomnography. Development of excessive daytime somnolence in weak subjects is a marker of preterminal muscular disease and heralds major vulnerability in the event of respiratory illness. Sitting positions in sleep, nocturnal cyanosis, morning drowsiness, headaches and vomiting, and even cor pulmonale attributed to nocturnal hypoventilation have been reported in patients with advanced neuromuscular disease. Appropriate ventilatory therapy may reverse the condition.

Nocturnal hypoventilation with hypoxemia and hypercapnia when uncorrected lead to blunting of peripheral and central respiratory chemoreceptor responses that determine a state of chronic alveolar hypoventilation.

NEUROMUSCULAR CONDITIONS WITH SLEEP DISORDER

Postpolio Syndrome

Survivors of the acute attack of poliomyelitis may develop a condition 20–30 years later characterized by progressive fatigue, joint pains, and weakness in muscles not previously affected that has been termed the postpolio syndrome. Sleep disturbances appear in 31% of patients, even in those without prior bulbar involvement. In the postpolio syndrome, central respiratory control and peripheral respiratory function may be affected. Physiological studies have shown delayed latencies of onset of muscle tone reduction, sawtooth waves, and rapid eye movements in REM sleep of patients with bulbar forms of poliomyelitis, suggesting neuronal pontine damage. Some patients present progressive deterioration of nocturnal sleep as sleep apnea episodes with oxygen desaturation events become increasingly frequent. Apneas are of the central, obstructive, and mixed variety. Some of the complaints typically attributed to the postpolio syndrome, such as increasing fatigue, may be the result of nocturnal respiratory dysfunction and thus potentially correctable with continuous positive airway pressure (CPAP) or bilevel positive airway pressure (BiPAP) applications. Sleep studies should be performed in all postpolio patients complaining of sleep disturbance and respiratory manifestations. Patients with kyphoscoliosis secondary to poliomyelitis often develop restrictive respiratory dysfunction, particularly if there is associated weakness of thoracoabdominal and respiratory accessory muscles.

Amyotrophic Lateral Sclerosis

Progressive degeneration of corticobulbar and corticospinal tracts and anterior horn cells determines the pattern of neuromuscular involvement in ALS. Several studies have reported sleep apnea events in patients with ALS, generally of the nonobstructive or mixed varieties, perhaps as a result of the inability to generate negative inspiratory gradients sufficient to overcome upper airway closing pressures. Response to noninvasive respiratory support with BiPAP apparatus has been favorable. Elimination of nocturnal respiratory distress and restlessness as well as alleviation of daytime somnolence and tiredness improve the quality of life.

Myasthenia Gravis

Patients with myasthenia gravis develop excessive muscular fatigability. It may involve the diaphragm and accessory respiratory muscles with resulting respiratory failure in unmedicated or uncontrolled patients. Sleep-related complaints in some patients include waking up with sensation of breathlessness, morning headaches, and daytime somnolence. Respiratory function may be altered during sleep, with CO_2 retention and respiratory failure serious enough to require ventilatory assistance. Polygraphic studies show an increased sleep apnea index with predominantly mixed and obstructive sleep apnea episodes, along with oxygen desaturation events of moderate severity. This is particularly evident during the REM stage, when the diaphragm is the only muscle that remains active in the exchange of air. Older patients with increased body mass index and abnormal daytime blood gas concentration are more vulnerable to the development of a diaphragmatic form of sleep apnea syndrome with oxygen desaturation. Daytime somnolence in a patient with myasthenia gravis should suggest abnormal breathing during sleep, even in the absence of abnormal daytime functional activity. The dysfunction usually responds to the administration of slow-release pyridostigmine at night, although patients receiving appropriate treatment with satisfactory daytime functional capacity may still have abnormal breathing during sleep. As in other neuromuscular conditions, polysomnographic evaluation is indicated and noninvasive ventilatory assistance should be considered.

Myotonic Dystrophy

Excessive daytime sleepiness and respiratory failure both during wakefulness and in sleep are commonly observed in patients with myotonic dystrophy. Hypersomnia may have features suggestive of narcolepsy, including sleep-onset REM periods. Hypersomnia may be aggravated by alveolar hypoventilation and the sleep apnea syndrome, but it is not reversed entirely with CPAP applications, suggesting that hypersomnia is in part an intrinsic disorder related to central nervous system disease not caused by sleep apnea.

Hypersomnia, apathy, mental decline, and slow alpha rhythms in subjects with moderately advanced disease have been linked to histological changes and dysfunction of the dorsomedial nuclei of the thalamus. The sleep-related breathing disorder in myotonic dystrophy may be another manifestation of central alteration. Nonobstructive sleep apneas and sleep-related alveolar hypoventilation are common and may contribute to increased somnolence. Early muscular weakness in patients with myotonic dystrophy affects craniofacial and mandibular growth, contributing to the development of obstructive sleep apnea by increasing airway resistance through a stenotic oropharynx. Hypersomnia in myotonic dystrophy may respond successfully to the administration of methylphenidate.

Muscular Dystrophies

Patients with Duchenne's muscular dystrophy develop restrictive lung disease as muscle weakness progresses and rib cage deformities appear. Studies of patients with moderately advanced disorder have reported nocturnal hypoventilation with profound desaturation during REM sleep despite normal awake minute ventilation. Others have described abundant fragmentation of nocturnal sleep, many sleep stage changes, and reduced REM sleep but no evidence of nocturnal hypoxia in patients with advanced muscular weakness and skeletal deformities. Daytime predictors of sleep hypoventilation in Duchenne's muscular dystrophy are a P_aCO_2 $\geqslant 45$ mmHg and a forced expiratory velocity of less than 40%. These patients should be tested with polysomnography, and consideration should be given to treatment with noninvasive positive pressure ventilation. On the other hand, preventive treatment with nasal intermittent positive pressure ventilation has not reduced survival of patients with Duchenne's muscular dystrophy with forced vital capacity between 20 and 50% of the predicted value.

Severe nocturnal respiratory failure has been described in patients with nemaline myopathy, a congenital myopathy with a relatively benign prognosis that affects all skeletal muscles including the diaphragm. Also, various combinations of nocturnal respiratory dysfunction have been reported in patients with congenital fiber-type disproportion syndrome, mitochondrial myopathy, and acid maltase deficiency.

GENERAL APPROACH

Patients with neuromuscular disorder may present with nocturnal restlessness, frequent unexplained awakenings, and loud snoring punctuated by episodes of wakefulness gasping for breath. Patients and relatives report difficulty awakening in the morning and prolonged sleep inertia that may interfere with morning activities. During daytime hours, these patients may present somnolence, fatigue, and inappropriate napping, which result in failure to thrive in the very young and declining school grades or work performance at later ages. More ominously, some patients develop nocturnal cyanosis, severe insomnia, morning lethargy, headaches, vomiting, and leg edema that indicate the occurrence of acute respiratory failure and cor pulmonale. Polysomnographic evaluation with the sleep apnea protocol, followed by a multiple sleep latency test when an intrinsic hypersomnia is also suspected, helps differentiate the various causes of sleep disturbance and serves to assess the severity of the disorder.

Nocturnal disruption with secondary excessive daytime somnolence may also occur as an independent abnormality translating nocturnal postural discomfort in a weak, incapacitated, and sometimes deformed patient.

SUGGESTED MANAGEMENT

Therapeutic goals should define whether therapy is directed at elimination of excessive daytime somnolence, improvement of nocturnal desaturation, reconstruction of sleep architecture, or correction of respiratory and heart failure. Positive pressure breathing corrects obstructive sleep apnea, improves hypoventilation, and assists diaphragmatic failure (Fig. 1). Supplemental oxygen via mask is recommended when positive air pressure therapy is insufficient to overcome mean levels of hypoventilation of 85% or less. BiPAP is better tolerated by patients with weak chest walls and failing diaphragm who cannot overcome expiratory forces. Supplemental oxygen via nasal cannula may be sufficient in some cases to correct REM sleep-related desaturations.

Tracheostomy is indicated in a few cases, but dependence and medical complications have to be weighed against the benefits obtained. Ethical considerations of prolongation of undignified life versus improvement of quality of life may have to be addressed in patients with terminal neuromuscular disease. Children younger than age 6 tolerate nasal ventilation poorly, so other therapeutic measures may have to be considered, including temporal use of tracheostomy.

Protriptyline (5–10 mg) at bedtime improves muscle tone and is of some value in patients with mild obstructive sleep apnea with weak pharyngeal walls. The REM sleep-inhibiting effect of protriptyline helps reduce REM sleep-related hypoventilation. There is evidence that methylphenidate controls hypersomnia in patients with myotonic dystrophy who do not respond to the application of CPAP.

—*Antonio Culebras*

See also–Amyotrophic Lateral Sclerosis (ALS); Cataplexy; Myasthenia Gravis; Myotonic Dystrophy; NREM (Non Rapid Eye Movement) Sleep; Postpoliomyelitis Syndrome; REM (Rapid Eye Movement) Sleep; REM Sleep Behavior Disorder; Sleep Disorders

Further Reading

Barthlen, G. M. (1997). Nocturnal respiratory failure as an indication of noninvasive ventilation in the patient with neuromuscular disease. *Respiration* 64, 35–38.
Culebras, A. (1996). Sleep and neuromuscular disorders. *Neurol. Clin.* 14, 791–805.
Culebras, A., Feldman, R. G., and Merk, F. B. (1973). Cytoplasmic inclusion bodies within neurons of the thalamus in myotonic dystrophy: A light and electron microscopy study. *J. Neurol. Sci.* 19, 319–329.
David, W. S., Bundlie, S. R., and Mahdavi, Z. (1997). Polysomnographic studies in amyotrophic lateral sclerosis. *J. Neurol. Sci.* 152, S29–S35.
Hukins, C. A., and Hillman, D. R. (2000). Daytime predictors of sleep hypoventilation in Duchenne muscular dystrophy. *Am. J. Respir. Crit. Care Med.* 161, 166–170.
Quera-Salva, M. A., Guilleminault, C., Chevret, S., *et al.* (1992). Breathing disorders during sleep in myasthenia gravis. *Ann. Neurol.* 31, 86–92.
Siegel, H., McCutchen, C., Dalakas, M. C., *et al.* (1999). Physiologic events initiating REM sleep in patients with the postpolio syndrome. *Neurology* 52, 516–522.
Steljes, D. G., Kryger, M. H., Kirk, B. W., *et al.* (1990). Sleep in postpolio syndrome. *Chest* 98, 133–140.
Van der Meche, F. G., Bogaard, J. M., van der Sluys, J. C., *et al.* (1994). Daytime sleep in myotonic dystrophy is not caused by sleep apnoea. *J. Neurol. Neurosurg. Psychiatry* 57, 626–628.
Wilson, D. O., Sanders, M. H., and Dauber, J. H. (1987). Abnormal ventilatory chemosensitivity and congenital myopathy. *Arch. Intern. Med.* 147, 1773–1777.

Neuromuscular Junction, Normal

Encyclopedia of the Neurological Sciences
Copyright 2003, Elsevier Science (USA). All rights reserved.

THE NEUROMUSCULAR JUNCTION (NMJ) is a functional unit consisting of highly specialized structures at the nerve terminal (presynapse) and at the muscle end plate (postsynapse) as well as the gap between them (synapse), across which electrochemical communication occurs. This highly evolved junction ensures highly reliable and efficient transmission over a wide range of conditions in the healthy individual. Because it is readily accessible and is found in a wide variety of species, it has been the subject of intensive investigation for many years. Although our knowledge of the NMJ is extensive, ongoing research continues to provide important insights into its detailed complexities. As individual motor axons within a peripheral nerve approach the muscle, they branch repeatedly, ultimately forming single lightly myelinated nerve fibers, each of which loses its insulating myelin just before dividing into several smaller branches known as the terminal spray. Each of these branches then terminates in a bulbous swollen tip (the terminal bouton), just above the specialized portion of an individual muscle fiber membrane known as the end plate zone. Each terminal bouton contains an abundance of small, rounded, membrane-enclosed vesicles arranged for quick release in a docking region known as the active zone. These vesicles are synthesized in the nerve cell body and transported by fast axonal transport to their final destination in the nerve terminal, and each contains 5000–12,000 molecules of the chemical neurotransmitter acetylcholine (ACh) (Fig. 1).

PRESYNAPTIC STRUCTURE AND FUNCTION

The presynaptic terminal also contains a network of ion channels and proteins that provide the machinery for vesicular release. As voluntary muscle activation is initiated, a signal travels from the corticospinal pathway to the origin of the motor axon (the anterior horn) selected by the upper motor pathways for activation. A depolarizing impulse then travels from the anterior horn down its motor axon, over the length of the axonal pathway, and down each branch of that axon, ultimately reaching the terminal boutons. As the depolarization wave moves over

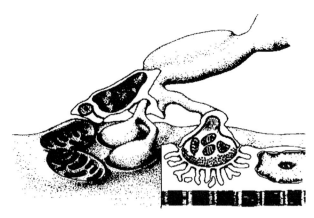

Figure 1
The neuromuscular junction. The muscle end plate is exposed on the far left (presynaptic elements removed) and intact terminal boutons are illustrated at the lower center (Schwann cell elements removed). A cross section of the pre- and postsynaptic elements is shown at far right, demonstrating (top to bottom) neurofilaments, mitochondria, synaptic acetylcholine vesicles, the synapse, primary synaptic clefts, muscle striations, and a muscle fiber nucleus [reproduced with permission from Jennekens, F. G. I., Veldman, H., and Wokke, J. H. J. (1993). Histology and pathology of the human neuromuscular junction with a description of the clinical features of the myasthenic syndromes. In *Myasthenia Gravis* (M. H. De Baets and H. J. G. H. Oosterhuis, Eds.), p. 101. CRC Press, Boca Raton, FL].

the terminal membrane, a number of voltage-gated calcium channels are opened, allowing calcium flux into the cell. Rising calcium levels then activate a network of proteins, triggering fusion of individual ACh vesicles with the terminal membrane and extrusion of their contents into the synapse. Functionally, the ACh vesicles can be categorized into two pools: an active pool, which is positioned and ready for immediate fusion and release, and a reserve pool, which must be mobilized toward the synaptic membrane before fusion and release can occur. The mechanics of vesicle mobilization, fusion, and release are complex and continue to be intensively studied. Vesicles in the reserve pool are connected to a network of specialized neurofilaments by the protein synapsin 1. After calcium entry into the cell, calcium calmodulin-dependent protein kinase (residing within the vesicle membrane) triggers phosphorylation of synapsin 1, enabling vesicle release from the network and subsequent mobilization. As the vesicle approaches the neuronal membrane, a series of interactions must occur between a number of vesicle membrane and other neuronal membrane proteins for docking and fusion. To date, the necessary vesicle proteins identified include synaptobrevin (also known as vesicle-associated membrane protein),

synaptotagmin, and synaptophysin. Important neuronal membrane proteins include syntaxin and SNAP-25 (soluble N-ethylmalemide-sensitive factor attachment protein-25). Other, less well-characterized cytoplasmic proteins are also likely involved, although the precise mechanistic details for each stage of vesicle mobilization, docking, and release have yet to be elucidated.

POSTSYNAPTIC STRUCTURE AND FUNCTION

Following vesicle fusion, ACh molecules are released and passively diffuse across the synaptic cleft (approximately 60 nm) toward the muscle fiber's end plate. The muscle end plate is an involuted structure containing numerous crests and valleys, with high concentrations of specialized nicotinic acetylcholine receptors (AChRs) concentrated on the shoulders of each crest. The AChR is a membrane-spanning protein containing five component subunits—alpha, beta, gamma, delta, and epsilon—arrayed in a circle around a central ion channel. The adult AChR contains two alpha subunits and one, beta, delta and epsilon subunit, whereas the embryonic AChR contains one gamma subunit instead of the adult epsilon. The embryonic gamma subunit is replaced in adult development or following denervation except in the extraocular muscles, in which the gamma subunits may persist into adulthood. The larger portion of each receptor extends above the membrane into the synaptic space and contains binding sites for two ACh molecules, located on each of the receptor's alpha subunits. Opening of the central ion channel only occurs when both AChRs are occupied. The receptors have a half-life of approximately 5 days at the junction following synthesis and transport and are removed via internalization and lysosomal digestion.

Following their arrival at the end plate, the ACh molecules within each vesicle successfully activate an average of 1000–2000 AChR ion channels in a given muscle fiber. The subsequent influx of sodium into the muscle fiber results in a localized area of electrical depolarization around the receptor site known as a miniature end plate potential (MEPP). During actual contraction, a large number of simultaneous MEPPs summate, creating a larger, global end plate potential that eventually reaches the muscle fiber's threshold for propagating a depolarization wave. This wave then travels over the entire muscle fiber, igniting a chain of events ultimately resulting in contraction of the muscle fiber. Following completion of depolarization, the ACh molecules are released from their receptors and hydrolyzed by synaptic acetylcholinesterase, preventing further receptor activation until the next wave of ACh release.

Significant structural and functional alterations in the NMJ may result from a variety of disease processes, including acquired and congenital myasthenia gravis and Lambert–Eaton myasthenic syndrome, which are detailed elsewhere in this encyclopedia.

—*Clifton L. Gooch*

See also–Acetylcholine; Lambert–Eaton Myasthenic Syndrome; Muscle Contraction, Overview; Myasthenia Gravis; Neuromuscular Disorders, Overview; Neuromuscular Transmission Disorders

Further Reading

De Baets, M. H., and Oosterhuis, H. J. G. H. (Eds.) (1993). *Myasthenia Gravis*. CRC Press, Boca Raton, FL.

Drachman, D. B. (1994). Myasthenia gravis. *N. Engl. J. Med.* 330, 1797–1810.

Gooch, C. L. (1997). Myasthenia gravis and Lambert–Eaton myasthenic syndrome. In *Neuroimmunology for the Clinician* (Y. Harati and L. A. Rolak, Eds.), pp. 263–299. Butterworth-Heinemann, Newton, MA.

Kandel, E., and Sieglebaum, S. (2001). Signaling at the nerve muscle synapse: Directly gated transmission. In *Principles of Neural Science* (E. Kandel, J. Schwartz, and T. Jessell, Eds.), 4th ed., pp. 187–205. McGraw-Hill, New York.

Lisak, R. P. (Ed.) (1994). *Handbook of Myasthenia Gravis and Myasthenic Syndromes*. Dekker, New York.

Rowland, L. (2001). Diseases of chemical transmission at the nerve–muscle synapse: Myasthenia gravis. In *Principles of Neural Science* (E. Kandel, J. Schwartz, and T. Jessell, Eds.), 4th ed., pp. 298–308. McGraw-Hill, New York.

Sanders, D. B. (1993). Clinical neurophysiology of disorders of the neuromuscular junction. *J. Clin. Neurophysiol.* 12, 169.

Sanders, D. B. (Ed.) (1994). Myasthenia gravis and myasthenic syndromes. *Neurol. Clin. North Am.* 12, 305–329.

Schonbeck, S., Chrestel, S., and Hohlfeld, R. (1990). Myasthenia gravis: Prototype of the antireceptor autoimmune diseases. *Int. Rev. Neurobiol.* 32, 175–200.

Neuromuscular Transmission Disorders

Encyclopedia of the Neurological Sciences
Copyright 2003, Elsevier Science (USA). All rights reserved.

NEUROMUSCULAR TRANSMISSION is a process that permits the central nervous system to control the movement of muscles in the body. Nerve impulses cause the release of a neurotransmitter, acetylcholine (ACh), into the junction between the nerve cell and the muscle cell. Diseases involving the neuromuscular junction are called neuromuscular transmission (NMT) disorders because they are caused by a dysfunction in the transmission of ACh at the nerve–muscle synapse. Depending on the site of dysfunction, NMT disorders are classified into three distinct groups: postsynaptic disorders, presynaptic disorders, and combined presynaptic and postsynaptic disorders.

Myasthenia gravis (MG), the most common and widely known postsynaptic disorder, occurs due to a decrease in the functioning ACh receptors induced by the ACh receptor antibodies. The best example of a presynaptic disorder is the Lambert–Eaton myasthenic syndrome (LEMS), which is commonly associated with carcinoma of the lung. The main defect in this disorder is the insufficient release of ACh at the presynaptic membrane induced by the antibodies against the voltage gate-dependent calcium channels. Another well-known presynaptic disorder is botulism. Botulinum toxin is known to inhibit the release of ACh. An example of a combined pre- and postsynaptic disorder is antibiotic-induced myasthenic syndrome, which is most commonly seen with aminoglycosides. These disorders can be diagnosed and differentiated from one another by the repetitive nerve stimulation (RNS) test and the single-fiber EMG (SFEMG).

REPETITIVE NERVE STIMULATION TEST

The RNS test is the most commonly used technique for studying NMT disorders because of its relative simplicity and rapid results. This test is performed by repetitive stimulation of any motor nerve with recording electrodes on innervating muscles. It assesses the physiological status of NMT by stimulating the nerve at various rates of supramaximal stimulation at rest and after exercise. Ideally, testing should consist of recording the compound muscle action potential (CMAP) from the muscle at rest, the CMAP after exercise, the response at the low rate of stimulation (LRS; 1–5 Hz), the response at the high rate of stimulation (HRS; 10–50 Hz), and post-tetanic (after HRS stimulation) or exercise responses. This ideal testing program can be easily applied to the distal muscles, such as those in the hand. The most commonly tested distal muscle is the abductor digiti quinti muscle. However, due to technical

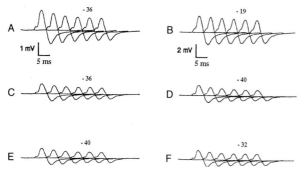

Figure 1
RNS responses in LEMS following Lambert's method at a rate of stimulation of 3 Hz: (A) at rest, (B) 10 sec after exercise, (C) 30 sec after exercise, (D) 1 min after exercise, (E) 2 min after exercise, and (F) 4 min after exercise. Note that there is a postexercise increase in amplitude (177% increase by ratio compared with the normal ratio of <115%) as well as a decremental response. Numbers above the responses represent the percentage of decrement (reprinted with permission from Oh, 1992).

difficulty, proximal muscle testing usually consists of recording the CMAP at rest and the response at LRS. The most commonly tested proximal muscles are the orbicularis oculi and trapezius muscles.

The most popular and commonly described RNS test in electromyography (EMG) textbooks is Lambert's method (Fig. 1). This method records the CMAP with a surface electrode from the abductor digiti quinti muscle, with the stimulating electrodes at the ulnar nerve at the wrist. The nerve is stimulated at the rate of 3 Hz according to the testing program. Some laboratories use the high rate of stimulation to rule out the presence of LEMS.

In normal muscles, there is no decremental or incremental response in the RNS test due to the wide range of the safety factor at the neuromuscular junction. A decrement greater than 8–10% is universally accepted as abnormal at the LRS. Normal values for the RNS tests vary depending on the rate of stimulation, the muscles tested, the techniques used, and the activation tests employed. Thus, one has to refer to the normal value for the specific muscle and technique. All parameters of the RNS test are helpful in the diagnosis of NMT disorders.

CMAP

The amplitude should be measured at rest and after exercise. The repetitive discharge must be recognized. A normal CMAP is indicative of a postsynaptic disorder, whereas a low CMAP indicates a presynaptic disorder. Repetitive discharges are indicative of one of the following disorders: excessive

acetylcholinesterase (AChE) medications such as pyridostigmine, organophosphate poisoning, or congenital MG type A or B. Postexercise facilitation (a significant increase in the amplitude after exercise) is pathognomonic of a presynaptic disorder (Fig. 1). Postexercise depression (a significant decrease in the amplitude after exercise) is associated with excessive AChE treatment, organophosphate poisoning, or myotonic syndrome.

RNS Test at LRS

The decremental response is sought in this test because an abnormal response at LRS is usually indicative of NMT block. Thus, the LRS is the most important parameter in the RNS test. In MG, the best diagnostic sensitivity is observed at LRS. A dramatic improvement in the abnormal decremental response with edrophonium is typical of MG. A decrement at the second response with a gradual increment (dip phenomenon) is pathognomonic of AChE toxicity.

RNS Test at HRS

The HRS is crucial in the differentiation between presynaptic and postsynaptic disorders because this is the single most important diagnostic test for LEMS. The decremental and incremental responses are obtained in this test. An abnormal decremental response is indicative of severe postsynaptic block. In mild postsynaptic block, the response at HRS is normal. A markedly abnormal incremental response (more than 100%) is pathognomonic of the following presynaptic disorders: LEMS, botulism, magnesium-induced weakness, and overlap myasthenic syndrome.

Post-tetanic Facilitation and Post-tetanic Exhaustion

Following brief tetanic stimulation, there is a short-lived electrophysiological improvement in the decremental response [post-tetanic facilitation (PTF)] followed by a prolonged electrophysiological worsening [post-tetanic exhaustion (PTE)] in MG. The post-tetanic response is representative of a physiological change occurring at the synaptic cleft at HRS: PTF represents a short-lived increase in ACh available at the postsynaptic receptor, improving an NMT block, and PTE may be due to receptor desensitization. PTF followed by PTE is observed in presynaptic and postsynaptic NMT disorders. Since this phenomenon represents a physiological change, technical artifacts cannot reproduce it. Thus, PTF followed by

PTE is pathognomonic of NMT disorders. On the basis of the patterns of abnormalities in the RNS test, one can differentiate between postsynaptic disorders, presynaptic disorders, and combined pre- and postsynaptic disorders.

In MG, the RNS test is positive in distal muscles in approximately 50% of cases (Fig. 2) and positive in proximal muscles in approximately 70% of cases. The classic pattern in MG is normal CMAP amplitude and decremental response at LRS. In LEMS, the RNS test is positive in 100% of cases. The classic pattern is low CMAP amplitude, decremental response at LRS, and incremental response at

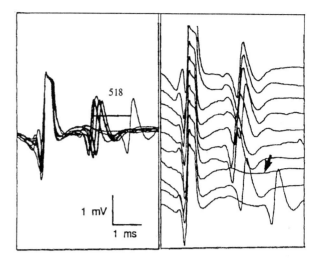

Figure 3
Abnormal jitter and blocking of the SFEMG in MG. The horizontal line and number indicate the range (R10) between the shortest and longest interpotential interval. The mean value of the consecutive interpotential interval difference (MCD) is 518 μsec (normal MCD, 53 μsec). The arrow indicates blocking of one single-fiber potential [reprinted with permission from Oh, S. J. (1993). *Clinical Electromyography: Nerve Conduction Studies*, p. 24. Williams & Wilkins, Baltimore].

HRS. In botulism, the classic pattern is similar to that of LEMS but less prominent in the degree of abnormality.

SINGLE-FIBER EMG

The single-fiber EMG, a relatively new test, is a selective recording technique in which a single-fiber EMG needle is used to identify and record action potentials from individual muscle fibers. This test assesses the microphysiological status of the end plates of muscles. This technique has proven to be of value in the diagnosis of MG and other NMT disorders.

The most characteristic finding is abnormal jitter, which is marked variability in the time interval between two potentials (Fig. 3). When jitter is markedly abnormal, blocking of one potential occurs. Jitter is abnormal in 88–100% of MG cases and in 100% of LEMS and botulism cases.

—*Shin J. Oh*

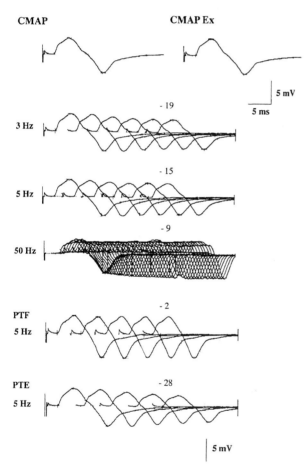

Figure 2
RNS response in FCU muscle following Oh's method. The RNS pattern is typical of mild MG: normal CMAP, decremental response at LRS, normal response at HRS, and post-tetanic facilitation (PTF) and post-tetanic exhaustion (PTE) phenomena. PTE, 5-Hz stimulation immediately after tetanic (50 Hz) stimulation; PTE, 5-Hz stimulation 4 min after tetanic stimulation [reprinted with permission from Oh, S. J. (1998). *Principles of Clinical Electromyography: Case Studies*, p. 482. Williams & Wilkins, Baltimore].

***See also*–Acetylcholine; Electromyography (EMG); Lambert–Eaton Myasthenic Syndrome; Myasthenia Gravis; Neuromuscular Disorders, Overview; Neuromuscular Junction, Normal**

Further Reading

Keesey, J. C. (1989). Electrodiagnostic approach to defects of neuromuscular transmission. *Muscle Nerve* **12**, 613–626.

Oh, S. J. (1988). *Electromyography: Neuromuscular Transmission Studies*. Williams & Wilkins, Baltimore.

Oh, S. J. (1992). Repetitive nerve stimulation test. *Methods Clin. Neurophysiol.* **3**, 1–15.

Sanders, D. B., and Stålberg, E. (1996). AAEM Minimonograph #25 Single-fiber electromyography. *Muscle Nerve* **19**, 1069–1083.

Stålberg, E., and Trontel, J. V. (1994). *Single Fiber Electromyography*, 2nd ed. Raven Press, New York.

Neuronal Ceroid Lipofuscinoses

Encyclopedia of the Neurological Sciences
Copyright 2003, Elsevier Science (USA). All rights reserved.

NEURONAL CEROID LIPOFUSCINOSES (NCLs), also known as Batten's disease, comprise a large group of neurodegenerative, lysosomal storage disorders that are inherited as an autosomal recessive trait and occur mainly in infancy and childhood. Eight forms of NCLs have been identified, with a frequency ranging in different countries from 0.1 to 7 per 100,000 live births. These disorders are prototypes of genetic conditions that interfere with neuronal and retinal functions but are not expressed or have only a minor role in the function of other cell types.

The NCLs provide two hallmarks of these disorders, namely, the age at onset followed by the loss of acquired brain function and presenting as neurodegenerative disorders. Early development in affected individuals, including speech and ambulation, may be normal, but after years or even a decade a continuous regression occurs. The important clinical concepts that have evolved from the general to specific provide an essential framework in guiding the necessary steps to reach a diagnosis among the increasing complexity of molecular genetics.

RESEARCH PROGRESS

Up to 1995, only four forms of NCLs were known, and the diagnosis was based on the age at onset, clinical signs, and pathological findings with specific lysosomal storage material of ceroid lipofuscins demonstrated at electron microscopy. The types of the disorders included (i) the infantile NCL (INCL) or Haltia/Santavuori disease, with granular osmiophilic deposits (GRODs); (ii) the classic late infantile NCL (cLINCL) or Jansky–Bielchowsky disease, with curvilinear (CV) profiles; (iii) the juvenile NCL (JNCL) or Spielmeyer–Vogt–Sjogren disease, with fingerprint profiles (FPs); and (iv) the adult NCL (ANCL) or Kufs' disease, with mixed profiles (CV and FPs, with or without GRODs). However, approximately 20% of disorders were clinically and pathologically atypical, with overlapping ages of onset and mixed profiles (CV, FPs, GRODs, and rectilinear complexes), and they did not fit the four recognized forms. With research progress, four additional forms have been identified: the Finnish variant (fLINCL), the early juvenile variant (vLINCL), the Turkish variant (tLINCL), and the northern epilepsy, which is known as progressive epilepsy with mental retardation. Six genes—*CLN1–CLN3*, *CLN5*, *CLN6*, and *CLN8*—have been associated with INCL, LINCL, JNCL, fLINCL, vLINCL, and progressive epilepsy with mental retardation, respectively. The gene locations of *CLN4*, associated with ANCL, and *CLN7*, associated with tLINCL, have not been identified.

The *CLN1* gene encodes palmitoyl protein thioesterase-1 (PPT-1), a lysosomal enzyme involved in depalmitoylation of proteins. The *CLN2* gene encodes a tripeptidyl peptidase-1 (TPP-1), a lysosomal enzyme acting as an aminopeptidase that removes tripeptides from the free N termini of proteins. The functions of four other proteins encoded by genes *CLN3*, *CLN5*, *CLN6*, and *CLN8* are unknown; however, their predicted amino acid sequences suggest that these proteins have transmembrane topologies. The pathological identification of distinctive lysosomal storage material (inclusions) (Fig. 1) remains a useful but not infallible guide to recognizing the eight different forms of NCL. Numerous mutations have been identified in genes *CLN1–CLN3*, *CLN5*, *CLN6*, and *CLN8*, and these are summarized in Table 1.

CLINICAL ASSESSMENT

After reviewing the history and clinical findings, the following questions should be addressed: Is this a progressive neurodegenerative disorder? Is this a lysosomal storage disorder? Can the child see? What is the developmental level of the individual? Have some previously acquired skills (cooing, babbling, few words, fluent speech, memory, pointing, imitating, using a spoon, sitting, and walking) been lost?

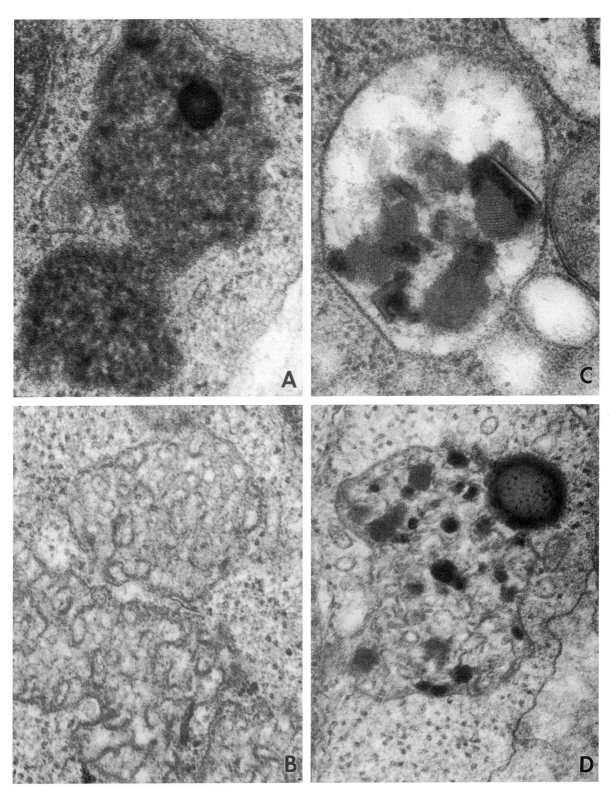

Figure 1

(A) Two large lysosomes composed of granular osmiophilic deposits in the cytoplasm of lymphocytes in a patient with infantile NCL. Magnification, × 105,000. (B) Three lysosomes composed of curvilinear profiles in cytoplasm of lymphocytes in a patient with classic late infantile NCL. Magnification, × 81,000. (C) Large vacuolated lysosome filled with fingerprint-like profiles and electrodense structures in a patient with juvenile NCL. Magnification, × 76,000. (D) Large lysosome composed of a mixed type of profiles (curvilinear and fingerprint) in a patient with early juvenile variant of late infantile NCL. Magnification, × 68,500.

Table 1 CLINICOPATHOLOGICAL, BIOCHEMICAL, AND GENETIC TESTING OF NCLs[a]

Form of NCL	Genetic symbol	Age of onset	Life expectancy (years)	Presenting symptoms	Electron microscopy	Enzyme activity assay	Gene location	DNA testing
Infantile[b]	CLN1	Birth to 37 years	10–56 +	Seizures, cognitive/motor decline, visual loss	GROD	PPT-1	1p32	223A→G
Classic late infantile	CLN2	2–8 years	15–46	Seizures, cognitive/motor decline, visual loss	CV/mixed	TPP-1	11p15	451C→T T523-1G→C 636C→T
Juvenile	CLN3	4–10 years	24–56	Visual loss, cognitive/motor decline, seizures	FP or mixed, vacuolated lymphocytes	Transmembrane	16p12	1.02-kb deletion
Adult	CLN4	15–50 years	33–64	Seizures, cognitive/motor decline Behavior abnormalities, cognitive/motor decline	Mixed	N/A	N/A	N/A
Finnish variant LINCL	CLN5	4–7 years	10–21.5	Cognitive/motor decline, seizures, visual loss	FP, CV, RL	Transmembrane	13q22	Tyr392STOP
Early juvenile variant LINCL	CLN6	18 months–8 years	?	Cognitive/motor decline, seizures, visual loss	CV, FP, RL	Transmembrane	15q21	214G→T 368G→A
Turkish variant LINCL	CLN7	1–6 years	?	Seizures, motor decline, visual loss	FP or mixed	N/A	N/A	N/A
Progressive epilepsy with mental retardation	CLN8	5–10 years	?	Seizures, cognitive decline	CV- or GROD-like structures	Transmembrane	8p23	Arg24Gly

[a] Abbreviations used: CV, curvilinear; FP, fingerprint profiles; GROD, granular osmiophilic deposits; LINCL, late infantile NCL; PPT-1, palmitoyl protein thioesterase-1; TPP-1, tripeptidyl peptidase-1; RL, rectilinear.

[b] Heterogeneity is most prominent in this form and overlaps with the onset of the other forms of NCL.

Sometimes, impairment of cognitive and motor skills may lead to behavioral disturbances that are misinterpreted as the cause. For example, it is not uncommon to attribute attention deficit or autism to visual loss. Ataxia and myoclonus are the leading signs in cLINCL. In JNCL, because of central scotomata, children appear to be looking out of the corners of their eyes, which are not in primary position; blindness should not be construed as lack of attention or hysteria when the child becomes emotionally distressed under pressure to perform an impossible task. Epilepsy is present in almost all forms of NCL but is the most obvious presenting symptom in cLINCL, associated with mutations within the *CNL2* gene. Myoclonus, often associated with giant visual or somatosensory evoked potentials, is the most distinctive epileptic manifestation and probably reflects discharges from dying neurons, a situation quite different from that of the more common seizure disorders. This important distinction is best demonstrated by positron emission tomography, which shows decreases in regional metabolic activity instead of focal increases associated with most epilepsies. As emphasized by Hughlings Jackson, the highest level of neuronal circuitry is the first affected in cerebral degeneration and results in abnormal behaviors.

PHYSIOLOGICAL ASSESSMENT

Impaired vision may be demonstrated by electroretinography and visual evoked potential studies. Electroencephalography (EEG) may be normal or show nonspecific disorganization in the early stages of cLINCL and JNCL. The EEG becomes flat after a few years in INCL and after two or three decades in JNCL. Multifocal epileptiform discharges are primarily found in cLINCL and are less common and more severe in JNCL. Generalized clonic–tonic seizures occur in JNCL cases but are overdiagnosed. They seldom occur in cLINCL and almost never in patients with INCL.

PATHOLOGY (ULTRASTRUCTURAL FINDINGS)

After determining the objective signs of visual impairment, the loss of acquired skills, and epilepsy, one should search for evidence of lipopigment storage. Considering the nature of the process, in the past a brain biopsy was preferred; however, since the 1970s simpler alternatives have become available. Electron microscopic studies of peripheral blood (buffy coat and leukocyte pellet) are the most convenient, but confirmation can be made in only 90% of cases. The most reliable studies are biopsies of skin or conjunctiva; these are more invasive but provide a wide range of cell types, including sweat glands, subcutaneous nerve bundles with Schwann cells, and endothelial cells, in which inclusions are more likely to be found. Electron microscopy is the mainstay of diagnosis for the eight forms of NCL; it can also identify other lysosomal storage disorders with overlapping clinical features, such as Sandhoff's disease and sialidosis. Lipopigment storage material presents with distinctive profiles: granular osmiophilic deposits in INCL, CV profiles in cLINCL, and FPs in JNCL. Inclusions are seldom widespread and may be inconspicuous. Mixed profiles have been associated with ANCL and the newly identified variants of LINCL (fLINCL, vLINCL, and tLINCL) and also with forms of progressive epilepsy with mental retardation. Pathologists experienced in the field should be consulted whenever the study appears inconclusive or negative.

ENZYME ACTIVITIES, MOLECULAR GENETIC STUDIES, AND TREATMENT

The PPT-1 in INCL and TPP-1 in cLINCL are the only forms associated with lysosomal hydrolases. It is important to perform molecular genetic studies, especially carrier detection studies of families, pheno/genotypic comparison, and prenatal diagnosis, to search for common and uncommon mutations. This information provides a first step toward devising rational therapies, even if one succeeds in "replacing the mutant gene" in large populations among the billions of neurons of the central nervous system. The search for treatment by enzyme or gene replacement and new pharmaceutical agents is under way. Useful antiepileptic drugs may exacerbate epilepsy, which is not easy to differentiate from the supposedly natural course of the disease. Many other common medications may have undesirable side effects, presumably depending on their ability to bind neuronal membranes. More research on the pharmacology of NCLs is necessary, especially as more animal models become available.

—*Krystyna E. Wisniewski, Michel Philippart, and Nanbert Zhong*

***See also*–Lysosomal Storage Disorders**

Acknowledgments

This study was supported in part by the New York State Office of Mental Retardation and Developmental Disabilities and by Grant NS/HD38988 from the National Institutes of Health, National Institute of Neurological Disorders and Stroke.

Further Reading

Camp, L. A., Verkruyse, L. A., Afendis, S. J., *et al.* (1994). Molecular cloning and expression of palmitoyl-protein thioesterase. *J. Biol. Chem.* **269**, 23212–23219.

Constantinidis, J., Wisniewski, K. E., and Wisniewski, T. M. (1992). The adult and a new late adult forms of neuronal ceroid lipofuscinosis. *Acta Neuropathol. (Berlin)* **83**, 461–468.

Uvebrant, P., and Hagberg, B. (1997). Neuronal ceroid lipofuscinosis in Scandinavia. Epidemiological and clinical pictures. *Neuropediatrics* **28**, 6–8.

Vines, D., and Warburton, N. J. (1999). Classical late infantile neuronal ceroid lipofuscinosis fibroblasts are deficient in lysosomal tripeptidyl peptidase I. *FEBS Lett.* **443**, 131–135.

Wheeler, R. B., Sharp, J. D., Schultz, R. A., *et al.* (2002). The gene mutated in variant late-infantile neuronal ceroid lipofuscinosis (CLN6) and in nclf mutant mice encodes a novel predicted transmembrane protein. *Am. J. Hum. Genet.* **70**, 537–542.

Williams, R. E., Topçu, M., Lake, B. D., *et al.* (1999). CLN7 Turkish variant late infantile NCL. In *The Neuronal Ceroid Lipofuscinoses (Batten Disease)* (H. H. Goebel, *et al.*, Eds.), pp. 114–116. IOS Press, Amsterdam.

Wisniewski, K. E., Zhong, N. (Eds.) (2001). Batten disease: Diagnosis, treatment, and research. *Adv. Genet.* **45**.

Wisniewski, K. E., Zhong, N., and Philippart, M. (2001). Pheno/genotypic correlations of neuronal ceroid lipofuscinoses. *Neurology* **57**, 576–581.

Neurons, Overview

Encyclopedia of the Neurological Sciences
Copyright 2003, Elsevier Science (USA). All rights reserved.

NERVE CELLS or neurons are cells specialized for receiving and sending signals. At least in the human body, nerve cells are always connected to some extent to other nerve cells. In other words, they form networks. This greatly increases the complexity of their responses. Another general feature of nerve cells is that the environments in which they occur are protected so that their exposure to molecules in the blood or interstitial tissues is restricted.

Nerve cells are composed of a cell body and a variable number of cytoplasmic extensions or processes. The processes are extremely important to the function of nerve cells since they determine their connectivity. They are the major site for receiving signals and virtually the only site for sending signals. Those processes that are specialized for receiving signals are called dendrites. The single process that serves to send signals out is called the axon. It usually branches, especially in its preterminal course. The cell body contains the nucleus with the genome as well as cytoplasmic molecular mechanisms for making and modifying proteins, mechanisms for producing energy from blood-borne molecules, mechanisms for breaking down and recycling unneeded molecules, and mechanisms for transportation of organelles and molecules.

Signals are transmitted from one nerve cell to another at particular sites called synapses. The input side of a synapse tends to occur on a small swelling of the terminal axon. The dendrites of nerve cells are studded with synapses, most of which are found on minute cytoplasmic protrusions called dendritic spines (Fig. 1). Synapses are also present on the cell body. Transmission at the majority of synapses is by release of a chemical messenger. The signals that the nerve cell receives at such a synapse are of two general types—those that increase neuronal excitability and those that inhibit it. The synapses on the cell body are mostly inhibitory, whereas those on the dendrites are excitatory. Synapses can be visualized with a light microscope by tagging with antibodies to proteins localized only at synapses. By electron microscopy, a synapse can be identified as a cluster of small vesicles close to the membrane of a presynaptic process (usually an axon) that is in close apposition to the thickened membrane of a postsynaptic process. The majority of synapses connect an axon to a dendrite, but a variety of unconventional synapses exist, such as axoaxonal,

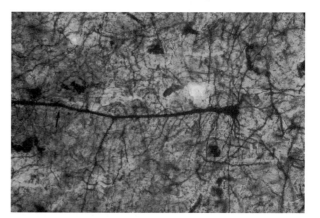

Figure 1
A large pyramidal cell from the cerebral cortex stained by a modified Golgi stain, which stains all the processes of this neuron except the axon and leaves neighboring neurons unstained. Dendritic spines can be seen on some of the dendrites.

dendroaxonal, and dendrodendritic. At sites at which the membrane of one neuron is immediately adjacent to another, it is possible for synapses to occur where transmission is electrical. Transmission of a signal across a synapse, from the presynaptic process to the postsynaptic process, is effected by the release of a transmitter molecule and its binding to a receptor specific for that molecule. More than 50 different molecules have been identified as transmitters in the brain. They are classified into two general types: those that react directly with an ion channel to open or close it and those that produce their effects by starting a chain of molecular events, such as activation of a cytoplasmic second messenger. The effects of this second type of transmitter tend to be more prolonged and less locally restricted than those of the first type.

The cytoplasm of dendrites contains ribosomes, which constitute the machinery for translating messenger RNA into protein. Messenger RNA from a particular subset of genes, labeled by a particular nucleotide sequence, is carried into the dendrites along the surface of microtubules. This makes possible the generation of specific proteins on the dendritic side of the synapse, perhaps in response to repeated activation of the synapse. Such a sequence of events probably underlies the long-term facilitation of synapses in response to activity. A submembranous actin cytoskeleton at the base of dendritic spines allows them a certain degree of motion. The dendritic tree of a large neuron thus has a large capacity for combining the effects of many inputs and modifying its own response to them. When the summation of these inputs is excitation, depolarization of the cell membrane may reach the trigger zone of the axon at the axon hillock, provoking an all-or-none response in the axon known as the axon potential.

The distinctness of the axon hillock varies in different types of neurons. It is cone shaped, connecting the cell body to the initial segment of the axon (Fig. 2), and filled with organelles similar to those in the rest of the cell body. The axon hillock has an unusually high concentration of voltage-sensitive sodium channels and therefore serves as a trigger zone for the action potential.

Ribosomes, which are numerous in the cell body and dendrites, are sparse in the initial segment of the axon and absent in the rest of it. This means that proteins and other membrane components needed in the axon must be transported from the cell body. Electron microscopy has shown that the main

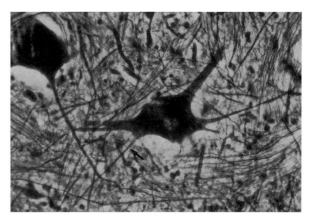

Figure 2
This large motor neuron from the anterior horn of the spinal cord was stained by Bodian's stain, which particularly stains neurofilaments. Small dendritic arborizations are not seen. The section is much thicker than that shown in Fig. 1. The axon is indicated by the arrow.

components in an axon are neurofilaments and microtubules, along with some vesicles and smooth endoplasmic reticulum. Fast anterograde axonal transport and retrograde transport involve attachment of vesicles to microtubules by specific motor molecules (kinesin and dynein). Neurofilaments, which move with slow axonal flow, probably lend physical stability to axons.

As mentioned previously, the axon serves to send a stereotyped signal, the action potential, which propagates along the axon to the terminals, where it activates the mechanism that causes synaptic vesicles to discharge into the synaptic gap. The action potential is therefore not the output signal. It is a message from one part of the neuron to another to activate the output signal. However, the action potential may be able to slightly modify the output signal by its rate of repetition. The output signal is transmitted by the release of a chemical messenger. Some nerve cells can produce more than one type of chemical messenger.

There are many varieties of neurons, and they can differ in a number of ways, such as the input they receive, the chemical transmitter or transmitters they discharge from their axon terminals, their size, the number of dendrites and their branching pattern, and the presence and number of dendritic spines. The axon of some neurons ends locally, no further from the cell body than its dendrites, such as interneurons in the cerebral cortex. Other cells, such as large pyramidal cells in the cortex, have an axon that may be 0.5 m in length. Motor cells of the anterior gray matter of the spinal cord send their axon out of the central nervous system to form a special type of synapse with skeletal muscle cells. Neurons of the dorsal root ganglia have a peripheral process with all the typical properties of an axon, which receives signals from specialized sensory endings and conducts them past the cell body to a central process that goes through the nerve roots to synapses in the spinal cord. This axon is connected to its cell body only by a slender convoluted process, although during embryonic development of these cells there is a stage at which the central and peripheral axonal processes exit directly and separately from the cell body.

—*Stirling Carpenter*

See also–Axons; Central Nervous System, Overview; Dendrites; Nervous System, Neuroembryology of; Vertebrate Nervous System, Development of

Further Reading

Kandell, E. R., Schwartz, J. H., and Jessell, T. M. (Eds.) (1995). *Essentials of Neural Science and Behavior.* Appleton & Lange, Norwalk, CT.
Sotelo, C., and Triller, A. (1997). The central neuron. In *Greenfield's Neuropathology* (D. I. Graham and P. L. Lantos, Eds.), 6th ed., pp. 3–61. Arnold, London.

Neurooncology, Overview

Encyclopedia of the Neurological Sciences
Copyright 2003, Elsevier Science (USA). All rights reserved.

NEUROONCOLOGY is the study of primary central nervous system tumors and the metastatic and nonmetastatic neurological complications of systemic cancer. This includes the diagnosis and treatment of primary spinal and all intracranial tumors. In the systemic cancer patient, this encompasses all neurological dysfunction, such as stroke, metabolic encephalopathy, and paraneoplastic disease, in addition to the common metastatic processes, such as brain, leptomeningeal, and epidural spinal cord metastases.

—*Lisa M. DeAngelis*

See also–Analgesia, Cancer Pain and; Brain Tumors, Clinical Manifestations and Treatment; Brain Tumors, Genetics; Central Nervous System Tumors, Epidemiology; Pain, Cancer and; Spinal Cord Tumors, Treatment of (see also specific entries in the Neurooncology section; e.g., Pituitary Tumors)

Neuroophthalmology

Encyclopedia of the Neurological Sciences
Copyright 2003, Elsevier Science (USA). All rights reserved.

NEUROOPHTHALMOLOGY is a hybrid field that combines the knowledge bases of clinical neurology and ophthalmology to diagnose and treat visual, pupillary, eyelid, and eye movement disorders. Practitioners must have an excellent command of the anatomy of the central visual pathways, brainstem, skull base, and orbit and of the physiology of both eye and brain. They must be comfortable with the techniques of the neurological and ophthalmological examinations. Neuroophthalmologists have generally completed residency training in either neurology or ophthalmology before obtaining a year or more of specialized fellowship training in the field. Rare and unusual disorders that defy diagnosis by general neurologists and ophthalmologists are often encountered. Other conditions may pose no diagnostic challenge, but specialized management skills can be applied to ensure optimal care.

Neuroophthalmologists diagnose and treat disorders of optic nerve function, including optic neuritis, ischemic optic neuropathy, and optic nerve tumors. They often take part in the management of patients with papilledema, such as from idiopathic intracranial hypertension (pseudotumor cerebri), or extrinsic optic nerve compression, such as from pituitary adenoma. Complex afferent problems with wide differential diagnoses that encompass both eye and brain disease include transient monocular and binocular visual loss, unexplained persistent visual loss, and positive visual phenomena (e.g., hallucinations). The pupils and eyelids are often the focus of neuroophthalmic attention. Asymmetries of pupil size (anisocoria) may raise serious diagnostic considerations, such as cerebral aneurysm or carotid artery dissection, that require urgent evaluation. Eyelid drooping (ptosis) or spasm may render a patient functionally blind by obstructing vision. Ocular motility disturbances, particularly those causing double vision (diplopia), also fall under the purview of the neuroophthalmologist. Such problems include cranial neuropathies (third, fourth, and sixth cranial nerves), myasthenia gravis, orbital disorders, and central eye movement disorders such as internuclear ophthalmoplegia and skew deviation. Involuntary eye movements, including nystagmus, are seen for diagnosis and treatment. Finally, patients with facial pain, especially when centered around the eye, are often referred to a neuroophthalmologist when routine management efforts fail.

A range of specialized diagnostic and therapeutic services are provided by neuroophthalmologists, including visual field interpretation, ocular motility assessment, and botulinum toxin injections for blepharospasm and hemifacial spasm. Electrodiagnostic procedures such as visual evoked potentials and electroretinography may also be offered, and practitioners who are residency trained in ophthalmology may deliver a range of ophthalmic surgical services.

—*Mark J. Morrow*

See also–Neurotology (see also specific Neuroophthalmology entries; e.g., Pupils; Retina; Visual Fields)

Further Reading

Leigh, R. J., and Zee, D. S. (1999). *The Neurology of Eye Movements*, 3rd ed. Oxford Univ. Press, New York.

Miller, N. R., and Newman, N. J. (Eds.) (1998). *Walsh and Hoyt's Clinical Neuro-ophthalmology*, 5th ed. Williams & Wilkins, Baltimore.

Trobe, J. D. (2001). *The Neurology of Vision*. Oxford Univ. Press, New York.

Neuropathic Pain Syndromes

Encyclopedia of the Neurological Sciences
Copyright 2003, Elsevier Science (USA). All rights reserved.

NEUROPATHIC PAIN has been defined by the International Association for the Study of Pain as "pain caused by injury to or dysfunction of the nervous system." Common examples of neuropathic pain include nerve root injury (radiculopathy) as part of low back or neck pain syndromes, postherpetic neuralgia, painful diabetic neuropathy, traumatic nerve injury, multiple sclerosis, and pain after thalamic stroke. It is estimated that 1–3 million people in the United States suffer from neuropathic pain. Because of its bizarre and distinct features compared to "normal" pain, neuropathic pain has been the subject of rich descriptions dating at least as far back as those of Silas Weir Mitchell in the 19th century. Mitchell saw numerous Civil War soldiers who suffered from extreme pain syndromes as a consequence of musket wounds to their nerves, which he managed in the Philadelphia General Hospital. His descriptions of the phenomenology of these syndromes and multiple treatment approaches uncannily parallel present-day descriptions, and it is fair to say that little has been discovered about the management of neuropathic pain that he did not discuss in detail in the 1860s. In fact, a number of treatment approaches that are considered especially modern in fact were among Mitchell's standard treatments, including acupuncture and long-term opioid therapy, the latter having been made possible by the introduction of crystallized morphine and the hypodermic needle in the previous decades.

A number of clinical features make neuropathic pain stand out. The pain is often severe or excruciating. Studies in which patients who have experienced multiple types of pain are asked to rate their relative severity indicate that neuropathic pain is among the most severe pain that human beings can experience. The quality of the pain is also distinct in that it is frequently described as burning or like electricity. The name of one of the most characteristic neuropathic syndromes, causalgia, in fact was coined by Mitchell from the Greek word *causos*, to burn. The lightest touch or other nonpainful stimulation may provoke exquisite pain in the neuropathic patient, a phenomenon called allodynia; stimulation that is normally mildly painful, such as a pinch or pressure, may cause severe pain (hyperalgesia). The severity of the pain may cause patients to adopt extreme behaviors in search of relief, such as constant immersion of the affected part in ice water or refusing to wear clothing over the affected area. The relatively poor responsiveness of neuropathic pain to opioids was observed by Mitchell and remains an active area of research. Mitchell clearly described the suspicions of other observers that these afflicted patients must be at least partially insane, a stigma that endures to the present day despite advances in our understanding of the pain.

Several classification schemes have evolved for neuropathic pain. A simple anatomical schema classifies neuropathic pain as central (caused by damage to the central nervous system, i.e., the brain or spinal cord) or peripheral (caused by damage to the peripheral nervous system, i.e., the nerve root, plexus, or peripheral nerve). Some syndromes are classified into both categories; for example, postherpetic neuralgia, which is frequently associated with damage to both nerve root and the adjacent spinal cord. Other syndromes, such as reflex sympathetic dystrophy, are not easily classifiable according to the simple central vs peripheral dimension because the location of the pathological process is speculative.

Another classification scheme is based on etiology, in which the categorization is based on the nature of the initiating insult. Examples include traumatic, metabolic, inflammatory, and vascular causes. A similar but more detailed diagnostic classification system invokes the specific initiating disease or disorder, such as diabetic neuropathy, inflammatory demyelinating polyneuropathy, postsurgical neuropathy, and traumatic spinal cord injury. It has long been noted, however, that patients with different kinds of neuropathic pain may have quite distinct symptoms, alone or together. For example, some patients complain predominantly of burning, whereas others complain of shooting, hypersensitivity to touch, cold, etc. It has been taken on principle that distinct qualities of symptoms must reflect different underlying pain mechanisms, and that the ultimate development of effective therapies for neuropathic pain must depend on a classification based on mechanism.

Understanding of the pathophysiological basis of neuropathic pain has increased dramatically in the past few decades, an era of dramatic advances in pain research in general. A quantum leap forward in neuropathic pain research occurred with the development of animal models of neuropathic pain. Preclinical research has identified a plethora of potential pathophysiological underpinnings of neuropathic pain, in some cases with correlates demonstrated in humans. For example, after injury to a peripheral nerve, the nerve endings may become hypersensitive to stimulation and may fire spontaneously when normally they would be quiet. This process is known as peripheral sensitization and probably underlies some types of neuropathic pain and allodynia. In other cases, injury to a peripheral nerve, such as amputation of the nerve, results in the formation of a tangled ball of immature nerve fibers—a neuroma. Devor and others have demonstrated spontaneous firing of action potentials from such neuromas apparently due to accumulation of sodium channels either on the neuroma or at the dorsal root ganglion of the nerve near the spinal cord.

If a nerve or group of nerves (e.g., in a whole limb) are amputated, the nervous system is completely deprived of input from that set of nerves (so-called deafferentation) and may become spontaneously hyperactive; the excessive nerve firing from these hyperactive central neuronal pools may cause pain. Such central hyperactivity has been demonstrated by electrical recordings from the human spinal cord during surgery for brachial plexus avulsion and from the human thalamus during surgery for pain from spinal cord injury. A striking example of pain after deafferentation is phantom limb pain, a common occurrence after amputation in which the patient continues to experience pain in the limb that is no longer there. Such pains may persist after amputations of body parts other than limbs, including the breast, anus, and teeth. The mechanism of phantom pain is uncertain but may involve central imprinting of pain memories.

An important concept regarding the mechanism of neuropathic pain is central sensitization. In this situation, injury to a peripheral nerve causes a persistent barrage of "pain signals" into the spinal cord from the nerve. Certain spinal cord neurons respond to excessive peripheral input by becoming hypersensitive; in turn, this plastic change in structure and function may initiate and sustain neuropathic pain. In some cases, this central sensitization is sufficient to sustain pain on its own; in other cases, continued peripheral input is required. The pharmacology of central sensitization appears to depend in many cases on activation of glutamate receptors (especially NMDA-type receptors) in the spinal cord, among other mechanisms. An interesting consequence noted in preclinical studies of central sensitization is that such pain is relatively resistant to opioid analgesia, but this resistance is reversed by administration of NMDA receptor antagonists, a strategy that has motivated intensive drug development efforts.

In recent years, researchers such as Woolf and Max have noted that the disadvantage of etiologic or diagnosis-based classifications is that the precise mechanism of pain may be the same in different diseases. For example, a patient with diabetic neuropathy may have shooting pains due to spontaneous discharges from damaged neurons (ectopic activity); this mechanism may be shared by a patient with postherpetic neuralgia with shooting pains, and it would presumably respond to similar treatments, despite the different diseases of origin. Conversely, one patient with postherpetic neuralgia may have allodynia due to peripheral sensitization, whereas another may have allodynia due to central sensitization, even though they share the same disease of origin. Moreover, the two patients with the same disease would probably require different analgesic approaches. This concept of mechanism-based treatment is currently being hotly debated. Although few doubt that ultimately this is the rational approach, it is clear that current technology does not permit accurate patient classification by mechanism. Therefore, clinicians must use trial-and-error treatment approaches, as in the time of Mitchell.

A particularly striking form of neuropathic pain is known as complex regional pain syndrome (types I and II), which is perhaps better known by its older but more colorful names, reflex sympathetic dystrophy (RSD) and causalgia (mentioned previously). These syndromes are characterized by severe, constant pain, usually in a limb; extreme allodynia; and, most notably, autonomic or trophic changes, such as swelling, excess sweating, abnormal hair growth, changes in color and temperature of the limb, and atrophy of skin, subcutis, muscle, and bone. When this syndrome follows minor trauma to the limb, it is known as RSD; when it follows a recognizable nerve injury, it is known as causalgia. No pain syndrome has aroused more controversy than RSD and causalgia. For at least a century, cases akin to RSD have been described in the literature that are clearly psychogenic. However, Mitchell described causalgia after musket wounds to nerves, which is clearly an organic problem. Whether some or all patients with RSD have psychogenic issues that at least partly account for their illness remains actively debated. Many patients with these syndromes enjoy resolution of their pain after blockade of the sympathetic nerves supplying the affected limb, which gave rise to the notion that the sympathetic nervous system is involved in the pathophysiology of this syndrome. However, even this remains unclear and continues to be debated.

Treatment of neuropathic pain is in many ways analogous to the treatment of chronic pain in general, albeit with important differences. The most important first obligation is to ensure that an accurate diagnosis is achieved with whatever tests are appropriate, although in many cases an accurate diagnosis will be elusive. The purpose of an accurate diagnosis is to ensure that primary treatment of the underlying disorder is provided and also to provide prognostic and other information that follows from the diagnosis. Examples of diseases for which determining the correct diagnosis is very important include entrapment neuropathies, which can be cured by surgical release; inflammatory peripheral neuropathies, which can be cured or palliated by a number of medical approaches; spinal radiculopathy due to metastatic cancer; and diabetic amyotrophy, which has no specific treat-ment but, unlike other types of diabetic neuropathy, has a favorable prognosis for spontaneous remission.

The second obligation is to help the patient set appropriate goals of treatment. Neuropathic pain, like other types of chronic pain, is frequently associated with substantial secondary complications of pain, including mood disorders (depression and anxiety), physical dysfunction, social withdrawal, and occupational distress. Setting realistic goals of treatment is paramount, such as reduction of pain, restoration of the ability of the patient to accomplish activities of daily living, and reduction of psychosocial distress. The critical balance for the physician is to set realistic expectations (cures are rare) but to maintain the hopes of the patient and family for successful disease management. A useful approach is to be realistic by explaining that a cure is unlikely (but not impossible) and that with persistence on the part of both patient and doctor, satisfactory control of pain and restoration of lifestyle are likely. Neurologists are frequently guilty of abandoning the patient as soon as the diagnosis is made (or the tests are done), when the patient very much needs the neurologist's help. This may in part be due to discomfort in dealing with one's own uncertainty and feelings of inadequacy as a physician in circumstances in which clear paths to success, especially if success is viewed as a cure, are rarely obvious. It is important to remember that Weir Mitchell, and centuries of physicians before him, had fewer effective remedies than we have today but performed an invaluable service to his patients; we can provide at least as much.

The third imperative of care is symptom reduction. There is no need to wait until the diagnosis is made; contrary to popular notions, effective analgesia does not interfere with diagnostic tests for neuropathic pain. Nonpharmacological therapies, such as cold, heat, liniments, and behavioral strategies, are safe but are not usually very effective, and the mainstay of treatment is pharmacotherapy. The classic medical treatment of neuropathic pain consists of the tricyclic class of antidepressants. Several have been shown to be effective, including amitriptyline, doxepin, nortriptyline, and desipramine (in order of most to least side effects). These medications have the advantages of durability of response and lack of addictive potential. They have a number of important liabilities. First, the onset of effect is 2–4 weeks. Second, they require titration to the effective dose, typically starting with 10–25 mg at bedtime and increasing every few days to a week until an effective dose is reached or side effects become intolerable. Typical side effects include dry mouth, constipation, sedation, dizziness, sexual side effects, and tachycardia. Although sedation may be useful for many patients if dosed at night, generally these side effects are troublesome, and the agents with the fewest side effects should be chosen first. Patients may respond idiosyncratically to the tricyclics and respond to one and not another. Therefore, systematic trials of multiple medications may be required, and each trial may take months. Interestingly, the serotonin-reuptake inhibitor antidepressants, such as fluoxetine (Prozac), do not have much effect on neuropathic pain.

It has long been observed, and has been one of the great clues to the mystery of neuropathic pain, that medications that treat epilepsy also can be effective for neuropathic pain. In recent years, gabapentin (Neurontin), an anticonvulsant, has emerged as a competitor to the tricyclics. Efficacy appears similar, but gabapentin has the distinct advantage of improved tolerability and no significant drug–drug interactions. The only disadvantage is that it must generally be dosed three times a day. It also must be titrated to effect, which is the case with all medications for neuropathic pain.

Other medications for neuropathic pain include other anticonvulsants, baclofen, mexiletene, and topical treatments such as the lidocaine patch. Opioids have been studied in several controlled clinical trials and appear to be at least as effective as other treatments—perhaps more. However, the opioids have not been examined carefully in long-term trials, and presumably they have the same liabilities as in other long-term treatment situations and so are not considered a first-line option except when rapid control of severe pain is necessary.

Experience in the treatment of neuropathic pain has given rise to the notion of rational polypharmacy in the treatment of chronic pain in general. Many investigators have observed that patients tend to obtain better relief with well-tolerated doses of multiple medications that act by different mechanisms than by single medications maximally dosed. Therefore, the management of neuropathic pain requires continuing medications that produce partial efficacy and adding other medications in continued therapeutic trials. Needless to say, success requires meticulous documentation of the pain relief achieved in these trials and can be frustrating for both doctor and patient.

Interventional treatments are also available for neuropathic pain. Completely implanted electrical spinal cord stimulators have been used for neuropathic pain for more than 30 years, and due to modern technology they are straightforward and safe to implant. Interestingly, spinal cord stimulation appears to be effective for neuropathic pain and pain due to ischemia (such as in chronic angina or peripheral vascular disease) but not for somatic pain (e.g., arthritis or cancer). Completely implanted pumps for the spinal administration of morphine and other analgesics have also been widely available for decades and can be effective for otherwise intractable neuropathic pain. Patients who cannot be successfully managed after reasonable trials of medical therapy should be referred to a pain management center for consideration of interventional treatment in addition to the multidisciplinary treatment often available in such settings.

Neuropathic pain is a striking syndrome that may occur in the setting of a variety of disorders. Rapid progress is being made in determining the mechanisms of neuropathic pain and developing treatments targeted to specific mechanisms. In the meantime, treatment is empirical and must frequently be multidisciplinary. The keys to treatment, as with all complex chronic medical illnesses, are accurate diagnosis, prompt and systematic palliative treatment, and a healthy dose of compassion and support.

—*Nathaniel Katz*

See also–Analgesics, Non-Opioid and Other; Complex Regional Pain Syndrome; Intercostal Nerve; Mitchell, Silas Weir; Neck and Arm Pain; Nerve Injury; Neuropathies, Diabetic; Opioids and Their Receptors; Pain, Basic Neurobiology of; Radiculopathy

Further Reading

Alo, K. M., Holsheimer, J. (2002). New trends in neuromodulation for the management of neuropathic pain. *Neurosurgery* 50, 690–703.

Baron, R., and Wasner, G. (2001). Complex regional pain syndromes. *Curr. Pain Headache Rep.* 5, 114–123.

Katz, N. (2000). Neuropathic pain in cancer and AIDS. *Clin. J. Pain* 16, S41–S48.

McQuay, H. J. (2002). Neuropathic pain: Evidence matters. *Eur. J. Pain* 6, 11–18.

Woolf, C. J., and Mannion, R. J. (1999). Neuropathic pain: Aetiology, symptoms, mechanisms, and management. *Lancet* 353, 1959–1964.

Neuropathies, Amyloid

AMYLOIDOSIS is a term used to describe a relatively heterogeneous group of disorders in which amyloid is deposited in various organs and tissues. The deposition of amyloid in peripheral nerves results in amyloid neuropathy. Amyloid is an insoluble proteinaceous material that has certain staining properties on histological preparation, most notably a positive staining for Congo red dye and an apple-green birefringence when examined under polarized light microscopy. Electron microscopy and x-ray diffraction have revealed that amyloid is a fibrillar protein that has a β pleated sheet configuration. This configuration is believed to be responsible for its typical staining features.

The amyloid protein is not uniform among the various forms of amyloidosis. This observation has led to a classification of the amyloid disorders based on the precursor plasma proteins that form the amyloid protein fibrils. Amyloid neuropathy does not occur in all forms of amyloidosis. The two most important forms of amyloidosis that are associated with amyloid neuropathy are AL amyloidosis and ATTR or familial transthyretin-associated amyloidosis. In AL amyloidosis, the amyloid protein is composed of immunoglobulin light-chain fragments that may be seen in plasma cell dyscrasias or more often as an idiopathic disorder termed primary systemic amyloidosis. In ATTR, the amyloid protein is composed of a mutant or abnormal form of transthyretin, a serum transport protein.

AL AMYLOID NEUROPATHY

The neuropathy associated with AL amyloidosis represents the most common form of amyloid neuropathy. AL amyloidosis has an annual incidence rate of approximately 8.9 per million, tends to occur in older patients as evidenced by its median age of onset of 64 years, and has a male predominance of 2:1. Although AL amyloidosis often presents as a multisystem disease due to amyloid deposition in other organs besides peripheral nerves, in approximately 40% of patients the neuropathy may be the presenting and most prominent clinical manifestation. Nevertheless, in 60% of patients the medical syndrome often heralded by weakness and weight loss as well as the nephrotic syndrome, cardiomyo-

pathy, or malabsorption dominate the clinical picture, with the neuropathy being a relatively unimportant mild component to the illness. The medical syndrome of AL amyloidosis often includes congestive heart failure, hepatomegaly, and massive proteinuria with edema. Other less common clinical features include macroglossia presenting as enlargement and stiffness of the tongue, "raccoon eyes" due to periorbital purpura, hypoadrenalism, hypothyroidism, hyposplenism, and nail dystrophy. The central nervous system is not involved.

The clinical features of amyloid neuropathy typically conform to a predominantly sensory neuropathy, especially in the early phases of the disorder. Typical sensory symptoms, including numbness and paresthesias, occur in a length-dependent distribution beginning in the toes and feet and later in the fingers and hands as the disease progresses. In some patients, the neuropathy conforms to a small-fiber neuropathy in which the small sensory fibers subserving pain and thermal sensations are predominantly affected. In this setting, the clinical picture is one of severe pain often described as a burning sensation along with aching, stabbing, and shooting pains. The neurological examination will usually disclose loss of sensation to various sensory modalities, including light touch, pain, and thermal, vibratory, and joint position sense. The distribution of the sensory loss follows the distal-to-proximal gradient of the sensory symptoms. Autonomic nerve involvement is common and may result in a wide array of autonomic symptoms, including constipation and diarrhea, postprandial bloating, altered sweating, erectile dysfunction, and urinary bladder dysfunction. More advanced autonomic nerve involvement typically causes postural lightheadedness or syncope due to orthostatic hypotension. On rare occasions, autonomic dysfunction may dominate the clinical picture with minimal or no sensory symptomatology or signs. As the neuropathy progresses, motor fiber involvement may occur, although usually the syndrome remains a predominantly sensory disorder. In approximately 20% of patients typical clinical features of carpal tunnel syndrome may occur manifested by intermittent tingling and numbness in the hands. Regardless of the type of neuropathy that develops in the early stages of AL amyloidosis, there is a tendency for significant progression with sensory, motor, and autonomic features.

Approximately 90% of patients with AL amyloidosis have a monoclonal (M) protein in the serum or monoclonal light-chain protein in the urine when tested with serum and urine protein electrophoresis with immunofixation. It is likely that patients who are not found to have an M protein may still have one but it is in such a low concentration that it cannot be detected even with these sensitive methods. Standard laboratory testing will often reflect abnormalities of the medical illness, such as nephrotic syndrome, cardiac disease, and malabsorption. Electrodiagnostic examination typically reveals changes of a distal axonopathy characterized by low or absent sensory responses and mild slowing of motor conduction velocities. With progression of the neuropathy, amplitudes of the motor responses may be reduced and the needle electrode examination may disclose changes of active and chronic motor fiber loss in a distal-to-proximal gradient.

The diagnosis of amyloid neuropathy depends on documenting the presence of amyloid in peripheral nerve or other tissues. Biopsy of the sural nerve is often performed and almost always documents the presence of amyloid. Typically, amyloid is noted in the endoneurium and in the perivascular regions of the epineurium on Congo red or cresyl violet stains. An apple-green birefringence is also sought when the Congo red-stained deposits are examined under polarized light microscopy. The diagnosis of amyloidosis can also be established with biopsy of other tissues, including abdominal fat pad, rectum, and gingiva, and the other organs that may be involved, including kidney, liver, intestine, and endocardium. Often, amyloid is sought from the relatively simple and less invasive biopsies of abdominal fat pad and rectal mucosa that together detect amyloidosis in approximately 90% of patients. The precise classification of amyloidosis can only be achieved by identifying the specific amyloid protein. This is accomplished by utilizing immunochemical methods that use antibodies directed against the major amyloid fibril precursor proteins. Although it has been surmised that amyloid deposition in peripheral nerve is the pathogenic mechanism of the neuropathy, it has been observed that amyloid deposition may be relatively modest compared to the degree of axon loss. These observations have led to speculation that amyloidosis may cause neuropathy via other mechanisms, such as vascular and direct pressure changes. However, it is likely that amyloid induces a neuropathic effect by direct caustic damage to nerve fibers and ganglion cells.

Unfortunately, there is no satisfactory therapy for AL amyloid neuropathy. This is due in part to the difficulty in preventing further amyloid deposition in peripheral nerves as well as the fact that amyloid fibrils are insoluble and thus may not respond to treatments designed solely to halt the deposition of amyloid in peripheral nerve. Management of amyloid neuropathy is primarily symptomatic and supportive. Aggressive management of the painful component is usually accomplished with a variety of drugs effective for neuropathic pain. For management of autonomic symptoms, medications that may control orthostatic hypotension, urinary bladder dysfunction, and altered gastrointestinal motility are used. In addition to supportive treatment, new therapies have emerged that are designed to halt the progressive deposition of amyloid. The rationale for these therapies assumes that the pathophysiology of AL amyloidosis is similar to that of multiple myeloma, a disorder related to a clonal proliferation of plasma cells in the bone marrow. Thus, therapies effective for multiple myeloma may also benefit AL amyloidosis. One such therapy utilizes cycles of prednisone (a corticosteroid) and melphalan (an alkylating agent). The response rate for this type of therapy is approximately 20%, but improvement in multiorgan dysfunction has been reported. Newer therapies involving high-dose melphalan therapy coupled with allogenic bone marrow transplantation or peripheral blood stem cell rescue have provided promising results. However, more study is needed to determine the efficacy and utility of these therapies. Prognosis of AL amyloidosis has been traditionally regarded as poor, with a median survival of approximately 18 months. In patients presenting with congestive heart failure due to early cardiac involvement, median survival is 4 months. A more favorable prognosis is expected when neuropathy dominates the clinical picture and in the setting of normal renal function and small numbers of clonal plasma cells in the bone marrow. In most patients death occurs within 4 years from the time of diagnosis, usually due to cardiomyopathy or a combination of other multiorgan failure.

FAMILIAL AMYLOID POLYNEUROPATHY

Familial amyloid polyneuropathy (FAP) is an autosomal dominant inherited disorder that has traditionally been described as several different types, including the Portuguese, Japanese, and Swedish types. These three types share similar clinical features but have different ages of onset. The Portuguese type has variable onset in the third and fourth decades, whereas the Japanese type has onset between 25 and

35 years of age and the Swedish type after 55 years of age. However, the biochemical defect in all three types is the production of an abnormal or mutant form of transthyretin. Thus, these types are referred to as ATTR or familial transthyretin-associated amyloidosis. Transthyretin, formerly called thyroxin-binding prealbumin, is a tetrameric protein with four identical subunits that functions as a transport protein for thyroxin- and retinol-binding protein. Numerous substitutions of single amino acids in transthyretin may result in FAP, but the most common substitution is methionine for valine at position 30. The clinical disorder associated with this particular mutation has been termed FAP type 1 or the Portuguese, Japanese, and Swedish types. In addition to transthyretin mutations, FAP may also result from rare mutations of apolipoprotein A-1, a high-density lipoprotein, and gelsolin, a ubiquitous cytoplasmic protein that interacts with actin filaments. The clinical features of FAP type 1 ATTR neuropathy are similar to those of AL amyloid neuropathy. Symptoms and signs of sensorimotor neuropathy and autonomic neuropathy are commonly encountered in ATTR amyloidosis. In FAP type 2, the Indiana type, the typical transthyretin mutation is Ser84 or His58. In this disorder, patients typically present in middle life with carpal tunnel syndrome and vitreous opacities. The associated sensorimotor and autonomic neuropathies are relatively mild. FAP type 3, the Iowa type, is associated with an abnormal apolipoprotein A-1. This disorder shares many features with FAP type 1, but carpal tunnel syndrome is not commonly observed and the autonomic neuropathy is less prominent. FAP type 4, the Finnish type, is caused by an abnormal gelsolin. This disorder presents with an unusual clinical syndrome of progressive cranial neuropathies and a peculiar thickening of the facial skin. The associated sensorimotor and autonomic neuropathies tend to be mild. Although the clinical features of the neuropathy in ATTR amyloidosis, particularly FAP types 1 and 3, are similar to those seen in AL amyloidosis, there are certain clinical distinctions seen in the systemic manifestations of the amyloidosis. In ATTR amyloidosis there is a tendency for earlier onset, usually in the third or fourth decade, and a slower progression. In addition, cardiac involvement is more variable and less uniform, renal involvement is less common, and macroglossia is not seen. Despite these differences, it is often difficult to differentiate AL amyloidosis from familial amyloidosis based solely on the clinical features.

The diagnosis of amyloidosis in FAP is pursued in the same fashion as in AL amyloidosis. In the presence of a family history and in the absence of a monoclonal protein, additional testing for genetic factors is obtained. Transthyretin can be assessed by isoelectric focusing of the serum, which can identify a mutant or variant form of transthyretin from wild-type transthyretin. The presence of a variant transthyretin should be pursued with genetic testing to identify the site of the mutation.

The prognosis for ATTR amyloidosis is generally better than that for AL amyloidosis. The typical survival is 12–15 years, with longer survival associated with later age of onset. Treatment of ATTR amyloid neuropathy involves the same supportive and symptomatic therapies used for AL amyloid neuropathy. Because transthyretin is synthesized in the liver, liver transplantation has been utilized for the treatment of ATTR amyloidosis. Although this form of therapy is relatively new and long-term results are still being evaluated, liver transplantation does result in the disappearance of the mutant transthyretin from the blood and improvement in the neuropathy. Timing of liver transplantation is critical. Surgery is not recommended in asymptomatic patients, but once symptoms occur, surgery should be performed soon because progression of the neuropathy may be relatively rapid in some patients.

—*Robert W. Shields, Jr.*

***See also*–Amyloidosis; Neuropathies, Diabetic; Neuropathies, Iatrogenic; Neuropathies, Idiopathic; Neuropathies, Instrumental; Neuropathies, Nutritional; Neuropathies, Overview; Neuropathy, Toxic**

Further Reading

Buxbaum, J. N., and Jacobson, D. R. (2001). The amyloidoses. In *Williams Hematology* (E. Beutler, M. A. Lichtman, B. S. Coller, T. J. Kipps, and U. Seligsohn, Eds.), 6th ed., pp. 1305–1316. McGraw-Hill, New York.

Dhodapkar, M. V., Bellotti, V., and Merlini, G. (2000). Amyloidosis. In *Hematology, Basic Principles and Practice* (R. Hoffman, E. J. Benz, S. J. Shattil, B. Furie, H. J. Cohen, L. E. Silberstein, and P. McGlave, Eds.), 3rd ed., pp. 1416–1432. Churchill Livingstone, New York.

Falk, R. H., Comenzo, R. L., and Skinner, M. (1997). The systemic amyloidoses. *N. Engl. J. Med.* 337, 898–909.

Gertz, M. A., Lacy, M. Q., and Dispenzieri, A. (1999). Amyloidosis. *Hematol. Oncol. Clin. North Am.* 13, 1211–1233.

Sezer, O., Eucker, J., Jakob, C., *et al.* (2000). Diagnosis and treatment of AL amyloidosis. *Clin. Nephrol.* 53, 417–423.

Neuropathies, Autonomic

Encyclopedia of the Neurological Sciences

AUTONOMIC NEUROPATHIES are peripheral neuropathies that involve peripheral autonomic nerve fibers either predominantly or exclusively. When classed by size, most of the autonomic neuropathies belong to the small fiber group. Small fibers conduct pain, temperature, and autonomic function. Hence, many neuropathies produce both distal pain and autonomic dysfunction because the underlying mechanism targets nerves that are small. Examples include some forms of diabetic neuropathy, autonomic neuropathy associated with HIV, and that associated with Fabry's disease. Other neuropathic processes, such as amyloidosis or porphyria, involve all fiber sizes and still carry a predilection for autonomic nerves. Most autonomic neuropathies are characterized by axonal loss, but some, such as Guillain–Barré syndrome, are commonly demyelinative.

Autonomic neuropathies frequently figure in another classification scheme—that of autonomic disorders in general. A brief review of the classification of dysautonomias (Table 1) will also aid in placing the peripheral autonomic disorders in perspective. In primary dysautonomias, a well-defined structural abnormality of the autonomic nervous system directly produces symptoms. Examples include multiple system atrophy and diabetic autonomic neuropathy. In contrast, secondary dysautonomias include diseases in which autonomic function appears to play a major role in symptom production but may be reactive to a nonautonomic pathophysiological source. Examples include the postural tachycardia syndrome and reflex sympathetic dystrophy.

MANIFESTATIONS OF AUTONOMIC NEUROPATHY

Much of our understanding of the frequency and sequence of the symptoms associated with autonomic neuropathy comes from our knowledge of diabetes. Thus, the sequence mentioned here may not apply in its entirety to other neuropathies to the extent that they progress by a mechanism different than diabetes. However, in most neuropathies, one can assume a process that involves the longest fibers first and the most proximal fibers and most robustly innervated organs last. Sexual dysfunction in men is one of the earliest symptoms of autonomic dysfunc-

Table 1   CLASSIFICATION OF DYSAUTONOMIAS

Primary dysautonomias
  Peripheral nervous system
    Autonomic neuropathies
      Acquired
      Inherited
    Pure autonomic failure
  Central nervous system
    Cervical or thoracic myelopathy
    Hypothalamic lesions
      Infiltrative
      Postconcussion
      Post-heat stroke
    Diffuse
      Lewy body disease
      Multiple system atrophy
Secondary dysautonomias
  Cardiovascular syndromes
    Orthostatic intolerance
    Postural tachycardia syndrome
    Cardiovasodepressor syncope
    Raynaud's phenomenon
    Mitral valve prolapse
  Focal and organ-specific syndromes
    Reflex sympathetic dystrophy
    Bladder urgency–frequency
    Irritable bowel syndrome
    Segmental hypohidrosis
    Hyperhidrosis

tion. At this point, one may find abnormalities in the response to deep breathing, but cardiovascular symptoms are absent. As the disease progresses, constipation may set in, along with dry eyes and dry mouth. Orthostatic intolerance may be present, but true orthostatic hypotension does not occur until late in the disease, when the bladder may fail and upper gastrointestinal symptoms may occur as well due to gastroparesis. These may be associated with weight loss so severe as to prompt a search for malignancy.

DIAGNOSTIC TESTS OF AUTONOMIC NEUROPATHIES

Testing of the autonomic nervous system provides a critical link to understanding both the nature and the pathophysiology of autonomic disorders. Testing can localize the lesion to a postganglionic or preganglionic level and sometimes to spinal or supraspinal sites, assess the breadth of involvement across different autonomic branches and organ system innervations, measure severity of involvement, and guide treatment of orthostatic hypotension and syncope. Localization utilizes the tests of sweating, whereas the other tasks draw information from the cardiovascular tests.

Although there are multiple tests of sweating, two are most commonly employed: the thermoregulatory sweat test and the axon reflex sweat test. The axon reflex test ascertains the integrity of the postganglionic sudomotor axon by measuring the response of a distant sweat gland to iontopheresis of acetylcholine across the skin. In contrast, the thermoregulatory sweat test evaluates the entire thermoregulatory process, including afferent limb, central hypothalamic integration, and efferent limb through the spinal cord and nerves. Thus, a central nervous system process will spare the axon reflex (Table 2).

Of the myriad tests of cardiovascular function available, this entry notes one test of cardiac parasympathetic function, the cardiac response to deep breathing; one test of all cardiovascular autonomic functions, the Valsalva maneuver; and one test of vasomotor sympathetic function, the tilt-table test. The reader is referred to textbooks of autonomic function for details of testing. The tilt study can aid in understanding the pathophysiology of symptoms and can guide treatment. When orthostatic hypotension accompanies symptoms of lightheadedness, one might focus on increasing arterial pressure. In contrast, a postural tachycardia without true orthostatic pressure drop may respond to agents that change central autonomic tone. A decrease in pulse pressure (systolic pressure–diastodiastolic pressure) indicates a loss of available blood volume and is best treated with volume expansion. Finally, vasodepressor syncope often responds well to a β-adrenergic blocker.

DISORDERS ASSOCIATED WITH AUTONOMIC NEUROPATHY

Table 3 summarizes disorders associated with autonomic neuropathy.

Diabetes

Autonomic neuropathy occurs with high prevalence, both in type 1 and in type 2 diabetes. Extensive work

Table 2 TESTS OF SWEATING THAT DISTINGUISH NEURAXIS LOCATION

	Thermoregulatory sweat test	Axon reflex sweat test
Preganglionic lesion	Abnormal central pattern	Normal
Postganglionic lesion	Abnormal peripheral pattern	Low or absent

Table 3 DISORDERS ASSOCIATED WITH AUTONOMIC NEUROPATHY

Diabetes
Immune/inflammatory-mediated neuropathies
  Pure autonomic neuropathy acute pandysautonomia
  Paraneoplastic disorder
  Guillain–Barré syndrome
  Amyloidosis
  Sarcoidosis
  Lyme disease
  HIV
  Lambert–Eaton myasthenic syndrome
  Monoclonal protein associated
Toxins/deficiencies
  Metals
  Botulism A
  Drugs
    Isoniazid
    Metronidazole
    Taxol
    Antiretroviral agents
  Vitamin deficiencies (B_{12} and B_1)
Inherited disorders
  Porphyrias
  Fabry's disease
  Tangier disease
  Riley–Day syndrome
  Mitochondrial disorders
Disorders with less clearly defined etiology

has elucidated neither the cause of diabetic neuropathy in general nor a reason for the disproportionate involvement of autonomic fibers. Nonetheless, diabetic autonomic neuropathy continues to be a major source of morbidity for diabetic patients. Many physician visits relate to neuropathic complaints, including pain, orthostatic hypotension, and bowel and bladder complaints. In addition, an autonomic neuropathy carries a poor prognosis for diabetics. A 1980 study suggested that 5-year mortality was 50%. Current information suggests that autonomic neuropathy impairs survival for diabetics, although perhaps not at the rate of 50%.

The mechanism of this increase in mortality is unknown but may relate to an imbalance in the parasympathetic and sympathetic inputs to the myocardium, resulting in fatal arrhythmias or repolarization abnormalities reflected in an abnormal QT segment. Clearly, improved glycemic control results in a lower frequency of neuropathy in general and autonomic neuropathy in particular.

From a clinical perspective, diabetic autonomic neuropathy presents two distinct patterns. The more common type is a slowly progressive, chronic neuropathy, with distal-to-proximal gradient and involvement of both somatic and autonomic fibers. Somatic complaints such as distal weakness, numbness, or pain predominate, and autonomic complaints must often be elicited by direct questioning. These usually include sexual dysfunction, distal loss of sweating, and loss of cardiac parasympathetic control on testing. If the disease progresses, constipation may ensue, along with thermoregulatory dysfunction and, eventually, orthostatic hypotension. However, patients with this type of diabetic autonomic neuropathy often do not present to an autonomic specialist because their autonomic complaints are usually overshadowed by somatic neuropathy and other organ system problems. This type of neuropathy usually occurs in patients with long-standing diabetes and is more likely with poor glycemic control, suggesting accumulation of glycosylated proteins or other metabolites as the major mechanism.

In contrast, the second type of diabetic autonomic neuropathy is subacute, progressing rapidly over days to weeks, and bears no relation to the duration of diabetes. In fact, this type of neuropathy frequently occurs with the onset of the disease and may trigger the diagnosis. It may also accompany a change in glycemic levels (for better or worse), such as a switch from an oral agent to insulin. Significant weight loss is frequent (presumably due to gastroparesis) and may prompt a search for cancer. A typical clinical triad comprises change in treatment method, weight loss following weeks later, and onset of symptoms of autonomic neuropathy. In this regard, this type of diabetic autonomic neuropathy appears to share this clinical presentation with a group of focal diabetic neuropathies, including so-called diabetic amyotrophy (an L3–L4 segment radiculoplexopathy), abdominal and thoracic mono-radiculopathies, and the rarer upper extremity diabetic plexopathy. The autonomic neuropathy appears to have subtypes. A diffuse type with generalized cardiovascular and sudomotor denervation is most common, dominated by orthostatic hypotension, syncope, and intolerance to thermal variation. A focal type involves the bowel and bladder, with loss of sphincteric control or retention. Sensory or motor fibers may be affected, and an insensate bladder or rectum may be present.

The mechanism of this group of neuropathies is unclear. Evidence suggests an inflammatory- or immune-mediated process, and some authors have used corticosteroid treatment with success. From a practical clinical standpoint, I have employed a 2- or 3-week high-dose corticosteroid trial in these patients if the deficit is severe, it is still progressing (implying an active disease mechanism), and an endocrinologist is available to monitor sugar control. Treatment of specific autonomic symptoms is discussed later.

Immune-Mediated, Inflammatory, and Infiltrative Disorders

The autonomic nervous system becomes a target of the immune system in the following circumstances: in postinfectious processes, both acute (akin to Guillain–Barré syndrome for the motor system) and chronic; as part of an antibody-mediated paraneoplastic syndrome; due to a monoclonal antibody that targets a moiety present on autonomic nerves.

In acute inflammatory polyradiculoneuropathy (classic Guillain–Barré syndrome), the autonomic nervous system is commonly involved and may produce major fluctuations in blood pressure and heart rate, occasionally resulting in sudden death. The mechanism of these fluctuations is unknown. They may result from preganglionic demyelination/denervation and receptor supersensitivity within the ganglion, with loss of function and hypotension occurring frequently, and sudden bursts of hypertension from a supersensitive response to circulating transmitters. Alternatively, baroreceptor failure (due to denervation) would produce a similar clinical picture.

Acute pandysautonomia constitutes a disorder equivalent to Guillain–Barré syndrome but restricted almost entirely to the autonomic nervous system. Strength, sensation, and reflexes may be entirely preserved or minimally affected. Typically, the patient complains of symptom progression over a few days, including lightheadedness, constipation, and urinary retention. Orthostatic hypotension may be profound and autonomic testing demonstrates complete peripheral autonomic failure. A more chronic form of this disorder also exists, in parallel to the existence of both acute and chronic inflammatory demyelinating polyradiculopathy. The finding of antibody to ganglionic acetylcholine receptors may help confirm the diagnosis in difficult cases. In addition to support for autonomic failure, management should include modulation of the immune system with plasmapheresis (acute cases), intravenous globulin, or corticosteroids.

Both Guillain–Barré syndrome and acute pandysautonomia are thought to be postinfectious, although specific evidence for this etiology is only present in some cases. For example, approximately 20% of cases of Guillain–Barré syndrome are preceded by diarrhea with stool positive for campylobacter jejuni. It is likely that postinfectious autonomic syndromes constitute a very wide spectrum of disorders. For example, many cases of postural tachycardia syndrome are preceded by a clear history of upper respiratory infection. In some cases, anti-ganglionic cholinergic antibodies can be identified. In others, anti-α-adrenergic receptor antibodies are present. These would presumably impair vascular responsiveness, resulting in orthostatic intolerance.

Immune-mediated autonomic neuropathy may also occur as a paraneoplastic syndrome. The most common underlying cancers are small cell of the lung, breast, and lymphoma. Autonomic dysfunction may result from isolated peripheral involvement or may be part of a larger clinical picture including both peripheral and central dysfunctions along with brainstem or limbic encephalitis. In the majority of cases, an anti-Hu antibody is present. Treatment includes addressing the underlying cancer, supporting the failing autonomic functions, and consideration of immunomodulatory therapy if the neuropathy is particularly aggressive.

Although not strictly speaking a neuropathy, the immune-mediated, frequently paraneoplastic Lambert–Eaton myasthenic syndrome deserves mention. Antibodies to voltage-gated calcium channels prevent release of acetylcholine into the effector junctions, reducing the effectiveness of all peripheral cholinergic transmission at neuromuscular, muscarinic postganglionic autonomic parasympathetic, and nicotinic ganglionic autonomic synapses. The first two classes of synapse are most affected, and patients typically complain of weakness, dry mouth and dry eyes, constipation, and, occasionally, bladder problems. The most commonly associated tumors are lung, breast, and ovary. Electromyography (EMG) will show an incremental response to rapid repetitive stimulation. Commercial assays can determine the type and titer of antibodies. Treatment is similar to that of the previously mentioned paraneoplastic processes. In addition, symptoms may also respond to 3,4-diaminopyridine.

Diseases that infiltrate the nerve, such as amyloidosis and sarcoidosis, may also result in an autonomic neuropathy. For unknown reasons, amyloidosis has a particular predilection for the autonomic nerves. This predilection occurs both in the familial and in the sporadic types. The mechanism of this preferential dysfunction is particularly puzzling since the amyloid fibrils clearly involve the entire nerve, both large and small fibers, on biopsy. The amyloid protein is usually a λ light chain in the acquired form, and an abnormal prealbumin in the inherited forms. Patients may present renal failure, congestive heart failure, and a neuropathy typically producing orthostatic hypotension and other autonomic symptoms along with some entrapment mononeuropathies, frequently carpal tunnel syndrome. A myopathy may also be present. Diagnosis is made through pathological examination of involved tissue by rectal mucosa, abdominal fat aspirate, or kidney or nerve biopsy. Light chains are not always found in the urine or blood.

The neuropathy associated with other types of monoclonal proteins usually involves large fibers, and symptoms are primarily ataxia and sensory loss, not autonomic. This is particularly true for the IgM group, the most common monoclonal protein-associated neuropathies. IgG- and IgA-associated neuropathies occasionally produce autonomic symptoms, but when they are present one should exclude an associated amyloidosis and free light chain.

Although much less common in sarcoidosis, autonomic neuropathies of various types do occur. The most frequent manifestation of peripheral nervous system involvement in sarcoidosis is in the seventh cranial nerve, presumably due to the predilection of the disorder for the basal meninges. Patients with 10th cranial nerve involvement, cardiac atrioventricular nodal involvement, and peripheral autonomic neuropathy, with stocking distribution loss of sweating, have also been described. Treatment with corticosteroids is often beneficial.

Infectious Agents

A small-fiber neuropathy in association with abnormal autonomic testing has been reported in one case of Lyme disease. This disease should be considered part of the differential diagnosis of an autonomic neuropathy, although other peripheral manifestations of Lyme disease, such as polyradiculopathy and cranial neuropathy, are far more common.

A variety of neuropathies occur in HIV infection, including a distal progressive type involving all fiber types, mononeuritis multiplex, and selective large- or small-fiber neuropathies. The small-fiber subtype may present with either distal pain or autonomic symptoms as the primary complaint, although both complaints are usually present on review of symptoms. Patients with AIDS may have more severe autonomic involvement, with a fixed rapid resting heart rate, orthostatic hypotension, and sphincteric complaints. Evaluation of autonomic neuropathy in patients with HIV should be meticulous and exclude reversible causes such as B_{12} deficiency and drug-induced neuropathy, particularly due to antiretroviral agents such as didanosine (ddI), zalcitabine (ddC), zidovudine, and stavudine. ddI and ddC appear to be more commonly associated with distal painful small-fiber neuropathy, although their impact on autonomic fiber function is unknown. Once suspected to produce a neuropathy, a drug should be stopped for at least 12 weeks to assess for reversal of the process. Both vincristine and isoniazid can be associated with a distal neuropathy, but this usually involves large rather than small nerve fibers. Finally, metronidazole may also produce a well-described neuropathy involving small pain and autonomic fibers.

Toxins and Deficiencies

The heavy metals are frequently mentioned in casual discussions of differential diagnosis of autonomic neuropathy. However, lead, mercury, and arsenic generally produce primarily a somatic (large-fiber) neuropathy, despite the frequent presence of abdominal pain in the clinical presentation of acute lead and arsenic intoxications. Only gold and thallium intoxications produce a well-documented autonomic neuropathy. Gold intoxication usually results from excessive gold dose for rheumatoid arthritis. As this agent is abandoned in favor of newer drugs, this will likely become a disease of the past. A clinical clue to this toxin is the presence of myokymia. Like arsenic, thallium intoxication occurs primarily due to purposeful poisoning. A gastrointestinal syndrome occurs 1 or 2 days after ingestion. This is followed by distal limb pain and then weakness. Alopecia is an important clue, but it occurs late in the disease, after chelation could prevent progression.

Botulism, which is a disorder preventing release of acetylcholine at the effector junction, may mimic an acute autonomic neuropathy. Botulism is the most potent naturally occurring toxin, with 0.5 µg of ingested botulinum toxin often sufficient to produce weakness. Six to 24 hr after ingestion of food, in which the anaerobic growth of *Clostridium botulinum* occurred, diarrhea occurs, which may prevent the later neuromuscular symptoms, presumably by flushing out the toxin. Weakness and autonomic symptoms progress over 3–10 days following exposure. Extraocular movements are involved first,

followed by the limbs and respiratory muscles. Autonomic symptoms are primarily muscarinic cholinergic, with dry mouth, dry eyes, dry skin, constipation, and bladder dysfunction. One report suggests that of the two common types of botulism, type A produces more profound weakness and fewer autonomic symptoms and type B has the opposite effect. Typical of presynaptic neuromuscular junction disorders, EMG will show an incremental response to rapid repetitive stimulation. Treatment consists of administration of antitoxin followed by long-term support until recovery.

Although many medications can produce a neuropathy, significant autonomic involvement is limited to a few drugs. The most common are the antiretroviral agents previously discussed with HIV-induced neuropathy. In addition, metronidazole in relatively small doses can result in a small-fiber neuropathy with distal pain and autonomic symptoms. Orthostatic hypotension may be present. Reversal may take 3–18 months after discontinuation of the drug. Taxol, a plant alkaloid utilized against solid tumors (most often breast cancer), may produce a severe autonomic neuropathy, with full-blown orthostatic hypotension, severe constipation, and bladder dysfunction. Finally, vincristine and isoniazid produce neuropathies that usually involve large fibers but may occasionally include small fibers. Both drugs interfere with microtubule formation. When small fibers are involved, the main symptom is usually distal pain. Autonomic dysfunction is rare.

Some vitamin B deficiencies result in autonomic dysfunction, particularly B_1 (thiamine) and B_{12}. Wernicke's encephalopathy (B_1 deficiency) typically presents with a change in mental status, ataxia, and ophthalmoparesis, especially of the abducting eye muscles. These are so dramatic as to frequently overshadow the autonomic abnormalities, which include hypothermia, hypotension, and bradycardia, presumably mediated by dysfunction of brainstem or hypothalamic autonomic centers, where pathological abnormalities are rife. Malnutrition related to alcohol abuse or gastrointestinal disease is the most common etiology. Intravenous glucose administration may precipitate the onset of symptoms.

Vitamin B_{12} deficiency's best known neurological effect on peripheral and central large sensory fibers spawned the name subacute combined degeneration. Pathological abnormalities occur in the dorsal columns, in the dorsal root ganglia, and in the peripheral nerve due to degeneration of both centrally directed and peripherally directed axons of the dorsal root ganglion cells. Autonomic symptoms, particularly orthostatic hypotension, are increasingly described in the literature, precipitated by both anesthesia with nitrous oxide and in the absence of this agent. We have seen several patients with a postural tachycardia syndrome and low B_{12} levels, which resolved with B_{12} replacement. It is important to note that in this circumstance 2000 units bimonthly (4000 units/month) of B_{12} is probably required to replenish tissue levels.

Inherited Disorders

Inherited disorders constitute the last category of disease associated with autonomic neuropathy. Although the most common form of amyloidosis is acquired, an extensive literature records several types of familial amyloidosis. In all types, an autonomic neuropathy figures prominently.

Together, the genetic defects in heme synthesis are termed porphyrias. Some of these disorders manifest only cutaneous symptoms, whereas others, particularly (in order of frequency) acute intermittent porphyria, variegate porphyria, and hereditary coproporphyria, are punctuated by intermittent attacks of profound neurological deficit. Any factor or agent that increases hepatic metabolism, such as barbiturate drugs, fasting, hormonal changes, stress, or infection, may trigger attacks. Autonomic dysfunction to most end organs is a late hallmark of these attacks, coinciding with peripheral motor manifestations. A typical attack begins with abdominal pain; then central nervous system manifestations occur, such as seizures, psychosis, and even coma; and finally peripheral nervous system manifestations occur, including distal pain and weakness with minimal sensory loss, involving upper extremities first and then lower extremities, face, and respiratory muscles. Labile hypertension and bradycardia may require treatment.

α-Galactosidase deficiency (Fabry's disease) is an X-linked disorder that occurs mainly in young boys. Women carriers may also be affected in later years. This produces an accumulation of neutral glycosphingolipids in the kidney, blood vessels, lens, and nerves. Cardiovascular death is frequent. Telangiectasias in the mucosa and nail beds can lead to clinical suspicion, and reduced levels of α-galactosidase in white blood cells confirm the diagnosis. Distal neuropathic pain and parasympathetic glandular dysfunction (manifested as dry eyes, dry mouth, and loss of sweating) dominate the neurological picture. The only pathophysiological study found glandular hyposensitivity to parasympathetic agents, suggesting an intrinsic glandular process rather than denervation as the cause of the glandular dysfunction. This finding is compatible with the known glandular sphingolipid accumulation.

Another lipid accumulation disorder, Tangier disease, can also produce an autonomic neuropathy similar to that seen in Fabry's disease in that the pain and sensory complaints usually overshadow the autonomic problems. Neuropathy may present in three ways: relapsing–remitting demyelinating process resembling mononeuritis multiplex in distribution, syrinx-like process with proximal loss of pain and temperature sensation and preservation of other modalities (autonomic symptoms such as constipation and dry mouth may be present), and stocking distribution slowly progressive distal-to-proximal neuropathy. Other clinical features include splenomegaly and pathognomonic large orange tonsils due to deposition of cholesteryl esters. Diagnosis is confirmed by the absence or low levels of high-density lipoprotein. A mutation in the adenosine triphosphate-binding cassette transporter gene on chromosome 9q31 causes the disease.

Hereditary sensory autonomic neuropathy type III (Riley–Day syndrome or familial dysautonomia) consistently devastates autonomic function more than any other neuropathy. Affecting primarily Ashkenazi Jews, the disorder begins in early childhood with constipation, bouts of abdominal pain and pseudoobstruction, flushing of the skin, and episodes of sweating, which may relate to pain or other intercurrent illnesses. Orthostatic hypotension alternates with hypertensive spikes. Mentation remains normal. Diagnostic features include the absence of fungiform papillae; the absence of tears, which nonetheless respond excessively to cholinergic agonists; an absent histamine flare response; and little somatic neuropathy by EMG. Treatment is primarily supportive, with clonidine used for both blood pressure and abdominal complaints, and gastrointestinal surgical intervention for esophageal and lower gut problems.

Autonomic neuropathy is also a prominent feature of some mitochondrial disorders, such as mitochondrial neurogastrointestinal encephalopathy, with achalasia and pseudoobstruction perhaps due to involvement of the enteric plexus or the extrinsic autonomic fibers by the autonomic neuropathy. Reduced thymidine phosphorylase activity is diagnostic. Other clinical features include extraocular muscle dysfunction such as ptosis and opthtalmoparesis, leukoencephalopathy on magnetic resonance imaging, and a sensorimotor (somatic) peripheral neuropathy. Other mitochondrial encephalomyopathies may produce similar symptoms, and we have reported a family with such a disorder.

Diseases of Uncertain Etiology

It is curious that the disorders listed previously are encountered less frequently than a growing set of disorders whose etiology and precise involvement of the autonomic nervous system remain elusive. These include the extremely common postural tachycardia syndrome, chronic fatigue syndrome, and fibromyalgia. Various reports have suggested that an autonomic neuropathy contributes to these disorders, but this conclusion is far from clear. The postural tachycardia syndrome includes orthostatic symptoms along with a rapid heart rate in the standing position, with fatigue and reduced quality of life. A focal autonomic neuropathy involving venous capacitance vessels in the gut and lower extremities is one of the hypothetical etiologies. The role of the autonomic nervous system in fibromyalgia and chronic fatigue is more obscure. Other secondary dysautonomias listed in Table 1 are beyond the scope of this entry.

TREATMENT

When treating the orthostatic symptoms that accompany autonomic neuropathy, one should begin with nonpharmacological methods and progress to medications when required. Table 4 provides a partial list of both treatment types.

Another major issue in autonomic neuropathy is distal pain. This is usually "neuropathic" in nature and, hence, not highly responsive to standard pain relievers, such as nonsteroidal antiinflammatory agents or narcotics. Optimal management usually involves the use of a conditioning program such as water jogging (which desensitizes and strengthens simultaneously) along with an anticonvulsant, such as gabapentin or topiramate, combined with a tricyclic antidepressant, such as amitryptiline at bedtime or imipramine during the day, to match the period of symptom peak. The management of other problems, such as constipation, diarrhea, and bladder and sexual dysfunction, is beyond the scope of this entry.

CONCLUSION

Autonomic neuropathy comprises an eclectic group of disorders with diverse mechanisms but similar clinical

Table 4   INTERVENTIONS FOR ORTHOSTATIC SYNDROMES

Nonpharmacological methods
  Exercises
    Water jogging (water pressure increases venous return)
    Self-tilt (10 min, twice per day)
    Venous toning exercises, especially thigh and abdominal strengthening
  Increase available volume
    Salt load (until urinary spot sodium >150 mEq)
    Elevate the head of the bed on bricks
    Frequent small meals
    High-pressure (40–50 mmHg) thigh-high stockings with abdominal corset
Pharmacological
  Direct adrenergic
    Midodrine
    Fludrocortisone low dose (increases α-receptor sensitivity)
    Venlaflaxine
  Volume expansion
    NSAIDs
    Fludrocortisone high dose (>0.2 mg/day)
    Erythropoietin
  Modulate central autonomic tone
    β-Adrenergic blockade
    Serotonin-specific reuptake inhibitors
Medications to avoid
  α-Adrenergic antagonists, such as antihypertensives and agents that increase urine flow through the prostate
  Tricyclic antidepressants in high dose
  Diuretics
  If antihypertensives are needed, angiotensin system agents are preferred

presentations and clinical problems. Nonautonomic signs and symptoms can provide very useful clues to diagnosis and evaluation. For example, telangiectasias cause suspicion of Fabry's disease, ophthalmoparesis causes suspicion of a mitochondrial disorder, and onset of symptoms after a severe viral infection suggests a postinfectious immune-mediated process. Autonomic testing is critical in distinguishing central and peripheral autonomic nervous system disorders when the presentation is ambiguous and may guide management of orthostatic symptoms. Effective management tools are available for the two most common problems encountered in these patients— distal pain and orthostatic complaints.

—*Thomas C. Chelimsky*

See also–Autonomic Dysreflexia; Autonomic Nervous System, Overview; Diabetes Insipidus; Diabetes Mellitus; Neuropathies, Diabetic; Neuropathies, Iatrogenic; Neuropathies, Idiopathic; Neuropathies, Instrumental; Neuropathies, Overview; Neuropathy, Axillary; Neuropathy, Toxic

Further Reading

Axelrod, F. B. (2002). Hereditary sensory and autonomic neuropathies. Familial dysautonomia and other HSANs. *Clin. Autonomic Res.* **12**, 12–14.

Bradley, W. G., Karlsson, I. J., and Rassol, C. G. (1977). Metronidazole neuropathy. *Br. Med. J.* **2**, 610.

Diabetes Control and Complications Trial Research Group (1998). The effect of intensive diabetes therapy on measures of autonomic nervous system function in the Diabetes Control and Complications Trial (DCCT). *Diabetologia* **41**, 416–423.

Ewing, D. J., Campbell, I. W., and Clarke, B. F. (1980). The natural history of diabetic autonomic neuropathy. *Q. J. Med.* **193**, 95.

Hughes, P. J., Lane, R. J., Cutler, S. J., *et al.* (1993). Small-fiber dysfunction in a *Borrelia burgdorferi* infection. *Muscle Nerve* **16**, 221–222.

Jenzer, G., Mumenthaler, M., Ludin, H. P., *et al.* (1975). Autonomic dysfunction in botulism B: A clinical report. *Neurology* **25**, 150–153.

Kelly, J. J., Jr., Kyle, R. A., O'Brien, P. C., *et al.* (1979). The natural history of peripheral neuropathy in primary systemic amyloidosis. *Ann. Neurol.* **6**, 1–7.

Laiwah, A. C., Macphee, G. J., Boyle, P., *et al.* (1985). Autonomic neuropathy in acute intermittent porphyria. *J. Neurol. Neurosurg. Psychiatry* **48**, 1025–1030.

Low, P. A., Dyck, P. J., Lambert, E. H., *et al.* (1983). Acute panautonomic neuropathy. *Ann. Neurol.* **13**, 412–417.

McCombe, P. A., and McLeod, J. G. (1984). The peripheral neuropathy of vitamin B_{12} deficiency. *J. Neurol. Sci.* **66**, 117–126.

Silvieri, R., Veglio, M., Chinaglia, A., *et al.* (1999). The relation between QTc interval prolongation and diabetic complications. The EURODIAB IDDM Complication Study Group. *Diabetologia* **42**, 68–75.

Simpson, D. M., Katzenstein, D. A., Hughes, M. D., *et al.* (1998). Neuromuscular function in HIV infection: Analysis of a placebo-controlled combination antiretroviral trial. *AIDS* **12**, 2425–2432.

Truax, B. T. (1984). Autonomic disturbances in Guillain–Barré syndrome. *Neurology* **4**, 462–468.

Ueno, S., Fujimura, H., Yorifuji, S., *et al.* (1992). Familial amyloid polyneuropathy associated with the transthyretin Cys114 gene in a Japanese kindred. *Brain* **115**, 1275–1289.

Vernino, S., Low, P. A., Fealey, R. D., *et al.* (2000). Autoantibodies to ganglionic acetylcholine receptors in autoimmune autonomic neuropathies. *N. Engl. J. Med.* **343**, 847–855.

Neuropathies, Diabetic

Encyclopedia of the Neurological Sciences
Copyright 2003, Elsevier Science (USA). All rights reserved.

CURRENTLY, nearly 16 million people in the United States have diabetes mellitus. The prevalence of diabetes continues to increase at an alarming rate, especially in younger individuals. This is largely attributed to the increased rate of obesity: For every kilogram increase in weight, the rate of diabetes will increase approximately 9%. The health care cost associated with such increased prevalence and the diabetic complications will, indeed, be very high. Of the several long-term complications of diabetes mellitus, neuropathies are the major cause of costly morbidity and disabilities. Diabetes is the leading cause of peripheral neuropathy in the world, supplanting leprosy. There are currently less than 1 million people with leprosy, whereas it is estimated that the number of diabetics will increase to approximately 200 million worldwide during the next 20 years. At least half of these individuals are expected to develop one or several forms of diabetic neuropathies during the course of their illness. Diabetes is considered the major contributing factor to diabetic foot ulcers and nontraumatic leg amputations. The estimated cost of lower limb ulcer alone in the Medicare population (age 65 and older) in 1995 was $1.5 billion.

There are six major types of diabetic neuropathies: cranial neuropathies, truncal radiculopathy or thoracoabdominal neuropathy, proximal neuropathies (i.e., radiculoplexopathies), entrapment neuropathies, autonomic neuropathy, and diabetic symmetrical polyneuropathies. One or several forms of these neuropathies may coexist with other diabetic complications (i.e., retinopathy and nephropathy) in the same patient. Duration and severity of diabetes mellitus often parallel the severity of diabetic neuropathy, and other risk factors may influence its development, severity, and progression, including excessive alcohol and tobacco use, hyperlipidemia, hypertension, and peripheral vascular diseases. Because diabetes is a common disorder that may coincide with other conditions causing peripheral neuropathies, the mere association of neuropathic symptoms with diabetes mellitus is not sufficient for a diagnosis of diabetic neuropathy, and other causes of peripheral neuropathies must be excluded. Electrophysiological studies are important in the diagnosis and characterization of diabetic neuropathies.

DIABETIC CRANIAL NEUROPATHIES

The most commonly affected cranial nerve in diabetes is the third cranial nerve. Less frequently, fourth and sixth cranial nerve and, rarely, seventh nerve palsies may also occur.

In diabetic third nerve palsy, abrupt, intense, sharp, and retroorbital or periorbital pain precede the onset of ophthalmoplegia, usually with sparing of pupils. Most patients are older than 50 years of age. Ischemia and infarct of the nerve and, rarely, focal brainstem infarct are thought to be responsible for this syndrome. There are no specific laboratory abnormalities in this neuropathy, but imaging studies are required to exclude masses, aneurysms, or subarachnoid hemorrhage. Diabetic cranial third nerve palsy has a good prognosis with a full recovery in 3–6 months, but it rarely may recur. During the painful phase of the syndrome, analgesics are given for pain and eye patches are used to suppress diplopia.

DIABETIC THORACOABDOMINALNEUROPATHY (TRUNCAL RADICULOPATHY)

The predominant symptom of truncal radiculopathy is the gradual onset of pain, in middle or later life, in the lateral chest or abdominal walls that typically intensifies at night. There is usually loss or diminution of or increased skin sensation anterolaterally. Abdominal muscle weakness may result in abdominal wall protrusion, with electromyography (EMG) studies showing denervation of these muscles. Profound weight loss may be associated with the onset of pain. It is presumed that a vascular lesion of the intercostal nerve is the cause of the syndrome, although there is no pathological confirmation. The syndrome is self-limiting, with the recovery and resumption of normal weight and resolution of pain usually occurring within a few months. During the painful phase of the neuropathy, analgesics, tricyclic antidepressants, tramadol, or gabapentin may be tried. If these drugs are not helpful, repeated local application of a local anesthetic patch will substantially reduce the pain.

PROXIMAL DIABETIC NEUROPATHY OR DIABETIC POLYRADICULOPLEXOPATHY

This syndrome is also called diabetic femoral neuropathy, diabetic amyotrophy, or Burns–Garland syndrome. It occurs in older type II diabetic patients (mostly male), usually preceded or accompanied by substantial weight loss. Occasionally, it may be the presenting feature of diabetes mellitus leading to its discovery by appropriate blood tests. Patients complain of pain of variable intensity in the back, buttocks, and perineal and anterior thigh regions followed by weakness and atrophy of proximal and,

to a lesser extent, distal muscles a few days or weeks later. In some patients, numbness and tingling of the anterior thigh with reduced pain sensation occur. Often, the syndrome is asymmetrical, but a symmetrical and less painful form evolving over weeks to months is also recognized. In the asymmetrical form, the opposite leg may also become involved after weeks or months, with or without improvement of the original leg. In some patients, there is a significantly elevated sedimentation rate. Involvement of upper limbs is rare, and such involvement should always raise other possibilities, such as chronic inflammatory demyelinating polyneuropathy. In the asymmetrical form, because of severe radicular pain, weakness, and reduced reflexes in the affected leg, it is not uncommon for patients to undergo intensive radiological imaging studies or have unnecessary spinal surgeries. However, imaging studies and other evaluations may be necessary to exclude neoplastic infiltration of the lumbosacral plexus or necrotizing vasculitis. EMG study of the proximal diabetic neuropathy shows multiple nerve root involvement, especially L2–L4, with prominent fibrillation potentials in the muscles innervated by these roots but also, to a lesser extent, in distal muscles. Pathologically, a vascular–ischemic process, similar to microvasculitis with small mononuclear cell infiltration, is seen in proximal and distal sensory nerve biopsies. These findings have raised the possibility of an immune-mediated inflammatory process. It is not clear, however, whether these changes are a primary process or secondary to the neuropathy. Although there are reports of beneficial effects of immunomodulating therapies in proximal diabetic neuropathy, this condition is usually self-limiting with total or partial recovery within 1 or 2 years. Until controlled trials are carried out, these therapies will have a minor role in the treatment of this form of neuropathy because of the potential significant adverse effects of these treatments in the older diabetic population. The hyperglycemic effect of corticosteroids, the increased risk of infection and poor wound healing with the use of corticosteriod therapy, and thrombogenic and nephrotoxic effects of intravenous immunoglobulin (IVIG) in a patient population known to be at risk for these complications argue against the use of these treatments. Pain management with tricyclic antidepressants, tramadol, or anticonvulsants, rehabilitation and supportive devices, adequate control of diabetes, and reassurance of the spontaneous recovery from the condition are all needed for most patients.

DIABETIC AUTONOMIC NEUROPATHY

It is rare for autonomic neuropathy to occur without clinical or subclinical features of a somatic neuropathy; nearly all diabetics with autonomic neuropathy have varying degrees of sensory neuropathy that usually precedes the abnormalities of autonomic function. In long-standing diabetes, there is a greater possibility of autonomic nervous system involvement. Virtually every organ innervated by the autonomic nervous system may be affected by diabetic autonomic neuropathy, although the extent of involvement is highly variable. It is extremely rare for only one system or organ to be involved, and careful evaluation will always reveal clinical or subclinical involvement of one or more of the other organs. Both sympathetic and parasympathetic components of the autonomic nervous system are affected, involving cardiovascular, urogenital, gastrointestinal, pupillomotor, thermoregulatory, and sudomotor functions. In older diabetic patients, autonomic impairments are further complicated by a decline in autonomic function with age. The autonomic dysfunction, particularly cardiac autonomic neuropathy, has a profound effect on the management, prognosis, morbidity, and mortality of diabetes mellitus.

Pupillary dysfunction in diabetic autonomic neuropathy includes miosis, oval pupils, and a reduced normal hippus phenomenon. These abnormalities may be detected as early as 2 years after the diagnosis of diabetes and correlate with the duration and severity of diabetes mellitus and the presence of somatic neuropathy and other diabetic complications. Diabetic neuropathy can be associated with multiple gastrointestinal disorders, including esophageal dismotility, gastroparesis and delayed gastric emptying, gastric dismotility, impaired gallbladder contractility and emptying, constipation, diabetic diarrhea, internal rectal sphincter dysfunction, and fecal incontinence. Management of some of these dysfunctions can be challenging, requiring close cooperation between the gastroenterologist and the diabetologist.

There are several important cardiovascular autonomic dysfunctions in diabetic neuropathy that profoundly influence the patients' management and overall prognosis. The early involvement of the parasympathetic nervous system results in the frequent observation of resting tachycardia at 90–100 beats per minute.

There is also a circadian dysrhythmia, with the usual reduced nocturnal heart rate blunted. Prolon-gation of the QT interval and silent (painless) myocardial ischemia are the major causes of increased mortality attributed to cardiovascular autonomic neuropathy. Orthostatic hypotension, rarely severe or symptomatic, occurs in only 3% of patients. The contributing factors to the development of orthostatic hypotension include reduced total splanchnic and cutaneous vascular resistance secondary to the sympathetic neuropathy as well as diminished heart rate and cardiac output. These effects may be exaggerated by the vasodilating effect of insulin injection or postprandial hyperinsulinemia. Impaired distal limb vasomotor response results from the loss of vasoconstrictor tone due to failure of sympathetic postganglionic C fibers. This leads to peripheral vasodilation, increased blood flow, opening of the arteriovenous shunt, and distal edema.

The urinary dysfunction in diabetic autonomic neuropathy occurs in 27–85% of patients with long-standing diabetes. Impaired bladder sensation is usually the first symptom of urinary autonomic dysfunction. This is followed by gradual development of infrequent urination, increased bladder capacity, urinary retention, and urinary tract infections. With the complete failure of detrusor muscles (detrusor areflexia), incontinence may ensue.

Erectile dysfunction is three times more common in diabetics than in nondiabetic age-matched control males, occurring in 27–71% of patients. It is one of the earliest manifestations of diabetic autonomic dysfunction. Although diabetic autonomic neuropathy is the major or only cause of erectile problems, in approximately half of patients other factors, such as vascular disease and microangiopathy, hormonal alterations, and psychological factors, also play an important role, especially among older patients. In diabetic impotency, there is reduced synthesis and release of acetylcholine of the parasympathetic nerves of corpus cavernosum tissues. Drugs that inhibit the enzyme 5-cyclic guanosine monophosphate phosphodiesterase in the corporal tissue and thus enhance the vasodilating effect of nitric oxide, such as sildenafil, have been proven to be beneficial in the treatment of impotence.

As many as 92% of patients with diabetic neuropathy demonstrate different patterns of sweating abnormalities when sensitive tests are used. The most common sweating abnormality is reduced sweating in distal limbs, which may be associated with profound compensatory truncal hyperhidrosis. Some patients may have profuse, symmetrical sweating over the face, scalp, and neck within minutes of eating very strong-tasting, spicy, or sour foods that provoke salivation (gustatory sweating). This is thought to be due to aberrant reinnervation of facial territory supplied by the superior cervical ganglion.

When a diabetic patient with autonomic neuropathy develops hypoglycemia, the warning signs (e.g., sweating, tremor, and palpitation) may be absent or blunted (hypoglycemic unawareness); impaired glucose counter-regulation after hypoglycemia is thought to be due to disturbed adrenergic responses.

MONONEUROPATHIES

Nerves that are susceptible to pressure (median, ulnar, common peroneal, and lateral femoral cutaneous) may be even more vulnerable in diabetics. This is due to relative ischemia of the nerve by vascular compromise as well as endoneurial metabolic abnormalities. When appropriate, decompression of nerve at the carpal or cubital tunnel may be performed.

SYMMETRICAL POLYNEUROPATHY

This is by far the most common form of all diabetic neuropathies. Nearly all therapeutic trials and research on the pathogenesis and pathology of the diabetic neuropathies have been conducted on this form of neuropathy. It occurs in both type I and type II diabetes, being predominately a length-dependent sensory neuropathy with an insidious onset. Most patients have numbness and painless tingling sensation in distal lower limbs. Pain occurs in only 10% of patients. However, pain may be distressing and debilitating. In some patients, acute diabetic cachexia associated with severe, diffuse pain and profound weight loss may occur. The sensory symptoms may be the presenting feature of diabetes leading to its discovery. With advanced sensory abnormalities, mild distal weakness and atrophy may also develop. With involvement of smaller nerve fibers, some degree of clinical or subclinical autonomic neuropathy is usually present and foot ulcer may develop. The electrophysiological abnormalities also follow a length-dependent pattern, with distal sensory nerves being most sensitive and involved early. Some mild slowing of motor nerve conduction may be detected.

The pathophysiology of diabetic polyneuropathy is not fully understood, but both metabolic and vascular mechanisms play important roles and are influenced by genetic factors. Most of the current understanding of the pathogenesis of diabetic polyneuropathy and its experimental therapies has been derived from studies of various animal models of diabetic neuropathy. However, no ideal animal model exists for diabetic neuropathies, and extrapolation of knowledge gained from current models to the human diabetic neuropathy is limited. It is clear that hyperglycemia results in polyol accumulation in the nerve, initiating a cascade of events leading to nerve degeneration. Hyperglycemia also leads to accumulation of glycosylation end products in the blood vessels and nerve proteins as well as increased oxidative stress. Impairment of essential fatty acid metabolism by hyperglycemia leads to prostaglandin abnormalities and reduced vasodilating effect. Hyperglycemia may also lead to altered neurotrophic factors, including nerve growth factor and IGF. Because of the multifactorial nature of the pathogenesis of diabetic polyneuropathy, many experimental and clinical therapeutic trials exploiting virtually every aspect of its proposed pathogenesis have been conducted in the past 30 years. These have included several aldose reductase inhibitors to reduce polyol accumulation, myoinositol supplementation, free radical scavengers, recombinant human nerve growth factor, fatty acid supplementation, inhibitors of glycosylated end products, and vasodilating agents. Unfortunately, none of these have shown substantial clinical efficacy. The cornerstone of treatment remains the rigorous and sustained glycemic control to slow the progression of neuropathy. Controlled trials have shown the efficacy of tricyclic antidepressants, tramadol, and anticonvulsants (gabapentin and carbamazepin) in the management of pain of diabetic polyneuropathy. In using these drugs, the principle of "start low, go slow" should always be followed in order to achieve therapeutic success and to minimize side effects.

—*Y. Harati*

See also–Diabetes Insipidus; Diabetes Mellitus; Neuropathies, Amyloid; Neuropathies, Autonomic; Neuropathies, Nutritional; Neuropathies, Overview

Further Reading

Backonja, M., Beydoun, A., Edwards, K. P., *et al.* (1998). Gabapentin for the symptomatic treatment of painful neuropathy in patients with diabetes mellitus: A randomized controlled trial. *J. Am. Med. Assoc.* **280**, 1831–1836.

Diabetes Control and Complications Trial Research Group (1995). Effect of intensive diabetes treatment on nerve conduction in the Diabetes Control and Complications Trial. *Ann. Neurol.* **38**, 869–880.

Dyck, P. J., and Thomas, P. K. (Eds.) (1999). *Diabetic Neuropathy*, 2nd ed. Saunders, Philadelphia.

Harati, Y. (1992). Frequently asked questions about diabetic peripheral neuropathies. *Neurol. Clin.* **10**, 783–807.

Harati, Y. (1996). Diabetes and the nervous system. *Endocrinol. Metab. Clin. North Am.* **25**, 325–358.

Harati, Y. (2000). Diabetes and the autonomic nervous system. In *The Autonomic Nervous System, Part II* (O. Appenzeller, Ed.), revised series No. 31. Elsevier, Amsterdam.

Harati, Y., Gooch, C., Swenson, M., *et al.* (1998). Double-blind randomized trial of tramadol for the treatment of the pain of diabetic neuropathy. *Neurology* **50**, 1842–1846.

Mokdad, A. H., Ford, E. S., Bowman, B. A., *et al.* (2000). Diabetes trends in the US: 1990–1998. *Diabetes Care* **23**, 1278–1283.

Sindrup, S. H., and Jensen, T. S. (1999). Efficacy of pharmacological treatment of neuropathic pain: An update and effect related to mechanism of drug action. *Pain* **83**, 389–400.

Thomas, P. K., and Tomlinson, D. R. (1993). Diabetic and hypoglycemic neuropathy. In *Peripheral Neuropathy* (P. J. Dyck, P. K. Thomas, and J. W. Griffen, *et al.*, Eds.), pp. 1219–1250. Saunders, Philadelphia.

Vinik, A. I., and Park, T. S. (2000). Symptomatic treatment of painful neuropathies. *Diabetologia* **43**, 957–973.

Neuropathies, Entrapment

Encyclopedia of the Neurological Sciences

THE TERM entrapment neuropathy applies when a peripheral nerve is chronically compressed, typically at a vulnerable site, leading to local nerve injury. There are numerous vulnerable locations in which a nerve trunk can become entrapped for a variety of reasons and due to a variety of mechanisms. A distinction is made between acute nerve compression, which typically is produced by brief but significant pressure, and entrapment-type injury, which is typically produced from longer term (chronic), often intermittent, compression or nerve distortion. Some researchers further separate entrapment via internal distorting forces from simple external compression, but this distinction is less critical for this discussion. Both types of injury affect large, discrete nerve trunks. Most syndromes involve named, single peripheral nerves and are thus a type of mononeuropathy; however, compression can occur at higher levels prior to the emergence of a nerve from its supplying plexus. One prominent example is impingement on a segment of the brachial (arm) plexus as the nerves traverse the shoulder area (thoracic outlet syndrome) that can occur from an extra rib or fibrous band. Syndromes and specific nerve anatomy are detailed separately for each individual nerve, but a number of entrapment syndromes and vulnerable sites of simple nerve compression are listed in Table 1.

Table 1   SELECTED RECOGNIZED SITES OF NERVE ENTRAPMENT AND COMPRESSION

Upper extremity
Median nerve
 Wrist: carpal tunnel syndrome
 Finger: digital neuropathy
 Near elbow:[a] ligament of Struthers syndrome
 Pronator syndrome:[a] compressed by pronator teres muscle
Ulnar nerve
 Just below elbow: cubital tunnel syndrome
 Above elbow: repetitive compression, trauma
 Wrist: Guyon's canal
 Palm: deep ulnar nerve (pure motor)
Radial nerve
 Forearm: posterior interosseous nerve (pure motor), cyst, benign tumor
 Upper arm: spiral groove (staturday night palsy, superficial site circling bone)
 Axilla (armpit):[a] crutch injury
Lateral antebrachial cutaneous nerve (windsurfers)
Suprascapular nerve
 Top of shoulder blade (suprascapular notch): ligament, reduced tunnel size
Brachial plexus
 Thoracic outlet syndrome (extra rib, fibrous band)
 Others: axillary, musculocutaneous
Lower extremity
Peroneal nerve
 Below knee: fibular head, superficial site circling bone
 Ankle:[a] anterior tarsal tunnel
Tibial nerve
 Ankle: tarsal tunnel syndrome
 Foot: more distal plantar and digital neuropathies, multiple causes
 Behind knee:[a] popliteal fossa
Sciatic nerve
 Upper posterior thigh/pelvis: piriformis syndrome[a], hip surgery complication
Lateral femoral cultaneous nerve
 Lateral thigh: meralgia paresthetica, compressive belts, obesity
Others
 Obturator (childbirth)[a]
 Genitofemoral[a]
 Illioinguinal[a]
 Pudendal (childbirth)[a]
 Femoral (groin)[a]

[a] Uncommon or rare syndrome.

NEUROPATHIES, ENTRAPMENT

meThere are a variety of mechanisms that lead to nerve injury, with differing scenarios at each characteristic site. Some processes include simple pressure, but nerve stretch, bending, twisting, and local friction can also injure nerve fibers. Other offending forces that may compress nerves include fibrous bands, scar tissue, an abnormally increased or anomalous muscle, tissue swelling, tumors, and deformed bone. Descriptions of entrapment sites or injury are provided for many of the individual nerves in the body, although some are quite rare or occur only in special situations or with specific repetitive activities. Many are likely underrecognized because symptoms are not always prominent enough to prompt medical attention.

CLINICAL MANIFESTATIONS

Symptoms are dependent on the particular nerve and territories involved. Nerve trunks are composed of fibers from various types of nerve cells serving different functions. The proportion of each type of nerve cell varies from nerve to nerve and thus affects the expected manifestations from injury. Some nerve branches carry almost exclusively motor (strength) fibers, and compromise leads to weakness, muscle atrophy, and occasionally spontaneous muscle twitching, termed fasciculations. Conversely, sensory nerve injury leads to loss or altered sensation in the nerve territory downstream of the injury, for example, numbness, tingling, spontaneous pins and needle sensation, and loss of touch and temperature perception. Innocuous sensory stimuli can be altered and perceived as odd, tingly, or even unpleasant or painful. Autonomic (vegetative or unconscious functions) nerve injury leads to disruption of fibers with control over functions such as local blood flow and sweating, resulting in difficulties in regulation of local temperature and skin moisture. Most nerves are mixed with a combination of various fiber types; thus, injury produces a combination of symptoms and signs. Manifestations are also dependent on the portion of the nerve trunk compromised because differing modalities tend to travel through separate areas of the nerve trunk.

Pain, however, is often the most prominent symptom and a prime reason that patients seek medical attention. Frequently, the site of compression is locally uncomfortable or painful. However, discomfort can be perceived elsewhere as "referred pain" usually regionally or in a shared anatomical territory as the primary insult, for example, median nerve entrapment at the wrist producing pain in the forearm or upper arm. In some cases, the predominant site of pain can be an aid in locating the entrapment site. Tinel's sign results when a site of injury is tapped and leads to a shooting pain or numbness in the territory of the nerve in question. This sign is most commonly associated with carpal (wrist) tunnel syndrome, when tapping over the median nerve in the wrist leads to sudden pain and shooting numbness into the median innervated thumb, index, and middle fingers.

PREDISPOSING FACTORS

All individuals are not equally susceptible to nerve injury. Certain underlying diseases can predispose an individual to certain entrapment syndromes. However, simply having a disorder of peripheral nerves in general (axonal or demyelinating peripheral neuropathy), such as from diabetes, alcohol abuse, or another cause, will reduce the extent of compression necessary to cause nerve damage. There are also uncommon hereditary conditions that predispose to compression injury from minor levels of exposure. One such disorder, commonly known as hereditary neuropathy with liability to pressure palsy (HNPP) or localized hypertrophic neuropathy, leads to multiple and recurrent injury to nerves from subtle nerve trauma mostly at typical sites of compression. Interestingly, the gene for this defect is identical to a form of a more common and generalized hereditary motor and sensory demyelinating neuropathy known as Charcot–Marie–Tooth disease (CMT). Whereas HNPP is caused by a deletion of or missing *PMP22* gene on chromosome 17, CMT results from a duplicated section of the same gene. Thus, two very different appearing diseases, although both involve the peripheral nerve, result with different defects of the same gene. Although HNPP should be considered whenever there is an excessive number of entrapments that are not well accounted for, this disease is present in only a small number of patients.

Certain types of repetitive behavior can induce an entrapment from so-called "overuse." Athletes, musicians, hobbyists, and some occupations are potentially vulnerable to certain syndromes with chronic repetitive activities. The most common entrapment, carpal tunnel syndrome (CTS), may be hastened by repetitive hand activities, such as typing, bread kneading, sewing, and stereotypical job activities. However, there are many unusual activities that humans engage in that make a specific site more vulnerable. For example, wind surfers build unusually large, specific forearm muscles that can compress the lateral antebrachial cutaneous sensory nerve, leading to a disconcerting patch of forearm numbness. Sports as diverse as bowling and playing video games to football and baseball have characteristic nerve injury syndromes dependent on the repetitive activity or forms of external compression. Examples include handlebar compression of sites along the ulnar nerve at the wrist or palm in long-distance cyclists, palm (deep ulnar) nerve compression in weightlifters, shoulder nerve impingement in baseball pitchers, and finger (digital) nerve injury due to playing video games or carrying plastic grocery bags. Knowledge of the activity and clinical signs can often lead to a probable clinical diagnosis.

Not only the activity but also limb positioning can irritate peripheral nerve. For example, the ulnar nerve curves around the elbow and is relaxed with the arm straightened. When bent, the nerve is stretched and compressed by local connective tissues. Involuntary arm bending when asleep can exacerbate an underlying ulnar neuropathy.

Other medical conditions, such as rheumatoid arthritis or gout, can cause local tissue swelling or changes in bone shape that can impinge on a nerve if in a vulnerable spot. There are a number of human anatomical variations of vestigial muscle or fibrous bands that fail to degenerate as usual during normal development. These anomalous structures are typically of no consequence unless they are situated in the path of a peripheral nerve and lead to entrapment.

PATHOPHYSIOLOGY

Some knowledge of the normal components and physiology of peripheral nerve is necessary to understand how compression leads to disrupted function. Peripheral nerves are composed of fibers (axons) arising from nerve cells (neurons) that reside in the spinal cord or adjacent ganglia. Each individual neuron and axon serves a dedicated function that depends on the attached, linked structures. For example, motor (strength) fibers supply a set of muscle fibers; somatic sensory fibers (conscious sensation) supply one or more specialized sensory organs; autonomic fibers supply blood vessels, involuntary muscle, special sensors, or glands; and some fibers terminate as simple bare nerve endings (heat and pain sensation). Axons are grouped into subunits termed fascicles. Each fascicle is encircled

by supporting connective and vascular tissues (endoneurium) that serve numerous functions, including blood supply and protection. There is also a protective blood–nerve barrier in the capillaries, analogous to but less restrictive to circulating factors than the blood–brain barrier. Multiple fascicles are linked and encircled by additional connective tissue (perineurium) that forms a nerve trunk. This is a large surgically visible unit potentially vulnerable to compression. Both sets of connective tissue, endoneurium and perineurium, have invaginations and folds that protect the nerve from mild stretch injury. When stretched, the initial force will be buffered by the unfolding of these invaginations and not transmitted to the axons. However, additional stretch can damage nerve fibers. Nerves also have interesting structures termed Renaut bodies that are assumed to act as microscopic protective bumpers for the nerves. These structures are seen at common entrapment sites. One study on cadavers without known entrapment neuropathy found these structures in a majority of compression sites but not in other areas of the nerve.

Another important concept is that all axons are not equivalent. Large-diameter motor and some sensory fibers take advantage of a system of enhanced conduction velocity. Axons are wrapped in many layers of a lipid-based substance called myelin that serves to insulate short segments from electrical activity, essentially functioning as a tiny capacitor. Electrically active nodes separate myelin segments, where the majority of ion channels are congregated (nodes of Ranvier). The larger the axon diameter, the larger the myelin sheath needed to accomplish the effect. This arrangement forces a conducting impulse to jump from node to node, thereby speeding conduction by an order of magnitude. This rapid transfer of current down the axon is called saltatory conduction. A dedicated Schwann cell supplies each small sheath and a long series of myelin sheaths form a microscopic tube from neuron to axon target. These structures are vital not only for conduction but also as a path for regenerating nerves. This arrangement differs from the myelin sheath anatomy in the brain, where one cell can myelinate a number of different axons. Small-diameter fibers may have little (cold) or no myelin (warm, pain, and autonomic) and conduct uniformly slowly. The importance is that the primary pathology of chronically compressed or entrapped nerves is disruption of these myelin segments leading to pathology termed demyelination.

There has been considerable animal work to establish the pathological processes in both acute nerve crush and compression as well as chronic low-level compression more applicable to entrapment injury. The effect of severe but brief (acute) trauma to a nerve trunk differs from the effects of intermittent trauma over an extended period (weeks to years). For example, in one model of entrapment, bands are placed around a rabbit leg or other animal limb that slowly compress the peripheral nerve (rabbit sciatic) as the animal grows. Many of the basic concepts discussed are inferred from this type of animal work.

Sunderland and Seddon both described classification systems to indicate the extent of injury that are still conceptually useful. There has been a long-standing controversy regarding the relative importance of pressure on nerve fibers vs disruption of blood supply leading to nerve injury (ischemia). Nearly everyone has experienced a brief episode of reversible nerve compression. For example, after continual leg crossing for 20–30 min, most people develop symptoms of peroneal nerve compression with numbness, tingling sensation, or even weakness in the foot and leg. Also, one may have alternatively experienced numbness and tingling in the ring and little fingers after leaning on a bent elbow for an extended period. This phenomenon has been shown to be vascular in nature and quickly reversible in most settings with pressure relief. There is also no recognizable pathology if the nerve is microscopically examined. In a clever experiment, Lewis and others proved that this scenario is due to ischemia. Two cuffs were applied to a limb. The more distal (lower) cuff was inflated and left in place until a loss of sensation occurred. Then the higher (proximal) cuff was inflated and the distal cuff released. Symptoms persisted until the proximal cuff was released and then quickly abated. Symptoms continued despite a change in the site of compression, supporting a vascular cause.

If pressure is continual or there are a sufficient number of intermittent exposures, then a persistent loss of function can occur. In fact, a nerve can tolerate a high degree of uniform pressure but is relatively intolerant to an abrupt pressure gradient, such as the edge of a compressive cuff. Over time, this type of local compression will induce changes in the nerve and myelin sheaths. The mildest form of injury is termed neurapraxia. The earliest visible changes appear to be disruption of the blood–nerve barrier and thickening of the connective tissue and microvessels. However, the earliest nerve changes seen are asymmetry and retraction of the myelin sheath from the nodes. As noted previously, these changes seen in cuff experiments are limited to the edges of the compressive force where the pressure gradient is highest. Eventually, a segment of myelin can be lost. This type of structural damage leads to local slowing or failure of conduction across the compressed segment. The remainder of the nerve in both directions remains intact and will conduct normally if electrically stimulated. There is no primary destruction of axons or connective tissues, simply a failure of function. As noted earlier, myelinated nerves require activation of interspersed nodes to propagate conduction down an individual axon. Nodes under a compressed area are wider and leaky to current. Initially, this change will increase the time needed to reach the necessary voltage to stimulate an action potential, thereby slowing conduction. Eventually, if sufficiently disrupted, the threshold current for an action potential is not reached and conduction is terminated (conduction block). Large myelinated axons are unable to maintain conduction even for a short distance if the nodal system is disrupted. These manifestations of focal slowing and conduction block can be demonstrated with clinical electrophysiological techniques discussed later, and correlate well with the degree of microscopic demyelination. This type of focal slowing of conduction velocity is the hallmark of demyelination, but some degree of conduction block must be present for disruption of function.

If more severe compression is present, the nerve axon is disrupted (axonotmesis) and loses contact with more distal segments. Subsequently, the downstream axon will slowly degenerate over 5–7 days (Wallerian degeneration). Both the axon and the myelin sheaths break down and are removed; however, the Schwann cells and connective tissues remain. The doomed, degenerating axon remains electrically excitable for a period of time; thus, results of tests performed soon after injury may appear identical to those for neurapraxia and axonotmesis. After Wallerian degeneration is complete the two processes can be separated with clinical electrophysiological techniques. Although axons are disrupted, axonotmesis-type injuries do not irreversibly damage the surrounding connective tissue and blood vessels. This relative sparing lays the groundwork for nerve regeneration, which is not possible with central neurons and axons. The stump of the site proximal to the injury will sprout and attempt to retrace the path through new Schwann cell sheaths.

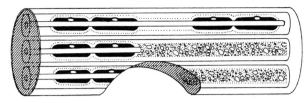

Figure 1

Illustration of variable types of nerve injury to different fascicles within the same nerve in a complex injury. Outline represents connective tissue sheath. Fascicles from top to bottom: focal demyelination with neurapraxia, axonotmesis with myelin sheath disruption and Wallerian degeneration with preserved connective tissue, and neurotmesis with additional connective tissue disruption [reproduced with permission from Stewart, J. D. (1986). Electrodiagnostic techniques in the evaluation of nerve compressions and injuries in the upper limb. *Hand Clinics* **2**, 677–687].

Trophic and nerve growth factors emanating from both the nerve stump and other tissues are essential for successful regeneration. Advancing new fibers grow approximately 1 mm/day but can be impeded by scar tissue or other factors. More severe injury (neurotmesis) separates the connective tissues at increasing levels of severity, reducing or eliminating the chance of spontaneous recovery. However, this type of extreme injury is not generally seen with entrapments and is limited to more forceful, traumatic processes. In actuality, many human conditions are likely a combination of processes (Fig. 1). It is not uncommon even with neurapraxia for there to be some signs of axonal degeneration. Also, the relative importance of direct pressure affecting axons vs small areas of ischemia related axon loss remains unresolved in practice. Many of the unpleasant symptoms related to an entrapment may be due more to transient vascular changes than to demyelination. Fixed loss of strength, muscle bulk, and sensation correlate well with the degree of demyelination, but intermittent sensory symptoms and pain do not. This discrepancy implies that fixed loss of function is due to demyelination or axon loss, and periods of spontaneous abnormal sensations (paresthesias) and pain are a result of intermittent ischemia. Paresthesias result from spontaneously generated activity in entrapped fibers under conditions of reduced blood flow. Surprisingly, these transient sensory phenomena are often more disturbing to the patient than mild loss of function.

DOUBLE CRUSH SYNDROME

Another ongoing controversy is whether one local nerve injury predisposes that nerve to an insult at a second remote distal site (double crush syndrome) (e.g., a pinched nerve in the neck making entrapment in the limb more likely). This vulnerability may be due to impairment of the cellular transport systems within the axon from the higher lesion. Although this concept is much discussed and has some direct physiological evidence, the importance to human disease is questionable.

CLINICAL NEUROPHYSIOLOGY

Although probable sites of entrapment can be suspected on examination, clinical neurophysiology can more definitively characterize the presence, type, severity, and location of the injury from entrapment. Nerve conduction studies (NCS) and electromyography (EMG) are methods employed. The underlying physiology discussed earlier can be routinely measured *in vivo*. Motor nerve conduction studies electrically stimulate peripheral nerves at various points along their course and record an evoked, summated waveform over a distal muscle termed a compound muscle action potential (CMAP). The amplitude and area of the recorded CMAP waveform, which approximately correlates to the number of stimulated axons and the precise time from stimulation to wave onset, are measured. When two different sites are stimulated, the time difference between the two responses is measured and, along with distance measures, a conduction velocity (CV) for a segment can be calculated. As noted earlier, focal demyelination is the hallmark of entrapment neuropathies. As an example, Fig. 2 shows a series of motor NCS in a patient with suspected ulnar neuropathy across the elbow. CMAP responses were induced at 2-cm intervals across the ulnar nerve course around the elbow and recorded over a distant small hand muscle. An abrupt disproportionate degree of slowing of calculated CV identifies the site of demyelination. Conduction block can also be identified as a sudden decrease in waveform amplitude and area when stimulating above the entrapment site. In this example, the waveform and conduction velocity abruptly change 2 cm above the elbow, with a 40% decrease in evoked amplitude and marked segmental slowing. The CMAP is the summation of many individual nerve axons; thus, this pattern implies a mixture of fibers—some with demyelination and others with conduction block. If a significant degree of Wallerian degeneration of axons has occurred, it will be reflected in lower amplitude and area in the responses below the block as well as

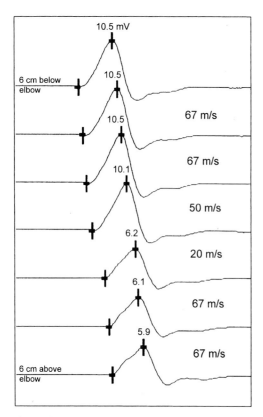

Figure 2
Ulnar motor nerve conduction study in a patient with ulnar mild fixed motor and sensory loss. Surface electrical stimulation was given from 6 cm below to 6 cm above the elbow in 2-cm increments. Amplitude is displayed above the waveforms (normal, >6.0 mV) and segmental velocity between waveforms (normal, >50 m/sec). Note the abrupt 40% decrease in amplitude and marked focal slowing of conduction velocity between the fourth and fifth traces.

in signs of loss of muscle fiber innervation (denervation) on EMG. When seen, this pattern implies at least some degree of axonotmesis, whereas pure conduction block or focal slowing with normal distal responses imply predominant neurapraxia, and a much improved chance of recovery.

The described techniques are routine and highly reliable in accessible systems such as the wrist and elbow. However, there are a number of less accessible sites that make electrical stimulation from the skin surface above and below a suspected entrapment site problematic. Because of difficulties regarding definitive proof, some syndromes remain controversial as to their frequency and, in some cases, their existence (e.g., a rare syndrome of sciatic nerve compression caused by an enlarged piriformis muscle in the pelvis as this large nerve exits into the thigh). Because of the deep location of this entrapment, it is problematic to

adequately perform routine electrical stimulation and local slowing typically cannot be confirmed. In this case, the diagnosis is presumptive and may prompt surgical decompression of variable benefit.

TREATMENT

The approach to treatment is dependent on the type and severity of compression. Fortunately, for the most common and easily identifiable syndrome, CTS, there are a number of effective therapies. In some cases, simply reducing or stopping a repetitive activity or posture can provide sufficient relief. In addition, there are a number of nonsurgical interventions that can be beneficial, such as wrist splints for CTS. Surgical decompression can be performed for many syndromes if other measures are insufficient or known to be ineffective for the compression site.

—*Louis H. Weimer*

See also–Carpal Tunnel Syndrome; Charcot–Mari–Tooth Disease; Median Nerves and Neuropathy; Neuropathies, Idiopathic; Neuropathies, Instrumental; Neuropathies, Overview

Further Reading
Dawson, D. M., Hallet, M., and Wilbourn, A. J. (Eds.) (1999). *Entrapment Neuropathies*, 3rd ed. Lippincott Raven, Philadelphia.
Stewart, J. D. (Ed.) (2000). *Focal Peripheral Neuropathies*, 3rd ed. Lippincott Williams & Wilkins, Philadelphia.

Neuropathies, Iatrogenic

Encyclopedia of the Neurological Sciences
Copyright 2003, Elsevier Science (USA). All rights reserved.

THE TERM IATROGENIC is derived from the Greek words *iatros* (healer) and *genic* (origin). As currently defined, iatrogenic neuropathies are undesired or unintended peripheral nervous system (PNS) lesions that patients sustain during the course of their medical care. They may be due to acts of comission or omission committed by anyone involved in the diagnosis or treatment, including not only physicians but also nurses, technicians, and pharmacists.

Almost every PNS structure in the human body can be damaged during the course of medical care and in a multitude of ways. The result can be mononeuropathies, multiple mononeuropathies, plexopathies, or generalized polyneuropathies. In this entry, some of the more commonly encountered iatrogenic PNS disorders are discussed.

The overall severity of an iatrogenic neuropathy (including its persistence) is determined by a number of factors, including the number and type of axons affected, the location of the abnormalities along the axons, and the pathophysiology of the disorder. The latter, in turn, depends on the nature of the underlying pathology. The pathology and pathophysiology of nerve lesions are discussed elsewhere in this encyclopedia. It is sufficient to note that most focal lesions result from axon loss, whereas a few are due predominantly to conduction block caused by demyelination. Similarly, most generalized disorders result from axon loss, whereas a few result from conduction slowing or block caused by demyelination.

CRANIAL NEUROPATHIES

Two cranial nerves sustain iatrogenic damage with some frequency—the VII (facial) nerve and the XI (spinal accessory) nerve. Iatrogenic facial neuropathies can occur along any segment of the nerve—intracranial, infratemporal, and extracranial—and nearly all are due to surgical procedures (e.g., acoustic neuroma removal). Axon loss underlies most of these and is frequently the result of nerve transection. Consequently, optimal therapy usually includes surgical exploration and nerve repair, if possible; recovery is often incomplete.

The majority of iatrogenic spinal accessory neuropathies involve solely the branch to the trapezius muscle; they occur during minor surgical procedures (e.g., lymph node biopsies) performed on the posterior triangle of the neck. Because the pathology is axon loss, and most of these do not recover spontaneously, often the appropriate treatment is surgical exploration and nerve repair, if possible, preferably performed within 3 or 4 months of onset.

BRACHIAL PLEXOPATHIES

The brachial plexus is one of the largest PNS structures and one of the most vulnerable. It is derived from the C5–T1 roots and passes from the base of the neck to the axilla. Anatomically, it consists of the following five components, from proximal to distal: roots, trunks, divisions, cords, and terminal nerves. Clinically, it is divided into two regions, supraclavicular and infraclavicular, because when the upper limb is at the side, the clavicle

overlies its third component (the divisions), whereas two of the remaining components (roots and trunks) are proximal, or supraclavicular, to the clavicle and the two others (cords and terminal nerves) are distal, or infraclavicular, to it.

At least three distinct types of iatrogenic supraclavicular plexopathies result from surgery. Classic postoperative paralysis is attributed to malpositioning of patients during operations performed under general anesthesia. It characteristically involves the upper trunk, resulting in arm and shoulder girdle weakness. The pathology is predominantly or solely demyelination, producing conduction block; consequently, recovery is usually prompt (within 4–6 weeks) and complete.

Postmedian sternotomy lesions are due to damage to the C8 anterior primary ramus (immediately before it contributes to formation of the lower trunk) caused by sternal splitting required to gain access to the heart during cardiac surgery. The distribution of the hand weakness, sensory loss, and sometimes pain is similar to that seen with ulnar neuropathies since the ulnar nerve is derived predominantly from the C8 root. However, some radial and median nerve-innervated muscles are also affected. The pathology most often is a combination of axon loss and demyelination causing conduction block. Usually, conservative treatment is indicated; most cases recover satisfactorily.

Surgery for disputed neurogenic thoracic outlet syndrome is typically performed to treat a highly controversial type of brachial plexopathy. The injury is almost always axon loss in type and involves the C8 and T1 roots. Pain and hand weakness are common permanent residuals.

Obstetrical paralysis is another supraclavicular plexopathy. Although considered an iatrogenic lesion, it can occur during childbirth when there are no medical personnel present. The most common presentation, referred to as Erb's palsy, is predominantly shoulder girdle weakness caused by C5–C6 root or upper trunk involvement. Less often, the C7 root or middle trunk also is affected. The underlying pathology most often is axon loss, frequently coexisting with demyelination causing conduction block. The appropriate treatment, operative versus conservative, is debated. Recovery is seldom complete; many patients are functionally one-armed as adults.

Radiation-induced brachial plexopathy usually involves the infraclavicular plexus, typically beginning with the lateral cord. In most instances, the radiation is directed toward the axillary lymph nodes to prevent spread of ipsilateral breast cancer. The pathology initially is demyelination causing conduction block, but axon loss gradually and inexorably supervenes. Most often, the first symptom is persistent paresthesias in one of the median nerve-innervated fingers. It may not appear until decades after the radiation therapy was given. The paresthesias slowly spread, and at some time progressive weakness occurs. Ultimately, after many years, the limb lacks movement and sensation. There is no effective treatment.

Iatrogenic infraclavicular plexopathies can occur during a variety of orthopedic procedures (e.g., shoulder arthroscopy and surgery for recurring anterior shoulder dislocations). The underlying pathology varies depending on the specific procedure, but axon loss usually predominates. The most appropriate treatment and the outcome also vary depending on the particular circumstances. A specific type of iatrogenic infraclavicular brachial plexopathy, medial brachial fascial compartment syndrome, results from axillary hematoma formation caused by axillary artery puncture with subsequent leakage of blood. It most often occurs following axillary arterograms or axillary regional blocks. The first symptom is almost always pain, which is soon followed by weakness in the terminal median nerve distribution. One or more other terminal nerves may also be involved, particularly the ulnar. These are characteristically severe axon loss lesions and there is little recovery. Operative decompression is beneficial only if it is performed within a few hours after onset of the symptoms.

LUMBOSACRAL (PELVIC) PLEXUS

In contrast to the brachial plexus, the pelvic plexus is seldom the site of iatrogenic injuries. Neoplasms are a far more common cause of pelvic plexopathies.

Radiation-induced pelvic plexopathies are late complications of treatment of various pelvic neoplasms, especially cervical carcinoma. Most often, the lumbar plexus is affected, often bilaterally. Progressive weakness of the quadriceps and thigh adductors as well as paresthesias are the most common symptoms. The underlying pathology is demyelination causing conduction block, but this gradually converts to axon loss over time. Consequently, the slowly progressive course is irreversible. There is no effective treatment.

A psoas compartment syndrome occurs in anticoagulated patients who bleed into the psoas compartment, which contains the lumbar plexus. Symptoms include pain, sensory loss, and marked weakness of quadriceps and thigh adductors. After a few hours, the underlying pathology is solely axon loss, and permanent residuals are common. The most appropriate treatment, operative versus conservative, is debated.

Ischemic lumbar plexopathies, unilateral or bilateral, can result from operations performed on the aorta and its major derivatives, particularly if cross-clamping is necessary. Clinical manifestations include weakness, pain, and sensory loss. Characteristically, the pathology is axon loss. There is no effective treatment and recovery is often poor.

Maternal paralysis presents in the postpartum period. It is due to compression of the lumbosacral trunk between the fetal head and the maternal pelvic brim during delivery. The main symptom is unilateral footdrop. The pathophysiology is conduction block caused by demyelination, so the prognosis is excellent.

LIMB MONONEUROPATHIES

Of the various types of PNS injuries, these are probably the most common type of iatrogenic neuropathy. Virtually any nerve may be damaged, at any location, depending on the circumstances, but injury to a major nerve trunk generally has the most serious clinical consequences.

The majority of upper limb iatrogenic mononeuropathies involve the ulnar, median, or radial nerves. Most iatrogenic ulnar neuropathies occur perioperatively, while the patient is under general anesthesia. They involve the elbow segment of the nerve and are attributed to malpositioning. The ulnar nerve is the most common PNS structure injured during surgical procedures. Typically, some combination of hand weakness, sensory deficit, paresthesia, or pain is noted in the early postoperative period. The underlying pathophysiology is remarkably variable, consisting of axon loss, demyelinating conduction block or conduction slowing, or any combination. Whenever axon loss is prominent, permanent residuals are typical. The value of surgical treatment is far less clear than with most other focal mononeuropathies.

Iatrogenic median neuropathies occur mainly at either the elbow region, due to invasive diagnostic or therapeutic procedures being performed in the antecubital fossa (e.g., venous infusions and cardiac catheterizations), or at the wrist, due to complications of carpal tunnel syndrome treatment. Typically, symptoms include weakness, paresthesias, and, with some of the proximal lesions, severe pain. The pathology is almost always axon loss. Surgery is often the most appropriate treatment. Even with surgery, however, suboptimal long-term results are common.

Most iatrogenic radial neuropathies occur in the midportion of the arm, at or near the spiral groove. Causes include improper positioning during surgical procedures, injuries during treatment of midshaft humeral fractures, tourniquet use, and misplaced intramuscular injections. Weakness (i.e., wrist drop and finger drop), sensory loss, and severe pain (with injection injuries) are characteristic symptoms. The pathology varies with the cause: axon loss with humeral fracture treatment and displaced intramuscular injections or demyelination causing conduction block with malpositioning. Axon loss lesions that do not recover spontaneously may require surgical exploration. The motor deficits can be ameliorated considerably by tendon transfers, but these should be performed only after nerve regeneration has failed to occur, and nerve repair is rejected.

Lower extremity iatrogenic nerve injuries most often involve the femoral, sciatic, and peroneal nerves. Iatrogenic femoral neuropathies have many causes, both intrapelvic and extrapelvic. Intrapelvic etiologies include traction or compression injuries due to retractor use during abdominal operations as well as ischemic injury during abdominal aneurysm repairs and whenever there is bleeding into the iliacus compartment in anticoagulated patients, producing a compartment syndrome. Most extrapelvic lesions occur at or near the inguinal ligament. Causes include various operations (e.g., herniorrhaphies) in which the nerve is stretched or, more often, sectioned; procedures in which the lithotomy position is employed and the leg is hyperflexed on the trunk (e.g., vaginal hysterectomies), producing compression damage; and various diagnostic and therapeutic procedures performed on the nearby femoral artery (arteriograms) that result in hematoma formation and secondary compartment syndromes. Regardless of cause, the main symptoms of these lesions are quadriceps weakness, sensory loss in a saphenous nerve distribution, and often pain. The pathology is usually axon loss, but with some lithotomy-induced lesions it is demyelination causing conduction block. Surgical exploration is indicated whenever spontaneous recovery does not occur. Whether very early surgical decompression should be performed for the iliacus compartment syndrome is debated.

Most iatrogenic sciatic neuropathies affect the proximal segment of the nerve in the gluteal or upper thigh region. Two of the most common causes are misplaced intramuscular injections and hip operations. The latter can manifest both immediate and delayed symptoms, depending on whether the nerve is damaged at the time of surgery (by traction, instrumentation, or inadvertent suturing) or whether it is injured later by compression resulting from postoperative bleeding and thus producing a gluteal compartment syndrome. Perioperative lesions can also result from patient positioning and from the application of a tourniquet around the midthigh. Regardless of cause, in most instances, the peroneal component is damaged more than the tibial component of the sciatic nerve. The pathology is almost always axon loss. Painful lesions may require surgical treatment. However, because of the nerve regeneration distances involved, motor function distal to the knee is seldom restored by surgical repair.

Iatrogenic common peroneal neuropathies frequently occur, most often due to external compression. Almost all affect the nerve segment at the fibular neck. Perioperative lesions result from faulty positioning (usually with the patient supine or in the lithotomy position) or from instrumentation. By definition, lesions due to the latter occur only when operations are performed on or near the knee (e.g., total knee replacements). With malpositioning, the pathology may be either axon loss or demyelination causing conduction block; in contrast, with instrumentation injuries, the pathology is invariably axon loss. Nonsurgical iatrogenic peroneal lesions result from pressure caused by plaster casts, leg braces, or tight bandages or from prolonged bed rest, particularly when patients are emaciated. The underlying pathology may be either axon loss or demyelination causing conduction block. Regardless of etiology, the major symptom is foot drop; pain is rarely mentioned. Most of these lesions recover with conservative treatment, although surgical repair may be required for those resulting from instrumentation.

MULTIPLE MONONEUROPATHIES

In relatively rare instances, two or more major nerves in a limb can sustain simultaneous iatrogenic damage. There are a number of causes, including intraarterial injections and the production of one or more compartment syndromes. Two other etiologies merit brief discussion: tourniquet paralysis and ischemic monomelic neuropathy. Tourniquet paralysis may involve major nerves of either the upper or the lower limbs. With upper limb involvement, there is simultaneous compromise of the radial, median, and ulnar nerves or, less often, the radial nerve alone. The pathophysiology characteristically is demyelination causing conduction block. With lower limb involvement, usually the sciatic nerve is affected alone and the pathology is almost always axon loss. Clinically, tourniquet paralysis is dominated by motor weakness. Treatment is almost invariably conservative; recovery is usually quite satisfactory, although often it does not begin until several months after onset.

Ischemic monomelic neuropathy (IMN) results from abrupt compromise of arterial blood flow in a limb. The nerve fibers in the more distal portion of the limb are injured in a length-dependent fashion; the damage is progressively more severe distally, and it is uniform at any particular limb level. Upper limb IMN characteristically involves the more distal portions of the median, ulnar, and radial nerves. Its cause is almost always iatrogenic: arteriovenous shunt placement at or proximal to the elbow, for dialysis purposes, in diabetic patients with renal failure. Lower limb IMN involves the more distal portions of the tibial, peroneal, and saphenous nerves. Among the iatrogenic causes are cannulation of the superficial femoral artery for cardiopulmonary bypass or for insertion of intraaortic balloon pumps. Burning pain in the hand or foot is the most prominent clinical feature, along with hand weakness with upper limb involvement. Restoring adequate arterial blood flow to the limb via various surgical procedures (e.g., arteriovenous shunt closure) is mandatory if it has not already been done. The long-term prognosis is favorable. The burning pain typically resolves slowly after several months.

DRUG-INDUCED POLYNEUROPATHIES

An appreciable number of medications can cause polyneuropathies, including drugs characterized as antiinflammatory and antirheumatic, antimicrobial, antineoplastic, and cardiovascular. The majority of drug-induced polyneuropathies are sensorimotor in type. However, several have unusual features. Thus, dapsone typically produces a "pure" motor neuropathy that is often more severe or limited to the distal upper limbs; zalcitabine and nitrofuradantoin can both cause sensorimotor polyneuropathies that persist for some time after drug discontinuance;

nitrofuradantoin can produce a fulminating polyradiculoneuropathy; and taxol can cause a pure sensory polyneuropathy in which painful dysesthesias, first involving the hands, may predominate. The pathology is characteristically axon loss. Typically, drug-induced polyneuropathy is treated with drug discontinuance; in most instances, recovery occurs, although occasionally it is incomplete.

CONCLUSION

Iatrogenic neuropathies are rather common, have many different causes, and may affect any portion of the PNS. Because their underlying pathology in the majority of cases is axon loss, recovery is often slow and may be incomplete.

—Asa J. Wilbourn

See also–Brachial Plexopathies; Lumbar Plexopathy; Mononeuropathy Multiplex; Neuropathies, Overview

Further Reading

Currier, D. S., and Garg, B. P. (1998). Neurologic complications of anesthesia. In *Iatrogenic Neurology* (J. Biller, Ed.), pp. 63–88. Butterworth-Heinemann, Boston.

Dropcho, E. J. (1998). Neurologic complications of radiation therapy. In *Iatrogenic Neurology* (J. Biller, Ed.), pp. 461–484. Butterworth-Heinemann, Boston.

Faden, A. I. (1998). Iatrogenic illness. *Neurol. Clin.* 16, 1–8.

Laycock, M. A. (1998). Drug-induced peripheral neuropathies. In *Iatrogenic Neurology* (J. Biller, Ed.), pp. 269–282. Butterworth-Heinemann, Boston.

Le Quesne, P. M. (1993). Neuropathy due to drugs. In *Peripheral Neuropathy* (P. J. Dyck and P. K. Thomas, Eds.), 3rd ed., pp. 1571–1581. Saunders, Philadelphia.

Wilbourn, A. J. (1998). Iatrogenic nerve injuries. *Neurol. Clin.* 16, 55–82.

Wilbourn, A. J. (1993). Brachial plexus disorder. In *Peripheral Neuropathy* (P. J. Dyck and P. K. Thomas, Eds.), 3rd ed., pp. 911–950. Saunders, Philadelphia.

Neuropathies, Idiopathic

Encyclopedia of the Neurological Sciences

IDIOPATHIC NEUROPATHIES refer to a group of acquired, sensory-predominant polyneuropathies (PNs) that remain of uncertain cause after potential etiologies have been excluded. In the literature, the term cryptogenic is occasionally substituted for idiopathic. Idiopathic sensorimotor neuropathies demonstrate clinical evidence of both sensory and motor nerve impairment, whereas motor nerves are clinically spared in idiopathic sensory neuropathies. Idiopathic sensory neuropathies may evolve into sensorimotor neuropathies with time. In addition, patients who have only sensory symptoms and signs on clinical evaluation may manifest evidence of motor nerve involvement on electrophysiological studies. These patients would be classified as sensorimotor neuropathies by most investigators.

Acquired chronic sensory and sensorimotor PNs are common in middle and late adulthood, with an estimated prevalence of more than 3%. The majority of acquired PNs are secondary to readily identifiable causes, such as diabetes, alcohol abuse, inflammatory diseases, and neurotoxic medications. However, once known etiologies are excluded, many neuropathies remain idiopathic (10–25% in recent series).

Idiopathic PN is in essence a diagnosis of exclusion, established after a careful medical, family, and social history, neurological examination, and directed laboratory testing. Such an approach is necessary to exclude the large number of known causes of sensory-predominant PN, including diabetes, chronic alcoholism, metabolic disturbances, endocrine abnormalities, connective tissue diseases, malignancy or amyloidosis, HIV or other infections, pertinent toxic or pharmacological exposures, and hereditary factors.

CLINICAL FEATURES

Patient Population

The onset of idiopathic sensory and sensorimotor PN is predominantly in the sixth and seventh decades, with a mean age between 50 and 60 years in prior studies. In a series of 93 patients compiled by one of the authors, the mean age of onset was 58 years, with a range of 37–94 years. Older studies have found that men are overrepresented in the idiopathic neuropathy population by as much as a 3:1 ratio (Table 1). This male predominance has not been observed in recent series.

Diagnostic Criteria

Diagnostic criteria for idiopathic sensory-predominant PN have been proposed. These criteria were based on clinical experience derived from a series of 93 patients. The authors identified these patients by the term chronic cryptogenic sensory polyneuropathy (CSPN). Inclusion criteria for CSPN require that there be a loss or alteration of sensation for at least 3 months beginning in distal limbs, usually with onset in feet before hands. There can be no presenting symptoms of weakness. Distal sensory loss on examination must be present in a symmetrical fashion and may include any of the following: loss of vibration, proprioception, light touch, pain (pinprick) sensation, or temperature. Hyporeflexia or areflexia may be present but are not required. Minimal weakness or atrophy is allowable in muscles supplying movement to the fingers and toes.

Results of electrophysiological studies and quantitative sensory testing are often, but not invariably, abnormal. Electrophysiological abnormalities indicate a primarily axonal process. Other laboratory studies, such as skin punch biopsy to measure intraepidermal nerve fiber density or autonomic testing, may provide evidence of peripheral nerve dysfunction when other testing is normal. Blood and urine testing should be normal. A monoclonal protein is allowed only in the setting of a monoclonal gammopathy of uncertain significance.

Exclusion criteria include any identifiable cause of PN; demyelination on nerve conduction studies (NCS); monoclonal gammopathies related to lymphoproliferative disorders, malignancy, or amyloidosis; and weakness at presentation other than toe and finger weakness.

Presenting Symptoms

Discomfort or pain is a common presenting symptom, reported by 65–80% of idiopathic PN patients. Numbness and tingling tend to be the most common symptoms, followed by a heavy feeling or weakness in the distal limbs. In pure sensory PN, numbness is the most common symptom, followed by paresthesias and burning. Approximately one-third to one-half of patients will have symptoms confined to their lower extremities. In the CSPN series, 42% of patients had symptoms restricted to the distal lower extremities for at least several months before hand involvement was noted. The average time for symptoms to spread to the upper extremities appears to be approximately 5 years. Autonomic and cranial nerve involvement is uncommon.

Physical Examination

On sensory examination, vibration is the primary modality most likely to be impaired, and it was reduced in 80% or more of patients in several large series. Pinprick was also reduced in 75–85% of patients, whereas light touch deficits varied in two series, ranging from 54 to 92%. Position sense tends

Table 1 IDIOPATHIC POLYNEUROPATHY PATIENT SERIES[a]

Reference	Total no. PN patients	No. idiopathic PN patients (%)	Male:female	Mean age at onset (years)	PN type (%) sm/sens/motor/other	NCS (%) ax/demyel/mix	Nerve bx (%) ax/demyel/mix
Matthews (1952)	46	32 (70%)[b]	N/A	N/A	N/A	N/A	N/A
Rose (1960)	80	45 (56%)	3:2	80% of patients >40 years old	N/A	N/A	N/A
Prineas (1970)	278	107 (38%)	2:1	40–50	84/6/10/0	CV slowing in all patients	N/A
Dyck et al. (1981)	205	49 (24%)	N/A	N/A	N/A	N/A	N/A
Fagius (1983)	91	67 (74%)	N/A	59	99/1/0	18/15/67[c]	N/A
Konig et al. (1984)	70	10 (14%)	N/A	72[d]	41/30/0/29	CV slowing in 84%	N/A
McLeod et al. (1984)	519	67 (13%)	3:1	51	64/25/11/0	94/6/0	100/0/0
Corvisier et al. (1987)	432	48 (11%)	N/A	65	66/0/0/34	N/A	41/48/11
Notermans et al. (1993)	~500	75 (10%)[e]	2:1	57	59/38/3/0	94/3/3	100/0/0
Mitsumoto et al. (1994)	35	17 (49%)	1:5	N/A	0/100/0/0	N/A	100/0/0
Gorson et al. (1995)		20	1:3	65	25/75/0/0	55/0/0; 45% normal	67/0/0; 33% normal
Holland et al. (1998)		32	1:1.6	~58	0/100/0/0	100% normal (by definition)	60/0/0; 40% normal
Wolfe et al. (1999)	402	93 (23%)	1:1	58	41/59/0/0[f]	100/0/0	93/7/0
Periquet et al. (1999)		104[g]	1:1.5	59	0/100/0/0	100/0/0 (Group 1 only)	N/A

[a] Abbreviations used: N/A, not available; sens, sensory; sm, sensori motor; ax, axonal; demyel, demyelinating; bx, biopsy.
[b] More than 50% of patients had acute onset.
[c] Includes all patients, including those with known causes of PN.
[d] Study included only patients older than age 60.
[e] Includes 22 patients from other centers.
[f] Patients with motor symptoms excluded from study.
[g] Group 1 and 2 patients included, 21 with known conditions.

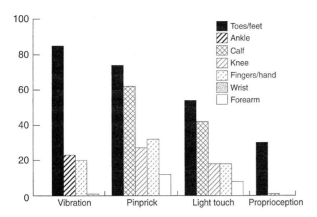

Figure 1
Sensory deficits on initial examination, portrayed as the percentage of all CSPN patients. The anatomical extent of the sensory deficit is depicted by bar graphs (modified from Wolfe *et al.*, 1999. Copyright 1999 American Medical Association).

to be least affected, being abnormal in only 20–30% of patients. Pinprick is the most sensitive modality in assessing the proximal extent of sensory loss (Fig. 1). Loss of pinprick and temperature sensation is universal in series of idiopathic small-fiber PN, whereas proprioception is almost always spared.

Approximately two-thirds of patients with idiopathic sensorimotor PN can be expected to have distal weakness and wasting. Although diagnostic criteria for the CSPN series excluded patients presenting with motor symptoms, 41% of these patients had mild distal weakness on examination and 15% had muscle atrophy. Foot weakness was present in 38%, hand weakness in 18%, and both foot and hand weakness in 15%. Therefore, hand weakness without foot weakness was rare.

Ankle deep tendon reflexes are absent in 50% to almost all idiopathic sensorimotor PN patients. Diffuse areflexia is uncommon in pure sensory PN but was observed in 25% of patients with sensorimotor PN. Patients with reduced deep tendon reflexes in the upper extremities almost always have reduced responses in the legs, again consistent with a length-dependent pattern.

ELECTROPHYSIOLOGICAL FEATURES

Nerve Conduction Studies

Chronic idiopathic PN is almost exclusively an axonal neuropathy (Table 1). NCS abnormalities should be expected in most idiopathic PN patients. In prior series, at least 75% of idiopathic PN patients

had abnormal NCS. As expected, sural sensory responses are most frequently affected and were abnormal in 70–85% of sensorimotor PN patients. Sensory and motor NCS abnormalities typically consist of reduced amplitudes with normal or minimal distal latency and conduction velocity changes. NCS abnormalities are observed in only 50% of patients presenting with painful, burning feet.

Electromyography

On electromyography (EMG), Wolfe *et al.* found abnormalities in 70% of CSPN patients who underwent needle examination. Fibrillations were present in 42% and neurogenic motor units in 63%. This is in agreement with small series of patients with pure sensory presentations. Therefore, patients with idiopathic PN who have only sensory signs commonly have motor involvement on electrophysiological studies. Most investigators would classify these neuropathies as sensorimotor, although EMG abnormalities restricted to intrinsic foot muscles may be considered equivocal evidence of motor nerve involvement.

LABORATORY FEATURES

Excluding Potential Causes

Before diagnosing a patient with idiopathic PN, it is mandatory to exclude identifiable causes of neuropathy. Laboratory studies should include at a minimum a complete chemistry battery and blood count, ESR, ANA, rheumatoid factor, vitamin B_{12} level, thyroid function tests, and serum protein electrophoresis with immunofixation electrophoresis. Other laboratory studies, such as 2-hr glucose tolerance testing, urine protein electrophoresis, and HIV serology, should be performed as clinically indicated.

Monoclonal Proteins and Autoantibodies

The frequency of monoclonal proteins in chronic idiopathic PN is as high as 10%, representing a monoclonal gammopathy of uncertain significance (MGUS) in most patients. Although some studies have demonstrated that patients with an IgM paraprotein may progress faster, with more sensory loss, ataxia, and weakness than those with an IgA or IgG monoclonal protein, there is significant clinical overlap between the different immunoglobulin classes, including late age of onset, generally slow progression, and predominantly distal, symmetrical sensory and motor involvement. Furthermore, PN patients with MGUS are difficult to distinguish on clinical and electrophysiological grounds from unclassified PN without a paraprotein, raising the possibility that the MGUS is coincidental in most patients.

Recent series have found anti-sulfatide antibodies in no or only a small percentage of patients with idiopathic PN.

Cerebrospinal Fluid

Cerebrospinal fluid (CSF) analysis is largely unremarkable in idiopathic PN when inflammatory neuropathies are excluded. The mean CSF protein from 73 patients in a 1993 study by Notermans *et al.* was 43 mg/dl. CSF was examined in 5 of 93 CSPN patients and was normal in 4. In our experience, CSF examination is of low yield in patients with chronic PN who remain unclassified after routine laboratory studies, have minimal motor involvement, and do not demonstrate demyelinating features on NCS. We do not routinely perform lumbar puncture in these patients.

Nerve Biopsy

Nerve biopsy tissue generally confirms the axonal nature of these idiopathic PNs. All 31 nerve specimens showed axonal degeneration in Notermans *et al.*'s 1993 series. There was no evidence of demyelination, inflammation, vasculitis, or amyloidosis. Myelinated fiber loss with axonal degeneration and regeneration were typical findings in other series. We argue that sural nerve biopsy is rarely helpful from a diagnostic or management standpoint in patients with an unclassified, predominantly sensory PN, and we do not recommend routine performance of nerve biopsies in these patients.

Quantitative Sensory Testing

Routine NCSs have several shortfalls in the assessment of idiopathic PN. NCSs are often normal in patients with primarily sensory PN. In addition, lower extremity sensory responses may be absent in normal subjects older than 60 years of age, complicating the interpretation of such a finding in elderly patients with idiopathic PN. Furthermore, NCSs are relatively insensitive to small-fiber dysfunction. In a large series, quantitative sensory testing (QST) for vibration and cold detection thresholds using the CASE IV system was slightly more sensitive than NCS, demonstrating abnormalities in 85% of patients (Table 2). QST was abnormal in 72% of patients in another large series. In a study of 32 patients with

Table 2   CLINICAL SUMMARY OF CSPN PATIENTS (*n* = 93)[a]

Gender	44 women, 49 men
Mean age at presentation	63.2 years (range, 37–94 years)
Mean duration of symptoms prior to evaluation	62.9 months (range, 3–240 months)
Mean follow-up period	12.5 months (range, 1–42 months)
Progression on examination	10 of 66 patients (15%)
Abnormal sensory NCS	77.0%
Abnormal motor NCS	59.6%
Abnormal needle EMG	70.3%
Abnormal QST	84.6%

[a] Abbreviations used: NCS, nerve conduction study; QST, quantitative sensory testing.

burning feet who had normal NCS, thermal thresholds were abnormal in 57% and vibration thresholds in 30% of patients. In all these studies, thermal thresholds were more likely to be abnormal than vibratory thresholds, illustrating the propensity for small-fiber involvement in idiopathic PN.

Skin Biopsy

Intraepidermal nerve fiber (IENF) density measurements on punch skin biopsy provide objective evidence of neuropathy, are less invasive than sural nerve biopsy, and have potential as an outcome measure in therapeutic trials. IENF was more sensitive than QST or sudomotor autonomic testing in a recent series, and it provided evidence of small-fiber neuropathy in three-fourths of patients with burning feet who had normal NCS. Although IENF density and small-fiber counts on sural nerve biopsy are concordant in most patients, skin biopsy appears to be a more sensitive tool than sural nerve biopsy in identifying small-fiber depletion. Although IENF has shown promise in the evaluation of idiopathic PN, this technique is not widely available and data collection can be time-consuming. Whether it will enter routine clinical practice remains unclear.

YIELD OF REEVALUATIONS

Reevaluations of idiopathic PN may eventually uncover a cause in a many patients. Dyck *et al.* found that intensive evaluation of referred unclassified neuropathies yielded an identifiable cause in a surprising 76%. Of 205 patients referred for evaluation, 42% had hereditary neuropathies, 21% inflammatory-demyelinating   polyradiculoneuropathies, and 13% other acquired neuropathies. Repeating laboratory studies on a routine basis, including serum agar gel and immunoelectrophoresis, was not informative. Differences in referral populations and the breadth of the initial workup are likely responsible for the contrasting yields of reevaluations.

Hereditary neuropathies may account for a large number of unclassified PN. Hereditary sensory neuropathies may occur without the emphasized features of foot ulceration, acral mutilation, and arthropathy, and when sporadic they are difficult to distinguish from idiopathic PN. Hereditary motor and sensory neuropathy (HMSN) type 2 should be considered when motor symptoms predominate and skeletal deformities are present. Muscle cramping in the legs and feet and the absence of paresthesias favor a hereditary neuropathy over other etiologies. Onset late in life does not exclude HMSN because it is estimated that 15% of patients with autosomal dominant HMSN type 2 present after the age of 50.

CLINICAL COURSE

The majority of patients with idiopathic sensory and sensorimotor PN follow a stable to slowly progressive course over years. A stable plateau phase is particularly characteristic of pure sensory PN. Independent ambulation is maintained in nearly all patients. However, walking canes and ankle bracing may be required over time in the sensorimotor population. The need for assistive devices in patients with pure sensory PN appears to be uncommon.

TREATMENT APPROACH

Pharmacotherapy of Neuropathic Pain

Most authorities agree that treatment of pain should be the primary focus of management in idiopathic sensory neuropathy. Treatment studies for neuropathic pain have been conducted mainly in diabetic and HIV-associated neuropathies and postherpetic and trigeminal neuralgias. Most rigorously studied are the tricyclic antidepressants and anticonvulsants.

Using a numbers-needed-to-treat methodology based on data from randomized, placebo-controlled, double-blinded trials, tricyclic antidepressants were recently recommended as first-line therapy for neuropathic pain. The leading alternatives were gabapentin, tramadol, and carbamazepine.

In a retrospective chart review, we found the tricyclic antidepressants amitriptyline and desipramine to be approximately equivalent in efficacy to carbamazepine for symptomatic relief of painful paresthesias and dysesthesias in idiopathic PN. As a whole, 29 of 59 patients (49%) responded to one of these agents. Similar success was found with gabapentin and mexiletine, although in a smaller number of patients. There is considerable variability in an individual's response to the different pharmacological agents and even to different drugs in the same class.

Patient Education

Perhaps of even greater importance than pharmacotherapy of neuropathic pain is patient education. Idiopathic PN patients are often anxious about their future since many have been told that their prognosis is bleak and that they will become physically incapacitated over time. Clearly, available literature supports the notion that the vast majority of patients remain stable or progress slowly, suffer limited motor disability, and remain independent. For those patients with pure sensory presentations, the prognosis may be even more favorable with long plateau periods. Simply informing patients of this natural history can provide considerable emotional and even physical comfort.

—*Zahid F. Cheema and Gil I. Wolfe*

***See also*–Neuropathic Pain Syndromes; Neuropathies, Iatrogenic; Neuropathies, Overview; Neuropathy, Toxic**

Further Reading

Asbury, A. K. (1987). Sensory neuronopathy. *Semin. Neurol.* **7**, 58–66.

Dyck, P. J., Oviatt, K. F., and Lambert, E. H. (1981). Intensive evaluation of referred unclassified neuropathies yields improved diagnosis. *Ann. Neurol.* **10**, 222–226.

Galer, B. S. (1995). Neuropathic pain of peripheral origin: Advances in pharmacologic treatment. *Neurology* **45**, S17–S25.

Gorson, K. C., and Ropper, A. H. (1995). Idiopathic distal small fiber neuropathy. *Acta Neurol. Scand.* **92**, 376–382.

Gosselin, S., Kyle, R. A., and Dyck, P. J. (1991). Neuropathy associated with monoclonal gammopathies of undetermined significance. *Ann. Neurol.* **30**, 54–61.

Grahmann, F., Winterholler, M., and Neundörfer, B. (1991). Cryptogenic polyneuropathies: An out-patient follow-up study. *Acta Neurol. Scand.* **84**, 221–225.

Holland, N. R., Crawford, T. O., Hauer, P., *et al.* (1998). Small-fiber sensory neuropathies: Clinical course and neuropathology of idiopathic cases. *Ann. Neurol.* **44**, 47–59.

Kissel, J. T., and Mendell, J. R. (1995). Neuropathies associated with monoclonal gammopathies. *Neuromusc. Disorders* **6**, 3–18.

McLeod, J. G., Tuck, R. R., Pollard, J. D., *et al.* (1984). Chronic polyneuropathy of undetermined cause. *J. Neurol. Neurosurg. Psychiatry* **47**, 530–535.

Mitsumoto, H., and Wilbourn, A. J. (1994). Causes and diagnosis of sensory neuropathies: A review. *J. Clin. Neurophysiol.* **11**, 553–567.

Notermans, N. C., Wokke, J. H. J., Franssen, H., *et al.* (1993). Chronic idiopathic polyneuropathy presenting in middle or old age: A clinical and electrophysiological study of 75 patients. *J. Neurol. Neurosurg. Psychiatry* **56**, 1066–1071.

Notermans, N. C., Wokke, J. H. J., van der Graaf, Y., *et al.* (1994). Chronic idiopathic axonal polyneuropathy: A five year follow up. *J. Neurol. Neurosurg. Psychiatry* **57**, 1525–1527.

Notermans, N. C., Wokke, J. H. J., van den Berg, L. H., *et al.* (1996). Chronic idiopathic axonal polyneuropathy: Comparison of patients with and without monoclonal gammopathy. *Brain* **119**, 421–427.

Periquet, M. I., Novak, V., Collins, M. P., *et al.* (2000). Painful sensory neuropathy: Prospective evaluation using skin biopsy. *Neurology* **53**, 1641–1647.

Pestronk, A., Li, F., Griffin, J., *et al.* (1991). Polyneuropathy syndromes associated with serum antibodies to sulfatide and myelin-associated glycoprotein. *Neurology* **41**, 357–362.

Sindrup, S. H., and Jensen, T. S. (2000). Pharmacologic treatment of pain in polyneuropathy. *Neurology* **55**, 915–920.

Wolfe, G. I., and Barohn, R. J. (1998). Cryptogenic sensory and sensorimotor polyneuropathies. *Semin. Neurol.* **18**, 105–111.

Wolfe, G. I., Baker, N. S., Amato, A. A., *et al.* (1999). Chronic cryptogenic sensory polyneuropathy: Clinical and laboratory characteristics. *Arch. Neurol.* **56**, 540–547.

Neuropathies, Instrumental

Encyclopedia of the Neurological Sciences
Copyright 2003, Elsevier Science (USA). All rights reserved.

INTEREST in the disorders that might interfere with the playing of a musical instrument and, indeed, might even be caused by the playing of that instrument has been increasing during the past 20 years. Most of these problems are primarily characterized by pain and can be classified as musculoskeletal. Nonetheless, because of the distribution and nature of the presenting symptoms, the possibility of a focal peripheral neuropathy must often be considered. Additionally, occupational cramps or focal limb dystonias, occasionally in association with a nerve entrapment, are not uncommon in instrumentalists. These will not be further discussed here.

A peripheral neuropathy is a disorder of that portion of the nervous system that lies outside the confines of the brain and spinal cord. This process may be generalized, typically affecting the most distal segment of nerves in the feet or hands, or localized to a single nerve trunk or branch thereof, in which case it may be characterized as a focal (or mono-) neuropathy. Although localized injury to a nerve can be the result of cutting, tearing, or stretching, the vast majority are associated with entrapment of the nerve as it passes through a narrowed channel bounded by bony structures, fibrous bands, bulky muscles, or enlarged arteries on its way to or from its ultimate destination. Strictly speaking, these points of entrapment are differentiated from those sites at which the nerve is potentially susceptible to external compression (such as the ulnar nerve at the elbow or "funny bone"), but the terms compression and entrapment neuropathy are often used synonymously.

CLINICAL PRESENTATION

Focal neuropathies typically develop insidiously and present clinically with pain, sensory disturbance, and weakness. The pain may be at the site of compression or may be distributed anywhere along the course of the nerve. Sensory symptoms, such as numbness, tingling, pins and needles, burning, or even itching, are usually in the cutaneous distribution of the nerve that is compressed. Muscle weakness or impaired motor control are often later effects. Because small fibers belonging to the autonomic nervous system are also contained in these nerve trunks, symptoms such as changes in sweating, skin temperature, or color and even hair or nail growth may be seen. It is the distribution of the pain, and, particularly, the localization of the sensory and motor disturbance, that allows the physician to suspect a diagnosis of a specific focal peripheral neuropathy. Precise localization of the point of compression is helped by the fact that each nerve has one or more points of high susceptibility to compression, by local signs such as tenderness or sensitivity to manipulation, and by specialized tests such as nerve conduction studies and needle electrode examination [collectively called electromyography (EMG)].

FREQUENCY OF ENTRAPMENT NEUROPATHY IN INSTRUMENTALISTS

There are no data to allow an accurate estimate of the frequency with which entrapment neuropathies occur in instrumental musicians. What can be stated is that among those instrumentalists who seek medical consultation for playing-related problems, compression neuropathies are commonly identified, although the frequency varies greatly in different reports. Among three neurologists seeing large numbers of musicians, the frequency of focal peripheral neuropathies reported ranged from 18 to 48%. In two large series from nonneurologists, the frequency was 7.2 and 4%, respectively. Although it cannot be claimed that focal peripheral neuropathies are more common among instrumentalists, there is reason to suspect that playing an instrument may influence the development of a focal peripheral neuropathy. For example, the left arm and hand are affected by playing-related problems two or three times more often than are the right arm and hand in bowed string players, but in our series of violinists and violists with ulnar neuropathy at the elbow, all 16 had left-sided involvement and only 1 had right-sided symptoms as well.

SPECIFIC NERVE ENTRAPMENT SYNDROMES IN INSTRUMENTALISTS

Carpal Tunnel Syndrome

Compression of the median nerve in the carpal tunnel is the most common entrapment neuropathy in all populations and is similarly frequent in musicians. Women are more likely to be affected than men and carpal tunnel syndrome (CTS) most typically occurs in the fifth and sixth decades of life. Characteristic features include pain, often in the hand and wrist but also more proximally, and paresthesias, usually but not invariably localized to the thumb through ring fingers. Pain, numbness, and tingling typically awaken the patient at night and will often occur with specific positions and activities, including playing an instrument. The symptoms may be provoked by specific maneuvers on examination. Some sensory disturbance can be identified in the distribution of the median nerve in most but not all patients. Weakness and muscle atrophy are less common. Specific electrodiagnostic testing confirms the diagnosis in most patients. In a personal series, CTS was identified in 52 instrumentalists, including 32 women and 20 men ranging in age from 17 to 79 years (mean, 44 years). There is a suggestion of greater susceptibility among keyboard players. Initial treatment may consist of splinting the wrist at nighttime, modifying hand activity, anti-inflammatory medication, and local corticosteroid injection. Definitive treatment usually consists of surgical release of the nerve by severing

the dense ligament that forms the roof of the carpal tunnel, and this is successful in the vast majority of cases.

Ulnar Neuropathy

Entrapment of the ulnar nerve at the elbow is generally considered the second most common focal peripheral neuropathy of the upper extremity. Pain may be noted at the elbow or in the hand, and sensory symptoms are common, affecting the little finger and usually the ulnar half of the ring finger. Weakness and muscle atrophy may be identified in some cases, affecting particularly finger movements critical for all instrumentalists. Traditionally, both prolonged elbow flexion and repetitive elbow flexion and extension have been considered predisposing factors, as has external compression, as may occur when leaning on one's elbow. In my series, there are 52 musicians with ulnar neuropathy, including 27 women and 25 men; average age is 40 years. Ulnar neuropathy appears to be particularly common among string instrumentalists, especially violinists and violists. Furthermore, it almost invariably occurs in the left arm, suggesting—based on the way that these instruments are played—that prolonged flexion with or without supination of the forearm is more important in provoking this entrapment neuropathy than repetitive flexion and extension at the elbow. All 16 violinists or violists in this group with ulnar neuropathies had left-sided involvement and only 1 had symptomatic right ulnar neuropathy as well.

The diagnosis is suspected from the sensory distribution and observed weakness. It is more difficult to confirm by electrodiagnostic testing than CTS. Nonoperative treatment may include splinting of the elbow to minimize or prevent flexion, especially during sleep; modification of playing time and position may be helpful in some instrumentalists. The type of surgical procedure to be carried out is controversial but commonly involves translocating the nerve toward the anterior side of the elbow. Outcome is generally favorable regardless of the specific operative approach.

Other Focal Neuropathies

Cervical radiculopathy may be considered a focal mononeuropathy at the level of the spinal canal or exit foramen. The common symptom is pain from the neck radiating to the upper extremity either proximally or distally, depending on the specific root involved, usually C6 or C7. Men are more likely to develop cervical radiculopathies than women and are generally older than those affected by either CTS or ulnar mononeuropathy. There is no evidence that violinists or violists are more susceptible, despite what might be intuitively suspected from the position required for playing these instruments. Diagnosis is suspected from the distribution of pain and the pattern of sensory, motor, and reflex changes. EMG and magnetic resonance imaging of the spine are useful diagnostic studies. Nonoperative treatment is favored, including modification of neck position during playing of the instrument. This may be facilitated by adaptive changes in the instrument (e.g., a higher shoulder rest or chin rest on a violin). Intractable pain or progressive neurological impairment may mandate surgical decompression.

Radial mononeuropathies are very uncommon in my experience but have been reported among instrumentalists. Symptoms include pain in the forearm and weakness of finger (or wrist) extension. Digital mononeuropathies, sometimes related to local compression against the instrument, particularly the left index finger in flautists, are not uncommon. Pain and numbness of one side of the finger result. They are best managed by changing position or adapting the instrument to diffuse the pressure. A variety of other focal neuropathies, including cranial nerve branches compressed between the mouthpiece of a brass instrument and the dental ridge, have been described. These typically produce numbness and sometimes motor dysfunction of a portion of the lip.

The problem of thoracic outlet syndrome (TOS) should be at least considered in this context. This is an extremely controversial disorder that may or may not represent localized nerve compression. A rare form of neurogenic TOS presents with clear sensory and motor findings. Much more commonly, patients describe pain and paresthesias, usually along the ulnar aspect of the forearm and hand, typically provoked by certain positions or maneuvers, some of which are characteristically assumed in playing an instrument. The neurological examination is almost invariably normal. Women are much more commonly affected than men, and among instrumentalists this is typically a disorder of the second and third decades. Validated clinical criteria for diagnosis are lacking and no diagnostic test has been shown to be satisfactory for confirming the presence of TOS. Given the difficulties in establishing a diagnosis, even if one agrees that it represents nerve entrapment, conservative treatment should be the rule. Modification of faulty posture, stretching of tense neck and upper trunk muscles, and avoidance of provocative positions will suffice in the majority of cases. Occasionally, a surgical approach may be required; this evokes debate both regarding whether it should ever be done and regarding the particular approach to be utilized. Proponents, however, point to very favorable surgical results despite unquestioned occurrence of some complications in a few cases.

CONCLUSION

In summary, instrumental musicians are subject to the common entrapment neuropathies that affect the general population. However, there may be some predisposition to certain entrapment syndromes, and the specific instrument played may determine both the type of entrapment and the lateralization of symptoms. Treatment may not differ greatly from that in the general population, but the extraordinary demands for neuromuscular control required to play an instrument may occasionally dictate that definitive treatment, including surgery, be elected at an earlier rather than later stage, before any significant nerve injury occurs. This can sometimes lead to a difficult therapeutic decision for instrumentalists, since they are typically loathe to consider surgical management except as a last resort.

—*Richard J. Lederman*

See also—Carpal Tunnel Syndrome; Neuropathies, Entrapment; Neuropathies, Overview; Radiculopathy; Ulnar Neuropathy

Further Reading

Charness, M. E. (1992). Unique upper extremity disorders of musicians. In *Occupational Disorders of the Upper Extremity* (L. H. Millender, D. S. Louis, and B. P. Simmons, Eds.), pp. 227–251. Churchill Livingstone, New York.

Dawson, D. M., Hallett, M., and Wilbourn, A. J. (1999). Nerve entrapments in musicians. *Entrapment Neuropathies*, 3rd ed., pp. 443–450. Lippincott–Raven, Philadelphia.

Dawson, W. J. (1995). Experience with hand and upper-extremity problems in 1000 instrumentalists. *Med. Probl. Perform. Art.* 10, 128–133.

Hochberg, F. H., and Lederman, R. J. (1995). Upper extremity difficulties of musicians. In *Rehabilitation of the Hand: Surgery and Therapy* (J. M. Hunter, E. J. Mackin, and A. D. Callahan, Eds.), 4th ed., pp. 1795–1808. Mosby, St. Louis.

Lederman, R. J. (1998). Neurological problems of performing artists. In *Performing Arts Medicine* (R. T. Sataloff, A. G. Brandfonbrener, and R. J. Lederman, Eds.), 2nd ed., pp. 47–71. Singular, San Diego.

Winspur, I. (1998). Nerve compression syndromes. In *The Musician's Hand: A Clinical Guide* (I. Winspur and C. B. Wynn Parry, Eds.), pp. 85–99. Dunitz, London.

Neuropathies, Nutritional

Encyclopedia of the Neurological Sciences
Copyright 2003, Elsevier Science (USA). All rights reserved.

FOR MANY centuries, nutritional disorders have been well-recognized causes of peripheral neuropathies and other ailments. Scurvy, one of the first diseases to be attributed to nutritional factors, was described in Eber's papyrus written in ancient Egypt (1500 B.C.) and later by Hippocrates (420 B.C.). This nonneurological disorder, caused by deficiency of vitamin C, is characterized by general malaise, multiple hemorrhages including periosteal hematomas causing joint and bone pain, and swollen and bleeding gums. In the 16th century, a French explorer, Jacques Cartier, reported that his crew had been cured of scurvy by an infusion of arbor vitae prepared by the inhabitants of Newfoundland. By the early 17th century, citrus fruits or juices were added to diets to prevent scurvy on the ships of the British East India Company. In 1853, James Lind, a British physician, described his experiments to cure scurvy in British sailors in his work *Treatise on Scurvy*. This publication is acknowledged to be the first description of controlled medical clinical trials.

In the late 1860s, the Japanese navy noted that approximately 40% of their seamen developed signs of beriberi, which is characterized by peripheral neuropathy, cardiomyopathy, or both. Director General Takaki of the Japanese Medical Service identified an association between beriberi and a diet containing large portions of polished rice. He attributed the disease to a lack of protein and recommended increasing the daily rations of vegetables, fish, meat, and barley. In 1875, no cases of beriberi were reported in the Japanese navy. Although these results were impressive, Takaki's conclusions were proven to be incorrect.

In 1886, Christian Eijkman was sent to a military hospital in Batavia, Dutch East Indies (which became Jakarta, Indonesia). Eijkman, a student of the bacteriologist Robert Koch, was part of a research team trying to identify the cause of beriberi. Fortuitously, he noticed that the chickens had a similar disorder characterized by gait impairment and edema. The chickens developed the illness during a five month period, after which the disorder disappeared rapidly. Eijkman noted that the chickens had been fed polished rice rather than the lower grade brown unpolished rice during this period. He reproduced the illness in chickens and in pigeons through a polished rice diet and subsequently cured the animals with unpolished rice or with the husks of rice. In 1912, Casamir Funk, a Polish biochemist, published his "vitamine theory" attributing scurvy, beriberi, pellegra, and rickets to a lack of "vital amines." Although these compounds were found not to be amines, the name vitamin was retained.

Pernicious anemia, which is due to deficiency of vitamin B_{12}, was originally described in 1822. The first experimental clue about the cause came in 1926 when George Minot and William Murphy, two physicians at Harvard Medical School, successfully treated 45 patients using a special diet that included daily servings of 120–240 g of lightly cooked liver. More than two decades later, vitamin B_{12} was isolated. For their insightful observations, Eijkman, Minot, and Murphy were recognized with Nobel prizes.

THIAMINE (VITAMIN B_1) DEFICIENCY

Thiamine deficiency causes two distinct neurological disorders: beriberi and Wernicke–Korsakoff syndrome. As previously noted, beriberi is characterized by a peripheral neuropathy that typically begins with painful paresthesias (sensations of pins and needles) in the feet spreading proximally and to the distal arms. Distal leg and arm weakness and atrophy develop and usually cause foot and wrist drop. Loss of autonomic nerve fibers leads to skin changes: atrophy, hair loss, and glossiness. Cranial nerves can be affected, causing weakness of the tongue, facial muscles, or larynx. The neuropathy can progress over weeks to months until treatment is initiated. When the disorder is restricted to peripheral neuropathy, it is referred to as dry beriberi, in contrast to wet beriberi, which has superimposed cardiomyopathy leading to edema. The neuropathy can be treated with oral thiamine (50 mg daily); however, therapy may not work unless initiated early in the course of the illness.

Wernicke–Korsakoff syndrome is actually two disorders that often overlap. Wernicke disease presents with abnormalities of eye movements, impaired gait, and mental status changes, whereas Korsakoff syndrome refers to cognitive changes characterized by short-term memory defects and a tendency to confabulate. These disorders are frequently accompanied by peripheral neuropathy.

Thiamine deficiency is most frequently encountered in countries in which polished rice is the major carbohydrate source. Individuals who are at higher risk of developing thiamine deficiency include alcoholics, patients on total parenteral nutrition, and people with anorexia nervosa. Additional factors that contribute to thiamine deficiency include hyperemesis gravidarum, gastric or small intestinal resection, and malabsorption syndromes.

The precise mechanisms by which thiamine deficiencies lead to beriberi and Wernicke–Korsakoff syndrome are uncertain. Thiamine is an important cofactor for several important metabolic enzymes, including transketolase, pyruvate dehydrogenase, α-ketoglutarate dehydrogenase, and pyruvate decarboxylase. Direct measurements of thiamine in body fluids are not reliable indicators of lack of thiamine. In patients with thiamine deficiency, erythrocyte transketolase activity is low and increases with addition of thiamine pyrophosphate. Elevated serum pyruvate is another indirect sign of thiamine deficiency.

NIACIN DEFICIENCY

Pellegra is derived from the Italian word *pelegra*, meaning dry skin. The disease is caused by niacin deficiency and is characterized clinically by the triad of dermatitis, diarrhea, and dementia. The skin changes consist of erythema and hyperkeratosis. Mental status changes, besides dementia, include confusion, depression and other mood changes, and altered sensorium. Spinal cord and peripheral nerve defects have been reported in patients with pellegra; however, these manifestations may have been due to other concomitant nutritional deficiencies. Pellegra is encountered in populations that rely on corn as a major food source.

Niacin (nicotinic acid and nicotinamide) is converted to nicotinamide adenine dinucleotide (NAD) and NAD phosphate (NADP), which are cofactors for more than 200 enzymes. Niacin is found in multiple foods, including meats, fish, legumes, and enriched grain products; however, it is also endogenously synthesized from the amino acid tryptophan. Therefore, to develop pellegra, patients must have a diet deficient in both tryptophan and niacin. Treatment with niacin, 40–250 mg daily, usually reverses most of the manifestations of pellegra.

PYRIDOXINE (VITAMIN B₆) DEFICIENCY AND TOXICITY

Pyridoxine is an unusual vitamin because either deficiency or excess of the compound cause periph-

eral neuropathies. The clinical manifestations of pyridoxine deficiency are anemia, peripheral neuropathy, and alterations of mood. The peripheral neuropathy causes distal limb sensory loss with painful paresthesia and burning feet, weakness, and loss of tendon reflexes. The changes in personality include depression, irritability, and confusion. Pyridoxine deficiency is often associated with isoniazid therapy for tuberculosis and with hydralazine treatment for hypertension. Pyridoxine deficiency is generally responsive to oral supplementation of 50–100 mg daily.

High doses of pyridoxine, usually more than 2 g daily over several weeks, can produce a sensory neuropathy with paresthesias, burning feet, and sensory ataxia. Pyridoxine in doses as low as 200 mg daily over longer periods has been reported to cause peripheral neuropathy. Pyridoxine can also cause a sensory neuronopathy due to toxicity to the dorsal root gangion cells.

Pyridoxal phosphate, the active metabolite of pyridoxine, is a cofactor of amino acid metabolism via transaminases. Deficiency of pyridoxine interferes with tryptophan biosynthesis, which in turn can cause niacin deficiency, producing secondary pellegra that is indistinguishable from primary pellegra. In addition, pyridoxine is required for synthesis of some lipids and neurotransmitters. The mechanism of pyridoxine neurotoxicity is unknown. A saturable transport mechanism is thought to protect the central nervous system from excess pyridoxine, whereas dorsal root ganglion cells are not so protected, thus accounting for the neuropathy and neuronopathy.

COBALAMIN (VITAMIN B₁₂) DEFICIENCY

Cobalamin deficiency is most commonly seen in the setting of pernicious anemia, an autoimmune disease caused by antibodies against intrinsic factor. Lack of intrinsic factor leads to malabsorption of vitamin B₁₂. Deficiency of this vitamin produces megaloblastic anemia and subacute combined degeneration of the spinal cord. Neurological features are evident in approximately 40% of patients with B₁₂ deficiency and classically present with the triad of myelopathy, peripheral neuropathy, and cognitive changes. Myelopathy can cause spasticity, hyperactive reflexes, urinary or fecal incontinence, and sensory symptoms. Sensory ataxia can impair gait. Neuropathy manifests as paresthesias and burning sensations of the hands and feet. Dementia with memory loss, psychosis, and mood disturbance are sometimes encountered. Neurological manifestations sometimes occur in the absence of hematological abnormalities.

Other causes of vitamin B_{12} deficiency include surgical resection of the stomach or ileum, inflammatory bowel disease, tapeworm (*Diphyllobothrium latum*) infestation, and strict vegetarian diets. All of these associated disorders lead to insufficient cobalamin uptake. Because body stores of vitamin B_{12} are relatively large and the vitamin is retained in the enterohepatic circulation, cobalamin deficiency usually develops more than 2 years after the onset of malabsorption.

Vitamin B_{12} is an important cofactor of methionine synthase, a cytosolic enzyme that catalyzes the reaction homocysteine + methyltetrahydrofolate → methionine + tetrahydrofolate. Methionine is converted to *S*-adenosylmethionine, which is required for methylation of phospholipids in myelin. Therefore, vitamin B_{12} deficiency causes demyelination. The deficiency can be confirmed by a low serum level; however, some patients have normal values. In virtually all patients, serum levels of homocysteine and methylmalonic acid are elevated and, therefore, are more sensitive indicators of cobalamin deficiency. Patients generally respond to intramuscular injections of vitamin B_{12}; however, patients with long-standing disease recover less well. Commonly, treatment consists of 1000 μg intramuscularly (im) of cobalamin daily for 5 days followed by 1000 μg im every month.

Nitric oxide exposure causes an acute form of vitamin B_{12} deficiency by oxidizing the cobalt center and inactivating methylcobalamin. The reduced form of cobalt is required to convert homocysteine to methionine, which in turn is required for proper formation of myelin as described previously.

VITAMIN E DEFICIENCY

In contrast to vitamin B deficiencies that can be caused by insufficient dietary intake, vitamin E deficiency is due to malabsorption. The neurological manifestations of vitamin E deficiency are diverse but typically include cerebellar ataxia and peripheral neuropathy. The neuropathy manifests as stocking-glove cutaneous sensory loss, severe loss of joint position and vibratory sensations, and areflexia. Other, less common, symptoms and signs are ptosis, ophthalmoparesis, nystagmus, dysarthria, and Babinski signs. The clinical presentation closely resembles hereditary spinocerebellar ataxias.

The diagnosis is confirmed by identifying low serum vitamin E levels. Malabsorption of vitamin E can occur in several conditions, such as cystic fibrosis, primary biliary atresia, inflammatory bowel disease, and extensive surgical resection of small intestine. Ataxia with isolated vitamin E deficiency (AVED) is an autosomal recessive vitamin E deficiency caused by mutations in the gene encoding α-tocopherol transfer protein. This protein normally incorporates vitamin E into low-density lipoproteins that are delivered to cells. AVED is clinically similar to Friedreich ataxia. Abetalipoproteinemia (Bassen–Kornzweig syndrome) is another autosomal recessive disorder associated with vitamin E deficiency. This disease begins in infancy with fatty diarrhea, abdominal distension, and growth retardation. Peripheral neuropathy and ataxia develop in the first year of life. Acanthocytes (red blood cells with spiny projections) and pigmentary retinopathy are two features that distinguish abetaliproteinemia from other forms of vitamin E deficiency. This disorder is due to mutations in the microsomal triglyceride transfer protein gene. This protein appears to be required for apolipoprotein B to be incorporated into lipoproteins.

Vitamin E is an antioxidant and free radical scavenger; therefore, lack of this vitamin probably causes increased susceptibility of neurons to oxidative damage. Oral supplementation of vitamin E, 400 mg twice daily, can prevent or reverse the progression of neurological dysfunction in patients with deficiency. In patients with abetalipoproteinemia or AVED, higher doses of vitamin E are typically given.

STRACHAN DISEASE

In 1888, Dr. Henry Strachan, a British Medical Officer stationed in Jamaica, reported 510 patients with a combination of "numbness" and "burning heat" in the hands and feet; impaired vision; hearing loss; pains in the joints and girdle; and skin lesions (cheilosis, angular stomatitis, genital and perirectal dermatitis, and trophic changes). The disorder is primarily a neuropathy that affects mainly optic and peripheral nerves. Dorsal root ganglion cells are primarily affected, with degeneration of the distal axons in both central and peripheral nervous systems. Similar outbreaks of Strachan disease were reported among inhabitants of Madrid during the Spanish Civil War, among prisoners of World War II, and in more than 50,000 Cubans in 1992 and 1993 after the loss of economic support from the former Soviet Union. Patients with this disorder generally improve with improved diet, vitamin supplementation, or both. Therefore, Strachan disease seems to be related to nutritional deficiency. Severely affected patients recover less well than mildly affected individuals. Although the disease is thought to be due to a lack of at least one vitamin B complex, the precise cause is unknown.

ALCOHOLIC NEUROPATHY

Chronic excessive ingestion of alcohol has been clearly associated with peripheral neuropathy; however, controversy exists as to whether the neuropathy is due to direct toxicity of alcohol, secondary nutritional deficiency, or both. Clinically, alcoholic neuropathy resembles dry beriberi. Symptoms usually begin in the feet with paresthesias and burning. Later, numbness, cramps, weakness, and sensory ataxia develop. On examination, patients have stocking more than glove sensory loss (particularly vibratory and proprioceptive senses), skin changes due to autonomic dysfunction, motor weakness, and areflexia. The skin is typically erthematous, atrophic, and shiny with loss of hair. Secondary skin ulcerations and neuropathic joint degeneration can develop. Orthostatic hypotension can be a manifestation of autonomic neuropathy. Muscle tenderness in the feet and calves is common. The reported frequency of neuropathy varies from 9 to 30% of hospitalized patients; however, up to 93% of ambulatory alcoholics have electrophysiological evidence of neuropathy. Pathological studies have revealed that the neuropathy is axonal. Ideally, treatment consists of abstinence from alcohol and improved nutrition. The neuropathy can improve slowly over many months; however, some patients have not improved despite apparently adequate treatment.

CRITICAL ILLNESS POLYNEUROPATHY

Patients treated in intensive care units (ICUs) sometimes develop an axonal neuropathy often called critical illness polyneuropathy. The patients typically have sepsis, multiorgan failure, or both. This predominantly motor neuropathy causes limb weakness but can also lead to respiratory muscle weakness. In fact, some patients are diagnosed because they have difficulty weaning from a ventilator. Facial muscles are sometimes mildly weak. Patients in ICUs sometimes develop a myopathy that can coexist with the neuropathy. The cause of critical illness polyneuropathy is unknown. Nutritional deficiency may contribute to this disorder; however, toxic, metabolic, and vasoactive compounds have been proposed as possible pathogenic factors. The neuropathy usually improves if the patient recovers from the underlying illness.

CONCLUSIONS

Peripheral neuropathies due to nutritional disorders are well-recognized conditions of great historical and scientific significance. For most of these disorders, specific associations between vitamin deficiencies or toxicity and neuropathy have been identified and have led to effective methods of prevention and treatments. In fact, these disorders are uncommon in developed countries with ample food supplies and food products enriched with vitamins. Despite impressive medical and scientific progress in understanding the nutritional neuropathies, the precise mechanisms leading to the nerve damage are not fully elucidated for many of these conditions.

—*Michio Hirano*

***See also*—Beri-Beri; Eating Disorders; Neuropathies, Overview; Neuropathy, Toxic; Thiamine (Vitamin B1); Vitamins, Overview**

Further Reading
Bolton, C. F., and Breuer, A. C. (1999). Critical illness polyneuropathy. *Muscle Nerve* 22, 419–424.
Green, R., and Kinsella, L. J. (1995). Current concepts in the diagnosis of cobalamin deficiency. *Neurology* 45, 1435–1440.
Healton, E. B., Savage, D. G., Brust, J. C., et al. (1991). Neurologic aspects of cobalamin deficiency. *Med. Baltimore* 70, 229–245.
Jackson, C. E., Amato, A. A., and Barohn, R. J. (1996). Isolated vitamin E deficiency. *Muscle Nerve* 19, 1161–1165.
Lincoff, N., Odel, J., and Hirano, M. (1993). "Outbreak" of optic and peripheral neuropathy in Cuba? *J. Am. Med. Assoc.* 270, 511–518.
Lindenbaum, J., Healton, E. B., Savage, D. G., et al. (1988). Neuropsychiatric disorders caused by cobalamin deficiency in the absence of anemia or macrocytosis. *N. Engl. J. Med.* 318, 1720–1728.
Roman, G. C. (1994). An epidemic in Cuba of optic neuropathy, sensorineural deafness, peripheral sensory neuropathy and dorsolateral myeloneuropathy. *J. Neurol. Sci.* 127, 11–28.
Schaumburg, H., Kaplan, J., Windebank, A., et al. (1983). Sensory neuropathy from pyridoxine abuse. A new megavitamin syndrome. *N. Engl. J. Med.* 309, 445–448.
Victor, M., Adams, R., and Collins, G. (1989). *The Wernicke-Korsakoff Syndrome and Related Neurologic Disorders Due to Alcoholism and Malnutrition.* Davis, Philadelphia.

Windebank, A. (1993). Polyneuropathy due to nutritional deficiency and alcoholism. In *Peripheral Neuropathy* (P. J. Dyck, P. K. Thomas, J. W. Griffin, P. A. Low, and J. F. Podulso, Eds.), Vol. 2, pp. 1310–1321. Saunders, Philadelphia.

Neuropathies, Overview

Encyclopedia of the Neurological Sciences

DISEASES of the peripheral nerve contribute substantially to the spectrum of neurological problems: The incidence of polyneuropathy in the United States is estimated to be 40 per 100,000 individuals, comparable to that of epilepsy or parkinsonism. Since not all patients seek medical attention, data regarding the etiologic composition of polyneuropathies are difficult to obtain. More than 2 million people suffer from this disorder in the United States. Many individuals with mild or subclinical neuropathy, whether genetically determined or acquired, are not subjected to evaluation or treatment. The largest and best documented neuropathy series originate from specialized centers or they are selected from biopsy cases and thus do not represent neuropathy in the general population. For example, leprosy, one of the leading causes of neuropathy in the world, has become extremely rare in the United States, but in endemic areas such as Africa and Asia prevalence exceeds 10 per 1000 individuals, with more than 500,000 cases detected each year. Authorities suggest that the disease first appeared in the Far East (before 600 BC), spread to Africa, and was then introduced in Europe. Spain and Portugal are the only endemic areas in Europe. In the United States, leprosy is indigenous to Hawaii and populations of Florida, Louisiana, and Texas.

The factors leading to the regression of leprosy are not fully understood but are presumed to be related to improved knowledge of its natural history and greater recognition of its clinical and pathological manifestations. Treatment may also play a role in its decline; however, the prevalence of leprosy was waning long before the introduction of sulfone therapy in 1941. In the early 1980s, estimates from the World Health Organization indicated a prevalence of 11–12 million cases of leprosy worldwide. The prevalence decreased to 0.9 million cases in 1996. In 1995, only 144 new cases of leprosy were reported in the United States.

While the prevalence of lepromatous neuropathy has declined steadily, diabetes mellitus has become the most common cause of peripheral neuropathy in the Western world. In a large cohort of diabetics, 8% had neuropathy at the time of diagnosis and 50% had neuropathy after 25 years. Future generations should see an improvement in these statistics with the advent of better methods of glucose control.

This entry summarizes the clinical approach to peripheral neuropathies, with emphasis on the underlying logic and the thought process used in evaluating neuropathy patients.

LOCALIZATION AND PATHOGENESIS

A disease process causing neuropathies can be classified on the basis of its two fundamental aspects: anatomical localization and pathogenetic mechanism of nerve injury. Neurogenic disorders include diseases that affect neuronal cell bodies (neuronopathies) and those involving their peripheral processes (peripheral neuropathies). The neuronopathies can be further subdivided into disorders of anterior horn cells, or motor neuron disease (e.g., poliomyelitis, amyotrophic lateral sclerosis, and spinal muscular atrophy), and sensory neuronopathies, or ganglionopathies (e.g., carcinomatous sensory neuronopathy, herpes zoster, and Sjögren's syndrome).

The peripheral neuropathies can be classified as those that initially affect axons, Schwann cells, and myelin. The axons of peripheral nerves are cytoplasmic extensions of the nerve cell bodies. Schwann cells that originate from the neural crest envelop multiple axons to form unmyelinated fibers or myelin sheath that encompasses individual myelinated fibers surrounded by a basal lamina. Peripheral nerve myelin is derived from the Schwann cell. The integrity of myelin sheath is dependent on both the Schwann cell and the axon. Death of the axon results in the prompt breakdown of myelin but not the Schwann cell. On the other hand, loss of myelin does not usually result in disruption of the axon. This principle is essential for understanding the difference between axonal and demyelinating peripheral nerve disorders. A demyelinated axon resumes normal impulse conduction after remyelination triggered by Schwann cell division occurs. Thus, disorders of the peripheral nerve can be broadly classified as myelinopathies that affect myelin and axonopathies that affect the axon.

The term myelinopathy refers to conditions in which the lesion primarily affects myelin or the myelinating (Schwann) cells. An immune-mediated acute inflammatory demyelinating polyneuropathy is one of the few frequently encountered diseases that primarily affects peripheral nerve myelin. Many of the demyelinating neuropathies are schwannopathies, in which the Schwann cell's metabolic functioning cannot maintain the myelin sheath. Toxic (amiodarone, perhexiline, and chloroquine induced) and infectious (leprosy and cytomegalovirus neuritis) myelinopathies are rare, as are hereditary disorders of Schwann cell lipid metabolism (metachromatic and Krabbe's leukodystrophy, adrenoleukodystrophy, and Niemann–Pick's and Farber's disease).

Segmental demyelination is damage to myelin sheaths that presents in a random, segmental fashion with sparing of axons. Electrophysiologically, it is represented by a conduction slowing that in the most severe cases evolves into a conduction block. Conduction block is an important expression of demyelination. A blocked axon displays a functional deficit as severe as that if the axon were transected. Although nerve transection and conduction block may show similar degrees of paralysis or sensory deficit acutely, they differ in terms of outlook, degree of muscle wasting, recovery time, and electrophysiological properties. For instance, in demyelinating neuropathies, conduction block is often transient, and remyelination may be rapid (days or weeks) and is frequently complete. This type of nerve injury is also called neuropraxia, which implies a reversible process. This is much more favorable and rapid than the course of recovery expected with transection of the nerve. The spectrum of demyelinating conditions includes primary traumatic damage to myelin sheaths (acute nerve compression), edema caused by myelinotoxic agents (hexachlorophene or triethyltin), and peeling and engulfment of myelin by activated macrophages at the nodes of Ranvier (Guillain–Barré syndrome).

Conditions that cause axonal degeneration with preservation of the cell bodies are referred to as axonopathies. These include both Wallerian degeneration and axonal atrophy and degeneration (Table 1). Wallerian degeneration is a result of physical interruption of an otherwise healthy axon when multiple axons are transected. Paralysis and anesthesia in the corresponding distribution immediately follow the injury. Degeneration of axons and myelin sheaths distal to the site of transection causes conduction failure, usually within days. Regeneration is slow, and recovery is variable and may be incomplete. In addition to direct trauma, other

Table 1 PATHOLOGICAL CLASSIFICATION OF NEUROPATHIC DISORDERS

Neuronopathies
  Somatic motor: anterior horn cell disease, amyotrophic lateral sclerosis, spinal muscular atrophy, progressive muscular atrophy, Kennedy's disease
  Somatic sensory: sensory ganglionopathies, Sjögren's syndrome, paraneoplastic syndrome, cisplatinum
  Autonomic hereditary dysautonomia
Demyelinating peripheral neuropathies
  Primary myelinopathies (Guillain–Barré syndrome, CIDP, multifocal mononeuropathy)
  Primary disorders of Schwann cells: schwannopathies, adrenoleukodystrophy, Krabbe's and metachromatic leukodystrophy, Farber's and Niemann–Pick disease, cerebrotendinous xanthomatosis
Axonopathies
  Distal: diabetic polyneuropathy, HIV-related distal sensory polyneuropathy
  Proximal: diabetic amyotrophy, prophyric neuropathy

causes such as nerve trunk ischemia may produce a picture of extensive distal degeneration frequently referred to as Wallerian-like degeneration. The term axonotmesis refers to the process that occurs when axons are interrupted by a crush lesion but the Schwann cell structure and endoneurial tissue remain intact. Axonal regeneration commences promptly and the growing axons reach proximal targets before distal sites of innervation. The term neurotmesis refers to a process in which an axon is severed and connective tissue is disrupted. Axon regeneration is limited due to damage of the connective tissue. This process not infrequently leads to neuroma formation and aberrant regeneration.

Axonal degeneration implies a distal axonal breakdown caused by a neuronal metabolic derangement. In distal axonopathy, a metabolic abnormality initially occurs in the cell body and/or throughout the axon. Eventual failure of axon transport results in degeneration of vulnerable distal regions of axons. Long and large-diameter fibers are usually first affected. Degeneration appears to advance proximally toward the nerve cell body (dying back) as long as metabolic dysfunction persists; its reversal allows the axon to regenerate along the distal Schwann cell tube to the appropriate terminal. Exogenous toxins, systemic metabolic disorders, and some inherited neuropathies are known to cause distal axonal degeneration of the peripheral nerve. However, the exact sequence of events in nerve tissue culminating in axonal degeneration as well as the distal vulnerability of these axons remain to be elucidated.

All motor axons, except the gamma efferents to intrafusal muscle fibers, are large to medium-sized myelinated fibers. Sensory fibers, however, are represented by the different-sized myelinated and un-myelinated fibers. In general, temperature and pain sensation are mediated by unmyelinated and small myelinated fibers, whereas proprioception, vibratory sense, and afferent limbs of the muscle stretch reflex are subserved by the largest myelinated fibers. Touch perception is mediated by both large and small fibers, and autonomic functions are conducted mainly by unmyelinated fibers.

Needless to say, the previously mentioned anatomical facts are of indispensable clinical utility. In small-fiber neuropathies, diminished cutaneous sensation, such as pain and temperature, is the dominant finding. It is often accompanied by burning painful dysesthesias and autonomic dysfunction. Touch is usually spared, along with motor function, balance, and muscle stretch reflexes. In contrast, large-fiber neuropathies are characterized by areflexia, imbalance from sensory ataxia, some degree of weakness, and minimal distal numbness. Determination of the fiber size involved in a pathological process is an essential step in pattern recognition of neuropathies outlined later.

DIAGNOSIS

The previously mentioned pathophysiological entities have specific clinical, electrophysiological, and, occasionally, pathological features that allow a clinician to classify a given patient's disease into one of the diagnostic categories previously discussed. Therefore, the initial step should be the determination of the site of the lesion, followed by an attempt to determine the cause of the disease. The spectrum of potential etiologies includes hereditary versus acquired neuropathies. Among the latter are those that are caused by metabolic derangement, those that are drug or toxin induced, those that are immune mediated, or those that are due to infectious causes (Table 2). Unfortunately, this investigation is frequently frustrating because it is not always possible to determine the cause of the neuropathic disorder and, as a result, to alter the natural evolution of the process.

What is the chance of making a diagnosis of peripheral neuropathy? In Dyck's series of 205 patients referred to the Mayo Clinic with undiagnosed peripheral neuropathy, the pathological type and etiology were determined in 76% of cases. These

Table 2 CLASSIFICATION OF NEUROPATHIES

Hereditary

Charcot–Marie–Tooth disease and related neuropathies

Hereditary sensory and autonomic neuropathies

Familial amyloid polyneuropathies

Peroxisomal defects: Refsum's disease, adrenomyeloneuropathy-galactosidase A deficiency, Fabry's disease

Lipoprotein disorders: Tangier's disease, β-proteinemia/familial hypo-β-lipoproteinemia

Acquired

Diabetic neuropathies

Immune-mediated neuropathies
   Guillain–Barré syndrome
   Chronic inflammatory demyelinating polyneuropathy
   Chronic neuropathies with antibodies to the myelin-associated glycoprotein

Neuropathies associated with vasculitis or inflammation of the blood vessels in the peripheral nerves

Neuropathies associated with monoclonal gammopathies

Neuropathies associated with neoplasms
   Sensory neuropathy associated with lung cancer
   Neuropathy associated with multiple myeloma
   Neuropathy associated with Waldenstrom's macroglobulemia, chronic lymphocytic leukemia, or B cell lymphoma
   Neuropathy associated with effects of radiation or caused by medications (vincristine and cisplatinum)

Neuropathy associated with amyloidosis

Neuropathy caused by infections (AIDS, cytomegalovirus, herpes zoster, hepatitis B or C, Lyme disease, leprosy, diphtheria)

Neuropathies caused by nutritional imbalance (deficiencies of vitamins B_{12}, B_1, B_6, or E; hypervitaminosis of B_6)

Neuropathy in kidney disease

Hypothyroid neuropathy

Neuropathies caused by alcohol and toxins

Neuropathies caused by drugs (vincristine, cisplatinum, taxol, nitrofurantoin, amiodarone, disulfiram, 2′,3′-dideoxycytidine and didanosine, dapsone)

Neuropathies caused by trauma and compression

Idiopathic neuropathies

data are comparable with those of the Dallas/San Antonio series reflecting the experience of 402 consecutive patients. In this series, 23% of patients were found to have neuropathies with no identifiable cause. The majority of these patients had a predominantly sensory polyneuropathy described in great detail. It is unclear whether this clinically uniform entity represents one discrete disorder or an etiologically heterogeneous group.

To successfully determine the site and cause of the lesion and, if possible, develop a plan for treatment, the clinician uses data from the history, neurological examination, and neurophysiological and laboratory studies.

HISTORY

There is a misperception that peripheral nerve disorders are so stereotyped in presentation that history and clinical findings provide very few clues to diagnosis. However, neuropathy specialists strongly believe that complete history and physical examination are the starting point in the evaluation of patients with peripheral neuropathies. History provides indispensable information that helps to direct the workup of the patient. Emphasis should be placed on social, occupational, and medical conditions predisposing to neuropathies. Identification of specific patterns of clinical abnormalities is crucial for making a differential diagnosis in each particular case.

Historical information important for diagnosis of peripheral nerve disorder includes the main complaint and history of the current illness, past medical history, family history, social history, chemical toxins, review of systems, and current medications.

The main complaints of most neuropathy patients present as some combination of weakness, sensory discomfort, and lack of coordination. Adjectives frequently used by patients to describe their disturbances include tingling, burning, dead, hot, icy, clumsy, and wooden. Although the best tool for determining a pattern of anatomical distribution of neuropathy is the neurological examination, the history may provide important clues. Patients with distal leg weakness complain of frequent tripping or difficulty walking on uneven surfaces. Skipping or walking or raising the knee to a height characteristic of a high-steppage gait are usually reported in association with a foot drop. Proximal weakness seen with acquired demyelinating neuropathies manifests as difficulty getting out of deep chairs or cars, climbing stairs, or rising from a squat position. In the upper limbs, proximal weakness usually causes the patient to have trouble reaching overhead to get things from shelves and also to have trouble shaving, combing hair, or brushing teeth. Complaints of worsening gait instability in darkness usually indicate proprioceptive loss. Some patients describe this impairment as "inability to find the feet in space." Autonomic involvement can cause lightheadedness upon standing up, bowel or bladder incontinence, urinary retention or constipation, sexual dysfunction, and trophic changes of the skin and its derivatives, including ulcer formation, easy bruisability, and altered healing.

The patient's age at the time of initial presentation of illness and duration of the symptoms are important for establishing a time course of neuropathy. Acquired neuropathies can be classified as acute (lasting up to 4 weeks), subacute (from 4 weeks to 2 months), and chronic (longer than 2 months). The time frame is crucial for the definition of some acquired demyelinating neuropathies. Guillain–Barré syndrome (GBS) evolves over 4 weeks or less, whereas chronic inflammatory demyelinating polyradiculoneuropathy (CIDP) progresses for more than 8 weeks. An intermediate or subacute demyelinating category has been described as a catchment for those between the 1- and 2-month time points. When a demyelinating neuropathy is suspected, establishing the accurate timing of illness progression is very important because treatment options vary for each neuropathy. For example, patients with an acute, monophasic illness such as GBS do not respond to oral steroids, whereas oral prednisolone is a valuable treatment modality for patients with CIDP, which frequently has a prolonged, fluctuating course. Appropriate questioning might also reveal subtle difficulties that have been present throughout patients' lives, indicating a hereditary nature of their neuropathies. Pertinent questions include the following: Were you athletic as a child? Were you able to keep up with your peers in a gym? Did you have funny-looking feet as a youngster? Did you have trouble with your shoes? Did you have pes cavus and hammertoe deformities surgically corrected later?

Lastly, medications should be reviewed carefully, including over-the-counter drugs and any nutritional and vitamin supplements and homeopathic substances.

The past medical history of the patient with neuropathy should focus on three key areas. Most important is the determination of the presence of any underlying systemic illness associated with peripheral neuropathy, such as diabetes, and other endocrine disturbances, connective tissue disorders, and renal and hepatic insufficiency. A history of surgery for cervical and lumbar laminectomies, thoracic outlet syndrome, and carpal tunnel release might influence the interpretation of neurological complaints and examination. If there is a history of multiple nerve entrapment, amyloidosis or HPNN should be considered. Foot and ankle surgeries may also indicate a hereditary process.

Family history is of paramount importance in a patient with peripheral neuropathy, and it requires specific questioning about every family member at least in an immediate family, including parents, children, and siblings. Information about walking abilities of the patient's relatives, their needs for a cane or wheelchair, and postural or foot deformities should be elicited. Frequently, other family members have been misdiagnosed with different types of "arthritis" or orthopedic disorders, when in fact the cause of their problems is a neuropathy.

Information about abuse of alcohol, tobacco, and recreational drugs is very important, although alcoholic neuropathy seems to be an overdiagnosed entity. Risk factors related to sexual preferences or drug use might be easily missed, especially at the time of the patient's initial evaluation. Even when risk factors are denied, the diagnosis of HIV-related painful neuropathy should not be entirely dismissed in a young man with an appropriate clinical picture.

Chemical exposure from toxic substances is another consideration. Despite the fact that only a small percentage of neuropathies are caused by toxic exposures, patients should be encouraged to generate a list of all suspected insulting agents. Nitrous oxide causes a condition reminiscent of cobalamin deficiency that is most likely seen among dentists and their assistants due to occupational exposure or recreational inhalation of the substance. It can also be abused in the form of whipped cream dispensers. Inhalation of industrial solvents such as methyl-*n*-butyl ketone and contact cements such as *n*-hexane was found to cause so-called glue-sniffers neuropathies in cabinetmakers and painters. Farmers, dry cleaners, welders, printers, firearms instructors, tree sprayers, and workers in the rayon, rubber, or plastics industry or those who manufacture batteries are also at potential danger of toxic exposure.

A review of systems will allow the identification of neuropathies related to primary disorders of other organs. For example, a constellation of joint deformities, pain, rash, and fever might prompt a rheumatological diagnosis that might explain the patient's peripheral neuropathy. Autonomic dysfunction can be due to diabetes, amyloidosis, or paraneoplastic process. Specific skin changes are likely to be reported with Fabry's or Refsum's disease. Questions about the respiratory status of a patient with neuropathy could lead to a discovery of sarcoidosis or lung cancer.

PATTERN RECOGNITION OF NEUROPATHIC DISORDERS

After a detailed history is obtained and a thorough neurological examination is performed, one can classify neuropathic disorders into several patterns.

Recognition of each pattern provides a limited differential diagnosis based on sensory and motor involvement and distribution of pathological signs. The final diagnosis is determined by utilizing pertinent elements of history and ancillary data. Many clinicians have used this approach in the past without being aware that they were doing so. Although it may seem oversimplified, the following approach of pattern recognition will usually get the clinician very close to the final diagnosis:

- *Pattern 1:* Symmetrical proximal and distal weakness with sensory loss. Differential includes inflammatory demyelinating polyneuropathies (GBS and CIDP).
- *Pattern 2:* Symmetrical distal weakness with sensory loss. Consider metabolic disorders, toxin- and drug-induced neuropathies, and hereditary etiology (Charcot–Marie–Tooth and amyloidosis).
- *Pattern 3:* Asymmetrical distal weakness without sensory loss. Search for motor neuron disease or multifocal motor neuropathy.
- *Pattern 4:* Asymmetrical distal weakness with sensory loss involving (i) multiple nerves: consider vasculitis, hereditary neuropathy with liability to pressure palsy, and infectious etiology, such as sarcoid, Lyme, HIV, or leprosy; or (ii) single nerves or anatomical regions: consider compressive neuropathy or radiculopathy.
- *Pattern 5:* Asymmetrical proximal and distal weakness with sensory loss. This is typically seen in polyradiculopathy or plexopathy related to diabetes mellitus, meningeal carcinomatosis, or lymphomatosis, and it could be idiopathic or hereditary.
- *Pattern 6:* Asymmetrical proprioceptive sensory loss without weakness. Consider sensory neuronopathy (ganglionopathy) due to cancer, Sjögren's syndrome, exposure to cisplatinum, vitamin B_6 toxicity, and HIV-related neuronopathy.
- *Pattern 7:* Symmetrical sensory loss without weakness that could be idiopathic, metabolic, or toxic.
- *Pattern 8:* Autonomic symptoms and signs with or without sensory or motor deficits. This can be encountered in neuropathies due to diabetes mellitus, amyloidosis, GBS, porphyria, HIV, and idiopathic pandysautonomia.

NEUROPHYSIOLOGICAL TESTS

After a clinical pattern of peripheral nerve involvement is recognized, ancillary tests must be performed to help reach a final diagnosis. Electrodiagnostic studies represent the next step in patient evaluation. They consist of nerve conduction studies (NCS) and needle electromyography (EMG). Electrophysiological data provide information about the distribution of neuropathy, supporting or refuting the findings from the history and neurological examination. They also allow the determination of whether the process involves sensory nerves, motor nerves, or both. Finally, theses studies can distinguish axonopathy from a primary myelinopathy.

An axonal pattern is usually determined by low compound muscle action potential (CMAP) amplitudes with relatively preserved distal latencies, conduction velocities, and F-wave latencies, along with fibrillations on needle EMG. Characteristics of a pure demyelinating neuropathy include slow conduction velocities, prolonged distal and F-wave latencies, relatively preserved amplitudes in the absence of conduction block or temporal dispersion, and the absence of spontaneous activity (fibrillations and positive waves) on needle EMG.

EMG can be extremely helpful in distinguishing between acquired and hereditary demyelinating neuropathy. In acquired demyelinating neuropathy, such as CBS and CIDP, there is segmental and multifocal slowing that follows an asymmetrical pattern and is frequently accompanied by conduction block and temporal dispersion. In contrast, not only is slowing in Charcot–Marie–Tooth type 1 hereditary neuropathy dramatic but also changes are uniform and nearly identical from side to side and conduction block or temporal dispersion are absent.

Both conduction block and temporal dispersion are electrophysiological indications of focal, segmental acquired demyelination. Conduction block represents a failure of propagation of the action potential across the demyelinated nerve segment. Partial conduction block is demonstrated on motor NCS when the CMAP amplitude and area become significantly smaller on proximal stimulation compared with distal stimulation. If no CMAP is obtainable on proximal stimulation, complete conduction block is indicated. Partial conduction block is considered when at least a 20–25% but preferably more than a 50% decrease in amplitude and area is found on proximal stimulation. Temporal dispersion reflects a delay, not a failure, of electrical transmission across a focal demyelinated segment of nerve. As a result, the negative phase of the potential elicited proximally will have a much longer duration, usually more than 15–30%.

If electrodiagnostic studies are normal, a neuropathy cannot be excluded because small myelinated fibers (Aδ) and unmyelinated C fibers are not assessed by usual nerve conduction studies. In some circumstances, quantitative sensory testing (QST) adds an important component to the assessment of the patient with neuropathy because it tests the function of the small fibers. By measuring temperature thresholds such as cold detection, heat detection, and heat pain, QST provides more precise information about sensory dysfunction in patients with distal limb pain and minimal, if any, findings on examination. In addition to heat pain nociception detection, QST also evaluates vibratory, warm, and cool thresholds. It is important to keep in mind, however, that QST has a number of limitations. It is a psychophysical test and therefore not truly objective. Poor performance may be willful or a result of inattention or poor understanding of instructions during the test. Abnormalities anywhere along the sensory pathways, related to either peripheral or central nervous system disease, may result in abnormal QSTs. Lastly, the importance of normative data in the clinical application of this technique should not be underestimated.

In some neuropathies, autonomic failure is a leading manifestation, and generalized neuropathy cannot be detected on examination or by nerve conduction studies. In these cases, autonomic testing is indispensable. It characterizes a lesion by assessing the involvement of sympathetic and parasympathetic fibers and determines the site of the lesion as either pre- or postganglionic. Autonomic function tests can also be useful in evaluating patients with distal painful small-fiber neuropathy. In these patients, distal sudomotor abnormalities detected by means of the quantitative sudomotor axon reflex test or thermoregulatory sweat test provide evidence of peripheral neuropathy. Access to an autonomic reflex laboratory is an obvious advantage for the evaluation of peripheral neuropathy; however, simple bedside tests, such as the measurement of pulse and blood pressure changes in supine and standing positions, should not be neglected. They are easy to perform and can serve as indicators of autonomic system involvement, for example, in a patient with suspected diabetic neuropathy or painful sensory neuropathy.

Thus, selectively using a battery of neurophysiological tests, the physician can objectively determine the presence of neuropathy; the fiber-type involvement, such as sensory (small and large fiber), motor, autonomic, or mixed; and the anatomical distribution. Then, the physician can speculate about an underlying cellular pathology.

LABORATORY DATA

The next step in the clinical evaluation involves laboratory studies. There are relatively few blood tests that should be ordered routinely in the evaluation of all, or almost all, patients with neuropathic disorders. Additional data can be obtained in selective cases when there is a strong clinical suspicion of a particular disorder. In a review of 402 consecutive patients evaluated at the University of Texas in Dallas and San Antonio, the only tests that contributed to the causative diagnosis of peripheral neuropathy were those for B_{12} levels, serum protein and immunofixation electrophoresis (SPEP and IFE), and serum glucose. Fasting and 2-hr postprandial glucose, glycosylated hemoglobin, and glucose tolerance tests are frequently done as part of a neuropathy workup and therefore deserve comment. Determination of the precise role and the best diagnostic test is a subject of continued investigation. In fact, peripheral neuropathy as a first sign of diabetes is rare. In a cohort of 117 patients diagnosed with painful peripheral neuropathy at the Neuromuscular Center at Ohio State University, none had diabetes based on fasting blood sugar and glycosylated hemoglobin. The most common variant of a neurogenic disorder presenting as an initial manifestation of diabetes is probably diabetic lumbosacral radiculoplexopathy, also called diabetic amyotrophy or Bruns–Garland's syndrome.

It is important to screen for monoclonal proteinemia in all patients with an undiagnosed peripheral neuropathy and perhaps atypically presenting motor neuron disease as well, particularly in the absence of upper motor neuron findings. An IFE is more sensitive than SPEP, so it should be obtained in all patients. Approximately 5–10% of patients with peripheral neuropathies or motor neuron disease have a serum monoclonal protein. Discovery of these proteins warrants a prompt search for myeloproliferative disorders, such as multiple myeloma, osteosclerotic myeloma, primary amyloidosis, lymphoma, leukemia, cryoglubulinemia, and Waldenstrom's macroglobulinemia. All idiopathic neuropathy patients with serum monoclonal proteins, as well as those without a serum monoclonal gammopathy suspected of having amyloidosis or myeloma, should undergo a 24-hr urine collection to try to detect a urinary monoclonal protein (so-called Bence–Jones

proteins). This is necessary because light chains may be found in the urine when no serum monoclonal protein is evident. If tissue is obtained, it should be stained for amyloid. Diagnosis depends on the demonstration of amyloid deposits in bone marrow aspirate (positive in approximately 50% of patients), fat aspirate (70%), rectal biopsy (80%), or nerve biopsy (80%). In patients who have a monoclonal protein in serum, bone surveys searching for osteosclerotic or osteolytic lesions and also bone marrow biopsy and aspirate may be indicated. Careful long-term follow-up is necessary in patients not found to have an underlying plasma cell dyscrasia. Most patients with a monoclonal gammopathy and peripheral neuropathy do not have an underlying lymphoproliferative disorder and are diagnosed as having a monoclonal gammopathy of undetermined significance (MGUS). The number of MGUS patients later diagnosed with malignancies from the initial neuropathy population is unknown; however, in the general population the number of people with MGUS who subsequently develop neoplastic disease is significant.

Neuropathy associated with MGUS can follow different patterns. Some patients can be classified into the CIDP group (pattern 1) and should be treated as having CIDP without gammopathy. Others (pattern 7) have no or minimal motor deficits in distal muscles. This condition is usually benign and requires symptomatic management. The role of paraproteins in the pathogenesis of neuropathy is debatable, although there are specific syndromes associated with certain defined antibodies that are contained within the paraprotein. The only patients with MGUS in whom binding of monoclonal protein to a specific antigen on the peripheral nerve has been demonstrated are those with an IgM monoclonal protein and antibodies directed against myelin-associated glycoprotein (MAG). However, only approximately 50% of patients with IgM paraproteins have MAG antibodies. In patients with IgG and IgA paraproteins, and in half of those with IgM, the role of the monoclonal protein in the neuropathy remains uncertain.

In terms of contributing to a specific new diagnosis, three antibody assays are especially valuable. The first is the anti-Hu antibody assay, which is used in cases in which carcinomatous sensory neuronopathy is suspected. Second is the anti-MAG antibody assay, which is useful for documenting patients with IgM paraproteins. The anti-MAG syndrome is particularly refractory to treatment, which requires consideration in planning a therapeutic strategy for the patient. A third assay, anti-GM1 antibody level, is potentially helpful in some patients with multifocal motor neuropathy. High titers of IgM anti-GM1 antibody justify a treatment trial with intravenous immunoglobulin, and this assay is particularly useful if electrodiagnostic data are inconclusive. However, the presence of anti-GM1 antibodies, especially of low titers, is nonspecific. In addition, GQ1b antibodies appear to be diagnostic for the Guillian–Barré variant of Fisher's syndrome.

Lumbar puncture is an informative diagnostic test, particularly for evaluation of possible demyelinating neuropathies. Although a high protein level may support a diagnosis of GBS, it is important to remember that most patients with this disorder have normal cerebrospinal protein levels for the first several days after onset. After 1 week, the cerebrospinal fluid (CSF) is remarkable for albumonocytological disassociation, with elevation of the protein content and minimal, if any, lymphocytic pleocytosis. In the proposed laboratory criteria, a CSF cell count of less than 10 lymphocytes/mm^3 protein is most supportive of the diagnosis, and a count higher than 50 cells/mm^3 casts doubt on the diagnosis. If there are more than 50 cells/mm^3, one should consider underlying HIV infection in addition to GBS, and HIV antibody assay should be performed. CSF cytological examination is necessary in suspected cases of polyradiculopathy related to meningeal carcinomatosis or lymphomatosis.

In most cases, it is difficult to provide a clinical diagnosis based on specific microscopic findings in the peripheral nerve biopsy. The repertoire of pathological changes in the nerve is relatively limited, potentially restricting the value of nerve biopsy. However, there are conditions in which nerve biopsy can be a source of pathognomonic information. Vasculitis, amyloidosis, sarcoidosis, giant axonal neuropathy, and leprosy are among the diagnoses that can be established by a nerve biopsy. The disease for which nerve biopsy is most useful is probably vasculitis since this is a treatable condition. The diagnosis of vasculitis needs to be confirmed histologically, and the nerve and adjacent muscle are often the most accessible and logical choice to biopsy in cases of suspected vasculitis complicated by peripheral neuropathy.

Although there are some disorders for which the nerve biopsy can show characteristic abnormalities, most of these diseases can be diagnosed by other means. For example, due to the advent of easily available molecular genetic blood tests for CMT-1A, hereditary neuropathy with liability to pressure palsy, and familial amyloidosis, less emphasis is placed on the characteristic nerve biopsy changes in these disorders. Thus, although sausage-shaped myelin enlargements or tomaculae can be demonstrated in hereditary neuropathy with liability to pressure palsy, this condition can now be identified through a molecular genetic blood test for the *PMP-22* gene deletion on chromosome 17p11.2. Infectious neuropathies such as leprosy can be more easily diagnosed by demonstrating acid-fast bacilli in skin rather than a nerve biopsy. Rarely, nerve biopsy can be justified to help determine the underlying pathologic process and thus the underlying diagnosis. Such instances include hereditary neuropathy, toxin exposure with recovery, or CIDP.

It is important to emphasize that nerve biopsies are not performed to address whether or not a patient has a peripheral neuropathy. This question is more appropriately answered by a combined approach emphasizing clinical and electrodiagnostic studies with support from quantitative sensory and autonomic testing and skin biopsies.

Skin biopsy for the evaluation of intraepidermal nerve fibers, a recently developed technique, is a useful test for predominantly small-fiber peripheral neuropathies that are relatively inaccessible to standard electrodiagnostic testing. The punch biopsy procedure of the skin carries a low risk of complications, and discomfort is minimal.

A typical indication is the complaint of painful feet in the absence of any objective signs of neuropathy on examination and nerve conduction studies. Loss of intraepidermal nerve fibers is characteristic of the distal painful sensory neuropathy. This intraepidermal nerve fiber population is not directly assessed by any other means of study. These are patients who particularly benefit from a skin biopsy, although there are other clinical settings in which skin biopsies may be helpful. For example, the technique has particular application as an outcome measure in disorders affecting the small myelinated and unmyelinated nerve fiber populations. Treatment regimens for small-fiber component of diabetic and AIDS-related neuropathies are appropriately evaluated by this method as well.

TREATMENT

Therapy of treatable neuropathies can be directed at the underlying disease process or it can be symptomatic. Symptomatic pharmacological therapy can be directed at pain control. Three broad categories of drugs can be used for neuropathic pain: tricyclic antidepressants, anticonvulsants, and antiarrhythmics. Tricyclic antidepressants, such as amitriptyline, nortriptyline, desipramine, and imipramine, are the first-line agents for most patients with neuropathic pain. Unfortunately, their use is often accompanied by intolerable anticholinergic and sedative side effects. Second-line pharmacological therapy includes the anticonvulsants carbamazepine and gabapentin. It is very important to begin with a low dose and to slowly increase the dosage to avoid side effects of oversedation and unsteadiness. If first- and second-line agents are ineffective or intolerable, we generally proceed to the antiarrhythmic drug mexiletine. It is important to give each drug a trial of at least 4–6 weeks before switching to another agent. Topical capsaicin was introduced as a therapy for neuropathic pain; it presumably acts by depleting substance P in unmyelinating primary afferent nerve endings. Another topical therapy is transcutaneous nerve stimulation, but it seems to be effective in only a minority of patients.

Orthostatic hypotension associated with autonomic neuropathies can be treated with fludrocortisone and the oral sympathomimetic agent midodrine. Midodrine is an α_1-adrenoreceptor agonist that increases blood pressure by producing arterial and venous constriction.

Other therapeutic modalities can stop or slow a disease process (pathogenetic treatment) or act on a cause of the illness (etiologic therapy). For example, for immune-mediated neuropathies a variety of immunosuppressive therapies are available, including oral and intravenous corticosteroids, azathioprine, cyclophosphamide, cyclosporine, intravenous immunoglobulin, and plasmapheresis. These options should be considered for acute and chronic demyelinating polyneuropathy, vasculitic neuropathy, and other neuropathies associated with definable connective tissue disease.

Leprous neuropathy is usually effective treated with a multidrug regimen, including dapsone, rifampin, and clofazimine. HIV-related neuropathies caused by cytomegalovirus are treated with intravenous ganciclovir and sometimes with steroids (in cases with a clear-cut vasculitic pattern). The effect of newer, highly active antiretroviral therapies on the incidence and severity of the various forms of neuropathy seen in HIV infection remains to be determined.

The most important vitamin-deficient states that can cause peripheral nerve disorders are cobalamin (vitamin B_{12}), α-tocopherol (vitamin E), and thiamin (vitamin B_1). Replacement therapy is indicated in all of these conditions, with the expectation of reasonable success in cases in which supplementation is instituted early during the course of illness. As a rule, the response is seen after at least several months of treatment, and recovery is slow.

—*Yelena Lindenbaum*

See also–Acute Motor and Sensory Axonal Neuropathy (AMSAN); Neuropathic Pain Syndromes; Pain, Overview

Further Reading

Barohn, R. J. (1998). Approach to peripheral neuropathy and neuronopathy. *Semin. Neurol.* **18**, 7–18.

Bromberg, M. B. (1991). Comparison of electrodiagnostic criteria for primary demyelination in chronic polyneuropathy. *Muscle Nerve* **14**, 968–976.

Brown, W. F., and Feasby, T. E. (1984). Conduction block and denervation in Guillain–Barré polyneuropathy. *Brain* **107**, 219–239.

Dyck, P. J., Oviatt, K. F., and Lambert, E. H. (1981). Intensive evaluation of referred unclassified neuropathies yields improved diagnosis. *Ann. Neurol.* **10**, 222–226.

Mendell, J. R., Periquet, I., Kissel, J. T., *et al.* (1998). Distal painful axonal idiopathic neuropathy: Criteria for diagnosis and distinction from other sensory neuropathies. *Neurology* **50**, A343–A344.

Mendell, J. R., Kissel, J. T., and Cornblath, D. R. (2001). *Diagnosis and Management of Peripheral Nerve Disorders*, Contemporary Neurology series. Oxford Univ. Press, Oxford.

Schaumburg, H. H., Berger, A. R., and Thomas, P. K. (1992). *Disorders of Peripheral Nerves*, Contemporary Neurology series. Davis, Philadelphia.

Yarnitsky, D. (1997). Quantitative sensory testing. *Muscle Nerve* **20**, 198–204.

Neuropathy, Axillary

Encyclopedia of the Neurological Sciences
Copyright 2003, Elsevier Science (USA). All rights reserved.

THE AXILLARY NERVE is an important upper extremity motor nerve known best because it innervates the deltoid muscle, which functions to raise the arm above the head. It also supplies the teres minor muscle and provides skin sensation to the lateral upper shoulder. The axillary nerve's motor fibers originate in the fifth and sixth cervical spinal cord segments and travel through the upper trunk and the posterior cord of the brachial plexus. The axillary nerve arises as the smaller of the two terminal branches of the posterior cord and then courses inferiorly and anterior to the subscapularis muscle to reach the quadrilateral space. This space is formed laterally by the surgical neck of the humerus, medially by the long head of the triceps, superiorly by the teres minor, and inferiorly by the teres major. The axillary nerve exits the quadrilateral space posteriorly, along with the posterior circumflex humeral artery, and then divides into anterior and posterior branches.

The posterior branch supplies the teres minor muscle and the posterior deltoid muscle, and it continues on as the upper lateral cutaneous branch supplying skin sensation to the upper lateral shoulder. The posterior deltoid extends (unbends) and externally rotates the arm. The teres minor muscle externally rotates the arm. The anterior branch supplies the anterior and middle deltoid muscles. The anterior deltoid flexes (or bends) and medially rotates the arm, and the middle deltoid abducts the arm or draws it away from the midline of the body.

CAUSES OF NEUROPATHY

Injury to the axillary nerve, also known as axillary neuropathy or palsy, causes weakness of the previously discussed functions of the deltoid and teres minor muscles. Although teres minor weakness impairs external rotation of the arm, this may be difficult to detect because the primary external rotator, the infraspinatus muscle, preserves this movement. The loss of skin sensation on the lateral upper shoulder with an axillary neuropathy varies from none to severe. The most common cause of axillary neuropathy is trauma to the shoulder region. Anterior dislocation of the shoulder and fracture of the neck of the humerus are particularly likely to cause a traction injury to the axillary nerve as it courses around the humerus. The axillary nerve may be injured in association with brachial plexus injuries involving the upper trunk, posterior cord, or more extensive plexus injuries. With a traction injury of the brachial plexus, the axillary nerve is especially prone to injury. The axillary nerve may be injured in the immune-mediated disorder known as idiopathic brachial plexopathy or neuralgic amyotrophy; occasionally, it may be the only nerve affected.

DIAGNOSIS

The diagnosis of axillary neuropathy is considered when physical examination shows weakness limited to the deltoid muscle and variable loss of sensation on the skin of the upper lateral arm. Electromyography (EMG) studies are performed to confirm the diagnosis and distinguish axillary neuropathy from other disorders that may have similar features. Fibrillation potentials in the deltoid and teres minor muscles, but not in other muscles, confirm the diagnosis of axillary neuropathy. Normal EMG results in specific muscle groups serve to eliminate other disorders from consideration. For example, a segmental or nerve root disorder can be excluded if EMG studies of the cervical paraspinal muscles are normal. Normal EMG studies of the supraspinatus and infraspinatus muscles exclude a suprascapular neuropathy. Normal EMG results in other muscles supplied by the fifth and sixth cervical cord segments help to exclude brachial plexus lesions, with the caveat that an isolated axillary neuropathy may occasionally be the only manifestation of an idiopathic brachial plexopathy.

TREATMENT

Treatment of axillary neuropathy is influenced by the specific cause. In all cases, physical therapy is indicated to maintain normal range of motion of the shoulder joint. Loss of motion at the shoulder joint due to deltoid muscle weakness can lead to a painful condition known as adhesive capsulitis, or a frozen shoulder, in which fibrotic tissue develops within the shoulder joint. This can be treated by progressive stretching exercises. It is preferable to prevent adhesive capsulitis from occurring by performing regular stretching and range of motion exercises. Patients with axillary nerve injury secondary to neuralgic amyotrophy usually require analgesic medication to help control pain early in the illness. Although recovery from neuralgic amyotrophy may take more than 1 year, the majority of patients have a good prognosis. Patients with traumatic axillary neuropathy should be followed for evidence of recovery. Spontaneous recovery often occurs after dislocation of the shoulder and fracture of the humerus. If recovery has not begun within 4 months of onset, and EMG studies do not reveal evidence of reinnervation, surgical exploration and nerve grafting should be considered. The prognosis for recovery after nerve grafting is generally good. If a penetrating injury causes complete laceration of the axillary nerve, exploration and nerve repair should be performed within several days of the injury.

—*Mark A. Ross*

See also–Musculocutaneous Nerve; Neck and
Arm Pain; Neuropathies, Overview

Further Reading

England, J. D., and Sumner, A. J. (1987). Neuralgic amyotrophy:
  An increasingly diverse entity. *Muscle Nerve* **10**, 60–68.
Liveson, J. A. (1984). Nerve lesions associated with shoulder
  dislocation: An electrodiagnostic study of 11 cases. *J. Neurol.
  Neurosurg. Psychiatry* **47**, 742–744.
Petrucci, F. S., Morelli, A., and Raimondi, P. L. (1982). Axillary
  nerve injuries—cases treated by nerve graft and neurolysis. *J.
  Hand Surg.*, 271–278.
Sunderland, S. (1991). *Nerve Injuries and Their Repair.* Churchill
  Livingstone, New York.
Toolanen, G., Hildingsson, C., Hedlund, T., *et al.* (1993). Early
  complications after anterior dislocation of the shoulder in
  patients over 40 years. *Acta Orthop. Scand.* **64**, 549–555.

Neuropathy, Toxic

Encyclopedia of the Neurological Sciences
Copyright 2003, Elsevier Science (USA). All rights reserved.

PERIPHERAL neuropathy is a potential side effect of a wide variety of pharmaceutical, occupational, and environmental agents. In North America, the overwhelming majority of instances of toxic neuropathy are iatrogenic; many inevitably accompany customary chemotherapeutic treatment regimens. Neuropathy from exposure to industrial or environmental agents is rare.

BASIC PRINCIPALS AND CORRELATED CLINICAL FEATURES

Distal Axonopathy (Central–Peripheral Distal Axonopathy)

Distal axonopathy is a common and thoroughly studied form of human neurotoxic disease. The neuropathological substrate is degeneration of distal regions of axons in the central and peripheral nervous systems. The nonspecific histopathological features of the axonal changes render nerve biopsy unhelpful in evaluation of an individual patient. In the peripheral nervous system degeneration appears to advance proximally toward the nerve cell body as long as exposure lasts; its reversal allows the axon to regenerate along the distal Schwann cell column to the appropriate terminal. A similar sequence often occurs in the distal ends of the long central nervous system axons, especially in the dorsal columns, although regeneration is poor.

Distal axonopathy is encountered following chronic or subacute exposure to many pharmaceu-

tical and occupational agents. Some cause severe systemic illness (arsenic and thallium), whereas others are well tolerated and patients appear healthy (acrylamide and pyridoxine). Most are associated with chronic low-level exposure and are characterized by insidious onset of sensory symptoms in the feet. A few have rapid onset and weakness is a prominent feature (*n*-hexane sniffers, dapsone, and organophosphates). Eventually, there is a stocking-glove pattern of acral sensory and motor dysfunction and loss of ankle tendon reflexes. Motor and sensory conductions are only moderately slowed, whereas sensory amplitudes are very diminished; cerebrospinal fluid protein levels are normal. Improvement generally commences at varying intervals following withdrawal from exposure; occasionally, symptoms and signs may intensify for several weeks (coasting) before recovery commences.

Demyelinating Neuropathy

Several agents (diphtheria toxin, amiodarone, and perhexiline maleate) are associated with demyelinating or mixed axonal–demyelinated features. Exposure to diphtheria toxin can result in a disabling, diffuse acute or subacute, predominantly motor neuropathy with areflexia that resembles Guillain–Barré syndrome.

Sensory Neuronopathy

Toxic sensory neuronopathy occurs when an agent produces widespread degeneration of sensory ganglion cells of peripheral and cranial nerves; this is accompanied by generalized sensory loss. Motor function is spared but individuals are disabled by sensory limb ataxia; recovery is poor. In humans, massive doses of pyridoxine and cisplatin have produced this condition. Sensory neuronopathies are readily produced in experimental animals by doxorubicin and methylmercury.

AGENTS ASSOCIATED WITH PERIPHERAL NEUROPATHY

Tables 1 and 2 list agents associated with peripheral neuropathy.

OCCUPATIONAL AND ENVIRONMENTAL AGENTS

Metals

Heavy Metals: Neuropathy from heavy metal exposure is extraordinarily rare in North American

Table 1   AGENTS STRONGLY ASSOCIATED WITH PERIPHERAL NEUROPATHY

Acrylamide	Lead
Allyl chloride	Methyl bromide
Amiodarone	Metronidazole
Arsenic	Misonidazole
2-t-Butylazo-2-hydroxy, etc.	Nitrous oxide
Capsaicin	Nucleoside analogs
Carbon disulfide	Organophosphates
Chloramphenicol	Perhexiline maleate
Cisplatin	Phenol
Colchicine	Podophyllotoxin
Dapsone	Pyridoxine
Diphtheria toxin	Rabies vaccine
Ethambutol	Suramin
Ethylene oxide	Taxoids
Gold salts	Thalidomide
Hexachlorophene	Thallium
n-Hexane	Vacor
Hydralazine	Vidarabine
Hydrazine	Vinca alkaloids
Hymenoptera stings	Nitrofurantoin
Karwinskia humboldtiana	Dimethylaminopropionitrile

medical practice; nevertheless, fruitless laboratory tests for metal toxicity are routinely ordered in the evaluation of patients with peripheral neuropathy. The problem is often compounded when moderately elevated levels of mercury or arsenic are detected, reflecting harmless, transient body burdens from environmental sources (e.g., shellfish ingestion). Such patients may receive needless and expensive chelation therapy.

Table 2   AGENTS PLAUSIBLY ASSOCIATED WITH PERIPHERAL NEUROPATHY

Cytarabine	Methaqualone
Carbamate pesticides	Methyl methacrylate
Ciguatoxin	Muzolimine
Cycloleucine	Naproxen
Disulfiram	Penicillamine
Ethionamide	Phenytoin
Gangliosides	Spanish toxic oil
Germanium dioxide	Sulfasalazine
Glutethimide	Sulfonamides
Tetrachloroethane	Trithiozone
Hexamethylmelamine	L-Tryptophan
Lidocaine, etc.	Zimeldine
Mercury	

Arsenic: Arsenic neuropathy usually results from ingestion of the trivalent (arsenite) form in suicide or murder attempts. Two types of neuropathy exist. Massive overdose causes immediate vomiting and circulatory collapse; one to 3 weeks later, subacute onset of sensory loss and variable weakness develop. In severe cases, an acute paralytic syndrome with demyelinating electrodiagnostic features occurs that eventually evolves into a distal axonopathy pattern. Systemic signs (Mees's lines, anemia, and skin changes) may not appear until after the onset of neuropathy. Recovery largely depends on the severity of neuropathy. Chronic low-level exposure causes the gradual onset of a predominantly sensory neuropathy with prominent position and vibration sense loss and painful paresthesias. Recovery is generally good following withdrawal. The efficacy of chelation therapy is unproven.

Lead: Lead produces a demyelinating neuropathy in experimental animals, whereas human nerve biopsies indicate axonal degeneration. Older reports describe distinct clinical patterns of weakness, including wrist drop, shoulder girdle weakness, intrinsic hand muscle atrophy, foot drop, and laryngeal paralysis; contemporary reports describe generalized weakness with few sensory signs. Treatment is usually reserved for individuals with high lead levels; it involves excretion of the mobilizable body burden by chelation with penicillamine, EDTA, or succimer.

Mercury: Elemental mercury and mercury vapor exposure is generally associated with tremor and emotional lability without evidence of neuropathy. The are rare anecdotal reports of a mild sensory axonal neuropathy following prolonged low-level exposure and one description of subacute, predominantly motor, axonal neuropathy in children.

Miscellaneous Agents

Ethylene Oxide: Ethylene oxide is a gas used in the sterilization of heat-sensitive medical instruments and biomedical materials. Chronic low-level exposure can cause distal axonopathy with acral numbness, sensory dysfunction, and loss of tendon reflexes. Experimental studies confirm that this is a distal axonopathy. Improvement follows termination of exposure. Usually, ethylene oxide exposure occurs via inhalation; however, excess residual ethylene oxide in dialysis tubing has been postulated to contribute to peripheral neuropathy. In some instances, cognitive impairment may accompany neuropathy.

Hexacarbons: *n*-Hexane and methyl *n*-butyl ketone (MnBK) are described together because both act through a common 1,4-γ diketone intermediary, 2,5-hexanedione, to produce peripheral neuropathy. *n*-Hexane is a solvent with wide industrial application in glues, thinners, and lacquers. Intoxication occurs following occupational exposure or inhalant abuse (glue sniffing). MnBK is inherently a more potent neurotoxin than *n*-hexane, but its use has been curtailed since it was implicated in a massive outbreak of toxic neuropathy in a fabric plant. Methyl ethyl ketone, although it does not cause peripheral neuropathy, is able to potentiate the effects of *n*-hexane or MnBK.

Peripheral neuropathy develops insidiously after exposure to either agent. Distal sensory loss predominates early but is soon overshadowed by severe weakness. Weakness may be so prominent as to cause orthopedic surgical procedures on patients who develop a "rubber knee syndrome" with minimal paresthesias. Subacute onset of severe ascending weakness following high-level exposure in glue sniffers may suggest a diagnosis of Guillain–Barré syndrome. Tendon reflexes are minimally affected; even in severe cases, usually only the Achilles reflex is lost. Improvement correlates with severity, and permanent deficits frequently result from prolonged high-level exposure. Coasting is especially common following withdrawal from exposure and may last for as long as four months. Nerve conduction is markedly slowed, which is unusual for an axonopathy. Nerve biopsy reveals multifocal paranodal, giant axonal swellings accompanied by myelin retraction; paranodal demyelination with secondary myelin changes is likely responsible for the unusual slowed nerve conduction. Spasticity and hyper-reflexia, reflecting corticospinal tract degeneration, may appear following recovery from neuropathy.

Organophosphates: The organophosphate (OP) pesticides currently deployed in North America are rarely associated with serious neurotoxicity, and then usually only following massive suicidal ingestions. Inhibition of acetylcholinesterase (AChE) is common to all OPs and is the basis for their use as pesticides; some OPs also cause a widespread central and peripheral distal axonopathy. Axonal dysfunction commences several weeks following exposure, a process referred to as organophosphate-induced delayed peripheral neuropathy (OPIDP). This process occurs independently from and is not related to the initial inhibition of AChE. Massive exposure to OPs causes rapid-onset muscarinic and nicotinic dysfunction and death results from pulmonary compromise—a combination of bronchoconstriction (muscarinic) and muscle paralysis (nicotinic). OPIDP follows OP exposure by 10–20 days; cramping of the calves, acral paresthesias, and distal weakness herald it. The course is subacute and maximal involvement occurs within two weeks of onset. Upon recovery from neuropathy, signs of myelopathy may appear. Some are left with residual lower limb spasticity and position sense loss. There is no specific treatment for OPIDP; the initial muscarinic effects may be blunted by atropine and pralidoxime administration.

PHARMACEUTICAL AGENTS
Chemotherapeutic Agents

Cisplatin: Cumulative doses of cisplatin exceeding 225–500 mg/m^2 cause a large-fiber, progressive sensory distal axonopathy that spares motor fibers. Position and vibration sense may be profoundly altered with little loss of pain and temperature sensation. Autonomic dysfunction, especially gastroparesis and vomiting, is frequent. Neuropathy from exposures less than 500 mg/m^2 is usually reversible; however, prolonged higher level exposure may result in a sensory neuronopathy with residual limb ataxia and loss of manual dexterity. Occasionally, the onset of cisplatin neuropathy is delayed and patients experience initial symptoms up to 4 months after drug withdrawal. It is then difficult to distinguish between cisplatin toxicity and neuropathy from the underlying malignancy.

Paclitaxel (Taxol): Symptoms of a predominantly sensory neuropathy appear soon after treatment in regimens using doses in excess of 200 mg/m^2. Initial symptoms of acral paresthesias and dysesthesias herald the onset of sensory loss accompanied by tendon reflex loss. Motor dysfunction has only been reported to follow prolonged, high-level administration. Myopathy may occur, especially with coadministration of other agents. Improvement usually occurs following cessation of therapy; however, neuropathy is frequently the dose-limiting factor in therapy.

Vincristine: Neuropathy usually commences in a stereotyped manner with sensory symptoms at onset. Paresthesias of the fingers (an uncommon initial locus for a distal axonopathy) usually herald neuropathy; later, they appear in the feet followed by variable degrees of distal sensory loss. Weakness, cramps, and clumsiness soon follow and are often severe; weakness eventually dominates the picture and is frequently disabling. Autonomic neuropathy with gastroparesis, constipation, and urinary retention is frequent. Trigeminal sensory loss occurs in 5–10% of cases. Neuropathy usually abates following dose reduction, allowing continued treatment.

Antimicrobials

Dapsone: Motor neuropathy (unusual for a toxic distal axonopathy) occasionally follows long-term, high-level treatment of pemphigus. Weakness may be diffuse but frequently affects the arms disproportionately; the median nerve is especially vulnerable. The appearance of hand weakness without sensory symptoms may lead to an erroneous diagnosis of motor neuron disease. Recovery is usually satisfactory following drug withdrawal.

Isoniazid: Isoniazid (INH) neuropathy is strongly dose dependent: Doubling the usual dose of 3 mg/kg per day results in an eightfold increase in neuropathy. Distal paresthesias, calf pain, and numbness begin three weeks to six months after onset of therapy, depending on dose and individual susceptibility. INH is deactivated by acetylation; individuals unable to acetylate normally (slow acetylators) develop higher levels of circulating INH and are more susceptible. Neuropathy can be avoided by coadministration of 100 mg of pyridoxine daily.

Nitrofurantoin: Chronic administration of nitrofurantoin, in conventional doses of 100 mg four times daily, may rarely cause a severe motor and sensory neuropathy in patients with renal dysfunction. An acute or subacute onset is common and may lead to an erroneous diagnosis of Guillain–Barré syndrome.

Miscellaneous Agents

Nitrous Oxide: Self-administration of nitrous oxide can cause megaloblastic anemia and myeloneuropathy indistinguishable from pernicious anemia. Moderate levels of abuse cause neuropathy; higher levels can produce myelopathy and optic atrophy. Neuropathy is heralded by acral paresthesias; numbness of the hands and feet and ataxia are common. At this stage, reflexes are attenuated and nerve conduction studies show mild slowing. Continued, self-administration results in spasticity and profound, poorly reversible, acral sensory loss.

Pyridoxine: Reversible sensory neuropathy of gradual onset is associated with prolonged oral consumption of high levels (> 500 mg daily) of pyridoxine. Onset of symptoms varies with the dose; daily intake of less than 1 g requires more than one year for symptom onset, whereas greater exposure produces neuropathy within months. The distal sensory neuropathy affects mainly the large-fiber functions of vibration and position sense; limb ataxia may mimic weakness because movements are misdirected and poorly controlled. An irreversible sensory neuronopathy syndrome has occurred in individuals given massive intravenous doses in excess of 100 g.

Amiodarone: This potent antiarrhythmic drug causes tremor, optic neuropathy, and peripheral neuropathy. Neuropathy is especially common and, although generally associated with prolonged dosing (longer than six months) at levels higher than 400 mg daily, has occurred at standard doses of 200 mg daily. Lower limb weakness, which may disable the patient, appears early and is followed by sensory dysfunction. Nerve conductions may be severely slowed, reflecting demyelination as well as axon loss. Recovery is satisfactory if the drug is withdrawn soon after symptoms commence.

Thalidomide: Thalidomide is increasingly studied as a possible immune modulator and oncological agent. Initial symptoms of thalidomide neuropathy are always sensory; usually, numbness and tingling occur in the feet and then in the hands. Insensitivity to pain and touch is profound; vibration and position senses are less affected. Weakness is variable, occurs later, and may involve proximal muscles. Neuropathy usually appears after approximately one year at doses of 25–50 mg, but it appears more rapidly with higher doses. Recovery is variable following withdrawal; sensory function may recover incompletely and slowly.

—*Herbert Schaumburg*

See also–Arsenic; Environmental Toxins; Lead; Mercury; Myopathy, Toxic; Neuropathies, Overview; Neurotoxicology, Overview; Organophosphates, Organochlorides, and Pesticides; Sensory Neuronopathy, Paraneoplastic

Further Reading

Albers, J. W., and Berent, S. (Eds.) (2000). *Clinical Neurobehavioral Toxicology*. Saunders, Philadelphia.

Brust, J. C. M. (1993). *Neurological Aspects of Substance Abuse*. Butterworth-Heinemann, Boston.

Rosenberg, N. L. (Ed.) (1995). *Occupational and Environmental Neurology*. Butterworth-Heinemann, Boston.

Schaumburg, H. H., Berger, A., and Thomas, P. K. (1991). *Disorders of Peripheral Nerve*, 2nd ed. Davis, Philadelphia.

Spencer, P. S., and Schaumburg, H. H. (Eds.) (2000). *Experimental and Clinical Neurotoxicology*, 2nd ed. Oxford Univ. Press, New York.

Neuropeptide Mediators of Neuro-Immune Communications

Encyclopedia of the Neurological Sciences
Copyright 2003, Elsevier Science (USA). All rights reserved.

IT WAS OBSERVED more than four decades ago that lesions in some structures of the central nervous system and stimulation of peripheral nerves supplying immune organs altered circulating levels and functions of lymphocytes in rodents. Studies during the past 30 years have begun to elucidate the mechanisms of such effects and establish the foundations of modern research in the field of neuroimmunology. Primary immune organs and lymphoid follicles in organs having extensive surface contact with the environment, such as lungs, the gastrointestinal (GI) tract, and skin, are heavily innervated with peptidergic nerves of adrenergic, cholinergic, nonadrenergic noncholinergic, and sensory subsets (Table 1). The thymic concentrations of some neuropeptides are higher than those in the central nervous system and they are localized in regions of greatest T cell content. Similarly, these peptides are located principally in T cell corridors of the spleen. More than 65% of mast cells and up to 30–40% of T cells in the GI tract bear peptidergic neural endings on their surface or are within one cell diameter of such endings. Of the peptides delivered neurally to immune cells, substance P (SP) and vasoactive intestinal peptide (VIP) predominate quantitatively at sites of immune responses. For example, SP and VIP are detected at nanomolar concentrations in lung fluids after intratracheal antigen challenge of immunized mice (Table 1). SP and VIP appear and disappear with distinctive and separate time courses, leading to a peak of SP in lung fluids 1 to 2 days after

Table 1   EVIDENCE FOR NEUROPEPTIDE MEDIATION OF NEURO-IMMUNE INTERACTIONS

Dense peptidergic innervation of thymus, spleen, and lymphoid follicles of GI tract, skin, and lungs

Peptidergic nerve endings on or very near mast cells and lymphocytes

Functionally relevant concentrations of substance P, vasoactive intestinal peptide, and some other neuropeptides at sites of immune responses

Immune cell expression of authentic functional receptors for substance P, vasoactive intestinal peptide, and some other neuropeptides

Potent effects of some neuropeptides on T cell, B cell, and macrophage activities *in vitro*

Effector and regulatory roles of some neuropeptides in animal models of immunity and immune-mediated inflammation

antigen challenge and a later plateau of maximal VIP concentration after 4 or 5 days.

The many effects of neurally delivered VIP and SP on immune cells are transduced by subsets of specific high-affinity G protein-coupled receptors (GPCRs), including the type 1 neurokinin (NK1) receptor for SP and types 1 and 2 VPAC receptors for VIP, the latter of which also recognize pituitary adenylyl cyclase-activating peptide (PACAP) of the same neuroendocrine peptide family. Immune cell expression of GPCRs for SP and VIP is regulated developmentally and by cellular activation. The relative levels of each neuropeptide receptor influence immune responses, as receptors for different neuropeptides and even different receptors for the same neuropeptide may mediate opposing effects. For example, VPAC1 predominates constitutively on mammalian mast cells, macrophages, and most T cells. Differentiation of mouse bone marrow-derived mast cells with stem cell factor increases expression of VPAC1 receptors and induces responsiveness of histamine release to VIP and PACAP. Resting peritoneal macrophages of mice and human blood monocytes express only VPAC1 receptors, and activation has little effect on this pattern. In contrast, the predominance of VPAC1 receptors relative to VPAC2 receptors on T cells is susceptible to regulation by T cell receptor (TCR) stimulation. The levels of VPAC1 receptors are higher on CD4$^+$ T cells than CD8$^+$ T cells in humans and mice, and TCR stimulation both increases expression of VPAC2 receptors and suppresses expression of VPAC1 receptors through transcriptional mechanisms. Enhancement of expression of CD4$^+$ T cell VPAC2 receptors is mediated in part by some cytokines in mice.

In several instances, an altered ratio of VPAC2 to VPAC1 receptors modifies the effect of VIP on T cells. Stimulation of T cell-increased adhesiveness, chemotaxis, and secretion of MMP-2 and MMP-9 by VIP is mediated by the VPAC2 receptors, but VPAC1 receptors may send opposite signals in some subsets of T cells. Thus, TCR-directed activation of T cells, which increases VPAC2/VPAC1, would increase chemotactic responsiveness to VIP as well as T cell capability for transmigration of basement membranes and tissues. The immunoregulatory roles of some other neuropeptides are modified by SP or VIP. SP prevents induction of synthesis of somatostatin neuropeptide by macrophages activated by different immune stimuli. Because SP enhances production of interferon (IFN)-γ, whereas somatostatin inhibits IFN-γ production, this effect of SP on somatostatin amplifies its recruitment of IFN-γ. Thus, immune cells bear GPCRs for SP, VIP, and some other neuropeptides, which are regulated by numerous immunological factors and transduce signals that significantly modify immune responses.

The postulated effects of neuropeptides on immunity until recently were based largely on *in vitro* observations because pharmacological probes that could be administered to animals lack specificity, potency, and often adequate bioavailability for *in vivo* studies. It was thereby concluded that the predominant neuropeptides SP and VIP would contribute oppositely to regulation of some aspects of immune cell functions, which may enhance the sensitivity of immunity to neuroregulation (Table 2). SP is stimulatory for most macrophage and T cell functions, whereas VIP is most often inhibitory of the same immune cell activities. SP is a potent monocyte/ macrophage chemotactic factor, enhances macrophage phagocytosis, and increases stimulus-sensitive production and secretion of immune cytokines. In contrast, VIP inhibits migration and phagocytosis by macrophages and suppresses generation of numerous cytokines with the exception of IL-10, for which secretion is strikingly augmented. Although both SP and VIP increase T cell adhesiveness, by increasing expression and/or activity of different surface proteins, opposite effects are observed on other T cell functions, including proliferation, production, and secretion of most cytokines and expression of cell surface proteins. There are too few data to derive conclusions about the effects of SP on migration of different subsets of T cells. B cell responses to SP and VIP, usually defined in T cell-dependent assays, include opposing influences on IgM production, shared enhancement of IgA generation, and distinctive suppression of IgG and augmentation of IgE by VIP (Table 2). The opposing effects of SP and VIP on cytokine generation by mast cells were observed at nanomolar levels, whereas the similar degranulating activity of both leading to histamine release was documented only at micromolar or higher concentrations.

The capacity of SP and VIP to modify integrated immune responses in mammals initially was examined only in a few systems with limited results. The simplest such investigations have consisted of documentation of short-term effects of intraperitoneal injection of 2–10 nmol of VIP per mouse on spontaneous and elicited generation of cytokines. For example, intraperitoneal instillation of 5 nmol of VIP per mouse results in 5- to 20-fold increases in IL-6 concentration in peritoneal fluid and serum after 2 to 3 hr. More complex studies have examined effects of SP or VIP in compartmentalized immune reactions shown to be associated with changes in SP, VIP,

Table 2   SUBSTANCE P AND VASOACTIVE INTESTINAL PEPTIDE EFFECTS ON IMMUNITY[a]

Target immune cell	Substance P	Vasoactive intestinal peptide
Mast cell	Enhances histamine and lipid mediator release; augments cytokine generation	Enhances histamine release; inhibits cytokine generation
Macrophage	Hemotactic; increases phagocytosis and cytokine production	Inhibits chemotaxis and phagocytosis; suppresses production of TNF-α, IL-6, IL-12; augments generation of IL-10
B lymphocyte	Stimulates IgA and IgM production	Decreases production of IgG and IgM; stimulates production of IgA and IgE
T lymphocyte	Increases adhesion and proliferation; stimulates production of IL-2 and IFN-γ; enhances expression of IL-2 receptor and of CD2 and CD45	Increases adhesion, MMP generation, and migration; suppresses proliferation; inhibits production of IL-2 and -10; augments production of IL-4, IL-5, and IFN-γ; reduces apoptosis

[a] Abbreviations used: MMP, matrix metalloproteinase; IFN, interferon; IL, interleukin; TNF, tumor necrosis factor.

Table 3   MAJOR ROLES OF NEUROPEPTIDES IN T CELL HOMEOSTASIS AND RESPONSES

Production/Differentiation/Survival	Migration/Tissue distribution	Immune responses

Thymus
  Enhance/accelerate CD4 production = VIP[a]
  Reduced CD4 apoptosis = VIP		

	Peripheral lymphoid tissues	
	Reduce apoptosis = VIP	
	T cell adhesion/chemotaxis/MMP production = VIP	
		SP + proliferation VIP−
		SP = B cell help/suppression = VIP
		SP + cytokine production VIP−

[a] =, Neuropeptide evoking effect; +, neuropeptide is stimulatory; −, neuropeptide is inhibitory.

and/or their receptors. For example, intratracheal antigen challenge of primed mice in a model of pulmonary delayed-type hypersensitivity evoked peak increases in mean lymphocyte counts in bronchoalveolar fluid of up to 20-fold on Days 4–6 after challenge and peak increases in cytokine concentrations of up to 50-fold on Day 1 for IL-2 and IFN-γ, Days 1 to 2 for IL-6, and Day 3 for IL-4. Concentrations of SP and VIP in bronchoalveolar fluids increased after intratracheal antigen challenge by up to 18-fold, with peaks on Days 1 to 2 and 4–7, respectively. The levels of mRNA encoding neuropeptide receptors in bronchoalveolar leukocytes increased to peaks on Days 2–4, with significant increases in T cell VPAC1, VPAC2, and NK-1 receptors and in macrophage VPAC1 and NK-1 receptors. To establish a critical role for SP in such responses, a daily intraperitoneal injection of a potent and bioavailable NK-1 receptor antagonist (CP-96,345) was given from Day 3 before antigen to the end of the study. This treatment reduced significantly the Day 5 peak accumulation of lymphocytes (by >55%) and macrophages (by more than 15%), whereas an inactive enantiomer of the NK-1 receptor antagonist had no effect. Thus, SP is required for optimal recruitment of T cells and possibly B cells into pulmonary parenchymal tissue mounting an immune response. VIP, through VPAC2 receptor-induced alterations in cytokines, promotes generation and functions of type 2 helper T cells (critical for allergy and inflammation) and reciprocally suppresses type 1 helper T cells (required for host defense and delayed-type hypersensitivity). Thus T cell-targeted VPAC2-transgenic mice have an allergic phenotype, whereas VPAC2-null mice have no allergies but enhanced delayed-type hypersensitivity.

In summary, SP and VIP are released and involved functionally in every phase of development, activa-

tion, and regulation of immune cells (Table 3). Viewed from the perspective of T cell involvement, VIP enhances and accelerates development of CD4$^+$ T cells by intrathymic actions and blunts apoptosis of thymocytes and T cells. VIP also evokes chemotactic migration of T cells from circulating pools into tissues, where it increases their survival. Some T cell immune functions are regulated bidirectionally by SP and VIP, including SP enhancement and VIP suppression of proliferation and cytokine generation, whereas others show shared effects of VIP and SP, as in regulation of antibody production (Table 3). Thus, immune cell production and maturation, predominant tissue localization, migration to sites of immune stimulation, and many aspects of specific immune responses are regulated by neuropeptides.

—*Edward J. Goetzl*

See also–Immune System, Overview; Neuroimmunology, Overview; Neuropeptides, Overview

Acknowledgment

This work was supported by National Institutes of Health Grant AI 34570.

Further Reading

Blum, A. M., Elliott, D. E., Metwali, A., et al. (1998). Substance P regulates somatostatin expression in inflammation. *J. Immunol.* 161, 6316–6322.
Dorsam, G., Voice, J. K., Kong, Y., et al. (2000). Vasoactive intestinal peptide mediation of development and functions of T lymphocytes. *Ann. N. Y. Acad. Sci.* 921, 79–91.
Goetzl, E. J., Adelman, D. C., and Sreedharan, S. P. (1990). Neuroimmunology. *Adv. Immunol.* 48, 161–190.
Goetzl, E. J., Banda, M. J., and Leppert, D. (1996). Matrix metalloproteinases in immunity. *J. Immunol.* 156, 1–4.
Goetzl, E. J., Voice, J. K., Shen, S., et al. (2001). Enhanced delayed-type hypersensitivity in mice lacking the inducible

VPAC2 receptor for vasoactive intestinal peptide. *Proc. Natl. Acad. Sci. USA* **98**, 13854–13859.

Kaltreider, H. B., Ichikawa, S., Byrd, P. K., et al. (1997). Upregulation of neuropeptides and neuropeptide receptors in a murine model of immune inflammation in lung parenchyma. *Am. J. Respir. Cell Mol. Biol.* **16**, 133–144.

Martinez, C., Delgado, M., Pozo, D., et al. (1998). VIP and PACAP enhance IL-6 release and mRNA levels in resting peritoneal macrophages: In vitro and in vivo studies. *J. Neuroimmunol.* **85**, 155–167.

McCann, S. M., Lipton, J. M., Sternberg, E. M., et al. (Eds.) (1998). Neuroimmunomodulation: Molecular aspects, integrative systems, and clinical advances. *Ann. N. Y. Acad. Sci.* **840**, 1–866.

Merrill, J. E., and Jonakait, G. M. (1995). Interactions of the nervous and immune systems in development, normal brain homeostasis, and disease. *FASEB J.* **8**, 611–618.

Schmidt-Choudhury, A., Meischner, J., Seebeck, J., et al. (1999). Stem cell factor influences neuro-immune interactions: The response of mast cells to pituitary adenylate cyclase activating polypeptide is altered by stem cell factor. *Regul. Peptides* **83**, 73–80.

Voice, J. K., Dorsam, G., Lee, H., et al. (2001). Allergic diathesis in transgenic mice with constitutive T cell expression of inducible vasoactive intestinal peptide receptor. *FASEB J.* **15**, 2489–2496.

Xia, M., Leppert, D., Hauser, S. L., et al. (1996). Stimulus-specificity of matrix metalloproteinase-dependence of human T cell migration through a model basement membrane. *J. Immunol.* **156**, 160–167.

Neuropeptides, Overview

Encyclopedia of the Neurological Sciences

NEUROPEPTIDES are peptides produced by cells within the nervous system. The term neuropeptide was coined by de Wied in the early 1970s upon the discovery that hormones, such as adrenocorticotropin hormone (ACTH), melanocyte-stimulating hormone (MSH), and vasopressin, induced complex behavioral effects in addition to their classic hypothalamic–pituitary endocrine actions. The subsequent isolation of the enkephalins in 1975 by Kosterlitz and coworkers and the discovery that the gut peptides, such as cholecystokinin (CCK), vasoactive intestinal peptide (VIP), and somatostatin, are produced in the brain led to an appreciation of the importance of neuropeptides in behavior and brain function in general.

Acting on specific peptidergic receptors, neuropeptides produce a myriad of highly specific physiological functions, including regulation of reproduction, growth, food and water intake, and electrolyte balance; control of respiratory, cardiovascular, and gastrointestinal functions; and modulation of sensibility and emotions. Due to highly advanced molecular biology techniques, novel neuroactive

peptides continue to be isolated from the central nervous system as well as from such diverse sources as plants, invertebrates, and frog skin. Recent discoveries include orphanin FQ or nociceptin, the endomorphins 1 and 2, and prolactin-releasing peptide. Many of these peptides were isolated only after the identification of their receptors, much like the prior discovery of the opioid receptors led to the isolation of the enkephalins. The diversity of neuroactive peptides is extensive. Some of the major families, their members, and their functions are shown in Table 1. Now that the complete sequence for the human genome has been unraveled, many more orphan receptors will undoubtedly be uncovered, followed by their endogenous ligands, which are likely to be novel neuropeptides.

SYNTHESIS OF NEUROPEPTIDES

Despite their wide range of structures, neuropeptides share many features. Generating neuropeptides is quite distinct from the enzymatic synthesis of the classic neurotransmitters. Almost all neuropeptides are formed from larger, precursor peptides. These precursor peptides are then sequestered into dense-core vesicles or secretory granules, in which they are processed through specific enzymatic proteolysis to yield active neuropeptides. The precursor peptides may contain a number of copies of the same neuropeptide or a number of biologically and structurally distinct peptides. For example, the pro-enkephalin precursor molecule contains six copies of [met^5]enkephalin and one of [leu^5]enkephalin (Fig. 1). The precursor for β-endorphin is an example of widely divergent peptides, including β-endorphin, α-melanocyte-releasing hormone (α-MSH), and adrenocorticotropin-releasing hormone (ACTH), that are generated from a single precursor.

The complexity of peptide processing is further illustrated by the ability of different neurons to contain proteases of differing specificities, thereby producing different peptide products from the same precursor. Alternatively, a peptide may be subjected to different post-translational modifications in different cells, such as glycosylation or phosphorylation. An example of this is the precursor molecule pro-opiomelanocortin (POMC) (Fig. 1), which gives rise to ACTH, melanotropins, and the opioid peptide β-endorphin. POMC mRNA can be found in the anterior and intermediate lobes of the pituitary, in the hypothalamus, and in various other brain regions as well as in the placenta and the gut, but the actual

Table 1   MAJOR FAMILIES OF NEUROPEPTIDES

Family	Member	Abbreviation	Function
Hypothalamic hormones	Oxytocin	OT	Sexual and social behaviors
	Vasopressin	VP/ADH	Renal function
Hypothalamic releasing and inhibiting hormones	Corticotrophin-releasing hormone	CRH	Initiates stress-induced release of ACTH and glucocorticoids
	Somatostatin	SS	Regulates secretion of growth hormone
	Growth hormone-releasing hormone	GHRH	Regulates secretion of growth hormone
	Thyrotropin-releasing hormone	TRH	Relsease of TSH and prolactin
	Gonadotropin-releasing hormone	GnRH	Pituitary and gonadal function
Tachykinins	Substance P	SP	Nociception; GI motility; anxiety and depression
	Bombesin		Nociception; GI motility
	Neurokinin α (substance K)	NKA	Nociception; GI motility bronchial contractions
	Neurokinin β	NKB	Nociception; GI motility; vasodilation via NO release
Opioids	Met and Leu-enkephalin		All involved in nociception, reinforcement and reward, neuroendocrine regulation, and increased food intake
	β-Endorphin		
	Endomorphins 1 and 2		
	Dynorphin		
	Nociceptin/orphanin FQ	OFQ	Nociception (hyperalgesia)
Neuropeptide Y and related	Neuropeptide Y	NPY	Increase in food intake and energy stores; inhibition of GI function
	Pancreatic polypeptide	PP	Inhibition of GI function
	Peptide tyrosine tyrosine	PYY	
Vasoactive intestinal polypeptide and glucagon family	Vasoactive intestinal polypeptide	VIP	Increase in GI motility; vasodilation
	Glucagon	GLU	Regulation of insulin secretion
	Glucagon-like peptide-1	GLP-1	Metabolism
	Pituitary adenylate cyclase-activating peptide	PACAP	Stimulation of adenylyl cyclase activity in endocrine organs
Other neuropeptides	Atrial natriuretic peptide	ANP	Diuresis; vasodilation
	Brain natriuretic peptide	BNP	Diuresis; natriuresis; weaker vasodilation effect
	Calcitonin gene-related peptide	CGRP	Body temperature; food intake
	Cholecystokinin	CCK	Satiety; opioid modulation
	Cocaine and amphetamine regulated transcript	CART	Feeding and body weight
	Cortistatin	CST	Sleep regulation
	Galanin		Feeding and body weight
	Gastrin		Gastric acid secretion
	Insulin		Glucose homeostasis
	Melanocortins		Weight gain
	Adrenocorticotropin-releasing hormone	ACTH	
	Melanocyte-stimulating hormone	MSH	
	Neuropeptide FF		Pain and opioid modulation
	Neurotensin		Satiety
	Prolactin-releasing factor	PRF	Prolactin release
	Secretin		Inhibition of gastric acid secretion and emptying
	Secretoneurin		Involved in nuerotransmission and inflammatory responses

peptides produced and released vary from region to region.

The release of neuropeptides from dense-core vesicles is calcium dependent, and neuropeptides are often released in conjunction with other neurotransmitters. Neuropeptides are generally inactivated through rapid extracellular degradation by various peptidases, many of which are highly selective.

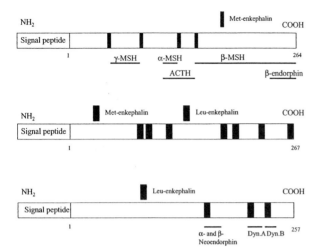

Figure 1
Schematic representation of the pro-opiomelanocortin (POMC), the proenkephalin, and the prodynorphin precursor proteins. ACTH, adrenocorticotropic hormone; MSH, melanocyte-stimulating hormone.

Unlike classic neurotransmitters, which are often recycled through uptake mechanisms, the replenishment of neuropeptides typically occurs via *de novo* synthesis.

DISTRIBUTION OF NEUROPEPTIDES IN THE CNS AND PERIPHERY

Neuropeptides were first described in the hypothalamus and the pituitary gland in connection with their endocrine functions. However, neuropeptides have now been identified in virtually all regions of the brain and spinal cord. Although present in the hypothalamus and pituitary, the neuropeptides somatostatin, substance P, insulin, CCK, the enkephalins, and VIP are also found in the dorsal horn of the spinal cord, the dorsal vagal complex, the amygdala, the nucleus accumbens, the periaquaductal gray, and the striatum. Many neuropeptides are also found in the peripheral nervous system. For example, the nerve plexi of the gastrointestinal tract contain CCK, VIP, substance P, the enkephalins, and somatostatin. However, a wide range of nonnervous tissues also contain these peptides, including the adrenal medulla, immune cells, testes, ovaries, pancreas, and placenta. Indeed, the highest concentration of the enkephalins, for example, is in the adrenal medulla.

During the mid-1980s, studies by Hokfelt and coworkers demonstrated the coexistence within a single neuron of both neuropeptides and classic neurotransmitters, with single neurons capable of coreleasing both at the same time. Neuropeptides often complement the actions of the neurotransmitter, as illustrated by the synergistic effects of the corelease of VIP and acetylcholine (ACh) or of calcitonin gene-related peptide (CGRP) and ACh. Alternatively, the neuropeptide and classic transmitter may also exert independent actions on different target cells.

TRANSPORT OF NEUROPEPTIDES

Neuropeptide transport systems are saturable and stereospecific and can be unidirectional or bidirectional, transporting peptides both in and out of the brain. In order for peripherally synthesized neuropeptides to exert central effects, they must first bypass highly active peptidases within the blood–brain barrier. Therefore, it has always been assumed that influx of neuropeptides from the periphery into the brain was not possible. However, there is increasing evidence suggesting that systemically administered peptides have potent central effects. Penetration of the blood–brain barrier by these peptides is largely dependent on their individual physicochemical properties.

NEUROPEPTIDE RECEPTORS

Many neuropeptides act through G protein-coupled receptors (GPCRs), which contain seven transmembrane domains that form a circular, or donut-like, structure on the surface of cells. The ligand-binding domains of many of the ligands of the GPCRs lie deep within the center of the "donut" formed by the transmembrane segments, whereas the G proteins interact with an intracellular portion of the receptor formed by the third cytoplasmic loop. When agonists bind, the receptor undergoes a conformational change that then influences the G protein and its interactions with the guanine nucleotides GDP and GTP. The G proteins represent the "middle management" by relaying messages from the receptor to modify levels of second messengers, such as cAMP or inositide phosphates, or by direct interactions with ion channels, thus transferring information.

Although the majority of neuropeptides bind to GPCRs, some neuropeptides act on different classes of receptors that are distinct from the G protein-coupled ones. For example, insulin acts on a tyrosine kinase-coupled receptor that contains a single transmembrane segment. The extracellular domain binds the hormone while the intracellular protein kinase catalytic domain phosphorylates target proteins within the cell, thereby conveying the message. Similarly, atrial natriuretic peptide binds to a guanylyl cyclase receptor in which the intracellular domain is the enzyme guanylyl cyclase, which is responsible for the synthesis of cyclic GMP.

OPIOID PEPTIDES AND THEIR RECEPTORS

The opioid peptides and their receptors provide an excellent example of neuropeptide systems. The enkephalins were discovered in 1975 by Kosterlitz and coworkers when they isolated two pentapeptides with opiate-like activity from porcine brain. These peptides were named methionine enkephalin (Tyr-Gly-Gly-Phe-Met) and leucine enkephalin (Tyr-Gly-Gly-Phe-Leu), and they differed only in the C-terminal amino acid. Both peptides mimicked the action of morphine in *in vitro* bioassays by inhibiting electrically stimulated contractions of smooth muscle. Two other families of opioid peptides are the endorphins and the dynorphins; other recently discovered peptides are nociceptin (also known as orphanin FQ), endomorphins 1 and 2, and the dermorphins and deltorphins, which were isolated from the skin of South American frogs.

The mammalian opioid peptides are generated from four precursor proteins: POMC, proenkephalin-A, prodynorphin (also known as proenkephalin-B), and pronociceptin. These proteins are processed at specific points to produce the various peptides (Fig. 1). [Met^5]enkephalin and [Leu^5]enkephalin are derived from proenkephalin-A, the dynorphins and α- and β-neoendorphin are derived from prodynorphin, and β-endorphin and the nonopioid peptides ACTH and MSH are derived from POMC. Pronociceptin gives rise to the peptide nociceptin/orphanin FQ.

Opioid peptides are widely distributed within the central nervous system and the periphery. Peptides derived from POMC are found in the arcuate nucleus and the nucleus tractus solitarius of the brainstem, the pituitary, and the pancreatic islet cells. The enkephalins and dynorphins share a similar localization, including a wide distribution throughout areas of the brain and spinal cord involved in pain perception, affective behavior, and motor control. Peptides derived from proenkephalin are also found in the adrenal gland and in neurons and nerve fibers in the gastrointestinal system.

Opioids act on receptors that belong to the superfamily of G protein-coupled receptors and comprise the μ, δ, κ, and opioid-receptor-like (ORL1) subtypes. Of the endogenous ligands, the enkephalins and endorphins bind to both the μ and δ receptors, whereas the dynorphins bind more selectively to the κ receptor. The dermorphins are highly selective for the μ receptor, as are endomorphins 1 and 2. As their name suggests, the deltorphins are highly selective for the δ receptor, and nociceptin/orphanin FQ is the endogenous ligand for the ORL1 receptor.

As indicated by their distribution, endogenous opioid peptides are responsible for the modulation of a vast range of physiological processes, including the production of analgesia, control of respiratory and cardiovascular functions, stress and immune responses, gastrointestinal function, and neuroendocrine control. Best known for their role in analgesia, the opioid peptides modulate synaptic transmission in nociceptive pathways and inhibit the responses of dorsal horn neurons to noxious stimuli. The synthesis and expression of these endogenous ligands in the brain and spinal cord are upregulated following tissue damage or inflammation. Interestingly, despite a structural similarity to dynorphin A, the pharmacological responses produced by the peptide nociceptin are often very different from and sometimes oppose the effects of other endogenous opioids. For example, when the peptide is administered supraspinally in the rat, it exhibits pronociceptive or antiopioid properties. In addition, nociception can elicit either an analgesic or hyperalgesic response depending on route of administration and species involved. Clearly, the opioid peptide family provides a prime example of how diverse and complex the functions of neuropeptides may be.

—*Claire Neilan and Gavril W. Pasternak*

See also—Basal Ganglia; G Proteins; Neurotransmitter Receptors; Neurotransmitters, Overview; Opioids and Their Receptors

Further Reading

Darlison, M. G., and Richter, D. (1999). Multiple genes for neuropeptides and their receptors: Co-evolution and physiology. *Trends Neurosci.* **22**, 81–88.

De Wied, D. (1969). Effects of peptide hormones on behavior. In *Frontiers in Neuroendocrinology* (W. F. Ganong and L. Martini, Eds.), pp. 97–140. Oxford Univ. Press, New York.

Hokfelt, T., Broberger, C., Xu, Z.-Q. D., *et al.* (2000). Neuropeptides—An overview. *Neuropharmacology* **39**, 1337–1356.

Strand, F. L. (1999). *Neuropeptides: Regulators of Physiological Processes*. MIT Press, Cambridge, MA.

Neuroplasticity
see Plasticity

Neuropsychiatry, Overview

THERE IS NO firm consensus as to what defines neuropsychiatry, but generally it involves a combination of psychiatric and neurological concepts and practices. It is logical that a merger of psychiatry and neurology would eventually occur since there is no debate that many mental illnesses, which psychiatrists deal with most directly, are the result of abnormal physical properties of the brain, which neurologists contend with most often. This merger of psychiatry and neurology formally occurred in 1987 when the *Textbook of Neuropsychiatry* was published by the American Psychiatric Press. The fourth edition of this textbook has evolved to include basic neuroscience principles and is called the *Textbook of Neuropsychiatry and Clinical Neurosciences.*

Specifically, neuropsychiatry may be defined as the assessment and treatment of patients with psychiatric symptoms that are related to explicit brain dysfunction or lesions. The latter includes conditions such as traumatic brain injury, cerebral vascular disease, seizure disorders, neurodegenerative diseases such as Alzheimer's disease and Parkinson's disease, schizophrenia, brain tumors, infectious and inflammatory diseases of the central nervous system, drug- and alcohol-induced mental disorders, and developmental disorders involving the brain. For example, schizophrenia, a disorder involving hallucinations, delusions, and cognitive problems, has been strongly associated with dopamine dysfunction, D_2 and 5-HT_{2A} receptor dysfunction, increased neuronal density in the dorsolateral prefrontal cortex, reductions in the neuronal number in the medial dorsal nucleus of the thalamus, and decreased lateral ventricle volumes. In summary, neuropsychiatry deals with psychiatric problems where measurable brain deficits exist.

—*Douglas L. Gelowitz*

See also–Diagnostic and Statistical Manual of Mental Disorders (DSM-IV); Freudian

Psychology; Neuropsychology; Psychiatry; Psychoanalysis; Psychotherapy

Further Reading

Arciniegas, D. A., and Beresford, T. P. (2001). *Neuropsychiatry—An Introductory Approach.* Cambridge Univ. Press, New York.
Ovsiew, F. (1999). *Neuropsychiatry and Mental Health Services.* American Psychiatric Press, Washington, DC.
Yudofsky, S. C., and Hales, R. E. (2002). *Textbook of Neuropsychiatry and Clinical Neurosciences,* 4th ed. American Psychiatric Press, Washington, DC.

Neuropsychology, Overview

DEFINITION AND USES

NEUROPSYCHOLOGY is the study of the relationship between brain function and behavior. The definition fits the principle of the synthesis of neurology and psychology, and it also describes the way in which neuropsychology developed. According to the Division of Clinical Neuropsychology of the American Psychological Association, a clinical neuropsychologist is a "professional psychologist who applies principles of assessment and intervention based upon the scientific study of human behavior as it relates to normal and abnormal functioning of the central nervous system." Behavioral neurologists and neuropsychiatrists may also use neuropsychological assessment in practice for clinical diagnosis or for research. These settings for neuropsychological practice, clinical and research, each incorporate the use of neuropsychology in various ways.

Clinical Use

Diagnosis—Localizing and Determining a Patient's Level of Impairment: In a clinical setting, neuropsychological assessment can be used to establish baseline capabilities of a patient and provide a comparison to observe longitudinal changes of recovery or decline. Knowing a patient's cognitive abilities and weaknesses assists with differential diagnosis among suspected disorders of similar origin or between psychogenic illness and neurogenic dysfunction.

Rehabilitation and Treatment Evaluation: By characterizing the type of deficits in a patient, the appropriate treatment can be determined. The knowledge of the extent of illness or impairment provides a resource base to design the best suited treatment method or the course of rehabilitation. Likewise, longitudinal neuropsychological assessment compared with baseline measures provides a strong tool to evaluate the efficacy of treatments administered.

Patient Care and Planning: Learning a patient's abilities and limitations results in a better understanding of the type of care required and expected level of functioning. This information affords the patient with knowledge about the extent of daily activity that may be dangerous or benign, such as whether the patient should return to work, requires a caregiver, or should drive a car. Neuropsychological measures may also provide a broader understanding of the progression of an illness or predict when a patient may return to normal daily functioning or activities.

Goals of Clinical Evaluation: The goals of clinical evaluation are to assess a broad range of skills and measure the functions of multiple brain regions. By using a battery of tests designed to assess global cognitive functioning, an examiner may determine the subject's cognitive strengths and weaknesses. The results of this testing provide information about the health of the brain areas that mediate the functions being tested. Of course, no single test can definitively describe the condition of specific neuroanatomical structures. However, results obtained from neuropsychological assessment can direct future neuropsychological, neurological, or psychiatric evaluation as needed. Similarly, a neuropsychological evaluation used in conjunction with other measures such as a neurological examination or brain images obtained by magnetic resonance imaging (MRI) can offer more insight for diagnosis and treatment.

Research Use

Characterizing Disorders and Understanding Behavioral Disorders: Research can improve the quality of testing with the evaluation of techniques, standardization of results, and development of more precise measures. The use of new measures or researching aspects of a disease can identify new behavioral aspects of the disease. Standardization through research provides age- and education-specific norms for clinical comparison assessment.

Relationship between the Brain and Behavior: The determination of behavioral deficits of a patient offers insight into the activity of the brain area that controls a specific function; likewise, areas known to be impaired can be used to analyze the functional and behavioral representation of the area and the resulting impairments. Animal experiments with induced lesions or human studies with localized lesions have been instrumental in the obtainment of the current knowledge of functional representation of the damaged anatomy. For example, Heinrich Kluver and Paul Bucy's 1938 experiment in which the temporal lobes of monkeys were removed and William Scoville and Brenda Milner's 1957 report of patient H.M.'s bilateral medial temporal lobe resection, which included the hippocampal formation, the amygdala, and other adjacent structures, were major contributors to the elucidation of the role of temporal structures in emotional processing and memory functioning.

Knowledge of various forms of aphasia and attention deficits has been obtained from lesion studies. Because of the ethical nature of lesion studies in humans, other options for studying anatomical behavioral roles are crucial. Many studies employ functional MRI, positron emission tomography, electrophysiological recording, and other imaging techniques. MRI is used in studies measuring the volumes of specific brain regions. This is a less invasive option for analysis of neuroanatomy in conjunction with the behavior and cognitive abilities of patients.

A battery of neuropsychological tests for clinical differential diagnosis generally includes measures for memory, language, visuospatial skills, executive functions, mathematical abilities, working memory, abstract reasoning, motor speed, and praxis. Within each of these domains, more distinct areas of functioning may be assessed to target specific disorders. For example, analysis for aphasia may include examination of many specialized areas of language, such as spontaneous speech, naming abilities, recognition of and response to verbal commands, repetition of phrases, reading comprehension, writing abilities, fluency, and verbal responses to printed and auditory stimuli. Detailed assessment of executive function might include measures of response inhibition, mental flexibility, novel problem solving, and conceptual reasoning. It is important that the battery collect information on a wide range of skills as well as on the patient's abilities and deficits. It is the pattern of results, rather than the impairments, that provides insight into the type of disorder a patient may possess.

HISTORY

As the emergence of a better understanding of the human brain developed, so did the development of the field of neuropsychology. Even before Phineas Gage's famous 19th-century accident, when an iron tamping rod was driven through his frontal lobes, scientists knew that there was a relationship between the human brain and human behavior. In the late 18th century, Franz Joseph Gall proposed that behavior emanated from the brain and that use of specific behaviors determined the size of the area of the brain that controls those functions. From these proposals came phrenology, the analysis of bumps on the skull that were considered to reflect overdeveloped brain regions and ultimately a person's behavior and personality. In the 19th century, Pierre Flourens, a French physiologist, argued against the ideas of phrenology using findings from his experiments. He is most noted for his work in animals, in which he removed regions of the brain and studied the subsequent behavioral changes. He found that the amount of damage determines the extent of loss of function, and he believed that the brain's recovery of function implied that there were no areas of specialization. There were exceptions to this argument, including his experiment ablating the brainstem of an animal, which led to the specific loss of respiration and death of the animal.

The next prominent work localizing brain and behavior was that of Pierre Paul Broca. Although he believed in the localization of function, Broca distinguished his ideas from those of Gall. Broca thought that specialization would occur not on the surface of the head but in the "convolutions" of the cortex, giving rise to the science of neuropsychology. In 1861, Broca published his findings of a patient, Leborgne, who had lost his ability to speak but could understand language. Broca's studies of this patient population led to the identification of the area of the brain that expresses language, the left posterior frontal lobe, which is now called Broca's area. This pattern of language deficits is now know as Broca's aphasia. Broca's work also allowed for the idea that the brain's functions can be lateralized to the left or right hemisphere. In 1870, Gustav Fritsch and Eduard Hitzig continued Broca's work in lateralization by showing that limb movement could be elicited in a dog by electrically stimulating the contralateral motor cortex. In 1876, Carl Wernicke published a paper describing another type of aphasia in which patients lose the ability to comprehend language but have the ability to speak. These patients possess lesions in the posterior temporal lobe, now known as Wernicke's area. From his own findings along with those of Broca, Fritsch, Hitzig, and Theodore Meinert, Wernicke developed the first hypothesis for language processing. He theorized that language is processed by sensory cortical areas for auditory and visual information, sent to the angular gyrus, and then sent to Wernicke's area for semantic recognition. The information is then transformed to motor representation in Broca's area. Based on this hypothesis, Wernicke predicted a third type of aphasia, conduction aphasia, in which the neural pathway that connects Wernicke's area to Broca's area (the arcuate fasciculus) is destroyed and the patient has difficulty speaking coherently.

By the early 20th century, localization of function of the brain was a widely accepted concept in the field. However, not all scientists accepted this strict concept, including Karl Lashley. His experiments with rats led him to argue that loss of behavioral functioning is directly related to the amount of tissue lost (mass action), resulting in the theory that the brain is a part of a dynamic system that responds to loss in various ways. In the 1960s, Russian psychologist and neurologist A. R. Luria combined the elements of localization of function and mass action to develop a more comprehensive theory of cortical processing. He postulated that the brain has three functional units: a unit for regulating tone; one for obtaining, processing, and storing information; and one for programming, regulating, and verifying mental activity. Although each component has a primary, secondary, and tertiary area that processes information in a hierarchical manner, he emphasized that the concerted effort of all three functional units is required for normal functioning of mental processes. Luria's theory was later shown to possess practical difficulties, but it provided the next group of neuroscientists with valuable concepts on which to develop better models. Although many of the hypotheses proposed in the past few centuries have been proven to be flawed, each idea initiated a better understanding of human cognition.

Current neuropsychological assessment techniques have evolved from two main traditions—American psychometric analysis and a more process-oriented, qualitative form of assessment. Ward Halstead was one of the predecessors of American psychometrics, using quantitative analysis of test results to assess patients. With the aid of his postdoctoral fellow, Ralph Reitan, his pioneering work on the effects of brain damage on cognition at the University of Chicago in the 1930s ultimately led to the development of the Halstead–Reitan Neuropsychological Test Battery. This battery was used for many years in the United States to assess "organicity" or brain damage in patients as well as provide empirical analysis. Although use of the entire battery may now be impractical due to its length and limitations, modified versions and revised selected tests are still being used today. Other neuroscientists, such as A. R. Luria and Edith Kaplan, believe that neuropsychological assessment should evaluate the way in which individuals perform tasks and develop responses rather than derive conclusions from achievement scores alone. Modern use of neuropsychological assessment, however, incorporates a combination of both quantitative and qualitative techniques. The prominent work of neuropsychologists such as those previously mentioned greatly influenced the development of the current field and furthered the practices of neuropsychological assessment.

COGNITIVE FUNCTIONS AND BRAIN REGIONS

The different areas of the human brain do not work as independent units, making testing of a specific domain quite difficult. For example, testing the function of the hippocampus via neuropsychological memory tests requires intact sensory processing to understand the test presented. Common visual episodic memory tests require the patient to copy a figure and redraw the figure from memory after a time delay. This test requires the patient to be able to visually process the task and to possess the motor skills to accurately complete the task. Likewise, many tests do not assess solely one domain of cognitive functioning. Visual memory tests that are also construction tasks assess spatial skills (a parietal function) of analysis along with the visual and motor components. Construction tests, such as the modified Rey–Osterreith test, can provide insight into deficits of attention, perception, or spatial function. Figure 1 is an example of a patient's copy of a complex figure.

The patient was diagnosed with Alzheimer's disease, which in many cases is known to affect the parietal lobes in addition to the hippocampus and other brain regions. Although the patient is able to perceive and reproduce the overall gestalt of the design, she is unable to correctly place details on the main figure, most noticeably the square-shaped flag on the left. The design is presented to the subject on a

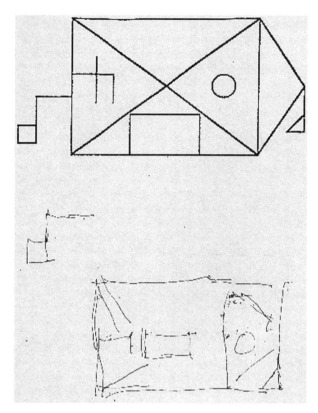

Figure 1
An Alzheimer's disease patient's copy of a complex figure.

typical $8\frac{1}{2} \times 11$-in. sheet of paper and the patient is asked to copy the drawing to the best of their abilities. Figure 2 is another example of a copy of the modified Rey–Osterreith from a patient diagnosed with diffuse Lewy body disease with a degree of dementia, similar to the Alzheimer's disease patient noted previously.

It is obvious from this reproduction that the patient does not have the ability to perceive or construct the general shape of the design, unlike the first patient. This patient recognized some of the details of the design, indicated by the copy of the circle and "h" figure on the left, but he was unable to correctly place them spatially on the drawing. Patients with Lewy body disease commonly have visuospatial and construction impairments. They may also have deficits in attention and executive functioning but often have relatively preserved memory.

Due to the many parallel pathways and connections that the brain uses to process information and perform cognitive functions, it is common to assess these functions using tests that target but are not limited to these domains. It is clear, then, that poor

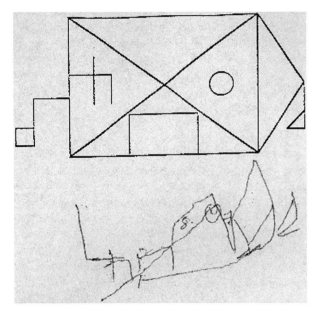

Figure 2
A copy of the modified Rey–Osterreith test from a patient diagnosed with diffuse Lewy body disease with a degree of dementia.

results on a measure of an individual's memory may be an indication of the health of the hippocampus but may also indicate dysfunction in other areas of the brain required to perform the test. By employing a visual memory test that includes a visuospatial construction component, the examiner may obtain information about the hippocampus in the temporal lobes and the parietal lobes (predominantly the right hemisphere). Another option for analyzing episodic memory function is to measure verbal memory or both visual and verbal memory for comparison. Verbal memory tests can simply entail recalling a specified list of words after a time delay. Comparing spontaneous recall and recognition of the words may provide insight into the type of memory deficit—encoding or retrieval.

There are also separate measures that target working memory function. Whereas episodic memory is a subset of declarative memory—a store of words, events, and facts that may be retrieved and stored for minutes, days, or years—working memory provides short-term rehearsal and storage of information during other cognitive processes. It is used when trying remember a phone number while searching for a pen and paper in a desk drawer. Such is an example of the phonological loop of working memory, with the other being the visuospatial system. The rehearsal of this phonological

(verbal) information is correlated to the left premotor cortex and Broca's area, whereas storage of the information is in the left parietal cortex. Conversely, the visuospatial subsystem of working memory stores information in the right parietal cortex. A common test to assess the phonological aspect of working memory is the recitation of a list of numbers in reverse order. The examiner begins with a list of two digits, asking the patient to state the list backward and gradually expanding the list until the patient fails on two trials of the same amount of numbers in a list. A visuospatial counterpart to this measure is the Wechsler Memory Scale-Third Edition spatial span, in which the patient touches spatially arranged blocks in reverse order of that in which the examiner touched the blocks. Because a majority of working memory requires attention using the central executive, another subcomponent of Alan Baddeley's model of working memory, much of working memory is located within the frontal lobes. Neuroimaging of patients while they perform neuropsychological tests that require a large amount of attention has shown that use of verbal memory and nonverbal working memory largely activates the frontal lobes, specifically the left and right dorsolateral prefrontal cortices, respectively.

Research has shown that 99% of right-handers demonstrate left hemisphere dominance with language. Because the extensive ability to communicate distinguishes humans from other animals, its seems appropriate that it is the most understood of all the neurobehavioral domains. Certainly, language has been the subject of intense study and experimentation during the past few centuries, as demonstrated by the work of Broca and Wernicke. There are many facets to language, and humans possess the potential to lose various nuances of these functions due to brain damage. Consequently, included in most neuropsychological batteries are measures of language and communication. The most common disorder of language dysfunction is aphasia. Testing for aphasia addresses the fluency of language output, naming, comprehension, repetition, articulation ability, and written language skills. Common tests of verbal comprehension are verbal commands for a patient to perform (e.g., "Point to your eye") or simple verbal questions (e.g., "Do you wear gloves on your feet?"). Similarly, these examples may be administered in written form to assess reading comprehension. Assessments of naming abilities usually include presentation of pictures or drawings of objects, animals, or famous people that range in familiarity to reflect difficulty levels. However, each test cannot identify a single type of aphasia or language dysfunction. Rather, it is the overall analysis of the deficits and skills that an individual possesses that directs a diagnosis. For example, Broca's aphasics present with nonfluent speech but relatively intact auditory comprehension; however, because of their syntactic impairment, they generally have difficulty comprehending grammatically complex phrases. Broca's aphasics also have poor repetition and naming skills. In contrast, Wernicke's aphasics have fluent speech with severe deficits in auditory comprehension, repetition, and naming. Patients with conduction aphasia, who have a lesion in the arcuate fasciculus, speak fluently and comprehend auditory information but have difficulty with naming and repetition. It is apparent that assessment of cognitive abilities requires many tests in many areas of functioning; even within a cognitive domain such as language, no single test can identify a disease.

Similarly, analysis of a person's executive capabilities is complex and requires measures of various domains. Exemplified by the tragic accident of Phineas Gage, who sustained injuries to his left and right prefrontal cortices, changes in personality and comportment can occur with damage to the frontal lobes. Previously known as a responsible and industrious railroad foreman, Phineas Gage became unreliable and was unable to maintain a job after surviving the explosion that forced an iron rod through his skull. His colleagues and family members noticed such a drastic change in his personality that he was "no longer Gage." Such an extreme example of a neurobehavioral response to tissue damage strikingly delineates some of the responsibilities of the frontal lobes. Gage's survival shocked the scientific community while sparking the current understanding of frontal involvement of cognition. For example, orbitofrontal lesions can cause disinhibition, inappropriate affect, distractibility, or im-

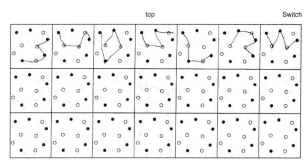

Figure 4
A design fluency test that measures mental flexibility and the ability to shift set.

paired judgment and insight. With lesions in the dorsolateral region, executive function impairments, stimulus-bound behavior, as well as perseveration are likely. In addition, apathy may be seen with lesions of the anterior cingulate circuit. However, traditional testing for these deficits is difficult when assessing functions such as an individual's personality or presentation of inappropriate affect. According to Lezak, there are four general components to testing executive functions: volition, planning, purposive action, and effective performance. She states that all of these functions are necessary for appropriate and socially responsible behavior, and that it is rare to find deficits in only one of these areas.

The execution of executive function tests employs the individual's ability to attend, perceive, and understand the task at hand, indicating the involvement of many levels of cognition. These tasks can also target inhibition, planning, and set shifting. Figure 3 shows an example of a patient's perseverative response to a design fluency task.

In this task, the subject is told to make a design using four lines to connect dots in each box. The subject has 60 sec to generate as many designs as possible. Each design must be different. This patient made only one correct design and repeated it six times during the evaluation, a clear example of perseveration. When prompted to make a different design, the patient attempted to create a novel figure and was genuinely surprised that each time she produced the same one. This patient was diagnosed with Huntington's disease, known to affect executive abilities as well as the more conspicuous motor dysfunction.

Another design fluency test that addresses mental flexibility and the ability to shift set also requires the subject to create designs using four lines (Fig. 4). In this case, each box contains filled dots and empty dots and the subject must draw lines connecting a

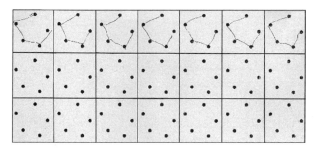

Figure 3
A patient's perseverative response to a design fluency test.

filled dot to an empty dot or vice versa, generating a novel design in each box.

As shown in Fig. 4, the patient had difficulty alternating between the two types of dots, evidenced by the second, third, and fourth designs. The sixth design is also a violation of the rules, containing five lines instead of four. As a result, this patient made only three correct designs, indicating impairment in executive abilities.

CONCLUSIONS

Localization of function has become a major part of neuropsychological assessment, but the fact that cognitive functions do not act independently makes direct quantitative extrapolation from test results difficult. Careful qualitative analysis of negative results may better delineate the type of impairments of a patient. It is clear that in the past few centuries, our understanding of cognitive functioning has increased greatly. It is also apparent that scientists have only just begun to explore the vast abilities of the mind. Just as neuropsychology has helped shape the development of cognitive theories, it will remain an important aspect of comprehending, diagnosing, and treating brain dysfunction. The multidisciplinary aspect of neuropsychology is partially responsible for its value in many environments and should make it a useful tool in the future.

Greater incorporation of neuropsychology in neuroscience as a whole is a likely prospect, as is its continued use in research and education. In addition, neuropsychology is likely to become more prominent in clinical settings for diagnosis and treatment. The role of computers is likely to increase since they are very suitable for assessment of reaction time and greatly enhance the standardization of test administration across sites. They are also invaluable for rapid scoring and interpretation of complex neuropsychological tests that yield multiple test scores and composite indices. Although the surge in computer applications is inevitable in this technologically driven society, there is no substitute for the qualitative analysis of an experienced professional. It is often necessary to obtain behavioral insight from a neuropsychologist to determine the source of deficits. It is not just the results from a test that give a diagnosis but also the type of results and the reason for an individual's performance observable only by another human.

—Sharon J. Sha and Joel H. Kramer

See also–Language, Overview; Learning, Overview; Localization; Memory, Overview; Neuropsychiatry, Overview; Psychotherapy, Overview (see also specific entries in the Neuropsychology section; e.g., Behavior, Neural Basis of)

Further Reading

Baddeley, A. (1992). Working memory. *Science* **255,** 556–559.

Corkin, S., Amaral, D. G., González, R. G., *et al.* (1997). H. M.'s medial temporal lobe lesion: Findings from magnetic resonance imaging. *J. Neurosci.* **17,** 3964–3979.

Cummings, J. L. (1993). Frontal–subcortical circuits and human behavior. *Arch. Neurol.* **50,** 873–880.

Damasio, A. R., and Damasio, H. (1992). Brain and language. *Sci. Am.* **267,** 89–95.

Damasio, H., Grabowski, T., Frank, R., *et al.* (1994). The return of Phineas Gage: Clues about the brain from the skull of a famous patient. *Science* **264,** 1102–1105.

Delis, D. C., Kaplan, E., and Kramer, J. H. (2001). *D-KEFS Examiner's Manual.* Psychological Corporation.

Filley, C. M. (2001). *Neurobehavioral Anatomy,* 2nd ed. Univ. Press of Colorado, Boulder, CO.

Goldman-Rakic, P. S. (1992). Working memory and the mind. *Sci. Am.* **267,** 111–117.

Kandel, E. R., Schwartz, J. H., and Jessell, T. M. (2000). *Principles of Neural Science,* 4th ed. McGraw-Hill, New York.

Kolb, B., and Whishaw, I. Q. (1996). *Fundamentals of Human Neuropsychology,* 4th ed. Freeman, New York.

Lezak, M. D. (1995). *Neuropsychological Assessment,* 3rd ed. Oxford Univ. Press, New York.

Maruish, M. E., and Moses, J. A., Jr. (1997). *Clinical Neuropsychology Theoretical Foundations for Practitioners.* Erlbaum, Mahwah, NJ.

Rezai, K., Andreasen, N. C., Alliger, R., *et al.* (1993). The neuropsychology of the prefrontal cortex. *Arch. Neurol.* **50,** 636–642.

Rozenwig, M. R., Leiman, A. L., and Breedlove, S. M. (1996). *Biological Psychology.* Sinauer, Sunderland, MA.

Scoville, W. B., and Milner, B. (1957). Loss of recent memory after bilateral hippocampal lesions. *J. Neurol. Neurosurg. Psychiatry* **20,** 11–21.

Zarske, J. A. (2001, February 14). Definition of a clinical neuropsychologist. Northern Arizona Neuropsychology website: http://www.nazneuropsychology.com/resource3.htm.

Neuroradiology, Diagnostic

Encyclopedia of the Neurological Sciences
Copyright 2003, Elsevier Science (USA). All rights reserved.

THE FIELD of neuroradiology can be broadly defined as the clinical application of neuroimaging tools to aid in the diagnosis and treatment of diseases affecting the nervous system. In diagnostic neuroradiology, neuroimaging procedures are used to answer specific questions raised by the neurological examination and history. For example, does a patient with a left-sided weakness and aphasia have an intracerebral hemorrhage? The management of this patient hinges on the answer to this question.

The proper use of neuroimaging tools and the interpretation of imaging data require knowledge of anatomy, imaging physics, physiology, and pathology. The anatomical location of a lesion dictates the possible causes. One critical distinction is whether a lesion is within the brain (intraaxial) or arising outside of the brain (extraaxial). Knowledge of imaging physics is also necessary. For example, the flow of blood or pulsation of cerebrospinal fluid can create apparent abnormalities on magnetic resonance imaging (MRI) scans that are artifactual (i.e., not caused by pathological tissue changes). In addition, the choice of the imaging tool depends on the clinical question. X-ray computed tomography (CT) is more reliable than MRI for the detection of acute subarachnoid hemorrhage (usually due to an aneurysm). Physiological parameters in normal and abnormal tissue also affect the images obtained with different neuroradiological techniques. These include blood flow, tissue water content and diffusion, magnetic susceptibility, and electron density. Finally, an intelligent listing of possible causes for an apparent lesion (the differential diagnosis) requires knowledge of different pathological entities. For example, herpes simplex virus should be considered for any lesion with edema and mass effect of the medial temporal lobe in an adult.

In this entry, the currently available imaging modalities used in modern neuroradiological practice are briefly reviewed. Similarly, the role of neuroradiology in the diagnosis and management of the broad categories of neurological disorders (vascular, infectious, etc.) is briefly discussed. The appropriate use of neuroradiological procedures is discussed in a final section.

DIAGNOSTIC NEURORADIOLOGY

History and Development

The first neurological applications of Roentgen's x-ray occurred soon after his discovery in 1895. Plain films of the skull and neck proved useful in the diagnosis and localization of foreign bodies. The use of plain films to diagnose intracranial disease, based primarily on changes observed in the skull or displacement of calcified structures such as the pineal gland, was pioneered in the first two decades of the 20th century. Although x-rays provided high-resolution images of electron-dense structures, such as bone or calcifications, diagnosis of abnormalities involving the contents of the skull was largely based on inference. The first major advance came with the observation that air introduced into the subarachnoid space allowed the visualization of the contour of the brain–air interface and, more important, was not toxic. This observation, initially made in a patient with traumatic pneumocephalus, led to the development of ventriculography and pneumoencephalography in the 1920s. These procedures were a central part of the armamentarium of the neuroradiologist until the advent of CT and MRI. The air-contrast procedures are now only historical notes, owing to the tremendous improvement in soft tissue definition and the noninvasive nature of CT and MRI.

Two other x-ray-based techniques that are still in current use are angiography (injection of a x-ray dense material into the blood) and myelography (injection of a x-ray dense material into the cerebrospinal fluid). Improvements in x-ray equipment and water-soluble contrast media supported the development of both procedures. Despite their invasive nature, the high resolution of x-ray images obtained with angiography or myelography is the primary reason that these procedures remain useful for the diagnosis of structural lesions in the age of CT and MRI.

Tremendous advances in computer technology led to the development of CT in the 1970s. CT images provide cross-sectional x-ray images of the brain, spine, and their coverings. It is from these radiological origins that the field of what may now be better termed "clinical or diagnostic neuroimaging" draws its name. MRI was introduced into clinical practice in the 1980s and represented a great leap forward in soft tissue contrast over CT.

These tools are primarily used for the definition of anatomy and structural lesions, such as hemorrhage, tumors, abscesses, and aneurysms. In addition to anatomical imaging, however, these and several other imaging modalities are also used for physiological measurements. Many of these applications, such as brain mapping with MRI techniques, remain investigational or research tools. Clinical applications of physiological imaging include Doppler ultrasound for the evaluation of arterial and venous pathology, positron emission tomography (PET) studies using fluorodeoxy glucose uptake for recurrent brain tumors or epileptogenic foci, and single photon emission computed tomography (SPECT) brain scans for relative blood flow.

IMAGING MODALITIES

Plain X-Ray Films

Plain x-ray films play a small role in modern neuroradiology. Although the resolution and detail obtained on plain films is greater than with CT or MR, the superior soft tissue contrast and multiplanar format of these techniques have led to the near complete retirement of plain radiography. The primary role of plain films in neuroradiology is in evaluation of bony pathology of the spine, particularly in the investigation of spinal trauma. In some trauma centers, CT has replaced plain films for the evaluation of the sinuses and for head trauma because the management of a patient with a skull fracture depends more on the presence or absence of intracranial pathology detected by CT than the simple presence or absence of a fracture.

Angiography

Conventional (x-ray) angiography provides high-resolution two-dimensional images of the arteries and veins of the head and neck (Fig. 1). Angiography is primarily used to identify abnormalities of these

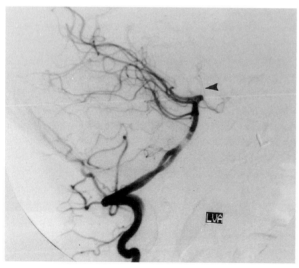

Figure 1
Conventional digital subtraction angiogram: lateral view of the head after injection of the left vertebral artery (LVA). Air and bony structures have been subtracted and all that remains on the image is the contrast media within the arteries. This is an early image in a series of images. Later images would show veins. Fine details, such as the perforating arteries of the thalamus, can be seen (arrowhead).

vessels, such as aneurysms, arteriovenous malformations, and atherosclerotic disease. It involves two major components: the introduction of contrast media into the vessel of interest and the acquisition of x-ray images before and after contrast injection. Conventional angiography provides the highest resolution and detail of normal and abnormal vascular anatomy of any of the currently available imaging tools. The limitations of this technique are primarily due to risks of placing catheters directly into the vessels of interest for the purpose of contrast media injection.

Myelography

Similar to angiography, myelography provides high-resolution images of the outlines of the thecal sac and its contents (normally nerve roots and spinal cord). It is primarily used to identify nerve root impingement from herniated intervertebral disk material. Contrast media is introduced into the cerebrospinal fluid of the subarachnoid space through a needle placed either in the lumbar spine or in the cervical spine (Fig. 2a). Conventional plain films, digital radiographs, or CT scans (Fig. 2b) are usually obtained after the injection of the contrast material. Myelography is generally reserved for patients in whom other less invasive imaging studies, such as CT and MR, are inconclusive.

Computed Tomography

CT provides cross-sectional x-ray images of the brain, spine, and their coverings. Although the resolution is less than that of plain films, the cross-sectional format and the soft tissue definition of CT are vastly superior (compare Figs. 2a and 2b). Hemorrhage within the skull is readily apparent, as are intracranial masses and ventricular enlargement. CT remains the procedure of choice for the diagnosis of acute hemorrhage, including both spontaneous and traumatic causes (Fig. 3a). Due to the availability of CT scanners in most emergency rooms and the ability to quickly scan unstable patients, CT plays a primary role in the evaluation of traumatic head injury and acute stroke. CT also remains particularly useful for the study of regions with important bony anatomy, such as the paranasal sinuses, the orbits, temporal bone and its contents, and the spine. Rapid scanning techniques have enabled the development of three-dimensional reconstructed images and CT angiography. The appropriate clinical uses for these special techniques are still under investigation.

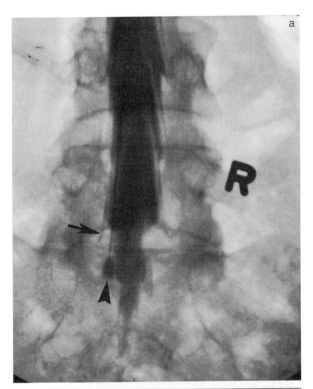

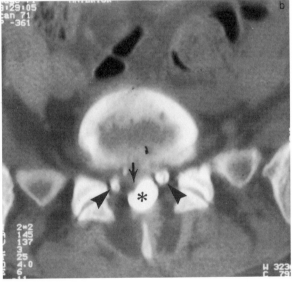

Figure 2
(a) Myelogram, anteroposterior projection: 48-year-old woman with radiating right leg pain in the distribution of the right S1 nerve root. Contrast media was injected through a needle placed in the L3/4 interspace (arrowhead indicates the contrast in the hub of the needle). Normal nerve roots are outlined by the contrast in the subarachnoid space. The left S1 nerve root (arrow) is outlined normally, whereas the right S1 nerve root is not seen. (b) CT scan after the myelogram at the L5/S1 level. Dense contrast is present within the cerebrospinal fluid-filled thecal sac (asterisk). Soft tissue is seen within the spinal canal, extending from the intervertebral disk, and indenting the thecal sac on the right (right and left are reversed on the CT relative to the myelogram) (arrow). The paired L5 nerve roots exit laterally without impingement. Both L5 nerve root sleeves are filled with contrast (arrowheads).

Magnetic Resonance

This technique does not require ionizing radiation, as do the preceding imaging tools. Rather, images are produced based on information regarding the differential effects of applied magnetic fields on different tissues. The MR signal from bone and air is minimal (signal void). Water-containing soft tissues are extremely well differentiated (e.g., gray matter from white) (Figs. 3b and 3c). Intravenous paramagnetic contrast agents are frequently used to help identify vascular structures and lesions with abnormal vascularity. Special noncontrast techniques have also been developed for MR angiography (Fig. 4) and myelography.

Owing to its superior soft tissue contrast (over CT) and three-dimensional capability, MR is the best technique for the evaluation of nearly all intra- and extraaxial lesions of the head and spine (Fig. 5). Consequently, MRI accounts for the majority of diagnostic neuroradiology procedures in most hospitals and outpatient clinics. Nevertheless, there are some situations in which MR is currently not the best tool, including the investigation of possible subarachnoid and intraparenchymal hemorrhage (CT), head trauma (CT), acute ventricular enlargement (hydrocephalus), and most bony abnormalities (CT). In addition, the study of abnormalities of the blood vessels is most accurately done with angiography. MR cannot be performed in patients with pacemakers or other devices or implants that may be affected by the strong magnetic fields.

Ultrasound

Ultrasound produces images from the differential ability of tissues to reflect sound waves back to the transducer. Gray-scale images are generated from this information. Sound waves are not transmitted well through bone or air. This limits the application of this noninvasive technology to investigations of the adult brain and spinal cord. Another widely used ultrasound method is the measurement of red blood cell velocity. The Doppler frequency shift is calculated from sound waves bouncing back from moving red cells in a blood vessel. Doppler ultrasound can be an extremely sensitive screening tool for the identification of narrowing or stenosis of the arteries of the neck (Fig. 6). For a given amount of blood flow, the velocity in a vessel will necessarily increase with reductions in vessel diameter. Transcranial Doppler sonography of the intracranial vessels is an important research tool for the investigation of cerebral hemodynamics. The Doppler techniques are the most common

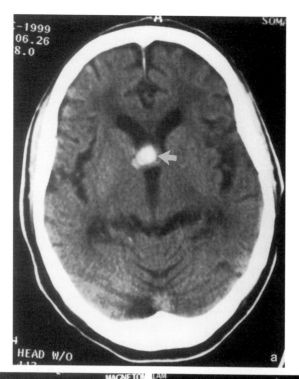

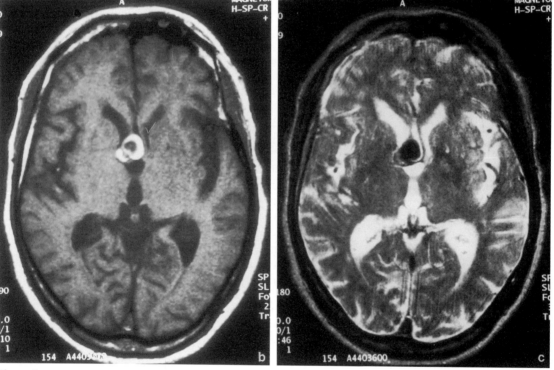

Figure 3

(a) CT scan of the head in an 89-year-old man with a hemorrhage associated with a cavernous hemangioma. This scan shows a high-attenuation (consistent with hemorrhage) mass near the midline in the region of the septum pellucidum (arrow). It is lobulated with a low-attenuation rim. Note the difference in attenuation (shown by different shades of gray) between the gray matter of the cortex and basal ganglia and the white matter. Cerebrospinal fluid in the ventricles and sulci is black, and bone is white. (b) T1-weighted axial MRI corresponding to Fig. 3a. Note the improved contrast between white and gray matter. The midline lesion shows increased signal on the periphery and reduced signal centrally. (c) T2-weighted image. Cerebrospinal fluid is white on T2-weighted images. Motion of the patient's head during the acquisition of this scan resulted in blurring of the image. The region of the cavernoma and hemorrhage is dark, representing signal loss due to distortion of the magnetic field. These findings are characteristic of blood products.

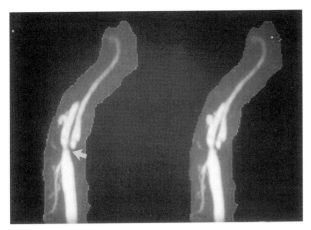

Figure 4
Magnetic resonance angiogram of a high-grade stenosis (arrow) of the origin of the internal carotid artery (courtesy of Drs. Willig and Turski, University of Wisconsin–Madison School of Medicine). (See color plate section.)

applications of ultrasound in adult neurological disease. Ophthalmological use of ultrasound for the investigation of the globe and retina is also common. In infants, before closure of the fontanels, ultrasound is a useful method for the diagnosis of intracranial pathology, such as hydrocephalus or hemorrhage.

Single-Photon Emission Computed Tomography

With SPECT imaging (and PET), the image is obtained from radioactivity coming from inside the patient rather than passing through the patient (as with CT or conventional x-ray techniques). The major advantage of this technology is that specific physiological processes can be imaged and measured by attaching radiotracers to different molecules. Clinical applications include the detection of cerebrospinal fluid leaks and the measurement of relative cerebral blood flow or blood volume.

Positron Emission Tomography

PET employs positron-emitting radiotracers rather than photon-emitting radiotracers, as with SPECT. Current clinical applications of PET include the evaluation of epileptogenic foci in patients with medically intractable seizure disorders and the distinction between recurrent brain tumor and radiation necrosis.

DISEASE CATEGORIES

A systematic approach to the review of anatomical imaging studies (primarily MR and CT) is a useful

exercise. If a lesion is identified, the purpose of most diagnostic procedures is to generate a list of the most likely causes in order to focus and guide subsequent patient care. After identifying the location and extent of a lesion (or lesions), the effect on adjacent normal structures (mass effect), the signal intensity (MR) or density (CT) of the lesion, as well as the presence and location of contrast enhancement should be described. This information is important in determining the nature of a particular lesion. For example, fat and blood products have distinctive signal characteristics on MRI. With this information in mind, the broad categories of pathological entities discussed in the following sections are considered, and then a list of possible etiologies is generated.

Neoplasms

The first issue in the neuroradiological evaluation of a tumor is determining the location of the lesion. The location of a neoplasm is critical in establishing the list of possible etiologies (the differential diagnosis). For example, a meningioma might be a possible cause for an extraaxial (of the skull or meninges) neoplasm, but not an intraaxial (of the brain

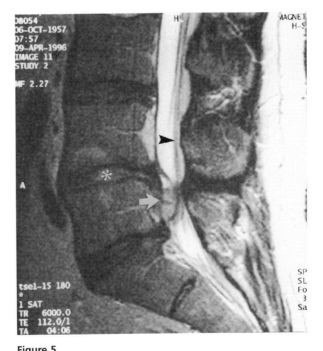

Figure 5
Sagittal T2-weighted image of the lower lumbar spine showing a large herniated disk from the L4/5 interspace. The cerebrospinal fluid is white, and nerve roots can be seen within the thecal sac (arrowhead). The extruded disk (arrow) is hanging down below the disk space (asterisk) and completely occupies the space of the canal.

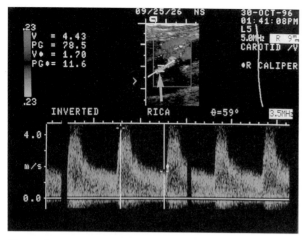

Figure 6
Color Doppler ultrasound of a high-grade stenosis of the right internal carotid artery. The Doppler cursor (arrow) is placed at the site of the highest velocity. The waveform on the lower aspect of the figure shows high peak systolic velocities, consistent with a high-grade stenosis, and high diastolic flow rates, characteristic of the low-resistance cerebral circulation. (See color plate section.)

parenchyma) tumor. In addition, some tumors are specific to certain locations, such as pituitary adenomas, germinomas of the pineal gland, and optic nerve gliomas. The second issue is to determine the extent of the mass and the structures involved by the tumor. Some tumors have no mass effect on surrounding structures and are found only by differences in tissue water content or contrast enhancement from normal surrounding brain.

Although some features on imaging studies are often suggestive of a specific type of neoplasm, the definitive distinction of different tumors from one another is usually not possible. This is particularly true of intraaxial tumors. Metastatic tumor and malignant gliomas often have a similar appearance. Biopsy is required for a tissue diagnosis. Important features to identify in the imaging investigation of tumors, in addition to the location and extent of the mass, include the presence of other parenchymal or meningeal lesions (suggesting metastatic disease) and secondary effects of the tumors, such as hydrocephalus or mass effect on critical structures.

The identification and localization of brain tumors are best accomplished with MRI. The superior tissue contrast afforded by this technique allows better definition of the tumor and its extent than CT provides. CT can be useful in situations in which the presence of hydrocephalus or hemorrhage is suspected. Another specific application of CT is to investigate the effect of a neoplasm on the bony

cranium or skull base. MR shows bone only as signal void (except for the cellular marrow). CT better determines bony remodeling or bone destruction.

Physiological imaging of brain tumors is currently limited to studies of tumor metabolism by PET. Some patients develop symptoms in a delayed fashion (months) after radiation to the brain (high-dose radiation is frequently used as an adjunct to surgical or chemotherapy for some brain tumors). The clinical and imaging appearance of radiation necrosis is similar to that of recurrent tumor. The two entities can be distinguished by the degree of uptake of fluorodeoxy glucose because recurrent tumors are metabolically active.

Infectious Disease

The imaging findings regarding infection of the central nervous system will depend on the location of the infection, the acuity of the infection, and, to a lesser extent, the specific pathogen. The immune status of the host will also affect both imaging findings and the likelihood of certain pathogens. Infections can invade the central nervous system in a limited number of ways, including direct extension of paranasal sinus infections through the bone to the epidural space, blood-borne to vessels (mycotic aneurysms or septic emboli) and secondarily to brain parenchyma (abscess), and into the subarachnoid space from either of these locations (meningitis).

Both CT and MR are commonly used to investigate patients suspected of having parenchymal or epidural abscesses. Parenchymal abscesses often appear similar to brain tumors, with central nonenhancing material (pus and cellular debris), a thick ring of enhancement (granulation tissue), and surrounding edema. An epidural abscess appears as fluid in the epidural space. Patients with meningitis are frequently found to have enhancement of the leptomeninges (pia and arachnoid).

Vascular Disease

Neuroradiology plays a role in imaging both the parenchymal consequences of vascular disease (ischemic stroke and hemorrhage) and the etiological causes of these events (aneurysms and vascular malformations, atherosclerotic disease, or other vascular causes).

The appearance of ischemic stroke on imaging studies changes over time. The first detectable change is restricted diffusion of water on special MR sequences. Increased tissue water can be seen within hours of ischemia on MR and less frequently on CT.

Currently, the primary use of imaging studies during the first few hours of a stroke is to make certain that the symptoms are not due to intracerebral hemorrhage. Within days, swelling of the infarcted tissue occurs, followed by atrophy and gliosis.

Emboli from atherosclerotic plaque are the most frequent cause of ischemic stroke. Severe stenosis at the common carotid bifurcation is common in patients presenting with ischemic symptoms. Surgical endarterectomy is highly effective in reducing the risk of future stroke in these patients. A smaller but significant benefit of endarterectomy has also been proven for patients with severe stenosis and no symptoms. For these reasons, patients with symptoms of ischemia or clinical evidence suggesting carotid stenosis are commonly evaluated with imaging tools to determine the presence and degree of narrowing of the arteries in the neck. Doppler ultrasound can be an excellent screening tool for this purpose. In laboratories with documented quality control (done by directly comparing Doppler results to angiography in a large number of patients), patients with normal or only mild degrees of stenosis can be reliably identified and excluded from further workup. Patients with increased velocities require angiography for the accurate measurement of stenosis. The relationship between blood velocity and luminal stenosis (the gold standard measurement on which the outcome for surgical endarterectomy was proven) is not linear. Many patients with high velocities have only mild stenoses. MR techniques for the evaluation of carotid stenosis are rapidly developing. These techniques are being evaluated for use as screening examinations as well. Other causes of ischemic stroke that can be identified by angiography include arterial dissection, venous thrombosis, and vasculitis.

The appearance of hemorrhage depends on several factors, including the location (intraparenchymal versus subarachnoid), the time from the initial hemorrhage to imaging, and the hematocrit. On CT, acute hemorrhage will appear dense (white), unless the patient's hematocrit is very low. During the following days and weeks, the density of the hematoma generally decreases. This process is more rapid in the subarachnoid space. On MR, parenchymal clot is evident within minutes on some experimental sequences, but it may take hours for distinctive signal characteristics to develop. The evolution of the signal from clot on MR primarily depends on the paramagnetic effects of different iron-bearing molecules related to hemoglobin. When hemorrhage is found on CT or MR, the images should be carefully reviewed for clues regarding the etiology. Evidence for an underlying tumor (including edema, evidence of prior bleeding, or contrast enhancement), vascular malformation, or other lesions (suggesting a multifocal process, such as septic emboli, vasculitis, or metastatic disease) can sometimes be identified and lead to a specific diagnosis.

Many causes of hemorrhage, including hypertensive hemorrhages and bleeding diatheses, cannot be distinguished on imaging studies. Important causes of hemorrhage that can be identified with angiography include aneurysms, vascular malformations, venous thrombosis, and vasculitis. MR techniques for the determination of venous thrombosis have been developed. Angiography, with its superior resolution, remains the procedure of choice for the diagnosis of all these lesions, with the possible exception of venous thrombosis.

Degenerative Disease

This category includes disorders that lead to the selective and progressive loss of neurons. One common neurodegenerative disorder is Parkinson's disease, which affects nigrostriatal neurons. Imaging does not often play a primary role in the diagnosis of these diseases, which are generally diagnosed by clinical examination and history. However, the pattern of neuronal loss and resultant atrophy observed on imaging studies such as CT or MR may suggest a specific and unsuspected disorder. Huntington's disease selectively affects the caudate nucleus, leading to focal atrophy. Wilson's disease leads to an abnormal increase in magnetic susceptibility effects in the basal ganglia.

Demylinating Diseases

Primary and secondary demylinating diseases damage or destroy myelin sheaths. The most commonly encountered of these diseases is multiple sclerosis (MS). Imaging plays an important role in the diagnosis and treatment of this disease. Focal regions of abnormal signal in the periventricular white matter of young patients are the most common finding. In a patient with a first or equivocal neurological deficit, distinctive periventricular lesions of different MR signal characteristics can strongly suggest the diagnosis of MS. The progression or regression of the lesions with medical therapy can be monitored with MR. Because many lesions are not clinically symptomatic, MR may provide a secondary endpoint for trials of therapy.

Dysmyelinating Disease

These diseases become manifest through abnormal production or maintenance of myelin. Many of these diseases have characteristic appearances on MR, including metachromatic leukodystrophy, adrenoleukodystrophy, and Canavan's disease.

Congenital

Congenital disorders include a broad range of developmental abnormalities, such as migrational disorders, neurocutaneous syndromes (e.g., neurofibromatosis), and severe developmental anomalies such as holoprosencephaly.

Trauma

Trauma to the head and spine from blunt injury (motor vehicle accidents or falls) or from penetrating injury (knifes and gunshot wounds) often requires investigation with imaging to assess the damage to internal structures. CT scans are used in the emergency room to detect intracranial hemorrhage and fractures of facial bones, skull, and spine. The information from these scans is used to determine if emergency surgery is necessary. Three-dimensional reformatted images are often useful for fracture investigation. Plain films are used to screen for cervical spine injury.

Spine

Degenerative disease accounts for most pathology encountered in the spine, including nerve root impingement by a herniated intervertebral disk, stenosis of the spinal canal, and other degenerative changes of the bone structures surrounding the thecal sac. MR, CT, and myelography all play a role in the investigation of degenerative disease. Myelography is useful for assessing nerve root impingement or spinal stenosis. Compression of the thecal sac or the dural sleeve surrounding a nerve root as it leaves the spinal canal can be identified with high resolution. CT scans can yield complementary information regarding the nature of the extradural compression (e.g., degenerative hypertrophy of a facet joint or a herniated disk). MR scans provide better soft tissue contrast. The investigation of intradural pathology is primarily done with MR.

Head and Neck

CT and MR are valuable extensions of the clinical examination for the investigation of head and neck tumors. They are frequently used to determine the local extent of carcinoma and to detect the presence of involved lymph nodes. This information is important for clinical staging and therapeutic planning. Another application is in the evaluation of cranial neuropathies. Structural lesions such as metastatic tumors to the skull base may be responsible for focal cranial nerve deficits.

EVALUATION OF DIAGNOSTIC TESTS

The goal of the practice of medicine is to improve the outcome of patients. This may be through prolonging meaningful life, relief of pain, or other improvement in the functional status of the patient. Increasingly, clinical trials of therapeutic interventions are being judged by their effect on patient outcome. Diagnostic tests are being held to a similar standard: Does the use of a particular imaging test to answer a particular clinical question lead to an improvement in patient outcome? The field of outcome-based research for diagnostic imaging is still in its infancy.

—Colin P. Derdeyn

See also–Angiography; Computerized Axial Tomography (CAT); Magnetic Resonance Angiography (MRA); Magnetic Resonance Imaging (MRI); Neuroimaging, Overview; Physiological Brain Imaging; Positron Emission Tomography (PET); Single-Photon Emission Computed Tomography (SPECT); Ultrasound, Carotid; Ultrasound, Transcranial Doppler

Further Reading

Connors, J. J., 3rd, and Wojak, J. C. (1998). *Interventional Neuroradiology: Strategies and Practical Techniques.* Saunders, Philadelphia.
Grossman, R. I., and Yousem, D. M. (1994). *Neuroradiology: The Requisites.* Mosby-Year Book, St. Louis.
Osborn, A. G. (1994). *Diagnostic Neuroradiology.* Mosby-Year Book, St. Louis.
Taveras, J. M., and Wood, E. H. (1964). *Diagnostic Neuroradiology.* Williams & Wilkins, Baltimore.

Neurosarcoidosis
see Sarcoidosis

Neurosyphilis

Encyclopedia of the Neurological Sciences
Copyright 2003, Elsevier Science (USA). All rights reserved.

SYPHILIS was initially described in Europe in the latter part of the 15th century. Its origin remains shrouded in mystery. Whether it was imported to Europe from the Americas during early exploration or whether it arose from a spontaneous mutation in an endemic treponeme remains the subject of historical controversy. Although known to be a communicable disease, the experiments of John Hunter resulted in confusion regarding the difference between gonorrhea and syphilis. Hunter infected himself with both *N. gonorrhoeae* and *Treponema pallidum*, thereby confusing the clinical distinction of these diseases.

Schaudinn and Hoffmann identified this almost transparent, spiral-shaped organism, which they called *Spirochaeta pallida*. Landsteiner's introduction of dark-field microscopy permitted observations of the organism in the meninges and brain, and at the same time serological tests for syphilis employing a basic lipoidal antigen were first reported by Wasserman, Neisser, and Bruck. However, a specific treponemal test, the *T. pallidum* immobilization, was not available until 1949.

The modern treatment of syphilis began in 1943 with the introduction of penicillin. Despite effective antibiotic therapy and the implementation of contact tracing, rates of syphilis at the dawn of the AIDS epidemic approached those observed in the years preceding World War II. Although the frequency of syphilis in the developed world has since begun to decline, it is an illness for which the physician must remain ever vigilant.

EPIDEMIOLOGY

Although the annual incidence of syphilis in the United States declined 18-fold from a peak of 72 cases per 100,000 in 1943 to 4 per 100,000 in 1956, the incidence increased dramatically during the early years of the AIDS epidemic. However, it has since declined. In 1998, a total of 6993 primary and secondary syphilis cases were reported to the Centers for Disease Control (CDC). Between 1990 and 1998, the primary and secondary syphilis rate declined 86% from 20.3 to 2.6 cases/100,000 population, which is the lowest level since reporting began in 1941. However, the illness affects certain groups within the U.S. population disproportionately. For instance, rates remain significantly higher in the South and among non-Hispanic blacks.

The frequency with which neurosyphilis complicates HIV infection likely parallels nationwide trends of syphilis prevalence. Initially, prevalence rates of neurosyphilis defined by a reactive cerebrospinal fluid

(CSF) Venereal Disease Research Laboratory (VDRL) test were between 1.0 and 2.0% for several large cohorts of HIV-seropositive individuals in the United States. This prevalence rate was substantially higher if only patients with serological evidence of syphilis were included. In one study, 9.1% of HIV-infected patients undergoing lumbar puncture because of a reactive serology and having no history of recent treatment for syphilis had a reactive CSF VDRL. Conversely, HIV seroprevalence is high in patients with syphilis, with rates varying between 15.7% for women and 27.5% for men. Neurosyphilis needs to be considered in the differential diagnosis of any neurological disease in an HIV-infected person.

PATHOGENESIS

Treponema pallidum, the bacterium that causes syphilis, is a long, slender, coil-shaped organism that measures 6–15 μm in length but only 0.15 μm in width, a dimension below the resolution of light microscopy. The organism has regular spirals numbering 5–20 and is actively motile, using a rotational screw-like activity, flexion, and back-and-forth motion. The organism has an amorphous coat of mucopolysaccharides, an outer membrane, an electron-dense peptidoglycan layer, and a cytoplasmic membrane revealed by electron microscopy. Three flagella extending from each end of the organism are located between the outer membrane and the electron-dense layer. These flagella twist around the body of the organism and provide the spiral shape of the organism and its mode of locomotion. Morphological, antigenic, and extensive DNA homology has been demonstrated between *T. pallidum* and the pathogens responsible for yaws and pinta, *T. pertenue* and *T. carateum*, respectively. Cultivation of *T. pallidum in vitro* is difficult and it is exquisitely fragile, rendering its study difficult. Animal studies are generally necessitated and the rabbit has proved to be the best animal model.

Following inoculation, the organism invades interstitial spaces and proliferates there. The organism has a relatively long doubling time of 30–33 hr. Soon after infection, a spirochetemia results with dissemination of *T. pallidum* to virtually every organ, including the central nervous system (CNS). Both humoral and cellular immunity play a role in the ensuing infection. Although antibodies to *T. pallidum* are detectable within 10–21 days of infection, the humoral response appears to be of little value in suppressing the infection. Effective control of the infection as evidenced by studies of rechallenge appears to reside with cellular immunity. Impairment of cellular immunity due to drugs, pregnancy, AIDS, etc., results in a more aggressive syphilitic infection than otherwise anticipated.

Detectable abnormalities of the CSF occur in 16–48% of all patients with early (primary or secondary) syphilis, indicating early invasion of the CNS by the organism. Viable treponemes are recoverable from the CSF in these early stages of infection. In the absence of the development of CSF abnormalities, neurosyphilis does not seem to occur. Merritt stated that "if the CSF is normal 2 or more years after infection, it will always remain so, and parenchymatous neurosyphilis will never develop," but the converse is not true because CSF abnormalities do not necessarily predict the development of neurosyphilis. In the Oslo study of the natural course of untreated syphilis, 9.4% of men and 5.0% of women ultimately developed neurosyphilis, and in the Tuskegee study 4% of survivors of untreated syphilis had neurosyphilis after a 20-year follow-up and 3% had it at 30 years. To date, there remains no satisfactory explanation for the lack of universal invasion of the CNS by T. pallidum, nor is there an explanation for the absence of neurosyphilis in the majority of individuals who manifest CSF abnormalities indicative of CNS invasion.

The pathology of neurosyphilis is the consequence of the invasion of the CNS by T. pallidum and the associated immunological response. In syphilitic meningitis, the earliest neurological complication of syphilis, invasion of the meninges by the spirochete results in an infiltration of the meninges by lymphocytes and, to a much smaller degree, plasma cells. This cellular infiltration may follow blood vessels into the brainstem and spinal cord along the Virchow–Robin spaces. Necrosis of the media and proliferation of the intima of small meningeal vessels accompanies T. pallidum invasion of the vessel walls.

Late stages of neurosyphilis can be classified as meningovascular and parenchymatous disease. In the former, the inflammation observed parallels that seen with syphilitic meningitis. The classic lesion is an endarteritis obliterans of medium and large vessels first described by Huebner in 1874. Fibroblastic thickening of the intima and thinning of the media characterize this lesion. Vasculitis in small vessels is referred to as Nissl–Alzheimer arteritis. The lesions of the brain and spinal cord occur as a secondary event. Gummas, which are thick, tough, rubbery lesions of fibrous trabecula with lymphocytic and plasma cell infiltration of the outer layers, varying in size from microscopic to mass-producing lesions, are occasionally noted.

The prototypical, although currently seldom seen, forms of neurosyphilis, tabes dorsalis and general paresis, typify parenchymatous neurosyphilis. The pathology of tabes dorsalis predominates in the dorsal roots and posterior columns of the lumbosacral and lower thoracic levels. Lymphocytic infiltration of the meninges occurs with these degenerative changes. The exact pathogenesis remains uncertain, but irreversible changes in the dorsal root fibers are believed to play a major role in the clinical manifestations of the disease. In general paresis, the brain is atrophic and the meninges thickened. The cerebral cortex, striatum, and hypothalamus are most severely affected. Neuronal loss and astrocytic and microglial proliferation are seen histopathologically. Treponema pallidum can be demonstrated in the cerebral cortex. Ependymal granulations are commonly observed and the meningeal inflammation is composed mainly of plasma cells.

CLINICAL FEATURES

Infection with T. pallidum is divided into several stages. Primary syphilis, the initial manifestation of infection, is an ulcerated, painless lesion with firm borders referred to as a chancre. This lesion develops at the site of epidermal or mucous membrane inoculation and is accompanied by regional lymphadenopathy. This lesion occurs approximately 3 weeks (range, 3–90 days) after infection, with time of latency dependent on the size of the inoculum. Although the lesion is a local manifestation, the spirochetes, even at this early stage, disseminate systemically as evidenced by the ability to transmit syphilis by blood donation from incubating seronegative donors and the presence of detectable T. pallidum in the CSF of a substantial percentage of infected persons.

Typically within 2–8 weeks of the appearance of the chancre, the features of secondary syphilis appear, characterized by a macular, maculopapular, or pustular rash that often involves the palms and soles, mucous patches, alopecia, diffuse adenopathy, iridocyclitis, hepatitis, periostitis, and arthritis. These features are attributable to the bacteremic phase of the illness and are accompanied by a brisk immune response.

Latent syphilis, a quiescent phase of syphilis that precedes the development of tertiary complications, is divided into early (<2 years of infection) and late (>2 years) stages to reflect the probability of recurrence of secondary syphilitic manifestations. Tertiary syphilis is characterized mainly by skin, osseous, cardiovascular, and neurological complications, with clinically apparent neurological complications affecting less than 10% of untreated patients.

Neurosyphilis is simply the occurrence of neurological complications due to infection with *T. pallidum*. It may occur during early or late syphilis. The spectrum of clinical illness associated with neurosyphilis is exceptionally broad. Virtually any region of the CNS may be involved, and it is not uncommon for some forms of neurosyphilis to overlap with others in a given patient.

The most common form of neurosyphilis currently diagnosed is asymptomatic neurosyphilis. Typically, serological evidence of syphilis prompts CSF analysis in the absence of neurological symptoms. These patients are at risk for developing symptomatic disease.

Among the symptomatic disorders of neurosyphilis, the earliest to manifest is syphilitic meningitis. Syphilitic meningitis often occurs within the first 12 months of infection and may be accompanied by features of secondary syphilis. Although the majority of patients with CSF abnormalities occurring in association with secondary syphilis are neurologically asymptomatic, approximately 5% of all patients with secondary syphilis will have acute meningitis. Confusion, lethargy, seizures, aphasia, and hemiplegia may be observed in association with syphilitic meningitis. Focal neurological findings are believed to be the consequence of associated vascular injury. As many as 40% of patients with secondary syphilis will exhibit headaches, meningismus, impaired vision, cranial nerve palsies (in descending order of frequency—VII, VIII, VI, and II), hearing loss, tinnitus, and vertigo in isolation or combination.

Meningovascular syphilis may affect the brain or spinal cord. It typically occurs 6 to 7 years after the initial infection, but it may occur as early as 6 months after the primary infection. Clinical manifestations are dependent on the area of the brain or spinal cord that is affected. The neurological manifestations include aphasia, hemiparesis, hemianesthesia, diplopia, vertigo, dysarthria, and a variety of brainstem syndromes. Many of the eponymous stroke syndromes of the brainstem described in the 19th century (e.g., Weber's, Claude's, and Nothnagel's) were descriptions of patients with meningovascular syphilis. In contrast to atherosclerotic cerebrovascular disease, these lesions were often very discrete due to the involvement of an isolated artery.

A large spectrum of spinal cord disorders are seen in association with syphilis (Table 1). Tabes dorsalis is the prototypical disorder, but it is very rare. Tabes is a parenchymatous form of neurosyphilis and typically has a latency from the time of infection of 15–30 years. The most distinctive and often heralding symptom is lightning-like pains that may be triggered by touch and most often affect the legs and abdomen. Pupillary abnormalities are observed in more than 90% of patients, with the hallmark abnormality being Argyll–Robertson pupils (miotic, irregular pupils exhibiting light-near dissociation). The gait is ataxic with a foot-stomping character due to an associated impaired position sense. Romberg initially described the sign that bears his name— imbalance on a narrow base with eyes closed—in a patient with tabes dorsalis. Impaired sensory perception leads to Charcot joints; painless swelling of joints, particularly the knees and ankles, due to repeated trauma; and perforating ulcers of the toes and soles of the feet. Lower extremity reflexes are absent, and sexual and sphincter dysfunction is observed.

Syphilitic meningomyelitis is perhaps the most common spinal syndrome currently complicating syphilis. It is characterized by slowly progressive weakness of the lower extremities accompanied by paresthesia. Eventually, bowel and bladder incontinence and paraplegia supervene. Spastic paraparesis or paraplegia and impaired sensory perception (disproportionate loss of vibratory and position sense) are found on physical examination. An acute infarction in the territory of the anterior spinal artery secondary to a syphilitic arteritis results in paraplegia with loss of pain and temperature sensation below

Table 1 SYPHILIS OF THE SPINAL CORD

Syphilitic meningomyelitis
Syphilitic spinal pachymeningitis
   Spinal cord gumma
   Syphilitic hypertrophic pachymeningitis
Spinal vascular syphilis
Syphilitic poliomyelitis
Tabes dorsalis
Miscellaneous
   Syringomyelia
   Syphilitic aortic aneurysm
   Charcot vertebra with compression of the spinal cord

the level of the lesion, with preservation of vibratory and position sense.

General paresis is a manifestation of parenchymatous neurosyphilis and, like tabes dorsalis, usually develops after a long (15- to 30-year) hiatus from the time of infection. In the preantibiotic era, general paresis accounted for a substantial percentage of psychiatric illness. In a recent study from South Africa, general paresis was found in 1.3% of all patients admitted for acute psychiatric care. Dementia and psychiatric disturbances, including emotional lability, paranoia, delusions of grandeur, hallucinations, and inappropriate behavior, are the hallmarks of general paresis. Tremors of the tongue and extremities, hyper-reflexia, hypomimetic facies, dysarthria, chorioretinitis, optic neuritis, and pupillary abnormalities including Argyll–Robertson pupils are seen. On cranial magnetic resonance imaging, frontal and temporal atrophy, subcortical gliosis, and increased ferritin in the basal ganglia have been seen in patients with general paresis.

Gummas of the nervous system are present as space-occupying lesions. Progressive focal neurological manifestations, seizures, and increased intracranial pressure complicate gummas of the brain. Brain computed tomography and cranial magnetic resonance often show a dural-based, enhancing lesion with associated mass effect. Gummas affecting the cervical spinal cord result in progressive quadriparesis, and those in the thoracic area result in progressive paraparesis.

Concomitant human immunodeficiency virus infection appears to significantly alter the natural history of neurosyphilis. Syphilis is more aggressive and may be more difficult to treat in the setting of immunodeficiency. These observations indicate the importance of the host's immune response in controlling this infection. The impairment in cell-mediated immunity may contribute to a more rapid progression of neurosyphilis in HIV-infected individuals than would otherwise be expected. However, serum nontreponemal (VDRL) titers at the time of presentation of neurosyphilis in the HIV-infected individual are typically high, averaging 1–128. Lukehart and colleagues demonstrated that *T. pallidum* could be isolated from the CSF of HIV-seropositive patients with primary, secondary, and latent syphilis following currently recommended CDC penicillin therapy. Syphilis should always be considered with acute and chronic meningitis in the HIV-infected patient. Unusual manifestations of syphilis reported in association with HIV infection include unexplained fever, bilateral optic neuritis with blindness, Bell's palsy, severe bilateral sensorineural hearing loss, syphilitic meningomyelitis, syphilitic polyradiculopathy, and syphilitic cerebral gumma presenting as a mass lesion.

In addition to the Argyll–Robertson pupil, other ophthalmological conditions associated with *T. pallidum* infection include interstitial keratitis, chorioretinitis, and optic atrophy. The latter is commonly unilateral and may occur with or without associated basilar meningitis. Otitic syphilis results in hearing loss (either acute or gradually progressive) and vertigo. Syphilitic damage of the eighth cranial nerve is a late manifestation of congenital syphilis, but it may occur with acquired illness.

DIAGNOSIS

There is no readily applicable gold standard for the diagnosis of neurosyphilis, and culturing this fragile organism from the CSF is cumbersome, of low sensitivity, and can be performed in only a few laboratories. In patients with neurosyphilis, the diagnosis is generally dependent on serological study. There are two categories of serological study: nontreponemal tests, which are flocculation tests using cardiolipin, lecithin, and cholesterol as antigen, and treponemal tests, which rely on specific treponemal cellular components as antigens. Nontreponemal tests include the VDRL test, rapid plasma reagin, Wasserman, and Kolmer tests. The treponemal tests include the fluorescent treponemal antibody absorption test, microhemagglutination assay, hemagglutination treponemal test for syphilis, and the treponemal immobilization test.

The presence of a reactive VDRL test in the CSF is quite specific, with rare reports of false positivity. The test is too insensitive, however, to exclude the diagnosis of neurosyphilis on the basis of a negative study. As many as one-fourth of patients with neurosyphilis are anticipated to have a negative serum VDRL. Its frequency of reactivity appears to vary with the clinical form of neurosyphilis, and its presence in asymptomatic neurosyphilis may be substantially lower than in symptomatic disease. The CSF VDRL is too insensitive to be relied on to exclude the diagnosis of neurosyphilis. For instance, in one study, *T. pallidum* was isolated from CSF in 12 (30%) of 40 patients with primary and secondary syphilis, but the CSF VDRL was positive in only 4 (33%) of these 12 patients. Therefore, measures other than a reactive CSF VDRL must be relied upon to establish the diagnosis of neurosyphilis. To date, there is no consensus regarding diagnostic criteria, and the physician should probably refrain from rigid adherence to narrow guidelines in making the diagnosis. However, a cardinal requirement for the diagnosis of neurosyphilis is a reactive serum treponemal test.

Neurosyphilis should be diagnosed in persons with reactive specific treponemal serologies occurring in association with a reactive CSF VDRL. A diagnosis of neurosyphilis should be considered in patients with serological evidence of syphilis and one or more of the following abnormalities in their CSF: a mononuclear pleocytosis, an elevated protein, increased IgG, or the presence of oligocional bands. Using these criteria, neurosyphilis is undoubtedly overdiagnosed. The value of the CSF FTA-ABS remains controversial. Unlike the CSF VDRL, which requires gross blood contamination of the CSF to be rendered falsely positive, small amounts of blood contamination may give rise to false-positive FTA-ABS test results. Furthermore, the FTA is a test for IgG antibody that may be of sufficiently small size to cross the blood–brain barrier and result in a false-positive CSF FTA-ABS. Various formulas using titers of specific treponemal tests from CSF and serum have been proposed but have not been widely adopted. Newer generation tests for syphilis and neurosyphilis, particularly those employing the polymerase chain reaction and monoclonal antibodies, may solve this dilemma, but further study is required before widespread application.

Coinfection with HIV considerably complicates the interpretation of CSF abnormalities because a mononuclear pleocytosis, increased protein, increased IgG, and the presence of oligoclonal bands may all attend HIV infection in the absence of neurosyphilis. A schema has been proposed for the diagnosis of neurosyphilis in the face of HIV infection (Table 2).

Although not diagnostic of neurosyphilis, radiological studies may be helpful in excluding other pathologies. The radiological manifestations of neurosyphilis include meningeal enhancement, hydrocephalus, gummas, periostitis, generalized cerebral atrophy, and stroke. Gummas are avascular, dural-based masses with surrounding edema that on magnetic resonance imaging are characteristically isointense, with gray matter on T1-weighted image and hyperintense on T2-weighted image. These lesions are typically densely contrast enhancing. Angiography of neurosyphilis is nonspecific. Large

Table 2 DIAGNOSING NEUROSYPHILIS IN THE FACE OF HIV INFECTION

Definite neurosyphilis
  +Blood treponemal serology (e.g., FTA-ABS and MHA-TP)
  +CSF VDRL

Probable neurosyphilis
  +Blood treponemal serology
  −CSF VDRL
  CSF monocuclear pleocytosis (>20 cells/mm^3)
  or
  −CSF protein (>60 mg/dl)

Neurological complications compatible with neurosyphilis, such as cranial nerve palsies, stroke, etc., or evidence of ophthalmic signs of syphilis (Argyll–Robertson pupils, optic atrophy, interstitial keratitis, and chorioretinitis)

Possible neurosyphilis
  +Blood treponemal serology
  −CSF VDRL
  CSF monocuclear pleocytosis (>20 cells/mm^3)
  or
  +CSF protein (>60 mg/dl)

No neurological or ophthalmological complications compatible with syphilis

vessels show segmental constriction or occlusion; smaller vessels, usually Sylvian branches of the middle cerebral artery, have focal stenoses with or without adjacent dilatation.

Neurosyphilis presents in variegate fashions and there is ample truth to the clinical adage of William Osier: "Know syphilis in all its manifestations and relations, and all things clinical will be added unto you." Neurosyphilis always needs to be considered in the differential diagnosis of the following disorders: acute meningitis; stroke, particularly in young people; progressive dementia; psychoses and behavioral disturbances; myelopathy; optic neuritis; chorioretinitis; and sensorineural hearing loss.

TREATMENT

Treponema pallidum is highly sensitive to penicillin. The treponemicidal level of penicillin is 0.03 μg/ml. Although the organism is capable of acquiring plasmids that produce penicillinase, there is no compelling evidence to suggest that penicillin loses its efficacy. When penicillin levels become subtherapeutic, the spirochetes begin regenerating within 18–24 hr. The CDC has recommended using 2.4 million units of benzathine penicillin intramuscularly at weekly intervals for 3 weeks in the treatment of neurosyphilis, but the recordable penicillin levels in the CSF during treatment fail to reach treponemicidal levels. The concentration of penicillin in the CSF is typically unmeasurable, probably not exceeding 0.0005 µg/ml, which is 1 or 2% of the serum levels. Furthermore, viable treponemes have been recovered from the CSF of individuals at the completion of therapy. Another recommended regimen that may also fail to achieve treponemicidal levels of penicillin in the CSF is procaine penicillin, 600,000 units intramuscularly daily for 15 days. Ideally, the treatment regimen for neurosyphilis should be 12–24 million units of crystalline aqueous penicillin administered intravenously daily (2–4 million units every 4 hr) for a period of 10–14 days. The penicillin should be administered at no less than 4-hr intervals to maintain the consistent levels at or above treponemicidal values. An alternative approach that achieves CSF treponemicidal levels is the daily oral administration of amoxicillin (3.0 g) and probenecid (0.5 g administered twice daily) for 15 days. In patients who are allergic to penicillin, erythromycin (500 mg four times daily for 30 days) has been recommended, but it does not diffuse readily into the brain and CSF and has no established efficacy in the treatment of neurosyphilis. Similarly, oral therapy with tetracycline yields very low CSF tetracycline concentrations and has unproven efficacy in the treatment of neurosyphilis. The successful use of intravenous ceftriaxone, 2 g daily for 10 days, and oral doxycycline, 200 mg twice daily for 21 days, has been reported.

The Jarisch–Herxheimer reaction, a systemic reaction to the rapid dissolution of treponemes, is characterized by the abrupt onset of fever and chills, headache, tachycardia, flushing, myalgias, and mild hypotension and may occur within several hours of the initiation of treatment in patients with meningovascular syphilis. Some authorities have recommended the administration of prednisone, 60 mg during the initial 24 hr, when symptoms of the Jarisch–Herxheimer reaction appear.

MONITORING THERAPY

Determining the adequacy of therapy depends on careful follow-up of the patient. Conversion of the serum VDRL or RPR to nonreactive should occur within 1 year after treatment of primary syphilis, within 2 years after treatment of secondary syphilis, and within 5 years after treatment of latent syphilis. This delay to reversion from a seropositive status reflects the duration and severity of the illness. Persistent seropositivity suggests persistent infection, reinfection, or a biological false-positive test.

The fixed neurological deficits of neurosyphilis may fail to improve with treatment, and some abnormalities, such as tabes dorsalis and optic atrophy, may worsen despite adequate therapy. Resolution of CSF abnormalities is the best determinant for the adequacy of treatment. Examination of the CSF within several days of the institution of penicillin treatment may be misleading because the CSF cell count may increase initially, particularly if accompanied by a Jarisch–Herxheimer reaction. However, the CSF should be examined at the termination of treatment to document a decrease in cell count, and it should then be examined at 6-month intervals for 2 or 3 years. The cell count should return to normal within 1 year of treatment (usually 6 months) and the protein concentration within 2 years. The disappearance of the CSF VDRL typically parallels its resolution in the serum and may be a less useful parameter of treatment adequacy than CSF cell count or protein concentration. Importantly, the CSF VDRL titers should not increase over time following effective therapy.

The potential for relapse of neurosyphilis following a course of recommended therapy suggests the potential need for secondary prophylaxis in treating neurosyphilis in the HIV-infected individual, as is employed in the management of some other CNS infections such as toxoplasma encephalitis and cryptococcal meningitis. In a study of 100 HIV-infected military personnel with syphilis, 4 of 7 persons with reactive CSF VDRL relapsed following high-dose intravenous penicillin. These relapses were often observed more than 12 months after initial therapy. However, these findings among HIV-seropositive patients have not been universally observed. The CDC has recommended that the initial therapy of intravenous aqueous penicillin be followed in HIV-infected individuals by weekly intramuscular injections of 2.4 million units of benzathine penicillin for 3 weeks. An alternative therapeutic course is the administration of a 30-day course of 200 mg doxycycline twice daily following the completion of intravenous therapy. Although secondary prophylaxis is extensively employed, further studies are warranted before secondary prophylaxis or some permutation of it can be broadly recommended. HIV-seropositive patients should be carefully monitored for relapse of neurosyphilis for 2 or more years following initial treatment.

PREVENTION

As a disease that is almost exclusively transmitted sexually, syphilis is preventable by sexual abstinence or a· monogamous relationship with an uninfected partner. As with AIDS, the chance of infection with *T. pallidum* is reduced significantly by the use of condoms. Only primary and secondary syphilis are considered to be contagious. Unless the disease recrudesces, as may be seen in early latent syphilis and which is the reason for its distinction from late latent syphilis, neither latent nor tertiary syphilis is considered contagious. In those individuals with primary, secondary, or latent syphilis, the manifestations of neurosyphilis can be avoided by the timely administration of adequate doses of penicillin.

—*Joseph R. Berger*

See also–HIV Infection, Neurological Complications of; Tabes Dorsalis

Further Reading

Berger, J. R. (1991). Neurosyphilis in human immunodeficiency virus type I-seropositive individuals. A prospective study. *Arch. Neurol.* 48, 700–702.

Blocker, M. E., Levine, W. C., and St. Louis, M. E. (2000). HIV prevalence in patients with syphilis, United States. *Sex. Transmitted Dis.* 27, 53–59.

Burstain, J. M., Grimpel, E., Lukehart, S. A., *et al.* (1991). Sensitive detection of *Treponema pallidum* by using the polymerase chain reaction. *J. Clin. Microbiol.* 29, 62–69.

Centers for Disease Control (1988). Recommendations for diagnosing and treating syphilis in HIV-infected patients. *MMWR* 37, 600–608.

Centers for Disease Control (1999). Summary of notifiable diseases, United States, 1998. *MMWR* 47, 1–93.

Clark, E. G. (1964). The Oslo study of the natural course of untreated syphilis: An epidemiologic investigation based on a re-study of the Boeck–Bruusgard material. *Med. Clin. North Am.* 48, 613–624.

Faber, W. R., Bos, J. D., Rietra, P. J., *et al.* (1983). Treponemicidal levels of amoxicillin in cerebrospinal fluid after oral administration. *Sex. Transmitted Dis.* 10, 148–150.

Flood, J. M., Weinstock, H. S., Guroy, M. E., *et al.* (1998). Neurosyphilis during the AIDS epidemic, San Francisco, 1985–1992. *J. Infect. Dis.* 177, 931–940.

Gordon, S. M., Eaton, M. E., George, R., *et al.* (1994). The response of symptomatic neurosyphilis to high-dose intravenous penicillin G in patients with human immunodeficiency virus infection. *N. Engl. J. Med.* 331, 1469–1473.

Harris, D. E., Enterline, D. S., and Tien, R. D. (1997). Neurosyphilis in patients with AIDS. *Neuroimaging Clin. North Am.* 7, 215–221.

Hollander, H. (1988). Cerebrospinal fluid normalities and abnormalities in individuals infected with human immunodeficiency virus. *J. Infect. Dis.* 158, 855–858.

Holtom, P. D., Larson, R. A., Leal, M. E., *et al.* (1992). Prevalence of neurosyphilis in human immunodeficiency virus-infected patients with latent syphilis. *Am. J. Med.* 93, 9–12.

Katz, D. A., Berger, J. R., and Duncan, R. C. (1993). Neurosyphilis. A comparative study of the effects of infection with human immunodeficiency virus [published erratum appears in *Arch. Neurol.* 1993 June, 50, 6141]. *Arch. Neurol.* 50, 243–924.

Lukehart, S. A., Hook, E. W., Baker-Zander, S. A., *et al.* (1988). Invasion of the central nervous system by *Treponema pallidum*: Implications for diagnosis and treatment. *Ann. Intern. Med.* 109, 855–862.

Malone, J. L., Wallace, M. R., Hendrick, B. B., *et al.* (1995). Syphilis and neurosyphilis in a human immunodeficiency virus type-I seropositive population: Evidence for frequent serologic relapse after therapy. *Am. J. Med.* 99, 55–63.

Polnikorn, N., Witoonpanich, R., Vorachit, M., *et al.* (1980). Penicillin concentrations in cerebrospinal fluid after different treatment regimens for syphilis. *Br. J. Vener. Dis.* 56, 363–367.

Roberts, M. C., Emsley, R. A., and Jordaan, G. P. (1992). Screening for syphilis and neurosyphilis in acute psychiatric admissions. *South Afr. Med. J.* 82, 16–18.

Rockwell, D. H., Yobs, A. R., and Moore, M. B. (1964). The Tuskegee study of untreated syphilis—The 30th year of observation. *Arch. Intern. Med.* 114, 792–798.

Tramont, E. C. (1976). Persistence of *Treponema pallidum* following penicillin G therapy. Report of two cases. *J. Am. Med. Assoc.* 236, 2206–2207.

Yim, C. W., Flynn, N. M., and Fitzgerald, F. T. (1985). Penetration of oral doxycycline into the cerebrospinal fluid of patients with latent or neurosyphilis. *Antimicrob. Agents Chemother.* 28, 347–348.

Zifko, U., Wimberger, D., Lindner, K., *et al.* (1996). MRI in patients with general paresis. *Neuroradiology* 38, 120–123.

Neurotology

Encyclopedia of the Neurological Sciences
Copyright 2003, Elsevier Science (USA). All rights reserved.

THE STUDY and practice of neurotology concerns conditions whose principal symptoms are dizziness, hearing loss, and tinnitus (spontaneous, illusory noises heard in one or both ears). Neurotologists are also sometimes called on to assess patients with peripheral facial palsy. Neurotology combines elements of neurology and otolaryngology/head and neck surgery; its practitioners must have an excellent command of the anatomy of the ear and skull base and the brainstem vestibular and auditory pathways as well as the physiology of the relevant central and peripheral structures. Techniques of the neurological and otological examinations are employed, and specialized ancillary testing is often critical in diagnosis and management. Neurotologists usually begin their training with residency in neurology or otolaryngology and then complete an additional year or more of a dedicated fellowship.

A neurotologist most commonly diagnoses and treats dizziness and balance disturbances. Evaluating patients with these problems is often quite challenging since the differential diagnosis includes disorders of the central and peripheral vestibular system as well as common nonvestibular conditions, such as orthostatic hypotension and affective disorders. Assessment takes into account the patient's history, particularly those stimuli that provoke dizziness. Bedside examination focuses on hearing, eye movement, limb coordination, joint position sense (proprioception), gait, and standing balance. Electronystagmography assesses the vestibular system and the closely related smooth pursuit, optokinetic and saccadic systems by measuring ocular motor responses to head and visual stimulus motion and to warming and cooling of the ear (caloric testing). Posturography tests subjects' ability to balance themselves at baseline and with reduced or altered visual and proprioceptive inputs. Treatments for dizziness vary from physical (canalith repositioning) maneuvers that cure benign positional paroxysmal vertigo to medications and surgery for selected cases of Meniere's disease and perilymphatic fistula. Many neurotologists work with physical therapists who specialize in balance problems; physical therapy is often the most important component in the care of these patients.

Hearing loss and tinnitus are hallmarks of auditory dysfunction and are much more often of peripheral than central origin. The vast majority of acquired auditory problems, such as age-related (presbycusis) and noise-induced hearing loss, are fairly symmetrical and slowly progressive. Other common problems, such as conductive deficits from trauma and infection, may be asymmetrical or acute, but diagnosis is seldom difficult and highly specialized care is not required. Neurotological expertise is often desirable for patients with asymmetrical or acute hearing loss of unclear origin, especially when central or eighth nerve pathology is suspected. Audiometry and auditory evoked potentials are the cornerstones of diagnosis. As with many vestibular problems, magnetic resonance or computed tomographic imaging of the ear, eighth nerve, skull base, and caudal brain structures is often an essential part of the evaluation.

—*Mark J. Morrow*

See also–Neuroophthalmology (see also specific Neurotology entries; e.g., Hearing Loss; Tinnitus)

Further Reading

Baloh, R. W., and Halmagyi, G. M. (1996). *Disorders of the Vestibular System*. Oxford Univ. Press, New York.
Baloh, R. W. (1998). *Dizziness, Hearing Loss and Tinnitus*. Oxford Univ. Press, New York.

Neurotoxicology, Overview

Encyclopedia of the Neurological Sciences
Copyright 2003, Elsevier Science (USA). All rights reserved.

ALTHOUGH individual cases of lead poisoning were reported as early as 200 B.C., it was not until the 20th century that industrialization in the United States and Europe alerted physicians to the importance of health hazards related to fumes and chemicals. In order to meet this need, the new medical specialty of occupational and environmental medicine developed, and neurologists and neuroscientists are pivotal to this effort. In addition to the study and evaluation of environmental toxins, neurotoxicology encompasses analyses of adverse effects related to prescribed medications and drugs of abuse. Finally, with a greater understanding of the normal chemical interactions in brain, spinal cord, and peripheral nerve function, endogenous neurochemicals that are toxic have been discovered, specifically excitotoxins. These chemicals are produced by chemical reactions within nerve cells in response to injury or enzyme reactions called oxidative stress. Once produced, these excitotoxins can cause nerve cells to depolarize to the point of further damage, sometimes generating a cycle of continued toxicity.

Whereas exposure to environmental toxic materials appears to be of greatest danger among industrial and agricultural workers in direct contact with poisons, the ubiquity and ease of dissemination of many toxic materials results in exposure of large segments of the population. Modern societies have met serious scientific and political challenges in disposing of poisonous wastes, and pollution of water and atmosphere with industrial by-products is now common. In the United States, the handling of industrial chemicals has been the primary focus, and in Europe the handling or mishandling of nuclear waste has preoccupied public attention. The growing utilization of drugs in medical and recreational settings as well as accidental poisoning and suicide or homicide attempts are prime factors contributing to the current importance of neurotoxicology in modern medicine.

Toxins may affect the central or peripheral nervous system by several mechanisms. There may be interference with the energy production necessary to maintain normal neural structure and function. This interference occurs either by inactivation of enzymes or by interference with coenzymes of the vitamin B group essential to oxidative energy mechanisms. In these circumstances, toxic responses are directly related to the concentration of the toxin or to availability of the involved coenzyme. Second, the toxin may interfere with the function of nerves through involvement of the nutrient vessels. Additionally, exposure to foreign material may result in allergic or other immunological phenomena. In this case, the dose of toxin is not necessarily directly related to the severity of clinical symptoms. Fourth, toxins may affect the nervous system through their effects on neurotransmitters, which are endogenous molecules that transmit chemical information from one nerve cell to another. Neurotransmitters affected by neurotoxins include acetylcholine, dopamine, norepinephrine, γ-aminobutyric acid, and glutamate. Finally, there may be alterations in other body systems causing acid–base or ionic imbalances that affect the nervous system indirectly. Whereas molecular biological advances have affected research efforts primarily in the neurodegenerative diseases, applications are now being made in the study of susceptibility to toxins.

Identification of the responsible agent is simple when exposure history is clear, when a single chemical is involved, and when neurological symptoms are characteristic for the offending material. Often, however, these issues are vague or complicated since most toxic spills or exposures involve multiple products and subjects have many different levels of exposure. Furthermore, even with uniform exposure, subjects may show different susceptibilities due to their own preexisting medical conditions. For example, renal or hepatic disease slows the metabolism or breakdown of many toxic products within the body so that disorders of these systems will predispose subjects to toxic symptoms after only minimal exposure. In some cases, intoxication may mimic neurological entities, such as multiple sclerosis, amyotrophic lateral sclerosis, combined system diseases, Guillain–Barré syndrome, cerebellar degen-

eration, intracranial neoplasms, and nervous system infections. In other circumstances, preexisting neurological disease may be exacerbated or accentuated following exposure to offending materials. Because of the extensive variability of neural response to toxic agents, great resourcefulness on the part of the diagnostician is required for adequate recognition and therapy of nervous system intoxication.

The most common clinical presentation after toxin exposure is vague and not specific enough to diagnose a chemical cause. Poor concentration, short-term memory loss, depressed mood, anxiety, restlessness, and loss of interest in work and hobbies are very common but not distinctive enough to exclude other causes. Decreased libido, irritability, headaches, weakness, and sleep disturbances ranging from insomnia to somnambulism are also common but not specific. Such features indicate a general brain disturbance (encephalopathy) but cannot be used to solidly diagnose a relationship to toxins. Patients may also show signs of peripheral neuropathy (distal weakness, decreased sensation, and loss of reflexes), tremor, and incoordination and gait instability (ataxia); when these occur along with encephalopathy, toxic etiologies are frequently considered.

Regardless of the clinical presentation, the diagnosis of neurotoxicant-related damage is one of exclusion. Other causes of central and peripheral nervous system dysfunction must be ruled out and a history of significant exposure needs to be clearly substantiated. The neurological examination, objective neuropsychological tests, electrophysiological studies (electroencephalography and electromyolgraphy), and neuroimaging studies may all be useful in different contexts. It is extremely important to obtain tissue samples of products that are stored, and reference sources are available to advise diagnosticians on the best tissues for different toxins, whether blood, urine, hair, etc. Chemical laboratories are available for the analysis of chemicals to which subjects have been putatively exposed.

Because of the litigious environment, scientific and medical analyses are often juxtaposed with or even obscured by legal questions and financial issues of compensation.

Once health effects have been detected, it can be scientifically problematic to relate these in a causal fashion to a specific chemical exposure. Since biomarkers for many chemicals are either difficult to obtain or do not exist, it is often extremely difficult to determine the intensity of current and past exposure or even the presence of toxic exposure in a given individual. Also, for an accurate estimate of change due to a toxin, knowledge of baseline neurological functioning prior to exposure is essential but rarely available. Because of these problems, the scientific analyses available from most cases of putative toxic exposure are almost always inconclusive.

Evaluation of the direct toxic effects on the central nervous system must also be considered in the context of the emotional state and personality characteristics of the patient. Psychological disturbance may be a primary sequela or a secondary emotional reaction to chemical exposure. In addition, specific inherent personality characteristics may predispose an individual to develop physical, cognitive, and psychological symptoms even without any direct toxic effects on the nervous system. Certain individual expectations concerning the adverse health effects of suspected chemical exposure may result in enhanced awareness of normal bodily sensations. The degree to which an individual is hypersensitive to endogenous stimuli (normal bodily sensations) may determine the duration and intensity of symptoms.

—*Christopher G. Goetz*

See also–Myopathy, Toxic; Neuropathy; Toxic (see also specific entries in the Neurotoxicology section; e.g., Alcohol-Related Neurotoxicity)

Further Reading

Bolla, K. I. (1996). Neuropsychological evaluation for detecting alterations in the central nervous system after chemical exposure. *Regul. Toxicol. Pharmacol.* **24**, 548–551.

Bolla, K. I., and Cadet, J. L. (2003). Exogenous acquired metabolic disorders of the nervous system: Toxins and illicit drugs. In *Textbook of Clinical Neurology* (C. G. Goetz, Ed.), pp. 769–798. Saunders, Philadelphia.

Goetz, C. G. (1985). *Neurotoxins in Clinical Practice.* Spectrum, New York.

Hartman, D. (1988). *Neuropsychological Toxicology; Identification and Assessment of Human Neurotoxic Syndromes.* Pergamon, New York.

Neurotransmitter Receptors

Encyclopedia of the Neurological Sciences
Copyright 2003, Elsevier Science (USA). All rights reserved.

NEUROTRANSMITTER RECEPTORS are proteins that recognize specific neurotransmitter molecules and signal their presence to the cell. Many neurotransmitter receptors are also present on cells outside the nervous system. Due to the existence of multiple neurotransmitters, it is important that the receptor be able to recognize and distinguish the appropriate transmitter (Fig. 1). Recognition occurs when a neurotransmitter binds to the receptor in a way that activates it to produce a signal. The information represented by this recognition event must be transmitted to the neuron as a whole through a process referred to as signal transduction.

Neurotransmitter receptors can be viewed as a complex of parts with different functions. Although a neurotransmitter receptor may consist of a single protein, it is always in contact with other proteins that participate in the signal transduction process and can also change the receptor's neurotransmitter recognition properties. These changes can serve to terminate the signal, allowing the receptor to respond to new signals at a rapid, sometimes millisecond, rate. Other proteins associated with the receptor may help to propagate the signal into the cell or to produce adaptation at the level of neurotransmitter recognition.

Many signals are produced or mediated by neurotransmitter receptors. They can be broadly categorized as activation of enzymes within the

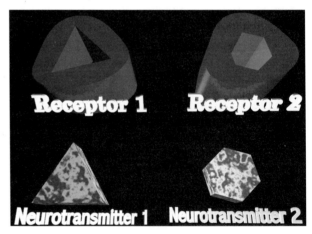

Figure 1
Every receptor has an endogenous neurotransmitter, and every neurotransmitter has specificity for a type of receptor. In this example, neurotransmitter 1 can associate with receptor 1 but not with receptor 2, whereas the opposite is the case for neurotransmitter 2. Because many more receptors exist than neurotransmitters, endogenous ligands can interact with many subtypes of receptors within a single family (e.g., acetylcholine and M_1–M_5 muscarinic acetylcholine receptors) but generally not with other families of receptors (i.e., acetylcholine does not interact with serotonin receptors).

neuron and conduction of ions into or out of the neuron. The immediate effect of these signals is to change the rate at which the neuron sends signals to other neurons. Less immediate effects include changes in the metabolic activity of the neuron, including changes in the expression of neuronal genes. A change in the rate at which a neuron sends signals to other neurons is largely determined by its electrical properties. These properties are strongly influenced by the movement of ions into and out of the neuron. Activation of neurotransmitter receptors that form ion channels opens the channel pore to allow the movement of ions either into or out of the cell. This changes the electrical potential of the neuronal cell membrane, which in turn determines whether or not it will send a signal down its axon. Ion channels that are not part of a receptor may also be activated by enzymes or their products, which are more directly connected to receptors lacking ion channel activity.

The signal transmission properties of the nervous system have been used to develop drugs that can mimic or influence the activity of neurotransmitters on their receptors. Much of the effort to understand neurotransmission is motivated by the need for drugs that can correct abnormal activity within the nervous system. Morphine is an example of a drug that acts directly on a neurotransmitter receptor (the μ opioid receptor) to produce analgesia. The recognition properties of receptors are critical for drug development because drugs are given systemically and permeate most parts of the body. A peculiarity of the nervous system is that there may be several receptors for the same neurotransmitter that can produce a different response to the same molecule. Drugs are often designed to be more selective for a specific receptor than the neurotransmitter that is normally recognized by it. The development of such compounds has increased our understanding of how neurotransmitters and their receptors work.

Neurotransmitter receptors are the means by which neurons receive signals from other cells and respond to them. Receptors can be seen as a complex of proteins working together to recognize neurotransmitters from other cells and transducing this signal into a change in which the neuron communicates with other cells.

NEUROTRANSMISSION

Neurotransmission begins with the binding of a neurotransmitter to a specific site on the receptor protein—the neurotransmitter recognition site. Recognition in this context means that there are physical and chemical interactions between the transmitter molecule and chemical groups on the protein receptor that do not occur with other molecules. These interactions can include negative or positive charge attractions, hydrophobic interactions between hydrocarbon groups, hydrogen bonding, and van der Waals interactions (nonbonded). The ability of proteins to selectively bind other molecules is an essential feature of enzyme as well as receptor function. Receptors, like enzymes, selectively bind molecules but differ in that they do not catalyze chemical changes in the bound neurotransmitter.

Proteins are flexible molecules capable of adopting many shapes referred to as conformational states. This capability results from the flexibility of the peptide and other chemical bonds present in the protein structure. Neurotransmitters must do more than simply attach to the receptor if a signal is to be generated. They must change the conformational state of the receptor so that the other parts of the receptor complex can detect the recognition event.

The tendency of a transmitter to remain bound instead of dissociating from its receptor defines its affinity for that receptor. A high-affinity interaction means that a transmitter will bind most of the receptors even if it is present at low concentrations. Conversely, a low-affinity interaction requires more transmitter to be available if the same level of receptor occupation is to occur. Changes in the conformational state of the receptor can either increase or decrease its affinity for the transmitter. Neurotransmitter receptors typically have at least two conformational states with either high or low affinity for the transmitter. The high-affinity state promotes binding of the transmitter and acquisition of its signal, whereas the low-affinity state promotes dissociation of the transmitter and termination of the signal. The conformational state of a neurotransmitter receptor is often regulated by its interaction with the signal transduction proteins complexed to it. Other mechanisms, such as the addition of phosphate groups to specific amino acids, can also regulate receptor affinity (Fig. 2).

The binding of a neurotransmitter to its receptor only initiates the transfer of a signal from one neuron to the other. The second stage is referred to as signal transduction, in which the recognition event triggers a change in the postsynaptic cell. The simplest form of signal transduction occurs when the receptor forms a hole or pore in the cell membrane.

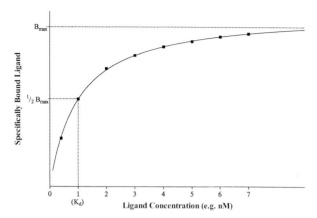

Figure 2

By labeling ligands with radioactive isotopes, their affinities and the density of available receptors can be measured, although this number may be very small (e.g., 20,000 receptors/cell). A radioligand saturation binding experiment is performed for this application. Known radioligand concentrations are incubated with tissue that expresses receptors for the ligand. After reaching equilibrium, the amount of radioligand that is specifically bound to the tissue is measured. When all the available receptors are bound to radioligand, saturation is reached and no further specific radioligand binding can occur. The amount of specifically bound radioligand at saturation is equal to the concentration of available receptors, referred to as the B_{max} value. The concentration of free radioligand required to bind half of the available receptors ($\frac{1}{2}B_{max}$) is its dissociation constant (K_d). The inverse of K_d is a measure of the ligand's affinity.

Binding of the neurotransmitter induces a conformational change in the receptor opening the pore or channel. Ions such as sodium, chloride, potassium, or calcium can flow through the open channel, depending on the selectivity of the channel and their relative concentrations inside and outside the cell, and change the membrane potential. The membrane potential may be increased (hyperpolarized) or decreased (depolarized) depending on which ions the channel conducts. Depolarization will increase the probability that the cell will transmit a signal down its axon, whereas hyperpolarization will inhibit it from doing so.

A second, more complex form of signal transduction involves the activation of receptor-associated enzyme proteins by the neurotransmitter-bound receptor. The principal class of such receptors is referred to as G protein-coupled receptors, which are described in more detail later. Because these receptor-associated enzymes can activate other cellular enzyme systems, the initial signal can be greatly amplified. Activation of these signal transduction systems can result in the opening of ion channels and changes in cellular metabolism.

NEUROTRANSMITTERS

Neurotransmitters are chemical compounds released by neurons after depolarization that act on other neurons to produce a response (Fig. 3). The response produced by a neurotransmitter is mediated by a neurotransmitter receptor capable of recognizing it. Neurotransmitters are the principal means by which neurons transfer information to each other. Characteristics of a neurotransmitter include its synthesis in the neuron, concentration in membrane-enclosed vesicles at presynaptic terminals, release by neuron terminal depolarization, induced activity at the postsynaptic terminal as a consequence of receptor binding, and removal from the synapse to terminate this effect. The defining characteristics of neurotransmitters have become less stringent due to evidence of some neurotransmitter release at nonsynaptic sites and because of the properties of

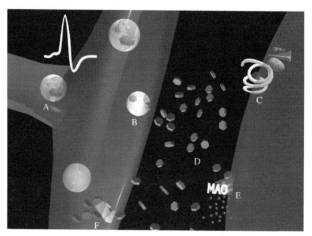

Figure 3

The synthesis, storage, action, and termination of norepinephrine, a representative brain neurotransmitter. (A) Norepinephrine is synthesized in the nerve cell and packaged into vesicles. In preparation for release, these vesicles are transported to the nerve terminal. (B) Upon arrival of an action potential at the axon terminal and the resultant calcium entry, vesicles fuse with the nerve terminal membrane, thereby releasing their contents into the synapse. (C) Released neurotransmitter diffuses across the synaptic cleft and can interact with postsynaptic receptor targets to cause excitatory or inhibitory postsynaptic potentials and/or stimulate second messenger systems. Termination of the response is accomplished by removing free neurotransmitter from the synapse. (D) Simple diffusion can carry the neurotransmitter out of the synapse, or (E) enzymes [e.g., monoamineoxidase (MAO)] can degrade or chemically modify the neurotransmitter, rendering it incapable of further action. (F) Finally, reuptake of neurotransmitter back into the presynaptic neuron or into surrounding cells can terminate the signal as well as recycle some of the neurotransmitter. (See color plate section.)

unusual neurotransmitter-like molecules such as nitric oxide.

There are many different neurotransmitter molecules (Fig. 4). They can be categorized as small molecules and much larger neuropeptides. The smallest neurotransmitter may be nitric oxide, with a molecular weight of 30, whereas the neurotransmitter peptide endorphin is composed of 30 amino acids and has a molecular weight of more than 3000—a 100-fold difference in size. Most neurotransmitters are localized to discrete parts of the nervous system, but three (adenosine, glutamate, and glycine) are present in every cell of an organism. Some neurotransmitters, including acetylcholine, norepinephrine, serotonin, and dopamine, can produce excitatory or inhibitory effects depending on the receptors on which they act. The diversity of structural and functional properties makes it difficult to categorize neurotransmitters.

The functional properties of a neurotransmitter differ in several important ways beyond the response produced at the postsynaptic site. Differences include their site of production within the neuron, the kinetics or time course of their response, and the method of removal from the synapse after release.

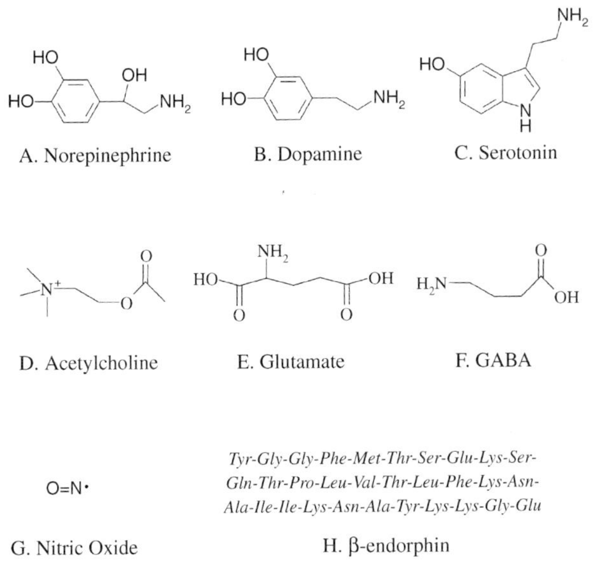

A. Norepinephrine B. Dopamine C. Serotonin

D. Acetylcholine E. Glutamate F. GABA

O=N·

Tyr-Gly-Gly-Phe-Met-Thr-Ser-Glu-Lys-Ser-
Gln-Thr-Pro-Leu-Val-Thr-Leu-Phe-Lys-Asn-
Ala-Ile-Ile-Lys-Asn-Ala-Tyr-Lys-Lys-Gly-Glu

G. Nitric Oxide H. β-endorphin

Figure 4
Examples of neurotransmitters representing the major families. (A) Norepinephrine, (B) dopamine, (C) serotonin, (D) acetylcholine, (E) glutamic acid, and (F) γ-aminobutyric acid (GABA) are small molecule neurotransmitters, where glutamic acid is also an amino acid neurotransmitter. (G) Nitric oxide is an unusual neurotransmitter in that it is an unstable soluble gas. (H) β-Endorphin is a much larger peptide neurotransmitter.

Small molecule transmitters, such as acetylcholine, epinephrine, norepinephrine, serotonin, and dopamine, are produced at the presynaptic terminal by local enzymes. All these except acetylcholine are produced from amino acid precursors, such as tyrosine (epinephrine, norepinephrine, and dopamine) or tryptophan (serotonin). Acetylcholine is produced by the acetylation of choline, a common nutrient. Peptide neurotransmitters such as enkephalin, dynorphin, cholecystokinin, and substance P are produced by the cleavage of much larger protein precursors primarily in the cell body of the neuron near its nucleus. The active neuropeptide products are packaged in secretory granules and then transported to their sites of release. One consequence of this difference between small and large neurotransmitters is that under conditions of high activity the neuropeptide supply at the presynaptic terminal can be exhausted.

The response kinetics for neurotransmitters differs depending on the type of receptor on which they act. Neurotransmitters acting on ion channel receptors such as glutamate (excitatory) and GABA (inhibitory) produce very fast responses (milliseconds). Glutamate and GABA also act on another class of receptors referred to as metabotropic or G protein-coupled receptors. These responses are much slower and can last for seconds to hours. The response mediated by an ion channel receptor results from the flow of ions (sodium, potassium, chloride, or calcium) that occurs when the transmitter opens the channel. Responses mediated by G protein-coupled receptors occur more slowly because they result from the activation of an extended series of enzymes.

There are two principal mechanisms by which neurotransmitters are removed from the synaptic space. The majority of neurotransmitters, including all neuropeptides and many small neurotransmitters, either diffuse away from their site of release or are destroyed by enzymes present on cell membrane surfaces. Acetylcholine is a classic example because it is very rapidly destroyed by acetylcholine esterase, which hydrolyzes the ester bond between the acetic acid and choline components of the neurotransmitter. Neuropeptides are degraded into their constituent amino acids by protease enzymes. Some small molecule neurotransmitters (e.g., norepinephrine, dopamine, and serotonin) are recaptured by the presynaptic terminal through a process called reuptake. Reuptake provides a means of recycling the transmitter so that high levels of neurotransmission can be maintained.

SIGNAL RECOGNITION

Receptors differ from other recognition proteins in that transmitter recognition generates a signal that is conveyed into the cell through the process of signal transduction. The activation of a receptor can result in the production of intracellular signaling molecules (e.g., cyclic adenosine monophosphate) called second messengers. The receptor informs the cell of the recognition event through signal transduction.

Neurotransmitter recognition occurs at specific locations or sites within the receptor structure. Single protein receptors such as G protein-coupled receptors have only one such site, whereas multimeric protein complex receptors such as ionotropic receptors have two or more for the same neurotransmitter. All neurotransmitter receptors have additional recognition sites on their internal cytoplasmic surfaces for the selective binding of intracellular proteins that participate in the signal transduction process. The neurotransmitter recognition site must allow access to extracellular neurotransmitters so that the receptor serves as a bridge through the membrane to link extracellular and intracellular events.

Neurotransmitter recognition by the receptor occurs through interactions between chemical groups (e.g., positively charged nitrogen, negatively charged carboxylate, uncharged hydroxyl, and other groups) of the transmitter and other chemical groups on the amino acid side chains of the receptor. The three-dimensional neurotransmitter key fits into the three-dimensional receptor lock through the spatial arrangement of these chemical groups. The interaction, or bonding, that occurs between these groups is relatively weak and reversible. This is necessary because the neurotransmitter must be able to dissociate from the receptor in order to terminate the signal and allow for new signals. Similar interactions occur on the opposite side of the receptor with effector proteins that convey the recognition event into the cell. Effector protein interactions with the receptor also have to be reversible.

Just as the insertion of a key into a lock changes the alignment of pins in the cylinder, recognition of a transmitter in a receptor changes the alignment of amino acids at the recognition site. Because amino acids of a receptor protein are linked into a continuous chain, the movement of a few amino acids has the potential to change the positions of many others. In this way, the conformation of the receptor protein (i.e., its overall three-dimensional shape) before transmitter recognition can change to a new conformation after recognition. This change can affect the recognition site of the effector protein at some distance from the transmitter recognition site and initiate effector activity. This kind of allosteric interaction between two distant positions on the receptor protein operates in both directions. The presence or absence of the effector protein also changes the alignment of amino acids at the neurotransmitter binding site. For a G protein-coupled receptor, the presence of the effector G protein complex increases the affinity of the neurotransmitter for its recognition site, whereas the binding of the neurotransmitter induces the activation and release of the G protein complex. Dissociation of the G protein complex leads to a reduction of neurotransmitter binding affinity and its dissociation to produce a feedback regulation of both sites. Similar effects also occur at ionotropic receptors but through different mechanisms.

NEUROTRANSMITTER RECEPTORS

Neurotransmitter receptors can be categorized into two classes. Extracellular ligand-gated ion channel receptors (ionotropic receptors) are complexes of four or more proteins surrounding a central pore that can be opened to allow ions to pass through. G protein-coupled receptors (metabotropic receptors) consist of a single protein complexed to other proteins that carry out the effector functions of the activated receptor. Both classes of receptors serve to mediate the response produced by the neurotransmitter in the postsynaptic cell. Receptors extend from the interior of the cell through the plasma membrane to the extracellular space. Neurotransmitter recognition occurs at the exterior side of the membrane. The signal represented by the recognition event is transferred into the neuron by a conformational change in the receptor protein (Fig. 5). The effect of this signal may be direct, through the opening of an ion channel, or indirect, through the activation of an associated G protein complex.

There are many more receptors than neurotransmitters. For example, the neurotransmitter serotonin is recognized by at least seven major receptor types, some of which are further categorized into multiple subtypes. The serotonin receptors are categorized into both ionotropic and metabotropic receptor classes and can mediate a large number of effects. A consequence of this diversity is that the signal given by the presynaptic neuron in the form of a particular transmitter can be interpreted in different ways by the postsynaptic cell. A neuron will signal many other neurons using the same neurotransmitter, but their response to that signal can be different.

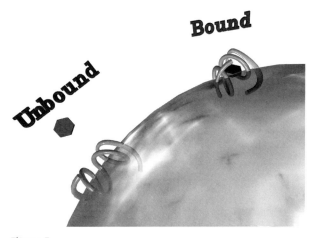

Figure 5

The act of neurotransmitter binding induces a conformational change in the three-dimensional structure of a G protein-coupled receptor. This bound versus unbound conformation permits intracellular signaling molecules, such as G proteins, to distinguish between an active and inactive receptor, thereby transducing the binding information into the cell.

IONOTROPIC RECEPTORS

Excitatory ionotropic receptors include the glutamate, nicotinic cholinergic, serotonin 5-HT$_3$, and purinergic receptors. Inhibitory ionotropic receptors include the GABA$_A$ and glycine receptors. The number of potential ionotropic receptors is very large because they are composed of multiple protein subunits, and most of these subunits exist in multiple forms. However, it is unlikely that the total number of potential permutations is ever expressed.

The ionotropic receptors can also be categorized into groups based on structural similarity rather than function properties. This leads to their division into three groups in which the number of membrane-spanning segments (transmembrane domains) of each subunit and the arrangement of subunits forming the ion channel are characteristic features. The first class consists of glutamate ionotropic receptors whose subunits have three full transmembrane domains and a loop that extends into the membrane from the cytoplasmic surface and then loops back without reaching the extracellular surface. These glutamate receptors are thought to be composed of four subunits surrounding the central channel. The second class of receptors includes the GABA$_A$ and glycine inhibitory receptors and the nicotinic cholinergic and serotonin 5-HT$_3$ excitatory receptors. All are characterized as having subunits with four transmembrane domains and are com-

posed of five subunits surrounding the ion channel. The third class of receptors consists of purinergic ionotropic receptors that recognize adenosine triphosphate (ATP) as a neurotransmitter. Subunits of these receptors have only two transmembrane domains. The number of subunits that combine to form the active receptor complex is unknown.

The excitatory or inhibitory effect produced by an ionotropic receptor depends on the ion or ions it conducts. Excitatory ionotropic receptors primarily conduct positively charged sodium ions from the outside of the cell into the interior. This depolarizes the cell in the area of the receptor and can lead to the generation of an action potential at the axon hillock if a sufficient number of other depolarization events occur (Fig. 6). In addition to sodium, some excitatory ionotropic receptors can conduct calcium ions. Calcium ion conductance does more than depolarize a neuron; it can activate a number of important cellular kinase enzymes (e.g., calcium–calmodulin kinase). Kinase enzymes regulate the activity of a large number of proteins, including receptors, voltage-gated ion channels, and other enzymes. They do so by adding phosphate groups to specific amino acids in proteins, including receptors. Thus, excitatory ionotropic receptors can have both fast depolarization and slower metabotropic effects.

Inhibitory ionotropic receptors conduct negatively charged chloride ions into or positively charged potassium ions out of the cell. Neurons have a

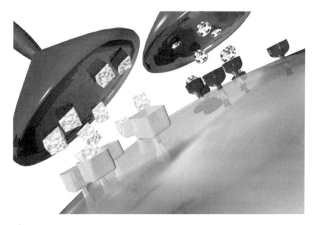

Figure 6

Neuronal axons that synapse onto another nerve cell may be of different types (cholinergic, serotonergic, glutamatergic, etc.). Receptors for each type of neurotransmitter must be expressed postsynaptically to receive these signals. In this way, the recipient cell of such varied information integrates and averages the incoming excitatory and/or inhibitory signals to determine if an action potential will be propagated to the next synapse.

negative potential across their membranes because there is a predominance of negative ions in the cell. The movement of chloride ions into or potassium ions out of the cell increases this negative potential and hyperpolarizes the cell. Consequently, the cell is less likely to reach its action potential threshold and is inhibited from producing an action potential.

Ionotropic receptors are responsible for the rapid transmission of information through the nervous system. Fast transmission is particularly important for transmitting sensory information into the central nervous system and for motor control of muscles.

Excitatory Ionotropic Receptors

The excitatory ionotropic receptors include glutamate, nicotinic cholinergic, serotonin 5-HT$_3$, and purinergic (ATP) receptors. These receptors represent all three ionotropic receptor classes and have limited structural similarities. All three can conduct sodium ions to induce depolarization, and some also conduct calcium ions. These receptors have a critical role in fast synaptic transmission that is characterized by a very rapid onset followed by the rapid desensitization or reduction of ion conductance to a low level as long as agonist is present. The conductance of calcium by some of these receptors is important for certain long-term changes in synaptic efficiency that underlies learning and memory.

By far the most abundant of the excitatory ionotropic receptors are those that recognize glutamate. These receptors are also likely the most abundant in the nervous system because nearly all neurons respond to glutamate stimulation. There are three basic types of glutamate receptors, which are classified according to their selectivity for the synthetic ligands N-methyl-D-aspartate (NMDA), α-amino-3-hydroxy-5-methyl-4-isoxazolepropionate (AMPA), and the naturally occurring neurotoxin kainic acid. These three divisions can be further subdivided based on their subunit composition, so there are many potential glutamate receptor subtypes.

NMDA receptors have unique pharmacological properties that distinguish them from other excitatory ionotropic receptors. For other receptors, the critical condition for activation is the presence of their neurotransmitter. In contrast, activation of NMDA receptors also depends on the presence of a cotransmitter glycine and depolarization of the membrane near the receptor. Glycine has its own recognition site on the NMDA receptor, and the presence of inactive antagonist competitors for this

site prevents activation of the receptor even when glutamate is present. The membrane voltage sensitivity of the NMDA receptor results from the presence of a site within the ion channel that binds the ion magnesium. When occupied by a magnesium ion, the channel cannot conduct ions and the receptor is inactive. Depolarization of the membrane near the receptor, normally by activation of another excitatory receptor, causes the magnesium ion to dissociate from its binding site to allow ion conductance. Thus, activity of NMDA receptors is dependent on several conditions independent of the presence of glutamate.

The number of subunits that combine to form a functional NMDA receptor has been a matter of dispute but is currently thought to be four. Five distinct subunits are identified for this receptor, and they are likely to combine at a ratio of 2:2. They are described as NR1, NR2A, NR2B, NR2C, and NR2D by one terminology. The subunits are unusually large, consisting of 939–1482 amino acids. The NR1 subunit is the most prevalent, whereas the NR2C and NR2D subunits are fairly rare.

The AMPA ionotropic glutamate receptor is widely distributed in the vertebrate nervous system, much like the NMDA receptors. AMPA receptors lack the conditional activation properties of the NMDA receptors. AMPA receptor tetramers are formed from four distinct subunits referred to as GluR1–GluR4. Each subunit can exist in two forms called flip and flop. The flip and flop variants differ from each other by a 38-amino acid sequence and result from alternative splicing of the subunit genes. These variants differ from each other in the response kinetic properties that they impart to the receptor complex by having different rates of desensitization.

A unique feature of the AMPA receptor B subunit is that it undergoes a process of RNA transcript editing that changes an amino acid in the protein sequence from glutamine (a neutral amino acid) to arginine (an amino acid with a positive charge in its side chain). Normally, gene DNA sequences correspond exactly to the final protein sequence because the RNA transcript is a copy of the DNA sequence. RNA editing occurs when an enzyme selectively changes a nucleotide in the messenger RNA so that the meaning of its codon (the triplet nucleotide sequence corresponding to a specific amino acid) changes from one amino acid to another. Because this amino acid position lies in the channel part of the receptor, it affects the ion selectivity of the channel. AMPA receptor channels having GluR2 subunits with glutamine can conduct calcium ions, whereas those having arginine in this position cannot conduct calcium. Most AMPA receptors have one or more GluR2 subunits that have been edited so they cannot conduct calcium.

Kainate glutamatergic ionotropic receptors are similar to AMPA receptors. There are subunits that form kainate receptors called GluR5–GluR7, KA-1, and KA-2. The pharmacology of kainate receptors is so similar to that for AMPA receptors that it is difficult to distinguish their responses to most glutamatergic drugs. Kainate receptors have different response kinetics and recover from desensitization approximately 10-fold more slowly than AMPA receptors. Like AMPA receptors, some kainate receptor subunits (GluR5 and GluR6) exist in RNA-edited forms that conduct calcium ions poorly.

Inhibitory Ionotropic Receptors

The GABA$_A$ and glycine ionotropic receptors share important features. Both conduct negatively charged chloride ions in response to neurotransmitter binding that results in an inhibitory hyperpolarization of the cell. They are characterized by subunits with four transmembrane domains, and the receptor complex consists of five such subunits. The subunits that form these receptors are not the same, and the number of different types of subunits is also different.

GABA$_A$ receptors are produced from four types of subunits referred to as α, β, γ, and δ. A receptor complex consists of two α, two β, and one γ or δ subunit. Molecular biology studies have identified six different α, three β, three γ, and one δ subunit. There could be more than 10,000 possible GABA$_A$ pentameric receptor combinations, but it is likely that more than 90% of the GABA$_A$ receptors present in brain are contributed by as few as 8 subunit combinations. The most common "subtype" of GABA$_A$ receptors has two α_1, two β_2, and one γ_2 subunit. This subtype is found in most parts of the brain on small interneurons that regulate the activity of larger excitatory neurons (Fig. 7).

GABA$_A$ receptors respond to a number of drugs and drug-like substances. The best known group of these is the minor tranquilizers called benzodiazepines. These drugs include clonazepam (Klonopin), used to treat epilepsy, and alprazolam (Xanax), used to treat anxiety. Sedatives such as the barbiturates and alcohol also act on GABA$_A$ receptors. These drugs are not recognized at the same site on the GABA$_A$ receptor as is the neurotransmitter GABA. Instead, they bind to different allosteric sites on

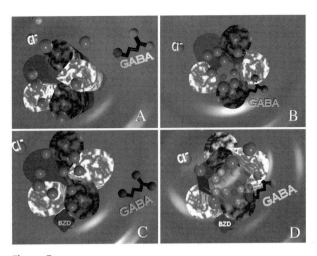

Figure 7
Ionotropic receptors (ligand-gated ion channels) are pore-forming proteins that can be activated and opened by neurotransmitter binding. (A) The γ-aminobenzoic acid (GABA) chloride channel is also the site of action of a group of drugs called benzodiazepines (BZDs) (e.g., alprazolam). (B) The receptor is composed of five subunits and allows influx of chloride into the cell when the neurotransmitter GABA binds to it. (C) BZD binding alone is not sufficient to open the channel. (D) The binding of both GABA and BZDs allows greater chloride influx than GABA binding alone. (See color plate section.)

the complex and modulate the effect produced by GABA.

The glycine ionotropic receptor complex differs from the GABA$_A$ receptor in that it is formed from different subunits and in a different order. There are four α subunits and one β subunit that can be combined to form the five-protein glycine receptor. These subunits consist of approximately 450 amino acids. They combine at a ratio of three α to two β subunits. Although there is substantial similarity (homology) between the amino acid sequences of GABA$_A$ and glycine receptor subunits, they are different.

There are some glycine ionotropic receptors in the brain, but their primary location is in the spinal cord, where they have an important role in regulating motor function. Strychnine is a selective antagonist of glycine receptors, meaning that it competes with glycine for binding to the receptor and prevents glycine-induced activation of the receptor.

G PROTEIN-COUPLED RECEPTORS

All G protein-coupled receptors share certain common features. They all bind a complex of three proteins (α, β, and γ), of which the α subunit binds guanyl nucleotide triphosphate (GTP). The G protein complex binds to the cytoplasmic face of the receptor, giving the complex access to the intracellular space of the cell. Like the ionotropic receptors previously described, G protein-coupled receptors extend through the cell membrane to the extracellular space, where they encounter neurotransmitters. Unlike ionotropic receptors, which are composed of several protein subunits combined to form an ion channel, G protein-coupled receptors consist of a single protein. The G protein-coupled receptor has a characteristic structure in which the protein chain passes through the membrane seven times, with the N-terminal end extending into the extracellular space outside the cell and the C-terminal end extending into the internal cytoplasm. This seven-transmembrane domain structure is another characteristic feature of these receptors.

G protein-coupled receptors can change the membrane potential but, unlike the ionotropic receptors, they must do this indirectly since they cannot conduct ions. Ion conductance changes produced by G protein-coupled receptor activation occur though the actions of the G protein complex on independent ion channels in the membrane. An important consequence is that membrane potential changes produced by G protein-coupled receptors occur more slowly than those of ionotropic receptors and for a longer period of time.

The G protein complex can be viewed as undergoing a cyclic activation and deactivation process that is catalyzed the G protein-coupled receptor (Fig. 8). The key to this cyclic process lies in the activity of the α subunit of the G protein complex. An inactive G protein-coupled receptor will bind the G protein complex. Neurotransmitter recognition by the receptor is transmitted to the bound G protein complex through a conformational change in the receptor protein. This causes a change in the guanyl nucleotide binding site of the α subunit that allows the dissociation of bound guanyl nucleotide diphosphate (GDP) and its exchange for GTP from the cytoplasm. The binding of GTP causes the entire G protein complex to disassociate from the receptor. The free G protein complex then breaks into two parts. One part, the βγ dimeric protein complex, remains in the membrane but moves away from the receptor. The freed GTP-bound α subunit also remains associated with the plasma membrane and comes into contact with intracellular enzymes that it can activate or inhibit. The three most important enzymes that the GTP-bound α subunit interacts with are adenylyl cyclase, phospholipase C, and phospho-

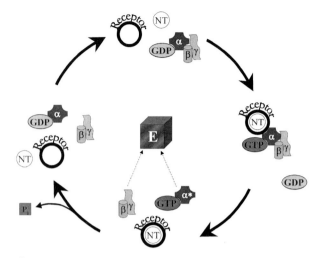

Figure 8
When activated, a G protein-coupled receptor catalyzes a cycle of events that results in the activation or inhibition of various effectors and downstream modulation of second messenger formation. Upon binding of a neurotransmitter, the receptor–G protein complex is activated. This allows for dissociation of guanosine diphosphate (GDP) from the α subunit of the G protein (Gα) and subsequent association of GTP. The Gβγ subunits, which are normally tightly bound to GDP-bound Gα, are released from GTP-bound Gα. In this way, both activated Gα and liberated Gβγ subunits are free to interact with effectors. Eventually, the GTPase activity of Gα hydrolyzes its bound GTP into GDP, allowing for reassociation with Gβγ and a resetting of the system for another round. The cycle can continue unabated until the neurotransmitter dissociates from its receptor.

lipase A$_2$. The nature of these interactions depends on the type of α subunit involved. The α subunit has GTPase enzyme activity that results in the hydrolysis of the terminal phosphate group from the bound GTP, converting it to GDP. This conversion results in the inactivation of the α subunit terminating the signal response initiated by the neurotransmitter-bound receptor. The GDP-bound α subunit regains its high affinity for the βγ complex to reform the complete G protein complex. This trimeric complex can then reassociate with a G protein-coupled receptor to start the whole process again.

A neurotransmitter-bound G protein-coupled receptor can initiate many cycles of G protein complex activation before the transmitter dissociates. This is part of the amplification of signal that is characteristic of G protein-coupled receptor activity. The signal is further amplified by the downstream interactions of the G protein complex subunits' many other effector molecules to form a cascade of protein-mediated changes in cell activity.

Each of the three subunits of the G protein complex exists in multiple forms. The G protein complex is defined by the α subunit. There are 23 distinct α subunits that can be categorized into four major groups referred to as $G\alpha_s$, $G\alpha_I$, $G\alpha_q$, and $G\alpha_{12}$ (Fig. 9). The $G\alpha_s$ protein stimulates the activity of the enzyme adenylyl cyclase to produce cyclic AMP from adenosine triphosphate. Cyclic AMP has many potential functions, including stimulating protein kinase enzymes that add phosphate groups to certain amino acids of specific proteins. The $G\alpha_I$ protein inhibits adenylyl cyclase activity. The $G\alpha_q$ protein activates the enzyme phospholipase C. This enzyme can hydrolyze the phospholipid phosphatidylinositol 4,5-bisphosphate in cell membranes to form two second messengers, inositol-1,4,5-trisphosphate (IP_3) and diacylglycerol (DAG). IP_3 acts on calcium channels within the cell to mobilize intracellular calcium ions, which in turn can activate several calcium-sensitive enzymes. DAG activates the enzyme protein kinase C, which regulates the activity of certain cellular proteins by adding phosphate groups to them. $G\alpha_q$ can also activate phospholipase A2, which can release another second messenger, arachidonic acid, from the membrane lipid phosphatidylinositol. The activity of the $G\alpha_{12}$ group of $G\alpha$ proteins is not well defined.

The β and γ subunits remain bound together during the G protein cycle, and this complex has its own activities. Currently, 5 β subunits and 11 γ subunits are known. The activities of free $\beta\gamma$ dimers are less well understood than those of the $G\alpha$ subunits, but it is known that they can open certain potassium channels to induce membrane hyperpolarization and can affect cyclic AMP formation by interacting with some of the adenylyl cyclase enzymes.

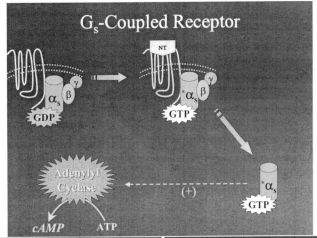

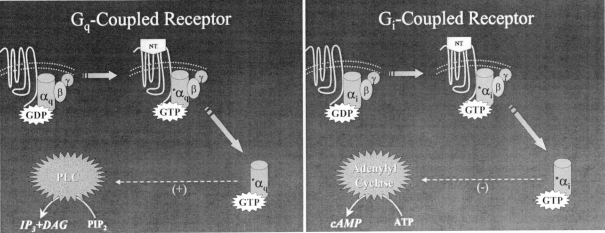

Figure 9

Three types of G protein-coupled receptors are demonstrated: adenylyl cyclase stimulatory (G_s), adenylyl cyclase inhibitory (G_i), and phospholipase C stimulatory (G_q). When the $G\alpha$ subunit is bound, activated by GTP binding (asterisk), it can interact with effectors and transduce neurotransmitter receptor activation into the cell.

G protein-coupled receptors are categorized into three major subclasses. The largest of these is the rhodopsin subclass, which includes receptors for acetylcholine, norepinephrine, dopamine, serotonin, and many neuropeptides. The second subclass is the secretin peptide receptor group. Neurotransmitter receptors in this subclass include receptors for the peptides calcitonin, corticotropin-releasing factor, and vasoactive intestinal peptide. Some of the receptors in this subclass are only found outside the nervous system, although most are present in both neural and nonneuronal tissues. The third subclass consists of the metabotropic glutamate and GABA$_B$ receptors. The three subclasses of G protein-coupled receptors are distinguished by major differences in their amino acid sequences, but they all share the common characteristics of having seven transmembrane domains and their ability to couple to G proteins. Because there are hundreds of different G protein-coupled receptors, only single representatives of each are described.

Muscarinic Acetylcholine Receptors of the Rhodopsin Subclass

Muscarinic receptors are so called because they can be selectively activated by the plant alkaloid muscarine to distinguish them pharmacologically from the ionotropic nicotinic acetylcholine receptors. They consist of five different subtypes referred to as M_1–M_5. The M_1, M_3, and M_5 receptors use the $G\alpha_q$ group of G proteins to activate phospholipase C, whereas the M_2 and M_4 receptors use the $G\alpha_i$ group to inhibit adenylate cyclase and stimulate ion conductance by certain potassium channels.

The muscarinic receptor subtypes are present in many tissues. In the nervous system, they are found in specific locations of most large structures of the brain, in the spinal cord, and in autonomic ganglia. They have important roles in the regulation of autonomic functions, such as breathing, heart rate, and glandular secretion, and have a critical role in the learning and memory functions of the central nervous system.

Like all G protein-coupled receptors, the muscarinic receptors have a seven-transmembrane domain structure in which the protein chain enters and exits the membrane seven times. The amino acid sequences of the transmembrane domains are highly similar (homologous) between the muscarinic receptors and have significant similarity to those of other rhodopsin subclass receptors. There is essentially no sequence homology to receptors of other G protein-

coupled receptor subclasses. There is much less homology between muscarinic receptors for those parts of the receptor sequence that extend outside of the membrane. The amino acid sequence extending from the N-terminal amino acid enters the membrane to form the first transmembrane domain, passes through the intracellular cytoplasm to form the first intracellular loop, and reenters the membrane to form the second transmembrane domain. Thus, there are three intracellular loops and three extracellular loops in addition to the extended extracellular N-terminal sequence and the extended intracellular C-terminal sequence. The transmembrane domains cluster to surround a central axis, and some appear to strongly interact. The extracellular loops do not appear to have an important role in acetylcholine recognition, which occurs in the space formed by the transmembrane domains (this is not the case for all other G protein-coupled receptors), but the intracellular loops have an important role in the recognition of the large G protein complex.

In addition to G protein complex binding, muscarinic and other G protein-coupled receptors bind at least two other important intracellular proteins, G protein receptor kinases and β-arrestins. G protein receptor kinases selectively phosphorylate serine or threonine amino acids in the third intracellular loop of muscarinic receptors. The addition of a phosphate group to these amino acids is strongly stimulated by acetylcholine binding. Phosphorylation of these amino acids promotes the binding of a β-arrestin protein that blocks G protein interactions by the receptor. This effectively inactivates the receptor (desensitization) and leads to its removal from the cell surface (internalization). Desensitization and internalization are elements of the signal termination process. Internalized receptors may be dephosphorylated in endosomes and returned to the cell surface through a process of receptor recycling, or they may be destroyed by proteolytic enzymes in lysomes (downregulation).

Vasoactive Intestinal Peptide Receptors of the Secretin Subclass

The vasoactive intestinal peptide (VIP) receptors are members of the secretin subclass of G protein-coupled receptors present at high density in the nervous system. Only two types of VIP receptors are known, and no subtypes or splice variants have been described. The human VIP-1 receptor consists of 457 amino acids, whereas the VIP-2 receptor has 438 amino acids. Both receptors have high affinity (equilibrium dissociation constants between 1 and 10 nM) for another endogenous peptide, pituitary adenylyl cyclase-activating polypeptide (PACAP). This suggests that both peptides may act as transmitters for these receptors in some tissues. The accepted abbreviations for the two VIP receptors, VPAC1 and VPAC2, reflect this potential overlap. PACAP also acts at a third secretin subclass receptor, PAC1, for which VIP has little affinity.

The VPAC1 and VPAC2 receptors have distinct distributions in the brain. VPAC1 receptors are located mostly in the cerebral cortex and hippocampus. VPAC2 receptors are concentrated in the deeper structures of the brain, including the thalamus, hypothalamus, and brainstem. The two receptors are only found together in the hippocampus. High concentrations of these receptors are seen outside the nervous system in the gastrointestinal system, lungs, and heart.

The recognition sites for VIP include amino acids of the transmembrane domain in addition to others of the extracellular N-terminal sequence, despite the large size of VIP (28 amino acids). Large peptide neurotransmitters for the rhodopsin subclass of G protein-coupled receptors also show a dependence on recognition by receptor amino acids present deep in the pocket formed by the seven-transmembrane domain core of these receptors. The VPAC1 and VPAC2 receptors couple to Gα_s-containing G protein complexes to stimulate adenylyl cyclase.

Glutamate Receptors of the Metabotropic Glutamate/GABA$_B$ Subclass

Glutamate serves as a neurotransmitter for a class of G protein-coupled receptors in addition to the ionotropic glutamate ion channel receptors. There are eight subtypes of metabotropic glutamate receptors (mGluR), identified as mGluR1–mGluR8, in the vertebrate nervous system. This diversity is further increased by the presence of four splice variants of the mGluR1 and two each for the mGluR5 and mGluR4 receptors. All these splice variants differ in the length of the cytoplasmic C-terminal tail of the receptor sequence. The mGlu receptors are classified into three groups determined by their protein sequence, pharmacology, and G protein interactions. Group 1 receptors include mGluR1 and mGluR5, group 2 receptors include mGluR2 and mGluR3, and group 3 receptors include mGluR4 and mGluR6–mGluR8.

The mGlu receptors are widely dispersed throughout the nervous system. They are often found on the presynaptic terminals of glutamatergic neurons, where they act as autoreceptors to regulate glutamate release. They are also found at postsynaptic sites, where they can regulate neuronal excitability and initiate other G protein-mediated effects.

mGlu receptors have several unusual structural features that distinguish them from other G protein-coupled receptors. They share significant sequence homology with the other members of this subclass, the GABA$_B$ receptors, but lack homology to receptors of the other two subclasses of G protein-coupled receptors. The mGlu receptors are much larger than other G protein-coupled receptors, with a very large N-terminal sequence and a large C-terminal tail. Unlike other G protein-coupled receptors that bind neurotransmitters in the space between the seven transmembrane domains, mGlu receptors recognize glutamate at a site formed in the extracellular space by the N-terminal chain. The extracellular parts of the mGlu receptors, including the extracellular loops connecting the transmembrane domains, have 19 cystines that can cross-link through dithio bridges to increase the rigidity of the protein structure. The N-terminal sequence is thought to form two clamshell-like halves surrounding a central glutamate recognition site. A distortion in the conformation of this extracellular structure could be transferred to the hinge region and further transmitted through the receptor to the G protein recognition site.

The mGlu receptors recognize at least two classes of G proteins. The group 1 receptors (mGluR$_1$ and mGluR$_5$) activate Gα_q-containing G protein complexes to stimulate phospholipase C. Both group 2 and group 3 mGlu receptors activate Gα_I-containing G protein complexes to inhibit adenylyl cyclase. Not all the effects of mGlu receptors can be linked to these two G protein families, and it is likely that other G protein effectors are involved.

The autoreceptor function of mGlu receptors on presynaptic terminals of glutamatergic neurons is an important means of regulating glutamate neurotransmission. Multiple subtypes of mGlu receptors can act as autoreceptors, and two mechanisms for this activity are hypothesized. One mechanism is the inhibition of voltage-gated calcium ion currents. Another possibility is that glutamate release is blocked by activation of presynaptic potassium channels to prevent depolarization of the presynaptic terminal. Currently, neither mechanism can be attributed to particular mGlu receptors, but all three groups of mGlu receptors can contribute to autoreceptor activity at different synapses.

There is little information on mechanisms related to mGlu receptor desensitization and downregulation. Several potential protein kinase phosphorylation sites are present at the cytoplasmic face of these receptors, but their participation in kinase activity has not been determined. The very large (300-amino acid) C-terminal tail of the receptor is unusual and may participate in regulating receptor sensitivity and movement in the membrane.

CONCLUSION

Neural activity depends on two modes of neurotransmission. The fast excitatory and inhibitory neurotransmission provided by ionotropic receptors enables us to perceive and respond to outside events in real time. However, it is equally important to distinguish what is critical in our perceptions from what is less critical and then to respond appropriately. This requires a different kind of neurotransmission that is more flexible and long-lasting, such as that provided by G protein-coupled receptors. Both forms of neurotransmission seem to be essential because they exist in nearly all forms of multicellular life.

Neurons receiving incoming waves of neurotransmitters are not passive recipients of this information. The message received is determined as much by the neurotransmitter receptors expressed by a neuron as the neurotransmitters it encounters. This concept helps to explain the observation that there are more types of neurotransmitter receptors than neurotransmitters.

Another important concept is that neurotransmitter receptors bridge extracellular and intracellular compartments in both directions. Events at the cytoplasmic face of the receptor influence neurotransmitter recognition, just as recognition influences effector activity.

How many neurotransmitter receptors are there? Currently, it is not known, but our ignorance is not likely to continue indefinitely, at least with regard to humans and a few other species. All neurotransmitter receptors are encoded in the genome, and they tend to have an important degree of similarity. A number of "orphan" receptors without known neurotransmitters have been identified through genetic screening methods. With the final sequencing of the human genome, it will be possible to identify more receptors by computer-assisted homology screening. Each new receptor is a potential drug target, and our ability to treat complex neurological and neuropsychiatric diseases will depend on our knowledge of neurotransmitter receptors.

—*Richard Knapp, Marc Rubenzik, Ewa Malatynska, Eva Varga, William R. Roeske, and Henry I. Yamamura*

See also–**Acetylcholine; Amino Acids; Basal Ganglia; Gamma Aminobutyric Acid (GABA); G Proteins; Neuropeptides, Overview; Neurotransmitters, Overview; Nicotinic Receptors; Sensory Receptors, Overview**

Further Reading

Nestler, E. J., Hyman, S. E., and Malenka, R. C. (Eds.) (2001). *Molecular Neuropharmacology: A Foundation for Clinical Neuroscience.* McGraw-Hill, New York.
Siegel, G. J., Agranoff, B. W., Albers, R. W., *et al.* (1999). *Basic Neurochemistry. Molecular, Cellular & Medical Aspects*, 6th ed. Lippincott Williams & Wilkins, Philadelphia.

Neurotransmitters, Overview

Encyclopedia of the Neurological Sciences

NEUROTRANSMITTERS are chemicals that are released from neurons to communicate through intercellular space. These chemicals are structurally diverse and include amines, amino acids, and peptides. Moreover, a given neuron may contain more than one transmitter. Neurotransmitters are usually produced and stored in the neurons from which they are released. Upon release into the intercellular space, they may interact with other neurons, nonneuronal cells, or even the cell of origin. These interactions occur through the binding of neurotransmitter molecules to specialized membrane proteins called receptors. Receptor binding leads to changes in membrane ion flux or intracellular metabolism that transmit information about neuronal activity to target cells.

NEUROTRANSMITTER HYPOTHESIS

The idea that neurons use chemicals to communicate is comparatively new, and evidence supporting this theory was first observed in the autonomic nervous system. In 1901, Langley showed that extracts from the adrenal gland mimicked the effect of sympathetic nerve stimulation. During the next decade, Elliott, Barger, and Dale found evidence pointing to epinephrine or a related amine as a humoral mediator in the sympathetic nervous system, and this was identified as norepinephrine by von Euler in 1946. Meanwhile, Dixon had proposed that a chemical resembling the plant alkaloid muscarine was responsible for vagal impulses, and Dale showed in 1914 that this substance might be acetylcholine.

The critical experiment required to prove chemical neurotransmission was performed in 1921 by Otto Loewi, who stimulated a frog's vagus nerve and observed that, as expected, the heart rate slowed. He then collected the fluid that perfused the heart, which he reasoned should contain any humoral factor that might be released by vagal stimulation, and applied it to a second heart. When this was done, the second heart slowed. The implication was that a chemical substance, which Loewi called Vagusstoff, was released from the stimulated vagus nerve of the first heart and reproduced the effect of nerve stimulation on a second, unstimulated heart. Subsequent experiments showed that sympathetic nerve stimulation also released a humoral factor, called Acceleransstoff by Loewi and sympathin by Cannon, that could mimic the effects of nerve stimulation.

During the intervening decades, criteria for neurotransmitter status have been developed and revised, additional neurotransmitter candidates have been identified, mechanisms for neurotransmitter release and inactivation have been elucidated, and neurotransmitter receptors and transporters have been cloned. Defects in neurotransmission have been implicated in a variety of neurological diseases, including botulism, Lambert–Eaton syndrome, myasthenia gravis, and Parkinson's disease, and knowledge about neurotransmitter systems has been widely exploited in drug discovery. Advances in the field of neurotransmitter research have been recognized by the awarding of eight Nobel prizes in physiology or medicine to Henry Hallett Dale and Otto Loewi (1936) for "their discoveries relating to chemical transmission of nerve impulses"; to Bernard Katz, Ulf von Euler, and Julius Axelrod (1970) for "their discoveries concerning the humoral transmitters in the nerve terminals and the mechanism for their storage, release, and inactivation"; and to Robert F. Furchgott, Louis J. Ignarro, and Ferid Murad (1998) for "their discoveries concerning nitric oxide as a signaling molecule."

CLASSIC NEUROTRANSMITTER CRITERIA

As the role of acetylcholine as a neurotransmitter, especially in the autonomic nervous system and at the neuromuscular junction, began to gain wide acceptance, the possibility was entertained that other transmitters existed as well. Therefore, acetylcholine became the model against which new neurotransmitter candidates would be judged, and key features of acetylcholine-mediated (cholinergic) transmission became established as criteria for canonical neurotransmitter status (Fig. 1).

First, neurotransmitters must be present in nerve terminals so they can be released in response to stimulation. This implies that they are synthesized in nerve terminals, presumably from precursors taken up by neurons. In the case of acetylcholine, the precursor is choline, which is converted to acetylcholine through the enzymatic action of choline acetyltransferase. A corollary of the requirement for neurotransmitter localization to nerve terminals is that the enzymes responsible for transmitter synthesis should be found there as well. Since the ability of neurons to communicate rapidly requires a preformed pool of transmitter molecules, nerve terminals must also possess sites for storing these molecules, which typically take the form of membrane-bound vesicles.

Second, neurotransmitters must be released in response to nerve stimulation. We now know that such stimulation activates sodium channels, which admit extracellular sodium into cells, leading to depolarization of the neuronal membrane. Depolarization, in turn, leads to opening of calcium channels, and the extracellular calcium that enters the nerve terminal through these channels triggers neurotransmitter release. Release occurs at specialized, active zones of the neuronal membrane and results from the

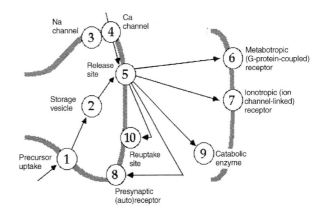

Figure 1
Synaptic pharmacology of classic neurotransmitters. Each numbered step in the process of neurotransmission also represents a potential target for drug action, as detailed in the text for individual neurotransmitter systems.

fusion of neurotransmitter-containing vesicles with the cell membrane, followed by exocytosis of their contents

Third, neurotransmitters must interact with target molecules, or receptors, on the surface of cells with which they communicate. Dale was the first to show that a given neurotransmitter (acetylcholine) could act through different receptors (nicotinic and muscarinic), and multiple receptors for a single transmitter are now known to be the rule. Neurotransmitter receptors are categorized into two classes: ionotropic receptors, which modulate ion fluxes, and metabotropic or G protein-coupled receptors, which activate chemical second messengers (Table 1). In some cases, receptors for a neurotransmitter can be found on the same neuron from which the transmitter is released. These autoreceptors help to regulate neurotransmitter release.

Fourth, neurotransmitters must be capable of inactivation to limit their actions in time and space, so mechanisms for inactivation must exist at or near their sites of release. Acetylcholine is inactivated by enzymatic breakdown, in which acetylcholinesterase is employed to regenerate choline. However, other transmitters are inactivated by removal from the synaptic cleft through reuptake into neurons or glia.

CLASSIC NEUROTRANSMITTERS

The classic, or canonical, neurotransmitters include acetylcholine; the amines norepinephrine, epinephrine, dopamine, serotonin, and histamine; and the amino acids glutamic acid, γ-aminobutyric acid (GABA), and glycine. Numerous drugs and several neurological disorders affect these transmitter systems (Tables 2 and 3).

Acetylcholine

Acetylcholine is synthesized from choline and acetyl coenzyme A by the action of choline acetyltransferase. The transmitter is stored in vesicles of nerve terminals and released into the synaptic cleft, where it can interact with nicotinic or muscarinic acetylcholine receptors. Acetylcholine is degraded extracellularly by acetylcholinesterase, which generates choline and acetate, the latter of which undergoes reuptake into neurons, providing the precursor for resynthesis of acetylcholine.

Acetylcholine is employed as the transmitter at the neuromuscular junction; in preganglionic, parasympathetic postganglionic, and sympathetic sudomotor fibers; and in central pathways arising in subcortical regions such as the septal nuclei and nucleus basalis and projecting to hippocampus and neocortex.

Neurological disorders associated with alterations in cholinergic transmission include botulism and the Lambert–Eaton myasthenic syndrome, which interfere with acetylcholine release, and myasthenia gravis, in which nicotinic receptors are subject to attack by autoantibodies.

Several therapeutic drugs act by modifying cholinergic transmission. Muscarinic acetylcholine receptor antagonists, such as trihexyphenidyl and benztropine, are used to treat Parkinson's disease and other movement disorders. Acetylcholinesterase

Table 1 NEUROTRANSMITTER RECEPTOR SUPERFAMILIES

	Superfamily	
	Class I	Class II
Subunits	Multiple	Single
Transmembrane segments	4	7
Speed of transmission	Fast (milliseconds)	Slow (seconds to minutes)
Receptor type	Ionotropic	Metabotropic
Transduction mechanism	Altered ion conductance (Na, K, Ca, Cl)	G protein-coupled second messenger production (cAMP, cGMP, Ca, IP_3, DAG)
Examples	Nicotinic ACh	Muscarinic ACh
	$GABA_A$	α- and β-adrenergic
	Glutamate—NMDA, AMPA	Dopamine D_1- and D_2-like
		5-HT (except $5-HT_3$)
		$GABA_B$
		Glutamate—metabotropic
		Cannbinoid CB1

Table 2 THERAPEUTIC DRUGS AFFECTING SYNAPTIC TRANSMISSION[a]

Site of action	Transmitter	Drug	Neurological disorder
Synthesis (increase)	DA	L-DOPA	Parkinson's disease
	5-HT	5-Hydroxytryptophan	Myoclonus
	Nitric oxide	Sodium nitroprusside	Hypertension
Storage (decrease)	NE, 5-HT, DA	Reserpine, tetrabenazine	Chorea
Release (increase)	DA	Amantadine	Parkinson's disease
	NE, DA	Dextromphetamine, methylphenidate	Narcolepsy
Reuptake (decrease)	NE, 5-HT, DA	Tricyclic antidepressants	Migraine, pain
	5-HT	Selective serotonin reuptake inhibitors	Migraine, pain
	GABA	Tiagabine, vigabatrin	Seizures
Breakdown (decrease)	ACh	Cholinesterase inhibitors—pyridostigmine, donepezil	Myasthenia gravis, Alzheimer's disease
	NE, 5-HT, DA	Monoamine oxidase inhibitors—selegiline, pargyline	Parkinson's disease, migraine
	NE, 5-HT, DA	Catechol-O-methyl transferase inhibitors—tolcapone	Parkinson's disease
Receptor (agonist)	DA (D_1 and D_2)	Ergot alkaloids	Parkinson's disease
	5-HT ($5-HT_{1B}$ and $5-HT_{1D}$)	Dihydroergotamine, triptans	Migraine
	GABA ($GABA_A$/BZ)	Clonazepam, lorazepam, diazepam	Seizures
	GABA ($GABA_B$)	Baclofen	Spasticity
	Opioid (μ)	Opioid analgesics	Pain
Receptor (antagonist)	ACh (muscarinic)	Benztropine, trihexyphenidyl	Parkinson's disease
	NE (β)	Propranolol	Migraine, tremor
	DA (D_2)	Haloperidol	Chorea
		Metoclopramide	Migraine
	5-HT ($5-HT_2$)	Methysergide	Migraine
	HA (H_1)	Diphenhydramine, meclizine	Vertigo
	GABA ($GABA_A$/BZ)	Flumazenil	Coma
	Glutamic acid (NMDA)	Amantadine	Parkinson's disease
	Adenosine (A_1)	Caffeine	Post-LP headache
	Opioid (μ)	Naloxone	Coma

[a] Abbreviations used: ACh, acetylcholine; BZ, benzodiazepine; DA, dopamine, HA, histamine; 5-HT, 5-hydroxytryptamine (serotonin); NE, norepinephrine.

inhibitors, which block the breakdown of acetylcholine and thereby increase transmitter concentrations at the synapse, are employed in myasthenia gravis (pyridostigmine) and Alzheimer's disease (donepezil).

Norepinephrine and Epinephrine

Norepinephrine and epinephrine (as well as dopamine) are catecholamines and are synthesized from the precursor amino acid tyrosine by a series of enzymatic steps. These involve the conversion of tyrosine to DOPA by tyrosine hydroxylase and of DOPA to dopamine by L-aromatic amino acid decarboxylase (in dopaminergic neurons) and subsequently of dopamine to norepinephrine by dopamine β-hydroxylase (in noradrenergic neurons) and of norepinephrine to epinephrine by phenylethanola-

mine-N-methyltransferase (in epinephrine-producing neurons and the adrenal medulla). Released norepinephrine binds to α- or β-adrenergic receptors, and its action is terminated by reuptake. Following this step, norepinephrine is broken down by monoamine oxidase (MAO) and catechol-O-methyl transferase (COMT) to produce 3-methoxy-4-hydroxymandelic acid as the principal metabolite.

Norepinephrine is the transmitter of sympathetic postganglionic fibers and of central pathways that originate in the locus coeruleus and project to cerebral cortex, cerebellum, spinal cord, and other regions. Epinephrine is the principal hormone produced by the adrenal medulla. A defect in norepinephrine synthesis has been implicated in pure autonomic failure.

Table 3 NEUROLOGICAL DISORDERS OF SYNAPTIC TRANSMISSION

Site of action	Transmitter	Disorder
Synthesis (decrease)	DA	Parkinson's disease
	NE	Pure autonomic failure
	GABA	Stiff-man syndrome
Release (decrease)	Acetylcholine	Botulism, Lambert–Eaton myasthenic syndrome
	Glycine, GABA	Tetanus
Receptor	Acetylcholine (nicotinic)	Myasthenia gravis
	Acetylcholine (muscarinic)	Mushroom (*Amanita muscaria*) poisoning
	Dopamine (D_2)	Antipsychotic drug-induced extrapyramidal syndromes
	Glycine	Strychnine poisoning
	Glutamic acid (NMDA)	Rasmussen's encephalitis
	Glutamic acid (multiple)	Domoic acid (blue mussel) poisoning

Drugs that alter adrenergic neurotransmission include agents that stimulate norepinephrine release and are used to treat narcolepsy (methylphenidate and dextroamphetamine) and antimigraine agents that inhibit norepinephrine reuptake (tricyclic antidepressants) or block β-adrenergic receptors (propranolol).

Dopamine

The synthesis of dopamine was discussed previously, and its enzymatic breakdown proceeds as described for norepinephrine, except that the major metabolite is homovanillic acid. Dopamine receptors are categorized as D_1-like and D_2-like, and they differ in the second messenger mechanisms to which they are coupled. The action of dopamine, like that of norepinephrine, is terminated by reuptake.

Dopamine is the neurotransmitter of three principal central pathways: the nigrostriatal tract, projecting from pars compacta of substantia nigra to caudate nucleus and putamen; the mesolimbic and mesocortical tracts, from the ventral tegmentum of midbrain to nucleus accumbens, olfactory tubercle, and neocortex; and the tuberoinfundibular tract, which stimulates prolactin secretion, from the arcuate nucleus to the median eminence.

Degeneration (as in Parkinson's disease) or pharmacological blockade (as in antipsychotic drug treatment) of the nigrostriatal dopamine pathway produce parkinsonism.

Drugs that modify dopaminergic transmission at a variety of sites are used to treat Parkinson's disease. These include L-DOPA, which provides the metabolic precursor for dopamine; amantadine, which acts in part by stimulating dopamine release; dopamine receptor agonists such as bromocriptine,

pergolide, lisuride, cabergoline, ropinirole, and pramipexole, which mimic the effect of dopamine at D_2-like receptors; and inhibitors of MAO (selegiline and pargyline) or COMT (tolcapone), which interfere with dopamine breakdown. Dopamine receptor antagonist drugs are used to treat chorea and other hyperkinetic movement disorders (haloperidol and phenothiazines) and migraine (metoclopramide).

Serotonin

Serotonin or 5-hydroxytryptamine (5-HT), an indoleamine, is synthesized from the amino acid precursor tryptophan through the action of tryptophan hydroxylase, which generates 5-hydroxytryptophan, and L-aromatic amino acid decarboxylase, which produces serotonin. The synaptic effect of serotonin is turned off by reuptake. Enzymatic breakdown depends on MAO and aldehyde dehydrogenase and yields 5-hydroxyindoleacetic acid. Serotonin acts through both ionotropic and G protein-coupled receptors.

The most prominent serotonergic pathway originates in the brainstem raphe nuclei and projects diffusely throughout the brain and spinal cord. A disorder of central serotonergic transmission has been proposed to underlie the pathophysiology of migraine.

The serotonin precursor 5-hydroxytryptophan has been used to treat myoclonus. Tricyclic antidepressants (e.g., amitriptyline) and selective serotonin reuptake inhibitors (e.g., fluoxetine), which block serotonin uptake and thus potentiate its effects, are used to treat a variety of pain syndromes. Serotonin $5\text{-}HT_{1B}$ and $5\text{-}HT_{1D}$ receptor agonist drugs, such as sumatriptan, rizatriptan, zolmitriptan, and naratriptan, are agents of choice for the acute treatment of migraine attacks.

Histamine

Histamine, or β-aminoethylimidazole, is produced from the amino acid precursor histidine by L-histidine decarboxylase. Its action is terminated by metabolic breakdown, which involves conversion to N-methylhistamine by histamine-N-methyltransferase and to N-methyl imidazole acetic acid by monoamine oxidase or to imidazole acetic acid by diamine oxidase. Histamine acts at G protein-coupled H_1–H_3 receptors. Histamine-containing neurons in the central nervous system are concentrated primarily in the hypothalamus and project widely to the brain and spinal cord.

Histamine H_1 receptor antagonists (antihistamines), such as meclizine, promethazine, and dimenhydrinate, are used to treat vertigo. The H_1 antagonist diphenhydramine is sometimes administered for acute dystonic reactions to antipsychotic drugs, but its therapeutic action in this setting is probably related to anticholinergic rather than antihistaminic effects.

Glutamic Acid

Glutamic acid, or glutamate, is the most abundant excitatory transmitter in the central nervous system. It is produced from α-ketoglutarate by the aminotransferases. Following its release, the action of glutamic acid is terminated by reuptake, predominantly into astrocytes. There, it is converted to glutamine, which is taken up into neurons and recycled to glutamic acid. Glutamic acid interacts with both ionotropic and G protein-coupled receptors. Ionotropic glutamic acid receptors are classified based on differences in their affinity for the glutamic acid analog N-methyl-D-aspartate (NMDA) as NMDA- or non-NMDA-preferring.

Glutamic acid-containing neurons are distributed widely throughout the central nervous system and include pyramidal cells of the cerebral cortex and cerebellar granule cells.

Autoantibodies directed against NMDA-preferring glutamate receptors have been implicated in Rasmussen's encephalitis, a rare inflammatory disorder manifested by seizures. Domoic acid, a toxin present in blue mussels, is thought to produce symptoms through its interaction with glutamic acid receptors. Excessive release of glutamic acid leading to neuronal cell death, termed excitotoxicity, appears to play a role in the pathophysiology of several neurological disorders, including stroke, epilepsy, head trauma, and perhaps neurodegenerative diseases such as amyotrophic lateral sclerosis and Huntington's disease.

The antiparkinsonian drug amantadine may act in part as an NMDA receptor antagonist. Other NMDA antagonists include the dissociative anesthetic ketamine and the recreational drug phencyclidine.

γ-Aminobutyric Acid

GABA is the most abundant inhibitory transmitter in the brain. Its synthesis depends on the enzyme glutamic acid decarboxylase (GAD), which converts glutamic acid to GABA. The synaptic action of GABA is terminated by reuptake, and it is subsequently metabolized by GABA transaminase. GABA binds to ionotropic $GABA_A$ receptors, which open chloride channels, and metabotropic $GABA_B$ receptors, which are coupled to G proteins that inhibit calcium channels.

GABA neurons are found throughout the brain and include inhibitory interneurons in many regions as well as cerebellar Purkinje cells. GAD deficiency causes pyridoxine dependency with seizures, an autosomal recessive disorder. Autoantibodies against GAD are found in stiff-man syndrome.

The anticonvulsants tiagabine and vigabatrin potentiate the effects of GABA by inhibiting its reuptake, whereas topiramate enhances $GABA_A$ receptor currents by an unknown mechanism. Benzodiazepine anticonvulsants and the benzodiazepine antagonist flumazenil act at sites on $GABA_A$ channels. The antispasticity drug baclofen binds to $GABA_B$ receptors.

Glycine

Glycine is a major inhibitory transmitter in the spinal cord. It is synthesized from serine by the enzyme serine hydroxymethyl transferase and its effects are terminated by reuptake. Glycine acts by binding to ionotropic receptors, including strychnine-sensitive receptors and strychnine-insensitive receptors, which are found on NMDA-preferring glutamic acid receptors. Glycine release is impaired in tetanus, and glycine receptor blockade is responsible for the symptoms of strychnine poisoning.

Others

Several additional molecules have been proposed as conventional (amine or amino acid) neurotransmitters, including adenosine, aspartic acid, and taurine.

NONCLASSIC NEUROTRANSMITTERS

Several molecules have a role in communication between neurons, although they differ from classically defined neurotransmitters in important respects. Thus, although classic transmitters are synthesized in nerve terminals, packaged in synaptic vesicles, released by exocytosis involving fusion of synaptic vesicles with the cell membrane, and bind to receptors on the postsynaptic membrane, nonclassic neurotransmitters depart from one or more of these features. Examples cited in the following sections are synthesized at least partly in the neuronal cell body (peptides), are synthesized in the cell membrane and released without vesicular packaging (endocannabinoids), or are released by passive diffusion (gases) and interact with intracellular proteins rather than membrane-bound receptors (Fig. 2).

Peptides

Numerous peptides, many found originally in other tissues, are present in the nervous system, where they are involved in interneuronal signaling. In some cases, a classic neurotransmitter and a neuropeptide coexist in and are released together from the same neuron. Neuropeptides include endocrine hormones and releasing factors such as corticotrophin-releasing hormone, gastrointestinal hormones such as cholecystokinin, neurokinins such as sub-

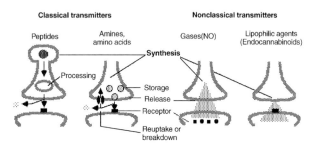

Figure 2
Comparative features of classic and nonclassic neurotransmission. Classic amine and amino acid transmitters are synthesized in nerve terminals, stored in and released from vesicles, act on membrane-bound receptors, and are inactivated by metabolic breakdown and reuptake. Peptides act in similar fashion, except they are synthesized at least partly in the cell body and are not known to undergo reuptake. In contrast, gaseous transmitters, such as NO, and lipophilic transmitters, such as endocannabinoids, are synthesized and immediately released without being stored in vesicles and can diffuse across membranes to activate intracellular effector proteins (e.g., soluble guanylate cyclase in the case of NO) or membrane receptors (e.g., CB1 cannabinoid receptors).

stance P, and opioid peptides such as the enkephalins and endorphins.

Amino Acids

As discussed previously, several amino acids appear to function as classic neurotransmitters, but a newer amino acid transmitter candidate, D-serine, is unconventional in certain respects. The most notable of these is that D-serine is released from glia rather than neurons, although it interacts with the strychnine-insensitive glycine receptor associated with neuronal NMDA receptors.

Endocannabinoids

Certain lipids related to arachidonic acid, including N-arachidonylethanolamide (anandamide) and sn-2-arachidonylglycerol, are neuronal signaling molecules that mimic the effects of $\Delta^9(-)$-tetrahydrocannabinol, the principal psychoactive constituent of marijuana.

Gases

The gases nitric oxide (NO) and carbon monoxide (CO) are unconventional transmitters that can diffuse across cell membranes to interact with intracellular effector proteins such as guanylate cyclase.

NO is produced in neurons by the enzyme neuronal NO synthase (nNOS) in response to stimuli that increase intracellular calcium levels. This process involves the conversion of arginine to citrulline. The NO that is liberated can act within the neuron that produced it or in other neurons or smooth muscle cells by binding to intracellular target proteins. One well-characterized target is soluble guanylate cyclase, which produces the intracellular second messenger cyclic GMP. The effects of NO are terminated by reaction with a wide array of substrates.

nNOS is distributed widely throughout the central and peripheral nervous systems. NO relaxes smooth muscle through its activation of guanylate cyclase, contributing to intestinal relaxation, vasodilatation, and penile erection. NO also has effects on neurons, where it appears to participate in long-term potentiation as well as excitotoxic neuronal injury. Clinically used nitrovasodilator drugs such as sodium nitroprusside and nitroglycerin act by releasing NO.

CO is produced by the enzyme heme oxygenase (HO) as a product of the conversion of heme to biliverdin. One isoform, HO2, is the main CO-producing enzyme in neurons. As in the case of NO, CO can act locally or diffuse into neighboring cells to interact with effector molecules such as soluble guanylate cyclase. HO2 is present in high concentrations in the brain and testes, and it is also found in the intestine. In contrast to NO, which helps to regulate penile erection, CO acts on the vas deferens to promote ejaculation.

—David A. Greenberg

See also—Acetylcholine; Amino Acids; Basal Ganglia; Dopamine; Endocannabinoids; Neuropeptides, Overview; Neurotransmitter Receptors; Nitric Oxide; Norepinephrine; Serotonin

Further Reading

Barañano, D. E., Ferris, C. D., and Snyder, S. H. (2001). Atypical neural messengers. *Trends Neurosci.* **24**, 99–106.

Catterall, W. A. (2000). Structure and regulation of voltage-gated Ca^{2+} channels. *Annu. Rev. Cell. Dev. Biol.* **16**, 521–555.

Hannah, M. J., Schmidt, A. A., and Huttner, W. B. (1999). Synaptic vesicle biogenesis. *Annu. Rev. Cell. Dev. Biol.* **15**, 733–798.

Insel, P. A. (1996). Adrenergic receptors—Evolving concepts and clinical implications. *N. Engl. J. Med.* **334**, 580–585.

Lin, R. C., and Scheller, R. H. (2000). Mechanisms of synaptic vesicle exocytosis. *Annu. Rev. Cell. Dev. Biol.* **16**, 19–49.

Liu, Y., and Edwards, R. H. (1997). The role of vesicular transport proteins in synaptic transmission and neural degeneration. *Annu. Rev. Neurosci.* **20**, 125–156.

MacDermott, A. B., Role, L. W., and Siegelbaum, S. A. (1999). Presynaptic ionotropic receptors and the control of transmitter release. *Annu. Rev. Neurosci.* **22**, 443–485.

Miller, R. J. (1998). Presynaptic receptors. *Annu. Rev. Pharmacol. Toxicol.* **38**, 201–227.

Sabatini, B. L., and Regehr, W. G. (1999). Timing of synaptic transmission. *Annu. Rev. Physiol.* **61**, 521–542.

Seal, R. P., and Amara, S. G. (1999). Excitatory amino acid transporters: A family in flux. *Annu. Rev. Pharmacol. Toxicol.* **39**, 431–456.

Shih, J. C., Chen, K., and Ridd, M. J. (1999). Monoamine oxidase: From genes to behavior. *Annu. Rev. Neurosci.* **22**, 197–217.

Neurotrophins

Encyclopedia of the Neurological Sciences
Copyright 2003, Elsevier Science (USA). All rights reserved.

THE NEUROTROPHINS are a family of growth factors that promote survival and maturation of neurons during the development of the nervous system. Neurotrophins also play important roles in the maintenance of the adult nervous system and its response to injury and disease.

HISTORY

The discovery of the prototypic neurotrophin, nerve growth factor (NGF), resulted from seminal experiments by Levi-Montalcini and Hamburger in the 1940s. They found that after removing the limb bud in the chick embryo, developing peripheral neurons innervating the limb bud died. These neurons were therefore dependent on their target, the limb bud, for their survival. With Stanley Cohen, they later characterized this target-derived neuronal survival factor as NGF. In addition to its role in survival, NGF also encourages outgrowth of axons from developing neurons; hence, it is a tropic as well as a trophic factor.

Initially, the effects of NGF were limited to peripheral nervous system neurons. A factor with similar neurotrophic and neurotropic actions on developing central nervous system neurons was purified from brain and termed brain-derived neurotrophic factor (BDNF). Comparison of the amino acid sequence of NGF and BDNF showed that the two neurotrophins were structurally related. Subsequently, two more factors were cloned based on their homology to NGF and BDNF: neurotrophin-3 (NT-3) and neurotrophin-4/5 (NT-4/5). A fifth neurotrophin, neurotrophin-6, has been cloned in fish.

FUNCTION

Development

Early work on the role of neurotrophins in the survival of developing neurons established the neurotrophic factor hypothesis. This hypothesis provides a model in which developing neurons compete for limited amounts of target-derived neurotrophin. Those neurons whose axons innervate target cells and receive neurotrophin will survive, whereas those without access to sufficient amounts of neurotrophins will die by apoptotic mechanisms.

Neurotrophins have been implicated in the regulation of developmental processes other than target-derived neuronal survival. Furthermore, neurotrophins can originate from sources other than the target, such as local sources around cell bodies. Precursor cells, both neuroblasts and nonneuronal precursors, depend on neurotrophins for both survival and proliferation. Differentiation and maturation of precursor cells and developing neurons are also influenced by neurotrophins. Neurotrophins also regulate sprouting of neuronal axons, local guidance of developing axons, and growth cone turning. Finally, neurotrophins have been shown to influence the formation of ocular dominance columns in the developing central nervous system. Together, the varied functions of neurotrophins underscore their importance in the construction of the nervous system.

Adulthood

The continued expression of neurotrophins through adult life indicates that their functions are not confined to developmental processes. Once mature, neurons lose their dependence on neurotrophins for acute survival and instead rely on neurotrophins for the maintenance of neuronal phenotype and function. Neurotrophins are also important in plasticity, which is the adult nervous system's ability to alter its structure and function in response to stimuli. Expression of neurotrophins increases upon neuronal activity, implicating these factors in activity-dependent processes such as synaptic plasticity. Neurotrophins modify both synaptic function (transmission) and structure (connectivity) in response to stimulus-dependent activity.

The maintenance of neuronal phenotype in the adult nervous system can be compromised by injury and disease. Neurotrophins protect neurons from endogenous toxic events that may be triggered by injury or disease, such as cell death induced by axotomy or glutamate excitotoxicity. In response to injury, neurotrophin expression is upregulated in both the peripheral and central nervous systems. The mechanisms of neurotrophin function in injury are not clear, but neurotrophins appear to be involved in axon regeneration and nerve repair in the peripheral nervous system and in the regrowth and/or reorganization of central neural connections.

As neurons age, their capacity to respond to neurotrophins diminishes and they are more susceptible to cell death. Lack of neurotrophin signaling may directly induce cell atrophy and changes in gene expression leading to apoptosis. Alternatively, decreased neurotrophin responsiveness, and hence neuroprotection, may render the aging neurons more vulnerable to insult and injury.

STRUCTURE AND SIGNALING

Factors, Receptors, and Pathways

The neurotrophin family of soluble growth factors comprises small polypeptides (12 to 13 kDa) that function as noncovalently associated homodimers. The tertiary structure of NGF reveals a tertiary fold

and a cysteine knot. Neurotrophins are found in all mammals and lower vertebrates.

Neurotrophins exert their effects on neurons by signaling through specific cell surface receptors—tropomyosin-related kinase (Trk) receptors and the p75 receptor. Trk receptors are transmembrane receptor tyrosine kinases that are necessary and sufficient for neurotrophin function. Particular Trk receptors bind each neurotrophin: TrkA binds NGF, TrkB binds BDNF and NT-4/5, and TrkC binds NT-3. Binding of the neurotrophin to Trk initiates intracellular signal transduction cascades that culminate in specific gene expression. Trk receptors can activate various second messenger pathways, including the mitogen-activated protein kinase pathways, the phosphoinositol 3-kinase pathway, and the phospholipase C-γ pathway. Which pathway is used influences the specific genes that are turned on and thus how the cell responds to the neurotrophin. Different signal transduction pathways have been implicated for the different functions of neurotrophins.

All the neurotrophins bind to the transmembrane receptor p75 (also known as the low-affinity NGF receptor). However, the role of p75 in neurotrophin function is quite complex and less well understood than that of the Trk receptors. P75 modulates Trk signaling by both direct association with Trks and through effects on Trk signal transduction. P75 is part of the tumor necrosis factor receptor family that controls cell survival by regulating apoptosis; thus, it is important for neurotrophin function in the context of cell death.

Signaling Location

The signal transduction pathways and the biological effects of neurotrophins differ depending on the location at which a neuron is stimulated. In general, neurons can be stimulated at either their axon endings (target derived) or locally at their cell bodies. In the classic view, the neurotrophin acts as a messenger produced by the target cell that signals survival to the neuron at its axon ending. The neurotrophin binds to its receptor at the axon ending and the neurotrophin/receptor complex is endocytosed into signaling endosomes. This signal is conveyed retrogradely through the axon to the cell body and culminates in changes in gene expression. Recent work, however, demonstrates that target-derived neurotrophins may not necessarily need to be endocytosed to promote survival, providing evidence for parallel signaling pathways for target-derived neurotrophic support. In addition to stimulating retrograde nuclear responses, neurotrophin signaling occurs locally at axonal endings. Local axonal neurotrophin signaling stimulates axon outgrowth rather than survival.

Presentation and signaling of neurotrophins at the cell bodies of neurons can also promote survival. However, the signal transduction cascades that are activated have been shown to differ when neurotrophins are presented to the axon endings versus when they are presented to the cell body. Specifically, different MAP-kinase species are activated by Trks at the cell body compared to those activated by retrograde Trk signaling. Therefore, the cell can interpret where the neurotrophin signal is originating.

In addition to target-derived or local neurotrophin actions that culminate in gene expression in neurons, neurotrophins can also act on the neuronal target. Neurotrophins can be anterogradely transported through axons and released from a neuron onto the dendritic spine of a postsynaptic neuron (target). Anterograde neurotrophin release and signaling play an important role in synaptic modulation. The fact that neurotrophins have different actions based on the localization of the receipt of the signal adds an additional layer of complexity to the neurotrophic factor hypothesis.

CONCLUSIONS

Research on neurotrophins started with a single factor (NGF) with survival effects on specific developing neurons and has progressed into a field involving many neurotrophins and neurotrophin receptors with diverse functions in both the developing and the mature nervous system. Although considerable progress has been made with regard to the signaling mechanisms and functions of neurotrophins, research has emphasized the immense complexity of the neurotrophin field. Many exciting and important aspects of the neurotrophins are likely to be uncovered in the future.

—*Anita Bhattacharyya and Clive Svendsen*

See also–Hematolymphopoietic Growth Factors; Neurotrophins, Developmental; Vertebrate Nervous System, Development of

Further Reading
Hamburger, V., and Levi-Montalcini, R. (1949). Proliferation, differentiation and degeneration in the spinal ganglia of the chick embryo under normal and experimental conditions. *J. Exp. Zool.* **111**, 457–502.

Heerssen, H. M., and Segal, R. A. (2002). Location, location, location: A spatial view of neurotrophin signal transduction. *Trends Neurosci.* **25**, 160–165.
Huang, E. J., and Reichardt, L. F. (2001). Neurotrophins: Roles in neuronal development and function. *Annu. Rev. Neurosci.* **24**, 677–736.
Lee, F. S., Kim, A. H., Khursigara, G., *et al.* (2001). The uniqueness of being a neurotrophin receptor. *Curr. Opin. Neurobiol.* **11**, 281–286.
MacInnis, B. L., and Campenot, R. B. (2002). Retrograde support of neuronal survival without retrograde transport of nerve growth factor. *Science* **295**, 1536–1539.
Patapoutian, A., and Reichardt, L. F. (2001). Trk receptors: Mediators of neurotrophin action. *Curr. Opin. Neurobiol.* **11**, 272–280.
Sofroniew, M. V., Howe, C. L., and Mobley, W. C. (2001). Nerve growth factor signaling, neuroprotection, and neural repair. *Annu. Rev. Neurosci.* **24**, 1217–1281.
Thoenen, H. (2000). Neurotrophins and activity-dependent plasticity. *Prog. Brain Res.* **128**, 183–191.

Neurotrophins, Developmental

Encyclopedia of the Neurological Sciences
Copyright 2003, Elsevier Science (USA). All rights reserved.

STUDIES by Hamburger and Levi-Montalcini in the 1930s–1950s revealed that during normal development of the nervous system, approximately 50% of neurons initially generated die. Thus, the demise of redundant neurons or "programmed cell death" is a feature of the normal itinerary of the developing nervous system. Their experiments with limb bud extirpation elegantly demonstrated the influence of the targets of innervation in neuronal development. Specifically, it was proposed that the target determines the size of its neural center by regulating neuronal death through a "metabolic exchange between the neurite and the substrate in which it grows." This hypothesis was confirmed in later experiments with mouse sarcomas and chick embryos, and a diffusible entity underlying initial effects they observed was named nerve growth factor (NGF).

The discovery of NGF led to the formulation of the neurotrophic factor hypothesis, which postulates that once a developing neuron has grown a process into its target, it competes with other developing neurons of the same type for a limited supply of a neurotrophic factor provided by the target. Decades of research involving NGF have led to the cloning and characterization of novel members of the NGF family of growth factors. This family, known as the neurotrophins (NTs), is composed of polypeptides, ~120 amino acids in length, structurally related to NGF and now includes the prototype NGF, brain-derived neurotrophic factor (BDNF), NT-3, NT-4/5, NT-6, and NT-7.

The regulation of neuronal function by the neurotrophins is far more complex than envisioned in the original hypothesis. It is now known that these molecules act on peripheral and central nervous system neurons and several other neuroectoderm-derived cellular populations to support their growth, differentiation, survival, and plasticity in the developing nervous system. In addition, the NTs contribute to the preservation and normal function of neurons in the mature nervous system as well as affect the electrophysiological properties of different neuronal populations by influencing properties such as neurotransmitter release. Although some of these effects require new gene expression, other effects do not. It has been shown that NTs can rapidly (within seconds) alter neurotransmitter release both at the developing neuromuscular junction and within the hippocampus, where they can influence long-term potentiation. Similar to their effects in blocking programmed cell death during normal development, the exogenous administration of NTs has also been shown to play a neuroprotective role against certain cellular insults, particularly those that incite apoptotic mechanisms of cell death during development. For example, although the administration of the NT BDNF is protective against CA1 neuronal cell loss in models of global ischemia in the adult brain, it is markedly neuroprotective following hypoxic-ischemic insults to the neonatal brain in which there is prominent apoptosis.

Understanding of the cellular mechanisms by which NTs signal progressed rapidly after the discovery of NT receptors. The effects of NTs are initiated by their binding to $p75^{NTR}$ (also called the low-affinity NGF receptor) and the trk family of cell surface tyrosine kinase receptors (trkA, trkB, and trkC). The trkA receptor was first isolated as a protooncogene from a colon carcinoma. It was later shown that trkA expression in the carcinoma was due to the abnormal fusion of the intracellular kinase domain of trkA with another gene resulting in aberrant expression. Normal expression of trkA was initially found most strongly in the peripheral nervous system (PNS); however, it is also expressed in select populations of central nervous system (CNS) neurons. TrkB and trkC are widely expressed in certain PNS and many CNS neurons.

Activation of the trk receptors by NTs results in receptor dimerization, autophosphorylation, and subsequent initiation of intracellular signaling cascades that in turn lead to changes in ion fluxes, phospholipid metabolism, neuronal membrane morphology, protein phosphorylation, and concentration changes of specific mRNAs and proteins. The dominance of particular intracellular signaling pathways (e.g., PI-3 kinase and MAP kinase) as well as the state of neuronal development (e.g., dividing neuronal precursor vs mature neuron) and exposure to specific insults can determine whether a neuron will respond in a particular fashion to a NT. The prosurvival and growth effects of NTs are mediated by trk receptors, and these effects do not require the $p75^{NTR}$. If the $p75^{NTR}$ is expressed along with a trk receptor in the same cell, NT actions are more potent. In contrast, there is evidence suggesting that if $p75^{NTR}$ is expressed by cells in the absence of trk receptors, NT-$p75^{NTR}$ binding can initiate cell death. This is likely due to the homology between $p75^{NTR}$ and the tumor necrosis factor (TNF) family of receptors, which can activate cell death pathways.

All known mammalian NTs are capable of supporting the growth and survival of subsets of dorsal root ganglion neurons. NT-6 and NT-7 have only been characterized in lower vertebrates but are thought to act similarly. However, the NTs differ in their sites of synthesis, developmental patterns of expression, and neuronal targets (Table 1). Moreover, BDNF and NT-3 are expressed in many cases by neurons that also express their receptors. Thus, it is likely that these NTs have both paracrine (local) and autocrine (self) actions.

Further diversification from the original neurotrophic factor hypothesis results from receptor infidelity. TrkA encodes a signal-transducing receptor for NGF, although at high concentrations NT-3 and NT-7 can also activate trkA. TrkB is activated by BDNF, but it can also be activated by NT-3. NT-3 primarily acts through trkC. NT-4/5 works primarily through trkB. In addition, some neurons are known to change their trk receptor expression during development, thus linking the sequential actions of NTs during the development of certain neuronal populations. Each trk receptor has different isoforms; however, trkB and trkC have both full-length and truncated isoforms. The full-length isoforms can mediate NT signaling, whereas the truncated isoforms lack an intracellular kinase domain. These truncated isoforms, although capable of binding NTs and heterodimerizing with

Table 1   NEUROTROPHINS AND THEIR RESPONSIVE NEURONS[a]

Neurotrophins	Responsive neurons
NGF	
PNS	Sympathetic
	Small sensory DRG
CNS	Basal forebrain cholinergic
	Striatal cholinergic
	Cerebellar Purkinje
BDNF	
PNS	Placode-derived sensory
	Specific DRG
	Nodose ganglion
	Spinal motor
CNS	Most cortical
	Most hippocampal
	Basal forebrain cholinergic
	Proprioceptive trigeminal
	Substantia nigra dopaminergic
	Retinal ganglion
	Facial motor
NT-3	
PNS	Sympathetic
	Specific DRG
CNS	Most cortical
	Most hippocampal
	Basal forebrain cholinergic
	Locus coeruleus
NT-4/5	
PNS	Sympathetic
	Specific DRG
	Nodose ganglion
CNS	Most cortical
	Most hippocampal
	Basal forebrain cholinergic
	Locus coeruleus

[a] Abbreviations used: PNS, peripheral nervous system; CNS, central nervous system; DRG, dorsal root ganglion.

full-length trk receptors, cannot signal. Their expression can suppress NT signaling through a dominant negative effect. This appears to be an important effect *in vivo*. BDNF and NT-3 can exert strong trkB- and trkC-mediated signaling in the developing brain; however, their signaling is markedly blunted during brain maturation secondary to expression of high neuronal levels of truncated trkB and trkC.

More has been learned about the specific functions of NTs and their receptors from targeted gene deletions in mice. Interestingly, most of the knockout mice for each of the NTs or receptors are lethal in either the embryonic or the early perinatal period. The NGF and trkA knockout mice have radically diminished numbers of dorsal root ganglia and trigeminal neurons, and the sympathetic ganglia vanish soon after birth. This is because NGF actions through trkA are required for the survival of both sympathetic neurons and small sensory dorsal root ganglion neurons that mediate temperature and pain sensation. TrkB knockouts have both sensory and motor neuronal deficiencies and die within the first 48 hr of life due to lack of appropriate feeding. Animals with homozygous deletion of the BDNF have a similar, although milder, phenotype to that of the trkB knockouts. There are both morphological and electrophysiological abnormalities that suggest roles for BDNF in synaptogenesis and neurotransmitter synthesis. NT-3 and trkC knockout mice have abnormal movements and posturing that is strikingly similar to that of the movement disorders seen in humans with large fiber sensory neuropathies. These mice are devoid of dorsal root ganglion neurons that regulate proprioception.

Constant secretion of NTs keeps cell survival signals activated and death signals inactive. However, under pathological conditions, the balance of survival and death signals may be tipped toward death. In some conditions, exogenous administration of NTs can keep intracellular survival signals activated (such as PI-3 and MAP kinase) and death signals suppressed, leading to neuronal survival. Recent evidence suggests that even in mature animals, exogenous NTs may stimulate dormant stem cells to differentiate and proliferate, thereby repopulating damaged nervous tissue with its pre-injury complement of neurons.

Impairment of the regulation of NTs or their receptors has been postulated to be relevant to neurodegeneration, neuropathies, pain, and cancer. Indeed, trials with NTs have been initiated to prevent neuronal death and maintain function in several human neurological diseases, including peripheral neuropathies, motor neuron diseases, spinal cord injury, and Alzheimer's disease. Diabetic neuropathy is characterized by degeneration of sensory fibers that mediate pain and temperature as well as degeneration of fibers that convey tactile sensation and proprioception. Experimental models of diabetic neuropathy have shown that retrograde axonal transport of NGF is impaired and that decreased availability of NGF may contribute to the pathogenesis. Subcutaneous injections of NGF in diabetic neuropathy have shown promising results, and human trials are in progress. BDNF and NT-3 promote motor neuron survival and are currently under investigation for treatment of spinal muscular atrophy and amyotrophic lateral sclerosis. Whether these NTs can stimulate survival of adult motor neurons as well as they stimulate survival of injured developing motor neurons is not clear. NGF may have promise for the reversal of the degeneration of basal forebrain cholinergic neurons that occurs in Alzheimer's disease. Basal forebrain cholinergic neurons supply almost all the cholinergic input to the cortex and hippocampus and are important in attention and memory. These neurons express the NGF receptors trkA and p75^{NTR}. Following axotomy, these neurons die. Administration of NGF directly or via gene therapy can rescue this death in both rodents and primates. Furthermore, NGF improves spatial memory in aged learning-impaired rodents. These kind of data have led to recent human trials in which genetically modified fibroblasts secreting NGF are transplanted into the brains of subjects with Alzheimer's disease. Conversely, indications for NT receptor antagonists in the nervous system include blocking inflammatory and pain states that are dependent on NTs and arrest of neoplasia in NT-dependent tumors.

The seemingly varied interactions between NTs and their receptors are clearly important in the establishment of appropriate neuronal signaling that regulates survival, synaptogenesis, synaptic plasticity, and electrophysiological changes. Because of their potent effects on specific neurons and the selective vulnerability of neuronal populations to various insults, such as ischemia, infection, trauma, and neurodegenerative disorders, it is hoped that the protective effects of NTs can be utilized to prevent or treat neurological disease. Clearly, there are potential problems with NT toxicity, such as the systemic pain syndrome caused by high doses of peripherally administered NGF. If delivery to or increased production of NTs (or their mimetics) to appropriate locations can be achieved without significant toxicity, these powerful molecules have potential to drastically alter the course of both acute and chronic neurological disease.

—Kara L. Arvin and David M. Holtzman

See also–Cell Death; Hematolymphopoietic Growth Factors; Neurons, Overview; Neurotrophins

Further Reading

Bredesen, D. E., and Rabizadeh, S. (1997). P75(NTR) and apoptosis—Trk-dependent and trk-independent effects. *Trends Neurosci.* 20, 287–290.

Chao, M. V. (1992). Neurotrophin receptors: A window into neuronal differentiation. *Neuron* 9, 583–593.

Cheng, Y., Gidday, J. M., Yan, Q., *et al.* (1997). Marked age-dependent neuroprotection by BDNF against neonatal hypoxic-ischemic brain injury. *Ann. Neurol.* 41, 521–529.

Eide, F. F., Vinig, E. R., Eide, B. L., *et al.* (1996). Naturally occurring truncated trkB receptors have dominant inhibitory effects on brain-derived neurotrophic factor signaling. *J. Neurosci.* 16, 3123–3129.

Kaplan, D. R., and Stephens, R. M. (1994). Neurotrophin signal transduction by the trk receptor. *J. Neurobiol.* 25, 1404–1417.

Kernie, S. G., and Parada, L. F. (2000). The molecular basis for understanding neurotrophins and their relevance to neurologic disease. *Arch. Neurol.* 57, 654–657.

Knusel, B., Rabin, S. J., Hefti, F., *et al.* (1994). Regulated neurotrophin receptor responsiveness during neuronal migration and early differentiation. *J. Neurosci.* 14, 1542–1554.

Smith, D. E., Roberts, J., Gage, F. H., *et al.* (2000). Age-associated neuronal atrophy occurs in the primate brain and is reversible by growth factor gene therapy. *Proc. Natl. Acad. Sci. USA* 96, 10893–10898.

Snider, W. D. (1994). Functions of the neurotrophins during development: What the knockouts are teaching us. *Cell* 77, 627–638.

Thoenen, H. (1995). Neurotrophins and neuronal plasticity. *Science* 270, 593–598.

Nicotinic Receptors

Encyclopedia of the Neurological Sciences

THE DIFFERENTIATION of acetylcholine receptors into subclasses based on the actions of the plant alkaloids muscarine and nicotine played an essential role in the development of concepts of neurotransmission in the central and peripheral nervous systems. Drugs that act on these muscarinic and nicotinic receptors play an important role in clinical medicine. The use of new molecular and pharmacological approaches to further differentiate cholinergic receptor subtypes and develop more selective drugs will likely lead to the development of more effective therapies in the future.

HISTORY

The work of Otto Loewi at the turn of the 20th century laid the foundation for not only the identification of neurotransmitters as chemical entities but also the conception of their mechanism of the brain through action on proteins that were labeled neurotransmitter receptors. The classic distinction between muscarinic and nicotinic receptors has been enriched by the understanding that muscarinic receptors are linked through G proteins to second messenger systems and tend to have slower action compared to nicotinic receptors. A variety of agents can block the often inhibitory consequences of the muscarinic receptor activity. Nicotinic receptors, on the other hand, are composed of a structurally related family of ion channels that are predominantly excitatory and active over a short period of time.

Historically, nicotinic receptors were first characterized at the neuromuscular junction by taking advantage of the large numbers of receptors found in a variety of species with modified organs associated, for example, with creating electrical discharges as a mechanism organism defense (e.g., in electric eels). The nicotinic receptors at the neuromuscular junction have been studied extensively in relation to human diseases such as myasthenia gravis. Here, autoimmune phenomena contribute to receptor dysfunction and the resulting muscle weakness.

Early studies in the central nervous system focused on the identification of muscarinic receptors. Five kinds of muscarinic receptors have been cloned, with the M1 receptor being more common in telencephalic areas. The identification of nicotinic receptors in the brain was delayed because appropriate pharmacological agents to characterize them were not available. However, it is now clear that both pre- and postsynaptic nicotinic receptors of various subtypes exist in the central nervous system and are important for motor function, pain, and cognition. The neuromuscular nicotinic receptor is the most extensively studied member of the superfamily of receptors.

STRUCTURE

Five subunits, labeled alpha, beta, gamma, delta, and epsilon, form the structure of the ion channel as various subtypes and in various combinations. Physical loops constituting intracellular and transmembrane components have been identified. The most common nicotinic receptor subtypes in the central nervous system are α_4, β_2, and α_7. The study of nicotinic binding sites in the central nervous system was assisted by the use of radioactively labeled nicotine and acetylcholine (with selective

blocking of muscarinic sites). Although the distribution of nicotinic receptors in the central nervous system remains to be fully elucidated, α_4 and β_2 units are distributed widely, whereas α_3, α_7, and β_4 are less abundant and located more in subcortical structures.

FUNCTION

Many nicotinic receptors appear to modulate neurotransmitter release through excitatory mechanisms. Presynaptic receptors or autoreceptors likely provide a feedback mechanism on transmitter release. The different subunit organizational patterns lead to different functional effects. The elucidation of these properties has been enhanced by the ability to express receptor combinations in cell lines. Nicotinic receptors have also been found to have binding sites in addition to the principal binding sites for the native neurotransmitter. A variety of modulatory sites have been proposed, perhaps the most interesting of which is a noncompetitive activator site or so-called allosteric modulating site.

From a systems perspective, nicotinic receptors have a role in directly stimulating not only postsynaptic neurons but also other functions. For example, nicotinic receptors are located on the blood vessels and can modulate blood flow.

Nicotine has many effects on central nervous system activity. A considerable amount of knowledge has been gained by studying nicotinic receptors in association with smoking (and other forms of drug abuse). Interestingly, exposure to nicotine by inhaling cigarette smoke increases the number of receptor binding sites. Nicotine has mixed agonist and antagonist properties. In addition to its addictive properties, nicotine affects weight and alters mood and cognition. Nicotine's effects on human beings *in vivo* are complex and include peripheral and central effects.

CLINICAL RELEVANCE

An understanding of the effects of nicotine on the brain has led to attempts to treat nicotine addiction as well as several neurological and psychiatric diseases. Various nicotinic chewing gums, patches, and other formulations can be used to diminish smoking behavior, particularly if associated with behavioral management.

Because nicotinic compounds can improve performance of animals with experimental lesions in the basal cholinergic forebrain, their role in cognition, particularly attention, has been studied intensively. Short-term administration of nicotinic compounds has been reported to improve cognition in humans. Galantamine, a cholinesterase inhibitor that also has nicotinic allosteric binding properties, was recently approved by the Food and Drug Administration for the treatment of Alzheimer's disease. It remains to be seen whether this property, which differentiates it from other available cholinesterase inhibitors, leads to any extra clinical benefit. However, such pharmacological probes will help us differentiate the cognitive enhancement properties of muscarinic and nicotinic cholinergic drugs.

The number of nicotinic cholinergic receptors is reduced in Alzheimer's disease and Parkinson's disease, including the Lewy body variant; thus, they are being explored as therapeutic targets in these conditions. Because in some cell culture systems nicotine has been shown to have a neural protective effect, perhaps through an amyloid or growth factor mechanism, nicotinic compounds might also be developed to slow progression of disease. In Parkinson's disease, nicotine may also affect the movement disorders because nicotinic receptors modulate dopamine release in basal ganglia.

Based on the association of smoking with psychiatric illness (e.g., schizophrenia) and some preliminary findings in animal tissues, nicotinic receptors have been proposed to play a role in the biological basis of psychosis and mood disorders. Nicotine has been shown to have effects on inflammatory bowel disorders, prostate function, and obstructive sleep apnea. Moreover, nicotine has weak analgesic effects, a characteristic that may be helpful in developing more effective treatments for pain.

CURRENT AND FUTURE ISSUES

Our understanding of nicotinic receptors and their role in brain function has increased greatly during the past 100 years. New molecular and genetic approaches for characterizing the various nicotinic cholinergic receptors provide the possibility that we may develop agents that are more selective for creating positive therapeutic benefits and avoid undesirable side effects. Selective agents that either block or enhance activity at specific nicotinic receptor sites may lead to more promising therapies for cognitive dysfunction, particularly those involving attention, such as attention deficit disorder, and various dementias, especially frontal lobe dementias. Moreover, understanding the role of cholinergic

transmission in motor systems may lead to more effective therapies for Parkinson's disease, Tourette's syndrome, and other movement disorders. Perhaps more is known about nicotinic receptors that any other receptor in the brain. However, this knowledge demonstrates the complexities that a systems neuroscience exposes in terms of understanding interactions between drugs and receptors in different neural systems.

—*Peter J. Whitehouse*

See also—Acetylcholine; Neurotransmitter Receptors; Smoking and Nicotine

Further Reading

Levin, E. D., and Simon, B. B. (1998). Nicotinic acetylcholine involvement in cognitive function in animals. *Psychopharmacology* **138**, 217–230.

Piasecki, M., and Newhouse, P. A. (Eds.) (2000). *Nicotine in Psychiatry: Psychopathology and Emerging Therapeutics.* American Psychiatric Press, Washington, DC.

Schmitt, J. D. (2000). Exploring the nature of molecular recognition in nicotinic acetylcholine receptors. *Curr. Med. Chem.* **7**, 749–800.

Nightmares

Encyclopedia of the Neurological Sciences
Copyright 2003, Elsevier Science (USA). All rights reserved.

A NIGHTMARE has usually been defined as "a frightening dream that awakens the sleeper." In recent times, the definition has sometimes been amended to "a long, frightening dream that awakens the sleeper from REM sleep." This amendment is to differentiate nightmares from night terrors, which are brief nondream/non-rapid eye movement (REM) experiences. This distinction is discussed here in terms of differential diagnosis. The traditional definition holds up well and is certainly the more useful one when a sleep laboratory is not immediately available.

NIGHTMARES VS NIGHT TERRORS

Although a nightmare is a certain type of dream and thus cannot be differentiated from a dream, it can be differentiated from certain other phenomena that are sometimes confused with it. This is where sleep laboratory studies are useful. Results of numerous studies indicate that the typical nightmare (a long, frightening dream) almost always occurs during REM sleep, most often from one of the longer (15 min or more) REM periods that occur toward the end of the night. This differentiates the nightmare from the night terror, which is not a dream but an awakening in terror. Night terrors occur almost always in the first half of the night during deep, non-REM sleep.

Night terrors are often confused with nightmares, and a patient complaining of having nightmares may be speaking of either phenomenon. The time of occurrence, length of the episode, and, if available, a laboratory sleep study can all help in making the diagnosis. The following is a simple question that almost always differentiates the two: "Are your nightmares dreams?" The person with ordinary nightmares will tend to answer "Yes, of course," whereas the person with night terrors will say "No, now that I come to think of it, I have ordinary dreams, and these episodes are something very different." Although nightmares are a subtype of REM dreams, night terrors appear to be something different. They have been called "disorders of arousal from slow-wave sleep." It has in fact been shown that a stimulus that produces a slight arousal from stage 3 or 4 sleep but not quite an awakening may sometimes induce a night terror episode. Thus, night terrors are quite similar to sleep walking and confusional arousals. All three of these can be produced by a partial arousal from slow-wave sleep.

FREQUENCY OF NIGHTMARES

Nightmares as defined previously are extremely common. Estimates suggest that at least half the population can remember having one or more nightmares in the past year. The frequency is definitely highest in children. Nightmares sufficiently severe so that parents mention them to physicians occur in approximately half of children 3–6 years old. My impression is that all children have at least a few nightmares, but they may or may not complain about them to their parents or pediatricians. Sometimes, they may not want to talk about them at all. Night terrors are less frequent, occurring in 2–5% of children and up to 1% of adults. There are other less common phenomena called hypnagogic hallucinations or hypnagogic nightmares. These are brief episodes that, in some cases, may be frightening, occurring while the person is half asleep. They occur frequently in patients with narcolepsy but only occasionally in patients who do not have this condition.

Many studies show nightmares to be more frequent in women than in men, but this result may be partially influenced by the reluctance of men to admit to having nightmares. A nightmare is seen by some males as a sign of weakness that should be suppressed or not mentioned. When men are asked repeatedly about nightmares in a supportive or nonthreatening environment, the difference in rates between men and women lessens considerably. There is still some difference, however, and this may be related to the higher frequency of physical and sexual abuse of women.

The prevalence of nightmares is highest in childhood and clearly decreases with age. However, the exact frequency of different ages varies in different studies and is not well established.

WHO HAS NIGHTMARES AND WHEN

There is a positive relationship between levels of anxiety and nightmares both across and within individuals. Nightmares tend to occur especially during anxious periods in an individual's life. Nightmares are also associated with certain personality patterns. Studies of persons who have frequent nightmares (one per week or more) for many years demonstrate that these persons have a pattern of features called "thin boundaries." These are people who can be described as open, sensitive, flexible, and vulnerable in various ways. They "let things through" in many senses of the term. They see the world in shades of gray rather than in black and white. They tend to spend a great deal of time daydreaming or in reverie, and they remember more dreams than average. The personality pattern called thin boundaries has physiological correlates as well and, to a certain extent, appears to run in families. It is probably based on genetic factors as well as early childhood experiences.

There is no question that nightmares are more frequent after traumatic events. However, it should be noted that this is often a perfectly normal phenomenon. For instance, after experiencing almost any kind of trauma (e.g., an escape from a fire, an attack, or a rape), it is not uncommon to dream, "I was overwhelmed by a tidal wave." Here, the nightmare appears to be picturing the emotional state of the person: "I am terrified, I am overwhelmed." It has been suggested that this picturing occurs in all dreams but is most easily recognized in nightmares after trauma. These nightmares should not be considered pathological, and they are sometimes viewed as functional: One function of dreaming may be the representation of emotion and the gradual making of connections with other events in one's life.

Sometimes, however, in persons who have experienced severe trauma, nightmares and other symptoms do not resolve over the weeks and months after trauma but remain constant and are very disturbing to the individual. These nightmares often appear to repeat the trauma experience, often with small changes. Here, the nightmares are one symptom of the condition posttraumatic stress disorder (PTSD).

WHAT PRODUCES NIGHTMARES

It has sometimes been thought that eating spicy foods will produce nightmares (the pepperoni pizza theory), but there is no evidence to support this. At one time, it was thought that suffocation (e.g., getting caught under the bed sheets) produced nightmares, but again there is little evidence to support this view. In fact, patients with obstructive sleep apnea, whose airways close off numerous times during sleep so that they repeatedly begin to suffocate, seldom report any nightmares.

What, then, does cause nightmares? As mentioned previously, there may be genetic and early environmental factors that produce a predisposition to nightmares; also, a traumatic or stressful event is likely to lead to nightmares. In addition, some medications have been shown to produce or exacerbate nightmares, including acetylcholinesterase inhibitors and, to a lesser extent, other cholinergic medication, dopamine agonists and related anti-Parkinson's drugs, and certain drugs used to treat hypertension, especially β-adrenergic blockers. Nightmares may also occur after sudden withdrawal of REM-suppressant drugs, benzodiazepines, alcohol, and barbiturates.

NIGHTMARES AS A SYMPTOM, NOT AN ILLNESS

As noted previously, a certain number of nightmares may be perfectly normal; in addition, nightmares may be related to certain personality characteristics. In neither of these cases should nightmares be a source for medical concern. However, a complaint of nightmares can be a symptom leading to the recognition of an underlying problem. For example, a sudden onset of nightmares in middle-aged or older persons taking a number of medications should lead

to a suspicion of a medication effect. If the onset of nightmares can be traced to the time when a new medication (e.g., a β-adrenergic blocker) was started, then a simple change of medications can be considered.

A very different situation occurs usually in a younger person—for instance, an anxious college student who has experienced much stress. If this person begins to experience severe nightmares along with anxiety, exaggerated or unrealistic fears or worries, etc., this may be a sign of a developing psychotic episode. If there is no medication or psychosis involved, some occurrence of severe nightmares indicates that one should ask in more detail about possible traumatic events occurring in the period just before the onset of nightmares.

TREATMENT OF NIGHTMARES

As is clear from the previous discussion, the nightmare in itself is not an illness or pathological condition requiring treatment. It is common, almost ubiquitous, and may even play a functional role after trauma. As mentioned, the nightmare can sometimes be a symptom of another condition requiring treatment. There are some situations, however, in which the nightmare is an important part of a condition requiring treatment. The condition known as PTSD is considered a serious mental illness. It is characterized by a history of severe trauma, and symptoms include nightmares as well as flashbacks, extreme sensitivity, and avoidance of emotional situations. A number of types of medication, as well as a number of types of psychotherapy, are used to treat PTSD.

In addition, some patients without PTSD may complain that their nightmares are frequent and severe and interfere with their sleep. In such cases, a number of different treatments have been found to be successful, but the treatment used depends on the clinical situation. It is certainly important to obtain a careful history, including a psychiatric history, before the treatment of nightmares. Successful treatments include psychodynamic therapy as well as special cognitive/behavioral treatments in which the patient writes out the nightmare, changes the ending, and rehearses the new less frightening version.

It is worth keeping in mind, however, that half of persons with severe frequent nightmares do not want treatment. Some of them say that they use the nightmares in their creative and artistic work, and others simply believe that nightmares have become part of them and they do not want them changed. It is extremely important for a physician or other professional attempting to treat nightmares to obtain a careful history and evaluation of the patient's overall state. In my experience, it is very uncommon for nightmares themselves to constitute an important problem that the patient wants to eliminate, although this does happen. More frequently, in adults and in children, nightmares may point to some other problem, physical or psychological, that may require treatment.

—*Ernest L. Hartmann*

See also—**Dreaming; Dreams, Significance of; Dream Therapy; Parasomnias; Post-Traumatic Stress Disorder (PTSD); REM (Rapid Eye Movement) Sleep; Sleep Disorders**

Further Reading

Hartmann, E. (1984). *The Nightmare: The Psychology and Biology of Terrifying Dreams.* Basic Books, New York.
Hartmann, E. (1991). *Boundaries in the Mind: A New Psychology of Personality.* Basic Books, New York.
Hartmann, E. (1998). *Dreams and Nightmares: The New Theory on the Origin and Functions of Dreams.* Plenum, New York.
Krakow, B., and Neidhardt, J. (1996). *Conquering Bad Dreams and Nightmares.* Berkeley, New York.

Nissl, Franz

Encyclopedia of the Neurological Sciences
Copyright 2003, Elsevier Science (USA). All rights reserved.

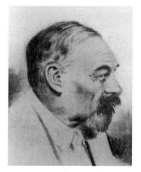

Franz Nissl (reproduced with permission from Haymaker, 1948).

FRANZ NISSL (1860–1919) was born in Bavaria, Germany, and his genius was recognized early in his career when he won the coveted first prize in his medical school at the University of Munich for his thesis titled *Pathological Changes of the Nerve Cells of the Cerebral Cortex.* Not only was this apparently an excellent paper but also it provided the direction for his future career, which he devoted to the study of the histology of the cerebral cortex and the correlation of microscopic structure with function in both health and disease. In his investigations for this seminal study, he used alcohol as a fixative for the tissues he studied instead of the fixative preferred at the time, which was Muller's solution of dichromate and sulfate. Nissl also substituted magenta red, and later methylene blue or toluidine blue, for the traditional carmine in the staining procedure.

After obtaining his medical examination in 1885, Nissl spent 3 years working in the district insane asylum in Munich, first as an assistant to von Gudden, and remaining there even after his mentor's death. In 1889, he was offered a position at the state asylum in Frankfurt, where Alois Alzheimer worked and shared his interest in neurohistological investigation. The two became close collaborators and friends, a relationship that endured for more than two decades, first in Frankfurt and later in Heidelberg. During this time period, Nissl published his historic three-part article in 1894 titled *The So-Called Granules in Nerve Cells*, which detailed the granular basophilic material in the cytoplasm of neurons that has come to be known as Nissl's substance, granules, or bodies. For neuropathologists at least, his name will be forever linked to this early contribution to the histopathology of the nervous system.

In 1895, at the urging of Kraepelin, Nissl went to Heidelberg, where he combined teaching, research, and consultative work. He became an adjunct professor in 1901. From 1904 to 1918, he served as professor of psychiatry and became director of the clinic following Kraepelin's departure in 1904 to Munich. While in that post, he published a paper on the neuron that favored the "nerve-net theory" and developed a procedure for quantitative measurement of albumin in the cerebrospinal fluid. Collaborations with Alzheimer resulted in a six-volume work on the histology of the cerebral cortex published in 1904. The best remembered aspect of their joint work, however, detailed features of general paresis of the insane. In his section, Nissl described the classic microscopic findings of neurosyphilis, including pachymeningitis, atrophy of the hemispheres, dilatation of the lateral ventricles, inflammatory infiltrates of lymphocytes and plasma cells, and "rod cells" in the cortex.

In 1918, Kraepelin invited Nissl to move to Munich to take a research position at a newly founded German psychiatric institute. However, after only 1 year there, spent with fellow great men of his day, Spielmeyer and Brodmann, Nissl unfortunately succumbed to a kidney ailment that had first plagued him during the early years of his medical studies. During the final 10 years of his life, he was intensively engaged in establishing connections between the cortex and thalamus, and he was working on thalamic–cortical projections in newborn rabbits at the time of his death. His unexpected demise prevented completion of this work. He died at age 58 in 1919.

On a personal level, Nissl never married and "never stopped work except for illness." He was said to be gnome-like, with bad posture and a tilting of his head, hypothesized to be an effort to minimize recognition of a large birthmark on his left face. During daytime hours he saw patients, who considered him their friend; at night he did his research, and still later at night he conversed with colleagues or played piano sonatas. His witty sayings were legendary, and his advice for the best way to preserve brain tissue (which he believed needed to stand 30 min before submersion in fixative) was "Take the brain out. Put it on the desk. Spit on the floor. When the spit is dry, put the brain in alcohol."

Despite his numerous accomplishments, like so many geniuses, Nissl occasionally despaired, was a fierce self-critic, and "labored over manuscripts that never went to press." Even on his deathbed, "Nissl, doubter of himself, deathless to the scientific world, kept complaining of what needed yet to be done."

—*Bette Kleinschmidt-DeMasters*

See also–Alzheimer, Alois (see Index entry Biography for complete list of biographical entries)

Further Reading

Haymaker, W. (1948). *A Guide to the Exhibit on the History of Neuropathology.* Army Institute of Pathology, Washington, DC.
McHenry, L. C. (1969). *Garrison's History of Neurology.* Thomas, Springfield, IL.
Rasmussen, A. T. (1970). In *The Founders of Neurology* (W. Haymaker and F. Schiller, Eds.), 2nd ed. Thomas, Springfield, IL.
Talbott, J. H. (1970). *A Biographical History of Medicine.* Grune & Stratton, New York.

Nitric Oxide

Encyclopedia of the Neurological Sciences
Copyright 2003, Elsevier Science (USA). All rights reserved.

A ROLE for nitric oxide (NO) as a biological messenger molecule has only recently been appreciated. In the nervous system, NO has dramatically altered our concepts regarding neurotransmission. Classically, neurotransmitters have been defined as molecules that are synthesized and stored in vesicles and released on demand to act at postsynaptic receptor proteins and whose action is terminated by enzymatic degradation or reuptake. NO is a small, labile, lipid-permeable free radical molecule. Therefore, NO cannot be contained within synaptic vesicles. NO is synthesized by NO synthase (NOS) and diffuses from its site of synthesis to targets in surrounding cells. NO forms covalent and noncovalent linkages with protein and nonprotein targets to elicit its biological effects. NO is inactivated by diffusion away from its targets and also forms covalent linkages to superoxide ion and scavenger proteins. NO does not use any of the conventional means for control of its biological actions. NO depends on its small size, reactivity, and diffusibility more than any other biological molecule to exert its biological effects. Thus, NO synthesis is the key to regulating its biological activity (Fig. 1).

NITRIC OXIDE SYNTHASE

NO is generated by three different isozymes of NOS to carry out many diverse biological functions. Inducible NOS (iNOS) is not normally expressed in healthy tissue but can be induced in response to injury or exposure to pathogens. In the immune system, NO generated by iNOS mediates, in part, the tumoricidal and bactericidal effects of macrophages. Most tissues in the body including the brain can also express iNOS. In blood vessels, NO generated by endothelial NOS (eNOS) is produced by endothelial cells to mediate blood vessel relaxation and inhibition of platelet aggregation. In the nervous system, NO generated by neuronal NOS (nNOS) was first recognized as a messenger molecule that mediates increases in cyclic GMP (cGMP) levels that occur after activation of glutamate receptors, particularly those of the N-methyl-D-aspartate (NMDA) subtype. eNOS and nNOS require calcium influx for activation. Both eNOS and nNOS can be regulated by protein phosphorylation, and nNOS activity is

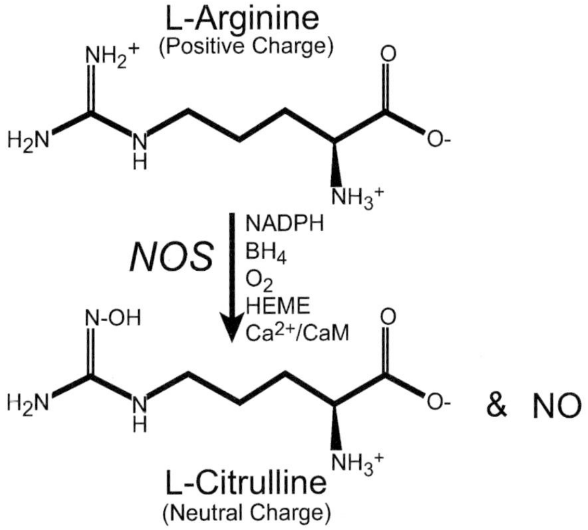

L-Arginine
(Positive Charge)

NH_2^+

H_2N

NH_3^+

NOS | NADPH
BH$_4$
O$_2$
HEME
Ca^{2+}/CaM

N-OH

H_2N

L-Citrulline
(Neutral Charge)

NH_3^+

& NO

Figure 1

Synthesis of NO. NO is formed from L-arginine through the enzymatic action of nitric oxide synthase (NOS), which requires reduced nicotinamide-adenine dinucleotide phosphate (NADPH), O$_2$, heme, Ca^{2+}, and calmodulin (CaM) and is accelerated by tetrahydrobiopterin (BH$_4$).

critically regulated by the phosphatase calcineurin. Additionally, nNOS can be regulated by interactions with other proteins. In the brain, nNOS is linked to the postsynaptic membrane near NMDA receptors via the postsynaptic density protein-95. Recently, two other nNOS-binding partners have been identified: a protein inhibitor of NOS and carboxyl-terminal PDZ ligand of NOS. eNOS and nNOS are constitutively expressed in healthy tissue. They can also be induced following injury or exposure to pathogens. In contrast, iNOS does not require influx of calcium for activation. Once synthesized, iNOS is catalytically active. The key to regulating iNOS activity is the regulation of protein expression. All three NOS isoforms share similar structural and catalytic domains, which has hampered the generation of selective pharmacological tools. Use of nonselective inhibitors *in vivo* will functionally inhibit all isoforms. Since NO generated by each isoform mediates different and varied biological actions, nonspecific inhibitors are poor candidates for drug therapy.

NITRIC OXIDE AS A NEURONAL MESSENGER

Immunohistochemical mapping reveals an association of nNOS with discreet neuronal structures and shows that the catalytic activity of nNOS accounts for NADPH diaphorase staining. Thomas and Pearse originally described NADPH diaphorase neurons by their ability to stain dark blue in the presence of nitroblue tetrazolium and NADPH but not NADH. These cells have the unusual property of being resistant to a variety of neurotoxic insults. Although the criteria for establishing a substance as a neurotransmitter are hotly debated, the formation of NO in discreet groups of neurons coupled with its ability to mediate and modify synaptic activity have solidified its place as a neurotransmitter. NO has many physiological functions in the nervous system. Through activation of cGMP-dependent protein phosphorylation cascades, NO may regulate neurotransmitter release. NO functions as the nonadrenergic, noncholinergic neurotransmitter of the gut, where it mediates relaxation of smooth muscles associated with peristalsis. Penile erections are mediated, in part, through the neurotransmitter action of NO. Cerebral blood flow is regulated through NO released from endothelial cells as well as autonomic nerves within the adventitia. NO also regulates cerebral blood flow through activity-dependent activation of NOS in neurons that influence small cerebral arterioles. The diffusion properties and the short half-life of NO make it an ideal candidate for playing a role in nervous system morphogenesis and synaptic plasticity. NO may perform a function in the development of the nervous system in that it is transiently expressed in the cerebral cortical plate during critical periods of neuronal development. NO may take part in the molecular maturation of adult spinal cord motor neurons, and it may have some responsibility in forming the initial pattern of connections in ocular dominance columns in the developing visual system. NO has also been suggested to play a prominent role in the activity-dependent establishment of connections in both the developing and regenerating olfactory neuronal epithelium.

Long-term potentiation (LTP) in the hippocampus and long-term depression in the cerebellum are forms of synaptic modulation. The role for NO in LTP has been controversial but has been clarified by genetic knockout of nNOS and eNOS. LTP is normal in nNOS knockout or eNOS knockout mice, but in double-knockout mice lacking both nNOS and eNOS, LTP in the stratum radiatum of the CA-1 hippocampal region is markedly reduced. However, LTP in the stratum oriens of the hippocampal CA-1 is unaffected. These investigations indicate that there are NO-dependent and NO-independent forms of LTP and that in certain circumstances NO may

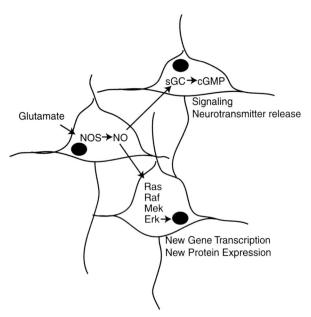

Figure 2

NO signaling between neurons. Glutamate activates the NMDA-preferring glutamate receptor, which stimulates neuronal NO synthase (NOS) via the scaffolding protein PSD-95 (not shown); this effectively couples calcium influx to neuronal NOS activation and NO production. NO diffuses from neurons in which NOS is activated and into surrounding neurons. NO can react with the heme center of soluble guanylyl cyclase (sGC), eliciting a conformational change and generating cyclic GMP (cGMP). NO can also activate the oncogene $p21^{Ras}$, perhaps by direct redox-sensitive activation or through activation of a NO-dependent guanine nucleotide exchange factor. This, in turn, activates a mitogen-activated protein kinase (MAPK) pathway involving the oncogene Raf, MAPK/extracellular signal-regulated kinase kinase (Mek), and extracellular signal-regulated kinase (Erk). This pathway can activate new gene transcription, leading to new protein synthesis.

function as a retrograde messenger in LTP. How NO participates in the synaptic plasticity of LTP is unknown. Ischemic preconditioning is another form of neuronal plasticity in which sublethal insults result in new gene transcription and protein expression that renders the brain resistant to subsequent lethal ischemia. NO plays a key role in preconditioning by activation of $p21^{ras}$ and stimulation of Raf, Mek, and Erk signaling (Fig. 2). The neuroprotective proteins expressed by activation of this pathway are not known.

MOLECULAR TARGETS OF NITRIC OXIDE

Because of its diatomic structure and free electron in a π orbital, NO can participate in several specific and complex chemical reactions. The reaction products

mediate the biological signaling of NO. As a radical, NO can donate electrons and react with transition metals, resulting in metal–nitrosyl complexes. Transition metals are contained in prosthetic groups of enzymes. The prototype enzyme in this class is guanylyl cyclase. NO modifies the heme moiety of guanylyl cyclase, resulting in a conformational change, activation, and generation of cGMP (Fig. 2). This was the first known target of NO. NO also increases prostaglandin production by activation of cyclooxygenase, another heme-containing enzyme. Numerous enzymes and proteins use iron to coordinate sulfide clusters (Fe–S). These proteins are also regulated by NO and include those in the mitochondrial respiratory chain, cis-aconitase, NADH succinate oxidoreductase, and NADH ubiquinone oxidoreductase. NO also stimulates the RNA-binding function of the iron-responsive element-binding protein in brain slices while diminishing aconitase activity. Proteins that contain zinc as the transition metal coordinating sulfide clusters, such as the zinc-finger transcription factors Sp1, EGR-1, vitamin D_3 receptor, and retinoid X receptor, are susceptible to NO modification and inhibition. S-Nitrosylation (S-NO) of proteins has recently been recognized as an important signaling mechanism following NO generation. However, under physiological conditions NO is a poor nitrosating species. Synthesis of S-NO is mediated by proteins with electron acceptors or metals to facilitate the formation of nitrosonium ions (NO^+) and subsequently S-NO. Additionally, reactions with oxygen to generate nitrogen oxide species can generate compounds such as N_2O_3 that can efficiently nitrosylate proteins under physiological conditions. This chemical modification of proteins is reversible and therefore fulfills important criteria for a signaling event. Proteins that are susceptible to regulation by nitrosylation are those containing disulfide bonds (S–S), mixed disulfide bonds (S–S–R), or cysteine sulfenic acids (RS–OH). S-Nitrosylation of proteins can be either stimulatory or inhibitory depending on the target protein. With a very fast reaction rate, NO can react with superoxide anion to form peroxynitrite (ONOO-), a potent oxidant and nitrating species. The functional consequence of ONOO-mediated attack on proteins is under investigation but appears in some cases to result in protein inactivation and subsequent cell death.

nNOS was disrupted and inactivated by homologous recombination to clarify its role as a messenger protein in the nervous system. This approach has advantages over pharmacological inhibition of NOS activity because it allows study of the neuronal enzyme independent of the other isoforms. Knocking out the gene for nNOS has a variety of important biological effects. Initial observations of the nNOS null mice indicated that there was marked enlargement of the stomach and hypertrophy of the inner circular muscle layer. This resembles the human disorder infantile pyloric stenosis. Recent studies indicate that nNOS null mice lack behavioral inhibition. nNOS null mice exhibit inappropriate sexual behavior by excessively mounting nonestrus females despite vocal protestation and cues from the females to stop. In addition, nNOS null males are overtly aggressive. They initiate attacks faster than wild-type controls. Their attacks are longer and of greater duration. They initiate more attacks and rarely adopt a submissive posture. These observations have been replicated with NOS inhibitors in normal mice, confirming a role for NO in the regulation of aggression. This disruption of normal mouse behavior in the nNOS null male mice is mediated in part through selective disruption of the serontonergic system.

NO AS AN ENDOGENOUS NEUROTOXIN

Under conditions of excessive formation, NO may be neurotoxic. NO's toxic actions are presumably triggered by activation of the NMDA receptor. Excessive glutamate receptor stimulation and the subsequent increase in intracellular calcium concentration are thought to initiate most forms of glutamate neurotoxicity. Abnormal activation of glutamate neurotransmission may contribute to neurodegenerative processes and diseases such as Alzheimer's disease, Huntington's disease, Parkinson's disease, epilepsy, and amyotrophic lateral sclerosis. In addition, the damage that follows focal cerebral ischemia leading to stroke is thought to occur due to excess glutamate acting on glutamate receptors of the NMDA subtype. Neurons grown in culture have served as an *in vitro* model for the study of excitotoxic processes. NOS inhibitors can block glutamate or NMDA excitotoxicity, and nNOS null neuronal cultures are resistant to excitotoxicity. Consistent with the notion that neuronally derived NO is neurotoxic, nNOS null mice are resistant to experimental stroke induced by permanent or transient occlusion of the middle cerebral artery. Initial confusion concerning the role of NO in experimental stroke was due to the use of nonspecific NOS

inhibitors. Genetically engineered mice null for eNOS, iNOS, or nNOS have clarified the role of NO in stroke and the respective roles of each NOS isoform. nNOS activation and overproduction of NO results in acute neurotoxicity. eNOS is critical for maintaining cerebral blood flow. Inhibiting eNOS or knocking out eNOS greatly exacerbate ischemic injury, whereas enhancing eNOS activity by administering the substrate L-arginine reduces infarct volume. iNOS mediates a secondary phase of neuronal injury 24–48 hr after the initial insult. Activation of iNOS has also been implicated in infectious encephalitis and in the cell injury that occurs in Parkinson's disease, multiple sclerosis, and AIDS dementia. Since inhibition of eNOS and nNOS in the brain can have opposing effects on neuronal survival, studies are under way to identify the

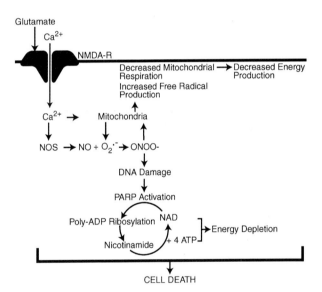

Figure 3

Mechanism of NO-mediated neurotoxicity. Acting via NMDA receptors (NMDA-R), glutamate triggers an influx of Ca^{2+}, which leads to superoxide anion (O_2^-) production in mitochondria and the production of NO in NOS-containing neurons. NO combines with superoxide anion to form peroxynitrite (ONOO-). Peroxynitrite damages mitochondrial enzymes, decreasing mitochondrial respiration and the production of ATP; peroxynitrite also damages the superoxide anion scavenger manganese superoxide dismutase (not shown), further increasing the production of superoxide anion. Peroxynitrite, which can diffuse across membranes, leaves the mitochondria and enters the nucleus, where it damages DNA and activates poly(ADP-ribose) polymerase (PARP). Massive activation of PARP leads to ADP ribosylation and depletion of nicotinamide-adenine dinucleotide (NAD). ATP is depleted in an effort to resynthesize NAD. In the setting of impaired energy generation due to mitochondrial dysfunction, this loss of NAD and ATP leads to cell death.

neurotoxic signal cascade initiated by NO. Recent investigations indicate that the major pathway by which NO may be toxic is through damage of DNA, with activation of the nuclear enzyme poly(ADP-ribose) polymerase (Fig. 3).

—*Ted M. Dawson and Valina L. Dawson*

See also–Neurotransmitters, Overview

Further Reading

Baranano, D. E., Ferris, C. D., and Snyder, S. H. (2001). Atypical neural messengers. *Trends Neurosci.* **24,** 99–106.

Bogdan, C. (2001). Nitric oxide and the regulation of gene expression. *Trends Cell. Biol.* **11,** 66–75.

Colasanti, M., and Suzuki, H. (2000). The dual personality of NO. *Trends Pharmacol. Sci.* **21,** 249–252.

Dawson, T. M., Sasaki, M., Gonzalez-Zulueta, M., *et al.* (1998). Regulation of neuronal nitric oxide synthase and identification of novel nitric oxide signaling pathways. *Prog. Brain Res.* **118,** 3–11.

Dawson, V. L., and Dawson, T. M. (1998). Nitric oxide in neurodegeneration. *Prog. Brain Res.* **118,** 215–229.

Lowenstein, C. J. (1999). NO news is good news. *Proc. Natl. Acad. Sci. USA* **96,** 10953–10954.

Marletta, M. A., Hurshman, A. R., and Rusche, K. M. (1998). Catalysis by nitric oxide synthase. *Curr. Opin. Chem. Biol.* **2,** 656–663.

Snyder, S. H., and Ferris, C. D. (2000). Novel neurotransmitters and their neuropsychiatric relevance. *Am. J. Psychiatry* **157,** 1738–1751.

Nodes of Ranvier

Encyclopedia of the Neurological Sciences
Copyright 2003, Elsevier Science (USA). All rights reserved.

LOUIS ANTOINE RANVIER (1835–1922), a noted French pathologist and physiologist, first described discontinuities or constrictions within the myelin sheaths of nerve fibers from the vertebrate peripheral nervous system. These constrictions are now termed nodes of Ranvier and are present at regular intervals along the length of all myelinated nerve fibers in both peripheral and central parts of the vertebrate nervous system.

Nodes of Ranvier are specializations of the axon that allow for rapid, jumping, or saltatory conduction of nerve impulses along the cell membrane. At nodes the axolemma is highly specialized in that it contains high concentrations of particular types of ion channels (e.g., voltage-sensitive sodium channels, sodium/potassium ATPase, Ca^{2+} ATPase, and the Na/Ca exchanger). The high concentration of so-dium channels (approximately $10,000/\mu m^2$), together with a low membrane capacitance at the internode resulting from the axon being myelinated, means that an impulse is actively generated at a node and that the impulse "jumps" from one node to the next along the length of a nerve fiber, thereby demonstrating saltatory conduction and increasing the rate of conduction of information along the length of the nerve fiber.

At the cellular level, nodes of Ranvier are specialized associations between the axons of nerve fibers and different types of supporting or glial cells. The types of glial cells differ between nodes in the peripheral and central parts of the nervous system. Furthermore, this distinction of cell types at nodes has allowed the recognition of a third type of node at the junction between the peripheral and central nervous system—the so-called transitional node of Ranvier.

The participating cells at peripheral, transitional, and central nodes of Ranvier may be most clearly visualized in longitudinal sections. These different cell types are classified as follows: peripheral—the axon and one Schwann cell on each side of the node (Fig. 1A); transitional—the axon, a Schwann cell on one side of the node, an oligodendrocyte on the other side, and an astrocyte (Fig. 1B) and central–an oligodendrocyte on each side of the node and a perinodal astrocyte (Fig. 1C).

There are a number of structural properties common to nodes of Ranvier at all three locations. A dense undercoating occurs on the axoplasmic aspect of the nodal axolemma (Fig. 1). This is currently interpreted as a specialization of the subaxolemma cytoskeleton serving to localize the high concentration of ion channels at the nodal axolemma. On the external aspect of the nodal axolemma there is a concentration of glycosoami-noglycans, termed the node gap substance, between glial cell processes and the axolemma within the nodal gap, which is the space between the terminal parts of the myelin sheath on either side of the node. Cytochemical studies have shown a high content of chondroitin sulfate glycosaminoglycans in the node gap substance. The node gap substance is thought to contribute to the localization of the high number of ion channels present within the nodal axolemma.

Within the axoplasm of axons is an organized, cellular cytoskeleton. Axonal microtubules are in-volved in transport of subcellular, membrane-limited particles along the length of the axon. Neurofila-ments are a type of cellular intermediate filament

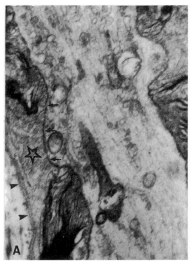

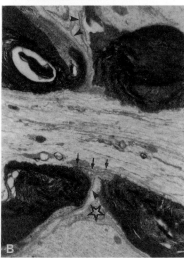

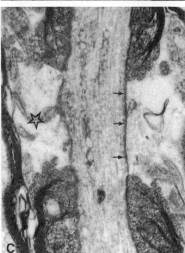

Figure 1
Longitudinal thin sections of a node of Ranvier from (A) the sciatic nerve of a rat, (B) a rat, and (C) the optic nerve of a guinea pig. (See text for details.) (Fig. 1B kindly provided by John P. Fraher.)

found only in neurons. Actin and spectrin filaments form a component of the subaxolemma cytoskeleton. Two major features characterize the cytoskeleton at nodes of Ranvier. First, microtubules outnumber neurofilaments by approximately three to one. Second, the number of neurofilaments is lower and the spacing between adjacent neurofilaments is less compared with those of internodes of the same axons. The reduced spacing between neurofilaments is thought to reflect the low degree of phosphorylation of neurofilament proteins at the nodes of Ranvier.

Some morphological features differ between peripheral, transitional, and central nodes of Ranvier. It is these, in addition to the relative position of the nodes, that have allowed distinction between the three types. In addition to the node gap substance, extracellular connective tissue elements occur at the nodal gap of peripheral and transitional nodes. These consist of a basal lamina (Figs. 1A and 1B, arrowheads) and small numbers of collagen type 3 or reticular fibers that form part of the endoneurium. These elements are currently believed to be synthesized by glial cells related to the nodal gap. Basal lamina and collagen fibers are not present in the nodal gap of central, myelinated nerve fibers (Fig. 1C).

In all three types of nodes, small finger-like cell processes (Figs. 1A–1C, stars) extend into the nodal gap. At peripheral nodes these processes are formed by Schwann cells and the processes extend into the nodal gap internal to the tube formed by the basal lamina on the external aspect of the myelin sheath (Fig. 1A). At transitional nodes both the Schwann cell on one side of the gap and an astrocyte extend processes into the nodal gap, again lying within the tube formed by the basal lamina (Fig. 1B). At central nodes, however, finger-like processes are not formed by the myelinating cells, the oligodendrocytes. Rather, such processes (Fig. 1C, star) are formed by a subtype of astrocyte, the so-called perinodal astrocyte.

Thus, although nodes of Ranvier are specialized for the same function at peripheral, transitional, and central parts of the mammalian nervous system, there are differences in the detailed cellular relations between nodes at these three regions that allow for their distinction using morphological criteria.

—*William L. Maxwell*

***See also*–Axons; Glia; Myelin; Nerve Injury; Oligodendrocytes**

Further Reading

Fraher, J. P. (1996). Nodal distribution and packing density in the rat CNS–PNS transitional zone. *Microsc. Res. Tech.* **34**, 507–521.

Ranvier, L. (1871). Sur la distribution des etranglements annulaires des tubes nerveux. *Compte Rendus Seances Soc. Biol.* **23**, 185–186.

Norepinephrine

Encyclopedia of the Neurological Sciences

NOREPINEPHRINE (also called noradrenaline) is a neurotransmitter in both the peripheral and central nervous systems. Norepinephrine produces many effects in the body, the most notable being those associated with the "fight or flight" response to perceived danger. The effects of norepinephrine and a related catecholamine, epinephrine (also called adrenaline), are mediated by the family of adrenergic receptors. The chemical structure of norepinephrine, as shown in Fig. 1, indicates that it is a catecholamine because it has both the catechol moiety (two hydroxyl groups on a benzene ring) and an amine (NH_2) group.

HISTORY

In the late 1940s, von Euler in Sweden and Holtz in Germany identified norepinephrine as the neurotransmitter of the mammalian sympathetic nerves and soon thereafter also found it to be a normal constituent of mammalian brain. Norepinephrine was subsequently shown to be a central neurotransmitter that can be visualized in the brain by fluorescent and immunohistochemical techniques.

NEUROCHEMISTRY OF NOREPINEPHRINE

Biosynthesis of Catecholamines

Norepinephrine is synthesized in neurons starting with the amino acid tyrosine, which is obtained from

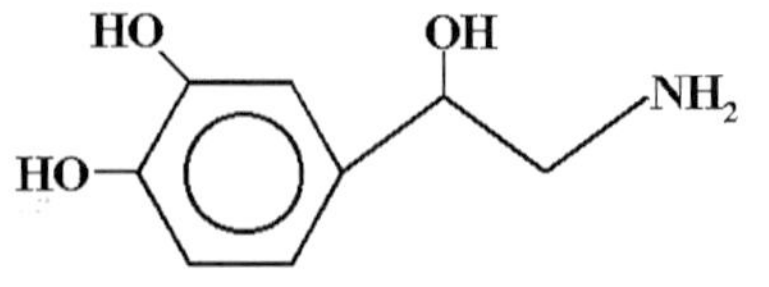

Figure 1
Structure of norepinephrine.

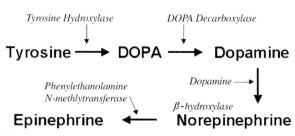

Figure 2
Biosynthesis of catecholamines.

the diet and can also be synthesized from phenylalanine. Tyrosine is converted to dihydroxyphenylalanine (DOPA) by the enzyme tyrosine hydroxylase; DOPA in turn is converted to dopamine in the cytoplasm. Dopamine, also a neurotransmitter, is taken up into vesicles and converted to norepinephrine by the enzyme dopamine β-hydroxylase. In the adrenal medulla and in a few brain regions, norepinephrine is converted to epinephrine by the enzyme phenylethanolamine N-methyltransferase. The biosynthesis of the catecholamines is summarized in Fig. 2.

Storage, Release, and Reuptake of Norepinephrine

Norepinephrine is stored in vesicles (also called storage granules) in the nerve terminals, which concentrate it and protect it from metabolism until it is released following nerve stimulation. The major mechanism by which the effects of norepinephrine are terminated is reuptake back into the nerve terminal by a high-affinity transporter. Norepinephrine can also be metabolized to inactive products. Inhibition of either of these processes results in an increase in the synaptic level of norepinephrine and a prolongation of its effects.

Metabolism of Norepinephrine

Norepinephrine is metabolized by the enzymes monoamine oxidase and catechol-O-methyltransferase to 3-methoxy-4-hydroxymandelic acid and 3-methoxy-4-hydroxyphenylglycol (MHPG). The major metabolite found in the blood and urine is MHPG, and levels of this metabolite are frequently used to assess the functional status of the noradrenergic system in human subjects.

ADRENERGIC RECEPTORS

Types and Subtypes of Adrenergic Receptors

Adrenergic receptors (also called adrenoceptors) mediate the effects of norepinephrine and epinephr-

Adrenergic Receptors

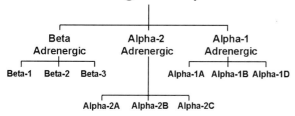

Figure 3
Classification of adrenergic receptors.

ine. Adrenergic receptors were originally classified in 1948 into two major types, α and β, based on their pharmacological characteristics (i.e., rank order potency of agonists in producing various effects). The current classification scheme, which is based on both pharmacological evidence and the molecular cloning of the nine different adrenergic receptors, includes three major types—α_1, α_2, and β—each of which is further divided into three subtypes (Fig. 3). Norepinephrine has similar affinities for all nine of the subtypes, with the exception that it is relatively weak (has low potency) at the β_2 subtype.

Location of Adrenergic Receptors

Although adrenergic receptors are found throughout the body in tissues innervated by both the peripheral and central nervous systems, a few locations are of special interest. α_1-Adrenergic receptors are found peripherally in some blood vessels, whereas α_2-receptors are located on platelets and on nerve terminals in both the peripheral and central nervous systems. In the heart, β_1-receptors predominate, whereas in the smooth muscles of the lungs, some blood vessels, and the uterus, β_2-receptors are relatively abundant.

EFFECTS OF NOREPINEPHRINE

Effects Mediated by the Autonomic Nervous System

The autonomic nervous system is divided into two components–the sympathetic nervous system and the parasympathetic nervous system. The final (postganglionic) nerves in the sympathetic system are adrenergic and thus release norepinephrine in end organs. The adrenal medulla, which is also part of the sympathetic system, releases epinephrine into the circulation. Activation of the sympathetic system, as occurs in response to perceived danger, results in the release of large quantities of norepinephrine and epinephrine. Norepinephrine acting at α_1-receptors causes constriction of cutaneous blood vessels, whereas epinephrine acting at β_2-receptors in the blood vessels of the skeletal muscles causes vasodilatation. Norepinephrine and epinephrine, acting at β_1-receptors, increase the force and rate of contraction of the heart, whereas epinephrine acting at β_2-receptors causes bronchodilatation and relaxation of smooth muscle in the uterus.

Effects Mediated by the Central Nervous System

In the central nervous system, the cell bodies of noradrenergic neurons are found primarily in the locus coeruleus in the brainstem. These neurons, however, project widely throughout the brain and spinal cord. The locus coeruleus, and hence norepinephrine, is an important regulator of a variety of physiological activities, including sleep/wake cycles, attention, orientation, mood, memory, and cardiovascular function, as well as autonomic and endocrine functions. Although adrenergic receptors are found throughout the brain, α_2-receptors are of particular importance because they regulate the

Table 1 DRUGS THAT MIMIC THE EFFECTS OF NOREPINEPHRINE

Receptor	Examples of drugs	Effect	Therapeutic indication
α_1	Phenylephrine	Vasoconstriction	Hypotension, nasal congestion
α_2	Clonidine, brimonidine	Lowers blood and intraocular pressure	Hypertension, glaucoma
β_1	Dobutamine	Increases heart rate	Cardiogenic shock
β_2	Albuterol, terbutaline, ritodrine	Relaxes smooth muscle in lung and uterus	Asthma, premature labor
Indirect acting	Amphetamine	Central nervous system stimulant	Narcolepsy, hyperactivity
Indirect acting	Desipramine, atomoxetine	Blocks norepinephrine reuptake	Depression
Indirect acting	Phenelzine	Inhibits norephinephrine metabolism by monoamine oxidase	Depression

Table 2   DRUGS THAT BLOCK THE EFFECTS OF NOREPINEPHRINE

Receptor	Examples of drugs	Effect	Therapeutic indication
α_1	Prazosin, terazosin	Vasodilatation	Hypertension, benign prostatic hypertrophy
α_2	Mirtazapine	Antidepressant	Depression
β_1	Propranolol, timolol	Decreases heart rate and intraocular pressure	Hypertension, angina, glaucoma
β_2	Atenolol, metoprolol	Decreases heart rate	Hypertension

release of norepinephrine as well as many other neurotransmitters.

DRUGS THAT MIMIC OR BLOCK THE EFFECTS OF NOREPINEPHRINE

Norepinephrine is rarely used clinically due to its rapid metabolism and many sites of action. Drugs that evoke responses similar to sympathetic nerve stimulation are called sympathomimetic drugs. They produce their effects either directly, by stimulating adrenergic receptors (adrenergic receptor agonists), or indirectly, by promoting the release of norepinephrine or by blocking its reuptake. Table 1 gives examples of various sympathomimetic drugs, with their mechanisms of action, the effects they produce, and common therapeutic indications.

Drugs that block the responses to sympathetic nerve stimulation and thus block the effects of norepinephrine are called adrenergic receptor antagonists. They have no direct effects on adrenergic receptors but act by blocking the effects of either released norepinephrine or an administered adrenergic receptor agonist. Table 2 gives examples of adrenergic receptor antagonists, with their receptor selectivity, the effects they produce, and common therapeutic indications.

—*David B. Bylund*

See also–Neurotransmitters, Overview

Further Reading

Ahlquist, R. P. (1948). A study of adrenotropic receptors. *Am. J. Physiol.* **153**, 586–600.

Bylund, D. B. (1988). Subtypes of α_2-adrenoceptors: Pharmacological and molecular biological evidence converge. *Trends Pharmacol. Sci.* **9**, 356–361.

Cooper, J. R., Bloom, F. E., and Roth, R. H. (1996). *The Biochemical Basis of Neuropharmacology*, pp. 226–292. Oxford Univ. Press, New York.

Frishman, W. H., and Kotob, F. (1999). Alpha-adrenergic blocking drugs in clinical medicine. *J. Clin. Pharmacol.* **39**, 7–16.

Hokfelt, T., Johansson, O., and Goldstein, M. (1984). Central catecholamine neurons as revealed by immunohistochemistry with special reference to adrenaline neurons. In *Handbook of Chemical Neuroanatomy, Vol. 2, Part 1: Classical Transmitters in the CNS* (A. Björklund and T. Hokfelt, Eds.). Elsevier, Amsterdam.

Liggett, S. B. (2000). Pharmacogenetics of beta-1- and beta-2-adrenergic receptors. *Pharmacology* **61**, 167–173.

NREM (Non-Rapid Eye Movement) Sleep

Encyclopedia of the Neurological Sciences
Copyright 2003, Elsevier Science (USA). All rights reserved.

THE POPULAR VIEW that behavioral quiescence is the first sign of resting [non-rapid eye movement (NREM)] sleep may be valid for the full-blown state of sleep but not for the preparatory period during which many animal species display complex motor behaviors directed to find a safe home for sleep. The defining signs of the period during which one falls asleep are peculiar changes in brain electrical activity [electroencephalogram (EEG)]. The EEG oscillations that define the transition from wakefulness to NREM sleep are associated with long periods of inhibition in neurons located in the thalamus, a deep structure in the brain and a gateway for most sensory signals in their route to the cerebral cortex. The consequence is that the incoming messages are blocked in the thalamus and the cerebral cortex is deprived of information from the outside world.

HUMORAL FACTORS IMPLICATED IN SLEEP ONSET

Some scientists who explore the mechanisms of sleep onset at the level of neurons regard the theories that implicate different humoral (chemical) substances in the onset of sleep as issuing from experiments lacking stringent methodological criteria or simply ignore those data. However, one must consider that the genesis and maintenance of the enduring behavioral state of NREM sleep are hardly attributable to only conventional neuronal mechanisms, which operate on short timescales. It is then conceivable that the commendable efforts of recording single neurons in order to understand how one falls asleep will only make sense when concerted studies on sleep humoral factors and on their actions upon neurons in critical brain areas will fully disclose the mechanisms of falling sleep. Currently, little is known about the effects of sleep-promoting chemical substances on neurons.

The notion of a humoral sleep factor was introduced at the beginning of the 20th century. The conclusion was that the need for sleep is due to a hypothetical substance accumulated when wakefulness is maintained over long periods of time. The terms sleep factor (SF) or sleep-promoting substance (SPS) are commonly used for chemicals that are hypothesized to promote sleep. The list of putative SFs is quite long. There are approximately 30 SFs and some models have proposed interactions between various substances that have the capacity to modify sleep for quite long periods. Some SFs are summarized here.

First, the delta sleep-inducing peptide (DSIP), termed so because initial reports claimed that it promotes sleep associated with EEG delta waves, may act through the modulation of endocrine systems and/or by direct action on lower brainstem or anterior hypothalamic neurons. The possible mechanism of DSIP is an antinociceptive action— that is, reducing noxious (pain) stimuli that produce alertness, thus favoring sleep onset. Second, the growth hormone-releasing factor (GRF) also belongs to the family of peptides. Its administration into cerebral ventricles produces EEG signs of NREM sleep and reduction of motor activity. The GRF-containing hypothalamic neurons may exert their action in promoting NREM sleep through an effect on the basal forebrain neurons that are implicated in sleep onset. Third, prostaglandins (PGs) D_2 and E_2 are endogenous substances that are hypothesized to induce sleep and wakefulness, respectively. The putative receptors of PGs were studied by autoradiography and the binding proteins were found in the posterior and anterior hypothalamus, which are postulated to be critical zones for regulating waking and sleep, respectively. Fourth, muramyl peptides (MPs) have a chemical structure that is similar to that of serotonin (5-HT), a neurotransmitter that was implicated in the generation of NREM sleep. Finally, one of the major factors accounting for sleep-inducing effects of prolonged wakefulness is adenosine (AD). Both upper brainstem and basal forebrain cholinergic (activating) neurons are under the tonic inhibitory control of endogenous AD. The conclusion of these experiments is that AD is a physiological SF that mediates somnogenic effects of prior wakefulness.

Clearly, a single neurochemical regulatory substance could not account for the genesis of the complex state of NREM sleep. In the future, the neuronal actions of SFs substances, which facilitate or promote sleep when injected into given brain areas, should be submitted to electrophysiological studies to shed light on chemically-modulated ionic currents of neurons located in brain areas involved in sleep regulation.

PASSIVE AND ACTIVE SLEEP

The concepts postulating that sleep is a passive phenomenon due to closure of cerebral gates (which leads to brain deafferentation or disconnection) or, alternatively, an active phenomenon promoted by inhibitory mechanisms arising in some cerebral areas have long been considered as opposing views. However, neurons with inhibitory influences (such as those located in the anterior hypothalamus) act on neurons that exert excitatory influences on the brain (such as those located in the posterior hypothalamus), and the final outcome of these relations is the disconnection of the forebrain. Therefore, the two (active and passive) mechanisms of sleep onset are probably successive steps within a chain of events, and they are complementary rather than opposed.

The idea that the diminution or cessation of sensory signals essentially causes sleep is supported by experiments reaching the conclusion that sleep results from the sudden withdrawal of sensory bombardment. Impairments of the state of vigilance, leading to hypersomnia, follow lesions of brainstem reticular neurons or some thalamic nuclei that represent the continuation of the brainstem reticular formation. Studies of patients with prolonged lethargy led to the conclusion that the brainstem–thalamic–cortical circuit contributes to the maintenance of alertness in mammals, especially primates. The role of some thalamic nuclei (called intralaminar) in regulating arousal is also highlighted by the fact that their activity increases during a task requiring alertness and attention in humans. Parallel extrathalamic pathways, through which brainstem reticular neurons influence the cerebral cortex, are relayed by histaminergic projections of posterior hypothalamic neurons and by cholinergic projections of the basal forebrain.

The basic mechanism of falling asleep is the transformation of a brain responsive to external signals into a closed brain. In humans, the onset of sleep is associated with functional blindness. The obliteration of messages from the outside world at sleep onset is due to inhibitory processes in the thalamus. It was demonstrated that the thalamic responses to stimuli applied to different pathways conveying signals from the external world are diminished from the very onset of drowsiness and that these responses are completely obliterated during further deepening of sleep. This occurs despite no measurable change in responses recorded from neural pathways before the thalamus. This demonstrates that the thalamus is the first relay station where reduction of afferent signals takes place when falling asleep. Thus, the cortex is deprived from the input required to elaborate a response and this process constitutes a necessary prelude for deepening the state of sleep.

The concept of active sleep, produced by inhibitory neurons, originated with the early clinical and anatomical studies showing that postencephalitic insomnia was associated with prominent damage in the preoptic area of the anterior hypothalamus. These observations were followed by experimental studies suggesting the antagonistic nature of the anterior (hypnogenic) and posterior (awakening) areas of the hypothalamus. Recently, it was shown that an inhibitory circuit links the anterior hypothalamus to the arousing areas located in the posterior hypothalamus, and that some neurons in discrete parts of the anterior hypothalamus are activated during NREM sleep. However, most neurons in the anterior hypothalamus display an increased rate of discharge during wakefulness. Moreover, the insomnia produced by anterior hypothalamic lesions does not imply that the anterior hypothalamic area is necessary for sleep. After insomnia, resulting from the irreversible lesion of anterior hypothalamic neurons, reversible (functional) inactivation of posterior hypothalamic neurons produces recovery of sleep. Thus, sleep can be restored by the removal of activating actions exerted by posterior hypothalamic histaminergic neurons, and there is no need to consider the "active inhibitory hypnogenic" properties of anterior hypothalamic neurons as indispensable for NREM sleep.

Rather than being generated in discrete brain regions, waking and sleep states are produced by complex chains of interconnected systems. Most experimental data argue against the notion of "center(s)" and instead favor the idea that waking and sleep states are generated by distributed systems. It follows that lesioning one sector of interconnected neuronal groups will not be followed by a permanent disturbance in a given state of vigilance but by compensatory phenomena due to the presence of remaining circuits consisting of neurons with properties similar to those of lesioned neurons.

BRAIN OSCILLATIONS DURING NREM SLEEP

Three types of brain rhythms characterize the state of NREM sleep: spindles, delta, and slow oscillations. Spindles (7–14 Hz) appear during early stages of sleep, sometimes preceding overt behavioral manifestations of sleep. They are generated in the thalamus even after the removal of the cerebral cortex. However, the cerebral cortex has a powerful role in the synchronization of spindles over widespread territories because in both animals and humans spindle sequences appear nearly simultaneously, and this synchrony is lost after removal of cortex. The thalamic neurons located in a peculiar (reticular) nucleus, which use a potent inhibitory neurotransmitter (GABA), can generate spindle oscillation even after disconnection from other thalamic nuclei and cerebral cortex. These neurons receive projections from thalamic relay neurons as well as cortical neurons. They do not have cortical projections but project back to thalamocortical cells and inhibit them (Fig. 1A). This is a simple recurrent inhibitory circuit. The pacemaking role of the thalamic reticular nucleus in the generation of sleep

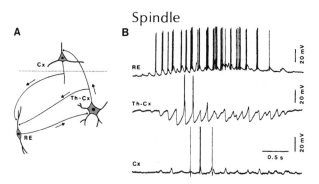

Figure 1

Spindle oscillations in thalamic reticular (RE), thalamocortical (Th-Cx, ventrolateral nucleus), and cortical (Cx, motor area) neurons of cats. (A) Circuit of three neuronal types. (B) Intracellular recordings of RE, Th-Cx, and Cx neurons in cats under barbiturate anesthesia (experiments performed in collaboration with M. Deschênes).

spindles was also demonstrated by loss of spindling in target thalamocortical systems after disconnection from the reticular nucleus. Spindles result from repetitive bursts of action potentials in thalamic reticular cells, which produce rhythmic inhibitory postsynaptic potentials in thalamic neurons with cortical projections, eventually leading to rebound spike bursts that are transferred to cortex (Fig. 1B). Spindles are primarily due to the decreased firing frequencies in thalamic-projecting brainstem activating neurons when the behavioral state of wakefulness shifts to sleep.

Delta oscillation (1–4 Hz) progressively appears and replaces spindles during late stages of NREM sleep. Delta oscillation has two components. One component is generated in the cerebral cortex as it survives complete destruction of the thalamus. The other component of this oscillation is stereotyped, clock-like, and is generated in the thalamus through the interplay between two ionic currents of thalamocortical neurons.

The slow oscillation (0.5–1 Hz) has a similar frequency in animals and humans. The cortical origin of the slow oscillation was demonstrated by its survival in the cerebral cortex after extensive destruction of the thalamus and its absence in the thalamus of animals whose cortex was ablated. Intracellular analyses showed that cortical neurons display a slow oscillation consisting of prolonged (0.4–0.7 sec) depolarizing and hyperpolarizing components. The long-lasting depolarization of the slow oscillation consists of excitatory potentials but also of fast inhibitory potentials, reflecting the action of synaptically coupled local cortical inhibitory neurons. The long-lasting hyperpolarization, interrupting the depolarizing phases, is a combination of potassium currents and the absence of neuronal activity in cortical and thalamic neuronal networks (disfacilitation). Both pyramidal neurons (which are excitatory and project to distant structures) and stellate neurons (which are inhibitory and are part of local circuits) display similar relations with the EEG components of the slow oscillation. During the depth-positive EEG wave of the slow oscillation, all cortical neurons are silent, whereas during the sharp depth-negative EEG deflection cortical neurons are mainly excited and discharge action potentials.

The systematization of sleep rhythms into three categories (spindles, delta, and slow) may be useful for didactic purposes, but these brain rhythms are not seen in isolation during NREM sleep but are

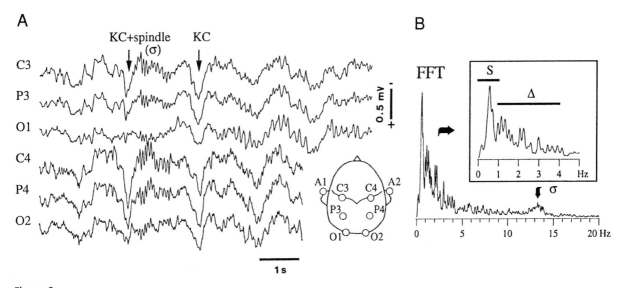

Figure 2
(A) The cortical slow oscillation groups thalamically generated spindles; the K complex (KC) in natural sleep. Scalp monopolar recordings with respect to the contralateral ear are shown (insert). Traces show a short episode from a stage 3 NREM sleep. The arrows point to two K complexes, consisting of a surface-positive wave followed (or not) by a sequence of spindle (sigma) waves. Note the synchrony of K complexes in all recorded sites. (B) Frequency decomposition of the electrical activity from the C3 lead into three frequency bands: slow oscillation (S, 0–1 Hz), delta waves (Δ, 1–4 Hz), and spindles (σ, 12–15 Hz) (recordings during human sleep were done in collaboration with F. Amzica).

grouped by the cortically generated slow oscillation. Thus, a cycle of the slow oscillation is often followed by a brief sequence of spindle waves. This combination of sleep rhythms produces the K complex, a major EEG feature in NREM sleep of humans (Fig. 2).

FUNCTIONAL ROLE OF NREM SLEEP OSCILLATION

What could be the role of spontaneously occurring oscillations in NREM sleep? During this sleep stage, the inhibition of thalamic neurons is effective in preventing the transfer of incoming signals from the outside world to cortex; thus, it ensures a safe sleep. However, this disconnection process may be just the tip of the iceberg. The rhythmic bursts of action potentials, which are associated with all three oscillatory types in NREM sleep, may prevent the metabolic inertia that would result from complete absence of discharges and would thus favor a quick passage from NREM sleep to arousal when danger is imminent. At variance with previous hypotheses, cortical neurons recorded from different areas have been found to be firing as actively when the animal is asleep as when the animal is alert, although their firing patterns change from one state to the other. Why are cortical neurons so busy when the brain is supposed to rest? One of the sleep mysteries lies in this question. During the state of NREM sleep, the rhythmic bursts of action potentials may reorganize and/or specify the circuitry, and they may also consolidate memory traces acquired during wakefulness. Repeated spike bursts occurring during spontaneous or evoked oscillations, like in NREM sleep, may lead to plasticity processes and self-sustained activity patterns, resembling those evoked in the late stages of stimulation. Such changes are due to resonant activities in closed loops, as in "memory" processes. These data indicate that slow wave sleep is not associated with a global annihilation of consciousness, but that some mental processes are active in this state. Indeed, dreaming mentation is not confined to REM sleep but also appears, with a different content (more logical and closer to real-life events) in slow wave sleep.

—*M. Steriade*

See also–Electroencephalogram (EEG); Periodic Limb Movements in Sleep (PLMS); Polysomnography, Clinical; REM (Rapid Eye Movement) Sleep; REM Sleep Behavior Disorder; Serotonin; Sleep, Overview; Wakefulness

Further Reading

Achermann, P., and Borbély, A. (1997). Low-frequency (<1 Hz) oscillations in the human sleep EEG. *Neuroscience* **81**, 213–222.

Amzica, F., and Steriade, M. (1997). The K-complex: Its slow (<1 Hz) rhythmicity and relation to delta waves. *Neurology* **49**, 952–959.

Jouvet, M. (1972). The role of monoamines and acetylcholine-containing neurons in the regulation of the sleep–waking cycle. *Ergebnisse Physiol.* **64**, 166–307.

Moruzzi, G. (1972). The sleep–waking cycle. *Ergebnisse Physiol.* **64**, 1–165.

Steriade, M. (1999). Coherent oscillations and short-term plasticity in corticothalamic networks. *Trends Neurosci.* **22**, 337–345.

Steriade, M. (2001). *The Intact and Sliced Brain.* MIT Press, Cambridge, MA.

Steriade, M., and McCarley, R. W. (1990). *Brainstem Control of Wakefulness and Sleep.* Plenum, New York.

Steriade, M., McCormick, D. A., and Sejnowski, T. J. (1993). Thalamocortical oscillations in the sleeping and aroused brain. *Science* **262**, 679–685.

Nystagmus and Saccadic Intrusions and Oscillations

Encyclopedia of the Neurological Sciences
Copyright 2003, Elsevier Science (USA). All rights reserved.

THE OCULAR MOTOR SYSTEM (OMS) is responsible for directing the eyes to a target of interest, maintaining fixation on that target, pursuing moving targets, and stabilizing the eyes during both head and body motion and movement of the background. When both the eyes and the visual scene are moving, it also maintains the percept of a stable world, preventing oscillopsia (the false perception of motion). The OMS is composed of many interacting feedback control subsystems that synergistically accomplish these diverse tasks. Each is responsible for specific types of eye movements. Saccades are fast eye movements that redirect the eyes from one target to another. Smooth pursuit movements are used to voluntarily pursue a moving target. The vestibuloocular reflex and optokinetic reflex stabilize the eyes in response to head or visual background movement, respectively. In addition, there are internal and external feedback loops controlling the extraocular muscles and pulleys and also fixation. When one or more of these subsystems becomes unstable due to either congenital or acquired conditions, an oscillation may result. Oscillations whose origins lie in subsystems that control slow eye movements are called nystagmus, of which there are many types. Alternatively, when the saccadic system is defective or unstable, saccadic intrusions and oscillations result.

The presence of either nystagmus or saccadic instability may indicate neurological abnormalities or may reflect nonsymptomatic congenital conditions. Specific types of oscillations may be diagnostic of the associated condition. The differential diagnosis requires accurate identification and characterization of the particular instability present. Eye movement recording can differentiate nystagmus types as well as saccadic intrusions and oscillations.

DEFINITIONS

Nystagmus can be classified into two broad categories, pendular and jerk. Pendular nystagmus is a sinusoidal oscillation with no prominent saccadic fast phases. Jerk nystagmus consists of an initial slow phase followed by a corrective saccadic fast phase. In some jerk waveforms the fast phases refoveate the target; in others, the slow phases are slowed or reversed by braking saccades. There are also combinations of pendular and jerk waveforms, which are called dual-jerk nystagmus. The specific waveforms of nystagmus (i.e., the shapes of the slow phases and the type of saccades imbedded in them) help differentiate nystagmus types and determine their etiology or relationship to associated neurological conditions. Also, the relative amplitudes and phases of the nystagmus in the two eyes or the conditions that elicit nystagmus help differentiate them. Saccadic intrusions are initiated by a saccade away from the target being fixated. They may appear singly or in small groups. When continuous runs of saccadic intrusions occur, they become saccadic oscillations.

NYSTAGMUS

There are many types of nystagmus, both spontaneous and induced, normal and abnormal. Only some of the more common, nonphysiological types are discussed in this entry.

Infantile Nystagmus

Several types of nystagmus may appear at birth or during infancy. Most are not symptomatic of severe neurological conditions. Fortunately, they can be diagnosed by their unique waveforms, characteristics, or interocular phase relationships. Unfortunately, an individual may have more than one type of infantile nystagmus, producing complex waveforms. Infantile nystagmus does not cause oscillopsia, the perception of a moving world.

The most common type is congenital nystagmus (CN). Several waveforms are pathognomonic for CN. Although individuals with CN may have strabismus or other deficits in the afferent visual system, these contributing factors are not the primary causes of CN. The many waveforms recorded in CN suggest at least two and probably three distinct causes for the oscillations in CN. Pendular CN is hypothesized to be the result of the failure to develop the damping that normally controls the inherent oscillation of the smooth pursuit system. Jerk CN has characteristic accelerating slow phases. Asymmetrical (a)periodic alternating nystagmus is a jerk CN that is probably caused by the same instability that produces the more periodic alternation seen in acquired nystagmus of vestibular origin. Finally, nonalternating CN with predominantly jerk waveforms may either be caused by another subsystem oscillation or result from a strong saccadic system acting on the same pendular oscillation responsible for the pendular waveforms.

The various idiosyncratic waveforms recorded in CN are a result of the interaction of the saccadic and fixation subsystems with the basic instabilities. This interaction facilitates target acquisition and maintained foveation, allowing good visual acuity despite the ocular oscillation. CN may damp at a specific gaze angle (null angle) or with convergence on a near target. These characteristics may be exploited therapeutically either optically, through the use of prisms, or surgically. Afferent stimulation of the ophthalmic division of the trigeminal nerve or of the neck damps CN in some individuals. This allows the use of soft contact lenses to damp the CN or electrical or vibratory stimulation of the forehead or neck. Finally, CN may be damped by lowering the responsiveness of the extraocular muscles. This is currently being done by tenotomy of the four horizontal recti tendons and reattachment at their original points of insertion on the globe. The nystagmus procedures that damp CN may be combined with strabismus procedures in patients who have both CN and strabismus.

A second type of infantile nystagmus is latent/manifest latent nystagmus (LMLN), which is always accompanied by strabismus. It is a jerk nystagmus (of both eyes) that beats in the direction of the fixating eye, regardless of the gaze angle and whether one eye is occluded or both are viewing (only one will be fixating due to the strabismus). LMLN has a linear slow phase that takes the fixating eye off target. When the slow phase velocity becomes too large for effective foveation, the ocular motor system switches from its normal, foveating saccade mode to a defoveating saccade mode (a rare instance in which the saccadic fast phases deliberately take the fixating eye off target). The fast phases take the eye past the target and slow phases then decelerate the eye toward the target, allowing the fixation subsystem to maintain target foveation at the low-velocity ends of the slow phases. Often, LMLN slow-phase velocity increases as gaze is directed in the direction of the fast phases (Alexander's law) and the OMS switches from one mode to the other, with the corresponding changes in the LMLN waveform.

Currently, correcting the strabismus surgically is the only therapeutic alternative; responsiveness of LMLN to tenotomy has not been demonstrated. However, by using a four-muscle approach to correcting the strabismus in patients who also have CN, the built-in effects of tenotomy on the latter may be appreciated.

Some individuals exhibit damping of their nystagmus with deliberate esotropia during fixation on a distant target; this is called the nystagmus blockage syndrome and is not the same as the convergence-induced damping seen in CN without strabismus. Blockage syndrome patients do have strabismus and CN that either damps due to the purposive esotropia or converts to a low-amplitude LMLN.

Finally, infants sometimes have mixtures of uniocular, grossly disconjugate, and variable-phase-difference pendular nystagmus. This is called spasmus nutans, and the pendular nystagmus is usually of a higher frequency and lower amplitude than CN; it is benign. However, the same type of nystagmus may be indicative of a brain tumor, and imaging is often required.

Acquired Nystagmus

The most common type of acquired nystagmus is gaze-evoked nystagmus (GEN), which is a jerk nystagmus. It is absent in primary position and is present only as gaze is directed laterally, it has fast phases that beat in the direction of gaze, and its amplitude increases with gaze eccentricity. GEN represents failure of the final, common, gaze-holding neural integrator, which is thought to be in the nucleus prepositus hypoglossi and the medial vestibular nuclei. Eccentric position signals leak exponentially toward zero, causing the eyes to follow the same course. GEN is most often associated with drug ingestion (e.g., sedatives, tranquilizers, and anticonvulsants) but may also indicate cerebellar dysfunction. GEN may also be associated with rebound and centripetal nystagmus.

Acquired pendular nystagmus is also common and usually is accompanied by oscillopsia. It may be present in more than one plane, with one predominating, or may be dissociated in the two eyes. In extreme cases, the movements may be totally disconjugate, resulting in a pendular vergence nystagmus. In some patients, the nystagmus stops momentarily after a saccade. Pendular nystagmus may be associated with demyelinating disease (e.g., multiple sclerosis), Pelizaeus–Merzbacher disease, or toluene abuse. It is thought to result from impaired visual connections to the cerebellum, leading to instability in reciprocal connections from the brainstem. Pendular nystagmus may accompany oculopalatal tremor or Whipple's disease.

Vestibular nystagmus (VN) is a jerk nystagmus with linear slow phases, suggesting a tonic imbalance in the vestibular push–pull tonic firing rate. Both peripheral and central disturbances can cause VN. As gaze is directed toward the fast phases, the nystagmus increases in amplitude (Alexander's law). Peripheral VN has a horizontal–torsional trajectory, beating away from the side of the lesion, and it is suppressed by visual fixation. Central VN is more complex, manifesting in downbeat, upbeat, torsional, or seesaw nystagmus. These variations of VN also display idiosyncratic waveforms and characteristics related to fixation and convergence. The associated neurological conditions are too numerous to mention.

Periodic alternating nystagmus (PAN) is a VN whose direction changes periodically, building up first in one direction and then in the opposite direction. Between these approximately 90-sec intervals of unidirectional jerk nystagmus are neutral intervals (usually short) of no nystagmus, pendular nystagmus, jerk nystagmus whose direction changes several times, upbeat or downbeat nystagmus, or square-wave jerks. The cause of PAN is thought to be a limit cycle instability in the velocity storage mechanism of the vestibular–optokinetic subsystems.

PAN is a vestibular dysfunction and can be temporarily stopped or reset by vestibular stimuli. PAN has been associated with a long list of neurological abnormalities, including those with cerebellar involvement, and also with visual loss.

Seesaw nystagmus is a vertically disconjugate, torsionally conjugate nystagmus associated with abnormalities of the chiasm (including congenital achiasma and hemichiasma) and the interstitial nucleus of Cajal. Its waveform may be pendular or jerk. Seesaw nystagmus may result from mesodiencephalic disease (e.g., stroke), parasellar masses, multiple sclerosis, Arnold–Chiari malformation, progressive visual loss, and other acquired or congenital conditions. It may represent a dynamic disorder related to the static disorder of dissociated vertical deviation.

SACCADIC INTRUSIONS AND OSCILLATIONS

There are several types of saccadic intrusions and oscillations. Fixation, even in normals, may be occasionally interrupted by saccadic intrusions that take the eyes off target for a short period of time. Target foveation may be restored either by a subsequent saccade or by a slow drift. Saccadic intrusions may occur in bursts of two to four intrusions. They do not cause oscillopsia.

Saccadic Intrusions

Square-wave jerks (SWJs) are intrusions that consist of two oppositely directed saccades that take the eyes off target and return them in approximately 200 msec. They are usually small (1–3°), but they may be larger. Because they are not corrected until a visual reaction time has elapsed, they are probably caused by spurious errors in the internal desired eye position signal driving the saccadic pulse generator. SWJs may appear in normals and the elderly and also with cerebellar syndromes, progressive supranuclear palsy, and hemispheric disease.

Square-wave pulses (originally called macro square-wave jerks, which was misleading) take the eyes off target and return them in 50–150 msec. They are usually larger than SWJs but may also be small; they may occur singly or in bursts. Unlike SWJs, their correction in less than the visual reaction time indicates that the internal desired eye position signal has not been disturbed and is used by the short-latency, efference copy mechanism to detect and correct the erroneous motor command. A possible site for the spurious signals generating square-wave pulses is within the pulse generator. Square-wave pulses may appear in multiple sclerosis.

Saccadic pulses take the eyes off target and are followed by a decelerating drift back to target. Double saccadic pulses are a couplet of back-to-back saccades with no intersaccadic latency that interrupt fixation. Because the eyes immediately drift back to the original fixation position after a saccadic pulse, the neural pulse that caused it is not integrated by the common neural integrator responsible for maintaining eye position. Thus, it may be presumed that the desired eye position signal was not changed and it prevented the integration to a new eye position. Runs of saccadic pulses occur in the abducting eye in internuclear ophthalmoplegia and may be mistaken for nystagmus (e.g., abduction "nystagmus").

Saccadic Oscillations

Runs of continuous SWJ are called square-wave oscillations. The following are possible causes of their generation: (i) the desired eye position signal remains disturbed or (ii) after the corrective, second saccade of each SWJ, the disturbance recurs. Either way, once a refractory period elapses after the return saccade of a SWJ, the cycle is repeated. Square-wave oscillations have been reported in progressive supranuclear palsy and acquired immunodeficiency disease.

Saccadic dysmetria is a postsaccadic, damped saccadic oscillation (hypermetria) or series of less than adequate saccades (hypometria). The intersaccadic intervals are approximately 200 msec. Hypermetria results from an increased gain (>1 but <2) in the saccadic subsystem, causing each saccade to overshoot by a fixed percentage of the desired amplitude until the required corrective saccades fall within a dead zone. If the gain is 2, a sustained oscillation results, and if it is >2, saccadic sizes increase. These latter oscillations are referred to as macro saccadic oscillations. Hypometria results from a low saccadic gain. Dysmetria is associated with cerebellar disease.

Runs of double saccadic pulses during fixation are called flutter. Postsaccadic bursts of double saccadic pulses are called flutter dysmetria, and multivectorial flutter is opsoclonus. The mechanism of flutter is probably within the saccadic pulse generator, resulting in an oscillation without intersaccadic latency. Flutter may appear in internuclear ophthalmoplegia and both it and opsoclonus may occur in brainstem encephalitis, paraneoplastic syndromes, or metabolic–toxic states. Opsoclonus can also occur in various types of cancer.

—L. F. Dell'Osso

***See also**–*Eye Movements, Saccades; Optokinetic Nystagmus; Vertigo and Dizziness

Further Reading

Dell'Osso, L. F. (1991). Nystagmus, saccadic intrusions/oscillations and oscillopsia. *Curr. Neuro-Ophthalmol.* **3**, 153–191.

Dell'Osso, L. F., and Daroff, R. B. (1999). Eye movement characteristics and recording techniques. In *Neuro-Ophthalmology* (J. S. Glaser, Ed.), 3rd ed., pp. 327–343. Lippincott Williams & Wilkins, Philadelphia.

Leigh, R. J., and Zee, D. S. (1999). *The Neurology of Eye Movements, Contemporary Neurology Series*, 3rd ed. Davis, Philadelphia.

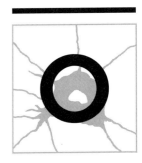

Obesity

Encyclopedia of the Neurological Sciences
Copyright 2003, Elsevier Science (USA). All rights reserved.

OBESITY [generally defined as a body mass index (BMI) > 30] constitutes one of the greatest single risk factors for the most prevalent chronic diseases, especially cardiovascular disease and diabetes, in developed countries throughout the world. Its effects on mental health and life satisfaction may be even more profound. Direct costs of obesity have consistently been estimated to account for approximately 5% of all health costs. Of particular concern, the incidence of obesity, in contrast to most chronic diseases, has increased dramatically during the past 20 years. For example, the NHANES surveys suggested that the prevalence of obesity in the adult population increased from 14.5% during the period 1976–1980 to 22.5% during the period 1988–1994. Similarly, the prevalence of obesity in 18-year-old Swedish military conscripts increased more than threefold between 1971 and 1995. Thus, unquestionably obesity constitutes a major and growing health risk.

Although in principle obesity can be reduced by simple changes in lifestyle (e.g., increase in exercise and especially a reduction in food intake), experience has amply demonstrated that despite the short-term efficacy of such programs to reduce body weight in highly motivated individuals, the reduction in body weight is almost never maintained so that long-term successful loss of body weight through diet and exercise is extremely rare. Currently, only surgical intervention (especially bariatric reduction of effective stomach size) appears to produce reliable long-term reductions in body weight, with similarly beneficial effects on diabetic symptoms. However, this potentially dangerous intervention is recommended only for extreme obesity entailing a BMI of more than 40.

Given the high prevalence and health consequences of obesity, the causes of this condition are of great interest. More precisely, it is of interest to account for individual variations in body weight—that is, why the vast majority of individuals in developed societies have equal access to food but exhibit dramatically different BMIs. Not surprisingly, genetic effects account for most of the variance in human BMI: A meta-analysis of the literature suggests that approximately 67% of BMI is due to genetic factors, although twin studies suggest up to approximately 80% of BMI is genetic. This may be usefully contrasted to Parkinson's disease, for example; several studies have failed to note any concordance for Parkinson's disease in identical twins.

On the other hand, in contrast to many diseases (e.g., Parkinson's disease) that are usefully considered as derangements in normal functioning, obesity may reflect genotypes that have in fact been selected for. Thus, from an evolutionary perspective, obesity in developed societies is thought to reflect a "thrifty genotype" that was selected for to produce efficient storage of nutrients during times of famine (a condition to which most human populations were routinely exposed until recently). An interesting monogenetic example of this phenomenon is that mice heterozygous for the obese gene survive prolonged fasting longer than wild-type mice, although mice homozygous for this gene are massively obese.

In this respect, alleles that lead to obesity may be analogous to alleles that lead to sickle cell anemia that have been selected for because heterozygous carriers are resistant to malaria. Furthermore, this selection process is dependent on environmental conditions (e.g., the availability of nutrition) that can change relatively quickly. Thus, populations that have been recently subject to famine conditions (which select for a thrifty genotype) develop a very high prevalence of obesity (with its associated diseases including diabetes) when conditions suddenly improve. It should be noted that although these effects are genetic, the manifestation of these genetic effects is highly dependent on the environment. For example, the population of the South Pacific island of Nauru exhibits a high prevalence of obesity on a Western diet, but under famine conditions the average BMI of this population might not be very different from the average BMI of any other population (although presumably natives of Nauru would survive famine better than other populations). Similarly, C57Bl/6J mice weigh approximately the same as A/J mice when on a standard lab chow diet, but when placed on a diet more similar to a typical Western diet (e.g., relatively high in fat), the C57Bl/6J mice become much more obese than the A/J mice.

It is generally appreciated that human obesity is a complex polygenic disease. However, mutations in five genes have been shown to produce obesity in a small number of humans: the leptin gene, the leptin receptor, the POMC gene, the melanocortin 4 gene, and the prohormone convertase 1 gene. Mutations in the melanocortin receptor appear to be by far the most common single-gene cause of human obesity. Furthermore, since mutations of leptin and the leptin receptor lead to reduced expression of hypothalamic POMC, the ligand for the MC4 receptor (α-MSH) is produced from the POMC precursor, and mutations in the prohormone convertase 1 gene lead to impaired processing of the POMC precursor, it can be generalized that all these forms of human obesity entail impaired production, processing, or responsiveness to the POMC product α-MSH. This generalization also applies to genetic obesity in mice. Thus, although obesity is a polygenic state, the melanocortin pathway may have an important role.

From a neurological perspective, an important issue is the role of the central nervous system in regulating body weight in general and in contributing to obesity in particular. It has long been known that damage to neurons in the medial basal hypothalamus (often referred to as the ventromedial hypothalamus) can produce obesity in humans and other mammals. However, like obesity due to single-gene defects, obesity due to hypothalamic damage is presumably rare. On the other hand, precise mapping studies with microlesions and chemical lesions have demonstrated that the specific hypothalamic area most effective in producing obesity is located between the ventromedial nucleus and the arcuate nucleus, an area that exactly overlaps with neurons that express POMC, the source of the ligand for the MC4 receptor. Furthermore, leptin receptors are expressed at their highest levels in this hypothalamic area, leptin produces maximum effect to reduce body weight when infused into this area, and lesions of this area block the effects of leptin. Thus, key gene mutations that are known to cause obesity in humans are either mainly or exclusively expressed in or act on hypothalamic neurons, damage to which also causes obesity, strongly supporting a major role of these hypothalamic neurons in causing obesity.

Although hypothalamic damage, or impairments in hypothalamic-active gene products, can clearly cause obesity, it remains to be established whether hypothalamic neurons play a major role in most forms of human obesity. From a clinical perspective, since most patients can relatively easily lose weight but can rarely keep the weight off, it is perhaps less important to understand how obese individuals become obese than to determine what is different between individuals who have never been obese and formerly obese individuals of the same weight. The key observation to account for this difference is that when either obese or lean individuals lose weight, their metabolic expenditures decrease to oppose further weight loss. Thus, formerly obese individuals will have lower metabolic rates than individuals who have never been obese with the same degree of adiposity so that formerly obese individuals will gain weight even if they consume the same number of calories as weight-stable individuals who have never been obese. The increase in body weight even when the number of calories consumed is the same as that consumed by weight-stable, lean individuals is also a characteristic of mice that are obese due to hypothalamic lesions or the same genetic defects as those that cause obesity in humans. These data suggest that the fundamental metabolic mechanisms that mediate obesity due to hypothalamic damage or single-gene defects may be similar to the mechanisms that mediate the far more common forms of obesity.

—*Charles V. Mobbs*

Further Reading

Albrecht, R. J., and Pories, W. J. (1999). Surgical intervention for the severely obese. *Baillieres Best Practice Res. Clin. Endocrinol. Metab.* **13**, 149–172.

Bray, G. A. (1989). 1989 McCollum Award Lecture. Genetic and hypothalamic mechanisms for obesity—Finding the needle in the haystack. *Am. J. Clin. Nutr.* **50**, 891–902.

Elmquist, J. K., Elias, C. F., and Saper, C. B. (1999). From lesions to leptin: Hypothalamic control of food intake and body weight. *Neuron* **22**, 221–232.

Flegal, K. M., Carroll, M. D., Kuczmarski, R. J., *et al.* (1998). Overweight and obesity in the United States: Prevalence and trends, 1960–1994. *Int. J. Obesity Relat. Metab. Disorders* **22**, 39–47.

Leibel, R. L., Rosenbaum, M., and Hirsch, J. (1995). Changes in energy expenditure resulting from altered body weight. *N. Engl. J. Med.* **332**, 621–628.

Maes, H. H., Neale, M. C., and Eaves, L. J. (1997). Genetic and environmental factors in relative body weight and human adiposity. *Behav. Genet.* **27**, 325–351.

Miller, W. C. (1999). How effective are traditional dietary and exercise interventions for weight loss? *Med. Sci. Sports Exercise* **31**, 1129–1134.

Mobbs, C., and Mizuno, T. (2000). Leptin regulation of proopiomelanocortin. *Front. Horm. Res.* **26**, 57–70.

National Task Force on the Prevention and Treatment of Obesity (2000). Overweight, obesity, and health risk. *Arch. Intern. Med.* **160**, 898–904.

Rosenbaum, M., Leibel, R. L., and Hirsch, J. (1997). Obesity. *N. Engl. J. Med.* **337**, 396–407.

Thompson, D., Edelsberg, J., Colditz, G. A., *et al.* (1999). Lifetime health and economic consequences of obesity. *Arch. Intern. Med.* **159**, 2177–2183.

Zimmet, P., Dowse, G., Finch, C., *et al.* (1990). The epidemiology and natural history of NIDDM—Lessons from the South Pacific. *Diabetes Metab. Rev.* **6**, 91–124.

Obsessive–Compulsive Disorder

Encyclopedia of the Neurological Sciences
Copyright 2003, Elsevier Science (USA). All rights reserved.

OBSESSIVE–COMPULSIVE DISORDER (OCD) is composed of obsessions and/or compulsions. OCD has an estimated lifetime prevalence in the general U.S. population of 2.5% and usually begins in childhood or the early twenties. The disorder is equally common in males and females, although the age of onset tends to be earlier for males.

Obsessions are recurrent and persistent thoughts, impulses, or images that are intrusive and inappropriate and that cause marked anxiety or distress in the affected individual. The person recognizes that the obsessions are a product of their own mind and are excessive or unreasonable (except in children). Obsessions are not simply excessive worries about real-life problems, and the person usually attempts to neutralize or suppress them with some other thought or action (compulsions). The affected individual is usually made extremely uncomfortable by just having the thought. Obsessions usually involve one of the following: contamination, pathological doubt, somatic concerns, need for symmetry, aggressive thoughts, blasphemous thoughts, and sexual thoughts. Multiple types of obsessions are found in most affected individuals and the obsessions may change over time.

Compulsions are behaviors (e.g., hand washing, ordering, and checking) or mental acts (e.g., praying, counting, and repeating words silently) that the person feels driven to perform in response to an obsession or according to rules that must be applied rigidly. The compulsions are aimed at preventing some dreaded event or situation or at reducing distress brought on by the obsession. However, compulsions are not connected in a realistic way with what they are designed to neutralize or prevent.

Compulsions are performed to decrease anxiety caused by obsessions. Compulsions may consume much of the waking hours of severely affected individuals. Typical types of compulsions include cleaning, rituals, checking, and hoarding. Cleaning compulsions are provoked in individuals by the obsession that real or imagined germs, dirt, or chemicals will "contaminate" them. Individuals with rituals must perform a series of complicated behaviors in an exact order or repeat them until they are done perfectly. Counting the number of syllables in a sentence or slats in a window shade are examples of rituals. Checking involves the obsession of harming oneself or others by forgetting to lock the door or turning off the gas stove. Some individuals may repeatedly retrace routes they drive to be sure they have not hit anyone or caused any accidents. Hoarding is one of the less common compulsions and it involves the constant collection of useless items, such as scraps, newspapers, clothing, containers, cans, stones, garbage, and even excrement, to the point that rooms are filled, doorways are blocked, and health hazards develop. This compulsion usually develops in response to the obsession that the item could possibly be needed in the future and the individual would be filled with regret if the item had been discarded. The hoarding subtype of OCD is considered particularly difficult to treat.

OCD SPECTRUM AND DIFFERENTIAL DIAGNOSIS

Disorders that share features of OCD include body dysmorphic disorder, hypochondriasis, the eating disorders, and the impulse-control disorders such as kleptomania, pyromania, pathological gambling, and trichotillomania (the pulling out of hair compulsion). All these disorders include recurrent thoughts that are difficult or impossible for the affected individual to resist. For example, in anorexia nervosa, the pathological fear of fatness could be considered an obsession and the extreme dieting and food rituals as the compulsions. Obsessive–compulsive "traits" have been theorized to be etiologically important in the development of psychiatric disorders.

Other disorders may mimic OCD. Tics and stereotyped movements are different than compulsions. Generally, the cognitive elements involved in compulsions are much more complex, whereas in tics and stereotypic movements the individual does not report any specific reason for the behavior, only a nonspecific tension that builds until the behavior is performed. Of note, Tourette's syndrome and OCD are frequently cooccurring disorders, and individuals with Tourette's should be routinely asked about the presence of obsessions and compulsions.

Schizophrenia is sometimes characterized by bizarre thoughts and fears (delusions) as well as stereotyped behaviors. However, although the individual with schizophrenia is distressed by the fears, having the fears or thoughts is usually not believed to be abnormal by the individual. Furthermore, the individual cannot believe that the delusions are irrational. In major depression, the depressed individual may have distressing, repetitive thoughts, but these are rarely resisted. In addition, depressive ruminations, in contrast to pure obsessions, are often focused on a past incident rather than on a current event or future events. Although it has a similar name, obsessive–compulsive personality disorder is actually quite different from OCD. Obsessive-compulsive personality disorder does not involve obsessions or compulsions; rather, it is characterized by a pervasive pattern of maladaptive orderliness, perfectionism, and control.

Finally, superstitions and repetitive checking behaviors are commonly encountered in everyday life.

The diagnosis of OCD is made only if they are time-consuming or result in significant psychosocial impairment or distress.

TREATMENT

Behavior Therapy

One of the most effective treatments is a type of behavior therapy known as exposure and response prevention, which is based on a positive-loop feedback theory of OCD. The disorder is believed to be the result of a perpetuated positive feedback loop between obsessions, which cause anxiety, and anxiety, which causes the development of further obsessions. Without the presence of compulsions, this cycle might exhaust itself when the individual eventually desensitizes to the anxiety. However, in OCD, the cycle continues because the compulsions decrease the anxiety just enough to prevent the desensitization process to occur. Exposure–response prevention disrupts this perpetuated cycle by focusing on decreasing compulsive behaviors.

During treatment sessions, patients are exposed to the situations that give rise to their anxiety and provoke compulsive behavior or mental rituals. However, patients are instructed not to engage in the compulsions. Subsequently, the anxiety arising from their obsessions lessens without their engaging in compulsions. For example, therapy for a compulsive cleaner who previously compulsively washed their hands after handling money might involve counting dollar bills without washing their hands. The treatment is generally conducted in a graduated, systematic manner, usually under the supervision of a therapist trained in behavior therapy, although there are self-help books with directions for self-guided treatment. Involvement of the individual's family or support system in this process can be invaluable.

Exposure–response prevention works well for patients whose compulsions focus on situations that can be recreated easily. A few engage in compulsive rituals because they fear catastrophic events that cannot be recreated conveniently. Therapy for these patients must rely more on imagined exposure to the anxiety-producing situations.

Various studies indicate that behavior therapy is successful for 50–90% of those with OCD. However, some patients will not agree to participate in behavior therapy because it is "embarrassing" and technically difficult. Affected individuals also frequently suffer from comorbid conditions that must also be treated.

Other types of psychotherapy, such as psychoanalysis or insight-oriented psychotherapy, have not been shown to be particularly effective in treating OCD. These patients frequently have a significant amount of anxiety and they benefit from support and reassurance, especially while undergoing behavior therapy. Psychoeducational and self-help support groups can be extremely helpful.

Medications

Numerous studies have demonstrated that highly serotonergic medications, including clomipramine and the selective serotonin reuptake inhibitors, are effective in the treatment of OCD. Medication treatment for OCD frequently requires higher dosages than for depression (e.g., 80 mg per day of fluoxetine is frequently required to treat OCD, whereas only 20 mg per day is the standard dose for depression). In addition, 2 or 3 months may be required for medications for OCD to reach optimal efficacy.

In general, medication therapy in OCD is not as dramatically effective as in, for example, major depression. Also, although approximately 50–60% of patients with OCD experience resolution or significant improvement of symptoms with a first-line drug, others require various combination or augmentation strategies before a satisfactory response is achieved.

Psychosurgery

Psychosurgery is generally reserved for intractable cases of OCD, but 50–85% of cases show improvement at 1-year follow-up after the psychosurgical procedure. Several procedures have been tried, including cingulotomy, subcaudate tractotomy, limbic leukotomy, and anterior capsulotomy, but none has been shown to be statistically superior to the others.

—*Descartes Li*

See also–Antianxiety Pharmacology; Anxiety Disorders, Overview; Bipolar Disorder; Borderline Personality Disorder; Delusions; Depression; Gilles de la Tourette's Syndrome; Impulse Control Disorders; Panic Disorder; Phobias; Schizophrenia, Biology of

Further Reading
Foa, E., and Wilson, R. (1991). *Stop Obsessing!* Bantam, New York.
Hyman, B. M., and Pedrick, C. (1999). *The OCD Workbook.* New Harbinger, Oakland, CA.

Occipital Lobe

Encyclopedia of the Neurological Sciences

THE OCCIPITAL LOBE encompasses the posterior portion of the human cerebral cortex and is primarily responsible for vision. The surface area of the human occipital lobe is approximately 12% of the total surface area of the neocortex of the brain. Direct electrical stimulation of the occipital lobe produces visual sensations. Damage to the occipital lobe results in complete or partial blindness or visual agnosia depending on the location and severity of the damage.

Vision begins with the spatial, temporal, and chromatic components of light falling on the photoreceptors of the retina and ends in the perception of the world around us. The occipital lobe contains the bulk of machinery that enables this process. However, our perception of the world is also affected by expectations and attention. Indeed, through extensive feedback to the occipital lobe and other lobes of the brain, especially the parietal and temporal lobes, general cognitive processes influence our visual perception.

VISUAL PATHWAYS: FROM THE RETINA TO THE OCCIPITAL CORTEX

The visual field is directly imaged on the retina by the optics of the eye; hence, the visual field topography translates into retinal topography (retinotopy), which is inverted due to the optical properties of the cornea and lens of the eye. Information from the retina leaves the eye through the optic nerve, which leads to the optical chiasm. Here, the fibers from the nasal side of the fovea in each eye cross over to the opposite side of the brain while the others remain on the same side. The result is that the mapping from external visual fields to the cortex is crossed. Visual information from the left half of the visual field (from both the right and the left eyes) goes to the right half of the brain (right hemisphere), whereas all the information from the right visual field goes to the left hemisphere. The vertical meridian representation of the two hemifields is joined via a large fiber system called the corpus callosum. From the optic chiasm there are two separate pathways that lead to the brain. The smaller one goes to the superior colliculus, a nucleus in the brainstem, which then projects to the thalamic pulvinar nucleus. The larger pathway goes through the lateral geniculate nucleus (LGN) of the thalamus and to the occipital cortex or primary visual cortex (V1).

MAPPING VISUAL AREAS: RETINOTOPY

Before the functions of the different areas are discussed, we first need to have an accurate map of the visual areas in the occipital lobe. Recently, our understanding of the functional organization of the human brain has greatly expanded due to the development of neuroimaging techniques [mainly functional magnetic resonance imaging (fMRI)] that allow direct noninvasive observation of patterns of brain activity in normal human subjects engaged in sensory, motor, or cognitive tasks. In particular, fMRI has been used to chart the retinotopic and functional organization of the visual cortex in the human brain. Visual field topography has been a primary source of information used to identify and map different visual areas in animals and humans. The mapping from the retina to the primary visual cortex is topographical in that nearby regions on the retina project to nearby regions in V1. In the cortex, neighboring positions in the visual field tend to be represented by groups of neurons that are adjacent to but laterally displaced within the cortical gray matter. This transformation preserves the qualitative spatial relations but distorts quantitative ones. Multiple horizontal and vertical meridian representations are arranged in approximately parallel bands along the cortical surface (Fig. 1, left). These vertical and horizontal meridian representations define the

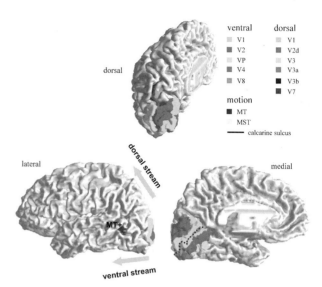

Figure 2
Retinotopic visual areas in the human visual cortex. These maps depict visual areas of a single subject obtained from fMRI scans performed at the Stanford University Imaging Center (courtesy of Brian Wandell and Alyssa Brewer).

borders between retinotopic regions. Perpendicular to these bands lie isoeccentricity bands (Fig. 1, right); however, the representation of the fovea is greatly expanded compared to that of the periphery. In humans, the foveal representation of low-level retinotopic regions converges in the occipital pole and as a person moves anteriorly, bands of mid- and peripheral eccentricity emerge.

In humans, V1 is located in the calcarine sulcus but can extend into the cuneus and lingual gyri (Fig. 2). The representation of the horizontal meridian is contained within the calcarine, such that the upper (dorsal) bank of the calcarine sulcus contains the lower visual field representation and the lower (ventral) bank contains the upper visual field representation. The border between V1 and V2d (dorsal) is marked by a lower field vertical meridian representation, and the border between V1 and V2v (ventral) is marked by an upper field vertical representation. V2d and V2v together provide a second complete representation of the visual field. In the dorsal part of the cuneus, the border between V2d and V3 is marked by another horizontal field representation. In a complementary fashion, in the ventral stream the border between V2v and VP is delineated by another horizontal meridian representation. Both V3 and VP contain a map of a quadrant of the visual field, and combined these areas provide a complete third hemifield representation. In dorsal

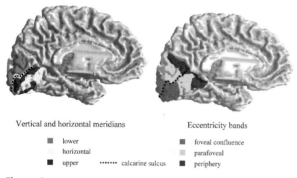

Figure 1
Retinotopic organization of the human visual cortex. Maps of the medial view of the occipital lobe of one subject obtained from fMRI scans performed at the Stanford Imaging Center. (Left) Vertical and horizontal visual meridians. These meridians can be used to define borders between retinotopic areas. (Right) Equal eccentricity bands in the human occipital lobe (courtesy of Brian Wandell and Alyssa Brewer).

visual cortex the border between V3 and V3a is marked by a lower visual field representation. V3a contains a complete hemifield representation, consisting of a lower horizontal and upper visual field representation. Anterior to V3a, an additional hemifield representation is mapped in V7. In ventral cortex the border between VP and V4v is defined by an upper vertical meridian. Researchers are currently debating the functional organization and naming conventions beyond V4v. Some have suggested that V4 consists of a complete hemifield representation comprising an upper horizontal and vertical representation, complementary to the representation in V3a in ventral cortex. Others have suggested an area beyond V4v, termed V8, that consists of an additional hemifield representation.

Beyond retinotopic cortex, the polar angle representation is cruder and the orderly representation of visual meridians is absent. However, the center/periphery organization extends into higher order visual areas. At the junction of the parietal, occipital, and temporal lobes is another visually responsive region that is strongly responsive to motion stimuli. This area is termed MT (Fig. 2), and adjacent to it are additional smaller motion responsive areas termed MST (Fig. 2).

Several other visually responsive areas have been identified in the occipital lobe and posterior temporal and parietal lobes. These include the kinetic occipital area (KO), which is responsive to motion boundaries, the lateral occipital complex (LOC), which is selective to objects, the fusiform face area (FFA), which is preferentially activated by faces, and the parahippocampal place area (PPA), which is activated by images of houses and scenes. Since these are higher level areas, the retinotopic representation in these regions is less preserved, and until recently these regions were defined based on their functional selectivity alone. However, the use of more sophisticated methods has revealed that a crude eccentricity organization extends even into higher order areas and correlates to the functional selectivity of these regions.

"WHAT" AND "WHERE" PROCESSING STREAMS IN THE HUMAN BRAIN

What does each area do? How do these regions subserve our visual perception and cognition? It has been suggested that these multiple visual areas are organized into two hierarchically functionally specialized processing pathways (Fig. 3): an occipito-

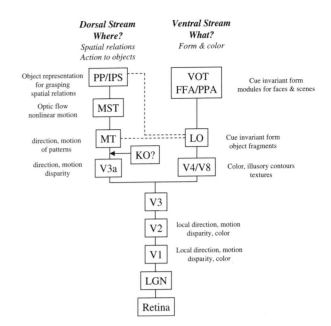

Figure 3
Schematic diagram of "what" and "where" processing streams in human visual cortex. Dashed lines indicate putative connections.

temporal pathway or ventral stream for object recognition and an occipitoparietal pathway or dorsal stream' for spatial vision and visually guided actions directed toward objects.

Areas along both the occipitotemporal and occipitoparietal pathways are organized hierarchically, such that low-level inputs are transformed into more useful representations through successive stages of processing. Virtually all visual-processing tasks activate V1 and V2. However, proceeding from one area to the next, the neuronal response properties become increasingly complex. Along the occipitotemporal pathway, for example, many V1 cells function as local spatiotemporal filters, responsive to oriented bars or to particular colors; in V2, cells may respond to illusory contours of figures; in V4, some cells respond only if a stimulus stands out from its background due to a difference in color or form; and in occipitotemporal regions, cells respond selectively to particular shapes. Similarly, proceeding from V1 to MT, new types of directional and motion selectivity emerge. For example, V1 is sensitive to the direction of motion of local components of a complex pattern, whereas MT is sensitive to the global motion of the same pattern.

Thus, much of the neural mechanism for both object vision and spatial vision can be viewed as "bottom-up" processes subserved by feedforward projections between successive pairs of areas within a pathway. However, anatomical studies have shown that each of these feedforward projections is reciprocated by a feedback projection. Projections from higher order processing stages to lower order ones may mediate "top-down" aspects of visual cognition, such as expectation, context, or attention, that affect our visual perception.

FUNCTIONAL SUBSYSTEMS

A further possible relation between anatomical structure and physiological maps is indicated by the hypothesis that there are separate neural pathways for processing information about different visual properties, such as motion, depth, color, and shape. Physiological and anatomical studies in the monkey brain indicate that this segregation of neural pathways begins in the retina, and different compartments within early visual areas project to different high-level areas. In the following sections, the processing that leads to the perception of motion, depth, color, and form in the human brain is discussed.

Motion

Objects in the world move relative to each other and to the viewer in a nearly ceaseless pattern of change. This activity provides a rich source of information about our environment. Motion processing encompasses different kinds of information, such as the derivation of the speed and direction of a moving target, the motion boundaries associated with an object, or the structure of an object determined from its coherent motion. Along the dorsal stream many regions are more active when subjects view moving vs stationary stimuli, including areas MT, MST, V3a, KO, parietal occipital cortex, and even low-level areas such as V1 and V2. Given the range of functions that motion processing subserves, this may not be surprising. Indeed, converging evidence suggests that some aspects of motion processing are localized in dedicated modules in the human brain.

The main motion-selective focus in the human brain is a region called MT+, located at the temporoparietiooccipital junction (Fig. 2). Human MT (Fig. 2) is selectively activated by moving vs stationary stimuli and exhibits high-contrast sensitivity. Comparison of coherent and incoherent motion of light points (in which dots move independently) reveals a significant change in activation within MT+ that increases linearly with the coherence of motion but reveals little change in early

visual areas, consistent with the idea of local processing of visual properties in early visual areas and global motion processing in later areas. Recently, several elegant studies have used the perceptual illusion of the motion aftereffect to show that human MT contains direction-selective neural populations. In addition, it has been shown that the activation of this area is enhanced when subjects attend to or tract motion. Thus, converging evidence from many labs shows that human MT+ response properties parallel both the response properties of single neurons and perception. This inference is further supported by clinical studies revealing that akinetopsia is associated with lesions in the vicinity of MT+.

In addition to MT+, other cortical sites such as V3a are activated by various types of coherent motion stimuli. Some regions (MST) seem to be correlated with the processing of optical flow information. Another specialized motion-related area, the KO area located posterior to MT, is involved in the processing of kinetic boundaries created by discontinuities in motion direction. KO is activated more strongly by kinetic gratings than by luminance-defined gratings, uniform motion, and transparent motion.

Another intriguing aspect of motion cue is related to the perception of biological motion or the motion of people and animals. Humans can perceive biological motion from impoverished visual displays in which points of light are attached to joints of a person moving in an otherwise dark room. From these sparse displays, people can discriminate the type of motion (running, dancing, etc.) as well as the sex of the mover. An area in a small region on the ventral bank of the occipital extent of the superior temporal sulcus, located lateral and anterior to human MT/MST, is selectively activated during viewing of point-light moving figures but not by the random movement or inverted motion of the same lights that comprised the point-light figures or by other biological motions such as hand, eye, or mouth movement.

Depth

Compared to the work that has been performed on motion and form processing, there are fewer studies concerning the processing of depth, surfaces, and three-dimensional (3D) structure. Like the processing of visual motion, the analysis of depth can involve both low-level cues, such as disparity, derived from the retinal images and high-level inferred attributes, such as the surfaces corresponding to retinal points with different disparities. In humans, experiments using random dot stereograms have shown a stream of areas that respond to these 3D stimuli: V1–V3, VP, V3a, and MT+. Of these, V3a appears to be the region most sensitive to changes in the disparity range, although all regions activated by random dot stereograms show a correlation between the amplitude of the fMRI signal and disparity. In contrast, other high-level areas, such as LOC, respond to random dot stereograms only when these stimuli include object-form, but these regions do not seem to be sensitive to the exact disparity values.

Color

The primate retina contains three classes of cones—the L, M, and S cones—that respond preferentially to long-, middle-, and short-wavelength visible light, respectively. Color appearance results from neural processing of these cone signals within the retina and the brain. Perceptual experiments have identified three types of neural pathways that represent color: a red–green pathway that signals differences between L and M cone responses, a blue–yellow pathway that signals differences between S cone responses and a sum of L and M cone responses, and a luminance pathway that signals a sum of L and M cone responses. Two main hypotheses have been proposed that link neural activity and color. One emphasizes regions in cortex that may play a special role in color perception, and the second emphasizes a stream of color processing stages beginning in the retina and extending into the cortex.

Human neuropsychological studies suggest that damage to a cortical region on the ventral surface of the occipital lobe, in the collateral sulcus, interferes with normal color processing. Recently, researchers used fMRI to measure color-related activity in the human brain. They measured the difference in activity caused by achromatic and colored stimuli. The area showing a significant change of activity was located in the collateral sulcus and is the same area implicated in achromatopsia. However, the retinotopic organization of this region is debated. Although the area associated with color signal tends to correspond with the foveal representation, some researchers refer to the area as V4, whereas others suggest the color-responsive area is beyond V4 and that it should be called V8.

Other results from several laboratories show that opponent color signals can be measured in a sequence of visual areas, including early visual areas. For example, for certain stimuli, the most powerful responses in area V1 are caused by lights that excite opponent color mechanisms. Measurements with contrast-reversing lights and simple rectangular patterns reveal powerful color opponent signals along the pathway from V1 to V2 and V4/V8. Moreover, moving stimuli, seen only by opponent color mechanisms, evoke powerful activations in motion-selective areas located in the lateral portion of the parietooccipital sulcus. Further research should reveal the processing stages and mechanism underlying color perception.

Form Perception and Object Recognition

The LOC, a cortical region located on the posterior aspect of the fusiform gyrus and extending ventrally and dorsally, responds more strongly when people view pictures of either common objects or unfamiliar 3D objects compared to when they view visual textures without obvious shape interpretations. Moreover, studies using event-related potentials recorded from electrodes placed directly on the cortical surface of patients before surgery found object-specific waveforms that show stronger activation for a variety of objects (e.g., cars, flowers, hands, butterflies, and letters) than for scrambled control stimuli. The location of these sites includes the LOC.

The LOC is largely nonretinotopic and is activated by both the contralateral and ipsilateral visual fields. It contains at least two spatially segregated subdivisions, a dorsal caudal subdivision LO (Fig. 4, lateral view) and a ventral occipital–temporal subdivision VOT (Fig. 4, ventral view). The LO is situated posterior to MT in the lateral occipital sulcus and extends into the posterior inferior temporal sulcus. The anterior ventral part of the LOC is located bilaterally in the fusiform gyrus and occipitotemporal sulcus. Each of these subdivisions contains a separate foveal representation. The fovea of LO is connected to the confluence of fovea of early visual areas, whereas the VOT contains a separate foveal representation located on the lateral bank of the collateral sulcus and extending into the fusiform gyrus. In ventral cortex there is a consistent relationship between eccentricity maps and object selectivity. Regions that are selective to faces overlap with the representation of the fovea, whereas regions that are selective to houses overlap a peripheral visual representation located in the collateral sulcus (Fig. 5). These experiments suggest that the entire object-selective region may be organized along an eccentricity axis that could be relevant to the way in which humans perceive different object categories.

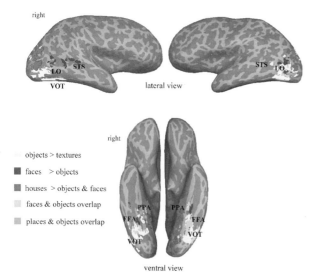

Figure 4
Object-selective regions in the human ventral processing stream. Object-, face-, and place-selective regions are depicted on the inflated brain of one subject. The brain was inflated using specialized software to enable visualization of regions buried inside sulci. Sulci are shaded dark gray and gyri lighter gray. LO, lateral occipital; VOT, ventral occipito-temporal and occipitotemporal sulcus; FFA, fusiform face area; PPA, parahippocampal place area; STS, superior temporal sulcus (experiments were conducted by Kalanit Grill-Spector and Nancy Kanwisher at the MGH imaging center, Charlestown, MA).

Any useful object-recognition system should be relatively insensitive to the precise physical cues that define an object (namely, cue invariance) and also be relatively invariant to the viewing conditions that affect the object's appearance but not its identity. That is, a good recognition system should have perceptual constancy. Indeed, recent studies reveal that the LOC is involved in the representation of shapes rather than the physical properties or local features in the visual stimulus. The LOC responded more strongly when subjects viewed objects defined by either luminance, texture, or motion cues rather than to control stimuli consisting of textures, stationary dot patterns, or coherently moving dots. The same regions were also selectively activated when subjects perceived simple shapes that were created via illusory contours, color contrast, stereo cues, texture boundaries, grayscale photographs of objects, or line drawings. Together, these results demonstrate convergence of a wide range of un-related visual cues that convey information about object shape within the same cortical regions, providing strong evidence for the role of the LOC in processing object shape.

Intriguingly, recent evidence suggests that some regions within the LOC might exhibit not only cue invariance but also modality invariance. In the vicinity of LO, and partially overlapping it, is a region activated more strongly when subjects touch objects but not when they touch textures. Thus, these regions may constitute a neural substrate for the convergence of multimodal object representations.

Although the LOC is activated strongly when subjects view pictures of objects, this does not by itself prove that it is the locus in the brain that performs object recognition. However, evidence from lesion studies demonstrates that damage to the fusiform and occipitotemporal junction results in a variety of recognition deficits. Also, studies in humans have shown that electric stimulation of similar regions interferes with recognition processes or, in some cases, can create an illusory percept of an object or a face. Recent fMRI experiments provide evidence that the activation of ventral occipital cortical regions is correlated to subjects' perception of objects, faces, and houses in a variety of experimental paradigms and tasks. Together, these findings suggest that these regions may be necessary (and perhaps even sufficient) for object recognition.

Within ventral occipitotemporal regions, several areas have been suggested as modules for representing and perceiving specific object categories, such as faces (FFA) and places (PPA) (Fig. 4). One of the most

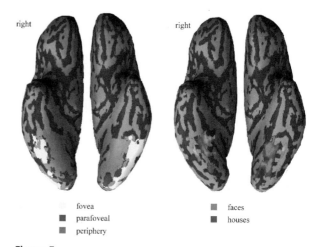

Figure 5
The relation of face and place areas to eccentricity bands. (Left) Eccentricity bands on the ventral view of an inflated brain. (Right) Face and place areas in the same subject. Note that the face area overlaps with foveal representations and the place area overlaps with peripheral representations (maps courtesy of Rafael Malach and Ifat Levy, Weizmann Institute of Science, Israel).

extensively studied areas in recent years is the FFA. The FFA responds much more strongly to a wide variety of face stimuli (e.g., front-view photographs of faces, line drawings of faces, cat faces, cartoon faces, and upside-down faces) than to various non-face control stimuli (e.g., cars, scrambled faces, houses, and hands). Other face-selective regions can be found in a more posterior occipital region partially overlapping LO and in a region near the posterior end of the superior temporal sulcus. The PPA, another category-selective region of cortex, responds strongly to a wide variety of stimuli depicting places and/or scenes (e.g., outdoor and indoor scenes and houses) compared to various nonplace control stimuli (e.g., faces or scrambled scenes). The following question arises: How many category-selective regions of cortex exist in the human visual pathway? Selectively activated focal regions of cortex were reported for other categories as well, including animals, tools, letter strings, and even body parts.

Although the basic response properties of the FFA and the PPA are generally agreed upon, what they indicate about the function of these regions is considerably less clear. Some researchers argue that the FFA and the PPA are cortical modules specialized for the recognition of particular object classes that are important in our everyday lives. Thus, the FFA is primarily involved in face recognition and the PPA is involved in scene perception. However, an important unresolved question concerns the functional significance of the responses in these regions to "non-preferred" stimuli, which have less significance than the optimal object class but clearly do have significance. The critical question is whether these lower responses reflect a critical involvement of these stimuli in the representation or recognition of other objects. One possibility is that each object is represented as the entire pattern of activity across all of these regions (LOC, FFA, and PPA), and that it is the distributed representation that forms the basis of object recognition. Another (nonexclusive) possibility, which I favor, is that the FFA, PPA, and LOC are in fact part of the same functional region, which is composed of a set of category-selective and/or feature-selective columns at such a fine scale that they cannot be resolved with fMRI, except for a few very large regions such as the FFA or PPA. Indeed, recent experiments support the idea that the PPA, FFA, and pFs may be part of the same functional area since there is a continuous mapping of eccentricity bands across all these regions. What is the basis of the functional organization in the ventral processing stream? Is it innate or learned? Is it dependent on the recognition task? Is it based on visual similarity? Future experiments will explore these alternatives.

CONCLUSIONS

Several general organization principles can be extracted from the data summarized in this entry. First, the occipital lobe is composed of a number of distinct visual areas. Second, several of these stages contain a retinotopic representation of the visual field. However, ascending through the processing stages the retinotopic mapping becomes coarser, whereas the functional properties of these areas become more complex. Third, all visual tasks activate an extended network of visual areas, including V1/V2. This is consistent with the idea that processing of visual information requires both local processing in lower visual areas and more complex operations extracting global attributes in high-level stages. Fourth, there is a general tendency of motion and depth processing to activate the dorsal processing stream extending into parietal and mid-temporal cortex, whereas color and form processing tend to activate the ventral processing stream, extending to ventral occipitotemporal areas. Finally, some specific cortical sites are preferentially activated by specific visual attributes (color, V4/V8; motion, MT +) or specific classes of stimuli and tasks (object recognition, LOC; faces, FFA).

Despite the rapid increase of our understanding of human visual areas in recent years, a question that remains largely unanswered is whether our subjective perceptual visual experience is a consequence of activity in the occipital lobe or whether the occipital lobe only extracts information about the visual world, which is then passed on to other brain areas that mediate awareness. Recent data suggest that there is a correlation between the activity in high-level areas in the occipital lobe and our awareness of the visual world. However, the available evidence is not sufficiently conclusive to determine whether the conscious experience relies exclusively on the occipital lobe or whether the occipital lobe is merely a part of a larger neural circuit that mediates visual awareness.

—*Kalanit Grill-Spector*

See also–Brain Anatomy; Cerebral Cortex; Motion and Spatial Perception; Perception and Perceptual Disorders; Retina; Vision, Color and Form; Visual Fields; Visual System, Central

Further Reading

Farah, M. J. (1990). *Visual Agnosia: Disorders of Object Recognition and What They Tell Us about Normal Vision.* MIT Press/Bradford Books, Cambridge, MA.

Grill-Spector, K., Kourtzi, Z., and Kanwisher, N. (2001). The lateral occipital complex and its role in object recognition. *Vision Res.* **41**, 1409–1422.

Kanwisher, N., Downing, P., Epstein, R., *et al.* (2000). Functional neuroimaging in visual recognition. In *The Handbook on Functional Neuroimaging* (R. Cabeza and A. Kingstone, Eds.). Cambridge Univ. Press, Cambridge, UK.

Mishkin, M., Ungerleider, L. G., and Macko, K. A. (1983). Object vision and spatial vision: Two cortical pathways. *Trends Neurosci.* **6**, 414–417.

Wandell, B. (1999). Computational neuroimaging: Color representations and processing. In *Cognitive Neuroscience* (M. Gazzaniga, Ed.). MIT Press, Cambridge, MA.

Zeki, S. (1995). *A Vision of the Brain.* Blackwell, Oxford, UK.

Occult Spinal Dysraphism
see Neural Tube Defects

Oculomotor Nerve (Cranial Nerve III)

Encyclopedia of the Neurological Sciences
Copyright 2003, Elsevier Science (USA). All rights reserved.

THE OCULOMOTOR or third nerve nuclear complex lies in the upper midbrain at the level of the superior colliculus, anterior to the sylvian aqueduct and periaqueductal gray (Fig. 1). Five extraocular muscles are innervated by the third nerve: the levator palpebrae superioris; the superior, inferior, and medial rectus; and the inferior oblique. It also supplies presynaptic parasympathetic input to the ciliary ganglion for pupillary constriction and accommodation. The oculomotor nuclear complex can be subdivided into multiple subnuclear regions. The medial rectus, inferior rectus, and inferior oblique subnuclei send efferent directives to the ipsilateral extraocular muscles, whereas the superior rectus subnuclei send efferent directives contralaterally through the opposite oculomotor nuclear complex to supply the contralateral superior rectus muscle (Fig. 2). The levator palpebrae superioris muscles are innervated by a single structure in the posterior superior aspect of the oculomotor nuclear complex and are both crossed and uncrossed. The

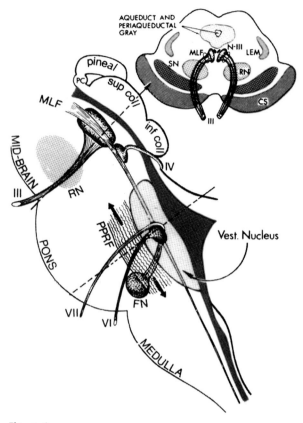

Figure 1
Diagrammatic axial and sagittal sections of the brainstem through the third nerve. N-III, oculomotor nucleus; MLF, medial longitudinal fasciculus; LEM, medial lemniscus; RN, red nucleus; SN, substantia nigra; CS, corticospinal tract; sup coll, superior colliculus [modified from Glaser, J. S. (Ed.) (1990). *Neuro-ophthalmology*, 2nd ed., p. 363. Lippincott, Philadelphia].

Edinger–Westphal nucleus lies in the anterior superior aspect of the oculomotor nuclear complex and supplies the parasympathetic innervation for the pupil (Fig. 2). The oculomotor efferent fibers pass through the red nucleus, substantia nigra, and cerebellar peduncles to enter the interpeduncular space anterior to the midbrain (Fig. 1). The paired oculomotor nerves pass inferior to the posterior cerebral artery and superior to the superior cerebellar artery before entering the posterior aspect of the cavernous sinus near the free edge of the cerebellar tentorium. Pupillomotor fibers lie in the dorsal medial aspect of the oculomotor nerve in its subarachnoid course. At the level of the anterior cavernous sinus or superior orbital fissure, the oculomotor nerve divides into a superior and inferior division before passing through the annulus of Zinn to enter the orbit. The superior division supplies the levator palpebrae superioris and the superior rectus;

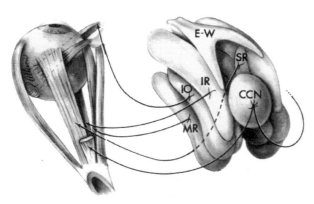

Figure 2
Oculomotor nuclear complex viewed from above, left posterior. E–W, Edinger–Westphal parasympathetic subnucleus; IR, inferior rectus; IO, inferior oblique; MR, medial rectus; SR, superior rectus; CCN, caudal nucleus to levator superioris [modified with permission from Glaser, J. S. (Ed.) (1990). *Neuro-ophthalmology*, 2nd ed., p. 363. Lippincott, Philadelphia].

the inferior division carries efferent directives to the medial rectus, inferior rectus, inferior oblique, and the presynaptic parasympathetic fibers to the ciliary ganglion (Fig. 2).

OCULOMOTOR NERVE PALSY: CLINICAL FEATURES

The oculomotor nerve may be disrupted at any point in its anatomical course: at the nucleus, within the midbrain, in the interpeduncular space, as it enters the cavernous sinus near the junction of the internal carotid artery and posterior communicating artery, in the cavernous sinus, at the level of the superior orbital fissure, and in the orbit. The precise location of the offending lesion can frequently be identified by documenting abnormalities in surrounding structures.

A complete isolated third nerve palsy will result in ipsilateral ptosis (a droopy lid) and an inability to elevate, depress, and adduct the eye (turn the eye in toward the nose), and the pupil will be fixed and dilated. If the lid is lifted, the eye will be seen to be "down and out." Incomplete oculomotor nerve palsies are extremely common and it is important to note whether or not the pupil is involved.

COMMON CAUSES OF ISOLATED OCULOMOTOR NERVE PALSY

Intracranial Aneurysm

A supraclinoid aneurysm at the junction of the internal carotid and posterior communicating artery is the most common cause of an isolated third nerve palsy if the pupil is dilated and fixed to a bright light. Twenty-seven percent of all intracranial aneurysms lie at the junction of the internal carotid and posterior communicating artery; 50% of these will develop a third nerve paresis. Retroorbital pain can precede the third nerve paresis by up to 2 weeks. High-resolution magnetic resonance imaging, magnetic resonance angiogram (MRA), or cerebral angiogram are mandatory; MRA may totally miss a small aneurysm and a transfemoral angiogram may be required. Rarely, an internal carotid posterior communicating artery aneurysm may present without pupillary involvement or subarachnoid hemorrhage; however, pupillary dysfunction will typically manifest within 7 days.

Vascular Oculomotor Nerve Paresis

Vascular disease, including hypertension and diabetes mellitus, is a very common cause for an isolated third nerve paresis without pupil involvement. Oculomotor nerve infarction secondary to vascular disease has been documented in the subarachnoid space, cavernous sinus, and midbrain. Eye pain may precede the onset of the third nerve paresis for up to 2 weeks prior to the onset of diplopia. Oculomotor paresis is not dependent on the degree of diabetic or hypertension control and commonly disappears within weeks to months. If objective signs of resolution are not apparent at 3 months, other etiologies must be considered.

Other Causes of Oculomotor Nerve Paresis

Tumor/Trauma: The most common tumor to present with an isolated third nerve paresis is a pituitary adenoma with lateral extension; parasellar tumors (e.g., craniopharyngioma and meningioma) and metastatic lesions have been reported to cause an isolated third nerve paresis with and without pupillary involvement. Pupil-sparing oculomotor (third) nerve palsies may be secondary to selective compression of the inferior portion of the oculomotor nerve without involvement of the dorsally placed pupillary nerve fibers, or the small pupillomotor fibers may be relatively spared due to slow tumor growth and chronic oculomotor nerve compression. When minimal trauma results in a third nerve palsy, with or without pupillary involvement, a parasellar mass (e.g., cavernous sinus meningioma) should be a consideration. The third nerve may be traumatically avulsed where it emerges from the brainstem or where it attaches to the dura as it enters the cavernous sinus.

Uncommon Causes: Less common causes for oculomotor dysfunction include brainstem infarction, carotid cavernous fistula, cavernous sinus thrombosis, cavernous sinus aneurysm, chemotherapy, collagen vascular disorders, dental anesthesia, heavy particle radiation, herpes zoster, internal carotid artery dissection, lymphoma, meningitis, migraine, monoclonal gammopathy, mucocele, multiple myeloma, nasopharyngeal carcinoma, neurosurgical procedures, oculomotor nerve tumor, pituitary apoplexy, pseudotumor cerebri, subdural hematoma, syphilis, temporal arteritis, and the Tolosa–Hunt syndrome.

Childhood: The differential diagnosis of an isolated third nerve paresis in childhood is different from that of adults and includes congenital disorders, trauma, ocular migraine, and inflammation. Aneurysm and vascular disease are uncommon diagnostic considerations.

—Thomas J. Carlow

See also–Abducens Nerve (Cranial Nerve VI); Accessory Nerve (Cranial Nerve XI); Facial Nerve (Cranial Nerve VII); Glossopharyngeal Nerve (Cranial Nerve IX); Hypoglossal Nerve (Cranial Nerve XII); Olfactory Nerve (Cranial Nerve I); Optic Nerve (Cranial Nerve II); Ptosis; Trigeminal Nerve (Cranial Nerve V); Trochlear Nerve (Cranial Nerve IV); Vagus Nerve (Cranial Nerve X); Vestibulocochlear Nerve (Cranial Nerve VIII)

Further Reading

Glaser, J. S., and Bachynski, B. (1990). Infranuclear disorders of eye movement. In *Neuro-ophthalmology* (J. S. Glaser, Ed.), 2nd ed., pp. 372–382. Lippincott, Philadelphia.

Lee, J. R., and Zee, D. S. (1999). *The Neurology of Eye Movements*, 3rd ed., pp. 361–368. Oxford Univ. Press, New York.

Miller, N. R. (1985). Topical diagnosis of neuropathic ocular motility disorders. In *Walsh and Hoyt's Clinical Neuro-ophthalmology* (N. R. Miller, Ed.), 4th ed., pp. 652–784. Williams & Wilkins, Baltimore.

Oculopharyngeal Muscular Dystrophy

Encyclopedia of the Neurological Sciences
Copyright 2003, Elsevier Science (USA). All rights reserved.

OCULOPHARYNGEAL muscular dystrophy (OPMD) is a late-onset, generally autosomal dominant, myopathy characterized by eyelid ptosis and dysphagia.

HISTORY

The first description of what is today called OPMD was made in 1915 by Taylor in a French Canadian family; he supposed a neuropathic pathogenesis, hence the name progressive vagus–glossopharyngeal paralysis with ptosis. In 1962, Victor *et al.* established the myopathic nature of the disease, its autosomal dominant inheritance, and coined its actual name. In the following decade, Barbeau described the large French Canadian cluster and suggested the existence of a founder effect in this population.

In 1980, Fernando Tome and Michel Fardeau identified on electron microscopy typical intranuclear inclusions (INIs) that became the morphological marker of OPMD. In 1990, we reported the existence of a second large cluster among the Jews originating from the Bukhara and Samarkand areas in Uzbekistan; the calculated prevalence of 1:700 in this population is probably the highest in the world.

In 1995, Bernard Brais and colleagues from the team led by Guy A. Rouleau demonstrated linkage of OPMD to chromosome 14q11 in three French Canadian families. This localization has subsequently been confirmed for other populations. In 1998, the same team from Montreal showed that short expansions of a $(GCG)_6$ repeat encoding for polyalanine, within the polyadenylation-binding protein 2 (*PABP2*) gene on 14q, are responsible worldwide for autosomal dominant OPMD. This finding of a new category of trinucleotide repeat diseases opened the era of molecular genetic studies among OPMD patients.

PREVALENCE

OPMD is found worldwide but is uncommon; there are, however, clusters with very high prevalence among French Canadians (1:1000), Bukhara Jews (1:700), and possibly Spanish Americans (in Colorado, New Mexico, and Arizona) as well as residents of the Montevideo area in Uruguay. In these populations there is evidence for founder effects.

GENETICS AND PATHOGENESIS

OPMD is produced by short expansions of a GCG repeat, encoding for polyalanine and located in the first exon of the *PABP2* gene on chromosome 14q11. Normally, there are six GCG repeats; seven repeats were found in Quebec among 2% of the population and in Japan among 1.1%, giving the $(GCG)_6$–$(GCG)_7$ genotype; whether this should be called polymorphism or recessive mutation is still debated since only one $(GCG)_7$–$(GCG)_7$ homozygote with mild OPMD features has been reported. $(GCG)_{8-13}$ expansions have been found in many different populations and in all the patients fulfilling the clinical and histological criteria for the diagnosis of OPMD.

$(GCG)_9$, which is the most common mutation, has been found in all three clusters with evidence for a founder effect. Its penetrance for heterozygotes is 1% before the age of 40, 6% before the age of 49, and 31% before the age of 59, and it reaches 100% at the age of 70.

In addition to heterozygotes $[(GCG)_6$–$(GCG)_9]$, homozygotes $[(GCG)_9$–$(GCG)_9]$ have been identified among French Canadians and Bukhara Jews and compound heterozygotes $[(GCG)_7$–$(GCG)_9]$ have been identified among the former.

OPMD is the first of a new kind of disease produced by triplet repeat expansions: The expansions are short and meiotically and mitotically stable, and the encoded peptide is an enlarged polyalanine domain rather than polyglutamate. It was suggested that PABP2, which is a strictly nuclear protein, acts as a carrier, introducing the enlarged polyalanine domains into the nuclei, which are subsequently damaged through a "toxic gain of function." This hypothesis was supported by the finding of PABP2 with enlarged polyalanine chains within INIs.

The cause of selective involvement of the levator palpebrae superioris and pharyngeal muscles in OPMD is unknown; it may be due to enhanced expression of the *PABP2* gene in these muscles.

HISTOPATHOLOGY

Because OPMD is a generalized muscle disease, most biopsies have been done from limb muscles (mainly deltoid and quadriceps), although the changes in extraocular and pharyngeal muscles may be more severe.

In addition to nonspecific myopathic changes, histochemical studies reveal small, angulated, mainly type 1 fibers and "rimmed vacuoles"; the latter are suggestive but not specific for OPMD and may also be found in inclusion body myositis (IBM).

The morphological hallmark of OPMD was described in 1980 by Tome and Fardeau using electron microscopy; it consists of INIs with an outer diameter of 8.5 nm, an inner diameter of 3 nm, and

up to 0.25 μm in length. They are strictly muscular and nuclear, occupy a clear area surrounded by chromatin, and are often disposed in tangles or palisades. The INIs of OPMD are different from the larger, cytoplasmic, and nuclear tubulofilamentous inclusions found in IBM. In skeletal muscles from heterozygotes, INIs are found in approximately 4.5% of nuclei; among homozygotes they are found in approximately 9.5% of nuclei and occupy a larger nuclear area. INIs have also been found in the biopsy of a patient with recessive $[(GCG)_7$–$(GCG)_7]$ OPMD. Recently, it was reported that INIs reacted with an antiserum raised against a synthetic PABP2 peptide fragment.

CLINICAL MANIFESTATIONS

Among heterozygotes $[(GCG)_6$–$(GCG)_{8-13}]$, the disease begins either with eyelid ptosis or dysphagia during the fifth or sixth decade. Dysphonia, correlated in severity with dysphagia, is also often an early sign. As a rule, ptosis affects all patients and is bilateral, although at the beginning some asymmetry may be noticed. To compensate the relentlessly progressive inability to open the eyes, patients contract frontal muscles, tilt their heads backward (the astrologist's posture), or use glasses with props. Due to early dysphagia, the patient is often the last to finish a meal; cold water swallowing time is prolonged beyond 7 sec for 80 cc as described by Bouchard. Severe dysphagia eventually leads to choking, recurrent aspiration pneumonia, and cachexia. After years of disease progression, some limitation of ocular movements may develop; it is usually mild and heterozygote patients rarely report diplopia. Weakness of facial muscles, especially orbicularis oculi, and proximal limb muscles are also late features. The advanced patient often looks terminally ill: emaciated, dysphonic, and dysphagic, with thin, dropping eyelids. However, most heterozygotes have normal life spans. There is no cardiac involvement.

Unusually severe OPMD phenotypes are found among homozygotes, compound heterozygotes, and possibly patients with the longer GCG expansions $[(GCG)_{11-13}]$. Among 10 $(GCG)_9$–$(GCG)_9$ homozygotes studied by Tome and Fardeau, OPMD began on average 20 years earlier (during the second or third decades), some patients had significant external ophthalmoparesis and marked muscle weakness, and 2 of them died of aspiration pneumonia before the age of 55.

Unusually mild OPMD has been reported in a recessive [(GCG)$_7$–(GCG)$_7$] patient, which may explain why this phenotype was not previously recognized despite a calculated prevalence of 1:10000 in Quebec.

Atypical OPMD syndromes have been described. Their common denominator is the lack of specific histological features for either OPMD or mitochondrial myopathies.

In addition to typical OPMD, an oculopharyngo-distal myopathy has been described in Japanese patients. It begins with ptosis and diplopia, progressing to complete extraocular palsy; there is severe facial involvement and the weakness is mainly distal. Two patients had bilateral optic atrophy, whereas two others had cardiomyopathy.

Myopathies with ocular and pharyngeal involvement beginning in childhood were described in two girls of French Canadian and African ancestry. Neither rimmed vacuoles nor typical INIs were found on muscle biopsies.

A probably autosomal recessive adolescent-onset oculopharyngeal somatic syndrome was described in two Greek siblings; they also had facial weakness, sternomastiod wasting, and respiratory failure requiring intermittent ventilator support. Muscle biopsy revealed vacuolar myopathy and in one patient atypical cytoplasmic and nuclear tubulofilamentous inclusions.

DIFFERENTIAL DIAGNOSIS

The main differential diagnosis is with myasthenia gravis, myotonic dystrophy, and mitochondrial myopathies. Myasthenia is sporadic, clinically fluctuative, and asymmetrical; diplopia may be an early complaint. Electrophysiological and immunological tests may confirm the diagnosis.

Myotonic dystrophy is also autosomal dominant but often manifests earlier, the muscular weakness is typically distal, and systemic features such as cataracts, frontal baldness, and cardiac arrhythmias or cardiomyopathy are present. Clinical and electrical myotonia help the diagnosis.

Most mitochondrial myopathies are sporadic and begin in childhood or adolescence, and external ophthalmoparesis may be an early feature. Short stature, pigmentary retinopathy, deafness, seizures, and cardiac conduction defects may be present; therefore, the name oculocraniosomatic syndrome was suggested for these conditions. Increased blood lactate and significant ragged red fibers on muscle biopsy confirm the diagnosis. Until recently, OPMD and mitochondrial myopathies were often classified together under the entity ophthalmoplegia plus. Since their inheritance and muscle histology are different and since extraocular muscle weakness is not a main feature of OPMD, this name is not justified.

DIAGNOSIS

The definite diagnosis of OPMD is made by finding either typical INIs on muscle biopsy or GCG expansions with the polymerase chain reaction. The genetic test is already available in Canada, Israel, and other countries.

TREATMENT

Until the future advent of genetic therapy, the treatment will remain palliative. Ptosis may be alleviated by using glasses with props; its surgical correction is done either by resection of the aponeurosis of levator palpebrae or by frontal suspension of the lids.

In early stages, when dysphagia is mainly for solid food, swallowing may be improved by changes in food consistency. When it becomes severe, crycopharyngeal myotomy will provide temporary relief.

—*Sergiu C. Blumen and Amos D. Korczyn*

***See also*–Muscular Dystrophy: Emery–Dreifuss, Facioscapulohumeral, Scapuloperoneal, and Bethlem Myopathy; Muscular Dystrophy: Limb–Girdle, Becker, and Duchenne; Myasthenia Gravis; Myotonic Dystrophy; Neuromuscular Disorders, Overview; Ptosis**

Further Reading

Arahata, K., Goto, K., and Uyama, E. (1998). Expanded *PABP2* gene product from intranuclear aggregates in oculopharyngeal muscular dystrophy. In *Proceedings of the Symposium in Honor of FMS Tome; Filaments and Myopathies, Paris*, pp. 30–31.

Blumen, S. C., Sadeh, M., Korczyn, A. D., *et al.* (1996). Intranuclear inclusions in oculopharyngeal muscular dystrophy among Bukhara Jews. *Neurology* **46**, 1324–1328.

Blumen, S. C., Nisipeanu, P., Sadeh, M., *et al.* (1997). Epidemiology and inheritance of oculopharyngeal muscular dystrophy in Israel. *Neuromusc. Disorders* **7**, S38–S40.

Blumen, S. C., Brais, B., Korczyn, A. D., *et al.* (1999). Homozygotes for oculopharyngeal muscular dystrophy have a severe form of the disease. *Ann. Neurol.* **46**, 115–118.

Bouchard, J. P., Gagne, F., Tome, F. M. S., *et al.* (1989). Nuclear inclusions in oculopharyngeal muscular dystrophy in Quebec. *Can. J. Neurol. Sci.* **16,** 446–450.

Brais, B., Xie, Y. G., Sanson, M., *et al.* (1995). The oculopharyngeal muscular dystrophy locus maps to the region of the cardiac α and β myosin heavy chain genes on chromosome 14q11.2–q13. *Hum. Mol. Genet.* **4,** 429–434.

Brais, B., Buchard, J. P., Xie, Y. G., *et al.* (1998). Short GCG expansions in the PABP2 gene cause oculopharyngeal muscular dystrophy. *Nat. Genet.* **18,** 164–167.

Brais, B., Rouleau, G. A., Bouchard, J. P., *et al.* (1999). Oculopharyngeal muscular dystrophy. *Semin. Neurol.* **19,** 59–66.

Drachman, D. A. (1968). Ophthalmoplegia plus: The neurodegenerative disorders associated with progressive external ophthalmoplegia. *Arch. Neurol.* **18,** 654.

Duranceau, A. (1997). Cricopharyngeal myotomy in the management of neurogenic and muscular dysphagia. *Neuromusc. Disorders* **7,** S85–S89.

Grewal, R. P., Jayaprakash, D., Karkera, D., *et al.* (1999). Mutation analysis of oculopharyngeal muscular dystrophy in Hispanic American families. *Arch. Neurol.* **56,** 1378–1381.

Olson, W., Engel, W. K., Walsh, G. O., *et al.* (1972). Oculocraniosomatic neuromuscular disease with "ragged-red" fibers: Histochemical and ultrastructural changes in limb muscles of a group of patients with idiopathic progressive external ophthalmoplegia. *Arch. Neurol.* **26,** 193.

Tome, F. M. S., and Fardeau, M. (1980). Nuclear inclusions in oculopharyngeal muscular dystrophy. *Acta Neuropathol.* **49,** 85–87.

Tome, F. M. S., and Fardeau, M. (1994). Oculopharyngeal muscular dystrophy. In *Myology* (A. G. Engel and C. Franzini-Armstrong, Eds.), 2nd ed., pp. 1233–1245. McGraw-Hill, New York.

Victor, M., Hayes, R., and Adams, R. D. (1962). Oculopharyngeal muscular dystrophy, a familial disease of late life characterized by dysphagia and progressive ptosis of the eyelids. *N. Engl. J. Med.* **267,** 1267–1272.

Olfaction
see Smell

Olfactory Nerve (Cranial Nerve I)

Encyclopedia of the Neurological Sciences
Copyright 2003, Elsevier Science (USA). All rights reserved.

ALL ANIMALS, from simple single-cell organisms to complex vertebrates, detect and react to chemicals/odors in their external environment, some at concentrations of only a few parts per million. These environmental odors are generally complex mixtures of individual chemicals/odorants; for example, coffee may contain as many as 1000 separate chemicals/odorants. Therefore, the olfactory system must be capable of detecting and identifying diverse odorant mixtures. Only the immune system surpasses the olfactory system in the ability to recognize a diverse array of molecules. Olfaction in higher animals is used for detection of food, identification of predators, kinship recognition, and mate selection. In fact, some mammals experience severe reproductive disadvantage if their olfactory system is compromised. In recent years, there has been considerable advances in our understanding of the molecular, anatomical, and neurophysiological mechanisms underlying function in the olfactory system.

CLINICAL IMPORTANCE

Deficiency in the sense of smell is a clinical condition that affects millions of individuals throughout the world. A loss or alteration in the perception of odors can have a serious impact on quality of life. Olfactory deficiencies can be classified as anosmia, the inability to detect all or specific odors; hyposmia, a general or specific decreased sensitivity to odors; or hyperosmia, a heightened sensitivity to general or specific odors. The most common form of olfactory deficit is hyposmia associated with aging, which afflicts millions of individuals older than 60 years of age. However, hyposmia and anosmia are also common following rapid high-velocity torsion of the head (e.g., whiplash in motor vehicle accidents) and in toxic injury to respiratory pathways. Hyperosmia and many forms of anosmia are usually associated with genetic deficits affecting a small number of individuals. Given the widespread prevalence of some form of olfactory deficit in the population, and the resulting impact of quality of life, it is important to understand how olfaction works in order to improve clinical treatments for olfactory dysfunction.

FROM MOLECULES TO RECEPTORS

Odorant molecules are detected by olfactory receptor neurons (ORNs), which are specialized sensory neurons located in a neuroepithelial sheet lining the caudal nasal cavity (Figs. 1A and 1B). Processes from these sensory neurons extend to the surface of the epithelium and end in six to eight sensory cilia that

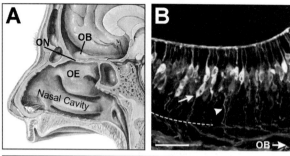

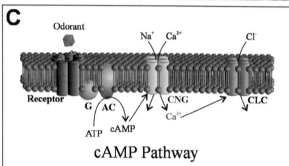

cAMP Pathway

Figure 1

(A) The lateral view of the human nasal region showing the olfactory epithelium (OE) lining the caudal nasal cavity and part of the brain. Axons from sensory neurons in the OE project through the cribriform plate forming the olfactory nerve (ON) and then terminate in the olfactory bulb (OB) [modified with permission from *Grant's Anatomy MEDICLIP Collection*, image HNC08021. Williams & Wilkins, Baltimore, 1999]. (B) High-power micrograph of a section of rodent OE stained for the olfactory marker protein, a robust label of mature olfactory sensory neurons. Olfactory receptor neurons (arrow) extend a single dendrite to the apical surface of the epithelium terminating in sensory cilia. The axons of these neurons extend from the base of the cell soma (arrowhead), pass through the basal lamina underlying the epithelium, and turn to course toward the OB. Scale bar = 25 μm. (C) Diagrammatic representation of the vertebrate cAMP signal transduction pathway as described in the text. G, G protein; AC, adenylate cyclase; CNG, cyclic nucleotide gated channel; CLC, chlorine channel.

interact with odorant molecules in the nasal air-spaces. Expressed within each cilium is the molecular machinery necessary for the detection of these odorant molecules (Fig. 1C). Olfaction begins with the binding of an odorant molecule to a complementary odorant receptor (OR) at the cilia membrane. ORs are members of the seven-transmembrane superfamily of receptor molecules. Each OR appears to be "tuned" to recognize a particular chemical moiety that may be present on a number of different odor molecules. The binding of an odorant to an OR triggers one of two signal transduction pathways. The first is a G protein pathway (Fig. 1C) in which the OR binds to an olfactory-specific G protein, G_{olf},

which in turn activates an adenylate cyclase type III molecule, leading to an increase in cyclic nucleotides, the opening of olfactory cyclic nucleotide gated channels (OCNCs), and the entry of calcium into the cilia. The increase in intracellular calcium triggers Na^+ and Cl^- conductances, leading to action potentials within the ORN that are propagated down the axon into the brain. The second is an phosphatydal inositol (IP_3) pathway in which the OR binds to a G protein, which then activates phospholipase C (PLC) to generate an increase in IP_3. The IP_3 second messenger also opens channels, leading to an influx of calcium into the cilia and triggering action potentials within the ORN. Evidence suggests that there is a prominent IP_3 transduction pathway in invertebrate animals, but the function and even the existence of this pathway in mammals are still controversial.

The family of olfactory receptor genes (ORGs) is estimated to consist of as many as 1000 genes, 3% of the ∼30,000 genes in the mammalian genome. Each ORN is thought to express only a single ORG, which can interact with a limited range of odorant molecules. The ORNs expressing the same ORG (an ORN–ORG cohort) are randomly distributed throughout one of four broad zones through the olfactory epithelium. A complex aroma, such as that of coffee, is likely to activate numerous ORN–ORG cohorts within the epithelium. The ability to detect and identify specific odors therefore becomes a computational problem that must be solved by olfactory parts of the brain.

CRANIAL NERVE I: THE OLFACTORY NERVE

The axons of ORNs form cranial nerve I, the olfactory nerve, which connects the olfactory epithelium to the olfactory bulb located in the anterior cranial fossa in man, specifically in the nucleus lateral to the gyrus rectus of the frontal lobe. Each ORN has a single axon that joins other ORN axons to form nerve fascicles in the lamina propria underlying the olfactory epithelium. These fascicles pass through the cribriform plate and terminate in the olfactory bulb. Unlike most cranial nerves, the olfactory nerve does not form a single "nerve" but rather comprises multiple fascicles that pierce the cribriform plate at multiple points to enter the olfactory bulb at dispersed loci. Individual axons of the olfactory nerve synapse on the dendrites of second-order neurons within globular structures of neuropil—glomeruli—surrounding the surface of the olfactory bulb. It was recently discovered that all the axons from ORNs expressing the same ORG converge onto two (or a few) glomeruli in the bulb (Fig. 2A). The location of these glomeruli is bilaterally symmetrical and invariant across animals. Therefore, each glomerulus may represented the summed activity of an ORN–ORG cohort whose individual members are randomly dispersed throughout the olfactory epithelium.

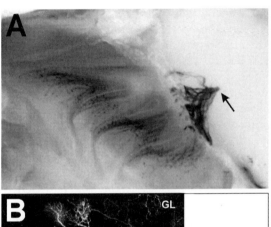

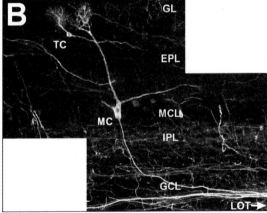

Figure 2
(A) Medial view of the nasal cavity or a P2-IRES-LacZ transgenic mouse showing the olfactory epithelium and olfactory bulb. Olfactory receptor neurons expressing the P2 odorant receptor gene coexpress β-galactosidase and were stained blue with an X-gal reaction. This cohort of receptor axons converge to a single glomerulus on the medial surface of the bulb (arrow). The corresponding lateral glomerulus is not visible in this preparation (reproduced with permission from Mombaerts *et al.*, 1996). (B) A single mitral cell (MC) and a single tufted cell (TC) retrogradely labeled by DiI. Both cells have an apical dendrite ending in a complex tuft within one glomerulus, and several lateral dendrites are visible extending from the mitral cell. Axons from these cells extend through the internal plexiform layer (IPL) toward the caudal bulb, where they form the lateral olfactory tract (LOT). GL, glomerular layer; EPL, external plexiform layer; MCL, mitral cell layer; GCL, granule cell layer.

OLFACTORY BULB

The olfactory bulb is a rostral outgrowth of the telencephalon with a cortical-like layered organization to various cellular and neuropil regions (Fig. 2). These layers consist of the nerve fiber, glomerular, external plexiform, mitral, internal plexiform, granule cell, and subventricular layers. Olfactory nerve axons surround the olfactory bulb, forming the nerve fiber layer. The olfactory axons leave the nerve layer to enter a glomerulus, in which they synaptically terminate on the dendrites of mitral cells, tufted cells, and periglomerular neurons within single glomeruli. Glial cell (astrocyte) processes encapsulate, and segregate, each glomerulus, each of which in turn is surrounded by the perikarya of juxtaglomerular cells. Many of the juxtaglomerular neurons surrounding glomeruli are GABAergic and/or dopaminergic. The projection neurons of the olfactory bulb are mitral cells in the mitral cell layer and tufted cells in the external plexiform and deep glomerular layer (Fig. 2B). Axons from mitral, middle tufted, and deep tufted cells pass through the internal plexiform and granule cell layers to project along the lateral olfactory tract to other regions of the central nervous system. A small number of tufted cells form the intrabulbar association system and synapse on granule cells in other areas of the same olfactory bulb. Granule cells, located within the granule cell layer deep to the mitral cell layer and within the mitral cell layer, make numerous reciprocal dendro-dendritic contacts with the lateral dendrites of mitral and tufted cells in the external plexiform layer (EPL). Granule cells have a long apical dendrite ramifying in the EPL; they also have short basal dendrites ramifying in the granule cell and mitral cell layers, but they lack an axon.

The projection of each ORN–ORG cohort to two or a few glomeruli suggests that each glomerulus represents a functional unit responding to a specific subset of odorant molecules. Thus, a complex odor will stimulate many ORN–ORG cohorts, which in turn will activate a distinctive pattern of glomeruli in the bulb that is unique to that odor. During the past several decades, a variety of experimental approaches, including 2-deoxyglucose incorporation, functional magnetic resonance imaging, and intrinsic optical signals, have shown that odors generate specific patterns of activity within the glomerular layer.

The flow of information in the olfactory system is from ORNs to the mitral/tufted cell and then to central cortical regions. However, this flow is significantly modulated at the following levels within the olfactory bulb:

1. *Presynaptic inhibition at the ORN to mitral cell synapse:* ORNs express both dopamine D_2 and $GABA_B$ receptors on their nerve terminals. These receptors are activated by dopamine and GABA, respectively, released from juxtaglomerular cells and function to presynaptically inhibit transmitter release from olfactory nerve terminals.

2. *Modulation by juxtaglomerular (JG) interneurons:* The many JG neurons surrounding each glomerulus are GABAergic interneurons. When activated by ORN input or dendrodendritic contact with mitral cell apical dendrites, they release GABA onto the dendrites of mitral/tufted cells within a glomerulus and between glomeruli.

3. *Lateral inhibition:* A form of lateral inhibition is mediated by the dendrodentric synapses between the mitral/tufted cells and the GABAergic granule cells. Excitation of mitral cells results in the activation of granule cells, which in turn may inhibit the same or other mitral cells. Lateral inhibition is a feature of both the visual and auditory sensory systems, in which it functions to enhance the signal-to-noise ratio. It is likely that the inhibitory circuits in the olfactory bulb play a similar signal-enhancing function prior to the output of the information to the primary olfactory cortex.

OLFACTORY CORTEX

Mitral/tufted cell axons exit the olfactory bulb along the lateral olfactory tract (Fig. 3) and innervate the anterior olfactory nucleus, piriform cortex, olfactory tubercle, taenia tecta, lateral entorhinal area, anterior

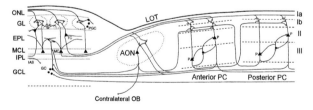

Figure 3
Diagrammatic representation of the olfactory bulb and piriform neural circuitry as described in detail in the text. ONL, olfactory nerve fiber layer; GL, glomerular layer; EPL, external plexiform layer; MCL, mitral cell layer; IPL, internal plexiform layer; GCL, granule cell layer; LOT, lateral olfactory tract; AON, anterior olfactory nucleus; IAS, intrabulbar association system; PGC, periglomerular cell; SA, short axon cell; TC, tufted cell; MC, mitral cell; GC, granule cell; P, pyramidal neuron.

hippocampal continuation, indusium griseum, and the periamygdaloid cortex, which are all present in the ventral brain. These brain regions are collectively known as the primary olfactory cortex (POC). Although our understanding of the peripheral mechanisms involved in olfaction is increasing rapidly, our knowledge of the functions of the various primary olfactory cortical regions is rudimentary. It is beyond the scope of this entry to discuss all the primary olfactory cortical regions in detail.

The POC is thought to regulate the function of the olfactory bulb via direct feedback connections that synaptically contact granule cells in the olfactory bulb (referred to as the centrifugal afferents). These centrifugal afferents are very dense and come from multiple sources. In general, the following anatomically distinct regions within the brain send either ipsilateral or contralateral centrifugal projections to the olfactory bulb: the anterior olfactory nucleus, piriform cortex, nucleus of the lateral olfactory tract, ventral hippocampi rudiment, dorsal peduncular cortex, medial diagonal band complex, hypothalamus, raphe nuclei, and the locus coeruleus. The anterior olfactory nucleus is the major source of contralateral innervation of the olfactory bulb via projections through the anterior commissure, and it also contributes to the ipsilateral innervation of the bulb. Centrifugal fibers appear to terminate on many olfactory bulb neuron types throughout all layers of the olfactory bulb, although the major targets of these fibers are the granule cells. The neurotransmitters and functions of the centrifugal fiber innervation have not been fully characterized; however, it is likely that the bulb receives primarily glutamatergic excitatory synaptic inputs from the primary olfactory cortex but also receives cholinergic, noradrenergic, GABAergic, and serotonergic innervation. Centrifugal afferents modulate the function of the olfactory bulb, but little is known about their specific role(s) in olfactory information processing.

In addition to the feedback connections with the olfactory bulb, the POC has extensive "associative" connections between POC structures on both the ipsilateral and contralateral hemispheres. Projections from the anterior olfactory nucleus and the piriform cortex through the anterior commissure form the major interhemispheric connections within the POC. The functional impact of these ipsilateral and contralateral associative circuits is poorly understood, but they could be involved in aspects of olfactory memory. The POC also has heavy extrinsic projections to the ipsilateral and contralateral hypothalamus and thalamus in addition to several other structures. Olfactory discrimination and cognition could arise via the POC to hypothalamus/thalamus to neocortex pathway; alternatively, virtually all of the POC comprises cortical structures and could be directly involved in aspects of olfactory cognition and memory.

ACCESSORY OLFACTORY SYSTEM

In addition to the main olfactory system described previously, most species also have an accessory olfactory system. The accessory olfactory system consists of the vomeronasal organ (VNO), a cylindrical tube lined by olfactory sensory neurons located in the dorsal septum. The VNO is primarily thought to be involved in the detection of pheromones (a substance secreted by an individual species, especially in the insect world, and perceived by smell by the same species and thatinfluences the behavior of the perceiver). Axons from ORNs in the VNO project down the medial side of the olfactory bulb to the accessory olfactory bulb located at the dorsocaudal part of the main olfactory bulb. The accessory olfactory bulb contains the same cell types and layers as the main olfactory bulb, but in a more "disorganized" arrangement. The mitral/tufted cells in the accessory bulb project to the anterior olfactory nucleus, the nucleus of the accessory olfactory tract, the bed nucleus of the stria terminalis, the medial amygdaloid nucleus, and the posterior cortical amygdaloid nucleus. Many of these cortical areas also project back to the granule cell layer of the accessory olfactory bulb. The presence of human pheromone cues is controversial. A recent study suggested that involuntary reproductive events (e.g., ovulation) can be modulated by a pheromone cue in man. However, the presence of a functional human VNO is widely debated, with recent reports indicating that there is no organized accessory olfactory bulb in man. It remains to be determined to what extent pheromone cues can influence human behavior.

—*M. T. Shipley and A. C. Puche*

See also–Abducens Nerve (Cranial Nerve VI); Accessory Nerve (Cranial Nerve XI); Facial Nerve (Cranial Nerve VII); Glossopharyngeal Nerve (Cranial Nerve IX); Hypoglossal Nerve (Cranial Nerve XII); Oculomotor Nerve (Cranial Nerve III); Optic Nerve (Cranial Nerve II); Smell; Taste; Trigeminal Nerve (Cranial Nerve V); Trochlear Nerve (Cranial Nerve IV); Vagus Nerve (Cranial Nerve X); Vestibulocochlear Nerve (Cranial Nerve VIII)

Further Reading

Buck, L., and Axel, R. (1991). A novel multigene family may encode odorant receptors: A molecular basis for odor recognition. *Cell* 65, 175–187.

Cajal, S. R. (1911). *Histologie du Systeme Nervous de l'Homme et des Vertebres*. Moloine, Paris.

Getchell, T. V., Bartoshuk, L. M., Doty, R. L., *et al.* (1991). *Smell and Taste in Health and Disease*. Raven Press, New York.

Gold, G. H. (1999). Controversial issues in vertebrate olfactory transduction. *Annu. Rev. Physiol.* 61, 857–871.

Johnson, B. A., Woo, C. C., and Leon, M. (1998). Spatial coding of odorant features in the glomerular layer of the rat olfactory bulb. *J. Comp. Neurol.* 393, 457–471.

Keverne, E. B. (1999). The vomeronasal organ. *Science* 286, 716–720.

Mombaerts, P., Wang, F., Dulac, C., Chao, S. K., Nemes, A., Mendelsohn, M., Edmondson, J., and Axel, R. (1996). Visualizing an olfactory sensory map. *Cell* 87, 675–686.

Monti-Bloch, L., Jennings-White, C., and Berliner, D. L. (1998). The human vomeronasal system. A review. *Ann. N. Y. Acad. Sci.* 855, 373–389.

Mori, K., Nagao, H., and Sasaki, Y. F. (1998). Computation of molecular information in mammalian olfactory systems. *Network* 9, R79–R102.

Mori, K., Nagao, H., and Yoshihara, Y. (1999). The olfactory bulb: Coding and processing of odor molecule information. *Science* 286, 711–715.

Rubin, B. D., and Katz, L. C. (1999). Optical imaging of odorant representations in the mammalian olfactory bulb. *Neuron* 23, 499–511.

Schild, D., and Restrepo, D. (1998). Transduction mechanisms in vertebrate olfactory receptor cells. *Physiol. Rev.* 78, 429–466.

Shipley, M. T., and Ennis, M. (1996). Functional organization of olfactory system. *J. Neurobiol.* 30, 123–176.

Stern, K., and McClintock, M. K. (1998). Regulation of ovulation by human pheromones. *Nature* 392, 177–179.

Yang, X., Renken, R., Hyder, F., *et al.* (1998). Dynamic mapping at the laminar level of odor-elicited responses in rat olfactory bulb by functional MRI. *Proc. Natl. Acad. Sci. USA* 95, 7715–7720.

Oligoastrocytoma
see Glial Tumors

Oligodendrocytes

Encyclopedia of the Neurological Sciences

ALTHOUGH neurons provide the conduit for electrical impulses, the main information currency in the central nervous system (CNS), their function depends on interactions with several other neural cell types. Foremost among these are oligodendrocytes that generate myelin, the fatty insulation around nerve fibers that facilitates rapid and saltatory conduction of action potentials. The number of oligodendrocytes present in the adult CNS results from close regulation of cell proliferation, survival, and differentiation by different growth factors during development. Oligodendrocytes and their precursors are major cellular targets in a variety of pathological conditions, including the autoimmune disease multiple sclerosis, ischemic insults, and CNS trauma.

DEVELOPMENT OF OLIGODENDROCYTES

Like other cells of the CNS, oligodendrocytes are derived from the neuroepithelial cells of the neural tube. Local cues induce some neuroepithelial cells to become specified to the oligodendrocyte lineage. The specified oligodendrocyte precursors then migrate throughout the developing nervous system, proliferate, and differentiate into mature oligodendrocytes (Fig. 1).

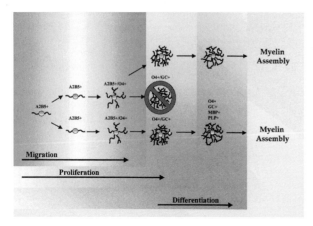

Figure 1

Overview of the development of oligodendrocytes. Immature bipolar oligodendrocyte precursors recognized by labeling with the mAb A2B5 proliferate extensively in response to PDGF, are highly migratory, and mature into multiprocessed pro-oligodendroblasts. Oligodendroblasts proliferate primarily in response to bFGF and can be recognized by labeling with mAb O4. Expression of the major glycolipid of myelin galactocerebroside (GC) and cessation of proliferation accompany differentiation of the precursors into oligodendrocytes. This is a particularly susceptible stage in the lineage, and in the absence of survival signals many of the cells die by apoptosis. Maturation of oligodendrocyte is accompanied by increased expression of myelin components (MBP and PLP) and assembly of the myelin sheath. (See color plate section.)

The initial specification of oligodendrocyte precursors requires ventrally derived signals in caudal regions of the emerging nervous system. One of the most important of these precursors is sonic hedgehog (Shh). Exposure of dorsal neuroepithelium to Shh results in the ectopic appearance of oligodendrocytes, whereas inhibition of Shh signaling blocks the appearance of oligodendrocytes throughout the CNS.

The proliferation of oligodendrocyte precursors is driven by several growth factors, including platelet-derived growth factor (PDGF) and fibroblast growth factor (FGF). Immature precursor cells respond primarily to PDGF, whereas more mature precursors respond primarily to bFGF. The response to these growth factors is mediated through distinct receptors. The major PDGF receptor on oligodendrocyte precursors is the PDGF-α receptor, and expression of this receptor provides a marker for oligodendrocyte precursors in the postnatal rat brain. The response to bFGF is mediated through different receptors depending on the maturity of the precursor cells. The magnitude of the proliferative response of oligodendrocyte precursors to individual growth factors is also influenced by additional signaling systems. For example, the chemokine GRO-1, although not an independent mitogen, acts synergistically with PDGF to enhance the proliferative response of oligodendrocyte precursors fourfold. In most cases, the source of these growth factors appears to be astrocytes of the presumptive white matter.

Immature oligodendrocyte precursors have diverse developmental potential. Extrinsic signals, such as the presence of serum or the cytokine cilary neurotrophic factor, promote these cells to differentiate into a distinct class of astrocytes termed type 2 astrocytes. Furthermore, rat optic nerve oligodendrocyte precursors have recently been shown to be capable of being reprogrammed to multipotential stem cells and to give rise to all major classes of neural cells under appropriate conditions *in vitro*.

Immature oligodendrocyte precursors are highly motile and migrate throughout the CNS. It is unclear how the migration of these cells is regulated. *In vitro* studies suggest that extracellular matrix proteins interacting with appropriate membrane-bound integrin receptors promote precursor cell migration, whereas growth factors such as PDGF may stimulate directional movement. The relevance of these migrational influences to the *in vivo* development of oligodendrocyte precursors is not clear.

CONTROL OF OLIGODENDROCYTE NUMBER: REGULATION OF DIFFERENTIATION AND SURVIVAL

Oligodendrocyte precursors differentiate into immature oligodendrocytes before they generate myelin (Figs. 1 and 2). Both cell intrinsic and cell extrinsic signals regulate this critical transition. *In vitro*, clonally related oligodendrocyte precursors differentiate at approximately the same time, suggesting the differentiation of these cells is in part regulated through an intrinsic clock that measures the number of cell divisions and/or elapsed time. Extrinsic signals also influence oligodendrocyte differentiation. Axonal signals promote the differentiation of oligodendrocyte precursors, and considerable circumstantial evidence suggests that axons provide a signal that initiates the process of myelination. Thyroid hormone also influences oligodendrocyte differentiation. Exposure to thyroid hormone elevates the number of mature oligodendrocytes and directly enhances the expression of myelin-specific genes.

Although oligodendrocyte precursors are highly proliferative, mature differentiated oligodendrocytes do not proliferate extensively; therefore, the regulation of oligodendrocyte precursor number is crucial for generating sufficient oligodendrocytes in the adult. The final number of oligodendrocytes that develop in a specific region of the CNS is closely correlated with the number of axons that require myelination. This matching of cell number is accomplished by regulation of cell proliferation and cell survival (Fig. 1). As in neuronal lineages, during

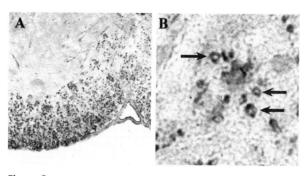

Figure 3

Developing myelin in the mouse spinal cord detected by antibodies to myelin basic protein (MBP). (A) Transverse section through the ventral region of the P7 mouse spinal cord. The myelin develops in a patchy manner, reflecting the differentiation and maturation of individual oligodendrocytes. (B) Higher power micrograph of an individual MBP-labeled oligodendrocyte in the developing spinal cord that is myelinating several adjacent axons (arrows). The MBP myelin sheaths cut in transverse section appear as dark circles with an unlabeled axon in the center. (See color plate section.)

development oligodendrocyte precursors are produced in excess and apoptosis and programmed cell death remove extraneous cells. *In vitro*, newly formed oligodendrocytes depend on PDGF for survival, whereas more mature oligodendrocytes depend on insulin growth factor-1 and the neurotrophin NT3 for survival. It seems likely that similar combinations of growth factors regulate oligodendrocyte survival during development in the intact CNS.

Oligodendrocyte precursors persist in the adult CNS, offering a potential source of cells for therapy and repair. Under normal conditions the proliferation of these adult cells is limited; however, in response to injury, or *in vitro*, adult oligodendrocyte precursors can proliferate extensively and generate large numbers of oligodendrocytes. Understanding how the proliferation and differentiation of these adult precursors are controlled will provide strategies for replacing oligodendrocytes lost during pathological conditions.

FUNCTION OF OLIGODENDROCYTES

The only known function of oligodendrocytes in mature CNS white matter is to generate myelin, which ensheaths axons (Fig. 3). Depending on the region of the CNS, a single oligodendrocyte may ensheath a large number of different axons. For example, in the optic nerve morphological studies suggest a single oligodendrocyte may wrap many different axons, whereas in ventral spinal cord one

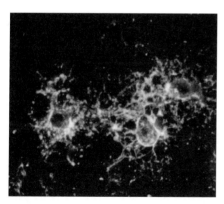

Figure 2

Differentiated oligodendrocytes can be identified in CNS tissue through expression of myelin-specific lipids. Three oligodendrocytes in the ventral spinal cord of the embryonic mouse are labeled with antibodies to a major glycolipid in myelin. These cells have a complex morphology with many processes projecting into the surrounding neuropil.

oligodendrocyte may associate with a single large-diameter axon.

The unique composition of the myelin sheath lends it insulating properties and allows for its unambiguous identification. Myelin consists of large amounts of cell membrane containing a high proportion (70–80%) of lipid. Of these, the glycolipids galactocerebroside and galactosulfatide are the most abundant. Mutant animals lacking these lipids have abnormal formation and maintenance of myelin. Major proteins that comprise CNS myelin include proteolipid protein (PLP), its alternatively spliced isoform DM20, and myelin basic protein (MBP). PLP and DM20 are integral membrane proteins located in compact myelin and are essential for myelin formation. MBP is an extrinsic membrane protein located on the cytoplasmic surface, and it is required for myelin compaction. Several less abundant proteins are also associated with CNS myelin, including myelin associated glycoprotein, which may be important for axon/oligodendrocyte interactions, and myelin oligodendrocyte glycoprotein, which may be important for the maintenance of myelin. The functional properties of different myelin proteins are highlighted in relevant mutant animals. Mutations in PLP/DM20 are modeled in a number of mutants, such as jimpy or rumpshaker mice. These animals have characteristic tremors, severe hypomyelination, and increased cell death of oligodendrocytes. Mutations in MBP are modeled in shiverer mice, which have greatly reduced CNS myelin.

OLIGODENDROCYTES IN DISEASE

Several pathological conditions affect the integrity of CNS myelin and the survival of oligodendrocytes, including multiple sclerosis, the leukodystrophies, and ischemic and traumatic insults to the developing and adult CNS.

The most common demyelinating disease in man is multiple sclerosis (MS), in which there is progressive loss of myelin and oligodendrocytes in discrete regions or plaques. The initial cause of MS is unknown; however, both genetic and environmental factors appear to contribute to disease occurrence. The prevalence of MS is rare in some ethnic groups and familial occurrence increases the risk of MS. In general, the prevalence of MS within the population increases in northern latitudes. Demyelination during MS is relatively dynamic, with some remyelination. Within active MS plaques there is inflammation and lymphocyte infiltration, whereas myelin removal is accomplished by activated macrophages. The initial target in MS may be either the myelin sheath or the oligodendrocyte cell body. Loss of these components, however, results in local axonal pathology that also contributes to the functional loss associated with the disease. Several animal models of MS have been developed, including experimental allergic encephalomyelitis induced by immunization with myelin, or specific peptides of MBP or PLP, and infection with Theiler's murine encephalitis virus, both of which reproduce many of the characteristics of MS.

Genetically based myelin disorders known as leukodystrophies reflect either abnormal myelin synthesis or lipid storage. Frequently, the number of oligodendrocytes and the amount of myelin are dramatically reduced in affected individuals. Furthermore, the composition of the myelin is altered from normal with excessive accumulation of distinct lipids. Mutations in myelin proteins also result in myelin disorders. For example, mutations in PLP/DM20 underlie Pelizaeus–Merzbacher disease.

Myelin and oligodendrocytes are also vulnerable to environmental and traumatic insults to the CNS. Malnutrition, copper deficiency, or lead toxicity result in hypomyelination. Likewise, fetal ischemic insults or trauma to the developing and adult CNS result in a loss of oligodendrocytes and CNS myelin.

Oligodendrocytes or their precursors may be the cellular origin of oligodendrogliomas, a distinct type of CNS tumor. Oligodendroglioma cells share morphological and biochemical characteristics with oligodendrocyte precursors. Recent studies demonstrate disruption of the PDGF/GRO-1 regulatory pathway mediating oligodendrocyte precursor proliferation in oligodendrogliomas, and such disruptions may contribute to CNS tumorogenesis.

CONCLUSIONS

Oligodendrocytes and myelin are critical components for the functioning of the mature CNS. The development of these cells is regulated by a variety of growth factors that promote cell proliferation, migration, survival, and differentiation. Many pathological conditions result in a loss of myelin and oligodendrocytes in the mature CNS. The realization that the adult CNS contains significant numbers of multipotent neural stem cells and oligodendrocyte precursors raises the possibility of therapeutic intervention in a number of demyelinating diseases. A major challenge is to harness the potential of these stem cells to facilitate repair. Such a goal requires detailed understanding of the molecular mechanisms mediating oligodendrocyte development and maintenance.

—*Robert H. Miller*

See also—Cell Death; Central Nervous System, Overview; Multiple Sclerosis, Basic Biology; Myelin; Neurons, Overview; Nodes of Ranvier; Optic Nerve (Cranial Nerve II)

Further Reading

Barres, B. A., and Raff, M. C. (1994). Control of oligodendrocyte number in the developing rat optic nerve. *Neuron* **12**, 935–942.

Barres, B. A., and Raff, M. C. (1999). Axonal control of oligodendrocyte development. *J. Cell Biol.* **147**, 1123–1128.

Kondo, T., and Raff, M. C. (2000). Oligodendrocyte precursor cells reprogrammed to become multipotential CNS stem cells. *Science* **289**, 1754.

Miller, R. H. (1996). Oligodendrocyte origins. *Trends Neurosci.* **19**, 92–96.

Nave, K.-A. (1995). Neurological mouse mutants: A molecular–genetic analysis of myelin proteins. In *Neuroglia* (H. Kettenmann and B. Ransom, Eds.), pp. 571–587. Oxford Univ. Press, New York.

Pfeiffer, S. E., Warrington, A. E., and Bansal, R. (1993). The oligodendrocyte and its many cellular processes. *Trends Cell Biol.* **3**, 191–197.

Quarles, R. H., Morell, P., and McFarlin, D. E. (1995). Diseases involving myelin. In *Basic Neurochemistry* (G. J. Siegel, B. W. Agranoff, R. W. Albers, and P. B. Molinoff, Eds.). Raven Press, New York.

Raff, M. C. (1989). Glial cell diversification in the rat optic nerve. *Science* **243**, 1450–1455.

Oligodendrogliomas
see Glial Tumors

Ophthalmology
see Neuro-Ophthalmology

Ophthalmoplegia

Encyclopedia of the Neurological Sciences
Copyright 2003, Elsevier Science (USA). All rights reserved.

OPHTHALMOPLEGIA is paralysis of the muscles of the eyes and can be broadly classified as external ophthalmoplegia and internal ophthalmoplegia.

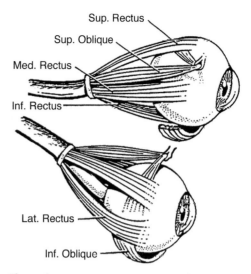

Figure 1
Each eye has six extraocular muscles.

External ophthalmoplegia is paralysis of the extrinsic muscles (Fig. 1) that move or rotate the eyes in different directions in the presence of normal pupillary responses. These muscles are known as the extraocular muscles and are under voluntary control. One or more of the extraocular muscles may be affected simultaneously. Each eye has six extraocular muscles, coupled in pairs (yoked), that enable them to move in a coordinated fashion and maintain alignment on a fixed object so that an image of that object falls on the most discriminating part of the retina, the fovea, of each eye simultaneously. This ensures binocular single vision (fusion), depth perception, and stereopsis (Fig. 2). If the visual axes are not aligned, the object is seen by noncorresponding (disparate) points of each retina and double vision (diplopia) results.

The extraocular muscles are innervated by the three cranial nerves on each side known as the ocular motor nerves: the third (oculomotor), fourth (trochlear), and sixth (abducens) cranial nerves. The sixth nerve innervates the lateral rectus muscle, and the fourth nerve innervates the superior oblique muscle. The third nerve innervates the remaining four extraocular muscles of each eye in addition to the levator palpebrae superioris, which elevates the upper lid to keep the eye open, the constrictor pupillae, which makes the pupil small, and the ciliary muscle, which changes the shape of the lens to allow the eye to focus on objects at different distances, such as when reading (accommodation).

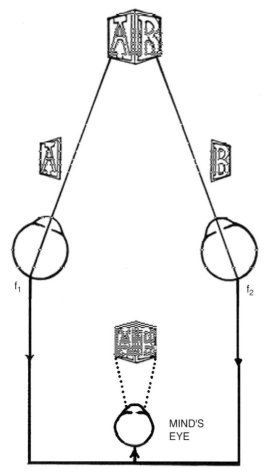

Figure 2
Binocular single vision (fusion), depth perception, and stereopsis.

Internal ophthalmoplegia refers to the combination of paralysis of the constrictor pupillae (iridoplegia), causing a large unreactive pupil, and the ciliary muscle (cycloplegia), causing impaired accommodation (poor near vision). These muscles are innervated by the autonomic nervous system and therefore are not strictly under voluntary control.

Sometimes the term total ophthalmoplegia is used to indicate loss of all functions mediated by the third (oculomotor) nerve; that is, a complete third nerve palsy, which is characterized by ptosis (drooping of the upper eye lid due to paralysis of the levator palpebrae superioris muscle), iridoplegia, cycloplegia, and paralysis of all the extraocular muscles supplied by the third nerve.

Any disorder that can affect the extraocular muscles, the ocular motor nerves, the neuromuscular junction (the connection between nerve and muscle), or the higher centers in the brain that control eye movements can cause ophthalmoplegia.

Diseases directly affecting the extraocular muscles include thyroid orbitopathy (Graves' ophthalmopathy), idiopathic orbital inflammatory disease (orbital pseudotumor), myopathies including mitochondrial disorders (chronic progressive external ophthalmoplegia), vitamin E deficiency, and congenital extraocular muscle fibrosis. Disorders affecting the neuromuscular junction include myasthenia (an immune-mediated disease), toxins such as botulism, tick paralysis, and certain curare-like anesthetic agents. The most common cause of ophthalmoplegia is damage to one or more of the ocular motor nerves along their course and may result from trauma (head injury and surgery), microvascular disease (diabetes and atherosclerosis), local infection or inflammation (chronic basal meningitis, sarcoid, and carcinoma), migraine (ophthalmoplegic migraine), or compression by a tumor or aneurysm. Such isolated ocular motor neuropathies, often referred to as ocular motor palsies, are frequently associated with eye pain and thus termed painful ophthalmoplegia. The Tolosa–Hunt syndrome is a particular form of painful ophthalmoplegia, also called superior orbital fissuritis, and is attributed to nonspecific granulomatous inflammation in the cavernous sinus–superior orbital fissure region. The pain is usually located in the periorbital region and described as severe gnawing and boring.

Diseases of the nuclear, paranuclear, and supranuclear gaze structures in the brain and brainstem also cause ophthalmoplegia. These include multiple sclerosis, vascular disorders such as stroke and vasculitis, encephalitis, paraneoplastic disorders, and tumors.

Internuclear ophthalmoplegia occurs with lesions of the neural pathway in the brainstem called the medial longitudinal fasciculus, which connects the third and sixth cranial nerve nuclei (Fig. 3) and impairs transmission of neural impulses to the ipsilateral medial rectus muscle. This results in partial or complete paralysis of adduction of the ipsilateral eye while preserving abduction of the contralateral eye. Such lesions can occur with a variety of disorders, especially multiple sclerosis and stroke.

Supranuclear ophthalmoplegia (supranuclear gaze palsy) occurs when the pathways from gaze centers in the cerebral hemispheres, which initiate voluntary eye movements, to the eye-movement

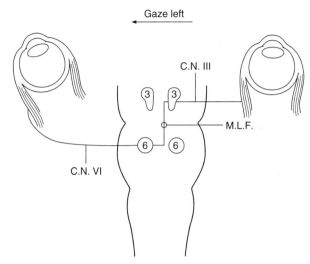

Figure 3
The medial longitudinal fasciculus (MLF), which connects the third and sixth cranial nerve (CN) nuclei. LE, left eye; RE, right eye.

generators in the brainstem are interrupted. Supranuclear ophthalmoplegia is characterized by loss of voluntary eye movements but sparing of reflex movements, such as vestibulo-ocular and optokinetic responses. Supranuclear gaze palsies occur classically in degenerative brain disorders such as progressive supranuclear palsy (PSP), with severe head injury or with stroke.

—*Patrick Lavin*

See also–Abducens Nerve (Cranial Nerve VI); Eye Movements, Overview; Migraine, Ophthalmoplegic and Retinal; Myopathy, Overview; Oculomotor Nerve (Cranial Nerve III); Progressive External Ophthalmoplegia (PEO); Trochlear Nerve (Cranial Nerve IV)

Further Reading

Lavin, P. J. M. (1998). The facial pain syndromes. In *An Atlas of Neuro-ophthalmology* (E. Rosen, S. Thompson, P. Eustace, and K. Cumming, Eds.). Mosby, St. Louis.

Lavin, P. J. M. (2000). Diplopia, nystagmus and other ocular oscillations. In *Neurology in Clinical Practice* (R. B. Daroff, G. M. Fenichel, C. D. Marsden, and W. G. Bradley, Eds.), 3rd ed. Butterworth, Boston.

Lavin, P. J. M., and Donahue, S. (2000). Neuro-ophthalmology: The efferent visual system. Gaze mechanisms and disorders. In *Neurology in Clinical Practice* (R. B. Daroff, G. M. Fenichel, C. D. Marsden, and W. G. Bradley, Eds.), 3rd ed. Butterworth, Boston.

Miller, N. R., and Newman, N. J. (Eds.) (1998). *Walsh and Hoyt's Clinical Neuro-ophthalmology*, 5th ed. Williams & Wilkins, Baltimore.

Opioids and Their Receptors

Encyclopedia of the Neurological Sciences

OPIUM has been a source of drugs used to relieve pain since ancient times. Opium contains a number of alkaloids, including morphine and codeine (Fig. 1), two of the most widely used painkillers in medicine. Despite their extraordinary utility in the control of pain, these drugs have a number of liabilities and side effects. In addition to their addictive potential, they also produce other undesired physiological effects, including respiratory depression and the inhibition of gastrointestinal transit (i.e., constipation). After defining the structure of morphine and codeine, chemists started to synthesize analogs in the hope that these would retain the painkilling qualities without the undesired actions. Although they have been only modestly successful, the thousands of agents that were made provided a great deal of information regarding the actions of these drugs, including the strict structure–activity relationships necessary for opioid activity. Medicinal chemists were able to define "rules" regarding the chemical structure of the drugs that had to be observed to maintain analgesic activity. These rules required certain chemical groups in specific positions. These rigid structural requirements implied a very specific recognition site, or receptor, long before they were identified biochemically. The first studies biochemically demonstrating opioid receptors were reported in the 1970s and measured the binding of the drug to

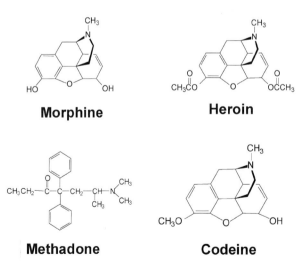

Figure 1
Structures of opiates.

a specific recognition site on the membrane of nerve cells (neurons). It is now known that the opioid receptors are in the G protein receptor family (G proteins are so called because they bind the guanine nucleotides).

The explosion in molecular biology has provided important insights into the receptors through which drugs act. Although there are many general categories of receptors, the G protein-coupled family of receptors is one of the largest, comprising more than 400 different receptors that have been cloned and their amino acid sequences determined. These receptors share many features. Foremost are their mechanisms of transduction, or how they communicate to the cell when they have been activated. They all physically interface with one of a series of G proteins that convey the "activation" of the receptor to a variety of biochemical and/or electrophysiological targets. In addition to these functional similarities, the G protein-coupled receptors are also structurally similar. They are all integral membrane proteins, meaning that they are located within the cell membrane. Indeed, G protein-coupled receptors are composed of a single long string of amino acids that goes through membrane seven times, with the amino terminus located on the outside and the carboxy terminus on the inside of the cell (Fig. 2). These seven spans are arranged in a donut-like shape, with the drugs binding to the cavity in their center.

ENDOGENOUS OPIOIDS

Classic studies of opioid action firmly established the ability of these drugs to relieve pain and documented their other actions. However, it was not clear why the brain should contain a receptor for morphine, a compound made in the poppy plant. This question was answered in 1970s with the identification of a series of peptides with opioid actions (Table 1). There are several classes of endogenous opioids, including the enkephalins, dynorphin A, and β-endorphin. Although these peptides are derived from the proteolytic processing of different precursors, the sequence of the first five amino acids of most of the opioid peptides corresponds to the sequence of one of the enkephalins. However, additional peptides have also been identified, including the endomorphins, which have actions similar to those of morphine and a number of related peptides. The pharmacology of many of the extended enkephalins other than dynorphin A and β-endorphin remains unknown. In addition, a number of

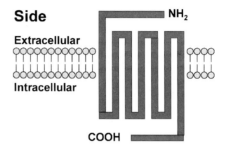

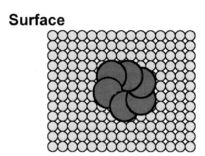

Figure 2
Schematic of G protein receptors. G protein-coupled receptors traverse the membrane seven times, with the amino terminus on the outside of the cell and the carboxy terminus on the inside. When viewed from the surface, these transmembrane domains orient themselves into a donut-like shape, with a pocket in the middle in which the ligand binds.

related peptides do not interact directly with opioid receptors but have been associated with homologous receptors such as orphanin FQ/nociceptin, which labels the ORL1 receptor.

PHARMACOLOGICAL CLASSIFICATION

With the synthesis of a wide range of opiates, it quickly became apparent that there was more than one class of opioid receptor. The receptors selective for morphine were termed mu, whereas a second receptor selective for the opioid ketocyclazocine was termed kappa. The discovery of the enkephalins and the other endogenous opioids greatly changed the concept of opioid receptors. Soon after the identification of the enkephalins, another class of receptors selective for this peptide were discovered and termed delta, whereas dynorphin A was identified as the endogenous ligand for the kappa receptors. However, many other opioid peptides have been described, raising the possibility that they too may have their own receptors that have not yet been identified. β-Endorphin is an excellent example. Studies from a number of laboratories imply a discrete receptor for this opioid peptide, termed epsilon. There is

Table 1 OPIOID AND RELATED PEPTIDES

Opioid/peptide	Sequence
[Leu^5]enkephalin	**Tyr-Gly-Gly-Phe-Leu**
[Met^5]enkephalin	**Tyr-Gly-Gly-Phe-Met**
Peptide E (amidorphin)	**Tyr-Gly-Gly-Phe-Met**-Lys-Lys-Met-Asp-Glu-Leu-Tyr-Pro-Leu-Glu-Val-Glu-Glu-Ala-Asn-Gly-Gly-Glu-Val-Leu
BAM 22	**Tyr-Gly-Gly-Phe-Met**-Lys-Lys-Met-Asp-Glu-Leu-Tyr-Pro-Leu-Glu-Val-Glu-Glu-Glu-Ala-Asn-Gly-Gly
BAM 20	**Tyr-Gly-Gly-Phe-Met**-Lys-Lys-Met-Asp-Glu-Leu-Tyr-Pro-Leu-Glu-Val-Glu-Glu-Glu-Ala-Asn
BAM 18	**Tyr-Gly-Gly-Phe-Met**-Lys-Lys-Met-Asp-Glu-Leu-Tyr-Pro-Leu-Glu-Val-Glu-Glu-Glu
BAM 12	**Tyr-Gly-Gly-Phe-Met**-Lys-Lys-Met-Asp-Glu-Leu-Tyr
Metorphamide	**Tyr-Gly-Gly-Phe-Met-Arg-Val**
Dynorphin A	**Tyr-Gly-Gly-Phe-Leu**-Arg-Arg-Ile-Arg–Pro-Lys–Leu-Lys-Trp-Asp-Asn-Gln
Dynorphin B	**Tyr-Gly-Gly-Phe-Leu**-Arg-Arg-Gln-Phe-Lys-Val-Val-Thr
β-Neoendorphin	**Tyr-Gly-Gly-Phe-Leu**-Arg-Lys-Tyr-Pro-Lys
β-Neoendorphin	**Tyr-Gly-Gly-Phe-Leu**-Arg-Lys-Tyr-Pro
β_h-Endorphin	**Tyr-Gly-Gly-Phe-Met**-Thr-Ser-Glu-Lys-Ser-Gln-Thr-Pro-Leu-Val-Thr-Leu-Phe-Lys-Asn-Ala-Ile-Ile-Lys-Asn-Ala-Tyr-Lys-Lys-Gly-Glu
Endomorphin-1	Tyr-Pro-Trp-Phe-NH$_2$
Endomorphin-2	Tyr-Pro-Phe-Phe-NH$_2$
Orphanin FQ/ nociceptin	**Phe-Gly-Gly-Phe**-Thr-Gly-Ala-Arg-Lys-Ser-Ala-Arg-Lys-Leu-Ala-Asp-Glu
Orphanin FQ2	Phe-Ser-Glu-Phe-Met-Arg-Gln-Tyr-Leu-Val-Leu-Ser-Met-Gln-Ser-Ser-Gln
Nocistatin	Thr-Glu-Pro-Gly-Leu-Glu-Glu-Val-Gly-Glu-Ile-Glu-Gln-Lys-Gln-Leu-Gln

considerable controversy regarding this receptor and its identification and characterization.

Mu Receptors

Morphine has played a pivotal role in opioid research and in the treatment of pain. The receptors that bind morphine with highest affinity and mediate most of its actions are termed mu (Table 2). These actions include the relief of pain, respiratory depression, and inhibition of gastrointestinal transit. Binding studies in the brain have clearly demonstrated mu receptors and revealed very discrete distributions among various brain regions. These distributions are consistent with regions known to be important in the control of pain. However, the functions of the mu receptors found in brain regions unrelated to pain modulation are unknown.

Two subtypes of mu receptors, mu$_1$ and mu$_2$, were proposed more than 20 years ago. Although both receptors bind morphine with high affinity, they can be readily distinguished by their binding selectivity and pharmacology. Whereas a number of mu-selective antagonists block the actions of both mu receptor subtypes, naloxonazine is a mu$_1$-selective antagonist that has proven valuable in classifying the actions of these two mu receptor subtypes. Nalox-

onazine-sensitive mu$_1$ receptor actions include the analgesic actions of morphine within the brain. Mu$_2$ receptors, on the other hand, mediate other morphine actions, including some of morphine's more problematic side effects, such as inhibition of gastrointestinal transit that contributes to the constipation associated with opioids and also respiratory depression. The presence of two mu receptors responsible for different actions raises the possibility of the development of drugs with selective actions and fewer side effects. However, such agents have not yet been developed.

Mu receptors have been cloned (MOR-1). The amino acid sequence indicates that the receptor is a member of the G protein-linked receptor family. This family of receptors has seven transmembrane regions and interacts with the G proteins that communicate the signal to a number of biochemical pathways, leading to the vast array of physiological actions. Mu receptors, like the other opioid receptors, activate inhibitory G proteins that diminish the activity of enzymes such as adenylyl cyclase and ion channels. The cloned receptor selectively binds opiates such as morphine with high affinity and is functionally active when expressed in cells. Reduction in the levels of these mu receptors using antisense techniques *in vivo*

Table 2 OPIOID RECEPTOR SUBTYPES AND THEIR ACTIONS[a]

Receptor	Clone	Action
Mu	MOR-1	Sedation
Mu$_1$		Supraspinal and peripheral analgesia
		Prolactin release, feeding
		Acetylcholine release in the hippocampus
Mu$_2$		Spinal analgesia, respiratory depression
		Inhibition of gastrointestinal transit
		Dopamine release by nigrostriatal neurons
		Guinea pig ileum bioassay, feeding
Kappa		
Kappa$_1$	KOR-1	Analgesia
		Dysphoria
		Diuresis
		Feeding
Kappa$_2$	(KOR-1/ DOR-1 dimer)	Unknown
Kappa$_3$		Analgesia
Delta	DOR-1	Mouse vas deferens bioassay, feeding
		Dopamine turnover in the striatum
Delta$_1$		Supraspinal analgesia
Delta$_2$		Spinal and supraspinal analgesia

[a] Some actions assigned to general families have not been correlated with a specific subtype.

indicates that the cloned mu receptor is important in the production of morphine analgesia. This correlation was further confirmed in animals in which the gene encoding the mu receptor was disrupted, producing a "knockout." In these knockout animals, morphine lost all analgesic activity.

Recently, a number of additional mu opioid receptors have been cloned that originate from the same gene (Fig. 3). Termed splice variants, these mu receptors share the same sequence as that of most of the initial receptor. The only differences concern the tip of the receptor inside the cell, on which the amino acid sequences differ due to the presence of alternatively spliced exons within their mRNA. They all show the same high affinity and selectivity for morphine and mu drugs as the initial cloned receptor, but they display different regional distributions within the brain. Most areas have one or another variant, although some regions contain more than one, such as the dorsal horn of the spinal cord (an important pain-processing region). However, even within the dorsal horn the receptors are located on different cells. The relationship between these splice variants and subtypes defined with naloxonazine remains unclear.

Kappa Receptors

Kappa receptors were initially defined with the opiate ketocyclazocine, and three subtypes have been identified. Dynorphin A is the endogenous ligand for the kappa$_1$ receptor, which has been studied most extensively. Kappa$_1$ drugs are effective analgesics, particularly at the spinal level, and they appear to lack some of the side effects seen with morphine-like

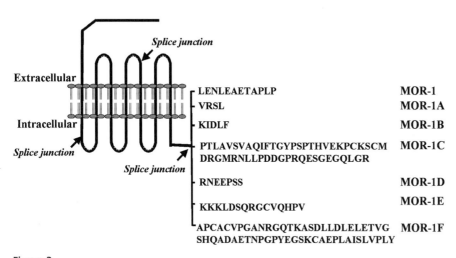

Figure 3

Schematic of the mu receptor splice variants of MOR-1. MOR-1, the first cloned mu receptor, contains four exons, with the last one (exon 4) encoding only 12 amino acids at the carboxy terminus. The shown variants contain the same first three exons as MOR-1, but instead of exon 4 they contain a variety of alternatively spliced exons that generate different amino acids at the amino terminus. The amino acids present in each of the splice variants downstream from the sequence encoded by exon 3 are given using letter abbreviations.

agents, such as respiratory depression. However, kappa$_1$ drugs have been reported to be unpleasant, with a high incidence of dysphoria and psychotomimetic effects. There are some clinical analgesics currently in use that work, in part, through kappa$_1$ receptors, but no selective drugs have made it to market. Interestingly, the highly selective kappa$_1$ drugs produce an intense diuresis.

Kappa$_1$ receptors have been cloned (KOR-1) from a number of species, including man. Like the mu receptor, kappa$_1$ receptors belong in the G protein family and are homologous to the mu receptor, as expected. When expressed, these cloned kappa$_1$ receptors show the same binding affinities and selectivities as previously demonstrated in brain. Like mu receptors, antisense and knockout studies have confirmed the importance of these cloned receptors in mediating the analgesic actions of kappa$_1$ analgesics.

Kappa$_2$ receptors are less well understood. They initially were defined in receptor binding studies. However, these studies required a complex combination of drugs to define the binding that could not be replicated *in vivo*. Thus, their pharmacology has remained unclear. Recently, evidence has suggested that the kappa$_2$ receptor may actually be a dimer composed of a kappa$_1$ receptor physically associated with a delta receptor. This receptor subtype needs to be studied further.

Kappa$_3$ receptors were initially discovered with the drug naloxone benzoylhydrazone. Like the other opioid receptors, kappa$_3$ receptors mediate analgesia and can be easily distinguished from the others by antagonists and antisense paradigms in animal models. A number of clinically available drugs have kappa$_3$ activity. Although the kappa$_3$ receptor has not been cloned, it appears to be closely related at the gene level to the orphanin FQ/nociceptin receptor (ORL$_1$).

Delta Receptors

Following the discovery of the enkephalins, a novel enkephalin-selective receptor, termed delta, was demonstrated in the mouse vas deferens bioassay and then the brain. Delta receptors can also elicit analgesia, but no delta-selective drugs are available clinically. However, thousands of analogs have been examined in animal studies and used to define delta pharmacology. Delta drugs do not have the same side effect profile as that of mu drugs and may be advantageous clinically. Like the other classes, subtypes of delta receptors, termed delta$_1$ and delta$_2$,

have been proposed based on antagonist studies. Although their pharmacology has not been completely evaluated, evidence suggests that delta$_2$ receptors mediate analgesia spinally and in the brain, whereas delta$_1$ receptors elicit analgesia primarily in the brain.

The delta receptor was the first opioid receptor cloned (DOR-1). Indeed, its sequence was used to isolate and identify the others. It is a G protein receptor highly similar to the others and its relevance to delta pharmacology was established using antisense and knockout strategies. However, the correlation of the cloned receptor with the pharmacologically defined subtypes is not entirely clear, although the cloned receptor appears to be most like the delta$_2$ receptor. Delta receptors have a distinct regional distribution within the brain. They can also couple with other receptor classes to form novel subtypes; for example, the combination of a delta receptor and a kappa$_1$ receptor forms the kappa$_2$ receptor.

Others

There are a number of other endogenous opioid peptides, which raises a question as to whether they also have their own receptors. Many investigators believe that β-endorphin has its own receptor, termed epsilon, but this remains controversial. Some of the other opioid peptides may also have their own receptors. Although sigma receptors were originally classified as opioid, recent work indicates that they are unique and not a member of the opioid receptor family. The sigma$_1$ receptor has been cloned and it is not even a member of the G protein-coupled receptor family.

—*Gavril W. Pasternak*

See also–Analgesics, Non-Opioid and Other; Heroin; Substance Abuse

Further Reading

Evans, C. J., Keith, D. E., Jr., Morrison, H., *et al.* (1992). Cloning of a delta opioid receptor by functional expression. *Science* 258, 1952–1955.
Kieffer, B. L. (1999). Opioids: First lessons from knockout mice. *Trends Pharmacol. Sci.* 20, 19–26.
Law, P.-Y., Wong, Y. H., and Loh, H. H. (2000). Molecular mechanisms and regulation of opioid receptor signaling. *Annu. Rev. Pharmacol. Toxicol.* 40, 389–430.
Pasternak, G. W. (1993). Pharmacological mechanisms of opioid analgesics. *Clin. Neuropharmacol.* 16, 1–18.
Pasternak, G. W., and Reisine, T. (1995). Opioid analgesics and antagonists. In *The Pharmacological Basis of Therapeutics* (J. G. Hardman and L. E. Limbird, Eds.), 9th ed. McGraw Hill, New York.

Oppenheim, Hermann

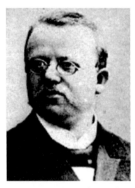

Hermann Oppenheim (reproduced with permission from the Louis D. Boshes Archives, University of Illinois at Chicago).

HERMANN OPPENHEIM (1858–1919) was a leading German neurologist of Jewish faith who strongly supported the development of neurology as an independent medical specialty. He was born in Warburg, Germany. His father was a rabbi and served as head of the district council. Oppenheim was an outstanding pupil, who studied medicine in Gottingen, Berlin, and Bonn. His doctoral thesis was on the physiology and pathology of urea excretion. In 1882, he became an intern at the Maison de Sante in Schöneberg near Berlin; then, he moved to the psychiatric clinic of the Royal Charite Hospital in Berlin in 1883. The head of the department and his teacher was Carl Westphal. Oppenheim published extensively on a diverse variety of neurological subjects, including syringomyelia, pseudobulbar palsy, bulbar paralysis, tabes dorsalis, neuritis, alcoholic paralysis, and lesions of the optic chiasm and traumatic neuroses. He was known for his ability to accurately localize lesions prior to neurosurgery (e.g., lesions of acoustic neuromas or spinal tumors). His skill in this area helped foster the growth and development of neurosurgery because clinical localization was an essential prerequisite in an era before the development or widespread use of arteriography, myelography, and other forms of neuroimaging. He published several articles with his neurosurgical colleagues, including M. Borchardt and F. Krause, on the results of neurosurgical operations. In 1889, he formulated the term "traumatic neurosis," hypothesizing this disorder to be based on organic microchemical brain changes not yet detected. This controversial theory won almost no support among his neurological or psychiatric contemporaries and colleagues.

Despite the clear support of the medical faculty at the Charite, Oppenheim failed to receive appointment as professor, which may have been due in part to the ingrained anti-Semitism prevalent at the time. Disappointed, Oppenheim left the Charite' and built a private neurological center that became well-known in Germany and abroad. He was appointed as a *Titularprofessor* in 1893.

In 1894, he published *Lehrbuch der Nervenkrankheiten* (*Textbook of Nervous Diseases*), which was reprinted in several editions and was translated into English (1911), Russian, Italian, and Spanish. It was one of the leading neurological textbooks in the era between the publication of Gowers' *Manual of Diseases of the Nervous System* (1886–1888) and S. A. K. Wilson's *Neurology* (1940).

Oppenheim was a founder member of the Society of German Neurologists and became president of this society in 1912. The unanimous rejection of his theory about traumatic neurosis led to his resignation of the presidency in 1916.

Oppenheim is remembered eponymously for his descriptions of amyotonia congenita, dystonia musculorum deformans, bilateral trigeminal neuralgia associated with multiple sclerosis, and characteristic personality changes (*Witzelsucht*) in frontal lobe lesions. He wrote comprehensive monographs on brain tumors, bulbar palsy without anatomical changes (myasthenic paralysis), encephalitis, brain abscesses, syphilis of the central nervous system, and both traumatic neurosis and war neurosis. His bibliography contains more than 220 publications.

Oppenheim died in 1919 at the age of 61 years due to a myocardial infarct. For more than 30 years, Oppenheim helped establish the identity of neurology in Germany. He believed that neurology should be an autonomous medical specialty, and he worked for this goal throughout his career. This explains why, in his obituary, A. Simons called Oppenheim "the undisputed leader of German neurology."

—*Rolf Malessa*

See also–Westphal, Carl (see Index entry Biography for complete list of biographical entries)

Further Reading

Harig, G. (1988). Zur Stellung und Leistung jüdischer Wissenschaftler an der Berliner Medizinischen Fakultät. *Charite'-Annalen.* 8, 213–214.

Simons, A. (1919). Hermann Oppenheim. *Z. ärztl Fortbild* **16**, 1–7.

Zülch, K. (1960). Hermann Oppenheim (1858–1919). In *Studium Berolinense* (H. Leussink, E. Neumann, and G. Kotowski, Eds.), pp. 285–289. De Gruyter, Berlin.

Optic Chiasm and Tract

Encyclopedia of the Neurological Sciences
Copyright 2003, Elsevier Science (USA). All rights reserved.

THE OPTIC CHIASM is a small (approximately 13 mm wide and 8 mm long), diagonally oriented (from a lateral view of the brain), X-shaped structure that lies on the undersurface of the brain above the pituitary gland (Fig. 1). It is formed by the decussation of the two optic nerves that carry axons of the retinal ganglion cell projections of each eye as they travel forward to the brain to transmit visual information. Each optic nerve contains slightly more than 1 million retinal ganglion cell axons. More than half of the axons of each optic nerve originate in the nasal retina and cross to the opposite side within the optic chiasm, whereas less than half originate in the temporal retina and pass through the optic chiasm without crossing over to the opposite side (Fig. 2). Therefore, the optic chiasm contains crossing visual

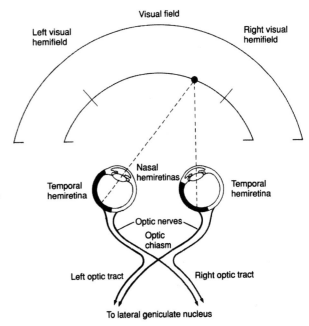

Figure 2
In the optic chiasm, the fibers of the nasal retina (i.e., the temporal visual field) of each eye cross, whereas the fibers of the temporal retina (i.e., the nasal visual field) of each eye proceed uncrossed. Thus, each optic tract contains visual fibers from the same hemifield of each eye [from Mason, C., and Kandel, E. R. (1991). Central visual pathways. In *Principles of Neural Science* (E. R. Kandel, J. H. Schwartz, and T. M. Jessel, Eds.), 3rd ed. Elsevier, New York. Reproduced with permission of The McGraw-Hill Companies].

fibers from the nasal retina of each eye and uncrossed visual fibers from the temporal retina of each eye.

As the visual fibers emerge from the posterior chiasm, they form the optic tracts. Due to the crossing arrangement within the chiasm, each optic tract contains visual fibers from the same side of the retina of each eye. That is, the right optic tract contains fibers from the temporal retina of the right eye and nasal retina of the left eye, and the left optic tract contains fibers from the temporal retina of the left eye and nasal retina of the right eye (Fig. 2). In this way, the same visual field from each eye (i.e., homonymous) is transmitted to the opposite visual cortex, located in the occipital lobe of the brain.

The retinal ganglion cell axons that pass through the optic chiasm and each optic tract synapse within the paired lateral geniculate nuclei that lie on either side of the upper brainstem. The lateral geniculate nuclei function as the relay station for visual information traveling from the retina to the visual cortex of the occipital lobe (Fig. 3).

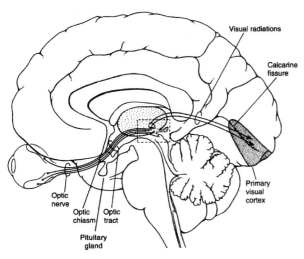

Figure 1
The optic chiasm, formed as the two optic nerves intersect and join together, is shown lying just under the surface of the brain but above the pituitary gland [from Mason, C., and Kandel, E. R. (1991). Central visual pathways. In *Principles of Neural Science* (E. R. Kandel, J. H. Schwartz, and T. M. Jessel, Eds.), 3rd ed. Elsevier, New York. Reproduced with permission of The McGraw-Hill Companies].

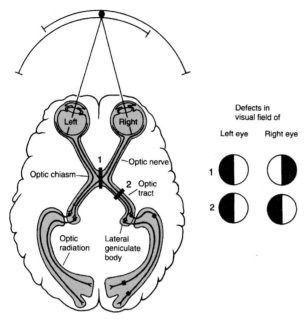

Figure 3
Due to the anatomical arrangement of the visual pathway, lesions of the optic chiasm and optic tract will generally produce characteristic patterns of visual field loss. The defect indicated for injury of the optic chiasm is referred to as a bitemporal hemianopia, whereas that corresponding to injury of an optic tract is a homonymous hemianopia [from Mason, C., and Kandel, E. R. (1991). Central visual pathways. In *Principles of Neural Science* (E. R. Kandel, J. H. Schwartz, and T. M. Jessel, Eds.), 3rd ed. Elsevier, New York. Reproduced with permission of The McGraw-Hill Companies].

The optic chiasm and tracts receive their blood supply from branches of the circle of Willis, major arteries at the base of the brain that surround these structures. The pituitary gland, a major organ responsible for hormonal metabolism, lies below the optic chiasm within the bony confines of the sella turcica at the base of the skull (Fig. 1). The cavernous sinus—a venous compartment that contains the three ocular motor nerves, the first division of the trigeminal nerve, oculosympathetic neurons, and a segment of the carotid artery—is positioned on either side of the optic chiasm. In clinical practice, it is important to recall these relationships because mass lesions may arise from them and compress the visual pathways.

CLINICAL CORRELATIONS

The major way to clinically assess the functional integrity of the optic chiasm and tracts is by assessing the visual field of each eye. The anatomical arrange-

ment of the optic chiasm and tracts ensures that visual information from each side of the visual field is transmitted to the opposite side of the brain. For example, when an object appears in the right visual hemifield, the nasal retina of the right eye and temporal retina of the left eye are stimulated (Fig. 2). The nasal retinal ganglion cell axons from the right eye cross in the chiasm to the left optic tract and the temporal retinal ganglion cell axons from the left eye pass uncrossed into the left optic tract. In this way, visual information from each eye is transmitted to the left visual cortex in the occipital lobe. Therefore, injury to either optic tract affects the opposite visual field of each eye, which is a clinical sign referred to as homonymous hemianopia (Fig. 3).

Since the optic chiasm contains crossing fibers from each nasal retina, injury to it will affect the temporal visual field of each eye. This clinical sign is referred to as bitemporal hemianopia (Fig. 3). Although it is not completely understood why the crossing fibers are preferentially susceptible to damage, it may be that they are relatively vulnerable to stretch injury from mass lesions or vascular compromise.

Gross abnormalities of the visual field can be detected in a face-to-face (patient-to-examiner) series of maneuvers, referred to as confrontational visual field testing. For example, if the patient cannot accurately count the examiner's fingers when they are quickly presented randomly in the right visual hemifield of each eye as the patient faces the examiner, this indicates a right-sided homonymous hemianopia. In addition, there are a variety of commercially available visual field testing devices, some automated and computerized and others that rely on a technician to explore the visual field, that are far more sensitive and quantitative for detecting and measuring abnormalities.

Besides trauma, mass lesions are the largest group of disorders that injure the optic chiasm and tracts. Of these, the most common include tumors of the pituitary gland, referred to as pituitary adenomas (Fig. 4). Other common neoplasms that injure these structures include meningiomas and craniopharyngiomas. In children, especially those with neurofibromatosis type I, tumors of the anterior visual pathways (e.g., chiasmal glioma) are an important cause of visual loss due to compression or infiltration of the neural pathways of vision. Benign cystic masses may arise from the region of the sella turcica to compress the optic chiasm. Cerebral aneurysms arising from the circle of Willis that

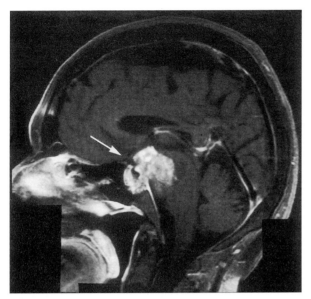

Figure 4
Magnetic resonance image of a side view (sagittal orientation) of the brain showing a large tumor arising from the pituitary gland (arrow). The optic chiasm cannot be seen because it is engulfed by the mass.

Optic Nerve (Cranial Nerve II)

Encyclopedia of the Neurological Sciences
Copyright 2003, Elsevier Science (USA). All rights reserved.

BY VIRTUE of its position as the second collection of fibers from the anterior/rostral end of the brain, the optic nerve has been labeled cranial nerve II. Notwithstanding this terminology, the optic nerve is distinguished from all other cranial nerves by several important anatomical and physiological properties; it is not a peripheral nerve at all. The optic nerve is in fact a white matter tract. It derives its myelin from oligodendrocytes and not Schwann cells; hence, it is prone to diseases of the central nervous system and not those of the peripheral nervous system.

The optic nerve carries approximately 1.2 million axons that derive from the retinal ganglion cells of the ipsilateral eye. By comparison, the acoustic nerve carries only approximately 30,000 fibers. Given the demands for high visual resolution, it should not be surprising that the optic nerve has been estimated to comprise 38% of all fibers that enter or exit the brain.

Retinal ganglion cells differentiate and contribute fibers that form the precursor of the optic nerve at approximately 5 weeks of gestation. These fibers grow back and reach the optic chiasm by approximately week 7. At this point, there are approximately 4 million axons in the primitive optic nerve. At approximately 16 weeks, many of these fibers begin to undergo apoptosis, reducing their number to that found in maturity. This initial overproduction and subsequent dying back may add to the specificity of retinal ganglion cell connections.

Converse to the direction of growth of the retinal ganglion cell axons, myelination begins at the optic chiasm at approximately 13 weeks of gestation and progresses toward the eye, reaching the lamina cribosa of the optic disk at birth or soon thereafter. Technically, the optic nerve now consists of fibers (axons with myelin sheaths).

RETINA

Visual transduction begins at the retina. However, unlike the simplistic analogy of "film in the back of the camera," a great deal of information processing occurs in the neural layers of the retina. At a minimum, there is temporal and spatial modulation of the signal between the percipient elements (rods

have not ruptured may present clinically by producing visual loss due to compression of the optic chiasm or tracts. Certain strokes can cause unilateral optic tract injury and produce homonymous hemianopia. Because of the strong association between mass lesions and visual field abnormalities referable to optic chiasm and tract injury, computed tomography or magnetic resonance imaging (Fig. 4) are usually one of the first steps employed to evaluate a patient with bitemporal hemianopia or homonymous hemianopia.

—*Daniel M. Jacobson*

See also–Brain Anatomy; Circle of Willis; Optic Nerve (Cranial Nerve II); Visual Fields

Further Reading

Glaser, J. S. (1990). Topical diagnosis: The optic chiasm. In *Neuro-ophthalmology*, 2nd ed., pp. 171–211. Lippincott, Philadelphia.
Hoyt, W. F. (1970). Correlative functional anatomy of the optic chiasm. *Clin. Neurosurg.* 17, 189–208.
Kline, L. B. (1998). Anatomy and physiology of the optic tracts and lateral geniculate nucleus. In *Walsh and Hoyt's Clinical Neuro-ophthalmology* (N. R. Miller and N. J. Newman, Eds.), 5th ed., pp. 101–120. Williams & Wilkins, Baltimore.
Slamovits, T. L. (1998). Anatomy and physiology of the optic chiasm. In *Walsh and Hoyt's Clinical Neuro-ophthalmology* (N. R. Miller and N. J. Newman, Eds.), 5th ed., pp. 85–100. Williams & Wilkins, Baltimore.

and cones), through the midretina (bipolar cells, horizontal cells, and amacrine cells), and to the inner retina (retinal ganglion cells). The final common pathway of the system comprises retinal ganglion cells whose axons converge, somewhat like the spokes of a wheel, into a 1.8-mm-diameter disk that forms the anterior end of the optic nerve. It is likely that there are two or more classes of retinal ganglion cells in man. More than 90% of the fibers are so-called P cells, which project to the parvocellular layers of the lateral geniculate nucleus (LGN). These cells are highly concentrated at the fovea (the portion of the retina that corresponds to fixation). In contrast, M cells project to the magnocellular layers of the LGN and are more linearly distributed across the retina.

As a consequence of this arrangement and the distribution of the photoreceptors (the cones are concentrated in the foveal area and the rods dispersed more peripherally), vision is most acute centrally not only in terms of acuity but also in terms of color vision and contrast sensitivity. As one moves progressively away from the central retina, there is a nonlinear decrease in sensitivity of several visual parameters. A large number of ganglion cells reflect this high density of photoreceptors at the fovea and form a bundle of axons that project directly to the temporal aspect of the optic disk. This papillomacular nerve fiber bundle is distinct from other axons, which reach the optic nerve head by a more arcuate course. The superior and inferior bands of axons never cross an imaginary horizontal midline that divides the retina into upper and lower halves.

Approximately 120 million rods and 6 million cones send input into the 1.2 million retinal ganglion cells whose axons form the optic nerve. There is attrition of both photoreceptors and retinal ganglion cells in the human retina in aging (especially after age 60) and disease.

The retinal ganglion cell axons form the nerve fiber layer, which is the innermost (anterior) component of the retina. The nerve fiber layer maintains a certain degree of retinotopy as it traverses the retina and then turns 90° posteriorly through the optic disk into the optic nerve. This retinotopy appears to become tighter as one proceeds posteriorly, but the fibers become disorganized again near the optic chiasm. At the optic chiasm, the fibers that derive from the nasal retina (approximately 53 or 54% of the total) decussate, whereas the fibers that derive from temporally located retinal ganglion cells remain ipsilateral in the chiasm and optic tract.

OPTIC NERVE HEAD

The optic nerve head, or papilla, constitutes the beginning of the optic nerve. Funduscopically, this appears as a yellow-orange disk that often has a small empty space centrally, termed the optic cup. At the optic nerve head, the 1.2 million nerve fibers gather and exit the globe. The optic nerve head does not represent the center of the visual field. It is located approximately 3 mm nasal to the fovea and hence produces a blind spot approximately 15° temporal to center. The optic nerve head is approximately 1.75 mm in horizontal diameter and 1.92 mm in vertical diameter.

The retinal nerve fibers must turn 90° while progressing posteriorly into the optic nerve. As they do so, they pass through stacks of perforated collagen plates termed the lamina cribrosa. The lamina cribrosa acts as a sieve that permits the axons to exit the eye while sealing in vitreous fluid that is maintained at a relatively high pressure (on average, 16 mm of mercury). This seal is maintained by specialized glial cells that surround the columns of axons as they pierce through the fenestrations of the collagen plates. More posteriorly, these bundles of nerve fibers are separated by well-defined collagen septae. Immediately behind the lamina cribrosa, the axons that constitute the optic nerve become myelinated. As a consequence, the diameter of the optic nerve increases from approximately 1.8 to 3.5 mm posterior to the lamina.

The sclera, which provides the structural support for the eye, blends into the dura mater as the outer meningeal cover of the optic nerve. In contrast, the arachnoid and the pia mater stop at the level of the posterior lamina cribrosa, resulting in a cul-de-sac for the subarachnoid space (Fig. 1).

OPTIC NERVE

The optic nerve runs from the eye to the optic chiasm. The retinal ganglion cell axons that constitute the nerve continue to project past the optic chiasm to terminate in various visual nuclei in the brain. The portion designated the optic nerve thus has anatomical, but not physiological, meaning. With this in mind, the optic nerve can be further divided into four segments. The intraocular segment includes the optic nerve head and is 1 mm in length. The intraorbital segment is free to move loosely in a bed of fat and runs for approximately 25 mm. The intracanalicular optic nerve is approximately 9 mm long and runs

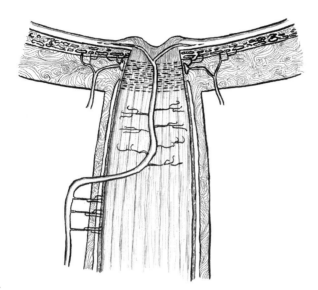

Figure 1
The optic nerve is covered by meninges. The dura mater is the outer meningeal cover of the optic nerve and it blends into the scleral covering of the eye. In contrast, the arachnoid and the pia mater of the optic nerve stop at the level of the posterior lamina cribrosa, resulting in a cul-de-sac for the subarachnoid space. The optic nerve fibers form approximately 1000 bundles with approximately 1000 axons in each bundle. Collagen septae separate these bundles. The ophthalmic artery and opthalmic vein run alongside the proximal optic nerve until they are 10–12 mm from the back of the eye, at which point they cross the arachnoid space and pia and pierce the nerve to a central position at the lamina cribrosa.

through a bony canal, sharing space with its blood supply, the ophthalmic artery. The intracranial optic nerve is approximately 16 mm long and ends at the optic chiasm. The optic nerve becomes wider as it courses posteriorly. The intraorbital optic nerve is approximately 3.5 mm in diameter anteriorly and approximately 5 mm in diameter in the posterior orbit. This is largely due to the thickening of connective tissues that form the septae. These septae, as well as the tough surrounding meninges, provide supple but strong support to the optic nerve, which must remain flexible in the orbit.

The optic nerve head has several anatomical and physiological features that make it vulnerable to damage. Glaucoma causes optic nerve damage through increased intraocular pressure. Anterior ischemic optic neuropathy is a consequence of reduced blood flow within the tight confines of the scleral canal. Since the intraorbital segment of the optic nerve is more than 25 mm long and the distance between the back of the globe and the orbital apex is less than 20 mm, there is linear "redundancy" of the

intraorbital optic nerve. This allows the nerve to easily move from side to side as the eye moves. It also allows the nerve to slip to the side when there is penetrating injury to the orbit. Finally, this slack allows for approximately 7 or 8 mm of proptosis before injury occurs to the nerve or the back of the globe.

The intraorbital optic nerve is fairly well protected. However, diseases that may affect any portion of the optic nerve, such as optic neuritis, occur here as well. The intracanicular segment is vulnerable because of its position in the optic nerve canal. Fractures of the sphenoid bone cause direct crush or sheer injury (traumatic optic neuropathy). Problems that lead to brain swelling may cause the optic nerve to compress its own blood supply in the tight confines of the canal (posterior ischemic optic neuropathy). The intracranial optic nerve may be subject to compressive injury from masses in the parasellar area, including pituitary adenomas or aneurysms of the ophthalmic artery.

The ophthalmic artery derives from the carotid artery at the anterior end of the carotid siphon. It slips into an infranasal position and runs along the optic nerve in its intracranial, intracanicular, and intraorbital course. A number of small penetrating vessels originate from the ophthalmic artery and join the pial circulation of the nerve. Approximately 12 mm posterior to the globe, the major portion of the ophthalmic artery traverses the subarachnoid space and enters the inferior aspect of the optic nerve. It then turns anteriorly and, together with the central retinal vein, runs into the eye through the middle of the optic nerve head, becoming the central retinal artery. The central retinal artery is not a significant contributor of circulation to the anterior optic nerve head. Instead, this region is supplied primarily by branches from an arterial complex that forms a ring (the circle of Zinn–Haller) around the optic nerve head. This arterial complex is fed by three or four short posterior ciliary arteries and by bridging vessels from the choroidal circulation (Fig. 1).

Blunt trauma may injure the intracanalicular portion of the nerve, either directly or by sheering branches of the ophthalmic artery that join the pial blood vessels. The dural covering of the optic nerve fuses with the periostium of the optic canal. The arachnoid and the subarachnoid space is continuous with that of the brain. This intracanalicular portion of the optic nerve is most vulnerable on its medial side, where the bony wall of the optic canal is very thin or may not exist at all; there may be only optic nerve sheath and mucosa separating the optic nerve from the ethmoid sinus. As the intracanalicular nerve exists the canal to become the intracranial nerve, there is a stiff falciform fold of dura superiorly that may notch the nerve in the settings of trauma or brain swelling.

The optic nerve partially decussates at the optic chiasm and joins the ipsilateral fibers from the other side to form the optic tract. In man, most of these fibers project to the LGN. However, just posterior to the optic chiasm, some fibers emanate from the tracts superiorly to enter one of three nuclei of the hypothalamus: the supraoptic, paraventricular, or suprachiasmatic nuclei. More posteriorly, a fascicle of axons branches off the optic tract to form the brachium of the superior colliculus, terminating in the optic tectum and pretectal nuclei. In the LGN, layers 1, 4, and 6 receive afferents from the contralateral eye and layers 2, 3, and 5 receive afferents from the ipsilateral eye. There are at least two types of retinal ganglion cells that project in a segregated fashion to the LGN. M cells terminate in layers 1 and 2 (magnocellular) of the LGN, and P cells terminate in layers 3–6 (parvocellular) of the LGN. This segregation continues past the LGN relay to the visual cortex. Anatomical separation of fibers has a physiological counterpart, with M cells relating more to high contrast sensitivity, low spatial frequency, and motion stereopsis and P cells subserving low contrast sensitivity, high spatial frequency, color, and high spatial resolution.

—Alfredo A. Sadun

***See also*–Abducens Nerve (Cranial Nerve VI); Accessory Nerve (Cranial Nerve XI); Facial Nerve (Cranial Nerve VII); Glossopharyngeal Nerve (Cranial Nerve IX); Hypoglossal Nerve (Cranial Nerve XII); Oculomotor Nerve (Cranial Nerve III); Olfactory Nerve (Cranial Nerve I); Oligodendrocytes; Optic Nerve Disorders; Retina; Trigeminal Nerve (Cranial Nerve V); Trochlear Nerve (Cranial Nerve IV); Vagus Nerve (Cranial Nerve X); Vestibulocochlear Nerve (Cranial Nerve VIII)**

Further Reading

Bruesch, S. R., and Arey, L. B. (1942). The number of myelinated and unmyelinated fibers in the optic nerve of vertebrates. *J. Comp. Neurol.* 77, 631.

Chou, P. I., Sadun, A. A., and Lee, H. (1996). Vasculature and morphometry of the optic canal and intracanalicular optic nerve. *J. Neurol. Ophthalmol.* 16, 325.

Chou, P. I., Sadun, A. A., Chen, Y. C., *et al.* (1996). Clinical experiences in the management of traumatic optic neuropathy. *J. Neurol. Ophthalmol.* 16, 325.

Collelo, R. J., and Schwab, M. E. (1994). A role for oligodendrocytes in the stabilization of optic axon numbers. *J. Neurosci.* 14, 6446.

Curcio, C. A., Millican, C. L., Allen, K. A., *et al.* (1993). Aging of the human photoreceptor mosaic: Evidence for selective vulnerability of rods in central retina. *Invest. Ophthalmol. Vis. Sci.* 34, 3278.

Hubel, D. H., Wiesel, T. H. N., and LeVay, S. (1977). Plasticity of oxular dominance columns in monkey striate cortex. *Philos. Trans. R. Soc. London Biol. Sci.* 278, 377.

Johnson, B. M., Miao, M., and Sadun, A. A. (1987). Age-related decline of human optic nerve axon populations. *Age* 10, 5–9.

Jonas, J. B., Gusek, G. C., and Naumann, G. O. H. (1988). Optic disc, cup and neuroretinal rim size, configuration and correlations in normal eyes. *Invest. Ophthalmol. Vis. Sci.* 29, 1151.

Kurosawa, H., and Kurosawa, A. (1985). Scanning electron microscopic study of pial septa of the optic nerve in humans. *Am. J. Ophthalmol.* 99, 490.

Livingston, M. S., and Hubel, D. H. (1987). Psychophysical evidence for separate channels for the perception of form, color movement, and depth. *J. Neurosci.* 7, 3416.

Livingstone, M., and Hubel, D. (1998). Segregation of form, color, movement, and depth: Anatomy, physiology, and perception. *Science* 240, 740.

Minckler, D. S. (1989). Histology of optic nerve damage in ocular hypertension and early glaucoma (Summary). *Surv. Ophthalmol.* 33, 401.

Onda, E., Cioffi, G. A., Bacon, D. R., *et al.* (1995). Microvasculature of the human optic nerve. *Am. J. Ophthalmol.* 120, 92.

Osterberg, G. (1935). Topography of the layer of rods and cones in the human retina. *Acta Ophthalmol.* 6, 1–103.

Provis, J. M., van Driel, D., Billson, F. A., *et al.* (1985). Human fetal optic nerve overproduction and elimination of retinal axons during development. *J. Comp. Neurol.* 238, 92.

Sadun, A. A., Johnson, B. M., and Smith, L. E. H. (1986). Neuroanatomy of the human visual system: Part III. Retinal projections to the superior colliculus and pulvinar. *NeuroOphthalmology* 6, 363.

Van Buren, J. M. (1963). *The Retinal Ganglion Cell Layer*, p. 130. Thomas, Springfield, IL.

Optic Nerve Disorders

Encyclopedia of the Neurological Sciences

THE OPTIC NERVE is a 50-mm-long central nervous system white matter tract myelinated by oligodendrocytes. A large branch of the ophthalmic artery enters the inferior portion of the nerve approximately 10 mm behind the globe to become the central retinal artery. This vessel supplies blood to most of the retina, but only insignificant amounts to the optic nerve head. The optic nerve head is primarily supplied by the circle of Zinn–Haller, a collection of anastomotic arterioles arising from the posterior ciliary arteries, and the pial and peripapillary choroidal circulation. Approximately 25 mm of the nerve is located in the orbits, with the proximal portion surrounded by the origins of the recti muscles (the annulus of Zinn). The optic canal is 4–10 mm long and runs through the sphenoid bone. This canal contains the optic nerve, the ophthalmic artery, branches of the sympathetic plexus, and the meninges that form the optic nerve sheath. The dural covering and the periosteum of the optic canal are fused and the arachnoid is continuous, allowing the optic nerve to be surrounded by cerebrospinal fluid. The nerves are fixed at the intracranial opening of the canal, with the inferior surface of the frontal lobe above them. The optic nerves join at the chiasm in the floor of the third ventricle. The 15- to 20-mm intracranial length of the nerve rises at approximately a 45° angle from the anterior clinoid process.

Most of the visual loss from optic nerve disorders occurs acutely, although compression can cause slow loss. Typically, there is loss of the central visual field, reduced visual acuity, color vision loss, and an afferent pupillary abnormality in the involved eye. Visual evoked potential (VEP) testing demonstrates prolonged latency in demyelinative disorders. In primarily axon loss lesions, a typical VEP finding is an absent, attenuated, or dispersed potential of abnormal morphology. Contrast sensitivity is reduced. The optic nerve head may be normal or swollen and usually develops atrophy after several weeks following acute damage. The presence or absence of pain, the patient's age, extent of recovery over time, and imaging findings are all important in establishing the correct diagnosis.

OPTIC NEURITIS

Optic neuritis is the most common optic neuropathy in the 18- to 45-year-old age group. In high-risk populations, it occurs in approximately 3 per 100,000 individuals per year. In lower risk populations, the annual incidence is approximately 1 per 100,000. It presents in 92% of patients as a painful loss of vision, often worse with eye movement. Visual loss may progress over 1 or 2 weeks and usually begins to improve within 1 month. There is usually excellent visual recovery. In 77% of cases, optic neuritis occurs in females. Papillitis (optic disk swelling) is present in 35% of cases, and some visual abnormality is present in 67% of patients. In monosymptomatic optic neuritis, vision recovers sooner with the administration of intravenous methyl prednisolone followed by prednisone compared to oral prednisone or placebo. After 30 days, patients typically have very good recovery of visual acuity. Visual acuity rarely worsens following discontinuation of steroids (2%). Recurrent optic neuritis occurs more often in patients treated with oral prednisone alone than in those treated with intravenous steroids or placebo (although this result is unexplained and controversial), indicating that this type of treatment should be avoided. Neurological events sufficient to diagnose a patient as having clinically definite multiple sclerosis (CDMS) develop at a slower rate among monosymptomatic optic neuritis patients taking intravenous methyl prednisolone during the first 2 years of follow-up. After 2 years, however, differences between treatment groups are not significant.

In monosymptomatic optic neuritis, magnetic resonance imaging (MRI) is superior to all other CDMS prognostic indicators (Table 1). If MRI is

Table 1 PERCENTAGE OF MONO-SYMPTOMATIC OPTIC NEURITIS PATIENTS WHO DEVELOP CLINICALLY DEFINITE MULTIPLE SCLEROSIS AFTER SPECIFIC TIME INTERVALS ACCORDING TO BASELINE MRI[a]

Time after entry	Baseline MRI		
	Normal (N = 202)	One or two lesions (N = 61)	Three or more lesions (N = 89)
6 months	1.0	6.8	17.2
1 year	2.6	14.0	25.6
2 years	4.9	19.7	31.7
3 years	9.3	27.7	43.1
4 years	13.3	35.4	49.8
5 years	16	37	51

[a]Excludes patients with probable or definite MS at time of study entry.

normal at baseline, the risk of developing MS at 5 years is 16%. If there are three or more periventricular white matter abnormalities, the risk of developing MS at 5 years is 51%. Patients with a normal MRI and a lack of pain, mild visual acuity loss, severe disk edema, disk or peripapillary hemorrhage, or macular exudates have a very low risk of CDMS. Usually, there is only mild disability after 5 years in patients who go on to develop MS. A benefit has been reported for starting anti-MS medication (β-interferon-1α) in patients with monosymptomatic optic neuritis and an abnormal MRI scan. Chest x-ray, blood tests, and lumbar puncture are not usually necessary to evaluate patients with typical clinical features of optic neuritis.

ANTERIOR ISCHEMIC OPTIC NEUROPATHY

Nonarteritic anterior ischemic optic neuropathy (AION) is the most common cause of acute optic nerve disease in patients older than 50 years. Approximately 6000 new cases occur annually in the United States. It usually presents as severe, sudden, painless loss of vision in one eye. It is associated with pale swelling of the optic nerve head in the involved eye (Fig. 1). The other eye often has a small cup to disk ratio, implying that anatomy contributes to the disorder. AION is thought to be due to occlusion of small branches of the posterior ciliary arteries. The unaffected eye can become involved later in up to 40% of cases.

Within 6 months, in approximately 40% of patients visual acuity improves by three lines. Average age of onset is 64 in smokers and 70 in nonsmokers. Approximately 70% of patients have a history of hypertension, diabetes, or tobacco use. Acute nonarteritic AION is always associated with disk elevation due to ischemia.

A key symptom to differentiate AION from optic neuritis is the absence of pain in the former. Approximately 90% of patients with optic neuritis usually recover most of their vision, whereas only approximately 40% of AION patients recover three lines of vision.

TEMPORAL (GIANT CELL) ARTERITIS

Giant cell arteritis (GCA) is a condition of the elderly. It usually occurs after age 70. The incidence increases with age, from 2.3 per 100,000 among patients in the sixth decade of life to 44.7 per

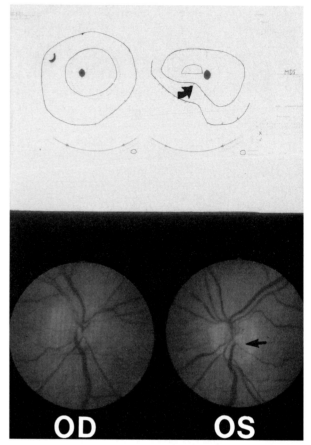

Figure 1

A 68-year-old man had sudden onset of painless visual loss in the right eye (OD). The inferior altitudinal defect is shown on visual field plot (top, arrow). The right optic nerve is edematous. The left optic nerve has a cup to disk ratio of less than 0.1 (bottom, arrow). These are typical features of nonarteritic anterior ischemic optic neuropathy. (See color plate section.)

100,000 in the ninth decade. If left untreated, it can rapidly cause blindness or infarction of other tissues, including the brain. Systemic features include jaw and tongue claudication, scalp tenderness, headache, fever, malaise, weight loss, anorexia, anemia, and joint aches. The sedimentation rate is usually elevated, although it may occasionally be normal. Visual loss is usually severe. When there is optic disk edema, it tends to appear pallid or "milky" (Fig. 2). Visual loss in GCA can also present with no optic disk edema as a retrobulbar optic neuropathy. Nonarteritic AION patients typically have a small cup to disk ratio in the unaffected eye (Fig. 1), whereas the disks of patients with GCA can be of any size. Thus, a large cup to disk ratio in the unaffected eye of a patient with AION should raise

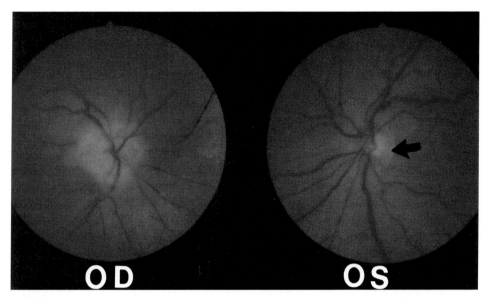

Figure 2
Milky swelling of the right optic nerve in an 80-year-old patient with giant cell arteritis (compare the disk appearance to that in Fig. 1). Note that the normal left eye has a cup to disk ratio of 0.4 (arrow). (See color plate section.)

the suspicion of GCA (Fig. 2). The rate of visual loss and the clinical picture in arteritic AION with GCA can be quite similar to those of the nonarteritic form. Only approximately 5% of patients with AION have temporal arteritis. The sudden onset of visual loss with optic disk edema, typical systemic complaints, and elevated sedimentation rate usually allow GCA to be diagnosed. A 2.5-cm temporal artery biopsy with up to 50 serial sections should be done to confirm the diagnosis. Steroids (1–1.5 mg/kg prednisone per day) should be started immediately, without waiting for biopsy, because the arterial pathology will remain diagnostic for weeks (Fig. 3). Some authors suggest using high doses of solumedrol (10–15 mg/km per day intravenously) at the onset of therapy.

Even with a good clinical response, steroids must be tapered slowly over months. Steroids should be reduced slowly enough to avoid recurrence of systemic symptoms and keep the sedimentation rate relatively low. If steroid side effects appear, methotrexate can be added to speed the taper.

COMPRESSIVE AND INFILTRATIVE OPTIC NEUROPATHY

Compressive optic neuropathy can be associated with proptosis, diplopia, disk edema, and visual loss. It may be caused by masses, metastatic infiltration, or thyroid orbitopathy. Proper imaging of the entire optic nerve from globe to chiasm is essential. Although computed tomography (CT) scan is popular for imaging the orbit, MRI is excellent for demonstrating occult compression when surface coils with fat suppression and contrast techniques are used. The brain should also be imaged with MRI in suspicious cases. Treatment may include surgery, radiation, and chemotherapy, depending on pathology.

HEREDITARY OPTIC NEUROPATHY

Hereditary optic neuropathy comprises a group of inherited disorders that usually present as painless visual loss. Imaging is typically negative. The most important of these disorders is Leber's hereditary optic neuropathy (LHON). Men are afflicted with this condition much more commonly than women (9:1 ratio). LHON usually strikes between ages 15 and 35 and begins with painless visual loss in one eye.

At onset, Leber's can be confused with optic neuritis. However, there is rarely pain. When there is no major improvement in vision and the second eye becomes involved weeks to months later, with visual loss usually approximately 20/200, the diagnosis becomes more clear. In the acute phase, there is usually some optic disk edema with vessel tortuosity,

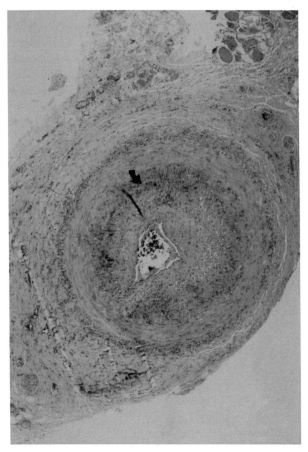

Figure 3
Positive temporal artery biopsy performed 3 weeks after starting steroids. There are numerous lymphocytes present in the internal elastic lamina (arrow), a pathognomonic sign of arteritis. (See color plate section.)

hemorrhage, and exudates. LHON is caused by mitochondrial DNA mutations, usually located at the 11778, 3460, and 14484 positions. Visual loss usually remains severe, although slow improvement can occur. The mitochondrial defect influences prognosis, with that at 11778 having the worst prognosis and that at 14484 the best. Treatment has been unsatisfactory. Avoiding tobacco, alcohol, and environmental toxins by patients at genetic risk has been recommended.

OTHER CAUSES OF OPTIC NEUROPATHY

Traumatic optic neuropathy is a complication of head injury and may occur even when external signs of damage are minor. In unresponsive patients, this diagnosis is often made on the basis of an afferent pupillary deficit. CT scanning is done to search for periorbital fracture and bleeding. MRI can be helpful in some cases. Currently, no therapy is of undisputed value. For this condition, the intravenous administration of methyl prednisolone in a 30 mg/km loading dose followed by 15 mg/km every 6 hr for 24–48 hr has been suggested by some authors. Optic canal decompression surgery using transethmoid or trans-sphenoidal approaches has occasionally been helpful.

Nutritional deficiency optic neuropathy can be caused by chronically reduced intake or malabsorption of nutrients such as thiamine and vitamin B_{12}. Toxic optic neuropathy can be caused by exposure to methanol, ethylene glycol, and ethambutol or by heavy, chronic use of tobacco and alcohol. A history of exposure should be sought and other optic neuropathies should be carefully eliminated.

Congenital anomalies of the optic disk include optic disk hypoplasia, drusen, optic nerve pits, and congenital optic atrophy. These can be associated with central nervous system and systemic malformations.

—David I. Kaufman

***See also*–Giant Cell (Temporal) Arteritis; Oligodendrocytes; Optic Nerve (Cranial Nerve II)**

Further Reading

Beck, R. W., Cleary, P. A., Trobe, J. D., *et al.* (1993). The effect of corticosteroids for acute optic neuritis on the subsequent development of multiple sclerosis. *N. Engl. J. Med.* **329**, 1764–1769.

Jacobs, L. D., Beck, R. W., Simon, J. H., *et al.* for the Champs study group (2000). Intramuscular interferon beta-1a therapy initiated during a first demyelinating event in multiple sclerosis. *N. Engl. J. Med.* **343**, 898–904.

Kaufman, D. I., Trobe, J. D., Eggenberger, E. R., *et al.* (2000). Practice parameter: The role of corticosteroids in the management of acute monosymptomatic optic neuritis. *Neurology* **54**, 2039–2044.

Kelman, S. E. (1998). Ischemic optic neuropathies. In *Clinical Neuro-Ophthalmology* (N. R. Miller and N. J. Newman, Eds.), 5th ed., pp. 549–598. Williams & Wilkins, Baltimore.

Miller, N. R., and Newman, N. J. (1997). *Walsh and Hoyt's Clinical Neuro-Ophthalmology*, 4th ed. Williams & Wilkins, Baltimore.

Newman, N. J. (1998). Hereditary optic neuropathies. In *Clinical Neuro-Ophthalmology* (N. R. Miller and N. J. Newman, Eds.), 5th ed., pp. 741–773. Williams & Wilkins, Baltimore.

ONTT Study Group (1997). Five year risk of multiple sclerosis after optic neuritis. Experience of the ONTT. *Neurology* **49**, 1404–1413.

Steinsapir, K. D., and Goldberg, R. A. (1998). Traumatic optic neuropathies. In *Clinical Neuro-Ophthalmology* (N. R. Miller and N. J. Newman, Eds.), 5th ed., pp. 715–739. Williams & Wilkins, Baltimore.

Optokinetic Nystagmus

Encyclopedia of the Neurological Sciences
Copyright 2003, Elsevier Science (USA). All rights reserved.

OPTOKINETIC NYSTAGMUS refers to the nystagmus induced by full-field visual motion. The term refers to the series of eye movements that occur when a subject attempts to fixate on a series of moving targets in the visual field. Optokinetic nystagmus, which is characterized by a jerk nystagmus whose slow component is in the direction of the moving targets and whose fast component is in the opposite direction, is a normal, physiological response, although stimuli for it are infrequent in daily life. The stimulus for optokinetic nystagmus, full-field visual motion, occurs normally whenever the head is moved in a lighted environment. The vestibulo-ocular reflex and the optokinetic system work synergistically to produce appropriate eye movements in this setting.

One common circumstance in which optokinetic nystagmus can be observed is during vehicular travel (e.g., while looking out the window from a moving train). In a clinical or research setting, optokinetic nystagmus is best induced by a moving, full-field stimulus such as projected stripes or a motor-driven visual surround. Strictly speaking, optokinetic nystagmus cannot be induced properly at the bedside since the stimulus (drum or tape) does not encompass the full visual field. Although nystagmus will occur when subjects observe small, patterned moving targets, in this case it is the pursuit system that generates the response rather than the optokinetic system. When the optokinetic system is properly activated, a perception of self-motion will be induced, which is called circularvection. Otokinetic nystagmus can be induced in the horizontal, vertical, or torsional direction depending on the stimulus. When inducing optokinetic nystagmus, the instructions given to the subject are critical. Examples include "count each stripe as it moves past," "look at each stripe as it moves past," or "stare at the stripes." Remarkably, each of these subtly different commands produces a different amount of eye movement.

The neural pathways underlying optokinetic nystagmus include the same pathways that are important for ocular pursuit, as well as the accessory optic system. At the onset of the optokinetic nystagmus response, the pursuit system contributes most significantly. If a subject is in complete darkness when the optokinetic stimulus stops, nystagmus will continue, which is called optokinetic after nystagmus.

The clinical usefulness of optokinetic nystagmus is limited since an assessment of ocular pursuit usually provides the same information. However, a left–right asymmetry in optokinetic nystagmus can be the result of a unilateral cerebral lesion. Also, optokinetic nystagmus has been used to determine whether blindness is psychogenic; the presence of optokinetic nystagmus implies that the apparently blind person can actually see. Optokinetic movement can also be used to test visual acuity in infants and can be used as a means of observing convergence–retraction nystagmus in some patients with midbrain abnormalities.

—*Joseph M. Furman*

***See also*–Bárány, Robert; Eye Movements, Saccades; Nystagmus and Saccadic Intrusions and Oscillations**

Organic Acid Disorders

Encyclopedia of the Neurological Sciences
Copyright 2003, Elsevier Science (USA). All rights reserved.

ORGANIC ACIDS (OAs) comprise a group of carbonic acids physiologically occurring as intermediates in a variety of intracellular metabolic pathways, such as catabolism of amino acids, mitochondrial ß-oxidation of fatty acids, the tricarboxylic acid cycle, and neurotransmitters, as well as cholesterol biosynthesis. Organic acid disorders (OADs) are caused by autosomal recessive inherited deficiencies of single enzymes in the outlined metabolic pathways and appear with a cumulative frequency of 1:2500 newborn; thus, they are the most common, life-threatening inborn errors of metabolism. The diagnostic hallmark of all OADs is an accumulation of characteristic OAs (and their corresponding acylcarnitines) upstream of the genetic block. OAs can be detected by gas chromatography–mass spectrometry (GC-MS) in blood, urine, and cerebrospinal fluid, and acylcarnitines can be detected by tandem mass spectrometry (MS-MS) in dried blood spots. Because OAs have different metabolic origins, the term organic acid disorders is based on the same diagnostic approach and does not reflect a common nosology. Neurological manifestations are especially common in OADs (e.g., in branched-chain OADs) or

Table 1 CLASSIFICATION OF ORGANIC ACID DISORDERS WITH NEUROLOGICAL MANIFESTATION

OAD subgroup	Disease	Enzyme	Gene
Cerebral	Glutaric aciduria type I	Glutaryl-CoA dehydrogenase	19p3.2
	4-Hydroxybutyric aciduria	Succinic semialdehyde dehydrogenase	6p22
	N-Acetylaspartic aciduria	Aspartoacylase	17p13-pter
	L-2-Hydroxyglutaric aciduria	?	?
	D-2-Hydroxyglutaric aciduria	?	?
	Mevalonic aciduria	Mevalonate kinase	12p24.1
Branched chain	Methylmalonic acidurias	Methylmalonyl-CoA mutase	6p12–21.1
	Propionic aciduria	Propionyl-CoA carboxylase	α: 13q32
		(α, β chains)	β: 3q21–22
	Maple syrup urine disease	Branched-chain α-keto acid dehydrogenase	E1$_α$: 19q13.2–q13.2
		(E1$_α$, E1$_β$, E2 subunits)	E1$_β$: 6p22–p21
			E2: 1p31

even the predominant feature in a subgroup of OADs that is termed cerebral (Table 1).

CEREBRAL ORGANIC ACID DISORDERS

Cerebral OADs characteristically present with progressive neurological signs and symptoms, such as macrocephaly, ataxia, myoclonus, extrapyramidal signs, and metabolic "stroke," but only exceptionally with acidosis, hypoglycemia, myopathy, or pancreatitis, the classic signs of OADs. This subgroup includes glutaric aciduria type I, 4-hydroxybutyric aciduria, N-acetylaspartic aciduria (Canavan's disease), L-2- and D-2-hydroxyglutaric acidurias, and mevalonic aciduria.

Glutaric Aciduria Type I

Glutaric aciduria type I (GA-I), first described in 1975, occurs with an estimated frequency of 1:40,000 newborns but has a higher frequency (up to 1:300 newborns) in genetically homogeneous communities, such as the Amish community in Pennsylvania or the Saulteaux-Ojibway Indians in Canada. It is caused by autosomal recessive inherited deficiency of glutaryl-CoA dehydrogenase (GCDH), a mitochondrial key enzyme in the catabolic pathways of the amino acids L-tryptophan, L-lysine, and L-hydroxylysine that catalyzes the decarboxylation and dehydrogenation of glutaryl-CoA to crotonyl-CoA. Approximately 100 disease-causing mutations in the GCDH gene, localized on chromosome 19p13.2, have been described, with R402W being the most frequent mutation in Caucasians, accounting for 10–20% of alleles. Deficiency of GCDH results in an accumulation of the marker metabolites

glutaric, 3-hydroxyglutaric, and glutaconic acids as well as glutarylcarnitine in body fluids, which can be detected by GC-MS or MS-MS. Because a subgroup of GA-I patients reveals only slight elevations of glutaric acid in urine despite severe disease progression, repeated quantitative urinary OA analysis or even specific determination of 3-hydroxyglutaric acid by stable isotope dilution techniques must be performed. GCDH activity can be determined in skin fibroblasts, amniocytes, and chorion biopsies.

Affected newborns and infants initially present with minor neurological signs and symptoms of hypotonia, irritability, and jitteriness. An important clue to diagnosis is the finding of macrocephaly, which is not necessarily present at birth but develops in 75% of affected infants between the ages of 3 and 6 months. Neuroimaging in this period typically reveals frontotemporal atrophy, widening of the Sylvian fissure(s) due to reduced opercula, subdural hemorrhages (often misdiagnosed as battered child syndrome), and delayed myelination, reflecting delayed cerebral maturation. If not diagnosed and treated early, GA-I is complicated by signs and symptoms of acute encephalopathy in 75% of affected patients, commonly occurring between the ages of 6 and 12 months and precipitated by acute febrile illness or even routine vaccinations. These encephalopathic crises result in irreversible destruction of vulnerable regions of brain, predominantly affecting the striatum and subsequently leading to a loss of previously acquired motor skills and the development of permanent dystonic/dyskinetic movement disorders with relatively well-preserved intellectual function. If the underlying metabolic disorder remains undiagnosed, additional cerebral systems are slowly and progressively destroyed. Growing evidence points to an excitotoxic sequence in GA-I as the underlying cause of neurodestruction, with 3-hydroxyglutaric acid acting as an endogenous neurotoxin via stimulation of N-methyl-D-aspartate receptors. However, genotype–phenotype correlation is poorly understood in GA-I, and the outcome of the disease depends on the development of acute encephalopathy rather than on residual enzyme activity or genotype. Treatment consists of a tryptophan- and lysine-restricted diet with reduction of natural protein intake as well as supplementation with L-carnitine. During intercurrent illness, the intravenous glucose, L-carnitine, electrolytes, and insulin are administered on an emergency basis. Since neurological deterioration in GA-I patients is preventable by appropriate treatment prior to onset of an encephalopathy, early diagnosed and treated children develop adequately, whereas patients who have an acute encephalopathy are severely handicapped and may die later in childhood.

4-Hydroxybutyric Aciduria

4-Hydroxybutyric aciduria, first identified in 1981, is a rare neurometabolic disorder with approximately 150 diagnosed patients worldwide. It is caused by an autosomal recessive inherited deficiency of succinic semialdehyde dehydrogenase (SSADH), which catalyzes the last step (succinic semialdehyde to succinic acid) in the catabolism of the inhibitory neurotransmitter γ-aminobutyric acid (GABA). Deficient SSADH, encoded by the SSADH gene that is localized on chromosome 6p22, gives rise to the upstream metabolite 4-hydroxybutyric acid (GHB), which accumulates in cerebrospinal fluid and is excreted in the urine. It can be detected by urinary organic acid analysis but isotope dilution analysis may be required for reliable diagnosis, especially in older patients because of the age-dependent decline of urinary excretion of GHB. SSADH activity can be determined in lymphoblasts, amniocytes, and chorion biopsies. The GABA metabolite GHB, which was initially employed as an agent for induction of anesthesia in children, possesses a variety of neuromodulatory features based on its interactions with dopamine, $GABA_A$, $GABA_B$, NMDA, and opiate receptors in the central nervous system. Illicit use of GHB revealed partial resemblance of the neurological manifestations in 4-hydroxybutyric aciduria. The clinical phenotype of 4-hydroxybutyric aciduria is notably heterogeneous, even within sibships. Psychomotor retardation and hypotonia invariably occur.

Behavioral problems, ocular motor apraxia, seizures, hyporeflexia, ataxia, and hyperkinesia can also be present. Based solely on clinical grounds, these features could be consistent with a variety of cerebellar syndromes or encephalopathies in childhood, and in the absence of accurate organic acid analysis 4-hydroxybutyric aciduria would not likely be a strong candidate in the differential diagnosis. An experimental therapeutic approach for affected children is the use of the antiepileptic drug vigabatrin, an inhibitor of GABA transaminase, which may result in increased alertness, improved attention span, ataxia, and better manageability. Vigabatrin has consistently increased GABA and decreased succinic semialdehyde and GHB concentrations in the cerebrospinal fluid.

N-Acetylaspartic Aciduria (Canavan's Disease)

N-Acetylaspartic aciduria (Canavan's disease), first described in 1989, is a neurodegenerative disease that is caused by deficient aspartoacylase (N-acetylasparaginase) and is biochemically characterized by the accumulation and increased urinary excretion of N-acetylaspartic acid (NAA), which can be detected by GC-MS. The diagnosis is confirmed by the enzymatic analysis of skin fibroblasts. Canavan's disease is found in all populations, but there is a higher frequency in the Ashkenazic Jews. The frequent missense mutation E285A in the aspartoacylase gene, localized on chromosome 17p13-pter, accounts for 80% of alleles in the Ashkenazim and for 60% of alleles in patients of non-Jewish origin.

In healthy individuals, NAA is found exclusively in high concentrations in brain tissue, but its biological function remains unclear. Canavan's disease presents with progressive neurological symptoms and signs starting at age 2–4 months. Progressive macrocephaly, hypotonia with prominent head lag, seizures, and the loss of previously acquired skills are regularly found. As the disease progresses, affected children develop optic nerve atrophy, pyramidal signs, and finally a decerebrate state. Neuroimaging studies show symmetrical leukodystrophic changes with loss of arcuate fibers of the cerebral white matter, and neuropathological studies show spongiform degeneration, particularly of the cortex and subcortical white matter. There is no known effective treatment. The prognosis of infantile Canavan's disease is fatal, whereas milder disease courses have been described in some patients.

L-2-Hydroxyglutaric Aciduria

As in the case of Canavan's disease, L-2-hydroxyglutaric aciduria is characterized by progressive loss of myelinated arcuate fibers and a spongiform encephalopathy. However, the time course and clinical features are different. In the first 2 years of life, mental and psychomotor development appear normal or only slightly delayed. Thereafter, progressive mental retardation, seizures, ataxia, and variable extrapyramidal signs become the most obvious clinical findings. By adolescence, patients are bedridden and severely mentally retarded (IQ 40–50). The neuroimaging findings in L-2-hydroxyglutaric aciduria are characterized by progressive loss of cerebral arcuate fibers, progressive cerebellar atrophy, and signal changes in the basal ganglia. L-2-Hydroxyglutaric acid is found to be highly elevated in all body fluids and can be detected by GC-MS combined with stereospecific chromatographic differentiation of L-2- from the stereoisomeric D-2-hydroxyglutaric acid. The pathogenesis of L-2-hydroxyglutaric aciduria is unknown. There is no specific therapy, but the seizure disorder can generally be controlled by the administration of standard antiepileptic medications.

D-2-Hydroxyglutaric Aciduria

Patients with D-2-hydroxyglutaric aciduria exhibit a variable phenotype and have been classified into two subgroups based on clinical and neuroradiological findings. Severely affected children present in early infancy, with the onset of encephalopathy manifested by severe psychomotor retardation, intractable seizures, cerebral visual failure, hypotonia, and cardiomyopathy. Neuroimaging studies of patients in this group show enlarged lateral ventricles, subependymal cysts, enlarged frontal subarachnoid spaces and subdural effusions, and signs of delayed cerebral maturation. Moderately affected children show variable symptoms, including mental retardation, macrocephaly, and hypotonia. Neuroimaging findings may show delayed cerebral maturation, ventriculomegaly, or subependymal cysts. The biochemical hallmark of this disease is the accumulation of D-2-hydroxyglutaric acid in all body fluids, which can be detected by GC-MS. Moreover, increased GABA and total protein concentrations are often found in cerebrospinal fluids. The underlying inherited defect in D-2-hydroxyglutaric aciduria is unknown. There is no known specific therapy.

Mevalonic Aciduria

Mevalonic aciduria, first described in 1986, inherited as an autosomal recessive trait, is a disorder of the peroxisomal cholesterol and nonsterol isoprene biosynthesis caused by mevalonate kinase deficiency. Mevalonate kinase catalyzes the phosphorylation of mevalonic acid, the product of the reduction of 3-hydroxy-3-methylglutaryl-CoA to 5-phosphomevalonic acid. Because cholesterol biosynthesis is regulated by feedback inhibition of its product cholesterol, this feedback loop is lost in mevalonate kinase deficiency, resulting in exorbitant accumulation and urinary excretion of mevalonic acid, which can be detected by GC-MS. Pathogenesis of mevalonic aciduria remains unclear, but clinical symptoms seem related to lack of cholesterol and other isoprenoids rather than to accumulation of mevalonic acid. The clinical presentation is variable. The most severely affected patients die in infancy with profound developmental delay, dysmorphic features, cataracts, hepatosplenomegaly, lymphadenopathy, anemia, thrombocytopenia, diarrhea, and malabsorption. Patients may also develop retinitis pigmentosa. Hematological findings also include variable and sometimes marked leukocytosis. The overall presentation may be mistaken for a myeloproliferative disorder. The intellectual impairment appears to be stationary, in contrast to progressive ataxia and dysarthria, in which it is paralleled by cerebral atrophy. A characteristic feature of mevalonic aciduria is recurrent crises with fever, lymphadenopathy, increase in the size of liver and spleen, arthralgia, edema, and morbilliform rashes without metabolic derangement. In between crises, standard chemical investigations are normal except for elevated serum creatine kinase in most patients. A rational treatment is not available and the prognosis is doubtful.

BRANCHED-CHAIN ORGANIC ACID DISORDERS

Branched-chain OADs comprise a group of neurometabolic disorders resulting from inherited defects of specific enzymes mainly involving the catabolism of branched-chain amino acids. This subgroup includes methylmalonic acidurias, propionic aciduria, and maple syrup urine disease, so named because of the sweet odor. Unlike for cerebral OADs, these patients present with classic metabolic symptomatology, such as acidosis, hypoglycemia, myopathy, or pancreatitis, but in addition develop characteristic neurological symptoms. There are three schematic presentation groups: a severe neonatal-onset form with metabolic abnormalities; a chronic, intermittent, late-onset form; and a chronic, progressive form presenting with hypotonia, failure to thrive, and developmental delay.

Methylmalonic Acidurias

Methylmalonic acidurias comprise a group of diverse inherited disorders that appear with a cumulative prevalence of 1:50,000 in Caucasians, with the common biochemical sign being methylmalonic acid accumulation in body fluids. Isomerization of L-methylmalonyl-CoA to succinyl-CoA is catalyzed by the mitochondrial enzyme methylmalonyl-CoA mutase (MCM), which is dependent on adenosylcobalamin as its cofactor. Classic methylmalonic aciduria is caused by mutations in the MCM gene (6p12–21.1), whereas it can be alternatively caused by defects in the biosynthesis of adenosylcobalamin or by deficient cobalamin transport. Residual activity of deficient MCM corresponds to mutations in the MCM gene as well as to severity of clinical presentation, reflecting a genotype–phenotype correlation in methylmalonic acidurias. Clinically, classic methylmalonic aciduria presents with severe neonatal metabolic crises, progressive failure to thrive, feeding problems, recurrent vomiting, dehydration, hepatomegaly, lethargy, seizures, and developmental delay. Furthermore, symmetrical necrosis of the globus pallidus is increasingly recognized in affected patients. In most cases, these lesions result from acute stroke-like events and are manifested by extrapyramidal signs. In other patients, neurological symptoms progress slowly over several years, resulting from poor metabolic control. Methylmalonic acid is considered to inhibit brain energy metabolism by several mechanisms, thus facilitating or primarily causing neuronal damage in methylmalonic acidurias. Diagnosis is based on the urinary detection of elevated methylmalonic acid concentrations and related metabolites (propionic acid, 3-hydroxypropionic acid, and methylcitrate) by GC-MS as well as increased concentrations of glycine and alanine (possibly also homocystein and methionin) by quantitative amino acid analysis. MCM activity can be investigated in skin fibroblasts. Classic methylmalonic aciduria is treated by restriction of isoleucine, valine, methionine, and threonine and by supplementation of L-carnitine. Cobalamin-dependent methylmalonic acidurias respond to substitution with vitamin B_{12}. The prognosis of classic methylmalonic aciduria is doubtful despite therapy, whereas vitamin B_{12}-reponsive methylmalonic acidurias have a reasonable outcome.

Propionic Aciduria

Propionic aciduria is one of the more common inherited disorders of OA metabolism, with a prevalence in Caucasians of 1:40,000 newborn. It is inherited as an autosomal recessive trait and is characterized by a deficiency of propionyl-CoA carboxylase (PCC). PCC is a biotin-dependent, heterotetrameric or heterohexameric enzyme consisting of α and β chains that carboxylyzes propionyl-CoA to methylmalonyl-CoA. The most frequent disease-causing mutations comprise deletions in the PCCB gene (3q21–22), encoding for the PCC β chain. Deficient PCC gives rise to propionic acid and other abnormal metabolites, such as methylcitrate, 3-hydroxypropionate, and propionylglycine, which can be detected by GC-MS. Elevated propionic acid interferes with a variety of metabolic pathways. Pathophysiologically relevant actions of propionic acid are an inhibition of N-acetylglutamate synthase, an enzyme of the urea cycle, resulting in hyperammonemia in metabolic crises, as well as a reduction of activity of cytochrome c oxidase and Krebs cycle enzymes, resulting in reduced ATP synthesis and lactic acidemia. Propionic aciduria frequently presents with severe metabolic acidosis, ketosis, lactic acidemia, hyperammonemia, hyperglycinemia, and hyperglycinuria. Neurological symptoms and signs are frequent, including the development of chorea and dystonia associated with basal ganglial hypodensities in neuroimaging studies, suggesting selective vulnerability of basal ganglia, particularly the globus pallidus, to disordered propionate metabolism. Furthermore, affected patients show developmental delay and mental retardation and seizures secondary to cerebral atrophy. Long-term treatment is based on the dietary restriction of isoleucine, valine, methionine, and threonine as well as supplementation with L-carnitine. Moreover, the facilitation of adequate emergency treatment of neonatal metabolic crises prior to confirmation of therapy is of utmost importance. Despite early diagnosis and treatment, the neonatal-onset form is still complicated by early death in infancy or childhood, whereas patients with the late-onset form reach adulthood, though often they are handicapped by severe extrapyramidal movement disorders.

Maple Syrup Urine Disease

In maple syrup urine disease (MSUD), branched-chain amino acids (leucine, isoleucine, and valine) and their corresponding α-keto acid derivatives are increased in physiological fluids due to inherited deficiency of the thiamin-dependent branched-chain α-keto acid dehydrogenase complex (BCKD), consisting of subunits $E_{1\alpha}$, $E_{1\beta}$, E_2, and E_3. Five different forms of the disease have been delineated, which differ with respect to age of onset, clinical severity, biochemical manifestations, residual enzyme activity, and responsiveness of BCKD to its cofactor thiamine. The classic form of MSUD presents in the neonatal period with poor feeding, irritability, lethargy, and progressive neurological deterioration, including alternating hypertonia and hypotonia with dystonic extension of the arms. The intermediate form of MSUD develops slowly, with progressive failure to thrive, developmental delay, and/or seizures. The intermittent form, which may present with seizures, stupor, or coma, is likely to be precipitated by increased protein intake or intercurrent illnesses. The clinical symptomatology of the fourth type is a thiamine-responsive form of MSUD, in which the metabolic disturbance is ameliorated by pharmacological doses of thiamine, similar to that seen in the intermediate form. The fifth type of MSUD is the deficiency of lipoamide dehydrogenase (E_3 deficiency) and is manifested after the neonatal period with failure to thrive, hypotonia, developmental delay, movement disorder, and progressive neurological deterioration.

Neuroimaging studies of patients with untreated MSUD show a characteristic pattern of diffuse generalized cerebral edema as well as localized edema affecting the cerebellar deep white matter, dorsal brain stem, cerebral peduncles, the posterior limb of the internal capsule, and the posterior aspect of the centrum semiovale. Hypomyelination is suggested and hypodensities may be present in the globus pallidus and the thalamus. Prominent neuropathological signs of untreated MSUD include cerebral atrophy and myelin deficiency, in addition to spongy degeneration and moderate astrocytic hypertrophy of the white matter. In the cerebellum, necrosis of granular cells and extensive neuronal loss are apparent in the pontine nuclei and substantia nigra. Electroencephalographic (EEG) abnormalities include comb-like rhythms (5–9 Hz) of spindle-like sharp waves over the central regions with multiple shifting spikes and sharp waves and burst suppression. The neuroradiological, neuropathological, and EEG findings of MSUD patients are characteristic. Diagnosis is confirmed by detection of an accumulation and increased urinary excretion of ∂-keto acids and branched-chain amino acids using GC-MS and quantitative amino acid analysis. Emergency therapeutic measures include forced anabolism to facilitate accumulated leucine and other branch-chain amino acids into protein, by infusions of electrolytes, glucose, and insulin, followed by long-term treatment with dietary restriction of branched-chain amino acids and substitution of thiamine if beneficial. Children

Table 2 ORGANIC ACIDS AS ENDOGENOUS NEUROTOXINS

Disease	Organic acid	Suggested neurotoxic effects
Glutaric aciduria type I	3-Hydroxyglutaric acid	NMDA receptor stimulation
		Phosphocreatine depletion
		Inhibition of glutamate decarboxylase
	Glutaric acid	Inhibition of synaptosomal glutamate uptake
		Inhibition of glutamate decarboxylase
D-2-Hydroxyglutaric aciduria	D-2-Hydroxyglutaric acid	NMDA receptor stimulation
		ATP synthase inhibition
Methylmalonic acidurias	Methylmalonic acid	Inhibition of succinate dehydrogenase
		Pyruvate decarboxylase
		β-Hydroxybutyrate dehydrogenase
		Transmitochondrial malate shuttle
Propionic aciduria	Propionic acid	Inhibition of N-acetylglutamate synthase
		Cytochrome c oxidase
Maple syrup urine disease	α-Keto isocaproic acid	Induction of glial and neuronal apoptosis
		Reduced cell respiration

ORGANIC SOLVENTS

diagnosed and treated early (i.e., before 5 days of age) have a satisfactory prognosis.

EXCITOTOXIC PATHOGENIC MECHANISMS IN ORGANIC ACID DISORDERS

The pathogenesis of the presented OADs is still poorly understood. Consequently, treatment of neurological symptoms is mostly restricted to symptomatic approaches. There is increasing evidence that some OAs act as endogenous neurotoxins by inhibition of mitochondrial energy metabolism (respiratory chain, β-oxidation of fatty acids, and tricarboxylic acid cycle), stimulation of N-methyl-D-aspartate receptors, and inhibition of physiological detoxification systems such as the urea cycle (Table 2). The organic acids are no longer exclusively considered as diagnostic metabolites of organic acid disorders but may serve as clues to their pathophysiology. Since understanding the pathogenesis is the prerequisite for developing rational neuroprotective strategies in OADs, it is hoped that this will improve current therapeutic regimens.

—*Stefan Kölker and Georg F. Hoffmann*

See also–Amino Acid Disorders

Further Reading

Chuang, D. T., and Shih, V. E. (1995). Disorders of branched chain amino acid and keto acid metabolism. In *The Metabolic and Molecular Bases of Inherited Disease* (C. R. Scriver, A. L. Beaudet, W. S. Sly, and D. Valle, Eds.), 7th ed., pp. 1239–1277. McGraw-Hill, New York.

Fenton, W., and Rosenberg, L. E. (1995). Disorders of propionate and methylmalonate metabolism. In *The Metabolic and Molecular Bases of Inherited Disease* (C. R. Scriver, A. L. Beaudet, W. S. Sly, and D. Valle, Eds.), 7th ed., pp. 1423–1449. McGraw-Hill, New York.

Gibson, K. M., Hoffmann, G. F., Hodson, A. K., *et al.* (1998). 4-Hydroxybutyric acid and the clinical phenotype of succinic semialdehyde deydrogenase deficiency, an inborn error of GABA metabolism. *Neuropediatrics* 29, 14–22.

Goodman, S. I., and Frerman, F. E. (1995). Organic acidemias due to defects in lysine oxidation: 2-ketoadipic acidemia and glutaric acidemia. In *The Metabolic and Molecular Bases of Inherited Disease* (C. R. Scriver, A. L. Beaudet, W. S. Sly, and D. Valle, Eds.), 7th ed., pp. 1451–1460. McGraw-Hill, New York.

Hoffmann, G. F., and Gibson, K. M. (1996). Disorders of organic acid metabolism. In *Handbook of Clinical Neurology* (H. W. Moser, Ed.), Vol. 22, pp. 639–660. Elsevier, Amsterdam.

Jouvet, P., Rustin, P., Taylor, D. L., *et al.* (2000). Branched chain amino acids induce apoptosis in neural cells without mitochondrial membrane depolarization or cytochrome c release:
Implications for neurological impairment associated with maple syrup urine disease. *Mol. Biol. Cell* 11, 1919–1932.

Kölker, S., Ahlemeyer, B., Krieglstein, J., *et al.* (2000). Maturation-dependent neurotoxicity of 3-hydroxyglutaric and glutaric acids in vitro: A new pathophysiologic approach to glutaryl-coA dehydrogenase deficiency. *Pediatr. Res.* 47, 495–503.

Surtees, R. A. H., Matthews, E. E., and Leonard, J. V. (1992). Neurologic outcome of propionic acidemia. *Pediatr. Neurol.* 8, 333–337.

Van der Knaap, M. S., Jakobs, C., Hoffmann, G. F., *et al.* (1999). D-2-Hydroxyglutaric aciduria: Biochemical marker or clinical disease entity? *Ann. Neurol.* 45, 111–119.

Wajner, M., and Coelho, J. C. (1997). Neurological dysfunction in methylmalonic acidaemia is probably related to the inhibitory effect of methylmalonate on brain energy production. *J. Inherit. Metab. Dis.* 20, 761–768.

Organic Solvents

Encyclopedia of the Neurological Sciences
Copyright 2003, Elsevier Science (USA). All rights reserved.

ORGANIC SOLVENT is a general term for chemical compounds or mixtures that extract, dissolve, or suspend non-water-soluble materials. Most are liquids and may be simple or complex in their structure. When individuals develop neurotoxic signs from organic solvent exposure, they have usually been poisoned by accident in the workplace, although deliberate intoxication can occur. Characteristics that typify solvents include high volatility (easy evaporation), lipophilia or high solubility in fat, lack of objectionable odor, and a propensity to cause some chemical dependency. Breakdown or metabolism of solvents often results in the production of other chemicals, called intermediate compounds, and these can also have toxic effects.

Several chemicals are included in the category of organic solvents. Some are listed in Table 1, with the usual neurotoxicological syndrome associated with exposure. In the painting industry, in which solvents are used in paints as well as in the cleaning fluids used in preparation and cleanup, mixtures of solvents (e.g., turpentine) can be associated with both acute intoxication and possibly chronic conditions such as memory loss, poor mental concentration, and depression. Some authors have alluded to a "painter's encephalopathy" to encompass such conditions, but the existence of this syndrome as a specific occupational disorder has been debated.

—*Christopher G. Goetz*

Table 1   ORGANIC SOLVENTS OF NEUROLOGICAL IMPORTANCE

Organic solvent	Usual route of exposure	Neurological signs
Ethylene glycol	Inhalation Accidental or purposeful drinking	Restlessness, followed by somnolence and coma Cessation of breathing Seizures
Formaldehyde	Accidental Purposeful dipping of cigarettes or marijuana in formaldehyde, then smoking	See Methanol

Benzene	Accidental fume inhalation
	Purposeful ingestion in suicide attempts
	Benzene intoxication can be seen as part of pharmacological treatment of chronic leukemias
		Acute intoxication
		    Euphoria with inhalation
		    Ataxia, muscle twitching
		    Seizures, paralysis
		Chronic intoxication
		    Tingling and weakness of extremities (peripheral neuropathy)
		    Hand weakness (median nerve neuropathy)
		    Seizures

Toluene	Accidental or purposeful inhalation	Exhilaration, fatigue Confusion and poor memory Psychotic behaviors Tremor and shaking Unsteadiness in walking Weakness and tingling in the extremities (peripheral neuropathy)
n-Hexane	Accidental or purposeful inhalation	Weakness and tingling in the extremities (peripheral neuropathy) Parkinsonism
Methyl-N-butyl ketone	Usually purposeful inhalation	Weakness and tingling in the extremities (peripheral neuropathy)
Tetrachlorethane	Accidental inhalation	Narcotic-like effects, somnolence, decreased respirations, coma
Trichlorethylene	Accidental and purposeful inhalation	Cranial (especially trigeminal nerve) and peripheral neuropathies Blindness from optic neuropathy Anxiety, insomnia, fatigue

Turpentine and nonspecified solvent mixtures	Accidental inhalation or ingestion
	Purposeful inhalation or ingestion
		Acute intoxication
		    Headache, fatigue, confusion
		Chronic intoxication
		    Fatigue, memory loss, sleep disruptions, depression
		    Weakness and tingling sensations in the extremities from neuropathy (Huffer's neuropathy)
		    Gait instability and poor coordination
		    Rarely muscle damage

Carbon tetrachloride	Accidental inhalation and purposeful ingestion in suicide attempts	Headaches, drowsiness Peripheral neuropathy and blindness from optic nerve damage

See also–Environmental Toxins; Methyl Alcohol; Organophosphates, Organochlorides, and Pesticides

Further Reading

Anetseder, M., Hartung, E., Klepper, S., *et al.* (1994). Gasoline vapors induce severe rhabdomyolysis. *Neurology* **44**, 2393–2395.

Filley, C. M., Heston, R. K., and Rosenberg, N. L. (1990). White matter dementia in chronic toluene abuse. *Neurology* **40**, 532–534.

Karlson-Stiber, C., and Persson, H. (1993). Ethylene glycol poisoning: Experiences from an epidemic in sweden. *J. Toxicol. Clin. Toxicol.* **31**, 499–500.

Pastore, C., Marhuenda, D., Marti, J., *et al.* (1994). Early diagnosis of n-hexane-caused neuropathy. *Muscle Nerve* **17**, 981–986.

Pezzoli, G. (1989). Parkinsonims due to n-hexane exposure. *Lancet* 2, 874.

Tetrud, J. W., Langston, J. W., and Irwin, I. (1990). Acute and persistent parkinsonism associated with ingestion of petroleum product mixture. *Ann. Neurol.* 28, 296.

Organophosphates, Organochlorides, and Pesticides

Encyclopedia of the Neurological Sciences
Copyright 2003, Elsevier Science (USA). All rights reserved.

ORGANOPHOSPHATES are powerful inhibitors of two important enzymes, acetylcholinesterase and pseudocholinesterase. In humans, the former enzyme is found in nervous tissue, specifically in brain, spinal cord, and myoneural junctions, at pre- and postganglionic parasympathetic synapses, and at preganglionic and some postganglionic sympathetic nerve endings of the portion of the nervous system known as the autonomic nervous system. Excess acetylcholine causes overstimulation and then depolarization blockade of the receptors for the important neurochemical or neurotransmitter acetylcholine. Most major organophosphate poisoning has been reported to occur with parathion, methylparathion, or derivatives. Subacute or chronic intoxication can be seen especially in farmers and industrial workers. Clinically, intoxication may range from latent, asymptomatic poisoning to a life-threatening illness. Toxicity is usually graded by serum cholinesterase activity. Decreases of 10–50% may not even be clinically detectable, but when levels are moderately depressed (20% normal), sweating, cramps, tingling of the extremities, and mild weakness of the swallowing musculature occur. At 10% normal, consciousness becomes depressed and myosis develops with no pupillary response to light. The intoxicated subject may become cyanotic from respiratory weakness, and pooled secretions may obstruct the airway. Although symptoms generally abate after removal of the causative agent, the resolution may be very slow; headaches and weakness may persist for 1 month and eye discomfort has been reported 5 months after exposure.

For treatment, pralidoxine is usually used intravenously to reverse the acute cholinergic alterations. The major action of this drug is to reactivate organophosphate-inhibited acetylcholinesterase ac-tivity. Pancuronium improves the neuromuscular transmission defect most likely by blockade of cholinergic receptors. High-risk groups for periodic intoxication are farmers and rural inhabitants. A study of 98 persons with regular contact to insecticides showed reductions in cholinesterase activity in 30%, despite no specific complaints.

Neuropathy can develop several days or even weeks after exposure to organophosphates. In these cases, acute cholinergic toxicity is followed after several days with a delayed, progressive weakness including foot drop, absent ankle jerk, and muscle weakness. Examples of responsible compounds are tri-aryl phosphate, nipafox, trichlorfon, and methamidophos, as well as triorthocresyl phosphate. There is no correlation, however, between the potency of acute cholinergic effects and the likelihood of neuropathy. The pathophysiology of this later onset neuropathy does not appear to relate to effects on the cholinergic system, and the mechanism appears to relate to a two-step phosphorylation and "aging" of the protein called neuropathy target esterase. Finally, there is a third organophosphate syndrome, termed intermediate, that involves weakness of the extremities and respiratory and swallowing muscles developing between 24 and 96 hr after toxin exposure. This condition has been most frequently reported in India and Sri Lanka, and the chemical mechanism of the toxic signs has not been studied extensively.

Triorthocresyl phosphate (TOCP) is an especially important compound related to organophosphate insecticides, and it induces a specific form of toxicity. The neurotoxicity of TOCP was recognized early in the 20th century when peripheral neuropathy accompanied phosphocreosote therapy for tuberculosis. In the 1920s, the epidemic of ginger paralysis in the southern United States created new interest in the neurotoxicity of TOCP, and the large number of intoxicated patients clarified the characteristic pattern of the disease. Ingestion of the toxic oily substance in amounts approximating 1 g was followed 12 hr later by gastrointestinal upset, and 1 to 2 weeks later, a dramatic flaccid paralysis developed, beginning distally in the legs and often accompanied by aches and tingling paresthesias. With larger doses, the weakness spread to the intrinsic hand muscles, the pelvic girdle, and the thighs. Cranial nerves remained spared, and sensory involvement was markedly less than motor involvement. Although the syndrome appeared initially as a neuropathy affecting only peripheral nerves, residual signs of spasticity and ataxia emphasized the marked involvement of the central nervous system. Although cholinergic overactivity may be important to the predominantly gastrointestinal prodrome, it is unlikely to play a significant pathogenic role in the delayed neurotoxicity of TOCP. Pathological studies suggest that TOCP exerts a direct toxic effect on axons by altering structural components of axonal and synaptic vesicle membranes. The primary axonal degeneration becomes apparent at approximately Day 8 and correlates well with the onset of clinical paresis. The axons of the peripheral nerve and those of the longest spinal cord tracts are similarly affected.

The chlorinated hydrocarbon insecticides, with dichlorodiphenyltrichloroethane (DDT) as the prototype, share many toxic properties, although individual variations exist. They are all highly soluble in fats and oils, and most are extremely enduring in the environment, making chronic toxicity a serious ecological and clinical problem. Pregnant women pass organochlorines to the fetus, and for humans, contaminated food provides 80% of organochlorine exposure. As a group, these compounds are primarily toxic to the nervous system, the major manifestations being tremor and convulsions. Another syndrome of concern is the neurobehavioral effects in children born to mothers with high exposure. Finally, intentional suicide by organochlorines and other pesticides is an important clinical entity, and in England and Wales pesticides have accounted for 44 of approximately 4000 poisoning deaths.

DDT is associated with acute and chronic neurotoxicity. Acutely, the patient develops a metallic taste in the mouth, and within 1 hr dryness of the mouth and extreme thirst develop. Drowsiness or extreme insomnia, burning of the eyes, and a gritty sensation within the lids follow. Some degree of night blindness may be evident, concentration becomes difficult, and prominent aching of the limbs, muscular spasms, tremors, stiffness, and pain in the jaw develop thereafter. After chronic low-dose exposure, isolated weakness such as a wrist drop due to a mononeuropathy, optic atrophy, or a diffuse polyneuropathy involving weakness and tingling sensations of the distal extremities can occur. When these symptoms result from exposure of the skin to DDT, they may be limited to the limb or limbs that were in immediate contact with the toxin. With chronic high-dose exposure, generalized convulsions, coma, and death have been reported. There is no specific antidote for DDT, and supportive measures and anticonvulsants are the therapeutic mainstays. After chronic expo-

sure, diphenylhydantoin may be additionally effective in reducing fat sequestration of DDT.

Toxaphene, a chlorinated derivative of camphene, and endosulfan (Thiodan) are regularly used insecticides, both associated with tremor and seizure activity. The toxicity of chlordane is similar, but focal seizures have been reported with unusual frequency with this toxin. Chlordecone (Kepone) has not been reported to induce seizures but causes a dramatic irregular tremor, maximal when the limb is static and unsupported and only minimally increased with intentional acts. In more severe cases, the tremor is evident at rest. Additionally, irregular, jerking eye movements, called opsoclonia, have developed with chlordecone toxicity—an effect not reported with other chlorinated hydrocarbon insecticides. The clinical syndrome of pseudotumor cerebri—headaches, increased intracranial pressure, and visual obscuration—has also been reported in workers exposed to high levels of this compound. Muscle and nerve biopsies performed on patients exposed to chlordecone suggest a toxic derangement of the Schwann cells that cover the peripheral nerves. There is an accumulation of electron-dense particles in Schwann cell cytoplasm, marked decreases in the density of unmyelinated fibers, and relative sparing of larger myelinated fibers. In a chlordecone exposure incident in Virginia, more than half of the active employees of a plant in which chlordecone was manufactured became moderately ill. A few required hospitalization for months, but severe toxic signs generally abated when patients were removed from the toxic environment. However, 4 years later, several workers continued to show incapacitating tremor.

Tetrachlorethane is among the most dangerous of all chlorinated hydrocarbons, and although its use is restricted, it is still used (under the names Alanol, Cellon, Emaillet, Novania, Tetralen, and Westron). It exerts a prolonged narcotic effect when subjects are acutely exposed to high doses. More commonly, poisoning results from chronic exposure to vapors; in such cases, headache, anorexia, and eventual paresthesias and muscle atrophy develop. Liver damage is especially prominent, and secondary encephalopathy may be the prominent neurological picture.

Picrotoxin and strychnine are additional pesticides with severe neurological toxicity. Both are central analeptic agents and cause seizures as their major toxic manifestation. Picrotoxin has been shown to block presynaptic inhibition in neurons and blocks several types of inhibitory synapses in lower animals. Evidence suggests that the agent is an antagonist to the neurochemical γ-aminobutyric acid. The initial symptoms of picrotoxin intoxication consist of burning sensations in the pharynx and esophagus, abdominal pains, nausea and vomiting, salivation, and diarrhea, followed by headache and giddiness. Sleepiness, rapidly followed by stupor, and, occasionally, loss of consciousness and coma develop. Within 20 min to 3 hr, severe trembling and generalized seizures occur, and in fatal cases death occurs from asphyxia or gastrointestinal hemorrhage. With oral intoxication, the stomach should be immediately emptied by lavage or by emetics such as apomorphine. The convulsions should be controlled by intravenous administration of barbiturates or other anticonvulsants.

Picrotoxin has been used therapeutically in the treatment of poisoning by central nervous system depressants, specifically barbiturates. Its narrow margin of safety, however, makes this drug the source of continued pharmacological controversy. Doses used in treating barbiturate overdose may reach 20 mg, a dose known to induce severe toxic effects.

Strychnine, in addition to its effect as a potent pesticide, is still a component of various tonics and cathartic pills. The lethal dose of strychnine seems to depend largely on absorption dynamics and individual susceptibility because as little as 20 mg has been fatal. The usual lethal dose is approximately 80 mg. The mechanism of action of strychnine appears to relate to an interference with central neural postsynaptic inhibitory mechanisms most prominently in the spinal cord and brainstem. Strychnine is known to act as a competitive inhibitor of the neurochemical glycine at its postsynaptic receptor sites. If taken by mouth, strychnine produces symptoms within 2 hr. Early, there is a sense of excitement and marked irritability. Mild paresthesias develop in the face or lower limbs, associated with stiffness and fasciculations or ribbling movements in the musculature throughout the body. The limbs, especially the lower extremities, become extended and rigid, whereas the arms occasionally become fixed in a flexed position. Involvement of the back muscles produces painful arching. The facial muscles are tonially activated in spasm, causing the patient to develop a characteristic forced smile called risus sardonicus, and jaw muscle contractions cause difficulties in speech and swallowing. Generalized, often severe, muscular spasms

may last from a few minutes to almost 30 min and are occasionally followed by a clonic convulsion of a generalized type. If the seizure is severe, the patient becomes comatose and cyanotic, with rapid irregular pulse and shallow respirations, often of the Cheyne–Stokes variety. Throughout this anguish, the subject remains intellectually clear, except for short periods of unconsciousness accompanying the more severe convulsions. The course is usually rapid, and if patients die, they usually do so within the first 24 hr. However, if victims can be kept alive for a period of 18 hr, complete recovery almost invariably occurs. Treatment is supportive and centers on respiratory control and prevention of seizures. Short-acting barbiturates and, recently, diazepam have been successful. The treatment otherwise resembles that for tetanus, with placement of the subject in a completely quiet and darkened room that is maximally free from external stimuli that can precipitate the massive spasms. If the patient is seen early enough after ingestion, the stomach may be emptied by emetics or lavage, and potassium permanganate may be instilled as a chemical antidote. It may be necessary to use a general anesthetic to control seizure activity. Morphine and apomorphine should be used with extreme caution because of the possibility of additive effects on depression of breathing centers in the lower brainstem.

—*Christopher G. Goetz*

See also–Environmental Toxins; Neurotoxicology, Overview; Organic Solvents

Further Reading

Besser, R., Vogt, T., and Gutmann, L. (1990). Pancuronium improves the neuromuscular transmission defect of human organophosphate intoxication. *Neurology* 40, 1275–1277.
Goetz, C. G., Kompoliti, K., and Washburn, K. (1996). Neurotoxic agents. In *Clinical Neurology* (R. J. Joynt and R. C. Griggs, Eds.), Vol. 2, pp. 1–112. Lippincott-Raven, Philadelphia.
Hall, R. H. (1992). A new threat to public health: Organochlorines and food. *Nutrition Health* 8, 33–43.
Senanayake, N. (1982). Acute polyneuropathy after poisoning by a new organophosphate insecticide. *N. Engl. J. Med.* 306, 155–157.
Spigiel, R. W., Gourley, D. R., and Holcslaw, T. L. (1981). Organophosphate pesticide exposure in farmers and commercial applicators. *Clin. Toxicol. Consult.* 3, 45–50.
Thompson, J. P., Casey, P. B., and Vale, J. A. (1995). Deaths from pesticide poisoning in England and Wales 1990–1991. *Hum. Exp. Toxicol.* 13, 437–445.

Orthostatic Hypotension

Encyclopedia of the Neurological Sciences

MAINTENANCE of upright posture is possible by instantaneous cardiovascular adaptation that depends primarily on an intact autonomic nervous system. When this system fails, as may occur in any neuropathy compromising autonomic nerves, orthostatic hypotension ensues. The incapacitating nature of orthostatic hypotension underscores the importance of cardiovascular autonomic reflexes for normal life. Severely affected patients are completely disabled, able to stand for only a few seconds before syncope ensues. Even though treatment remains suboptimal, orthostatic hypotension is arguably the symptom of autonomic impairment most amenable to treatment. These patients are hypersensitive to pressor agents because of baroreflex impairment and receptor upregulation. Therefore, some of the features of their autonomic impairment can be used to their benefit.

PATHOPHYSIOLOGY

When a normal individual stands, up to 700 ml of blood pools in the legs and lower abdominal veins. Venous return decreases, resulting in a transient decline in cardiac output. The reduction in central blood volume and arterial pressure is sensed by cardiopulmonary volume receptors and arterial baroreceptors. Afferent signals from these receptors reach vasomotor centers in the brainstem. Efferent fibers from these centers reduce parasympathetic output and increase sympathetic outflow. Norepinephrine is released from postganglionic sympathetic nerve terminals at target organs, resulting in an increase in heart rate and cardiac contractility, partial restoration of venous return and diastolic ventricular filling by venoconstriction, and an increase in peripheral resistance by arteriolar vasoconstriction. As a net effect of these adaptive mechanisms, upright cardiac output remains reduced by 10–20% compared to supine, systolic blood pressure is reduced by 5–10 mmHg, diastolic blood pressure increases by 2–5 mmHg, mean blood pressure remains almost unchanged, and heart rate increases by 5–20 beats per minute.

DEFINITION

Orthostatic hypotension is arbitrarily defined as a decrease in systolic blood pressure of at least 20 mmHg or diastolic blood pressure of at least 10 mmHg within 3 min of standing. It is best characterized clinically as any decrease in arterial blood pressure that produces symptoms such as lightheadedness, blurred vision, weakness, fatigue, cognitive impairment, and pain in the back of the neck, finally leading to transient loss of consciousness. Symptoms never occur while supine but usually occur shortly after standing and are always relieved immediately on sitting or lying down. Failure to meet these criteria should cause the physician to rule out other causes of syncope (e.g., seizures, arrhythmias, or transient ischemic attacks). If patients have symptoms suggestive of but do not have documented orthostatic hypotension, repeated measurements of blood pressure should be performed. Occasionally, patients may have delayed orthostatic hypotension, which is only apparent after they stand for 10–30 min.

DIAGNOSIS

Whenever one encounters a patient with orthostatic hypotension, it is important to first rule out conditions or medications that can induce orthostatic hypotension (Table 1). These can occur in subjects with an intact autonomic function. In these cases, orthostatic hypotension is usually accompanied by a compensatory increase in heart rate. Therefore, it is important to measure both blood pressure and heart rate for an adequate interpretation. It is also possible that the conditions enumerated in Table 1 can precipitate orthostatic hypotension in patients with borderline autonomic function. In this case, heart rate may increase on standing but not enough to compensate for the decrease in blood pressure.

The diagnosis of autonomic impairment can be made easily with simple measurements of heart rate

Table 1 CONDITIONS AND MEDICATIONS THAT MAY PRECIPITATE OR WORSEN ORTHOSTATIC HYPOTENSION

Volume depletion
Prolonged bed rest/deconditioning
Alcohol
Diuretics
Tricyclic antidepressants
Phenothiazides
Venodilators (nitrates)
Antihypertensives (alpha-blockers, guanethidine)
Insulin

and blood pressure (Table 2). Although no single test completely differentiates patients with autonomic failure from age-matched control subjects, together they provide a reliable indicator of the presence and severity of cardiovascular autonomic impairment.

Two additional factors may precipitate hypotension in patients with autonomic failure. First, meals lower blood pressure dramatically in patients with primary autonomic failure and therefore may provoke symptomatic postprandial orthostatic hypotension. Second, insulin lowers blood pressure in diabetic patients with autonomic neuropathy and has no effect in those without autonomic neuropathy. The frequency and magnitude of these problems may be small in most patients but may be of importance in some.

MANAGEMENT

In general, a stepwise approach to treatment according to the severity of the symptoms is preferable (Table 3). Table 3 provides general guidelines; treatment should be individualized. Some recommendations may actually be contraindicated

Table 2 ASSESSMENT OF AUTONOMIC FUNCTION: BEDSIDE PHYSIOLOGICAL TESTS

Posture
  Measure blood pressure (BP) and heart rate (HR) after patient has been supine 15 min and standing 5 min. Express as supine−standing values.
  Normal response: systolic BP, 0 to −20 mmHg; diastolic BP, −10 to 5 mmHg; HR, 0–15 beats/min.
Sinus arrhythmia (SA) ratio
  Have patient breathe deeply six times per minute while monitoring HR.
  Measure longest R–R interval during expiration and shortest R–R interval during inspiration. Take average of six breaths.
  SA ratio = R–R_{exp}/R–R_{insp}; normal response, ≥ 1.2.
Valsalva ratio
  Use 6- to 12-ml syringe barrel as mouthpiece connected to sphygmomanometer.
  Ask patient to blow mercury column to 40 mmHg for 15 sec while monitoring HR in continuous strip. Repeat four times.
  Make sure effort is barred by thorax and not mouth (e.g., by introducing a pin-size leak in the mouthpiece).
  Measure shortest R–R during strain and longest R–R after release.
  Valsalva ratio = R–$R_{release}$/R–R_{strain}; normal response, ≥ 1.4.
Cold pressor test
  Measure baseline BP and HR. Have patient place hand in ice water for 1 min. Measure BP and HR after 1 min.
  Normal response: increase in systolic BP >15 mmHg.

Table 3 STEPWISE APPROACH TO MANAGEMENT OF ORTHOSTATIC HYPOTENSION

Remove aggravating factors
Medical treatment
  Liberalize salt intake, salt supplements
  Head-up tilt during the night
  Waist-high support stockings
  Exercise as tolerated
Pharmacological treatment[a]
  Fludrocortisone
  Short-acting pressor agents

[a] See Table 4.

in a given patient. The first approach must always be to eliminate any of the conditions enumerated in Table 1 that may induce orthostatic hypotension. The suggestions for management described previously are relevant to patients with documented autonomic impairment.

Nonpharmacological Therapy

In patients with persistent symptoms, conservative nonpharmacological therapy is indicated. Patients with autonomic failure are unable to conserve sodium, and liberalization of sodium intake is generally recommended. These patients have exaggerated nocturnal diuresis with relative hypovolemia and worsening of orthostatic hypotension early in the morning. Elevating the head of the bed with 6- to 9-in. blocks can reduce nocturnal diuresis. This simple step may improve orthostatic hypotension in the morning. During the day, wearing waist-high, custom-fitted elastic support stockings will exert pressure on the legs and reduce venous pooling. It is important to avoid wearing support stockings while supine because they may contribute to diuresis and supine hypertension.

It has recently been discovered that intake of 16 oz. of water results in an acute (within 30 min) and transient (approximately 60 min) increase in blood pressure in patients with autonomic failure. This pressor effect can be substantial and can be used to alleviate orthostatic hypotension. It is commonly recommended that patients drink 16 oz. of water approximately 15 min before getting out of bed in the morning, when symptoms are at their worst.

Pharmacological Therapy

Some patients may require pharmacological therapy in addition to nonpharmacological therapy. At this stage, the goal of treatment is to minimize symptoms rather than to normalize an upright blood pressure. Therapy is usually initiated with fludrocortisone acetate at a low dose (0.1 mg/day) and increased slowly to 0.4 mg/day if needed. A weight gain of 1 or 2 kg and mild ankle edema may be desirable in these patients. However, hypokalemia, supine hypertension, and pulmonary edema may occur, and patients must be monitored carefully. Fludrocortisone will not be effective unless it is given in conjunction with increased salt intake (e.g., 1-g sodium chloride tablets taken with meals). Fludrocortisone will worsen supine hypertension and should be used with caution in patients suffering from this complication.

Most patients with severe autonomic impairment also require short-acting pressor agents. The goal in using these drugs is to provide patients with periods during which they can remain upright rather than to try to keep severely afflicted patients symptom free throughout the day. Most of the agents listed in Table 4, if effective in a given patient, will increase blood pressure for 2 or 3 hr. In general, these agents are best given before periods of exertion as needed rather than at fixed (e.g., tid) intervals. This approach may reduce the likelihood of side effects and the development of tolerance that reduces their long-term efficacy. Patients should also avoid lying down for 4 or 5 hr after taking these drugs to prevent supine hypertension. These drugs have negligible effects in healthy subjects; the increase in blood pressure seen in patients with autonomic failure is a reflection of their extreme hypersensitivity to most pressor and depressor agents. For this reason, treatment should be started at very small doses and should be individualized. This is best done by measuring blood

pressure at 15- to 30-min intervals for 2 or 3 hr after administration of the first dose of each drug.

Treatment of Related Conditions

Autonomic failure can be associated with low-production anemia and inappropriately low serum erythropoietin levels. If other causes of anemia are ruled out, patients can be treated with recombinant erythropoietin (25–50 U/kg sc three times per week). Erythropoietin has been shown to improve upright blood pressure, and its use may be warranted for this reason alone rather than as a treatment for anemia.

Many patients may also have supine hypertension resulting from preexisting essential hypertension or as part of their autonomic failure. In some patients, significant hypertension may be present even in the seated position. During the day, supine hypertension is best managed by simply avoiding the supine position. At night, it is often necessary to give vasodilators at bedtime, after which the patient should be advised against getting up during the night without assistance. Hydralazine hydrochloride (25–100 mg) and low doses of nitrates as transdermal preparations (e.g., 0.1 mg/hr Nitro-Dur applied at bedtime and removed on arising) or short-acting calcium channel blockers (e.g., 10 mg nifedipine) are often useful.

—*Italo Biaggioni and Horacio Kaufmann*

See also–**Autonomic Nervous System, Heart Rate and; Neuropathies, Autonomic; Postural Orthostatic Tachycardia Syndrome (POTS); Syncope**

Table 4 PHARMACOLOGICAL AGENTS IN THE TREATMENT OF ORTHOSTATIC HYPOTENSION

Agent	Dose	Side effects
Sodium chloride	2 g/day	Nausea, diarrhea
Fludrocortisone (Florinef)	0.1–0.4 mg/day	Hypokalemia, congestive heart failure, supine hypertension
Midodrine (Proamitine)	5–10 mg[a]	Scalp itching, goose bumps
Yohimbine (Yocon)	5.4 mg[a]	Nervousness, tremor

[a] A dose of these short-acting pressor agents, given before exertion, will improve orthostatic symptoms for 2 or 3 hr. In general, administration of more than three doses/day is discouraged to avoid side effects and developments of tolerance.

Further Reading

Jordan, J., Shannon, J. R., Biaggioni, I., *et al.* (1998). Contrasting actions of pressor agents in severe autonomic failure. *Am. J. Med.* 105, 116–124.

Jordan, J., Shannon, J. R., Grogan, E., *et al.* (1999). A potent pressor response elicited by drinking water. *Lancet* 353, 723.

Kaufmann, H. (1997). Syncope. A neurologist's viewpoint. *Cardiol. Clin.* 15, 177–193.

Shannon, J. R., Jordan, J., Diedrich, A., *et al.* (2000). Sympathetically mediated hypertension in autonomic failure. *Circulation* 101, 2710–2715.

Vagaonescu, T. D., Saadia, D., Tuhrim, S., *et al.* (2000). Hypertensive cardiovascular damage in patients with primary autonomic failure. *Lancet* 355, 725–726.

Wright, R. A., Kaufmann, H., Perera, R., *et al.* (1998). A double-blind, dose–response study of midodrine in neurogenic orthostatic hypotension. *Neurology* 51, 120–124.

Osler, William

Encyclopedia of the Neurological Sciences
Copyright 2003, Elsevier Science (USA). All rights reserved.

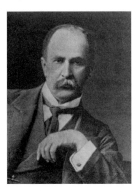

William Osler (courtesy of the National Library of Medicine).

THE NAME William Osler (1849–1919) evokes an image of a dynamic, thoughtful, multifaceted, disciplined individual who made extraordinary contributions to the development of medicine, both in the United States and throughout the world. To this can be added Osler's contributions to the field of neurology, particularly child neurology. At the time he was active, the fields of pediatrics and neurology were just beginning to develop in the United States. Osler's bibliography includes more than 1400 papers, monographs, and notes exploring almost every subspecialty; of these, it has been estimated that approximately 200 works deal with neurology and more than 100 with pediatrics. Osler's clinical research and writings in these areas concentrated on the field of child neurology, including such topics as cerebral palsy, chorea, tics, muscular dystrophy, and childhood migraine.

Born in 1849 in Bond Head near Toronto, Canada, Osler was the eighth child in a family of nine children. Osler received his early education first at nearby backwoods grammar schools and later at boarding schools at Barrie and Weston. Osler entered Trinity College in Toronto in 1867 intent on following his father's footsteps into the ministry, but at the beginning of his second year he decided to enter medical school. In 1870, he transferred from Toronto to McGill University in Montreal, and following his graduation in 1872 he spent 2 years studying in Great Britain and Europe, where he met William Macewen, Charles Darwin, Burdon Sanderson, Rudolf Virchow, and other eminent scientists.

Soon after Osler's return to Canada in 1874, he was appointed lecturer in the Institutes of Medicine at McGill. During a decade on the McGill faculty, he began the extensive postmortem and histological studies that underpinned his later writings. In 1884, due largely to the efforts of S. Weir Mitchell and H. C. Wood, Osler was appointed professor of clinical medicine at the University of Pennsylvania. Then in 1889, he began a new position as chief of medicine at the newly established Johns Hopkins Hospital in Baltimore, where he wrote his classic *Principles and Practice of Medicine* (1892) and described hereditary hemorrhagic telangiectasia. From the time he left Johns Hopkins in 1905 until his death on December 29, 1919, Osler was regius professor of medicine at Oxford University. This last move was dictated in part by his health and the ever-increasing burden of teaching, writing, and clinical duties.

Osler's many contributions to internal medicine and his fame as a teacher and clinician have largely obscured his contributions to neurology. However, his bibliography reflects an interest in the nervous system that spanned both clinical and theoretical topics and was sustained throughout his career. Osler disproved the notion that the brains of criminals are anatomically distinct, and another early paper touched on the mind–brain question that was then being debated. His early interest in brain anatomy is evidenced by his study of the comparative neuroanatomy of the seal.

Osler published numerous papers on clinical neurology and neuropathology, including several on stroke, intracranial aneurysm, brain tumors, and spinal cord disorders. Osler described the three forms of "muscular atrophy" known at the time—pseudohypertrophic muscular dystrophy, Erb's disease, and Duchenne's disease. He also contributed to the growing literature on Friedreich's ataxia and facioscapulohumeral muscular dystrophy, and he studied the significance of cranial bruits in children, concluding that the finding is usually of no significance. Although many of these articles were routine case reports of little lasting significance, others, such as his paper on Jacksonian epilepsy and cerebral localization (based on a pathological study of a girl with a glioma), were more important. Osler also contributed numerous editorials and book reviews related to neurological topics as well as chapters on neurological subjects in textbooks written by William Pepper and Francis X. Dercum.

In 1885, Osler was elected to membership in the Philadelphia Neurological Society, which had been founded the previous year. Weir Mitchell was the first president of the society and remained president during Osler's time in Philadelphia. Osler regularly attended the society's meetings and showed a keen interest in neurology. Soon after Osler's arrival in Philadelphia, he was appointed to the staff of the Philadelphia Orthopedic Hospital and Infirmary for Nervous Diseases. Here, Osler initiated much of his work on the neurological disorders of children, although some of his experience was not published until after he left Philadelphia. At the infirmary, Osler worked closely with Weir Mitchell, his son John K. Mitchell, Morton Sinkler, and Morris J. Lewis. Osler continued to perform numerous autopsies and gave special attention to the study of lesions of the brain, spinal cord, and the thoracic viscera. In 1888, Osler was elected to the American Neurological Association.

Osler called attention to the association between acquired chorea and endocarditis. Two additional articles detailed his accumulating experience with 410 cases of chorea at the infirmary, but the monograph summarizing this work on chorea was not completed until after his move to Baltimore. This book was dedicated to William Gowers. Although Richard Bright had noted the association between heart disease and chorea, it was Osler, among others such as Sturges, who solidly established it. Osler also reported in detail two families with Huntington's chorea, including one autopsy in which he mentioned ventricular dilatation but not atrophy of the caudate nucleus.

A series of articles in *Medical News* on childhood cerebral palsy summarized Osler's experience with 120 children from the infirmary. These articles formed the basis for his classic monograph on cerebral palsy, *The Cerebral Palsies of Children*, which was dedicated to S. Weir Mitchell. Osler's publications on cerebral palsy appeared at approximately the same time as the work of Gowers. Like Gowers, Osler emphasized the diverse causes of childhood hemiplegia. Osler classified his patients with nonprogressive upper motor neuron dysfunction according to the distribution of their weakness (hemiplegia, diplegia, and paraplegia) and separated the children with congenital dysfunction from those whose weakness was acquired later in childhood. The monograph contains numerous case descriptions and emphasizes signs, symptoms, and etiology. Osler also included some sketches of

neuropathological material correlating the clinical and pathological findings.

Osler wrote on numerous other topics of pediatric neurological interest, including several papers on sporadic cretinism, neuritis in typhoid fever, bacteria and tuberculous meningitis, Tourette's syndrome, and myotonia congenital. The first edition of Osler's *Principles and Practice of Medicine* was published in 1892 and contained approximately 300 pages devoted to the nervous system. Among the topics emphasized were his studies of 460 children with epilepsy as well as others with pediatric migraine headaches.

Even after Osler's death in 1919, his association with the nervous system continued. Osler left his brain to the Wistar Institute in Philadelphia for study. Osler's interest in neurology spanned his entire career in medicine but was especially keen during his years in Philadelphia, where he encountered and was stimulated by many of the great American neurologists of his day. In turn, Osler, through his prolific writings and leadership, stimulated others in the field and greatly enhanced the development of neurology in the United States in the 20th century.

—*Stephen Ashwal and E. Steve Roach*

See also–Gowers, William; Mitchell, Silas Weir; Osler–Weber–Rendu Syndrome; Penfield, Wilder (see Index entry Biography for complete list of biographical entries)

Further Reading

Ebers, G. C. (1985). Osler and neurology. *Can. J. Neurol. Sci.* **12**, 236–242.

McHenry, L. C. (1993). William Osier—A Philadelphia neurologist. *J. Child Neurol.* **8**, 416–422.

Mills, C. K. (1927). *Dr. William Osler in Philadelphia. Sir William Osler Memorial Volume.* International Association of Medical Museums, Philadelphia.

Osler, W. (1892). *The Principles and Practice of Medicine Designed for the Use of Practitioners and Students of Medicine.* Appleton, New York.

Roach, E. S., and Ashwal, S. (1990). William Osler. In *The Founders of Child Neurology* (S. Ashwal, Ed.), pp. 325–333. Norman, San Francisco.

Robbins, B. H., and Cristie, A. (1963). Sir William Osler the pediatrician. *Am. J. Dis. Child.* **106**, 124–129.

Rogers, F. B. (1959). Neurology in Philadelphia: Personalities and events. *Philadelphia Med.* **55**, 84–90.

Rogers, F. B. (1970). Osler and Philadelphia. *Trans. Studies Coll. Phys. Philadelphia* **38**, 118–123.

Osler–Weber–Rendu Syndrome

Encyclopedia of the Neurological Sciences

OSLER–WEBER–RENDU syndrome, also known as hereditary hemorrhagic telangiectasia (HHT), is a group of autosomal dominant inheritable disorders characterized by telangiectasias, recurrent epistaxis, and a family history of the disease. HHT occurs in all ethnic populations with a prevalence that ranges from 1 in 2500 to 1 in 50,000 individuals. HHT affects both males and females and its penetrance is age related and is approximately 97%. The homozygous condition is thought to be lethal *in utero* or perinatally. Recently, mutations in the gene *endoglin* on chromosome 9 and *ALK1* (activin receptor-like kinase-1) on chromosome 12 have been associated with HHT.

The clinical manifestations of HHT are caused by aberrant vascular structures, including telangiectasias and arteriovenous malformations (AVMs). In HHT, telangiectasias and AVMs may develop in the nasal and oral mucosa, skin (lips, tongue, trunk, and extremities), gastrointestinal tract (stomach, duodenum, small bowel, colon, and liver), lung, and central nervous system (brain and spinal cord). The criteria for diagnosing HHT reflect the variable manifestations of the disease and require that only two of the following conditions be present to establish a diagnosis of HHT: recurrent epistaxis, telangiectasias in a location other than the nasal mucosa, autosomal dominant inheritance, or visceral involvement.

The nonneurological manifestations of HHT are caused by telangiectasias and AVMs located in the nasal mucosa, skin, lung, and gastrointestinal tract. Telangiectasias of the nasal mucosa are the most common manifestation of HHT and may cause severe epistaxis in some individuals. The telangiectasias that develop on the skin usually result in only minor bleeding. Pulmonary AVMs create direct right-to-left shunts that may produce cyanosis, exertional dyspnea, clubbing, and secondary polycythemia. Telangiectasias and AVMs that occur in the stomach, duodenum, small bowel, and colon are a late manifestation in HHT and can present with significant upper or lower gastrointestinal bleeding. Hepatic AVMs may cause nodular hepatic fibrosis and left-to-right shunts that result in high-output cardiac failure.

Neurological manifestations of HHT will develop in approximately 10% of patients with HHT, and a majority of the neurological manifestations will present in the third or fourth decade of life. The neurological manifestations of HHT include migraine, headache, stroke, brain abscess, intracerebral hemorrhage, subarachnoid hemorrhage, seizure, and portosystemic encephalopathy. In a study of HHT patients with neurological manifestations, 61% experienced neurological manifestations secondary to pulmonary AVMs, 36% experienced manifestations secondary to vascular malformations of the brain or spinal cord, and 3% experienced manifestations secondary to portosystemic encephalopathy caused by hepatic AVMs.

The neurological manifestations of pulmonary AVMs result from a right-to-left shunt created by the vascular malformation. The right-to-left shunt causes hypoxemia and polycythemia hyperviscosity. It also permits the passage of peripheral venous emboli and septic emboli into the cerebral circulation.

Brain and spinal cord vascular malformations that have been described in HHT include telangiectasias, AVMs, saccular aneurysms, and a carotid-cavernous fistula. Vascular lesions located in the brain may rupture and cause subarachnoid, intracerebral, or intraventricular hemorrhage. The clinical presentation of this hemorrhage depends on its extent and location but could involve headache, visual disturbances, seizure, ataxia, or motor deficits. Spinal cord vascular lesions associated with HHT are usually AVMs and have been observed in cervical, thoracic, and lumbar sections of the spinal cord. Symptoms of these lesions are due to mass effect and compression of the surrounding cord by the lesion or from hemorrhage.

Patients with HHT who present with neurological symptoms or signs must be screened for both central nervous system (CNS) lesions and pulmonary AVMs since these lesions are the most frequent cause of neurological complications in this disease. Magnetic resonance imaging and cerebral angiography are the most effective methods for detecting CNS lesions in HHT. High-resolution spiral chest computer tomography is the most sensitive method for detecting pulmonary AVMs.

In patients with HHT, pulmonary and CNS vascular malformations that are symptomatic or enlarging should be aggressively treated. Endovascular embolization of pulmonary AVMs using coils or balloons is currently the standard treatment, although surgical ligation or resection can be utilized. The therapy employed for CNS vascular lesions depends on the nature of the lesion, its location, and the experience of the institution performing the intervention. Central nervous system vascular lesions have been successfully treated using endovascular coiling and embolization, neurovascular surgery, and stereotactic radiosurgery.

—*James E. Conway and Daniele Rigamonti*

See also—Arteriovenous Malformations (AVM), Surgical Treatment of; Capillary Telangiectasia; Osler, William

Further Reading

Guttmacher, A. E., Marchuk, D. A., and White, R. I. (1995). Hereditary hemorrhagic telangiectasia. *N. Engl. J. Med.* **333**, 918–924.

Haitjema, T., Westermann, C. J. J., Overtoom, T. T. C., *et al.* (1996). Hereditary hemorrhagic telangiectasia (Osler–Weber–Rendu disease). *Arch. Intern. Med.* **156**, 714–719.

Perry, W. H. (1987). Clinical spectrum of hereditary hemorrhagic telangiectasia (Osler–Weber–Rendu disease). *Am. J. Med.* **82**, 989–997.

Roman, G., Fisher, M., Perl, D. P., *et al.* (1978). Neurological manifestations of hereditary hemorrhagic telangiectasia (Rendu–Osler–Weber disease): Report of 2 cases and review of the literature. *Ann. Neurol.* **4**, 130–144.

Shovlin, C. L. (1997). Molecular defects in rare bleeding disorders: Hereditary haemorrhagic telangiectasia. *Thromb. Haemostas.* **78**, 145–150.

Osteitis Deformans
see Paget's Disease

Otology
see Neuro-Otology

Oxidative Metabolism

Encyclopedia of the Neurological Sciences
Copyright 2003, Elsevier Science (USA). All rights reserved.

OXIDATIVE METABOLISM is the major biochemical means for producing energy in eukaryotic cells. In the presence of adequate oxygen, mitochondria generate the majority of cellular energy in most cell types by oxidizing carbohydrates and fats. The mitochondrial respiratory (electron transport) chain is the common final pathway for energy production. Mitochondria, via the respiratory chain, generate energy by the process of oxidative phosphorylation (OXPHOS), in which the reduction of oxygen to water is coupled to the production of the high-energy phosphate compound adenosine triphosphate (ATP). Electron transport between respiratory chain complexes is coupled to the extrusion of protons across the inner mitochondrial membrane by proton pump components of the respiratory chain. An electrochemical gradient ($\Delta\Psi$) across the inner mitochondrial membrane, which is alkaline and negative on the side of the mitochondrial matrix and acidic and positive externally, is thus produced. Protons flow across the inner membrane into the mitochondrial matrix through ATP synthase (complex V), which utilizes the energy thus produced to synthesize ATP from adenosine diphosphate (ADP) and inorganic phosphate (P_i).

The oxidation of carbohydrates begins in the cytoplasm with the formation of pyruvate by the glycolytic pathway. Pyruvate diffuses through the outer mitochondrial membrane and is metabolized to acetyl-CoA and reduced nicotine adenine dinucleotide (NADH) by the pyruvate dehydrogenase complex, located in the inner mitochondrial membrane. Acetyl-CoA enters the tricarboxylic acid (TCA) cycle, resulting in the formation of three NADH molecules and one reduced flavin adenine dinucleotide ($FADH_2$) molecule as well as the production of a molecule of ATP (via guanosine triphosphate). In addition to the $FADH_2$ formed by the TCA cycle in the oxidation of succinate to fumarate by succinate dehydrogenase (complex II), $FADH_2$ is also generated by acyl-CoA dehydrogenases in the fatty acid oxidation cycle and by the action of glycerol phosphate dehydrogenase, which is part of the glycerol phosphate shuttle. NADH is also formed in the fatty acid oxidation cycle by 3-hydroxyacyl-CoA dehydrogenases in the conversion of 3-hydroxyacyl-CoA compounds to their ketoacyl-CoA derivatives. NADH and $FADH_2$ donate electrons to the mitochondrial respiratory chain, with subsequent production of energy in the form of ATP. Electrons derived from NADH enter the respiratory chain via complex I. Electrons from $FADH_2$ enter via either coenzyme Q_{10} (ubiquinone) or succinate dehydrogenase (complex II). Protons are pumped across the mitochondrial inner membrane by complexes I, III, and IV. These ions then reenter the mitochondrial matrix through complex V (ATP synthase); such reentry is coupled to the formation of ATP. Because three protons are pumped across the mitochondrial inner membrane for each NADH oxidized by the respiratory chain and two for each $FADH_2$ oxidized, NADH oxidation results in the formation of three molecules of ATP, and $FADH_2$ oxidation results in the formation of two molecules of ATP. The yield from the complete oxidation of glucose is 36 ATP molecules (Table 1).

Fatty acids, derived from adipose tissue triglycerides, are converted to coenzyme A esters in the cytosol and then enter the mitochondria through enzymatic reactions involving carnitine. Long-chain fatty acyl-CoA molecules are converted to acylcarnitine derivatives by the outer mitochondrial membrane enzyme carnitine palmitoyltransferase-1 (CPT-1). The acylcarnitines are then transported across the inner mitochondrial membrane to the mitochondrial matrix by a translocase and are subsequently metabolized to acyl-CoA and free carnitine by CPT-2. The released acyl-CoA then enters the fatty acid oxidation cycle. With each turn of the fatty acid oxidation cycle, one molecule each of acetyl-CoA, NADH, and $FADH_2$ are generated. Acetyl-CoA may either enter the TCA cycle, if carbohydrate and fat degradation are in balance, or be used for ketone body formation, if fat degradation predominates. Acyl-CoA dehydrogenases catalyze the initial step in fatty acid oxidation and contain noncovalently bound FAD. Electrons generated by the acyl-CoA dehydrogenase reaction are transferred to the coenzyme Q_{10} (ubiquinone) component of the respiratory chain by the concerted actions of the electron transport flavoprotein (ETF) and electron transport flavoprotein–ubiquinone oxidoreductase (ETF-QO). Thus, electrons from fatty acid oxidation can enter the respiratory chain through complex I (from the oxidation of NADH), complex II (from oxidation of succinate in the TCA cycle to generate $FADH_2$), or coenzyme Q_{10} (from ETF and ETF-QO).

In addition to the intramitochondrial reactions in which reducing equivalents are generated for eventual use in energy production by the mitochondrial respiratory chain, NADH formed in the cytoplasm can also be oxidized by mitochondria. NADH formed in the cytoplasm can enter mitochondria by two shuttles—the glycerol-3-phosphate dehydrogenase shuttle and the malate–aspartate shuttle—and subsequently donate electrons to mitochondrial respiratory chain complex I.

Although the major components of oxidative metabolism—namely the TCA cycle, fatty acid oxidation cycle, and respiratory chain—are often discussed separately, it should be emphasized that proper functioning of each pathway is interdependent on the normal function of the others. Indeed, succinate dehydrogenase is a central enzyme in both the TCA cycle and the respiratory chain. The respiratory chain represents the final common pathway for the production of energy by oxidative metabolism.

Table 1 ATP YIELD FROM THE COMPLETE OXIDATION OF GLUCOSE[a]

	ATP yield per glucose
Glycolysis: glucose to pyruvate (cytosolic)	
Phosphorylation of glucose	−1
Phosphorylation of fructose 6-phosphate	−1
Dephosphorylation of two molecules of 1,3-diphosphoglycerate	+2
Dephosphorylation of two molecules of phosphoenolpyruvate	+2
Two NADH formed in oxidation of two molecules of glyceraldehyde 3-phosphate	
Conversion of pyruvate to acetyl-CoA (mitochondrial)	
Two NADH are formed	
Tricarboxyclic acid (TCA) cycle (mitochondrial)	
Metabolism of two molecules of succinyl-CoA yields two molecules of GTP	+2
Six NADH are formed in the oxidation of two molecules of isocitrate, α-oxoglutarate, and malate	
Two $FADH_2$ are formed in the oxidation of two molecules of succinate	
Oxidative phosphorylation (mitochondrial)	
Two NADH from glycolysis[b]	+4
Two NADH formed in the oxidative decarboxylation of pyruvate	+6
Two $FADH_2$ formed in the TCA cycle	+4
Six NADH formed in the TCA cycle	+18
Net yield per glucose	**+36**

[a] Modified from Stryer, L. (1988). Biochemistry, 3rd ed., p. 344. Freeman, New York.

[b] Each NADH from glycolysis yields only two ATP because of the cost of transferring cytosolic NADH into the mitochondria via, e.g., the glycerol phosphate shuttle. Otherwise, each NADH yields three ATP and each $FADH_2$ yields two ATP (see text).

MITOCHONDRIAL EVOLUTION

Mitochondria are thought to have evolved from aerobic bacteria that underwent endocytosis by primitive eukaryotic cells approximately 1.5 billion years ago. The first living cells likely arose approximately 3.5 billion years ago in an environment lacking oxygen but rich in organic molecules. The earliest energy-producing metabolic pathways are thought to have resembled present-day anaerobic fermentation, a process in which partial oxidation of an energy-rich organic molecule (e.g., glucose) is linked to the production of NADH and ATP. NADH is reoxidized to NAD^+ by the conversion of pyruvate to lactate by the enzyme lactate dehydrogenase.

With time, waste products from bacteria producing energy from fermentation accumulated and actually changed the environment. Early bacteria likely excreted various organic acids, including lactate, formate, acetate, propionate, butyrate, and succinate. The excretion of these organic acids lowered the environmental pH, producing selective pressure for the evolution of transmembrane proton pumps to protect bacterial cells from the harmful effects of intracellular acidification. Two types of proton pumps evolved. The first type of pump is hypothesized to have used ATP hydrolysis to power itself. However, as nonfermentable organic acids accumulated in the environment, the supply of geochemically produced fermentable nutrients was depleted. This additional change in the environment favored bacteria that did not require ATP for proton pumping, instead allowing ATP to be used in other essential cellular reactions. This selective pressure may have been responsible for the evolution of membrane-bound proteins that used different redox potentials to transport electrons to each other, creating energy for proton pumping. The next major step in the evolutionary process was the combination of these two types of proton pumps into a single type of bacteria. The electron transport pump would function as usual, transferring electrons down an electrochemical gradient and using the energy generated to create a proton gradient. Protons could then flow through the ATP-driven type of pump, in effect driving it in reverse; instead of using ATP to pump protons, reverse proton flow would provide the energy necessary to form ATP from ADP and P_i. Bacteria possessing both types of pumps would be at a tremendous selective advantage.

The next evolutionary breakthrough occurred approximately 3 billion years ago with the appearance of cyanobacteria, which are primitive photosynthetic bacteria. Such organisms flourished and produced large quantities of reduced organic compounds. Because they used water as the electron source for carbon dioxide reduction, oxygen entered the environment for the first time. Oxygen levels in the atmosphere began to increase approximately 1.5 billion years ago (Fig. 1). With this increase in atmospheric oxygen, bacteria could then use oxidative metabolism to synthesize ATP. A cytochrome oxidase was added to the preexisting electron transport chain, allowing oxygen to serve as the final electron acceptor. Mitochondria are postulated to have arisen by the endocytosis of a bacterium containing such an electron transport chain, complete with a cytochrome oxidase, by a primitive eukaryotic cell.

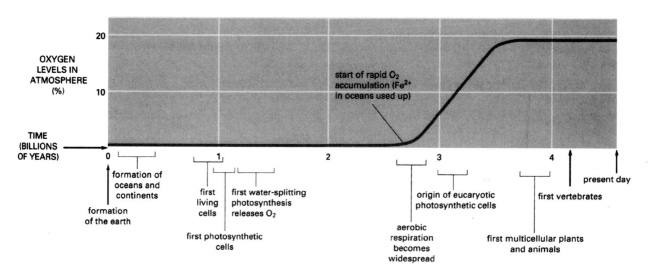

Figure 1

Evolution of eukaryotic cells (reproduced with permission from Alberts *et al.*, 1994, p. 701).

MITOCHONDRIAL BIOLOGY AND BIOCHEMISTRY

Mitochondria are bounded by a relatively smooth outer membrane and a highly convoluted inner membrane, which form an internal matrix space and an intermembrane space. The mitochondrial matrix space contains hundreds of enzymes, including the components of the TCA and the fatty acid oxidation cycles. The matrix also contains the mitochondrial genome (2–10 copies/mitochondrion), unique mitochondrial transfer RNAs (tRNAs) and ribosomal RNAs (rRNAs), and enzymes involved in the replication of mtDNA and processing of mitochondrial mRNA. The mitochondrial respiratory chain is embedded in the inner mitochondrial membrane and consists of multisubunit enzymes, designated complexes I–V. The respiratory chain complexes are protein–lipid structures that also contain specialized compounds that are directly involved in electron transport, namely transition metal compounds (hemes, iron–sulfur clusters, and protein-bound copper), flavins [flavin mononucleotide (FMN) and FAD], and a quinoid compound (coenzyme Q_{10}). Electrons enter the respiratory chain via complexes I and II and are then transferred to the mobile carrier coenzyme Q_{10}. The electrons then flow sequentially through complex III, cytochrome c, and complex IV and finally reduce oxygen to form water. Protons are pumped from the mitochondrial matrix to the intermembrane space by complexes I, III, and IV and flow back into the matrix through complex V (ATP synthase). Complex V synthesizes ATP from ADP and P_i. ATP then exits the mitochondrial matrix via an inner membrane protein, adenine nucleotide translocase (ANT), and enters the cytoplasm through an outer membrane protein, the voltage-dependent anion channel (VDAC; porin).

The respiratory chain is encoded by the coordinated interaction of two genomes, the nuclear and mitochondrial. With evolution, transfer of most of the mtDNA sequences to the nucleus has occurred, resulting in shrinkage of the mitochondrial genome to its current size of 16,569 base pairs. Drift of the mitochondrial genetic code has also taken place; mitochondrial genes have their own unique genetic code, making them unrecognizable to the transcriptional and translational systems outside the mitochondria. Thirteen respiratory chain subunits, 22 tRNAs, and 2 rRNAs are encoded by the mtDNA, whereas the remaining ~73 subunits, proteins

important in maintaining respiratory chain stability, ribosomal proteins, mtDNA regulatory factors, and DNA and RNA polymerases, are encoded in the nucleus.

Transcription of mtDNA creates a polycistronic RNA. A nuclear-encoded endonuclease then cleaves the RNA transcript into its constituent tRNAs, rRNAs, and mRNAs. The 13 OXPHOS subunits are synthesized from nine monocistronic and two bicistronic mRNAs. The remainder of the mitochondrial proteins and OXPHOS subunits are encoded by nuclear genes, synthesized in the cytoplasm, and imported into mitochondria, taking their place in the outer mitochondrial membrane, intermembrane space, inner membrane, or matrix. Peptides destined for the mitochondria typically contain an amino-terminal-targeting sequence of 12–30 amino acids that is subsequently cleaved by specific mitochondrial matrix proteases. Cytosolic chaperone proteins are also required for correct targeting of precursors to mitochondrial import receptors. Mitochondrial matrix precursor proteins and precursors to OXPHOS components enter the matrix through translocation channels in the inner membrane. The inner membrane multiple conductance channel (MCC) has been postulated to be the pore through which precursor proteins enter the mitochondrial matrix. Mitochondrial matrix heat shock proteins (hsp 70 family) then direct the folding and assembly of multimeric matrix enzymes and inner membrane respiratory chain complexes.

Complex I (NADH Dehydrogenase; EC 1.6.5.3)

NADH dehydrogenase (complex I) is a protein composed of 42 subunits, 7 of which are encoded by the mitochondrial genome. Complex I transfers electrons to coenzyme Q_{10} after the electrons have passed through a series of redox groups, including FMN and six iron–sulfur clusters. Complex I is subdivided into three distinct polypeptide groups—the flavoprotein fragment, the iron–protein fragment, and the hydrophobic protein fragment. The flavoprotein fragment contains FMN, six iron atoms, and three polypeptides with molecular weights of 51, 24, and 10 kDa, respectively. The 51-kDa fragment contains FMN and is the NADH binding site. The iron–protein fragment contains the coenzyme Q_{10} binding site and a further 9 or 10 iron atoms. The hydrophobic protein fragment contains the six iron–sulfur clusters, which transfer electrons to coenzyme Q_{10}.

Complex I spans the inner mitochondrial membrane. The energy generated from the oxidation of NADH to NAD^+ and the transfer of electrons through the redox reactions is used to transfer protons from the mitochondrial matrix to the intermembrane space. The NAD^+ generated by complex I is used in numerous metabolic reactions by NADH-linked dehydrogenases, including components of the fatty acid oxidation cycle (short-, medium-, long-, and very long-chain acyl-CoA dehydrogenases and short- and long-chain 3-hydroxyacyl-CoA dehydrogenases), pyruvate dehydrogenase, TCA cycle enzymes (isocitrate, α-ketoglutarate, and malate dehydrogenases), β-hydroxybutyrate dehydrogenase (which functions in ketone body metabolism), and amino acid catabolic enzymes such as glutamate dehydrogenase. Cytosolic reactions dependent on the NAD^+ generated by complex I include the glycolytic enzymes glyceraldehyde 3-phosphate dehydrogenase and lactate dehydrogenase. The malate–aspartate shuttle carries reducing equivalents generated by NADH production in cytosolic reactions across the inner mitochondrial membrane because the membrane is impermeable to NADH. The shuttle donates electrons to mitochondrial matrix NAD^+, generating NADH, which is subsequently oxidized by complex I. It is easy to understand the widespread metabolic consequences of impaired complex I activity, given its central position in metabolic pathways responsible for catabolism of glucose, fatty acids, and amino acids.

Complex II (Succinate Dehydrogenase; EC 1.3.5.1)

Succinate dehydrogenase (complex II) represents a key component of both the mitochondrial respiratory chain and the TCA cycle. It catalyzes the dehydrogenation of succinate to fumarate, with the electrons generated being donated to the mobile inner membrane electron carrier coenzyme Q_{10}. Complex II contains four subunits, all of which are encoded by nuclear genes, and it is localized to the mitochondrial matrix side of the inner mitochondrial membrane. It is the only respiratory chain complex to be solely coded for by the nuclear genome. Because it does not span the inner mitochondrial membrane, it is not involved with proton translocation and the formation of a proton gradient. The four subunits are a 70-kDa FAD-containing polypeptide (Fp), a 27-kDa iron–sulfur protein containing three iron–sulfur clusters, and two smaller anchoring peptides contain-

ing b-type hemes. Despite its relatively small size, complex II plays a critical role in energy metabolism.

Complex III (Cytochrome bc_1 Complex; EC 1.10.2.2)

The cytochrome bc_1 complex (complex III) spans the inner mitochondrial membrane and translocates protons to the intermembrane space. It mediates the transfer of electrons from coenzyme Q_{10} to cytochrome c, the two mobile electron carriers in the respiratory chain. Complex III is composed of 11 polypeptide subunits, only 1 of which (cytochrome b) is encoded by the mitochondrial genome. Electron transfer is primarily carried out by cytochrome b, cytochrome c_1, and a nonheme iron–sulfur protein. Cytochrome c_1 interacts directly with the mobile electron carrier cytochrome c.

Complex IV (Cytochrome c Oxidase; EC 1.9.3.1)

Cytochrome c oxidase (complex IV) transfers electrons from reduced cytochrome c to oxygen, forming water. Complex IV spans the inner mitochondrial membrane and translocates protons to the intermembrane space. Complex IV is composed of 13 subunits, 3 of which (subunits I–III) are encoded by the mitochondrial genome. The cytochrome c binding site is contained in subunit II, and subunit III may participate in proton translocation. The complex IV redox centers consist of hemes a and a_3 and copper atoms.

Complex V (ATP Synthase; EC 3.6.1.3)

ATP synthase (complex V) synthesizes ATP from ADP and P_i, utilizing the electrochemical gradient formed by proton pumping by complexes I, III, and IV. Two segments, F_0 and F_1, comprise complex V. The F_0 segment translocates protons from the intermembrane space back into the mitochondrial matrix, and the F_1 segment sits at the end of a stalk connecting it to F_0 and catalyzes the synthesis of ATP. The ATPase 6 and 8 subunits are encoded by the mitochondrial genome, whereas the remaining 14 subunits are encoded by the nuclear genome.

MITOCHONDRIAL ION CHANNELS

Proper function of the mitochondrial respiratory chain is dependent not simply on an intact respiratory chain; outer and inner mitochondrial membrane channels responsible for the bidirectional flow of nucleotides and essential ions are also crucial for normal oxidative metabolism. The voltage-dependent anion channel (VDAC) is selective to different ions depending on the transmembrane voltage. At low transmembrane voltage, anions including adenine nucleotides, phosphate, and chloride can pass. VDAC is open for cations and various uncharged molecules during times of high transmembrane voltage. The adenine nucleotide translocator (ANT) catalyzes the exchange of ATP produced by the mitochondrial respiratory chain with cytoplasmic ADP across the inner mitochondrial membrane. At least three tissue-specific ANT isoforms exist. Patients with defects in these channels have been reported.

MITOCHONDRIAL METAL HOMEOSTASIS

It has become evident that the function of the mitochondrial respiratory chain is dependent on normal processing and homeostasis of metal ions. Friedreich ataxia is usually caused by an abnormal GAA triplet expansion in the first intron of the *frataxin* gene. Frataxin is a nuclear encoded intra-mitochondrial protein, although its function is not clear. Frataxin mutations result in a loss of mtDNA and a severe respiratory chain defect associated with an abnormal elevation of intramitochondrial iron concentration. A mutation in another nuclear gene involved in mitochondrial iron homeostasis, *ABC7*, has been associated with X-linked sideroblastic anemia and ataxia. The Wilson disease protein localizes to the trans-Golgi network, and a modified, likely cleaved, form of this protein is located in mitochondria. Mutations result in intramitochondrial accumulation of copper, mtDNA deletions, and abnormal respiratory chain function. Although the exact mechanisms have not been elucidated, these examples highlight the importance of intramitochon-drial metal homeostasis for proper functioning of the mitochondrial respiratory chain.

—*Gregory M. Enns*

See also–Ion Channels, Overview; Mitochondrial Encephalomyopathies, Overview

Further Reading

Alberts, B., Bray, D., Lewis, J., *et al.* (1994). Energy conversion: Mitochondria and chloroplasts. *The Molecular Biology of the Cell*, pp. 653–720. Garland, New York.

Allikmets, R., Rashkind, W. H., Hutchinson, A., *et al.* (1999). Mutation of a putative mitochondrial iron transporter gene (ABC7) in X-linked sideroblastic anemia and ataxia (XLSA/A). *Hum. Mol. Genet.* **8**, 743–749.

Bakker, H. D., Scholte, H. R., Van den Bogert, C., *et al.* (1993). Deficiency of the adenine nucleotide translocator in muscle of a patient with myopathy and lactic acidosis: A new mitochondrial defect. *Pediatr. Res.* **33**, 412–417.

Bradley, J. L., Blake, J. C., Chamberlain, S., *et al.* (2000). Clinical, biochemical and molecular genetic correlations in Friedreich's ataxia. *Hum. Mol. Genet.* **9**, 275–282.

DiMauro, S., Bonilla, E., Davidson, M., *et al.* (1998). Mitochondria in neuromuscular disorders. *Biochim. Biophys. Acta* **1366**, 199–210.

Huizing, M., Ruitenbeek, W., Thinnes, F. P., *et al.* (1996). Deficiency of the voltage-dependent anion channel: A novel cause of mitochondriopathy. *Pediatr. Res.* **39**, 760–765.

Lutsenko, S., and Cooper, M. J. (1998). Localization of the Wilson's disease protein product to mitochondria. *Proc. Natl. Acad. Sci. USA* **95**, 6004–6009.

Saraste, M. (2000). Oxidative phosphorylation at the fin de siècle. *Science* **283**, 1488–1492.

Taanman, J.-W. (1999). The mitochondrial genome: Structure, transcription, translation and replication. *Biochim. Biophys. Acta* **1410**, 103–123.

Wallace, D. C., Lott, M. T., Brown, M. D., *et al.* (2001). Mitochondria and neuro-ophthalmologic diseases. In *The Molecular and Metabolic Bases of Inherited Disease* (C. R. Scriver, A. L. Beaudet, W. S. Sly, and D. Valle, Eds.), pp. 2425–2509. McGraw-Hill, New York.

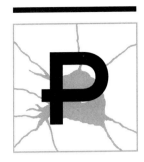

Paget's Disease

Encyclopedia of the Neurological Sciences
Copyright 2003, Elsevier Science (USA). All rights reserved.

OSTEITIS DEFORMANS, first described by Sir James Paget in 1877, is commonly referred to as Paget's disease of bone to differentiate it from Paget's disease of the breast. Two forms of osteitis deformans can occur. The monophasic form, also known as osteoporosis circumscripta, is associated with a steady and progressive softening of the affected bone. The biphasic form is characterized by bone resorption alternating with bone production. Any portion of the skeletal system may be affected, but there is a predilection for the axial skeleton and femurs.

INCIDENCE

Osteitis deformans, a skeletal disorder of adult life, is more common in males than females and in patients of European descent. Its incidence increases after 40 years of age, and it may affect more than 15% of the elderly. A family history of the disorder is present in 14% of patients. Its etiology is unknown, but viral, genetic, and environmental factors have been implicated.

SIGNS AND SYMPTOMS

Osteitis deformans manifests with a variety of neurological and orthopedic symptoms (Table 1). Compression of the brainstem due to basilar invagination can cause weakness, ataxia, spasticity, and hydrocephalus. Spinal cord compression due to narrowing of the spinal canal can produce quadriplegia or paraplegia. Radiculopathies associated with pain, sensory dysfunction, weakness, and fasciculations can be caused by narrowing of the spinal foramina.

Pain in the affected region is often the most common clinical manifestation of the disease. Ten to 20% of patients can be asymptomatic.

DIAGNOSTIC TESTING

Marked elevation of the serum alkaline phosphatase level (25–50% above normal) occurs in active osteitis deformans. Urinary levels of hydroxyproline are also elevated and parallel those of alkaline phosphatase. A significant elevation of these biochemical markers

Table 1 CLINICAL MANIFESTATIONS OF OSTEITIS DEFORMANS

General	Orthopedic	Neurological
Pain	Bone pain	Headache
Macrocephaly	Bone deformities	Cranial neuropathies
Leonine facies	Fractures and pseudofractures	Hydrocephalus
Poorly fitting dentures	Chronic ankle pain	Dementia
Bowed legs	Protrusio acetabuli	Seizures
Shortened stature	Coxa vara deformity	Ataxia
Simian posture	Arthritis of hip and knee joints	Sensory dysfunction
Waddling gait	Bone tumors	Weakness
High-output congestive heart failure		Spasticity
		Neurogenic claudication

indicates either active and extensive disease or intense activity in an area of monostotic involvement.

Plain radiographs demonstrate affected bones as enlarged with thickened cortices and areas of focal bone resorption and formation with a disordered trabecular pattern. Radiographs of the skull usually demonstrate areas of osteoporosis circumscripta affecting the skull vault. When the disease affects the base of the skull, basilar invagination may be detected. Bone scans and computed tomography can help visualize affected skeletal areas. Magnetic resonance imaging demonstrates basilar invagination, encroachment of neural structures, hydrocephalus, and narrowing of neural foramina.

TREATMENT

Because the cardinal manifestation of osteitis deformans is pain, the primary goal is analgesia. Pain may be due to intrinsic bony changes, increased metabolic activity in the affected areas, arthritic changes, neural compression, or a combination of all these factors. Therapy directed against the rapid rate of bone turnover is achieved with bisphosphonates, calcitonin, and mithramycin. Alendronate, clodronate, etidronate, pamidronate, and tiludronate are most commonly used. Salmon, eel, porcine, and human calcitonins are prescribed for the treatment of Paget's disease. Mithramycin effectively relieves bone pain in a few days. Combination therapy enhances the therapeutic effectiveness of the agents and also decreases the frequency of side effects. Neurological dysfunction has been reversed with the individual or combined use of calcitonin, mithramycin, and bisphosphonates. Single-agent therapy is less effective than combination therapy. Treatment is unnecessary in asymptomatic patients or in patients with monostotic involvement and normal levels of serum alkaline phosphatase.

Neurosurgical intervention is indicated for decompression of the brainstem, spinal cord, and spinal nerves in compressive syndromes refractory to medical therapy. Orthopedic interventions are indicated for the management of severe pagetic arthritis (shoulder, hip, or knee), osseous deformities (femur or tibia), pseudofractures or pathological fractures, and bone neoplasms. Before surgical intervention is attempted, medical therapy is essential to decrease the vascularity of the operative field.

—*Roberto Masferrer and Virginia Prendergast*

Further Reading

Ankrom, M. A., and Shapiro, J. R. (1998). Paget's disease of bone (osteitis deformans). *J. Am. Geriatr. Soc.* **46**, 1025–1033.
Delmas, P. D., and Meunier, P. J. (1997). The management of Paget's disease of bone. *N. Engl. J. Med.* **336**, 558–566.
Merkow, R. L., and Lane, J. M. (1990). Paget's disease of bone. *Orthop. Clin. North Am.* **21**, 171–189.

Pain, Assessment of

Encyclopedia of the Neurological Sciences
Copyright 2003, Elsevier Science (USA). All rights reserved.

PAIN research and therapy during the past century evolved from Descartes' concept of pain as a direct transmission system from "pain receptors" in the body tissues to a "pain center" in the brain. Injury or other pathology is assumed to lead inevitably to pain. As a result, the early history of pain measurement focused on the psychophysical relationship between the extent of injury and perceived pain. Various stimuli, such as electric shock or radiant heat, were applied to the skin and subjects in the laboratory provided estimates of pain intensity. Elegant psychophysical power functions were generated, and all studies of pain measurement until the publication of the gate control theory of pain concentrated exclusively on the measurement of pain intensity.

The gate control theory, together with the increasing emphasis on pain as a major clinical problem, led to the recognition that pain rarely has a one-to-one relationship to a "stimulus." Acute pain is sometimes proportional to the extent of injury, but the contribution of psychological factors reveals complex relations that are profoundly influenced by fear, anxiety, cultural background, and the meaning of the situation to the person. Chronic pain presents an even greater problem for the Cartesian psychophysical concept: Backaches often occur without any discernible organic cause, and postherpetic neuralgia persists long after peripheral nerve regeneration and healing of all tissue.

The new emphasis on the varieties of clinical pain and their variability led to new concepts of pain measurement. Instead of using stimuli such as radiant heat to obtain psychophysical standards to measure clinical pain, it became necessary to measure the subjective experience of pain without reference to external causes.

People suffering acute or chronic pain provide valuable opportunities to study the mechanisms of pain and analgesia. Therefore, the measurement of pain is essential to determine the initial intensity, perceptual qualities, and time course of the pain so that the differences among different pain syndromes can be ascertained and investigated. Furthermore, measurement of these variables provides valuable clues that help in the differential diagnosis of the underlying causes of the pain. They also help determine the most effective treatment, such as the types of analgesic drugs or other therapies, necessary to control the pain and are essential to evaluate the relative effectiveness of different therapies. Thus, the measurement of pain is important to determine pain intensity, quality, and duration; to aid in diagnosis; to help decide on the choice of therapy; and to evaluate the relative effectiveness of different therapies.

DIMENSIONS OF PAIN EXPERIENCE

Since the beginning of the 20th century, research on pain has been dominated by the concept that pain is purely a sensory experience. However, pain also has a distinctly unpleasant, affective quality. It becomes overwhelming, demands immediate attention, and disrupts ongoing behavior and thought. It motivates or drives the organism into activity aimed at stopping the pain as quickly as possible. To consider only the sensory features of pain and ignore its motivational–affective properties is to look at only part of the problem. Even the concept of pain as a perception, with full recognition of past experience, attention, and other cognitive influences, still neglects the crucial motivational dimension.

These considerations led Melzack and Casey to suggest that there are three major psychological dimensions of pain: sensory–discriminative, motivational–affective, and cognitive–evaluative. These dimensions of pain experience are subserved by physiologically specialized systems in the brain. The sensory–discriminative dimension of pain is influenced primarily by the rapidly conducting spinal systems. The powerful motivational drive and unpleasant affect characteristic of pain are subserved by activities in reticular and limbic structures that are influenced primarily by the slowly conducting spinal systems. The cognitive–evaluative dimension of pain, which involves neocortical or higher central nervous system processes such as evaluation of the input in terms of past experience, exerts control over activity in both the discriminative and motivational systems.

It is assumed that these three categories of activity interact with one another to provide perceptual information on the location, magnitude, and spatio-temporal properties of the noxious stimuli; motivational tendency toward escape or attack; and cognitive information based on past experience and probability of outcome of different response strategies. All three forms of activity could then influence motor mechanisms responsible for the complex pattern of overt responses that characterize pain.

THE LANGUAGE OF PAIN

Clinical investigators have long recognized the varieties of pain experience. Descriptions of the burning qualities of pain after peripheral nerve injury or the stabbing, cramping qualities of visceral pains frequently provide the key to diagnosis and may even suggest the course of therapy. Despite the frequency of such descriptions, and the seemingly high agreement that they are valid descriptive words, studies of their use and meaning are relatively recent.

Anyone who has suffered severe pain and tried to describe the experience to a friend or to a doctor often finds themselves at a loss for words. The reason for this difficulty in expressing pain experience is not because the words do not exist. There is an abundance of appropriate words. Rather, the main reason is that, fortunately, they are not words that we have occasion to use often. Another reason is that the words may seem absurd. We may use descriptors such as splitting, shooting, gnawing, wrenching, or stinging as useful metaphors, but there are no external objective references for these words in relation to pain. If we talk about a blue pen or a yellow pencil, we can point to an object and say "that is what I mean by yellow" or "this color of the pen is blue." However, what can we point to in order to tell another person precisely what we mean by smarting, tingling, or rasping? A person who suffers terrible pain may say that the pain is burning and add that "it feels as if someone is shoving a red-hot poker through my toes and slowly twisting it around." These "as if" statements are often essential to convey the qualities of the experience.

If the study of pain in people is to have a scientific foundation, it is essential to measure pain. If we want to know the effectiveness of a new drug, we need numbers to indicate that the pain decreased by some amount. However, although overall intensity is important information, we also want to know whether the drug specifically decreased the burning quality of the pain or if the especially miserable, tight, cramping feeling is gone.

PAIN RATING SCALES

Until recently, the methods used for pain measurement treated pain as though it were a single unique quality that varied only in intensity. These methods include the use of verbal rating scales (VRSs), numerical rating scales (NRSs), and visual analog scales (VASs). These simple methods have all been used effectively in hospital clinics, and they have provided valuable information about pain and analgesia. VRSs, NRSs, and VASs provide simple, efficient, and minimally intrusive measures of pain intensity that have been used widely in clinical and research settings in which a quick index of pain intensity is required and to which a numerical value can be assigned.

Verbal and Numerical Rating Scales

Verbal rating scales typically consist of a series of verbal pain descriptors ordered from least to most intense (e.g., no pain, mild, moderate, and severe). The patient reads the list and chooses the one word that best describes the intensity of his or her pain at the moment. A score of zero is assigned to the descriptor with the lowest rank, a score of 1 is assigned to the descriptor with the next lowest rank, etc. Numerical rating scales typically consist of a series of numbers ranging from 0 to 10 or 0 to 100, with endpoints intended to represent the extremes of the possible pain experience and labeled "no pain" and "worst possible pain," respectively. The patient chooses the number that best corresponds to the intensity of his or her pain at the moment. Although VRSs and NRSs are simple to administer and have demonstrated reliability and validity, the advantages associated with VASs make them the measurement instrument of choice when a unidimensional measure of pain is required. However, this may not be true when assessing chronic pain in the elderly.

Visual Analog Scales

The most common VAS consists of a 10-cm horizontal or vertical line with the two endpoints labeled "no pain" and "worst pain ever" (or similar verbal descriptors). The patient is required to place a mark on the 10-cm line at a point that corresponds to the level of pain intensity they presently feel. The distance in centimeters from the low end of the VAS to the patient's mark is used as a numerical index of the severity of pain.

VASs for pain affect have been developed in an effort to include domains of measurable pain experience other than the sensory intensity dimension. The patient is asked to rate the unpleasantness of the pain experience (i.e., how disturbing it is to them). Endpoints are labeled "not bad at all" and "the most unpleasant feeling imaginable."

VASs are sensitive to pharmacological and non-pharmacological procedures that alter the experience of pain and correlate highly with pain measured on verbal and numerical rating scales. Instructions to patients to rate the amount or percentage of pain relief using a VAS (e.g., following administration of a treatment designed to reduce pain) introduce unnecessary bias (e.g., expectancy for change and reliance on memory) that reduces the validity of the measure. A more appropriate measure of change may be obtained by having patients rate the absolute amount of pain at different points in time, such as before and after an intervention.

A major advantage of the VAS as a measure of sensory pain intensity is its ratio scale properties. In contrast to many other pain measurement tools, equality of ratios is implied, making it appropriate to speak meaningfully about percentage differences between VAS measurements obtained either at multiple points in time or from independent samples of subjects. Other advantages of the VAS include (i) its ease and brevity of administration and scoring, (ii) its minimal intrusiveness, and (iii) its conceptual simplicity, providing that adequately clear instructions are given to the patient.

Standard VASs also have several limitations and disadvantages, including difficulty with administration in patients who have perceptual motor problems, impractical scoring method in a clinical setting in which immediate measurement of the patient's response may not be possible, and the occasional patient who cannot comprehend the instructions. The major disadvantage of VASs is the assumption that pain is a unidimensional experience that can be measured with a single item scale. Although intensity is, without a doubt, a salient dimension of pain, it is clear that the word "pain" refers to an endless variety of qualities that are categorized under a single linguistic label and not to a specific, single sensation that varies only in intensity or affect. The development of VASs to measure pain affect or unpleasantness has partially addressed the problem, but the same shortcoming applies within the affective domain. Each pain has unique qualities. Unpleasantness is only one such quality. The pain of a toothache is obviously different from that of a pin-prick, just as the pain of a coronary occlusion is uniquely different from the pain of a broken leg. To describe pain solely in terms of intensity or affect is like specifying the visual world only in terms of light flux without regard to pattern, color, texture, and the many other dimensions of visual experience.

THE MCGILL PAIN QUESTIONNAIRE

Melzack and Torgerson developed procedures to specify the qualities of pain. The result was the McGill Pain Questionnaire (MPQ; Fig. 1), a multidimensional clinical and research tool for studies of the effects of various methods of pain management. The MPQ consists of 78 words categorized into three

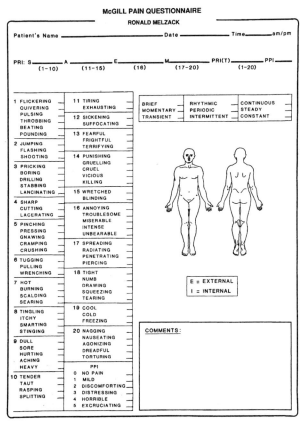

Figure 1
McGill Pain Questionnaire. The descriptors are classified into four major groups: sensory, 1–10; affective, 11–15; evaluative, 16; and miscellaneous, 17–20. The rank value for each descriptor is based on its position in the word set. The sum of the rank values is the pain rating index (PRI). The present pain intensity (PPI) is based on a scale of 0–5 (reproduced with permission from Melzack, 1975).

major classes and 20 subclasses. The classes are (i) words that describe the sensory qualities of the experience in terms of temporal, spatial, pressure, thermal, and other properties; (ii) words that describe affective qualities in terms of tension, fear, and autonomic properties that are part of the pain experience; and (iii) evaluative words that describe the subjective overall intensity of the total pain experience. Each subclass has a descriptive label and consists of a group of words that were considered by most subjects to be qualitatively similar. Some of these words are undoubtedly synonyms, others seem to be synonymous but vary in intensity, whereas many provide subtle differences or nuances (despite their similarities) that may be of importance to a patient who is trying desperately to communicate to a physician.

In addition to the list of pain descriptors, the questionnaire contains line drawings of the body to show the spatial distribution of the pain, words that describe temporal properties of pain, and descriptors of the overall present pain intensity (PPI).

The descriptor lists of the MPQ are read to a patient with the explicit instruction that they choose only those words that describe their feelings and sensations at that moment. Three major indices are obtained:

- *The pain rating index (PRI) based on the rank values of the words:* In this scoring system, the word in each subclass implying the least pain is given a value of 1, the next word is given a value of 2, etc. The rank values of the words chosen by a patient are summed to obtain a score separately for the sensory (subclasses 1–10), affective (subclasses 11–15), evaluative (subclass 16), and miscellaneous (subclasses 17–20) words and also to provide a total score (subclasses 1–20). Figure 2 shows MPQ scores (total score from subclasses 1–20) obtained by patients with a variety of acute and chronic pains.
- *The number of words chosen (NWC).*
- *The PPI—the number–word combination chosen as the indicator of overall pain intensity at the time of administration of the questionnaire:* The PPI is recorded as a number from 1 to 5, where each number is associated with the following words: 1, mild; 2, discomforting; 3, distressing; 4, horrible; and 5, excruciating.

The most important requirement of a measure is that it be valid, reliable, consistent, and, especially, useful. The MPQ appears to meet all these

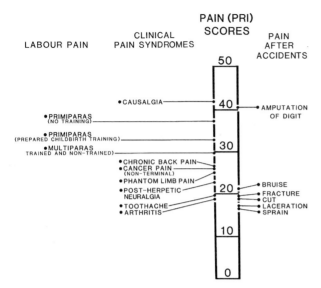

Figure 2
Comparison of pain scores using the McGill Pain Questionnaire.

requirements and provides a relatively rapid way of measuring subjective pain experience. When administered to a patient by reading each subclass, it can be completed in approximately 5 min. It can also be filled out by the patient in a more leisurely way as a paper-and-pencil test, although the scores may differ somewhat. Since its introduction in 1975, the MPQ has been used in more than 350 studies of acute, chronic, and laboratory-produced pains. It has been translated into several languages and has also spawned the development of similar pain questionnaires in other languages.

Because pain is a private, personal experience, it is impossible for us to know precisely what someone else's pain feels like. No man can possibly know what it is like to have menstrual cramps or labor pain. Nor can a psychologically healthy person know what a psychotic patient is feeling when they say they have excruciating pain. However, the MPQ provides insight into the qualities that are experienced in a reliable and valid manner.

SHORT-FORM MCGILL PAIN QUESTIONNAIRE

The short-form MPQ (SF-MPG) was developed for use in specific research settings when the time to obtain information from patients is limited and when more information is desired than that provided by intensity measures such as the VAS or NRS. The SF-MPQ consists of 15 representative words from the

sensory ($n = 11$) and affective ($n = 4$) categories of the standard, long-form (LF-MPQ). The PPI and a VAS are included to provide indices of overall pain intensity. The 15 descriptors making up the SF-MPQ were selected on the basis of their frequency of endorsement by patients with a variety of acute, intermittent, and chronic pains. An additional word, splitting, was added because it was reported to be a key discriminative word for dental pain. Each descriptor is ranked by the patient on the following intensity scale: 0 = none, 1 = mild, 2 = moderate, and 3 = severe. The SF-MPQ correlates very highly with the major PRI indices (sensory, affective, and total) of the LF-MPQ and is sensitive to clinical change brought about by various therapies.

DESCRIPTOR DIFFERENTIAL SCALE

The Descriptor Differential Scale (DDS) was developed to remedy a number of deficiencies associated with existing pain measurement instruments. The DDS was designed to reduce bias, assess separately the sensory intensity and "unpleasantness" (hedonic) dimensions of pain, and provide quantification by ratio-scaling procedures. The DDS consists of two forms that measure separately the sensory intensity and unpleasantness qualities of pain. Each form consists of 12 verbal descriptors, where each descriptor is based on a 21-point scale with a minus sign at the low end and a plus sign at the high end. The patients rate the magnitude of the sensory intensity or unpleasantness of the pain they are experiencing. The magnitude of pain endorsed by the patient in relation to each descriptor is assigned a score of 0 (minus sign) to 20 (plus sign), where a score of 10 represents pain intensity or unpleasantness equal to the magnitude implied by the descriptor. Total mean scores may be obtained for the sensory intensity and unpleasantness dimensions by averaging the patient's scores on each 12-item form. The DDS has been demonstrated to be differentially sensitive to pharmacological interventions that alter the sensory or unpleasantness dimensions of pain.

BEHAVIORAL APPROACHES TO PAIN MEASUREMENT

Recent research on the development of behavioral measures of pain has produced a wide array of sophisticated observational techniques and rating scales designed to assess objective behaviors that accompany pain experience. Techniques that have demonstrated high reliability and validity are especially useful for measuring pain in infants and preverbal children who lack language skills, adults who have a poor command of language, or when mental clouding and confusion limit the patient's ability to communicate meaningfully. In these circumstances, behavioral measures provide important information that is otherwise unavailable from patient self-report. Moreover, when administered in conjunction with a subjective, patient-rated measure, behavioral measures may provide a more complete picture of the total pain experience. However, behavioral measures of pain should not replace self-rated measures if the patient is capable of rating their subjective state and such administration is feasible.

The subjective experiences of pain and pain behaviors are presumably reflections of the same underlying neural processes. However, the complexity of the human brain indicates that although experience and behavior are usually highly correlated, they are far from identical. One person may be stoic so that their calm behavior belies their true subjective feelings. Another patient may seek sympathy (or analgesic medication or some other desirable goal) and in so doing exaggerate their complaints without also eliciting the behaviors that typically accompany pain complaints of that degree. These individual differences point to the importance of obtaining multiple measures of pain and should keep us aware that since pain is a subjective experience, the patient's self-report is the most valid measure of that experience.

PHYSIOLOGICAL APPROACHES TO PAIN MEASUREMENT

Profound physiological changes often accompany the experience of pain, especially if the injury or noxious stimulus is acute. Physiological correlates of pain may serve to elucidate mechanisms that underlie the experience and thus may provide clues that may lead to novel treatments. Physiological correlates of pain experience that are frequently measured include heart rate, blood pressure, electrodermal activity, electromyographic activity, cortical evoked potentials, and, recently, brain imaging techniques, such as functional magnetic resonance imaging, positron emission tomography, and magnetic source imaging. Despite high initial correlations between pain onset and changes in these physiological responses, many habituate with time despite the persistence of pain. In

addition, these responses are not specific to the experience of pain per se and occur under conditions of general arousal and stress. Studies that have examined the general endocrine–metabolic stress response to surgical incision indicate that under certain conditions it is possible to dissociate different aspects of the stress response and pain. This indicates that although there are many physiological and endocrine events that occur concurrently with the experience of pain, many appear to be general responses to stress and are not unique to pain.

CONCLUSION

Pain is a personal, subjective experience influenced by cultural learning, the meaning of the situation, attention, and other psychological variables. Approaches to the measurement of pain include verbal and numeric self-rating scales, behavioral observation scales, and physiological responses. The complex nature of the experience of pain suggests that measurements from these domains may not always show high concordance. Because pain is subjective, the patient's self-report provides the most valid measure of the experience. The VAS and the MPQ are probably the most frequently used self-rating instruments for the measurement of pain in clinical and research settings. The MPQ is designed to assess the multidimensional nature of pain experience and has been demonstrated to be a reliable, valid, and consistent measurement tool. A short-form MPQ is available for use in specific research settings when the time to obtain information from patients is limited and when more information than simply the intensity of pain is desired. The DDS was developed using sophisticated psychophysical techniques and is designed to measure separately the sensory and unpleasantness dimensions of pain. It has been shown to be a valid and reliable measure of pain with ratio scale properties and has recently been used in a clinical setting. Behavioral approaches to the measurement of pain also provide valuable data. Further development and refinement of pain measurement techniques will lead to increasingly accurate tools with greater predictive powers.

—Joel Katz and Ronald Melzack

See also–Pain, Basic Neurobiology of; Pain Management, Multidisciplinary; Pain Management, Psychological Strategies; Pain, Overview; Sensation, Assessment of

Acknowledgments

This work was supported by an Investigator Award to J.K. from the Canadian Institutes of Health Research (CIHR), CIHR Grants MCT-38144 and MOP-37845 (J.K.), and Grant A7891 from the Natural Sciences and Engineering Research Council of Canada (R.M.).

Further Reading

Gracely, R. H., and Kwilosz, D. M. (1988). The Descriptor Differential Scale: Applying psychophysical principles to clinical pain assessment. *Pain* **35**, 279–288.

Huskisson, E. C. (1983). Visual analogue scales. In *Pain Measurement and Assessment* (R. Melzack, Ed.), pp. 33–37. Raven Press, New York.

Jensen, M. P., and Karoly, P. (1992). Self-report scales and procedures for assessing pain in adults. In *Handbook of Pain Assessment* (D. C. Turk and R. Melzack, Eds.), pp. 135–151. Guilford, New York.

Melzack, R. (1975). The McGill Pain Questionnaire: Major properties and scoring methods. *Pain* **1**, 277–299.

Melzack, R. (1987). The short-form McGill Pain Questionnaire. *Pain* **30**, 191–197.

Melzack, R., and Casey, K. L. (1968). Sensory, motivational, and central control determinants of pain: A new conceptual model. In *The Skin Senses* (D. Kenshalo, Ed.), pp. 423–443. Thomas, Springfield, IL.

Melzack, R., and Torgerson, W. S. (1971). On the language of pain. *Anesthesiology* **34**, 50–59.

Melzack, R., and Wall, P. D. (1965). Pain mechanisms: A new theory. *Science* **150**, 971–979.

Price, D. D., Harkins, S. W., Rafii, A., *et al.* (1986). A simultaneous comparison of fentanyl's analgesic effects on experimental and clinical pain. *Pain* **24**, 197–203.

Pain, Basic Neurobiology of

Encyclopedia of the Neurological Sciences

THE SENSATION OF PAIN is fundamental to survival. Paradoxically, it is useful because it is so unpleasant. Normally, pain sensation is tightly coupled to the presence or threat of tissue injury. The normal threshold for heat pain, between 45 and 50°C, is the temperature at which proteins begin to coagulate. Pain provides such strong incentive to move away from harm that it is difficult not to withdraw from a sudden painful stimulus. Individuals without normal pain sensation, either congenitally or acquired, often have repeated injuries leading to amputations and infections, and sometimes death.

Virtually all animals experience unpleasant responses to dangerous stimuli, and in even the lowest organisms, these are tightly coupled to escape reflexes and to interneurons that allow animals to "learn" to avoid this danger in the future. The most fundamental functions of the nervous system are to avoid painful stimuli that threaten survival and to seek out pleasurable stimuli, such as food, that enhance survival. Pain that lasts a few days or weeks after an injury is useful; it discourages use of the injured area and allows it to heal. Normally, pain resolves as tissues are repaired and inflammation resolves. If pain becomes chronic, major medical, psychological, and social problems ensue.

There are two categories of chronic pain. Nociceptive/inflammatory pain is acute or chronic pain associated with tissue damage. An example is arthritic joint pain due to chronic inflammation and joint destruction. In chronic inflammatory pain, the sensory nervous system is working properly. Neuropathic pain is pathological pain that occurs in the absence of, or out of proportion to, tissue injury. The major injury is to the pain pathways. These become electrically hyperexcitable and send action potentials to the brain that are interpreted as tissue injury, even when there is none. A common example is sciatica, in which pain is perceived as radiating down the back of the leg when, in fact, the injury is usually in the back, to a nerve root exiting the spine. The presence of neuropathic pain is a fundamental sign of neurological injury, and like a motor deficit, its location and characteristics can be used to localize and characterize neural lesions.

Chronic pain is not a diagnosis but a description of a symptom complex. The most common symptom is ongoing (or stimulus-independent) pain that occurs without any contact with, or use of, the painful area. In contrast, various stimuli can produce stimulus-evoked pain. Pain evoked by a usually innocuous stimulation (such as light touch) is referred to as allodynia (Fig. 1). Allodynia can occur after acute, inflammatory, or neuropathic pain; can be provoked by mechanical, thermal, or chemical stimuli; and can be produced by different mechanisms in different circumstances. Many of us have experienced allodynia to touch after sunburn, and neuropathy patients often complain that they cannot bear the touch of bedclothes on their allodynic feet. Pain patients may also feel hyperalgesia, or excess pain after a minor painful stimulus. A clinical example is severe pain from needle prick. The pain response can be qualitatively abnormal (hyperpathic), with a prolonged duration or unusual sensory quality. The term lancinating pain refers to sudden paroxysms of severe

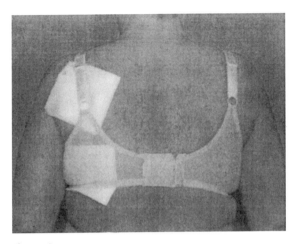

Figure 1
A postherpetic neuralgia patient with gauze pads placed under her brassiere straps to relieve allodynia.

pain that usually last only seconds to minutes. The pain is often described as "stabbing" or "lightning-like." A zone of primary hyperalgesia can surround an injured area; it is attributable to peripheral mechanisms. More distant secondary hyperalgesia (e.g., in the territory of a different peripheral nerve or spinal segment) is mediated in the central nervous system (CNS). Primary hyperalgesia has been described for both mechanical and thermal stimuli, whereas secondary hyperalgesia appears to be present for mechanical but not thermal stimuli.

It used to be expected that serious illness would be accompanied by chronic pain. It is now appreciated, though, that pain can often be ameliorated even if the underlying disease cannot. As with other chronic diseases, such as asthma and chronic heart failure, different mechanisms contribute to the presence of pain, and understanding these mechanisms offers the hope of developing new effective and specific treatments. In the United States, the Joint Commission on Accreditation of Healthcare Organizations recently mandated that every hospital implement a plan for evaluating and treating pain. There are clear benefits in reduced morbidity and health care costs, from reducing postoperative pain and decreasing length of stay after surgeries. The benefits of good pain management are self-evident.

The goal of this entry is to briefly review the underlying neuroanatomical and molecular substrates for normal and pathological pain processing. The recent explosion in molecular neurosciences has not spared the pain field, and only the most superficial overview of clinically relevant mechanisms can be attempted here.

NEUROBIOLOGY OF ACUTE PAIN

Properties of Primary (Peripheral) Nociceptive Neurons

The nociceptive pathways begin with primary somatosensory afferent neurons that transduce different types of potentially noxious energy into action potentials and transmit them to the CNS. Virtually all of the many sensory neurons that penetrate into the epidermis are nociceptors, as are all tooth-pulp and corneal neurons. There are different types of nociceptors, each specialized to fire in response to specific types of stimuli. Stimuli can be broadly categorized into mechanical, thermal, or chemical types. Different subtypes of neurons are activated by energy of particular intensity, frequency, or characteristics. Thinly myelinated Aδ nociceptive fibers provide information about the location, intensity, duration, and nature of a painful stimulus. Their impulses reach consciousness earliest to produce "first pain" and to provoke reflex withdrawal. The more abundant unmyelinated C fibers are associated with the affective-motivational response to painful stimuli. Because they are unmyelinated, C fibers conduct more slowly and produce the more diffuse and persistent sensation called "second pain." Many C fibers are polymodal and can respond to multiple types of stimuli. C fibers tend to be the predominant source of chronic and visceral pain.

Under normal conditions, most nociceptors do not fire until the stimulus approaches levels that can cause actual tissue damage. Approximately half of cutaneous Aδ and one-third of C fibers appear not to fire at all under normal conditions (silent or sleeping nociceptors) and only activate under conditions of tissue injury or inflammation. Some of these mechanoinsensitive afferents encode histamine-induced itch. Similar fibers have been found in the knee joint, cornea, and viscera. The transducers of cold pain appear to be located in or near the walls of cutaneous blood vessels. Psychophysical studies of human subjects have shown that activation of individual nociceptive primary afferents does not necessarily produce a sensation of pain, so spatial and temporal summation within the CNS may be necessary as well.

Nociceptive terminals bear a myriad of receptors on their axolemmae, including those for bradykinin, prostaglandins, leukotrienes, histamine, serotonin, substance P, thromboxanes, platelet-activating factor, protons, and free radicals. Some of these chemical stimuli can produce action potentials, whereas others lead to sensitization or easier firing after a mechanical or thermal stimulus. Many have proinflammatory paracrine effects and result in the release of other molecules from inflammatory cells that can directly stimulate nociceptive action potentials. It is clear that the primary afferent nociceptors participate in, and are strongly influenced by, tissue inflammation.

In the past few years, new information has emerged about the transient receptor potential (TRP) family of ion channels that transduce heat pain among other stimuli. VR_1, the polymodal vanilloid receptor, mediates the burn sensation produced by capsaicin in hot chili peppers. Noxious heat ($>43°C$), lipids, and protons (present during injury and inflammation) also activate the VR_1 molecule. Studies of the sensory properties of VR_1 knockout mice have contributed to our understanding of normal and pathological sensory function. Molecular studies of other sensory transducers are also under way. Nociceptive fibers have efferent as well as afferent activity. When activated by injury or inflammation, they can release paracrine molecules such as substance P and calcitonin gene-related peptide (CGRP). These contribute to vasodilation and to sensitization of nearby nerve endings.

Nonnociceptive sensory signals (e.g., touch, position, vibration, and proprioception) are relayed by other types of primary afferents, including the thickly myelinated and rapidly conducting $A\delta$ fibers. These usually ascend the dorsal columns of the spinal cord to the nuclei gracilis and cuneatus in the brainstem.

Peripheral Nociceptive Axons

Primary afferent somatosensory neurons are bipolar, with one axon extending from the periphery to the cell body located in the peripheral nervous system (PNS) and the other from the cell body into the CNS. Within peripheral nerves, axons are enrobed by Schwann cell processes or myelin. Schwann cells (as well as other endoneurial cells, such as fibroblasts, macrophages, and mast cells) contribute profoundly to neural function and probably influence nociception in ways that are not yet appreciated. They are immunologically active and play a critical role in axonal development, differentiation, injury, and regeneration. They contain receptors for and synthesize many neuroactive molecules. They modulate concentrations of molecules in the adaxonal environment. By virtue of their very small diameter, most nociceptive neurons are unmyelinated (C fibers) or only thinly myelinated. Thus, they are among the more slowly conducting sensory neurons

(approximately 1 m/sec). Most peripheral nerves contain sympathetic afferents and efferents as well as somatic axons. Segmental reflexes between the two systems cause the autonomic components of pain, especially visceral pain. These include muscle guarding, changes in vascular tone, and sweating.

The Basis of Visceral Pain

Pain in deep somatic and visceral structures is generated by substantially different mechanisms than those for the skin. Touch, exquisitely developed in the skin, is rudimentary in many internal organs, presumably because they are in constant contact with neighboring tissues but not often contacted by external objects. Therefore, deep pain is diffuse and poorly localized. Similarly, there is little need for receptors for pain from cutting or burning. In contrast, internal tissues are sensitive to hypoxia and ischemia with its attendant acidosis, and the hollow viscera and organ capsules are sensitive to distension. Acute visceral pain seems to more commonly produce widespread autonomic effects, such as sweating, pallor, tachycardia, and hypotension. Referral of pain from deep to superficial structures (e.g., from ischemia myocardium to the arm or jaw, or from the diaphragm to the shoulder) is based on convergence of somatic and visceral neurons within the spinal cord. Far less is known about mechanisms of visceral than cutaneous pain, presumably because of the difficulty accessing tissues. Most basic science studies of visceral pain are conducted using animal models. Studies commonly involve creating visceral pain by distending or inflaming the uterus or colon and recording the electrical activity of the dorsal horn.

Cell Bodies (Perikarya) of Primary Nociceptive Neurons

The cell bodies of primary somatosensory neurons lie just outside the CNS in the sensory ganglia. The trigeminal, or Gasserian, ganglion contains the cell bodies of the trigeminal neurons that subserve facial sensation, and the spinal dorsal root ganglia (DRG) contain the cell bodies of the somatosensory neurons that innervate the rest of the body. Within individual ganglia, nociceptive neurons (C and $A\delta$) tend to have smaller cell bodies than nonnociceptive sensory neurons. Selective immunolabeling has established that more than 12 types of peptides are found in varying proportions of DRG cell bodies. The more commonly expressed neuromodulators include CGRP, vasopressin, oxytocin, and substance P. The functional significance of these localizations and colocalizations is only beginning to be understood, attesting to the complexity of nociceptive processing. Signals ascending from the periphery are modified in the sensory ganglia before spreading to the central axon of the primary afferent neuron that projects into the CNS. The sensory ganglia are outside the blood–nerve barrier and thus vulnerable to systemic influences.

Central Axons of Primary Nociceptive Neurons

These axons are vulnerable to compression at the neural foramen from herniated intravertebral disks, bony osteophytes, or thickened ligaments. Some central axons travel for long distances within the CNS, where they are vulnerable to diseases that affect the spinal cord. Central primary afferent axons are probably more involved in neuropathic pain than is realized because most conditions that affect the peripheral axon (e.g., distal axonopathy) affect the central axon as well. Many discussions of the effects of injury to the peripheral nociceptive axon do not consider the fact that injured primary afferent sensory neurons may be disconnected from their central target by the same disease process that affects the peripheral axon. This central–distal peripheral axonopathy has been demonstrated in autopsy studies of patients with painful diabetic polyneuropathy.

A clinically important feature of nociceptive neuroanatomy is that incoming central afferent axons trifurcate and send collateral axons several segments up and down the spinal cord in Lissauer's tract. This oft-forgotten fact explains why so many patients with lesions of peripheral nerves or roots also develop pain in adjacent, seemingly uninvolved areas. Also note that some primary afferents enter the spinal cord through the ventral, rather than dorsal, roots.

Organization of the Dorsal Horn

Somatotopic organization provides information about the localization of painful stimuli. For instance, lateral portions of the foot project to medial portions of the dorsal horn. Somatic afferents appear to project only to the ipsilateral half of the spinal cord, although the increasing number of articles attesting to bilateral effects of unilateral nerve injury suggests that indirect pathways (perhaps glial) remain to be described. Visceral afferents may project bilaterally or to the region near the central canal.

Dorsal horn neurons that respond to both gentle and noxious stimuli are known as wide-dynamic-range (WDR) neurons, whereas those responding only to noxious stimuli are known as high-threshold or nociceptive-specific neurons. Different types of primary afferents project to discrete Rexed laminae within the dorsal horn. The bulk of C fibers project to the nociceptive-specific projection neurons in outer laminae II and lamina I (substantia gelatinosa). WDR neurons, which receive input from low-threshold mechanoreceptors (among others), tend to be located deeper within the dorsal horn in laminae IV–VI. Many terminate in lamina V. Visceral afferents often project deeply to laminae VII and VIII. In the trigeminal system, the nucleus caudalis is equivalent to lamina I of the spinal dorsal horn. Processing here seems to be similar. Woolf and colleagues provided strong evidence that, in rats with nerve injury, allodynia may involve sprouting of central axons of Aβ touch fibers onto second-order pain-processing projection neurons in the more superficial laminae.

Excitation of Dorsal Horn Neurons by Nociceptive Peripheral Neurons

Relatively few studies of dorsal horn physiology and pharmacology have been conducted in tissues from humans, much less from actual pain patients. It is widely assumed that findings derived from the study of rats and a few nonhuman primates apply to humans as well; this assumption needs to be tested. Nociceptive neurons form monosynaptic excitatory synapses onto secondary projection neurons in the superficial layers of the spinal or trigeminal dorsal horn as well as polysynaptic inhibitory synapses that involve segmental inhibitory interneurons. Both acute and chronic pain are associated with an augmentation of dorsal horn excitation.

Primary afferents release more than 12 neurotransmitters and neuromodulators onto their postsynaptic targets. Some produce responses that last milliseconds, whereas others induce changes that last seconds or minutes. Glutamate is the fast-acting neurotransmitter that appears to mediate most direct excitatory synapses from primary afferents onto spinal neurons. Aspartate is present as well. The postsynaptic effects of glutamate involve both activation of ligand-gated ion channels and complex effects mediated through G protein-coupled receptors. A multiplicity of subtypes of AMPA/kainate and NMDA receptors has been implicated. Because of the complexity of these pathways, it has proven difficult to effectively and specifically block excitatory nociceptive transmission in the dorsal horn.

Afferent terminals in the dorsal horn also contain a plethora of neuromodulatory peptides, including CGRP, substance P, neuropeptide Y, neurokinin A, gastrin-releasing peptide, somatostatin, vasoactive intestinal polypeptide, and galanin, as well as endogenous opiates such as dynorphin and enkephalin. There is no clear pattern of colocalization or clear correspondence between specific types of sensory stimuli and release of specific peptides. These peptides tend to be released in response to prolonged trains of stimuli and may contribute to the changes in properties that underlie central sensitization and other modulations of the response to injury. Central afferent terminals contain receptors for neuromodulators that influence their synaptic activity. Binding of opioids, for instance, appears to decrease synaptic activity and may act to dampen pain responses. Binding of neuropeptide Y and GABA may have a similar effect.

Inhibitory Synapses onto Second-Order Nociceptive Neurons

Primary afferents also have profound inhibitory effects on second-order spinal pain neurons. These involve at least one intercalated segmental interneuron that is excited by primary afferent nociceptors and forms an inhibitory synapse on second-order dorsal horn pain neurons. This type of circuitry is typical in sensory systems and helps to limit spatial and temporal spread of the response to an incoming action potential. It is widely assumed that enhanced excitatory neurotransmission between first- and second-order pain neurons underlies neuropathic pain, as it does for acute and inflammatory pain. However, there is increasing experimental evidence that the hyperactivity of dorsal horn pain neurons that underlies chronic pain states can also be triggered by diminished input from primary nociceptive afferents. This may diminish segmental inhibitory circuits and result in a net excitation of second-order pain neurons.

Other primary afferents, such as low-threshold mechanoreceptors, can also indirectly inhibit spinal pain projection neurons. This explains the relief obtained from rubbing a painful area (and probably from scratching an itch as well). The effectiveness of dorsal column and peripheral nerve stimulators for treating chronic pain may be mediated by triggering inhibitory interneurons as well. Glycine and GABA

appear to be the primary inhibitory neurotransmitters in the dorsal horn. Baclofen, a GABA$_B$ agonist long used to treat spasticity, has been shown to have some efficacy against neuropathic pain in animal models and human patients. Conversely, pharmacologically antagonizing spinal GABA or glycine can produce the onset of hyperalgesia in animals, in the absence of any injury or painful stimulation. Intraspinal opioids derive much of their effect by augmenting segmental inhibitory circuits.

Descending monoadrenergic projections in the dorsolateral cord from areas such as the nucleus raphé magnus, the lateral tegmentum, and the locus coeruleus also inhibit second-order pain neurons, contributing to the considerable modulation of pain signals in the spinal cord. These comprise the diffuse noxious inhibitory control (DNIC) pathways. The raphé nuclei use serotonin as a neurotransmitter, whereas the locus coeruleus and lateral tegmental cells use norepinephrine. Tricyclic antidepressants probably derive at least part of their antihyperalgesic effects from enhancing these descending inhibitory inputs. Endogenous opiates, such as dynorphin, enkephalins, and endorphins, activate these descending antinociceptive pathways as well. Cholecystokinin has also been implicated. Higher functions, emotions, and other components of consciousness modulate dorsal horn processing and possibly primary afferent function via these descending pathways.

Ascending Projection Pathways

After considerable integration and processing, most pain signals from the dorsal horn cross the spinal midline in the anterior commissure to travel in the anterolateral quadrant to the reticular formation in the brainstem or to the thalamus. This medial zone of decussation of nociceptive fibers is vulnerable to compression or disruption by syrinxes of the central spinal canal. These produce pain in corresponding dermatomes and often spare motor function since the motor fibers lie laterally in the corticospinal tracts. The lateral spinothalamic tracts are the main (but not the only) ascending pain pathway. In the mid-20th century, neurosurgeons occasionally treated severe unresponsive pain in patients with limited life expectancies (e.g., due to cancer) by performing percutaneous lateral spinothalamic tractotomies. Success rates were approximately 75%. This remains a valid option in a few select cases today.

A complex somatotopic organization is maintained in the ascending pathways. Laminae I and V project to the lateral thalamic nuclei, where discriminative aspects of pain tend to be processed. Laminae I, IV, and VII project to the medial nuclei, where affective-motivational information is processed. Other ascending nociceptive pathways include the spinoreticular tract, which may be the ascending limb of the DNIC system, the spinomesencephalic tract, which may be involved in proprioception, and the spinohypothalamic tract. The spinoreticular tract is a primitive system essential to homeostasis and integration. The periaqueductal gray is its major target.

Pain Processing in the Brain

Much information has been obtained from neuroanatomical tracing and electrophysiological studies in experimental animals. The newer imaging modalities are providing important additional information, often from human subjects. In 1906, Dejerine and Roussy first described a central pain syndrome after stroke affecting thalamocortical pathways. Since then, it has become appreciated that lesions anywhere along the central pain pathways can produce central pain and disturbances of nociceptive function. It has also become clear that there is no single pain center in the brain. Afferent nociceptive fibers from the spinal and trigeminal systems project widely to the thalamus and brainstem, and the thalamus radiates to many areas of the brain. These are the neuroanatomical substrates for the pronounced motor, hormonal, emotional, and memory responses that accompany the perception of pain.

The spino- and trigeminothalamic tracts terminate in six major regions of the primate thalamus. The deep laminae of the spinal cord tend to project to the lateral thalamus and onto the somatosensory cortex, where the location of the painful stimuli can be determined and an appropriate motor response initiated. Lamina I also projects to the ventral medial nuclei, which project to the frontal cortex (especially the anterior cingulate gyrus) to convey the emotional concomitants of pain. The ventral posterior nuclei are somatotopically organized and project to primary and secondary somatosensory areas of the cortex. Spino- and trigeminobulbar projections feed back onto the dorsal horn but also affect homeostatic circuitry that is mediated by the brainstem.

NEUROBIOLOGY OF CHRONIC NOCICEPTIVE PAIN

Chronic nociceptive/inflammatory pain is readily understood by most clinicians because it involves temporal prolongation of the mechanisms of acute pain. The major source of neuronal hyperactivity continues to be the peripheral nociceptive neuron. Diagnosis is usually straightforward, and clinicians are often willing to prescribe pain medications since there is evidence of ongoing tissue injury. The prototype is the chronic arthritides, in which chronic joint pain reflects ongoing joint destruction. Medications that are effective for acute pain, including nonsteroidal antiinflammatory drugs (NSAIDs) and the opioids, are generally effective for chronic nociceptive pain as well. Combining palliative pain medications with disease-modifying treatments that remove the source of tissue injury is the best treatment for this type of pain. NSAIDs can have both actions. Chronic nociceptive/inflammatory pain differs from acute pain in that properties of injured neurons and associated nonneuronal cells change when pain is prolonged. Hyperalgesia can spread beyond the immediate area of injury. The benefits of hyperalgesia after injury are obvious; it forces the organism to limit use of an injured area and maximizes the opportunities for healing.

Effects of Tissue Injury on Nociceptive Transduction

Repeated activation of nociceptive pathways changes the properties of nociceptive primary afferent neurons. The most common clinical manifestation is the presence of hyperalgesia. Specifically, nociceptors can exhibit a lowered threshold for activation, recruitment of previously silent nociceptors, or an expansion of the area from which a single fiber can be activated (receptive field). These effects can increase by an order of magnitude the number of impulses that arrive to the spinal cord after injury.

Peripheral sensitization is mediated by the myriad receptors on the distal ends of primary afferents. Products released by injury and inflammation appear particularly likely to activate nociceptors or to decrease their threshold for activation. There are receptors for many products of tissue injury or inflammation (e.g., protons, histamine, bradykinins, prostaglandins, serotonin, and cytokines). Their activation increases the electrical excitability of afferent neurons so that they may fire spontaneously without a stimulus, fire more frequently or for longer, or fire after a usually subthreshold stimulus. Nociceptors show a shift in the stimulus-response curve for mechanical and thermal as well as chemical stimuli.

Stein and coworkers deciphered an elegant relationship between opioid receptors present on peripheral nociceptive terminals and endogenous opioids that are released by inflammatory cells. Opioid receptors have been detected on peripheral nociceptive terminals in rat and man. Following binding of an opioid, the excitability of the nociceptor and its transmission of action potentials is diminished, and its release of substance P, an excitatory proinflammatory neuropeptide, is diminished. Inflammatory cells that migrate to regions of tissue injury, including T and B lymphocytes, monocytes, and macrophages, have been shown to synthesize and release endogenous opioid peptides. Presumably, the paracrine effect acts to diminish nociceptive transmission in inflamed tissues. The discovery of peripheral opioid receptors has led to the use of intraarticular opioids during knee surgery. Because the effect is local, only minute doses are needed and systemic side effects are minimized.

Effects of Tissue Injury on Nociceptive Axons

Tissue injury and inflammation can profoundly alter the transmission of nociceptive action potentials. Since the propagation of action potentials is dependent on the ionic milieu around the axon, conduction will be altered if it is perturbed. Nociceptive neurons with thin or no myelin may be especially vulnerable to environmental changes. Additionally, pressure or stretch of axons from local injury or edema can cause neural hypoxia or myelin retraction. Sorkin and colleagues have shown that tumor necrosis factor-α, a potent inflammatory cytokine, can act directly on the midaxon to enable it to generate ectopic action potentials. Any injury that blocks axonal transport can cause signal-transducing molecules to be aberrantly inserted along the axon rather than at the distal end in the receptive field. This makes the axon ectopically capable of signal transduction.

Effects of Tissue Injury on Sensory Ganglia

The neuronal cell bodies within the spinal or trigeminal sensory ganglia integrate signals arriving from the periphery and then generate new action potentials that travel to the CNS. Since ganglia are outside the blood–nerve barrier, their electrophysiological properties are probably influenced by systemic conditions. Damage to the sensory ganglia (e.g., by compression at the spinal foraminae) can result in aberrant electrical hyperactivity originating from the ganglion itself. No doubt alterations in the chemical milieu can also perturb normal function.

Effects of Tissue Injury on the CNS

Injuries have distant as well as local effects. A zone of heightened pain sensitivity (hyperalgesia) typically surrounds an injured area. This encourages immobilization after an injury to facilitate healing. Severe injuries can produce whole-body symptoms, such as anorexia and lethargy. Although unpleasant, these aid recovery by decreasing overall activity and allowing resources to be diverted to healing. Samad and colleagues presented evidence that CNS prostanoids mediate these distant effects, and that induction of cyclooxygenase-2 (COX-2) mediates the CNS effects of tissue injury. These findings suggest that the generalized antiinflammatory effects of NSAIDs require that they penetrate into the CNS rather than just the injured tissues. The net effect of inhibiting CNS prostanoid production remains to be determined.

NEUROBIOLOGY OF CHRONIC NEUROPATHIC PAIN

Neuropathic pain is more complex than acute or inflammatory pain because the pain pathways are injured. The patient feels the pain in the tissues that are innervated by the damaged neurons, even though the painful area may be normal and the actual injury within the nervous system. Neurologists and neurosurgeons are uniquely qualified to localize and investigate the causes of neuropathic pain. Unfortunately, they currently comprise less than 10% of pain specialists, so many neuropathic pain patients never have their lesions properly diagnosed and receive palliative treatment only, rather than disease- or mechanism-specific therapies. The creation in 2000 of an American Board of Psychiatry and Neurology certificate of Added Qualification in Pain Management should encourage more neurology residents to pursue training in pain management.

In neuropathic pain, the normal mechanisms of nociception are perverted, which complicates diagnosis and treatment. Different mechanisms, both normal and pathological, are likely to be present within the same patient. As with other complex chronic diseases (e.g., asthma), patients may need several different medications, each influencing different contributing mechanisms. Despite the appeal of "molecular scalpels" that intervene precisely for maximum specificity and efficacy, the most effective medications for neuropathic pain remain the "dirty" drugs that intervene at several different points along the pain pathways. For instance, tricyclic antidepressants are sodium-channel blockers as well as potentiators of catecholaminergic neurotransmission (among other effects).

The most common clinical neuropathic pain syndromes are the small-fiber sensory polyneuropathies (e.g., diabetic and idiopathic), sensory mononeuropathies (usually from trauma), and sensory neuronopathies (e.g., shingles). Note that only neurological diseases that affect pain-processing neurons are likely to produce pain. Diseases that affect other types of sensory fibers, such as the large-fiber sensory neuropathies, tend to produce sensory ataxia instead. Central neuropathic pain syndromes can be produced by any injury or disease that affects central pain pathways. Central pain has been reported in stroke, multiple sclerosis, and parkinsonism, among others. In phantom limb pain, hyperexcitability of central pain neurons leads to the perception of pain in a limb or tissue that has been removed by surgery or due to trauma. Central causes of neuropathic pain are rare due to the protected position of the brain and spinal cord. Peripheral causes of chronic neuropathic pain are distressingly common.

Injury to Peripheral Nociceptive Axons

Polyneuropathies that affect the small-diameter peripheral nociceptive neurons are a common cause of neuropathic pain. Although diabetic sensory polyneuropathy is the best known, there may be even more patients with idiopathic small-fiber neuropathy, meaning that the cause of their painful neuropathy is not yet understood. Many patients

have mixed neuropathies. Motor or large sensory fiber involvement produces familiar signs on neurological examination and traditional diagnostic tests. Some patients have neuropathies limited to nociceptive neurons only, and they will have normal strength and reflexes as well as sense of touch, proprioception, and vibration. They often also have normal electromyographic and nerve conduction studies. Until recently, the only objective evidence of neurological damage was from sural nerve biopsy. These biopsies are performed in few patients, and most small-fiber neuropathy patients are hidden in the population. For instance, a proportion of patients carrying the descriptive labels "fibromyalgia" or "chronic fatigue syndrome" may well have occult small-fiber neuropathies. The lack of objective evidence of disease results in additional problems because requests for pain medication or disability benefits may not be heeded.

At the end of the 20th century, small skin or epidermal biopsies began to be used by neurologists to provide a window into the peripheral somatosensory nervous system. These biopsies are immunolabeled with anti-PGP9.5 antibody, a pan-axonal marker that permits quantitation of epidermal nerve endings using light microscopy (Fig. 2). All published skin biopsy studies of patients with painful neuropathies have demonstrated loss of epidermal neurites, usually severe, although the presence or absence of pain was not usually an outcome measure. There were similar findings in the sensory neuronopathy postherpetic neuralgia and in some traumatic mononeuropathies. Loss of peripheral nociceptive nerve endings might be useful as a diagnostic marker for

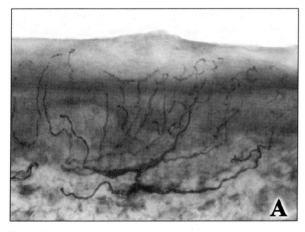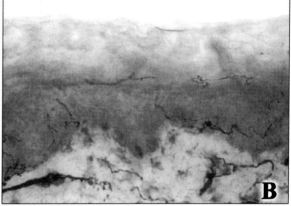

Figure 2
PGP9.5 immunolabeled nerve endings within punch skin biopsies. Representative labeled vertical skin-biopsy sections from a normal subject (A) and a subject with painful small-fiber neuropathy (B). Note the paucity of nerve endings in B.

peripheral neuropathic pain, although it remains to be seen whether the technique becomes widely available. For some patients, it can provide anatomical corroboration of a neuropathic pain syndrome.

The skin biopsy technique has also been found to be more sensitive than sural nerve biopsy for the diagnosis of painful neuropathies, presumably because it samples a more distal portion of axon than does sural nerve biopsy. It can be applied to areas outside of the sural nerve territory and can be repeated to follow disease progression or response to therapy. The major disadvantage is that skin biopsies are less suited for detecting demyelination. Since pain syndromes involve unmyelinated or thinly myelinated axons, this is not a major limitation.

It initially appears counterintuitive that the presence of neuropathic pain should be associated with a paucity of pain-sensing neurons. In some cases, injured truncated axons may be initiating pain messages more proximally, but in other cases (sensory neuronopathies and central peripheral distal axonopathies), measures of neurite density in the skin probably reflect the densities of central afferent axons synapsing on dorsal horn neurons. Electrophysiologists have shown that deafferented CNS sensory neurons become hyperexcitable probably due to loss of the spinal inhibitory interneurons.

Injury to Nerves or Nerve Roots

Mononeuropathies can cause chronic pain by several mechanisms. If regenerating axons do not find their distal target, tangles of nerve endings can form at the distal end of a proximal nerve stump. Since these then become the distal-most portions of the axons, sodium channels and other sensory transducers are inserted into the axolemma here. Pressure or tapping over a neuroma can be very painful. Demyelination can allow ephaptic spread of action potentials between adjacent axons. This is thought to underlie the severe lancinating pain that can sometimes be triggered by light touch (as in trigeminal neuralgia). Some painful mononeuropathies are due to nerve or root compression, and definitive relief can sometimes be obtained by prompt neurosurgical decompression. Milder cases can respond to medical treatments.

Injury to Sympathetic Axons

Nerve injuries often affect the postganglionic sympathetic axons that course among somatic axons. This explains the sometimes dramatic presence of edema and changes in skin color and temperature in areas of nerve injury and neuropathic pain. In its most flagrant form, this is known as complex regional pain syndrome (CRPS). Some individuals with nerve injury have trophic changes in hair, skin, and nails, and even in the metabolism of underlying bone, that reflect injury to the axons that normally innervate these structures.

The contribution of sympathetic efferents to neuropathic pain syndromes has been hotly debated. Tyrosine hydroxylase-containing axonal sprouts within the DRG of nerve-injured rats and human pain patients have been demonstrated by McLachlan and coworkers, but their functional significance is not known. In some patients, peripherally administered adrenergic agonists acquire the ability to trigger pain, and it was hypothesized that they were the source of pain. The term sympathetically maintained pain was coined, and some chronic pain patients were treated with sympatholytic medications such as clonidine or with surgical sympathectomy. Unfortunately, these interventions only rarely provide significant relief, and in recent years it has become apparent that abnormal sympathetic activity, although often associated with nerve injury, is not a major cause of pain in most patients. Hence, the replacement of the term "reflex sympathetic dystrophy" by the more neutral term "CRPS" in 1994. However, given the plasticity of the electrophysiological properties of primary afferent nerve endings, it is likely that secretions of nearby sympathetic efferents, along with those of remaining abnormal primary afferents, immune cells, keratinocytes, and other local nonneural cells, influence the function of injured somatosensory afferents.

Injury to Sensory Ganglia

Neuronal cell bodies within sensory ganglia are electrically active and generate action potentials. These properties can be altered by mechanical or biochemical abnormalities. Both the spinal and trigeminal ganglia are surrounded by bone and are vulnerable to compression. Additionally, sensory ganglia are outside of the blood–brain (or nerve) barrier and thus likely to be influenced by circulating neuroactive molecules such as cytokines. Some diseases attack sensory neuronal cell bodies directly. Sjögren's disease and several paraneoplastic syndromes can cause sensory neuronopathy, but by far the most common one is shingles (herpes zoster), which has the highest annual incidence of any neurological disease.

Shingles is a focal reactivation of the varicella-zoster virus (VZV) that produces varicella in

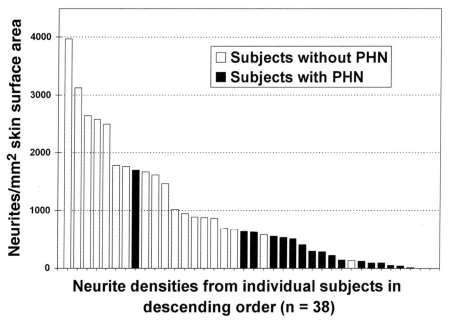

Figure 3
Density of epidermal innervation in previously shingles-affected skin from subjects with PHN (black bars) and without (open bars). These data suggested that preserving a minimum density of innervation was associated with remaining pain-free after shingles. [Reproduced with permission from Oaklander, A. L. (2001). The density of remaining nerve endings in human skin with and without postherpetic neuralgia after shingles. *Pain* **92,** 139–145.]

children. After chicken pox, the virus becomes dormant in sensory ganglia and can reactivate if immunity wanes with aging or immunosuppression. When the virus reactivates, it produces a stroke-like zone of death of neuronal cell bodies and surrounding satellite cells. Both the central and peripheral sensory axons undergo Wallerian degeneration, sometimes causing bystander damage to adjacent motor axons as well. Approximately 15% of patients will be left with postherpetic neuralgia (PHN), a common cause of chronic neuropathic pain. Since the risk of shingles and PHN after shingles is proportional to the patient's age, shingles and PHN are a major health threat to the geriatric population. The immunosuppressed are also at increased risk of shingles. Shingles receives little attention from neurologists, perhaps because the only visible lesion is dermatological, but it is a neurological emergency that requires immediate and aggressive intervention to minimize or prevent chronic neurological damage and disability.

Shingles and PHN are studied by those investigating mechanisms of neuropathic pain and used for clinical trials of new medications. C. P. N. Watson's autopsy studies demonstrated that patients with PHN after shingles, but not those without PHN, had dorsal horn atrophy at spinal segments affected by prior shingles. This extended several segments up and down the cord, probably providing the anatomical correlate for the secondary zone of allodynia and hyperalgesia that surrounds the dermatome of actual shingles involvement. Recently, skin biopsy studies have suggested that PHN pain may only ensue among shingles patients with the fewest remaining nociceptive neurons (Fig. 3). Thus, there is evidence that degeneration of entire sensory neurons, as well as of distal axons, is associated with the presence of neuropathic pain.

Effects of Peripheral Neural Injury on the Dorsal Horn

Injury or death of peripheral nociceptive neurons profoundly influence their postsynaptic targets in the dorsal horn. There is evidence that many damaged primary afferent nociceptors lose contact with their postsynaptic target cells within the dorsal horn. Surprisingly, the decrease in incoming action potentials leads to some of the same consequences as does hyperexcitability of primary afferents after tissue injury. When second-order dorsal horn neurons are deprived of peripheral input, they increase their gain to maximize input from the remaining peripheral fibers. Although this helps to maintain normal function, if extreme, it can lead to spontaneous activity of dorsal horn neurons or to prolonged bursts of firing after minimal input from the periphery. These changes contribute to hyperalgesia and ongoing neuropathic pain. Death of C fibers can lead to sprouting of remaining A fibers onto nociceptive second-order neurons in the superficial layer of the dorsal horn. This anatomical plasticity is the most likely explanation for allodynia in neuropathic pain.

Some of the electrical hyperexcitability of deafferented dorsal horn projection neurons (described in animals and patients by Loeser) is probably related to death or malfunction of the inhibitory interneurons, whose function was described earlier. Dorsal horn atrophy has been reported in PHN patients and in experimental animals. Basbaum and Wall described expansion of the receptive field—the area in which stimulation of the periphery can trigger an action potential—of deafferented dorsal horn neurons. This may represent the formation of new anatomical synapses, although immediate expansions after tissue injury may represent "unmasking" of normally silent synapses. This reorganization in nociceptive processing underlies interesting sensory phenomena that can be observed in patients with injury to sensory fibers.

Effects of Peripheral Neural Injury on the Brain

Less is known about the effects of peripheral neural injury on higher centers, but there is increasing evidence that peripheral nerve injuries perturb nociceptive signal processing all the way up to the rostral-most centers. Thalamic recordings from pain patients by Lenz and others have shown increased electrical activity in areas of thalamus that process input from body parts perceived as painful, but normal levels of excitability in adjacent regions of thalamus receiving input from non-painful areas.

Newer imaging techniques, such as functional magnetic resonance imaging and positron emission tomography, have demonstrated widespread effects of peripheral injury in parts of the brain including the frontal lobes, thalamus, anterior cingulate, and periaqueductal gray. Surprisingly high levels of plasticity have been found within the primary and secondary somatosensory cortex of patients with various neuropathic pain syndromes. Patients with phantom pain after amputation have been shown to

have expansion of adjacent areas of the sensory homunculus into cortical territory that formerly subserved the missing body part. This explains why some patients are able to trigger phantom arm pain by stroking near their mouth. Interestingly, this phenomenon has been described 1 or 2 days after limb amputation, raising the question of whether there is unmasking of normally silent synapses rather than growth of new synapses. The effects of various pain medications on cortical plasticity need to be investigated. Plasticity within the cortex, and probably in other areas of the CNS as well, may underlie the gradual adaptation and recovery from chronic pain that some patients experience. It also highlights the importance of minimizing a patient's pain with aggressive treatment to dampen synaptic plasticity that might serve to potentiate the pain state. There are virtually no long-term outcome studies of neuropathic pain patients, with the exception of PHN, for which there continues to be slow reduction in the severity and prevalence of pain, even after many years. More long-term prospective studies are needed.

Spinal Cord Injuries

Neurological diseases that affect the spinal cord can injure spinal dorsal horn neurons or their central axonal projections. Conditions that affect the dorsal columns are less likely to produce pain than conditions affecting the lateral spinothalamic tracts, in which pain fibers ascend. Since sensory, but not motor, fibers decussate within the spinal cord, pain can be the major or only symptom of disease processes that affect the central regions of the spinal cord. Syringomyelia is the prototype. Patients with severe injury, such as from spinal cord trauma, can have mixed pain syndromes with both peripheral and central components.

Brain Injuries

Any type of lesion (e.g., tumor, infection, and demyelination) that affects pain pathways can cause pain. The pain is often perceived in or around a body area with sensory loss from the neural injury. Conversely, lesions of the dorsal column–medial lemniscal pathways appear neither necessary nor sufficient to cause central pain. Unfortunately, animal models of central pain are not widely studied, so much less is known about the mechanisms of central pain. Central neuropathic pain differs from peripheral pain in an intriguing way. The pain may not occur until months or, rarely, a few years after the neurological insult. This has been most convincingly demonstrated for post-stroke pain. The most likely explanation is that this delay is related to the slower rate of myelin clearance and tract degeneration in the CNS than in PNS, but this has not been rigorously examined. Nonetheless, it is important for neurologists to be aware of this potential for tardive central pain so as not to miss the correct diagnosis.

CONCLUSIONS

Although acute pain serves a vital and necessary function, chronic pain is a disaster from every perspective. Its medical, social, and economic consequences may at least be minimized by good pain management. It is important to determine whether a patient's pain is from somatic or neural injury and to pursue a firm anatomical diagnosis. Patients with neuropathic pain are less likely to be correctly diagnosed and treated than those with pain from an obvious tissue injury. Physicians need to improve their ability to evaluate pain patients and to treat neuropathic pain patients as they do other victims of neurological disease.

The advent of animal models of pain has greatly contributed to our understanding of pain mechanisms. They have provided explanations for puzzling effects, such as the presence of pain outside injured areas, the presence of pain without tissue injury, and the referral of pain to distant areas.

Increased efforts to study human pain patients are needed. Autopsy protocols need to be established to investigate pain-producing lesions, and human genetic studies of patients and families with disorders of pain processing need to be performed. Candidate genes and molecules identified in animal studies need validation in humans before starting large-scale clinical trials. These neuroscientific endeavors must be accompanied by educational efforts so that all physicians become comfortable with the diagnosis and treatment of patients with chronic pain.

—*Anne Louise Oaklander*

See also–Neuropathic Pain Syndromes; Pain, Assessment of; Pain Management, Multidisciplinary; Pain, Overview; Pain, Visceral

Further Reading

Brand, P., and Yancey, P. (1993). *Pain: The Gift Nobody Wants.* Harper Collins, New York.

Carlton, S. M., and Coggeshall, R. E. (1998). Nociceptive integration: Does it have a peripheral component? *Pain Forum* 7, 71–78.
Devor, M., Govrin-Lippmann, R., and Rappaport, Z. H. (2002). Mechanism of trigeminal neuralgia: An ultrastructural analysis of trigeminal root specimens obtained during microvascular decompression surgery. *J. Neurosurg.* 96, 532–543.
Mogil, J. S., Wilson, S. G., Bon, K., *et al.* (1999). Heritability of nonciception I: Responses of 11 inbred mouse strains on 12 measures of nociception. *Pain* 80, 67–82.
Oaklander, A. L. (1999). The pathology of pain. *Neuroscientist* 5, 302–310.
Phillips, D. M. (2000). Joint commission on accreditation of healthcare organizations pain management standards are unveiled. *J. Am. Med. Assoc.* 284, 428–429.
Wilcox, G. L., and Seybold, V. (1997). Pharmacology of spinal afferent processing. In *Anesthesia: Biologic Foundations* (T. L. Yaksh, *et al.*, Eds.). Lippincott-Raven, Philadelphia.
Woolf, C. J., Shortland, P., and Coggeshall, R. E. (1992). Peripheral nerve injury triggers central sprouting of myelinated afferents. *Nature* 355, 75–78.

Pain, Cancer and

Encyclopedia of the Neurological Sciences
Copyright 2003, Elsevier Science (USA). All rights reserved.

THE PROBLEM OF PAIN among cancer patients is endemic. Appropriate and effective clinical responses to this problem require that the physician appreciate the cause of the pain, its underlying mechanism, its natural history, and its significance. Since the seminal works of John Bonica, various attempts have been made to taxonomize cancer pain. The description of cancer pain syndromes has facilitated a better understanding of the causes of pain among cancer patients and enhanced the possibility of specific treatment approaches based on better understanding of the underlying pathological process.

Cancer pain syndromes are defined by the association of particular pain characteristics and physical signs with specific consequences of the underlying disease or its treatment. Syndromes are associated with distinct etiologies and pathophysiologies, and they have important prognostic and therapeutic implications. Pain syndromes associated with cancer can be either acute or chronic. Adverse consequences of cancer therapy, including surgery, chemotherapy, and radiation therapy, account for 15–25% of chronic cancer pain problems, and a small proportion of chronic pain experienced by cancer patients is caused by pathology unrelated to either the cancer or the cancer therapy.

ACUTE PAIN SYNDROMES

Cancer-related acute pain syndromes are most commonly due to diagnostic or therapeutic interventions, and they generally pose little diagnostic difficulty. Although some tumor-related pains have an acute onset (such as pain from a pathological fracture), most of these will persist unless effective treatment for the underlying lesion is provided.

Many investigations and treatments are associated with predictable, transient pain. For patients with a preexisting pain syndrome, otherwise innocuous manipulations can also precipitate an incident pain. Acute cancer pain syndromes may be caused by diagnostic interventions (e.g., a lumbar puncture headache), therapeutic interventions (e.g., postoperative pain), analgesic techniques (e.g., injection pain and capsaicin pain), or antitumor therapies.

Occasionally, cancer patients suffer from acute pain syndromes unrelated to diagnostic or therapeutic interventions. Of these, the most common are thromboses or acute painful infections (i.e., abscess or zoster).

CHRONIC PAIN SYNDROMES

Most chronic cancer-related pains are caused directly by the tumor. Data from the largest prospective survey of cancer pain syndromes revealed that approximately one-fourth of patients experienced two or more pains. More than 90% of patients had one or more tumor-related pains, and 21% had one or more pains caused by cancer therapies. Somatic pains (71%) were more common than neuropathic (39%) or visceral pains (34%). Bone pain and compression of neural structures are the two most common causes.

Bone Pain

Bone metastases are the most common cause of chronic pain in cancer patients. Cancers of the lung, breast, and prostate most often metastasize to bone, but any tumor type may be complicated by painful bony lesions. Bone metastases could potentially cause pain by any of multiple mechanisms, including endosteal or periosteal nociceptor activation (by mechanical distortion or release of chemical mediators) or tumor growth into adjacent soft tissues and nerves. Bone metastases most commonly occur in the axial skeleton. Multiple specific pain syndromes are recognized, depending on the site of bony involvement. Of these syndromes, the most critical are those

that indicate impending catastrophic outcomes, such as spinal cord compression or pathological fracture. The early recognition of pain syndromes due to tumor invasion of vertebral bodies is essential since pain usually precedes compression of adjacent neural structures and prompt treatment of the lesion may prevent the subsequent development of neurological deficits. Several factors often confound accurate diagnosis; referral of pain is common, and the associated symptoms and signs can mimic a variety of other disorders, both malignant (e.g., paraspinal masses) and nonmalignant.

Visceral Cancer Pain Syndromes

Visceral cancer pain syndromes are common. Pain may be caused by pathology involving the luminal organs of the gastrointestinal or genitourinary tracts, the parenchymal organs, the peritoneum, or the retroperitoneal soft tissues. Obstruction of hollow viscus, including intestine, biliary tract, and ureter, produces visceral nociceptive syndromes that are well described in the surgical literature. Pain arising from retroperitoneal and pelvic lesions may involve mixed nociceptive and neuropathic mechanisms if both somatic structures and nerves are involved.

Headache and Facial Pain

Headache in the cancer patient results from traction, inflammation, or infiltration of pain-sensitive structures in the head or neck. Early evaluation with appropriate imaging techniques may identify the lesion and allow prompt treatment, which may reduce pain and prevent the development of neurological deficits. The most common causes of chronic headache among patients with advanced cancer include intracerebral tumor, leptomeningeal metastases, and metastases to the base of the skull. The character of the pain and other coexisting clinical features may be suggestive of a specific syndrome. Moderate headache that is worse in the morning and is exacerbated by stooping, sudden head movement, or Valsalva maneuvers (cough, sneeze, or strain) suggests intracerebral tumor; headache associated with multifocal neurological symptoms, including cranial nerve lesions, suggests leptomeningeal metastases; and retroorbital pain associated with diplopia and proptosis suggests orbital metastases.

Neuropathic Pains Involving the Peripheral Nervous System

Besides spinal cord compression, the most common chronic neuropathic pain syndromes include brachial or lumbosacral plexopathy and painful peripheral neuropathy. Of the potential causes of plexopathy in cancer patients, the most common are tumor infiltration and radiation fibrosis.

Brachial Plexopathy: Plexus infiltration by tumor is the most prevalent cause of brachial plexopathy and is most common in patients with lymphoma, lung cancer, or breast cancer. The invading tumor usually arises from adjacent axillary, cervical, and supraclavicular lymph nodes (lymphoma and breast cancer) or from the lung (superior sulcus tumors or so-called Pancoast tumors). Pain is nearly universal and often precedes neurological signs or symptoms by months. In contrast, among patients with radiation plexopathy, pain is a relatively uncommon presenting symptom and when present is usually less severe.

Lumbosacral Plexopathy: Lumbosacral plexopathy in cancer patients is usually caused by neoplastic infiltration or compression. As with malignant brachial plexopathy, pain is the dominant symptom: It is usually the first symptom. Radiation-induced plexopathy also occurs, and occasional patients develop the lesion as a result of surgical trauma, infarction, cytotoxic damage, infection in the pelvis or psoas muscle, abdominal aneurysm, or idiopathic lumbosacral neuritis. Polyradiculopathy from leptomeningeal metastases or epidural metastases can mimic lumbosacral plexopathy, and evaluation of the patient must consider these lesions as well.

Painful Peripheral Neuropathy: Painful peripheral neuropathy in cancer patients is usually caused by neurotoxic chemotherapy agents, particularly the vinca alkaloids (especially vincristine), *cis*-platinum, and oxaliplatin. This syndrome typically presents with painful paresthesias in the hands and/or feet and signs consistent with an axonopathy, including "stocking-glove" sensory loss, weakness, hyporeflexia, and autonomic dysfunction. The pain is usually characterized by continuous burning or lancinating pains, either of which may be increased by contact. Uncommonly, peripheral neuropathy may be observed as a paraneoplastic phenomenon.

Chronic Pain Syndromes Associated with Cancer Therapy

Chronic treatment-related pain syndromes are associated with either a persistent nociceptive complication of an invasive treatment (e.g., a postsurgical abscess) or, more commonly, neural injury. In some cases, these syndromes occur long after the therapy is completed, resulting in difficulty in making the differential diagnosis between recurrent disease and a complication of therapy.

Chemotherapy-Induced Neuropathy: Chemotherapy-induced peripheral neuropathy caused by *cis*-platinum may continue to progress months after discontinuation of therapy and may persist for months to years. This is less common with vincristine or paclitaxol.

Steroid-Induced Avascular Necrosis: Intermittent or continuous corticosteroid therapy may result in the development of avascular necrosis of the femoral or humeral head. Involvement of the femoral head is most common and typically causes pain in the hip, thigh, or knee. Involvement of the humeral head usually presents as pain in the shoulder, upper arm, or elbow.

Gynecomastia with Hormonal Therapy for Prostate Cancer: Chronic gynecomastia and breast tenderness are common complications of antiandrogen therapies for prostate cancer.

Breast Surgery Pain Syndromes: Chronic pain of variable severity is a common sequela of surgery for breast cancer. The most common sites of pain are the breast scar region and the ipsilateral arm. Although chronic pain has been reported to occur after almost any surgical procedure on the breast (from lumpectomy to radical mastectomy), it is most common after procedures involving axillary dissection. The pain is usually characterized as a constricting and burning discomfort that is localized to the medial arm, axilla, and anterior chest wall. On examination, there is often an area of sensory loss within the region of the pain. The etiology of this pain syndrome is believed to be related to damage to the intercostobrachial nerve, a cutaneous sensory branch of T1–T3.

Post-thoracotomy Pain: Studies have identified several post-thoracotomy pain syndromes: The most common (63%) is prolonged postoperative pain that abated within 2 months after surgery. Recurrent pain, following resolution of the postoperative pain, is usually due to neoplasm. Pain that persists following the thoracotomy and then increases in intensity during the follow-up period is commonly caused by local recurrence of disease and infection. Overall, the development of late or increasing post-thoracotomy pain was due to recurrent or persistent tumor in more than 95% of patients.

Phantom Pain Syndromes: Phantom limb pain is perceived to arise from an amputated limb, as if the limb were still contiguous with the body. Phantom pain is experienced by 60–80% of patients following limb amputation but is only severe in approximately 5–10% of cases. Phantom pain syndromes have also been described after other surgical procedures. Phantom breast pain after mastectomy, which occurs in 15–30% of patients, also appears to be related to the presence of preoperative pain. A phantom anus pain syndrome occurs in approximately 15% of patients who undergo abdominoperineal resection of the rectum. Phantom anus pain may develop either in the early postoperative period or after a latency of months to years. Late-onset pain is almost always associated with tumor recurrence.

Breakthrough Pain

Transitory exacerbations of severe pain over a baseline of moderate pain or less may be described as breakthrough pain. Breakthrough pains are common in both acute or chronic pain states. These exacerbations may be precipitated by volitional actions of the patient (so-called incident pains), such as movement, micturition, cough, or defecation, or by nonvolitional events such as bowel distention. Spontaneous fluctuations in pain intensity can also occur without an identifiable precipitant. Breakthrough pains must be distinguished from exacerbations of pain associated with failure of analgesia. End-of-dose failure (of analgesia) is commonly observed as therapeutic levels of analgesic decline. This phenomenon is observed most commonly when the interval between scheduled doses exceeds the known duration of action of short half-life analgesics.

CONCLUSION

Adequate assessment is a necessary precondition for effective pain management. In the cancer population, assessment must recognize the dynamic relationship between the symptom, the illness, and major concerns related to quality of life. Syndrome identification and inferences about pain pathophysiology are useful elements that may simplify this complex undertaking.

—*Nathan I. Cherny*

See also–Analgesia, Cancer Pain and; Brachial Plexopathies; Facial Pain; Lumbar Plexopathy; Neuropathic Pain Syndromes; Pain, Basic

Neurobiology of; Pain, Postoperative; Pain, Visceral; Phantom Limb and Stump Pain

Further Reading

Bonica, J. J. (1953). *The Management of Pain.* Lea & Febiger, Philadelphia.

Caraceni, A., and Portenoy, R. K. (1999). An international survey of cancer pain characteristics and syndromes. IASP Task Force on Cancer Pain. International Association for the Study of Pain. *Pain* **82,** 263–274.

Cherny, N. I., and Portenoy, R. K. (1999). Cancer pain: Principles of assessment and syndromes. In *Textbook of Pain* (P. D. Wall and R. Melzack, Eds.), 4th ed. Churchill Livingstone, Edinburgh, UK.

Foley, K. M. (1987). Cancer pain syndromes. *J. Pain Symptom Manage.* **2,** 13–17.

Foley, K. M. (1987). Pain syndromes in patients with cancer. *Med. Clin. North Am.* **71,** 169–184.

Grond, S., Zech, D., Diefenbach, C., *et al.* (1996). Assessment of cancer pain: A prospective evaluation in 2266 cancer patients referred to a pain service. *Pain* **64,** 107–114.

Hartenstein, R., and Wilmanns, W. (1984). Clinical pain syndromes in cancer patients and their causes. *Recent Results Cancer Res.* **89,** 72–78.

Mercadante, S. (1997). Malignant bone pain: Pathophysiology and treatment. *Pain* **69,** 1–18.

Taddeini, L., and Rotschafer, J. C. (1984). Pain syndromes associated with cancer. Achieving effective relief. *Postgrad. Med.* **75,** 101–108.

Vecht, C. J., Hoff, A. M., Kansen, P. J., *et al.* (1992). Types and causes of pain in cancer of the head and neck. *Cancer* **70,** 178–184.

Pain, Deafferentation

Encyclopedia of the Neurological Sciences
Copyright 2003, Elsevier Science (USA). All rights reserved.

PAIN is necessary to maintain the physical integrity of animals; it is the subjective experience of the processing of nociceptive signals. The perception of physical pain normally is absent from consciousness until nociceptive stimuli exceed a threshold level. Signals from nociceptive receptors are conducted via the peripheral nerves to the spinal cord and brain. The pain system is hierarchically organized with neurons of the dorsal horn playing an essential role in primary integration; subsequent modulation occurs at multiple anatomical sites. Local and descending inhibitory neurons continuously modulate incoming nociceptive signals. The pain system's potential for marked plasticity underlies the emergence of deafferentation pain following injury; several molecular mechanisms are involved. Because the currency of nervous system activation is the action potential, all changes that influence the probability of neuronal firing are relevant to the experience of pain.

When peripheral nerve or central nervous system (CNS) connections are injured, pain signaling becomes destabilized. Abnormal pain experiences can occur either spontaneously or in response to minimal stimuli. The abnormal pain that occurs following loss of connections from nerves, spinal cord, or brain structures is known as deafferentation pain (DP). DP confers no apparent advantages and is maladaptive. Clinically, DP is difficult to treat and can cause considerable suffering.

The terms neuropathic pain and deafferentation pain are often used incorrectly to describe similar clinical problems. Both entities share some common mechanisms, but they are not identical. Deafferentation is simply a loss of afferent input and can result in pain after an interruption at any point in the pathway from sensory receptors to the cortex. In neuropathic pain, the primary injury is to the peripheral nerve (PN) and not to the CNS. Sensory processing from the nerve is abnormal, but connections are not necessarily physically interrupted. DP can arise from nerve injuries or from injuries that are entirely within the CNS, in the absence of nerve injury. Therefore, deafferentation can be considered peripheral dorsal root ganglion (DRG) or central (within the CNS). In addition, deafferentation can be self-limited (e.g., Guillain–Barré demyelination) or permanent (e.g., limb amputation). Deafferentation is commonly, but by no means universally, followed by pain.

CLINICAL FEATURES

Loss of intrinsic CNS connections accompanies conditions such as traumatic spinal cord injury, anterior spinal artery syndrome, spinal multiple sclerosis, intrinsic spinal tumors, thalamic strokes, and syringomyelia. Likewise, loss of afferent connections from PNs follows injury to the cauda equina or brachial plexus, herpes zoster, diabetic neuropathy, compressive radiculopathy, and arachnoiditis, and so on. "Phantom" pain following limb amputation is a classic DP state due to the loss of peripheral afferents. Surgical procedures that injure nerves can also cause DP, and dysesthesia following targeted nervous system lesions intended to reduce pain by creating deafferentation can complicate such procedures.

DP can occur spontaneously in the complete absence of peripheral stimuli or in response to minimal nociceptive stimuli (hypersensitivity). Nonnociceptive stimuli such as vibration, light touch, or even air movement can be perceived as painful (allodynia). Burning sensations and sudden lancinating pains are often described.

MECHANISMS OF DP

There is no simple classification for DP. After normal connections in the pain system are interrupted, abnormal sensory processing can activate the thalamic, cortical, and subcortical neurons that create the awareness and affective components of the conscious experience of pain. Because the system is plastic, hierarchical, and has several feedback loops, changes at one level give rise to changes at related loci.

The interruption that creates DP can occur (i) in the nerve or sensory terminal, sensory ganglion, spinal nerve root, or spinal gray matter; (ii) in an ascending or descending spinal cord or brainstem tract; (iii) in a subcortical structure such as the thalamus; or (iv) in the cortex (e.g., a parietal infarct).

In the intact pain system, unmyelinated C and myelinated Aδ afferent fibers terminate in the dorsal gray matter. Secondary or tertiary neuronal processes then ascend to the supraspinal levels, including the thalamic nuclei, brainstem, reticular nuclei, and hypothalamus. Tertiary or quaternary neurons project to the somatosensory cortex, cingulate gyrus, insula, and other cortical regions. Descending serotonergic or noradrenergic neurons can be activated to modulate segmental sensory processing. The spinothalamic system maintains a somatotopic organization from the dorsal horn to the thalamus and somatosensory cortex; however, other systems are organized more diffusely.

The general principle of DP is that the interruption of normal connections leads to abnormal spontaneous neuronal activity. A lowered threshold for activation, activation in response to nonnociceptive stimuli, and abnormal sensory integration have their basis in altered membrane properties, reorganized and novel connections, and altered gene expression.

INJURY TO NERVES

Injury to the nerve or sensory terminals alters the properties of both DRG and intrinsic spinal cord neurons. The primary synapses of C and A fibers, which terminate on neurons in spinal gray matter lamina I/II and lamina V, have been considered the "pain gate." In response to the nerve injury, the somatosensory nervous system is profoundly reorganized, with shifts in sensory receptive fields, membrane thresholds, and receptor functions and changes in the response characteristics of the central sensory neurons. Uncoupling the pain gate neurons from normal afferents results in abnormal spontaneous firing. Woolf et al. described neuroplasticity following PN injury with central terminals of Aβ fibers sprouting into those regions of the dorsal horn that normally receive only C fiber input. Nonnociceptive sensory inputs can then lead to the activation of second-order neurons that signal pain and may contribute to allodynia.

DRG neuron death following nerve or root injury results in peripheral deafferentation; apoptosis has been implicated. A loss of retrogradely transported trophic molecules, such as nerve growth factor, neurotrophin-3, and glial cell line-derived neurotrophic factor (GDNF), may be involved. Following nerve injury, other retrograde signals, such as increased interleukin-6, appear to prevent the death of DRG neurons. Therefore, neuron survival depends on the interaction of several mechanisms.

INJURY TO SEGMENTAL GRAY MATTER

The hypothesis that unregulated spinal neuronal discharge causes DP is supported by the discovery of spontaneous hyperactive neuronal discharges within the gray matter of patients with a chronic spinal cord injury. PN injury leads to transganglionic synaptic degeneration in the dorsal horn and may also cause the death of dorsal horn neurons involved in processing pain. Therefore, PN injury may either alter the function of spinal cord neurons or kill them, thereby resulting in central deafferentation. Widespread neuronal death within the local gray matter, in addition to the loss of afferent inputs, follows traumatic avulsion of nerve roots. Avulsion causes abnormal changes in many more dorsal horn neurons than does nerve transection.

The substantia gelatinosa (SG), lamina II of the spinal gray matter, is an essential structure for the integration of pain signals. The SG is the principal region of termination of unmyelinated C polymodal pain fibers. Local integrative function is evidenced by the colocalization of excitatory and inhibitory neurotransmitters and peptides, including dynorphin, enkephalin, γ-aminobutyric acid (GABA), glutamate, and substance P.

Substance P is released from C fibers in association with an intense nerve stimulation or injury. The activation of NMDA receptors is involved. An increase in intracellular calcium and a shift in resting potential may lower the activation threshold of SG interneurons. The expression of substance P receptor (VR1) is lost after dorsal rhizotomy. Receptor expression may be regulated by trophic factors, including GDNF delivered into the CNS by afferent fibers.

INJURY TO TRACTS

Like nerves, tracts consist of axon bundles. Axonal injury seldom leads to the death of the related cell body, but it does disconnect neurons from their normal targets.

The principal spinal sensory system implicated in DP is the spinothalamic tract (STT). Lesions of only the dorsal columns in experimental animals have not been associated with obvious DP. However, when such lesions occur in combination with a peripheral injury, abnormal pain occurs.

Descending systems from the hypothalamus, periaqueductal gray matter, and brainstem raphe magnus are implicated in DP. Their effects are mediated by serotonin and noradrenaline, possibly through GABAergic interneurons. Serotonergic terminations at pain afferent synapses in the dorsal horn can inhibit the transmission of nociceptive signals. Therefore, when they are interrupted, excessive nociceptive signals can be transmitted to supraspinal levels. GABA immunoreactivity decreases after nerve injury, and transplanted cells that secrete either GABA or serotonin can reduce pain after experimental nerve or spinal cord injury.

INJURY TO SUPRASPINAL STRUCTURES

DP may follow thalamic and cortical strokes. The thalamus, a relay for STT signals and a well-mapped stereotactic target, provides a window to study altered processing of pain signals using electrophysiological recording techniques. Thalamic changes in response to deafferentation include aberrant and spontaneous firing.

DATA FROM STUDIES OF MOLECULAR RECEPTORS AND SIGNALING MOLECULES

The advent of transgenic and gene knockout techniques facilitates elucidation of the molecular mechanisms that underlie DP. For example, studies using knockout animals have shown that protein kinase C gamma function is required for the development of allodynia after partial nerve injury. Interneurons in the inner layer of lamina II are implicated.

DATA FROM EXPERIMENTAL IMAGING STUDIES

Diagnosis of the cause of DP and the selection of a therapeutic approach are complex issues. Invasive and noninvasive studies, including deep brain and dorsal horn electrode recording, magnetoencephalography, positron emission tomography, functional magnetic resonance imaging (fMRI), and somatosensory evoked potentials, have been instructive regarding plastic changes in brain and spinal cord organization in patients with DP. For example, in upper extremity amputees with phantom pain, imagined movements of the amputated hand activated a much larger than normal region of the somatosensory cortex. Changes have also been observed in the cingulate gyrus and thalamus. Correlation of such abnormal activity with the patient's pain may improve both diagnosis and therapy.

DIAGNOSIS

Advanced imaging and neurophysiological studies are usually available only in research institutions. The cornerstone of diagnosis remains a skilled clinical examination and patient history. The patient's report of the qualities, intensity, and frequency of the pain and associated disabilities influence the choice of treatments.

TREATMENT

It is difficult to obtain long-term effective control of DP. Various pharmacological, neuromodulatory, and surgical strategies can be used. For initial therapy of both neuropathic pain and DP, antidepressant and antiepileptic drugs are preferred to narcotics. Antiseizure drugs stabilize abnormally excitable neuronal membranes, preventing aberrant firing. Gabapentin is widely used because it is well tolerated, easily titrated, has few drug interactions, and requires no laboratory monitoring. It appears to block activity at calcium channels, making neurons less likely to fire abnormally.

Transcutaneous electrical nerve stimulation and acupuncture have been mildly successful in treating DP. Augmented release of endogenous opiates by electrode stimulation of the periaqueductal gray matter is ineffective for DP. However, intrathecal morphine delivery has achieved long-term benefits in a number of patients who have failed other therapies. Intrathecal baclofen infusion is also reported to reduce DP.

Paradoxically, creating additional lesions of the CNS can be employed to treat some forms of DP. The discovery that anterolateral cordotomy could provide remarkable relief to some cancer patients led to the development of percutaneous radiofrequency cordotomy. Sectioning of the STT (cordotomy), however, has been associated with no long-term benefit. In fact, STT sectioning is a model for the creation for DP. Other surgical lesions that have been applied to reduce DP include stereotactic midbrain tractotomy and complete spinal cord transection.

Spontaneous abnormal activity in the dorsal horn contributes to DP following root avulsion injuries. In such cases, destructive lesions of the dorsal root entry zone (DREZ) carry a high probability of achieving a long-term reduction in pain. Unmyelinated pain fibers and myelinated proprioceptive sensory fibers are segregated as they enter the dorsal horn. Theoretically, pain afferents can be lesioned without destroying proprioceptive fibers while preserving some segmental sensation, minimizing additional deafferentation, and maximizing local inhibition. The Nashold DREZ modification involves the complete thermal destruction of the dorsal horn, including the neurons of the SG that are believed to fire spontaneously in DP. DREZ is the most effective ablation technique for DP. Several neuromodulatory techniques, such as dorsal column stimulation, thalamic stimulation, and motor cortical stimulation, have been successful in certain patients. In cancer patients with severe pain, a cingulotomy can remove the emotional content of pain without removing awareness that the pain is present. However, such lesions have not been very effective for DP.

CONCLUSION

DP is caused by a loss of connections in the CNS and maladaptive plasticity. Underlying mechanisms involve alterations in gene regulation, in the expression and function of membrane channels and receptors, in unmasking of silent connections, and in the formation of *de novo* connections. Diagnosis of the location of injury and the sites of aberrant neuronal activity is improving due to the advent of fMRI, other forms of functional neuroimaging, and recent scientific discoveries. Advances in pharmacotherapy and neuromodulatory techniques have improved clinical management. Current surgical techniques are effective in some patients; however, therapy needs to be improved considerably. Cellular transplantation and gene therapy strategies are under investigation.

—James D. Guest

See also–Congenital Insensitivity to Pain with Anhidrosis (CIPA); Nerve Injury; Neuropathic Pain Syndromes; Pain, Basic Neurobiology of; Pain, Overview; Sensation

Further Reading

Csillik, B., and Knyihar-Csillik, E. (1982). Reversibility of microtubule inhibitor-induced transganglionic degenerative atrophy of central terminals of primary nociceptive neurons. *Neuroscience* 7, 1149–1154.

Eaton, M. J., Plunkett, J. A., Martinez, M. A., *et al.* (1999). Transplants of neuronal cells bioengineered to synthesize GABA alleviate chronic neuropathic pain. *Cell Transplant* 8, 87–101.

Loeser, J. D., Ward, A. A., Jr., and White, L. E., Jr. (1968). Chronic deafferentation of human spinal cord neurons. *J. Neurosurg.* 29, 48–50.

Lotze, M., Flor, H., Grodd, W., *et al.* (2001). Phantom movements and pain. An fMRI study in upper limb amputees. *Brain* 124, 2268–2277.

Nashold, B. S., Jr. (1981). Modification of DREZ lesion technique. *J. Neurosurg.* 55, 1012.

Ovelmen-Levitt, J. (1988). Abnormal physiology of the dorsal horn as related to the deafferentation syndrome. *Appl. Neurophysiol.* 51, 104–116.

Sindou, M., Quoex, C., and Baleydier, C. (1972). Fiber organization at the posterior spinal cord–rootlet junction in man. *J. Comp. Neurol.* 153, 15–26.

Wall, P. D., and Gutnick, M. (1974). Properties of afferent nerve impulses originating from a neuroma. *Nature* 248, 740–743.

Woolf, C. J., Shortland, P., and Coggeshall, R. E. (1992). Peripheral nerve injury triggers central sprouting of myelinated afferents. *Nature* 355, 75–78.

Zhao, S., Pang, Y., Beuerman, R. W., *et al.* (1998). Expression of c-Fos protein in the spinal cord after brachial plexus injury: Comparison of root avulsion and distal nerve transection. *Neurosurgery* 42, 1357–1362.

Pain, Invasive Procedures for

Encyclopedia of the Neurological Sciences
Copyright 2003, Elsevier Science (USA). All rights reserved.

THIS ENTRY provides an overview of procedures that may be performed in a multidisciplinary pain management program. The description of each procedure is meant to provide the referring practitioner with general indications and techniques. Many of the procedures listed here should only be undertaken by specialists with specialized training and a complete understanding of patient selection, sterile technique, anatomy, pharmacology of local anesthetics, and potential adverse reactions.

HEAD AND NECK PROCEDURES

Sphenopalantine Block

Anatomy: The sphenopalantine ganglion is located in the pterygopalatine fossa posterior to the middle turbinate. It is composed of somatic, parasympathetic, and sympathetic fibers.

Indications: Injections of this ganglion may treat cluster and migraine headaches in addition to other facial pain syndromes.

Procedure: There are two main approaches to this procedure: the transmucosal and transramus approaches. The transmucosal approach is easiest and commonly done. The patient is supine with the head extended. A cotton tip swab soaked with a high concentration of local anesthetic (occasionally cocaine) with or without epinephrine is introduced into the middle turbinate. To promote maximal absorption, the swab is left in place for approximately 15 min. The transramus approach is performed with radiographic guidance. A spinal needle is advanced through the coronoid notch of the jaw to the pterygopalatine fossa immediately below the maxillary nerve.

Complications: With the transmucosal technique, mucosa bleeding and irritation can occur. Paresthesias from the maxillary nerve and injury to ipsilateral facial structures have been reported with the transramal approach. Local anesthetic toxicity may occur with both procedures.

Trigeminal Nerve Block and Gasserian Ganglion Block

Anatomy: The trigeminal nerve consists of the ophthalmic, maxillary, and mandibular branches that branch from the Gasserian ganglion within Meckel's cave.

Indications: This procedure can provide analgesia for acute pain conditions resultant from facial trauma, postoperative incisional pain, or pain from acute herpes zoster. This procedure can also be useful in the diagnosis of facial pain. Neurodestructive procedures of the trigeminal nerve can provide palliation of malignant pain syndromes. Neurodestructive procedures of the Gasserian ganglion are useful for trigeminal neuralgia or pain secondary to facial malignancies. Controversy exists regarding whether microvascular decompression should be used as an alternative first-line treatment for patients who are able to withstand posterior craniotomies. Patients with multiple sclerosis and trigeminal neuralgia demonstrate less efficacy from this procedure.

Procedure: The patient is supine with the mouth partially open. Following palpation of the coronoid process, local anesthetic is infiltrated with a 1.5-in. needle inserted fully to the hub. The solution is injected in 1-cc increments, aspirating before each injection. For the Gasserian ganglion, the procedure is performed under radiographic guidance with a 3.5-in., 22-gauge needle that is directed under the zygomatic arch until bone is felt. Using a submental view, the needle is inserted through the foramen ovale, sometimes causing paresthesias or encountering cerebrospinal fluid.

Complications: The highly vascular area surrounding the trigeminal nerve may lead to inadvertent vascular uptake and toxicity of local anesthetic. Neurolytic procedures may result in anesthesia dolorosa and dysethesias.

Greater Occipital Nerve Block

Anatomy: The dorsal ramus of the second and third cervical nerves innervates the obliquus capitis inferior, emerging beneath it to divide into a medial and lateral branch. The larger medial branch, known as the greater occipital nerve, ascends under the spinalis capitis and the trapezius muscle to join the occipital artery to the posterior and superior aspect of the scalp.

Indications: This procedure is used for treatment of occipital neuralgia after pharmacological therapy has failed or of migraine and muscle tension headaches involving the pain in the posterior occiput.

Procedure: The greater occipital nerve can be blocked by identifying the occipital prominence in the back of the head at the superior nuchal line. The needle is fanned during the injection to ensure complete anesthesia of the nerve. Neurolytic procedures have also been done for chronic posterior occiput pain, but with little evidence of long-term efficacy.

Complications: Rare complications include nerve injury, bleeding, and intravascular injection. Needles that are placed too deep might result in foramen magnum injection or spinal cord injury.

PERIPHERAL NERVE BLOCKS

General Technique for Peripheral Nerve Blocks

Generally, three approaches have been described to successfully block peripheral nerves. The first approach is the paresthesia technique, which uses anatomical landmarks or nerve stimulation. Eliciting paresthesias to determine appropriate needle location is controversial, especially in patients complaining about neuropathic pain. The second technique relies on landmarks to determine needle entry site. Either surface anatomy or radiographic guidance relying on bony landmarks are advocated, especially for deep nerve locations. Nerve stimulators are often used as a third technique to help identify precise locations. Low-frequency pulses and slow, methodical advancement of an insulated needle allow careful localization of the nerve with less chance of injury.

General Indications: Peripheral nerve blocks are used to identify and treat nerve pathology. Single injections can be used for preoperative identification of nerve entrapments. A series of nerve injections can treat neuropathic pain states such as entrapment neuropathies. Radiofrequency lesioning has also been used for peripheral nerve pain.

Complications: Complications are rare but can include persistent paresthesias and nerve palsies secondary to fluid injection within confined areas.

Brachial Plexus Block

Anatomy: The brachial plexus is formed by nerve fibers from the anterior rami of C5–T1, with occasional contributions from C4 and T2. The brachial plexus exits the lateral aspect of the cervical spine inferolaterally in conjunction with the subclavian artery. Both the nerves and artery course between the anterior and middle scalene muscles passing beneath the middle of the clavicle and above the top of the first rib in its course to the axilla.

Indications: This procedure is indicated for a variety of painful conditions, including acute herpes zoster, brachial plexus neuritis, shoulder and upper extremity trauma, RSD, and cancer pain. Several procedures may be performed with intermittent blockade or with an embedded catheter for continuous blockade.

Procedure: The brachial plexus may be accessed via the interscalene, supraclavicular, and axillary approach. Using surface anatomy and a nerve stimulator, the needle is positioned depending on the patient's report of paresthesia or muscle twitching. After identification of the nerve, the desired mixture is injected. Catheters have also been used to provide excess for prolonged infusions.

Complications: Major complications include neural trauma with resultant pain (persistent or exacerbated), intravascular injection, hematoma, and phrenic nerve blockade. Phrenic nerve palsy may have significant morbidity in patients with preexisting respiratory compromise and limited pulmonary reserve. Pneumothorax may result during blockade of the more proximal portions of the brachial plexus. Inadvertent injection of the epidural space and intrathecal injection are risks of interscalene block.

Median Nerve

Anatomy: The median nerve at the wrist is located deep between the tendons of the palmaris longus and flexor carpi radialis. The median nerve passes through the carpal tunnel into the hand and supplies sensation and motor control to the thumb, index finger, middle finger, and the radial portion of the ring finger.

Indications: This procedure is sometimes used for therapy of carpal tunnel syndrome.

Procedure: The wrist is flexed and the palmaris longus tendon is identified. A needle is inserted just proximal to the wrist and slowly advanced at an acute angle while being directed proximally. A paresthesia is often elicited.

Complications: Care must be taken to avoid trauma to the nerve. Persistent paresthesia from the block is the primary complication.

Intercostal Nerve

Anatomy: The intercostal nerves arise from the anterior division of the thoracic paravertebral nerve. The typical intercostal nerve consists of somatic and sympathetic components. The nerve supplies sensation to the dermatomal level as well as some sensory innervation above and below the level.

Indications: Intercostal nerve blocks are used to treat various painful chest conditions, including post-thoracotomy pain syndromes, intercostal neuralgias, and fractured ribs. Dermatomal pain syndromes from malignancies are also responsive to blockade and neurolytic procedures.

Procedure: The appropriate rib is palpated and a needle is inserted and makes contact with the rib, usually in the posterior axillary line. The needle is moved from the rib margin inferiorly to where the injection is performed. Care must be taken to avoid deep or uncontrolled penetration into the lung.

Complications: The foremost risk is a tension pneumothorax. A clinically significant pneumothorax can occur sometime after the procedure has been completed.

Femoral Nerve Block

Anatomy: The femoral nerve innervates the anterior thigh and medial calf. The femoral nerve is composed of the posterior branches of the L2–L4 nerve roots. The nerve descends between and provides innervation to the psoas and iliacus muscle as it courses below the inguinal ligament to enter the thigh. The nerve also innervates the sartorius, quadriceps femoris, pectineus muscle, and knee joint. It is a constituent of the neurovascular bundle of the femoral artery and vein, to which it is lateral.

Indications: Blockade is used for evaluation and treatment of femoral nerve neuralgias. Neurolysis of this nerve is sometimes used for treatment of malignant pain syndromes that are refractory to other treatment modalities.

Procedure: Below the inguinal ligament, the needle is inserted lateral and perpendicular to the femoral artery and advanced 0.75 in. The patient often reports a paresthesia. After careful aspiration, the desired solution is injected.

Complications: Bruising and ecchymosis may occur. Intravascular injection is a substantial risk.

Tibial Nerve Block

Anatomy: The tibial nerve is one of two major branches of the sciatic nerve. It provides sensation to the posterior portion of the calf, heel, and medial plantar surface of the foot. The tibial nerve begins in the popliteal fossa and descends between the two heads of the gastrocnemius muscle deep to the soleus and then medially between the Achilles tendon and the medial malleolus into the foot.

Indications: Tibial nerve blockade is useful for evaluation and treatment of foot and ankle pain. Injection of the tibial nerve at the ankle can be useful in the diagnosis and treatment of tarsal tunnel syndrome.

Procedure: The nerve is accessible to blockade in the posterior popliteal fossa and ankle. With the ankle approach, the leg is externally rotated and the posterior tibial artery is palpated between the medial malleolus and the Achilles tendon. A 25-gauge needle is introduced slowly toward the posterior groove of the medial malleolus. A paresthesia is often obtained at a depth of approximately 0.5 in. The needle is then slightly redirected and the desired solution injected.

Complications: The main complications of this block are postblock pain, hematoma, and ecchymosis. Because this block can elicit paresthesia, nerve damage is possible if the needle is not slightly withdrawn before injection.

Saphenous Nerve Block

Anatomy: The saphenous nerve is the largest branch of the femoral nerve and innervates the medial portion of the lower leg and the foot. The nerve travels with the femoral artery through Hunter's canal, and at the medial condyle of the distal femur it supplies the medial portion of the knee and the lower leg.

Indications: The saphenous nerve block is useful in managing medial knee and leg pain. This nerve can become entrapped within Hunter's canal as it courses through the adductor magnus muscle.

Procedure: Two approaches have been described, one at the ankle and the second above the knee joint. For the approach at the knee, the patient is supine with the leg externally rotated. After Hunter's canal is identified superior to the medial condyle of the femur, a needle is slowly advanced approximately 0.25–0.5 in. Either a paresthesia can be elicited or a nerve stimulator can be used for accurate identification of needle placement. Following appropriate positioning and aspiration, the desired solution is injected.

Complications: Because of the proximity of the greater saphenous artery, postprocedure hematoma

is common. Needle-induced trauma can lead to postprocedure paresthesia.

Lateral Femoral Cutaneous Nerve Block

Anatomy: The posterior division of L2 and L3 forms the nerve. The nerve courses through the psoas compartment laterally and inferiorly beneath the ilioinguinal nerve to exit at the level of the anterior superior iliac spine, where it descends beneath the fascia lata. The nerve provides sensation to the lateral thigh from the greater trochanter to knee.

Indications: The primary indication for this procedure is the evaluation and management of femoral nerve neuralgia or meralgia paresthetica.

Procedure: The nerve is blocked by placing a needle 1 in. medial to the anterior superior iliac spine and immediately below the inguinal ligament.

Complications: Increased localized pain is a common complication. Injection of the peritoneal cavity is possible with too deep placement of the needle.

Obturator Nerve Block

Anatomy: The primary innervation of the hip joint is the obturator nerve, which is composed of the posterior divisions of L2–L4. The nerve leaves the medial border of the psoas muscle and descends into the thigh along with the obturator vessels by the obturator foramen. The nerve also supplies motor fibers to the superficial and deep hip adductors as well as the posterior part of the knee joint.

Indications: This procedure is used to evaluate and treat pain and spasm originating from the hip joint and hip adductors. Neurolytic procedures are used for spastic conditions such as cerebral palsy.

Procedure: In a supine position, the pubic tubercle is identified. Using a point 1 in. lateral and 1 in. inferior, a spinal needle is introduced perpendicular until the superior pubic ramus is identified. The needle is then redirected laterally and inferiorly until it can be advanced 0.75 in. A paresthesia is sometimes elicited at this point. After aspiration, the solution is injected. Radiographic guidance or a nerve stimulator facilitate this procedure.

Complications: Significant complications, such as intraperitoneal and bladder injection, have occurred. Intravascular injection is possible.

Sciatic Nerve Block

Anatomy: The sciatic nerve innervates most of the distal lower extremity and foot. The largest nerve in the body is derived from the fusion of L4–S3. The nerve passes in front of the sacrum and piriformis muscle, where it leaves the pelvis via the sciatic notch. The sciatic nerve lies anterior to the gluteus maximus muscle. The sciatic nerve then courses down the leg near the lesser trochanter, where it lies posterior and medial to the femur.

Indications: This nerve block is used to treat and evaluate pain of the distal lower extremity. Neurolytic procedures can be used to palliate end stage oncology pain, such as distal pathological fractures or painful gangrene of the distal lower extremity. With a catheter placement, continuous blockade of this nerve is used for acute painful conditions.

Procedure: There are several different approaches to sciatic nerve blockade. Multiple approaches facilitate blockade in a large variety of clinical conditions and include anterior, lithotomy, and posterior techniques. The posterior approach requires the patient to be in a lateral or Sim's position. The upper leg is slightly flexed and the greater trochanter and ischial tuberosity are identified. The sciatic nerve lies halfway between these landmarks. A spinal needle is introduced at the landmark and slowly advanced until a paresthesia is noted, usually at a depth of 2 or 3 in. After the patient reports the paresthesia, the needle is slightly withdrawn and the desired solution is injected. Alternatively, a nerve stimulator can be used to identify the nerve.

Complications: The main side effects are localized pain and ecchymosis. If appropriate care is not taken, intranerve injection can lead to nerve damage and persistent paresthesia.

SPINAL PROCEDURES

Epidural Space Block

Anatomy: The epidural space is between the dura and the posterior longitudinal ligament anteriorly and posteriorly between the vertebral laminae and the ligamentum flavum. The vertebral pedicles and intervertebral foramina form the lateral limits of the epidural space. The superior limit of the epidural space is the fusion of the dura to the foramen magnum. The inferior limit is the sacrococcygeal membrane. The epidural space is made of fat, veins, arteries, and lymphatic and connective tissue.

Indications: Administration of a combination of depot steroid injections and local anesthetic is helpful in a variety of conditions, including radiculopathies, localized nonradiating spine pain, spondylosis, vertebral compression fractures, postherpetic neuralgias, and malignant pain syndromes secondary to localized metastasis. The injection of autogenous blood is used for treatment of spinal headaches.

Procedure: The cervical epidural space can be approached with the patient in a sitting, prone, or lateral position. Two techniques can be used to perform an epidural injection. The hanging drop technique requires slow advancement of an epidural needle until a drop of fluid placed at the end of the needle is drawn in, indicating entrance into the subatmospheric pressure of the epidural space. The loss of resistance technique advances the epidural needle with an attached glass syringe until a loss of resistance is felt as the needle passes through the ligament into the epidural space. Radiographic guidance may decrease misplaced injections due to false loss of resistance.

Complications: These injections should not be performed in the presence of local or systemic infections. Coagulation status must be normal to avoid epidural hematoma. Despite these precautions, epidural infection and hematoma can still occur. Other serious complications include spinal cord injury, total spinal anesthesia with resultant respiratory depression, hypotension, and cardiovascular collapse. With unrecognized intravenous injection, local anesthetic toxicity within the central nervous system (CNS), heart arrhythmias, and complete atony have occurred. Less serious complications include persistent paresthesia and worsened pain from needle trauma.

Selective Nerve Root Blocks

Anatomy: The cervical nerves exit the intraspinal canal through their respective foramen, which are located immediately below the transverse process. For C1 and C2, the nerves exit at approximately the midpoint of the vertebral body. The nerves are numbered for the vertebral body below their exit site, with the exception of C8, which does not have corresponding vertebrae. The rest of the spinal nerves exit below the respective transverse processes. The nerve divides almost immediately and gives off a branch to the facet joint. Immediately paravertebrally, the spinal nerve is accessible for blockade.

Indications: This procedure can be used for both diagnostic and therapeutic indications. Diagnostic procedures are indicated as a preoperative procedure when the precise origin of a radiculopathy is unknown. This procedure can also be used for treatment of radiculopathies. Because of the precise injection of therapeutic agent, this procedure can improve symptoms that were resistant to unguided epidural steroid injections. This technique has been used in neurolytic procedures or when an intraspinal approach for selective rhizotomies is necessary in patients with malignant pain syndromes.

Procedure: Radiographic guidance is required along with a small amount of radioopaque contrast for precise localization of the needle. Many different techniques have been described for this procedure. The needle is placed just below the transverse process and directed toward the neuroforamen.

Complications: Although rare, the most serious complications are either vertebral artery in the cervical area or intrathecal injection. Other complications include nerve root injury and possible paraplegia following trauma to the vasculature of the spinal cord. For neurolytic procedures, unintended loss of function is the primary complication, which can be minimized by using small volumes. Risk is increased due to close proximity to areas of the spinal cord controlling limb function.

Facet Joint Injection

Anatomy: The facet joints are formed by the articulations of the superior and inferior articular facets of the lamina of the adjacent vertebrae. The joints are true synovial joints and extensively innervated. Each joint receives innervation from above and below as well as from the level on which it is located.

Indications: Both clinical and radiological features of facet joint pain are nonspecific. An improved objective diagnostic approach may be provided by single photon emission computed tomography. Facet joints can refer pain to various areas of the trunk and upper extremities. Pain is generated by either arthritic degeneration of the synovial joint or acute inflammatory conditions such as trauma or rheumatic conditions.

Procedure: This procedure must be done under fluoroscopic guidance. Two approaches are described: injection into the capsule of the joint known as a medial bundle branch block (MBBB) and intraarticular joint injection. For an MBBB approach, the fluoroscopic beam is aligned obliquely to visualize the joint or AP position and the needle is advanced to the middle of the articular pillar, where the medial branch passes. With the intraarticular procedure, the joint surfaces are visualized by an oblique position of the fluoroscopic camera. The same approach can be used for neurolytic procedures commonly done with radiofrequency lesioning.

Complications: Major complications include injections into the vertebral artery in the cervical area and the pneumothorax in the thoracic area and also intrathecal and spinal cord injections. A temporary localized increase in pain is common.

Diskography and Intradiskal Electrothermaplasty

Anatomy: Spinal disks are found between each vertebral body of the spine (Fig. 1). The characteristics of cervical, thoracic, and lumbar disks vary, but common to each disk are a tough outer fibrous ring know as an annulus and the inner gelatinous nucleus pulposis.

Indications: This procedure is indicated to evaluate persistent pain after traditional diagnostic approaches, such as imaging or electromyography (EMG), have failed to determine an etiology. This

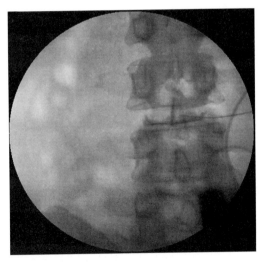

Figure 1
AP view of a normal-appearing disk during diskography.

test seeks to provoke pain that reproduces the patient's pain complaint. This is known as concordant pain. Discordant pain is pain that does not simulate the patient's pain. The procedure should be done on at least three levels, including an asymptomatic level for a control.

Procedure: In general, lumbar and thoracic disks are approached from the posterior lateral position under radiographic guidance. The cervical disk is approached from an anterior position slightly lateral to the midline. Water-soluble contrast is used to identify the appropriate needle location. Resistance to injection is noted along with any pain that the patient reports. A healthy disk is not painful, and some resistance is normal. A syringe attached to a pressure manometer is often used to avoid over-pressurization of the disk. Based on the patient's pain report, a second control disk is injected. If failure to elicit pain or discordant pain is reported, other levels may be done to identify the painful disk. Postprocedure computed tomography scan can detect extravasation of contrast, indicating a torn annulus. Although controversial, diskography may predict successful outcome in helping to determine surgical outcomes.

Complications: Increased pain from the procedure is common and self-limited. Significant complications include diskitis, trauma to the nerve roots, local damage to blood vessels, and epidural hematoma. In the thoracic area, pneumothorax is a risk.

Intradiskal Electrothermaplasty

Intradiskal electrothermaplasty is a newly described procedure for diskogenic back pain first proven by provocative diskography. This procedure is very similar to the approach used for diskography.

Complications: Complications are similar to those of diskography, with the additional risk of thermal damage to the spinal cord.

Vertebroplasty

Anatomy: The relevant anatomy consists of the vertebral body, which is located between the disk spaces of the lumbar and thoracic spine.

Indications: Vertebroplasty is performed on compression fractures of the vertebral column secondary to osteoporosis or malignancies.

Procedure: This procedure must be done under radiographic guidance. Often, monitored anesthesia care or conscious sedation are required. Methylmethacrolate is used to stabilize the body of the fractured vertebrae.

Complications: Many serious but rare complications have been reported for methylmethacrolate, including cement embolism, spinal cord injury by unrecognized injection into the epidural space, and somatic nerve injury from placement of the cannula.

AUTONOMIC NERVOUS SYSTEM

Sympathetic Blockade

These procedures are done for neuropathic pain syndromes that are either sympathetically mediated or have a sympathetic component. If a favorable response is obtained, a series of injections may elicit a therapeutic response that progressively increases in duration after each block. Especially in the treatment of complex regional pain syndromes, rehabilitation and the block can be effective. Sympathetic blocks are also used to treat the pain from acute zoster infections, arm limb syndromes following CVAs, and Raynaud's syndrome. No double-blind studies have been done for CRPS or other conditions. The urgent nature of addressing a patient's pain report will probably preclude controlled studies from ever being done. Many case series and anecdotal experience suggest an important role for these procedures.

Stellate Ganglion Block

Anatomy: The ganglion is located on the anterior surface of the longus colli muscle. The muscle lies anterior to the transverse processes of the seventh and first thoracic vertebrae.

Indications: Stellate ganglion blocks are used for blocking the sympathetic innervation to the face, neck, and ipsilateral arm.

Procedure: With the patient supine and chin extended, the medial edge of the sternocleidomastoid muscle is palpated on its medial border. The inferior cricothyroid notch is noted and, along with the carotid neurovascular bundle, is retracted medially. A needle is inserted until the transverse process is contacted. The needle is then withdrawn slightly, and appropriate solution is injected.

Complications: Complications of this procedure can occur from intravascular injection of local anesthetic into the carotid or vertebral artery, resulting in focal neurological deficits, convulsions, or cardiovascular arrest. Injection of the local anesthetic intraspinally can lead to a total spinal. Inadvertent local anesthetic blockade of the brachial plexus, recurrent laryngeal, or phrenic nerve is not uncommon. Pneumothorax is a known complication as well.

Superior Hypogastric Plexus Block

Anatomy: This plexus is in the retroperitoneal space anterior to L5–S1 vertebral bodies and contains visceral afferents from the pelvic viscera and part of the descending colon.

Indications: This procedure is indicated for pelvic pain syndromes of both visceral and myofascial origins, such as interstitial cystitis, endometriosis, pelvic adhesions, malignancies, chronic prostatitis, and other muscular structures of the pelvic floor. The block also has prognostic value for surgical presacral neurectomy. Neurolytic solutions can treat pain from pelvic malignancies.

Procedure: This procedure is usually performed under radiographic guidance. Either one or two needles are placed lateral to the lumbar spine, usually at the L3–L4 level. The needles are directed anteriorly to L5–S1 vertebral bodies. Injection of contrast demonstrates adequate coverage of the plexus.

Complications: The main complication is intravascular injection of iliac vessels.

Celiac

Anatomy: The celiac plexus is located in the retroperitoneal space immediately anterior to the aorta at L1 (Fig. 2). The plexus is composed of visceral afferents from the abdominal viscera, including the entire small intestine, liver, stomach, pancreas, and ascending and transverse colon.

Indications: Celiac plexus block is indicated for upper abdominal pain. This block has been used for treatment and diagnostic purposes. This block also treats the noncancer pain of acute pancreatitis. Neurolytic celiac plexus blocks are usually reserved for intraabdominal malignancies. Solutions used for blockade are bupivacaine with or without steroid and either 6–12% phenol or 50–100% alcohol.

Procedure: There are many approaches for blockade, including the anterior approach using ultrasound, the transgastric approach using endoscopy, and the posterior approach using radiographic

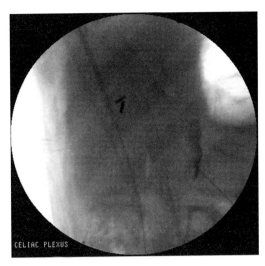

Figure 2
Lateral view of needle placement at L1 for celiac block.

guidance such as computed tomography or flouroscopy. Both single-needle transaortic and dual-needle approaches are common. In the transaortic technique, the patient is prone, with the spinal needle entrance 8 cm lateral to the midline below the 12th rib on the left. The needle is advanced until aortic pulsation is felt. The needle is inserted into the aorta, and blood return is noted. The needle is then advanced through the anterior side of the aorta and X-rays are obtained prior to injection of local or neurolytic solution. Care must be taken to avoid intravascular injection.

Complications: The procedure using local anesthetic has few complications if intravascular injection is avoided. If alcohol is used, there is usually an intense burning sensation in the upper abdominal area, usually requiring supplemental parenteral or intravenous analgesia. Phenol is a local anesthetic and has less pain associated with use. Orthostatic hypotension, diarrhea, and rare complications of somatic nerve root damage and paraplegia can occur.

Efficacy: Good pain relief is achieved in approximately 65% of patients who have cancer of the pancreas. Few data are available for upper abdominal pain of nonmalignant origin. The neurolytic block can last up to 6 months.

Paravertebral Sympathetic Lumbar

Anatomy: The lumbar sympathetic chain is composed of pre- and postganglionic fibers. The preganglionic fibers exit their respective neuroforamina and innervate the spinal ligaments and meninges. The chain is located at the anterolateral margin of the vertebral bodies.

Procedure: With the patient prone and under radiographic guidance, a spinal needle of sufficient length is introduced approximately 3 in. lateral to the spinous process. The needle is advanced at a 35–45° angle, slightly cephalad to the transverse process. AP and lateral views with contrast injection are obtained to ensure proper needle placement.

Complications: Complications include spinal nerve anesthesia, somatic nerve blockade, epidural or spinal anesthesia, and nerve root injury. Neurolytic blocks can cause somatic nerve dysfunction, spinal cord injury with resultant paralysis or paresis, and loss of bowel and bladder continence. Because of the proximity of the sympathetic chain, it is common for spinal nerves to be at least partially blocked following this procedure. Care must be taken with neurolytic solutions to avoid permanent nerve injury.

Efficacy: Sympathetic blockade is one of the main diagnostic and therapeutic procedures for sympathetic-mediated pain syndromes. Many studies show efficacy.

INTRAMUSCLAR PROCEDURES

Trigger Point Injections

Anatomy: Trigger point injections are characterized by areas of tender nodules or distinct bands of muscle, the palpation of which can reliably refer pain to consistent locations on the trunk or extremities. Trigger points are identified by applying pressure over the presumed location until the patient's pain is replicated.

Indications: Injection of trigger points may improve both the range of motion and the function of the affected area. This procedure may play a useful role in conjunction with a rehabilitation program.

Procedure: A trigger point can be injected with either a dry acupuncture needle or a needle filled with saline or local anesthetic with or without steroid. This procedure is often repeated during the rehabilitation program in order to treat recurrences. Recently, botulism toxin has been advocated for use during trigger point injections in order to treat resistant myofascial pain.

Complications: Following the procedure, the pain elicited from the trigger point area may temporarily worsen. Misdirected needles may puncture adjacent organs and blood vessels. Inadvertent intravascular injection of local anesthetic may precipitate seizures or systemic toxicity.

Efficacy: Well-controlled outcome studies are limited in part due to the lack of consistent criteria for the diagnosis of trigger points. Case series and small controlled studies have demonstrated short-term improvement. Case reports suggest that botulinum toxin is efficacious.

Piriformis Muscle

Anatomy: This muscle arises from the pelvic surface of the sacrum, the sacrotuberous ligament, and the posterior portion of the ilium. The muscle then courses through the sciatic foramen to insert into the upper border of the greater trochanter.

Indications: Patients presenting with this syndrome often complain of radiculopathy-like symptoms.

Procedure: The muscle in thin persons can often be palpated and with pressure will reproduce the symptoms. The muscle is approached in a similar fashion as the posterior approach to the sciatic nerve. A nerve stimulator or EMG can be used to increase accuracy.

Complications: With the sciatic nerve in the immediate vicinity, long-term anesthesia and paresthesia can occur. Local pain and irritation are the most frequent complications.

INTERVENTIONAL PROCEDURES

Spinal Catheters and Infusion Devices

Indications: Spinal infusions can be used to determine efficacy for long-term neuroaxial treatment of chronic pain via neuroaxial infusions. Epidural infusions have been used as interim therapy to facilitate rehabilitation for chronic pain conditions such as CRPS. Devices such as Port-a-Caths, fixed for programmable pumps, are used in cases in which extended infusions for more than 3 months are necessary. These devices are often used for treatment of cancer pain or other intractable pain syndromes.

Procedure: A large-gauge needle is inserted into the desired area with a loss of resistance technique for epidural placement or intrathecally for intraspinal catheters. Following placement of the needle, a catheter is advanced through the needle with radiographic guidance. After appropriate placement, the needle is withdrawn, and the catheter is fixed to the skin for temporary catheters or fixed to the posterior ligament of the spine for permanent catheters. There are two types of catheters and multiple techniques for implantation and anchoring. Some epidural catheters have Dacron sleeves that purport to reduce the incidence of infection migrating to the epidural space. Implantable systems such as epidural Port-a-Caths or implantable infusion pumps may decrease the risk of infection for long-term infusions. When these devices are used, a pocket must be formed, usually in the chest or abdominal wall. A specialized technique using a modified epidural needle and catheter known as epidural lysis of adhesions has been described.

Complications: Spinal cord injury and unrecognized catheterization of epidural veins can lead to inadvertent intravascular injection of local anesthetic into the epidural veins. Because of the delayed onset of epidural dilaudid and morphine, respiratory depression many hours after injection has been reported. With any exteriorized catheter, infection is a constant risk and appropriate care is required. The presentation of an epidural abscess with the potential of spinal cord compression requires appropriate clinical vigilance. Less serious complications include catheter leaks and medication side effects. Spinal opiates can cause nausea and vomiting, urinary retention, pruritus, sedation, and respiratory depression. These side effects are usually transient and can be symptomatically treated.

Neurostimulation

Indications: Electrical stimulation of the CNS has long been used for analgesia in neuropathic pain states (Fig. 3). Electrodes can be used for both peripheral and central stimulation. Epidural placement of multielectrode arrays can be effective for a variety of conditions, including neuropathic pain syndromes and pain from vascular insufficiency. Electrodes have also been implanted along peripheral nerves, such as the median, radial, sciatic, tibial, and peroneal nerves. Recent methods have used a suboccipital approach for occipital neuralgia and transsacral approaches for pelvic pain and bladder dysfunction. Deep brain stimulation has been used to

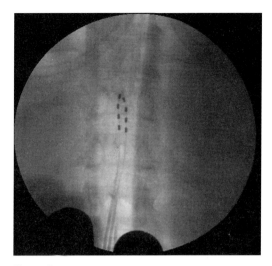

Figure 3
AP view of dual spinal cord simulators in place.

a limited extent for various central pain syndromes and Parkinson's disease.

Procedure: For peripheral nerve stimulator placement, surgical exposure of the nerve is required. A flat or paddle lead is place alongside the desired nerve. Fascial grafts are often used to protect the nerve. For epidural stimulation, the placement of the electrode is similar to the placement of epidural catheters. Trial stimulation determines efficacy prior to implantation of the system. Fixation of the electrode is important to avoid movement. There are two types of pulse generators—an external system that relies on radiofrequency current for power and a battery-operated implantable pulse generator. This portion of the device is implanted in the buttock, over the greater trochanter, or most commonly in the abdominal wall.

—Edgar L. Ross and Edward Michna

See also–Pain, Assessment of; Pain Management, Multidisciplinary; Pain Management, Psychological Strategies; Pulvinotomy; Rhizotomy

Further Reading
Abram, S. E. (2000). Neural blockade for neuropathic pain. *Clin. J. Pain* **16**, S56–S61.
Aldrete, J. A. (1997). Extended epidural catheter infusions with analgesics for patients with noncancer pain at their homes. *Reg. Anesth.* **22**, 35–42.
Arter, O. E., and Racz, G. B. (1990). Pain management of the oncologic patient. *Semin. Surg. Oncol.* **6**, 162–172.

Dellemijn, P. L., Fields, H. L., Allen, R. R., et al. (1994). The interpretation of pain relief and sensory changes following sympathetic blockade. Brain 117, 1475–1487.

Geurts, J. W., Van Wijk, R. M., Stolker, R. J., et al. (2001). Efficacy of radiofrequency procedures for the treatment of spinal pain: A systematic review of randomized clinical trials. Reg. Anesth. Pain Med. 26, 394–400.

Hogan, Q. H., and Abram, S. E. (1997). Neural blockade for diagnosis and prognosis. A review. Anesthesiology 86, 216–241.

Kim, P. S. (2002). Role of injection therapy: Review of indications for trigger point injections, regional blocks, facet joint injections, and intra-articular injections. Curr. Opin. Rheumatol. 14, 52–57.

Kinard, R. E. (1996). Diagnostic spinal injection procedures. Neurosurg. Clin. North Am. 7, 151–165.

McDonald, J. S., Pensak, M. L., and Phero, J. C. (1990). Thoughts on the management of chronic facial, head, and neck pain. Am. J. Otol. 11, 378–382.

Ten Vaarwerk, I. A., and Staal, M. J. (1998). Spinal cord stimulation in chronic pain syndromes. Spinal Cord 36, 671–682.

Ten Vaarwerk, I. A., Jessurun, G. A. J., De Jongste, M. J. L., et al. (1999). Clinical outcome of patients treated with spinal cord stimulation for therapeutically refractory angina pectoris. The Working Group on Neurocardiology. Heart 82, 82–88.

Pain Management, Multidisciplinary

Encyclopedia of the Neurological Sciences

MORE THAN 60 million Americans suffer from some type of persistent or recurrent acute pain sufficient to impact significantly on their lives. Despite major advances in knowledge of sensory physiology, anatomy, and biochemistry, along with the development of potent analgesic medications and other innovative medical and surgical interventions, pain relief for many pain sufferers remains elusive.

Pain is a complex, subjective phenomenon composed of a set of factors, each of which contributes to the interpretation of nociception (activation of sensory transduction in nerves by thermal, mechanical, or clinical energy impinging on specialized nerve endings) as pain. The complexity of pain is especially evident when it persists over extended periods of time because a range of psychological and social factors interact with the physical pathology to modulate reports of pain and subsequent disability. Thus, each individual uniquely experiences the perception of pain.

Not only does chronic pain adversely affect pain sufferers' physical and psychological well-being but also it costs billions of dollars to society in lost productivity, health care expenditures, and disability compensation. The health care costs of chronic pain patients for the one year preceding referral to a specialist in pain treatment range from $500 to $35,400, with an average of $13,284, excluding the costs of surgical procedures. Surgical procedures add substantially to health care expenses. For example, the most prevalent complaint of patients treated by pain specialists (40–60%) is some form of back pain. The cost for lumbar surgery (including surgery, anesthesiology, and hospitalization) is approximately $25,000, with a total of almost $5 billion spent annually on surgery for chronic back pain patients alone. Furthermore, health care use after surgery may increase for some patients because of iatrogenic complications. Serious complications that require additional surgery are relatively common.

There has been a growing epidemic during the past two decades of chronic pain and disability complaints in all industrialized countries. As health care costs for those who suffer from chronic pain have grown, it has become apparent that the traditional biomedical model provides an inadequate foundation for the delivery of effective health care. Multidisciplinary pain management evolved because it has proven to be more effective and less costly than the traditional methods of addressing chronic pain. During the past 25 years, specialized treatment facilities—multidisciplinary pain centers and clinics—have been established to treat patients with recalcitrant pain problems. More than 400 pain treatment facilities have been established in the United States, and there are an additional 1000 worldwide. The estimated average cost for an outpatient treatment by pain specialists in the United States is $8100. More than $1.5 billion is spent on specialized pain treatment annually.

CHARACTERISTICS AND GOALS OF MULTIDISCIPLINARY TREATMENT

There is no single model of a pain clinic. Specific details may vary with the patient population, medical and other health care disciplines involved, general philosophy, and combinations of therapeutic modalities used. The International Association for the Study of Pain describes four levels of pain treatment programs: multidisciplinary pain centers, multidisciplinary pain clinics, pain clinic, and modality-oriented clinic. The multidisciplinary pain centers and clinics (MPCs) are most comprehensive and differ only in the emphasis on education and research at multidisciplinary pain centers. Pain clinics, on the other hand, usually focus on a specific diagnosis (e.g., headache), and modality-oriented clinics are characterized by the emphasis on a treatment (e.g., nerve blocks).

Several epidemiological studies have compared the characteristics of people who have chronic pain in the community with those of patients treated at MPCs. Compared with persistent pain sufferers treated in the community, MPC referrals were more likely to

- Have work-related injuries
- Report greater health care use
- Report more constant pain
- Be taking opioids
- Have had surgery for their pain (mean, 1.7 operations)
- Report greater functional impairment
- Have lower levels of education
- Endorse more negative attitudes about the future
- Suffer greater levels of emotional distress

Up to 90% of patients treated at MPCs have at least one psychiatric diagnosis (50% are significantly depressed), more than 60% have more than one diagnosis, and up to 59% have significant personality disorders.

Traditional diagnostic processes have failed to identify a remediable cause of pain for many chronic pain sufferers treated at MPCs. These patients require comprehensive treatment because of the disruption of their lives associated with persistent pain. Indeed, these patients' health care providers must feel comfortable abandoning the search for a cure and instead accept palliation as a viable outcome. For the majority of these patients cure is unrealistic. The goal, then, is to improve the patient's ability to function, not to cure the disease that has led to pain. Hence, the diagnostic process must identify the areas of functional impairment and disability, and treatment must address all the factors that contribute to disability. In contrast to traditional medical therapy, patients cannot be passive recipients of the ministrations of providers. Such patients must accept responsibility and work to achieve the benefits of treatment.

There is no standard way for treatment at an MPC to be delivered. Each program incorporates a broad range of modalities and idiosyncratic components. However, several underlying concepts characterize MPCs (Table 1). One fundamental concept is the understanding that patients with complex pain

Table 1   CONCEPTS OF TREATMENT AT MULTIDISCIPLINARY PAIN CLINICS

Reconceptualization of the patients pain and associated problems from uncontrollable to manageable

Overt or covert efforts are made to foster optimism and combat demoralization

Flexibility is the norm, with attempts to individualize some aspects of treatment to patient needs and unique physical and psychological characteristics

Emphasize active patient participation and responsibility

Provide education and training in the use of specific skills, such as exercise, relaxation, and problem solving

Encourage patient feelings of success, self-control, and self-efficacy

Encourage patients to attribute success to their own role

problems are best served by a team of specialists with different health care backgrounds. Another concept is the realization that the report of pain is not just the result of body damage but has psychological and environmental origins as well. Equally important, MPCs treat not only the experience of pain but also associated patient distress, dysfunction, and disability.

The goals of multidisciplinary pain management are typically specific, definable, operationalizable, and realistic in nature. There are a number of general goals that are shared by MPCs, namely

- Identification and treatment of any unresolved medical problems
- Symptomatic improvement if not complete elimination
- Elimination of any unnecessary medications
- Restoration of physical functioning
- Reduction in inappropriate use of the health care system
- Restoration of social functioning and social reintegration
- Restoration of occupational functioning—return to work and usual activities
- Improvement in psychological functioning
- Enhancement of independence

The integration of multiple modalities and disciplines for treatment of pain has probably been the single most important advancement in modern care of the patient who suffers from chronic pain. The treatment team must be more than a group of professionals from different disciplines, each of whom is treating the patient simultaneously. The emphasis is on the person who is experiencing the pain and their social context and not just the anatomical part(s) involved. There must be constant communication among team members and mutual reinforcement of the overall treatment goals. Team members must reinforce each other's role and efforts, communicate respect for each other's skills with the patients, and maintain awareness of what other team members are doing. They must provide a consistent message to patients. The treatment team must build an alliance with the patient to instill motivation for and acceptance of self-management because in the majority of cases the treatments involved will not result in complete elimination of pain.

OUTCOMES

Given constraints on health care resources, there is a growing interest in accountability and evidence-based treatment outcome data. The effectiveness of pain treatment facilities has been the subject of much criticism, particularly among some third-party payers. Asking whether MPCs are effective, however, may be an unsuitable way to phrase the question of whether they are worthwhile. It might be more appropriate to broaden the question by asking how effective are pain treatment facilities compared to alternative treatments and on what outcome criteria. That is, we can ask how effective are pain treatment facilities compared to alternatives such as surgery on measures such as reduction in pain, reduction in medication and health care utilization, increased physical activity, closure of disability claims, and return to work.

Several reviews and meta-analyses on treatment outcome studies have evaluated the clinical and cost-effectiveness of MPCs. Despite the recalcitrance of the pain problems of the patients treated, the outcome data generally support the efficacy of MPCs on each of the criteria noted previously. MPCs and more conventional measures have approximately the same effect on reducing pain. However, MPCs appear to be more effective in significantly reducing consumption of prescription analgesic medication, reducing health care utilization, leading to closure of disability claims, increasing functional activities, and helping patients return to work. They have also been shown to be more cost-effective than patient education and physical therapy alone, surgery, prescriptions for long-term opioid medication, and implantable devices.

To illustrate the differences in treatment outcomes between MPCs that focus on rehabilitation and conventional alternatives, we can refer to more than 65 published studies that include 3089 patients. Based on the aggregation of outcomes (i.e., meta-analysis), 45–65% of patients treated at MPCs return to work following treatment compared to 20% of patients who return to work following surgery for pain and 25% who return to work following implantable pain control devices (e.g., spinal cord stimulators). There is little evidence to support the success of long-term use of opioids in improving patients' functional outcomes, including return to work.

Following treatment at MPCs, patients required one-third the number of surgical interventions and hospitalizations required by patients treated with conventional medical and surgical care. Treatment at MPCs resulted in closure of disability claims for one-half of those receiving disability at the time of treatment. Even at long-term follow-up, patients who were treated in pain rehabilitation programs appeared to function better than 75% of chronic pain patients treated by conventional, unimodal treatment approaches. It is also worth noting that conventional medical and surgical interventions can result in iatrogenic complications that may require additional costly treatment. However, there are no known equivalent problems noted for rehabilitation provided at MPCs.

Extrapolations from the data included in meta-analyses and recent studies indicate that not only are MPCs clinically effective but also they are cost-effective. Using the 3089 patients included in the meta-analysis mentioned earlier, savings in excess of $20 million would be achieved based on reductions in health care utilization and indemnity costs during the first year following treatment, even after factoring the cost of treatment at MPCs (average, $8100). Considering the average age of patients treated at MPCs is 45 years, the anticipated savings until age 65 would exceed $248 million. If we used the same assumptions for the estimated 175,000 patients treated at MPCs, then the financial savings would exceed $11 billion in the first year following treatment.

FUTURE DIRECTIONS

Most MPCs include a broad range of components within a single rehabilitation package. Further research is needed to isolate the shared components of various successful treatment programs. Studies are needed to answer the question, What treatments delivered in what ways are most effective for patients with what set of characteristics? Successful answers to this question will permit more clinically effective and cost-effective ways to treat the difficult population of patients with chronic pain.

—Dennis C. Turk

See also–Depression; Pain, Assessment of; Pain, Invasive Procedures for; Pain Management, Psychological Strategies; Pain, Overview

Acknowledgments

Preparation of the manuscript was supported in part by grants from the National Institute of Arthritis and Musculoskeletal and Skin Diseases (AR/AI44724) and the National Institute of Child Health and Human Development (HD33989).

Further Reading

College of Physicians and Surgeons of Ontario (2000). *Evidence-Based Recommendations for Medical Management of Chronic Non-malignant Pain*. College of Physicians and Surgeons of Ontario, Toronto.

Cutler, R. B., Fishbain, D. A., Rosomoff, H. L., Abdel-Moty, E., Khalil, T. M., and Steele Rosomoff, R. (1993). Does non-surgical pain center treatment of chronic pain return patients to work? A review and meta-analysis of the literature. In *Proceedings of the 7th World Congress of Pain, Seattle*, pp. 801–802. IASP Press, Seattle, WA.

Flor, H., Fydrich, T., and Turk, D. C. (1992). Efficacy of multidisciplinary pain treatment centers: A meta-analytic review. *Pain* **49**, 221–230.

Loeser, J. D., and Turk, D. C. (2001). Multidisciplinary pain management. In *Bonica's Management of Pain* (J. D. Loeser, S. H. Butler, C. R. Chapman, and D. C. Turk, Eds.), 3rd ed., pp. 2069–2079. Lippincott Williams & Wilkins, Philadelphia.

Marketdata Enterprises (1995). *Chronic Pain Management Programs: A Market Analysis*. Marketdata Enterprises, Valley Stream, NY.

Turk, D. C., and Gatchel, R. J. (1999). Multidisciplinary programs for rehabilitation of chronic low back pain patients. In *Managing Low Back Pain* (W. H. Kirkaldy-Willis and T. N. Bernard, Eds.), pp. 299–311. Churchill Livingstone, New York.

Turk, D. C., and Okifuji, A. (1997). Multidisciplinary pain centers: Boons or boondoggles? *J. Workers Compensation* **6**, 9–26.

Pain Management, Psychological Strategies

THE INTERNATIONAL ASSOCIATION for the Study of Pain defines pain as "an unpleasant sensory and emotional experience associated with actual or potential tissue damage or described in terms of such damage." This definition recognizes that pain is an emotional as well as a sensory phenomenon. Pain is the most common reason to see a physician, and epidemiological studies have independently documented that chronic noncancer pain is seen as an international problem of immense proportion.

Chronic pain influences every aspect of a person's functioning. Profound changes in quality of life are associated with intractable chronic pain. Significant interference with sleep, employment, social function, and daily activities is common. Chronic pain patients frequently report depression, anxiety, irritability, sexual dysfunction, and decreased energy. Family roles are altered, and worries about financial limitations and future consequences of a restricted lifestyle abound. Patients with chronic back pain generally present with a history of multiple medical studies yielding minimal physical findings.

CATEGORIES OF PAIN

Pain syndromes may be categorized according to the character and history of the symptom. There are four general categories of pain. Acute pain is typically self-limiting and resolved within 6 months (e.g., childbirth pain, postoperative pain, and pain after injury). Chronic episodic pain involves intermittent episodes that recur for more than 6 months (e.g., migraine headache, temporomandibular joint disorder, and sickle cell disease). Chronic noncancer pain involves pain persisting for more than 6 months (e.g., low back pain and fibromyalgia). Chronic progressive pain increases in severity and tends to be associated with malignancies or degenerative processes (e.g., cancer pain and rheumatoid arthritis).

GATE CONTROL THEORY

Ronald Melzack and Patrick Wall put forward a theory of pain in 1965 based on the understanding of neurophysiological pathways and pain mechanisms. They suggested that impulses from large myelinated nerve fibers had a way of closing down the transmission of impulses from small unmyelinated nerves (which transmit signals associated with pain). They also suggested that descending impulses from the brain could have the same effect of closing down nerve transmission from the periphery. They put forward the notion that pain perception can be affected not just by sensation but also by evaluative and affective systems. They proposed that pain messages are modified in the central nervous system so that the subjective pain experience is a result not only of physical sensation but also of emotional and mental (cognitive) factors. Thus, the gate control model of pain integrates the modulation of peripheral stimuli by cortical variables. Psychological and social factors are not just perceived as reactions to pain; they are an integral part of determining the perception and experience of pain.

Chronic pain represents a complex interaction of factors. The pain is often related to an initial somatic event but, over time, is increasingly influenced by the patient's personality, beliefs, and environment. Attempts to reliably distinguish between organic and psychogenic pain have been largely unsuccessful. Many practitioners incorrectly believe that chronic pain reflects either organic pathology or psychogenic symptoms. If physical findings are inadequate to account for a patient's report of chronic pain, then the pain is often perceived to be largely psychological. It is generally unwarranted, however, to assume that psychological factors are the primary cause of pain.

There are a number of commonly held but inaccurate assumptions regarding pain. These include the beliefs that pain is only a physical sensation, that chronic and acute pain are the same and require the same treatment, and that pain is proportional to injury severity. We now recognize that pain is a complex phenomenon that is neither solely organic nor purely psychological (imaginary).

PSYCHOLOGICAL ASSESSMENT OF CHRONIC PAIN

Important components of chronic pain that must be evaluated as part of a psychological assessment include pain intensity, emotional distress and coping, and activity interference. In addition, a behavioral analysis should be conducted, and information on psychosocial history, adverse effects of treatment, and health care utilization should be obtained.

Pain Intensity

Pain intensity can be measured by subjective numerical pain ratings, a visual analog scale (VAS), verbal rating scales, pain drawings, and combined standardized questionnaires. Despite its frequent use in measuring chronic pain, the VAS has the disadvantage of being time-consuming to score as well as having questionable validity for older patients.

Verbal scales not only measure pain intensity but also assess sensory and affective dimensions of the pain experience. These scales may consist of as few as 4 or as many as 15 words ranked in order of severity ranging from "no pain" to "excruciating pain." Verbal scales can also be used to measure pain description. The patient chooses from a list of words that best describe the pain experience (e.g., piercing, stabbing, shooting, burning, or throbbing).

Emotional Distress and Coping

Most chronic pain patients do not have a history of premorbid psychiatric disturbance but show reactive emotional distress in response to their pain. However, when present, major psychopathology is indicative of a poor prognosis for pain therapy. There is ongoing debate among mental health professionals about the best ways to measure psychopathology in chronic pain patients. Pain patients frequently endorse somatic complaints in response to their condition. Thus, there is always a need for caution in interpreting psychological tests in which somatic complaints are considered indicative of psychopathology in pain patients. The measures most commonly used to evaluate psychopathology and emotional distress in chronic pain patients include the Minnesota Multiphasic Personality Inventory-2, the Symptom Checklist 90-Revised, the Millon Behavior Health Inventory, the Illness Behavior Questionnaire, and the Beck Depression Inventory.

A person's beliefs about pain are important in predicting the outcome of treatment. Negative thoughts about an ongoing pain problem may contribute to increased pain and emotional distress, decreased functioning, and greater reliance on medication. Certain chronic pain patients are prone to maladaptive beliefs about their condition that may not be compatible with its physical nature (e.g., "This pain will make me lose my mind" and "Soon I will become an invalid"). The most popular tests used to measure maladaptive beliefs include the Coping Strategies Questionnaire, the Pain Management Inventory, the Pain Self-Efficacy Questionnaire, the Survey of Pain Attitudes, and the Inventory of Negative Thoughts in Response to Pain.

Activity Interference

The assessment of functional capacity and interference with activity is important since third-party payers frequently judge treatment outcome on the basis of improved function and a return to work. Reliable instruments used to measure function include the Sickness Impact Profile, the Short-Form Health Survey-36, the Multidimensional Pain Inventory, the Pain Disability Index, and the Oswestry Disability Questionnaire. Other functional measures include the Chronic Illness Problem Inventory, the Waddell Disability Instrument, and the Functional Rating Scale. Automated measurement devices, such as the portable up-time calculator and the pedometer, are useful to obtain accurate measures of activity. These devices should be used in conjunction with self-monitoring assessment techniques.

Clinical Interview

Although self-report psychometric tests offer reliable and valid ways to assess the pain experience, the most popular means of determining whether a patient is an appropriate candidate for therapy or participation in a pain management program is an initial interview. Before meeting with the patient, it is helpful to review all patient referral information, including discharge summaries, psychological testing results, past physician notes, and medical history reports. The following should be covered during the interview: relevant medical history, education and employment history, history of drug or alcohol abuse, history of psychiatric disturbance, and current perceived support. Preliminary demographic and medical history information can be obtained through the completion of a comprehensive questionnaire and clarified during the interview. Structured interview measures are available for the assessment of alcoholism and substance abuse (e.g., CAGE questionnaire, Michigan Alcoholism Screening Test, and the Self-Administered Alcoholism Screening Test) and for psychiatric diagnosis (Structured Clinical Interview for DSM [*Diagnostic and Statistical Manual of Mental Disorders*]), although validity in patients with chronic pain has not been extensively studied. Perceived support is an important variable in predicting positive treatment outcome, and whenever possible, the patient's family members and/or significant other should also be interviewed.

PSYCHOLOGICAL INTERVENTIONS FOR PAIN

Goals of Psychological Interventions

Patients with chronic pain who consult their primary care physicians, pain specialists, pain services, or pain management programs are usually experiencing a significant degree of psychological distress that requires intervention. The therapeutic aims of interdisciplinary interventions for chronic noncancer pain include decreased pain intensity, increased physical activity, decreased reliance on pain medication, a return to work, improved psychosocial functioning, and reduced use of health care services. Psychological interventions for chronic pain shift from a disease cure focus to an illness/symptom management focus. Emphasis is placed on active patient involvement, with realistic expectations for improvement and recovery. Most patients seek psychological treatments for their pain with the hope that they will diminish the pain. However, they should be told not to set total pain elimination as their primary goal. Instead, they should focus on other, more attainable goals, such as a gradual increase in function without causing a flare-up of their pain. Patients are often encouraged to participate regularly in exercise (including stretching, cardiovascular reconditioning, and weight training) and to increase their activity at a progressive rate under supervision. The goal is to gradually increase function without exceeding predetermined limits of pain and discomfort.

Multidisciplinary Approach

Chronic pain involves a complex interaction of physiological and psychosocial factors, and successful intervention requires the coordinated effort of a treatment team with expertise in a variety of therapeutic disciplines. Although some pain centers offer a single-treatment approach, most programs use a blend of medical, psychological, vocational, and educational techniques. Most interdisciplinary pain treatment programs have as their core staff one or more physicians, a clinical psychologist, and a physical therapist. Other health professionals who may play important roles include clinical nurse specialists, occupational therapists, vocational rehabilitation counselors, and alternative medicine specialists such as acupuncturists.

Multidisciplinary pain programs administered on an outpatient basis are often highly structured, time limited, and organized along a specific treatment schedule. The patient is expected to attend clinic sessions and to participate actively in all aspects of the program. These expectations must be made clear. To this end, patients frequently sign a treatment contract that details the general program requirements as well as their individual treatment goals. In addition to helping patients to understand exactly what is expected of them, such a contract provides a mechanism for identifying those patients who, prior to treatment, lack motivation or may have difficulty conforming to the structure of the program. Patients are asked to keep a daily written record of their pain intensity, medication use, and activity levels. The treatment of chronic pain, using a rehabilitation approach, must encompass a full range of psychological and social/behavioral interventions in order to adequately address those factors that are known to exacerbate and maintain pain, distress, and related disability. These interventions include education, progressive exercise, cognitive therapy, relaxation training, vocational counseling, group and family therapy, and relapse prevention.

Education

Most people with chronic pain have an inadequate understanding of the nature of their painful condition. It is important for them to be knowledgeable about their pain and the treatments designed for them. Many individuals fear that their pain is a signal that a more serious life-threatening condition, which may be as yet undiscovered, accounts for their pain. They need to understand that pain due to inflammation, adhesions, scarring, and muscle tension can sometimes be the problem and not necessarily a sign of an underlying disease. Chronic noncancer pain is better managed when the individual understands that there will be fluctuations in intensity, that medical interventions are palliative, and that what they do about the pain can be as beneficial as what is being done to them. Education can take the form of lectures, books, pamphlets, tapes, videos, and individual instruction.

Progressive Exercise

Most patients lose physical stamina and flexibility because of reluctance to exercise and a perceived need to protect themselves from additional physical injury. Some patients have been medically advised to restrict activity when pain increases. Patients with chronic pain need to know that exercise is important. Getting back to usual activities as soon as possible after an injury helps to prevent disability. Some stretching, cardiovascular activity, and weight training should be encouraged. Behavioral research suggests that compliance with exercise is best in a structured setting in which each person is monitored and given encouragement for their accomplishments. Graduated exercise with activity pacing is important. Unfortunately, some people with chronic pain discontinue a regular exercise regimen within 6 months

after a treatment program is concluded. For this reason, periodic follow-up is also important.

Cognitive Therapy

There are a number of objectives of cognitive therapy. The first is to help patients change their view of their problem from overwhelming to manageable. Patients who are prone to "catastrophize" benefit from examining the way they view their situation. What could be perceived as a hopeless condition can be reframed as a difficult but manageable condition over which they can exercise some control. A second objective is to help convince patients that the treatment is relevant to their problem and that they need to be actively involved in their treatment and rehabilitation. A third objective is to teach patients to monitor maladaptive thoughts and substitute positive thoughts. Persons with chronic pain are plagued, either consciously or unconsciously, by negative thoughts related to their condition. These negative thoughts have a way of perpetuating pain behaviors and feelings of hopelessness. Demonstrating how and when to attack these negative thoughts and when to substitute positive thoughts and adaptive management techniques for chronic pain is an important component of cognitive therapy. Most chronic pain patients need support in maintaining their gains. Important aspects of cognitive–behavioral therapy include giving specific homework assignments, offering appropriate examples to patients, helping to organize a daily routine and schedule, recruiting support from family members, encouraging outside activities and involvement, linking patients to appropriate resources, monitoring progress, and actively following patients after treatment.

Relaxation Training

Chronic pain patients tend to experience substantial residual muscle tension as a function of the bracing, posturing, and emotional arousal often associated with pain. Such responses, maintained over a long period, can exacerbate pain in injured areas of the body and increase muscular discomfort. For example, it is common for patients with low back pain or limb injuries to develop neck stiffness and tension-type headaches. Relaxation training can lead to pain reduction through the relaxation of tense muscle groups, the reduction of symptoms of anxiety, the use of distraction, and the enhancement of self-efficacy. In addition, this training can increase the patient's sense of control over physiological responses. In a pain management program, patients are taught and encouraged to practice a variety of relaxation strategies, including diaphragmatic breathing, progressive muscle relaxation, autogenic relaxation, guided imagery, and cue-controlled relaxation techniques. Hypnosis and biofeedback training are also commonly employed.

Vocational Counseling

The most relevant predictor of return to work is the duration of unemployment. After 6 months of unemployment due to chronic pain, the probability of return to work is 50%; the likelihood decreases to 10% after 1 year. Other factors negatively impacting the likelihood of returning to work include limited formal education, limited transferable skills, poor perceived social support, ongoing litigation, a poor relationship with the employer, and job dissatisfaction. The goal of vocational rehabilitation is a return to work. After an extended period out of work, patients become both physically and psychologically deconditioned to the demands and stresses of the workplace. Together, a vocational rehabilitation counselor and the patient can develop a plan that incorporates both long-range employment goals and short-term objectives based on medical, psychological, social, and vocational information. Vocational rehabilitation counselors are specialists in the assessment of aptitudes and interests, transferable skills, physical capacity, modifications in the workplace, skills training, and job readiness.

Many chronic pain patients receive workers' compensation benefits or social security disability income. Patients may fear that their benefits will be jeopardized if they return to work. A vocational rehabilitation counselor can help a patient negotiate with an employer a return-to-work trial that will not jeopardize the patient's income. Through counseling strategies and assessment tools, a patient's suitability for returning to work or retraining can be determined. Patients should be familiar with the Americans with Disabilities Act so that they know their rights regarding discrimination due to a pain-related disability.

Group Therapy

Group therapy presents an opportunity to discuss concerns or problems that patients have in common. The specific problem-solving strategies used may be the same as those in individual supportive therapy and cognitive–behavioral therapy. A group-based pain management program offers some distinct advantages over individual treatment. First, most pain patients have similar needs. Thus, information can be presented more efficiently to a group than to individuals. Second, group processes can help change behavior. Patients seem to benefit from interacting with other people with chronic pain. Group members can encourage each other to practice relaxation, exercise regularly, and maintain a positive attitude. Third, a structured time-limited program offers definite goals, rules, and end points. Patients know what they can realistically expect and are given clear feedback regarding their participation in the program's activities.

Family Therapy

Chronic pain significantly impacts all members of a family. Family members need to be educated about the goals of therapy and should have an opportunity to share their concerns. Moreover, active involvement of family members helps ensure the patient's long-term success. Therefore, both patients and members of their families should be invited to discuss their concerns and expectations and to express their feelings. In addition to enhanced communication, family members need to learn how to help the person in pain achieve and maintain goals and come to understand that they are not alone in dealing with that person.

Relapse Prevention

Most chronic pain patients need support after completing a pain treatment program in order to maintain the gains they have achieved. Patients should be encouraged to identify and anticipate situations that place them at risk for returning to previous maladaptive behavior patterns. They should also be encouraged to rehearse problem-solving techniques and behavioral responses that will enable them to avoid a relapse. The goals of relapse prevention are to help the patient maintain a steady level of activity, emotional stability, and appropriate medication use; anticipate and deal with situations that cause setbacks; and acquire skills that will decrease reliance on the health care system. Many techniques can be discussed for preventing a relapse, including setting specific short- and long-range goals; identifying situations that place the patient at risk for a flare-up; creating a relapse-prevention plan; reviewing pain management strategies; encouraging participation in booster sessions and follow-up support groups; including family members in treatment and follow-up; combining medical, psychological, and vocational therapies in a multidisciplinary setting; and offering professional support when needed. Relapse of a chronic pain condition is a multifactorial problem that can be only partially controlled. It is important to note that pain management requires changes in lifestyle. Patients tend to revert to negative pain behaviors and must plan ways to prevent themselves from doing so.

Effectiveness of Interdisciplinary Interventions

Psychological interventions received as part of a comprehensive multidisciplinary pain management program have been shown to be effective, with high ratings of helpfulness at a relatively low cost. Patients who complete a multidisciplinary pain program return to work or undergo vocational rehabilitation more often than do patients who do not enter a pain program. Multidisciplinary pain programs also produce marked subjective and functional improvements in chronic pain patients: Pain ratings decrease from admission to discharge, reliance on medication decreases, and physical functioning increases. These positive treatment outcomes are often maintained for years after discharge.

—*Robert N. Jamison*

See also–Pain, Assessment of; Pain, Invasive Procedures for; Pain Management, Multidisciplinary; Somatoform Disorders

Further Reading

Chapman, S. L., Jamison, R. N., Sanders, S. H., *et al.* (2000). Perceived treatment helpfulness and cost in chronic pain rehabilitation. *Clin. J. Pain* **16**, 169–177.
Fordyce, W. E. (Ed.) (1995). *Back Pain in the Workplace: Management of Disability in Nonspecific Conditions*. International Association for the Study of Pain, Seattle, WA.
Garofalo, J. P., and Polatin, P. (1999). Low back pain: An epidemic in industrialized countries. In *Psychosocial Factors in Pain: Clinical Perspectives* (R. J. Gatchel and D. C. Turk, Eds.). Guilford, New York.
Gatchel, R. J., and Turk, D. C. (Eds.) (1996). *Psychological Approaches to Pain Management: A Practitioner's Handbook*. Guilford, New York.
Jamison, R. N. (1996). *Mastering Chronic Pain: A Professional's Guide to Behavioral Treatment*. Professional Resource Press, Sarasota, FL.
Jamison, R. N. (1996). *Learning to Master Your Chronic Pain*. Professional Resource Press, Sarasota, FL.
Karoly, P., and Jensen, M. P. (1987). *Multimethod Assessment of Chronic Pain*. Pergamon, New York.
Nigl, A. J. (1984). *Biofeedback and Behavioral Strategies in Pain Treatment*. Spectrum, New York.
Philips, H. C., and Rachman, S. (1996). *The Psychological Management of Chronic Pain: A Treatment Manual*, 2nd ed. Springer, New York.
Turk, D. C., and Melzack, R. (Eds.) (1992). *Handbook of Pain Assessment*. Guilford, New York.

Pain, Overview

Encyclopedia of the Neurological Sciences
Copyright 2003, Elsevier Science (USA). All rights reserved.

PAIN may be defined as a set of behavioral manifestations resulting from activation in specific neural pathways or networks. The pathways may be subcategorized into known functional systems, such as sensory, autonomic, affective, or cognitive. The definition of pain by Donald Price is a useful one. It includes acute and chronic pain and reflects the basic behavioral components to pain or injury (i.e., a sensory experience that is an actual tissue damage or perceived body threat and an emotional reaction that is defined as aversive or unpleasant). However, it does not address objective measures of pain, reflecting a current lack of understanding of the complexity of neural networks.

Unfortunately, there is no known "cure" for many pain syndromes, particularly chronic pain conditions such as neuropathic pain, which often results in significant frustration among patients and their health providers. Indeed, many patients will seek out any alternative to get rid of their pain, which results in numerous unnecessary procedures and treatments. Without objective measures of pain—whether radiological, genetic, chemical, or immunological—clinical advances in providing directed therapies that provide complete relief will remain difficult if not elusive. For the most part, current therapies, including pharmacological, behavioral, or interventional therapies, are either unsubstantiated by appropriate clinical trials or are ineffective.

Pain remains a major clinical problem. Recent data from Australia indicate that the prevalence of chronic pain in the population is approximately 30%. Chronic pain following certain types of surgery is estimated to affect 20–50% of subjects. These data are driving new developments. The National Institutes of Health has initiated programs to define epidemiological, molecular, and other changes, recruiting increasingly more clinicians and scientists into the field. The World Health Organization has produced some fundamental changes in many countries by implementing basic approaches to the problem. Physicians and patients are becoming more educated about the problem. Thus, for example, our understanding of the frequency and cause of neuropathic pain following dental work is now better than it was in the past. New methods for classifying pain by basic neurobiological mechanisms will be helpful in clinical trials but are too cumbersome for busy outpatient clinics.

Pain patients continue to provide valuable information. Indeed, some fundamental understandings of pain systems are owed to patients who have suffered from spinal cord injuries from gunshot wounds. Howard Fields noted that patients with chronic neuropathic pain complain more of unpleasantness than pain. Central neural circuits clearly must account for this and provide insight into perhaps novel approaches to treating "unpleasantness" and suffering. Patients who have undergone cingulotomy (interruption of certain pathways within the brain) for chronic pain almost without exception state that "the pain is the same ... but I don't care."

THE NEW NEUROBIOLOGY

During the past few years, there has been a convergence of discoveries in both the neuroscience and clinical domains of pain. A number of significant advances have contributed to a proliferation of articles in the pain literature.

Research in five areas is providing significant incubation for this process: molecular and cellular biology, developmental biology, genetics, epidemiology, and neuroimaging. All these areas will dramatically influence how patients are evaluated and treated.

Molecular Biology

The promise of major advances in molecular biology and genomics has still to be evaluated in terms of producing targeted analgesics. A number of interesting drugs are under development, making their way through preclinical and clinical trials. However, molecular biology has produced major insights into the fundamental mechanisms of pain. The discoveries have been mainly related to changes in the dorsal ganglion neurons and in the dorsal horn of the spinal cord, which are critical areas for processing of pain signals. Candidate target genes include novel receptors, neurotransmitters, trophic factors (i.e., molecules that encourage nerve growth), channels, transcription factors, and immunological agents.

The capsaicin gene (vanilloid receptor, VR-1) has provided a mechanism for specific activation of nociceptors by heat and alterations in tissue pH. Specific drugs that act at the VR-1 receptor, such as resiniferatoxin, are currently in phase II trials and may have additional clinical applications when targeted directly at the spinal cord or dorsal root ganglion.

Defined neurotransmitter systems (e.g., endogenous opioid systems) appear to be very involved in pain processing. Specific receptor activation is associated with changes in neural function that may reduce subsequent response to a drug. The classic example is tolerance to opioids. Understanding of signal transduction from receptor to second messengers and subsequent neuronal changes in gene expression or structural changes has literally been revolutionized in the past decade. It has allowed for new approaches to develop opioid-related therapies that limit the development of tolerance, dependence, or addiction.

A renewed interest in trophic factors has occurred since the failed trials of nerve growth factor. Trophic factors are of fundamental interest because of their purported role following nerve damage. For example, brain-derived neurotrophic factor may function as a neurotransmitter/neuromodulator in the dorsal horn of the spinal cord. The factor is released from the central terminations in the dorsal horn of small-diameter afferents. The release produces increased excitability of dorsal horn cells, contributing to a process called central sensitization, wherein the central nervous system undergoes long-term changes that facilitate the pain state.

Following a serendipitous finding that the sodium channel blocker tocainamide produced amelioration of neuropathic symptoms in a patient treated with the drug for a cardiac arrhythmia and who also had neuropathic pain, recent work has defined a number of sodium channels, some of which are unique to small afferent fibers. The development of a drug that does not have the central nervous system (CNS) and cardiac effects of current agents such as mexiletine may result in higher-dose therapeutics without the risk of serious cardiac or CNS side effects. Behavioral analysis of knockout mice has demonstrated a striking role for specific voltage-gated sodium channels in noxious stimulation. Interestingly, these advances have also allowed for the evaluation of the mechanism of action of commonly used antidepressants for pain including amitriptyline, which has at least in part a sodium channel-blocking mechanism.

Developmental Biology

In the past decade, there has been a greater understanding that newborns feel pain when undergoing invasive procedures. The newborn nervous system is still immature and pain can produce long-term sequelae. The reason for this is that the immature nervous system is considered to have lower excitation thresholds resulting in increased levels of central changes, which may continue into adulthood as permanent alterations in structure and function.

Genetics

Exciting work, particularly from Jeffrey Mogil's group, has begun to define genetic contributions of different behavioral responses in rodents. Work in rodent models of acute and chronic pain response to analgesics has begun to define allelic variants that may underlie these differences. The process is a powerful one and should revolutionize our ideas about the etiology, susceptibility, progression, and specific analgesic response to a drug. Although most of this work has been performed using animals, in recent years these same tools have been applied to human trials in an attempt to link specific responses to a genetic background. In many ways, this is similar to some biopharma approaches that provide specific therapy to a particular patient based on the patient's genetic profile using pharmacogenetic screening (i.e., interindividual differences).

Epidemiology

Perhaps the most important advancement is the recent interest in supporting proper epidemiological studies. By defining the problem, the actions that will help more people quickly can also be defined. Recent data from Australia indicate that approximately 20% of the population suffers from chronic pain. Approximately 6% of patients undergoing molar tooth extraction develop neuropathic pain. A number of patients have pain following neural lysis. The true incidence of chronic postsurgical pain is not defined.

Neuroimaging

Pain is a sensory and emotional experience produced by noxious stimuli or by damage to the nervous system. Although there is no clinical test for pain, researchers have defined specific pathways and CNS structures involved in pain processing. Current understanding is derived from clinical descriptions and research in animals. Studies of pain have utilized electrophysiological techniques, ablation or electrical stimulation of CNS structures, and molecular markers of neuronal activity. These approaches have allowed researchers to map groups of cells within the nervous system in animal models of acute and chronic pain. Until recently, the most informative research methods were not applicable to experiments in humans. Noninvasive techniques that measure neuronal activity in humans, including magnetoencephalography and functional magnetic resonance imaging, are now being used to discern CNS pathways involved in pain. These approaches are being applied to acute or chronic pain states in humans and animals.

Pain neuroimaging research has significant translational abilities to pain cliniconeurobiology because the "pain signal" can be investigated in the brains of humans in acute and chronic pain conditions and the utility of human surrogate models of clinical pain can be evaluated. These advances will completely revolutionize the understanding of pain, including objective diagnosis and the mechanism of action of analgesics, and even provide prognostic data in patients with nerve damage. For example, work in neuroimaging on phantom limb pain has shown that the cortical plasticity observed to correlate with pain can be normalized using prosthetic stimulators of the stumps of amputated forelimbs. Such normalization is associated with a decrease in pain. In addition, earlier neuroimaging studies indicate a thalamic signal for neuropathic pain. This is an exciting area of study still in its infancy.

CURRENT PROBLEMS

Old technologies and old mind-sets are currently being used in therapeutic approaches. Indeed, age-old ideas about pain etiology continue to persist. For example, the idea that trigeminal neuralgia is produced or initiated by arterial pulsations or pressure was developed in the 11th century by the Arab physician Jurjani. Even today, there are no data to prove that this is true. Few treatments are effective for chronic pain patients. Physicians are still dependent on essentially five categories of drugs: opioids, NSAIDS, antiepileptics, antidepressants, and local anesthetics. Slightly different approaches for injecting a stable of drugs into different locations are used for pain relief, without much data supporting such an approach. The clinical approach is by and large a systematic trial-and-error use of drugs and interventional and behavioral treatments.

The notion of multidisciplinary approaches to pain therapy may be a respectable way of admitting that there is no specific effective treatment for most pain patients. This lack of knowledge is a problem that is being addressed by basic science in a more rapid manner than are clinical approaches and perhaps reflects difficulties in undertaking studies in patients with chronic pain.

Evidence-based approaches to understanding the efficacy of specific therapies have begun to define a basis for evaluating treatment outcomes. Such programs have been spearheaded by groups such as Henry McQuay's in Oxford. This group has advanced processes for evaluating pain studies, including trials that have fixed and clearly defined inclusion criteria (e.g., moderate or severe allodynia) and fixed and clearly defined outcomes or outcome measures (e.g., at least 50% pain relief).

THE FUTURE

In the future, it may be possible to diagnose and treat patients with pain in a similar manner as for bacterial pneumonia. An objective test will define the state of pain and a genetic profile will determine the most appropriate plan for therapy.

Translating Neuroscience Advances into Clinical Practice

Basic science has contributed a great deal to our understanding of pain. The translation into clinical success has not paralleled the new breakthroughs.

Genetically Determined Basis for Pain Therapy

The possibility of defining genetically based pharmacotherapies now seems possible. As noted previously, major advances in defining genetic bases for behavioral responses have been made. Pharmacogenetic screens would greatly modify treatment approaches. Of course, these advances would need to be paralleled by advances in pharmacotherapies; however, such screening may define classes of patients who may specifically respond to current analgesics. Already, differences between men and women with respect to responses to analgesics have been discovered.

Objective Definition of Pain

Objective definitions of pain, whether invasive or noninvasive, will be critical for providing specific diagnoses for neuroscience. Tissue banks have been started for skin, nerve, dorsal root ganglia, spinal cord, and even brain tissue. Objective decoding of neural circuitry using noninvasive imaging techniques holds the promise of defining the specific pain state and the response to therapy.

Different Time, Different Drug

Chronic pain is an evolving process. From basic and clinical science, there is good reason to believe that following nerve damage, for example, pain evolves over time and may ameliorate over time. Thus, animal models, including the spared nerve injury model, the spinal nerve ligation model, and the loose ligature model, indicate a progressive increase in tactile allodynia within 1 or 2 weeks. During this time course, different genes are expressed and regulated. Less is known about the chronic state. In humans, pain may persist for months to years (e.g., postherpetic neuralgia) and spontaneously regress. Our current understanding indicates that drugs that may inhibit alterations in connectivity may be useful in the perioperative period, whereas drugs that alter established central sensitization or spontaneous activity are useful during a later stage in the progression of manifestations resulting from nerve damage. In addition, some commonly used drugs (e.g., morphine) may produce neural death in spinal cord neurons.

Translating Clinical Observations into Neuroscience

The major advances in promoting pain clinics, training pain specialists, educating other physicians and surgeons about pain, and increasing the overall level of consciousness in the field provide opportunities for real advances. Clinical approaches can promote changes in many ways; for example, traditional approaches provide opportunities for clinical trials of novel analgesic agents. However, there are other opportunities, including those discussed in the following sections.

Serendipitous Clinical Observations

Unexpected clinical observations that provide unique insight into possible pain mechanisms should be further explored. There are many examples in the pain field, from surgical observations to serendipitous drug effects. The evaluation of findings such as pain crossing territories and pain in unexpected distributions has been slow. However, based on current understanding of neural processing, there is good evidence on how these processes occur.

Tissue Samples—Correlation with the Disease Process

The ethical collection of tissue for biomedical research has been a slow process in the pain field. However, tissues collected using approved methods allow for very important information to be evaluated in molecular and anatomical laboratories. Such data provide important and specific insights into the overlap, or lack thereof, of the animal and human condition in normal and disease states.

—*David Borsook*

See also–Pain, Basic Neurobiology of; Pain, Invasive Procedures for; Pain Management, Multidisciplinary

Further Reading

Anand, K. J., and Maze, M. (2001). Fetuses, fentanyl, and the stress response: Signals from the beginnings of pain? *Anesthesiology* 95, 823–825.

Blyth, F. M., March, L. M., Brnabic, A. J., *et al.* (2001). Chronic pain in australia: A prevalence study. *Pain* 89, 127–134.

Dannhardt, G., and Kiefer, W. (2001). Cyclooxygenase inhibitors—current status and future prospects. *Eur. J. Med. Chem.* 36, 109–126.

Ezzo, J., Berman, B., Hadhazy, V. A., *et al.* (2000). Is acupuncture effective for the treatment of chronic pain? A systematic review. *Pain* 86, 217–225.

Fields, H. L. (1999). Pain: An unpleasant topic. *Pain* 6, S61–S69.

Fields, H. L. (2000). Pain modulation: Expectation, opioid analgesia and virtual pain. *Prog. Brain Res.* 122, 245–253.

Hill, R. G. (2001). Molecular basis for the perception of pain. *Neuroscientist* 7, 282–292.

Price, D. D. (2000). Psychological and neural mechanisms of the affective dimension of pain. *Science* 288, 1769–1772.

Wilkinson, H. A., Davidson, K. M., and Davidson, R. I. (1999). Bilateral anterior cingulotomy for chronic noncancer pain. *Neurosurgery* 45, 1129–1134.

Woolf, C. J., and Max, M. B. (2001). Mechanism-based pain diagnosis: Issues for analgesic drug development. *Anesthesiology* 95, 241–249.

Pain, Pelvic

Encyclopedia of the Neurological Sciences
Copyright 2003, Elsevier Science (USA). All rights reserved.

CHRONIC PELVIC PAIN is a common and significant affliction of women during their reproductive years (mean age, approximately 30 years). In the United Kingdom, it is estimated to have an annual prevalence of 3.8% in women, which is higher than that of migraine (2.1%) and similar to that of asthma (3.7%) and back pain (4.1%). In a US study of women in primary care practices, 39% had pelvic pain at least some of the time and 12% had pain on more than 5 days per month or lasting 1 full day or longer each month. A Gallup poll in the United States found that 16% of women reported pelvic pain problems and that 11% limited home activity because of it, 16% took medications for it, and 4% missed at least 1 day of work per month because of it. Pelvic pain is estimated to account for 10% of all referrals to gynecologists and is the indication for 12% of all hysterectomies and more than 40% of gynecological diagnostic laparoscopies. Pelvic pain often leads to years of disability and suffering, with loss of employment, marital discord and divorce, and numerous untoward and unsuccessful medical misadventures. Clearly, pelvic pain is an important part of the practice of any clinician who provides health care for women.

Pelvic pain may be acute, recurrent, or chronic. If a woman has pain of more than 6 months' duration that is located primarily in the pelvis, she is diagnosed with chronic pelvic pain. Part of the rationale for this criterion is that after months of pelvic pain, pain can become an illness rather than a symptomatic manifestation of some other disease. The cyclic pain of dysmenorrhea and the episodic pain of dyspareunia are sometimes considered criteria for pelvic pain, but it is probably better to consider them separately because the diagnoses and treatments of dysmenorrhea and dyspareunia frequently differ from those of chronic pelvic pain. However, women with pelvic pain often have dysmenorrhea and dyspareunia as part of their symptom complex.

Chronic pelvic pain is a frustrating problem for most physicians, partially because the majority think of pain within the context of the classic Cartesian model. This model postulates that pain is the direct result of tissue trauma that activates specific neuroreceptors and neural pain fibers, and that the severity of pain is directly proportional to the severity of the traumatic insult. As a corollary, pain that is unassociated with identifiable tissue injury is regarded as spurious or psychogenic. Although this model is sometimes useful for acute pain, it is not applicable to chronic pain. Attempts to find enough organic pathology to explain chronic pain have routinely been frustrating, and somatic pathologies, such as endometriosis, adhesions, or leiomyomata, have at best an uncertain relationship to chronic pelvic pain when the scientific evidence is closely scrutinized. Considering chronic pain as solely a psychiatric disorder has also been frustrating and not supported by available scientific evidence. A biopsychosocial model is best used in caring for women with chronic pelvic pain.

Melzack and Wall's gate control theory is the model most frequently utilized in trying to understand chronic pain. In oversimplified terms, this theory states that afferent neural impulses from the periphery may be modulated by spinal and cortical signals (gates). The modulation may be either enhancement or diminution of the afferent impulse. The neurophysiological events that gate or modulate the pain impulse are influenced by numerous factors, both peripheral and central. The gates may be affected by the level of firing of the visceral afferent nerves; afferent input from cutaneous and deep somatic structures; endogenous opioid and nonopioid analgesic systems; and various central excitatory and inhibitory influences from the brainstem, hypothalamus, and cortex. This theory provides a neurological basis for the observation that various somatic and psychogenic factors may increase or decrease the perception of pain (such as anxiety, depression, physical activity, mental concentration, marital discord, etc.). Although neurophysiological and biochemical research has resulted in significant modifications of this theory since its original proposal, it still works as a good (but not the only) model for the clinical observations in chronic pain patients and provides a more productive approach to diagnosis and therapy than the classic Cartesian model.

There are some identifiable psychosocial characteristics of chronic pelvic pain patients. Psychological interviews suggest they are anxious and depressed and have low self-esteem and high dependency. Psychometric testing using, for example, the Minnesota Multiphasic Personality Inventory shows that chronic pelvic pain patients have a characteristic personality profile, with high scores on the hysteria, hypochondriasis, and depression scales. These personality profiles are noted in patients in whom organic pathology can be found and in those in whom no such pathology is noted. Such psychological changes tend to maintain or increase the level of pain, regardless of the degree of physical disease. Additionally, when pain treatment is successful, the high scores on hysteria, hypochondriasis, and depression revert to normal.

The clinical relevance of current pain theories is that diagnosis and treatment must integrate many influences: the patient's personality and affect,

cultural influences, stress, organic changes that may trigger nociceptive signals, sensory thresholds or gates, and the patient's cognition about pain. Clearly, for pelvic pain no clear distinction between psychological and physical causes of pain can be made, nor are attempts to make such a distinction useful. Rather than trying to establish organic versus functional etiologies, it is more useful to ask each patient if there is any physical disease or abnormality that requires medical or surgical treatment and if there is emotional or psychological distress that requires treatment.

DIAGNOSES AND ETIOLOGIES

Often, patients with chronic pelvic pain either lack a demonstrable organic injury that accounts for their pain or possess organic pathology that is of uncertain relationship to the pain. Therefore, in contrast to the usual search for one diagnosis or etiology to account for the pain, a more useful approach is to (i) evaluate the pain as a diagnosis, with the potential of several organic contributors, and (ii) assess the person with chronic pain as someone with a unique exposure history, taking into account the many factors that lead to the individual's biopsychosocial situation.

Women suffering chronic pelvic pain are a heterogeneous group, and the possible disorders that may cause or contribute to their pain are numerous and varied and include visceral and somatic diseases. Occasionally, one of these disorders is the only diagnosis and curative treatment is possible. More often, the pain is long-standing with numerous prior diagnoses and treatments, and a number of contributing factors may need evaluation and treatment. Therefore, a multidisciplinary approach is often ideal.

Women with chronic pelvic pain are no less likely than the rest of the population to develop acute and serious illnesses, such as appendicitis or cystitis. Thus, with acute exacerbation of pain it is important to review the symptoms and reevaluate the patient thoroughly to rule out the possibility of acute medical or surgical conditions and not just attribute the exacerbation to a flare-up of the woman's chronic pelvic pain.

GENERAL GUIDELINES WHEN OBTAINING THE PATIENT'S HISTORY

Quite often, the diagnostic approach to the woman with chronic pelvic pain is directed as much by the specialty of the evaluating physician as by the woman's clinical characteristics. Clearly, the diversity of potential etiological or contributing diagnoses demands a more general approach. Although the primary physician may not have the expertise to diagnose or manage all the possible diagnoses, he or she can do a thorough, explorative history that will direct further evaluation and requisite referrals.

The location of pain is a crucial part of the history. A useful technique at the initial interview and at intervals during care is to have the patient perform a "pain map" on a human anatomy diagram. Other pain locations are often revealed in this manner. For example, up to 60% of women with chronic pelvic pain also have headaches, and up to 90% have backaches. The location of chronic pain is sometimes, but not always, useful in differential diagnosis. Visceral pain is not as well localized as somatic pain, so patients with chronic pain and visceral pathology may have trouble localizing their pain. Lateral pelvic pain is commonly of adnexal or sigmoid colonic origin. Midline infraumbilical pain is often due to pathology of the uterus and cervix. Pain from the bladder or vagina may localize over the mons pubis, pubic bone, or groin. Lower sacral and midline pain may be from the uterosacral ligaments and posterior cul-de-sac. Complaints of pain both ventrally and dorsally often suggest intrapelvic visceral pathology, whereas dorsal low back pain only suggests an orthopedic or musculoskeletal somatic origin.

—*Fred M. Howard*

See also–Headache, Tension-Type; Pain Management, Psychological Strategies; Pain, Visceral

Further Reading

Howard, F. M. (1993). The role of laparoscopy in chronic pelvic pain: Promise and pitfalls. *Obstet. Gynecol. Surv.* 48, 357–387.
Jamieson, D. J., and Steege, J. F. (1996). The prevalence of dysmenorrhea, dyspareunia, pelvic pain, and irritable bowel syndrome in primary care practices. *Obstet. Gynecol.* 87, 55–58.
Mathias, S. D., Kuppermann, M., Liberman, R. F., *et al.* (1996). Chronic pelvic pain: Prevalence, health-related quality of life, and economic correlates. *Obstet. Gynecol.* 87, 321–327.
Reiter, R. C., Shakerin, L. R., Gambone, J. C., *et al.* (1991). Correlation between sexual abuse and somatization in women with somatic and nonsomatic chronic pelvic pain. *Am. J. Obstet. Gynecol.* 165, 104–109.
Zondervan, K. T., Yudkin, P. L., Vessey, M. P., *et al.* (1999). Prevalence and incidence in primary care of chronic pelvic pain in women: Evidence from a national general practice database. *Br. J. Obstet. Gynaecol.* 106, 1149–1155.

Pain, Postoperative

Encyclopedia of the Neurological Sciences
Copyright 2003, Elsevier Science (USA). All rights reserved.

PAIN is among the most common of patient complaints encountered by health professionals but remains poorly treated. Patients recovering from major surgery and trauma have historically experienced analgesic underadministration and inadequate pain relief. Undermedication has been related to a lack of physician and nursing education, misconceptions regarding opioid morbidity, and a reliance on demand dosing.

PATHOPHYSIOLOGICAL RESPONSES TO POORLY CONTROLLED PAIN

Pain may be defined as the conscious awareness of tissue injury. Pain perception (nociception) reflects activation of nociceptors following thermal, mechanical, or chemical tissue injury, afferent transmission to the spinal cord, and relay via dorsal horn to higher cortical centers. Along with ethical and humanitarian reasons for minimizing pain and suffering is the understanding that pain-related anxiety, sleeplessness, and release of stress hormones/catecholamines may have deleterious effects on postsurgical outcome. This is particularly true in elderly or critically ill populations. The following pathophysiological responses are associated with increased pain intensity and have adverse effects on key organ functions:

• *Peripheral sensitization:* Musculoskeletal injury is accompanied by release of bradykinin, serotonin, and prostaglandin. Prostaglandin stimulates the release of substance P, which in turn sensitizes additional nociceptors at sites adjacent to the injury. This process of recruitment and sensitization of peripheral nerve endings underlies hyperalgesia, an altered state of sensibility in which the intensity of pain sensation induced by noxious stimulation is greatly increased.

• *Neuroendocrine responses:* Nociceptive impulses alter the activity of the hypothalamus and adrenal cortex/medulla. These changes, termed the neuroendocrine or stress response to injury, are characterized by an increased secretion of catabolic hormones, such as cortisol, glucagon, and catecholamines, and lead to muscle wasting, impaired immunocompetence, and decreased resistance to infection.

• *Sympathoadrenal activation:* Surgical injury is associated with marked increases in plasma epinephrine and norepinephrine concentrations. Increased sympathetic tone has been associated with hypertension and hypercoagulability, which increase the risk of stroke and pulmonary embolus. These factors may also precipitate myocardial ischemia in patients with poorly compensated coronary artery disease.

• *Chronic pain:* Humoral and neurological alterations, including reflex motor and sympathetic tone in and around the site of injury, may increase postoperative discomfort and disability. Continued sensitization of nociceptors and alterations in spinal cord processing of noxious input (spinal sensitization) may worsen acute pain and may result in prolonged disability, impaired rehabilitation, and chronic pain.

VARIABLES INFLUENCING ACUTE PAIN MANAGEMENT

Although opioid analgesics are frequently administered on a milligram/kilogram basis, there is no evidence to link body weight and individual dose requirement. Age appears to be the most important variable in determining dose–response and the degree of pain relief attained following administration of opioid analgesics. The site, extent, and duration of surgery may dramatically influence both the intensity of postoperative pain and analgesic requirements. Patients with a history of chronic pain and opioid tolerance may also require increased amounts of drug to compensate for both baseline requirements and that needed to control pain following surgery.

Declines in cardiac, hepatic, and renal function are often associated with significant alterations in the volume of distribution, clearance, and excretion of most analgesic agents. Unless dose adjustments are made, agents that undergo hepatic clearance and biotransformation and renal excretion may have a significant prolongation of effect.

PAIN SERVICES AND THERAPEUTIC OPTIONS FOR POSTOPERATIVE ANALGESIA

Acute pain management services have been developed that include dedicated caregivers trained to formulate and provide safe and effective therapy. A pain service director or clinical nurse coordinator is responsible for the introduction and maintenance of specialized therapy and oversees development of standardized protocols and order sets and nursing education. Standardized protocols include the assessment and charting of pain scores as the fifth vital sign. Patients with high pain intensity scores (>5 on a 10-point visual analog scale) often require additional analgesics and follow-up assessment. Postoperative pain services are generally multidisciplinary and multidepartmental. Anesthesiologists, surgeons, nursing staff, and pharmacists play important roles in providing safe and efficient pain management.

PARENTERAL AND ORALLY ADMINISTERED ANALGESICS

Although dosing on demand or as needed by intramuscular and orally administered analgesic regimes remains the mainstay of acute pain management, many studies have documented inadequacies associated with such therapy. Deficiencies associated with dosing on demand or as needed include the findings that patients often wait too long to request pain relief, staff may not be able to immediately deliver medication, and therapeutic plasma concentrations may not be uniformly maintained. Traditional dosing on demand or as needed involves a sequence of events that inevitably delays analgesic administration, resulting in repetitive cycles of increasing pain (Fig. 1). Since the dose administered is relatively large and absorption is erratic and prolonged, the initial analgesic effect may be followed by excessive sedation and possibly respiratory depression.

Oral Analgesics

Oral administration of analgesics is a safe, simple, and cost-effective method of controlling acute pain that should be considered the therapy of choice for patients tolerating oral diet and experiencing moderate discomfort. Orally administered opioids, such as morphine and meperidine, are poorly absorbed and undergo significant enterohepatic metabolism. For this reason, onset is delayed, and duration is less predictable. Oxycodone has higher oral effectiveness because it is more reliably absorbed and less likely to undergo first-pass hepatic metabolism. Sustained-release opioid preparations including morphine and oxycodone require less frequent administration, avoid frequent peak and trough plasma levels, and provide greater analgesic uniformity. These preparations provide 8–12 hr of pain relief and are ideally suited for patients suffering

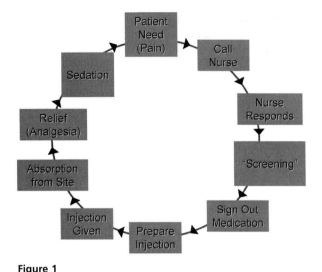

Figure 1
The traditional acute pain cycle as managed with intramuscular or intravenous doses of opioid analgesics as needed. Patient-controlled analgesia avoids pain dispensing by nurses as well as the uptake and distribution variables, thereby eliminating the cycle [reprinted with permission from Preble, L. M., Guveyan, J., and Sinatra, R. S. (1992). Patient characteristics influencing postoperative pain management. In *Acute Pain Mechanisms and Management* (R. S. Sinatra, A. H. Hord, B. Ginsberg, and L. M. Preble, Eds.), p. 144. Mosby-Year Book, St. Louis].

discomfort during rehabilitation. Less potent analgesics, including tramadol (a weak nonhabituating opioid) and a variety of nonsteroidal antiinflammatory drugs (NSAIDs), may be prescribed in patients with mild to moderate pain and as supplements for treated patients. Rofecoxib and celecoxib represent a new and potentially safer class of NSAID drugs termed the cyclooxygenase-2 (COX-2) inhibitors. Celcoxib and rofecoxib selectively block COX-2, thereby inhibiting prostaglandin synthesis following tissue injury; however, unlike other NSAIDs, they do not block COX-1, which maintains platelet function and gastric mucosal integrity. Both are contraindicated in patients with gastric bleeding and renal disease. Single doses of rofecoxib and celecoxib improved pain scores in patients recovering from spinal fusion; however, rofecoxib's effect on reducing pain intensity and intravenous (iv) morphine consumption was more prolonged. Neither coxib was associated with increases in perioperative blood loss.

Parenteral Therapy

Morphine effectively blocks pain following severe musculoskeletal injury and is commonly employed in patients recovering from orthopedic surgery.

Onset of analgesia occurs within 5 min after iv and 15 min following intramuscular administration, and the duration ranges from 2 to 4 hr depending on dose and site of administration. Administration of morphine may release histamine and has been associated with hypotension and biliary colic. Hydromorphone and fentanyl are useful alternatives. Bolus doses of fentanyl (50–200 µg) and iv infusions (50–200 µg/hr) are advocated for patients who remain intubated.

Ketorolac is a potent NSAID available as a parenteral formulation. Doses of 30–60 mg are equipotent to 10 mg of morphine. Ketorolac is not associated with sedation or respiratory depression; however, major side effects, including hemorrhage, gastric ulceration, and renal toxicity, may limit its usefulness. To minimize complications doses should be limited to 7.5–15 mg every 6 hr for a maximum of 48 hr.

INTRAVENOUS PATIENT-CONTROLLED ANALGESIA

Patient-controlled analgesia allows patients to titrate small doses of pain medication in amounts proportional to a perceived pain stimulus. The technique avoids cycles of excessive sedation and ineffective pain control observed with "by the clock" and "on demand" intramuscular dosing, and it limits variability related to inappropriate "screening" and drug absorption. Patients are allowed to control dose frequency (within prescribed limits) and compensate for individual differences in pain perception and alterations in pain intensity. Patients activate the pump by pressing a button and a preprogrammed amount of opioid (bolus dose) is then administered over 10–30 sec. A 6- to 12-min lockout interval prevents a second dose from being delivered.

The key to successful initiation of patient-controlled analgesia is the administration of an opioid "loading" dose (usually 5–15 mg of morphine or 0.5–3 mg of hydromorphone), which provides a baseline plasma concentration of analgesic. Morphine is the standard and most widely administered patient-controlled analgesia, although other opioids have been successfully employed (Table 1).

More sophisticated patient-controlled analgesia devices incorporate a continuous rate (basal) infusion plus patient-activated bolus doses on demand. This form of administration is generally offered to patients recovering from extremely painful

Table 1   DOSING GUIDELINES FOR IV PATIENT-CONTROLLED ANALGESIA

Opioid	Concentration	Loading dose	Incremental bolus dose	Lockout interval (min)	Basal infusion rate	Comments
Morphine	1 mg/ml	3–10 mg	0.5–1.5 mg	6–8	0.5–1.5 mg/hr	Major surgical pain
Meperidine (Demerol)	10 mg/ml	25–50 mg	5–15 mg	6–8	Not recommended	Useful for visceral pain; limit dose 600 mg/24 hr
Hydromorphone (Dilaudid)	0.2 mg/ml	0.5–1 mg	0.1–0.3 mg	6–8	0.1–0.3 mg/hr	Rapid onset; minimal side effects
Oxymorphone (Numorphan)	0.1 mg/ml	0.3–1 mg	0.1–0.2 mg	6–8	0.1–0.2 mg/hr	For severe pain
Fentanyl	20 µg/ml	30–100 µg	10–20 µg	5–6	10–20 µg/hr	Rapid onset; short duration of effect

procedures, individuals presenting with opioid tolerance, and cancer patients.

SPINAL OPIOID ANALGESIA

The administration of opioid analgesics into the spinal or epidural space (neuraxial analgesia) is an efficient and powerful method of controlling pain in a variety of clinical settings. Neuraxial opioids provide greater analgesic potency than similar doses administered parenterally, and they also provide high selectivity in that analgesic effects are maintained in the absence of motor or sympathetic blockade.

Single Boluses of Epidural or Intrathecal Opioids

Morphine was first to receive Food and Drug Administration (FDA) approval for epidural and intrathecal use and remains the most widely investigated and extensively used spinal opioid. A single intrathecal bolus (0.25–0.5 mg) or multiple boluses of epidural morphine (2.5–5 mg) are commonly utilized for control of pain following trauma and lower extremity orthopedic surgery. In general, analgesic onset is appreciated after 30–60 min, peak effect occurs at 90–120 min, and the duration ranges from 12 to 24 hr.

Continuous Epidural Analgesia

Continuous infusion of epidural opioids, or opioids plus dilute local anesthetics, allows more precise titration and extended duration of neuraxial analgesia. Continuous infusion techniques also provide therapeutic versatility since short-duration opioids such as fentanyl and dilute local anesthetic solutions may be administered.

Epidural infusions of morphine and hydromorphone offer effective and uniform analgesia; however, hydromorphone is associated with less sedation and pruritus. Lipophilic opioids are commonly administered as continuous epidural infusions since their rapid onset and short duration facilitate analgesic titration. Improved analgesic effectiveness may be achieved by combining epidural fentanyl with dilute solutions of bupivacaine.

Epidural infusion of local anesthetics such as ropivacaine or infusions of the α-adrenergic analgesic clonidine may be considered in patients who are exquisitely sensitive to opioid-related adverse events. However, these agents are associated with sensory/motor blockade, sympathetic blockade, and hypotension.

Patient-Controlled Epidural Analgesia

Patient-controlled epidural analgesia offers higher analgesic efficacy and lower dose requirements than iv patient-controlled analgesia while providing greater control and patient satisfaction than either single doses or continuous infusions of epidural opioids. The technique should be considered the therapy of choice for high-risk patients recovering from highly invasive procedures (e.g., thoracotomy, upper abdominal surgery, total knee replacement).

Hydromorphone and more lipophilic opioids such as fentanyl that offer greater titratability have become the agents of choice in this setting. Upon completion of surgery, infusions of epidural fentanyl (5 µg/ml) or hydromorphone (10–20 µg/ml) may be continuously administered and supplemented with extremely dilute concentrations of bupivacaine or ropivacaine. Local anesthetics are omitted from the epidural infusate in patients at risk for hypotension.

Patient-controlled epidural boluses of 2–5 ml every 6–10 min are also provided to minimize pain during movement and ambulation.

Adverse Events and Contraindications

Pruritus and nausea are the most common side effects associated with epidural or spinal opioids; however, respiratory depression is the most feared complication. Respiratory depression is most common in patients treated with morphine, elderly patients with COPD, and patients coadministered parenteral opioids.

Vigilant observation and documentation of inadequate respiratory effort, slow respiratory rate, or unusual somnolence represent the best form of monitoring. Prophylactic naloxone infusions (400 μg/liter) of 100–125 ml/hr have been advocated to reduce the risk of opioid-induced respiratory depression in elderly or debilitated patients while maintaining effective analgesia. Naloxone infusions are also advocated for reducing the severity of pruritus. Antiemetics, including droperidol, metaclopramide, and ondansetron, are administered to control symptoms of nausea and vomiting. Contraindications to spinal/epidural opioid analgesia include spinal fracture, infection at the insertion site, septicemia, coagulopathy, and administration of low-molecular-weight heparinoids for prophylaxis of deep venous thrombosis. The FDA issued an advisory about the potential risk of epidural hematoma in patients receiving regional (spinal or epidural) anesthesia and low-molecular-weight heparin.

NEURAL BLOCKADE FOR ACUTE PAIN MANAGEMENT

Peripheral neural blockade minimizes exposure to opioids and is ideally suited for patients sensitive to opioid-induced ileus and ventilatory depression. Infiltration techniques employ injections of local anesthetic at the site of surgery and offer 6–12 hr of postoperative analgesia. Injection into wound techniques require surgical infiltration of concentrated local anesthetic solutions into skin, subcutaneous tissues, and the joint capsule. Continuous infiltration techniques employ multihole 19-gauge catheters to continuously infuse either 0.125 or 0.25% bupivacaine under the skin and muscle layers of the incision and into injured bone.

Continuous brachial plexus blockade provides effective pain control for extended periods of time following shoulder and rotator cuff procedures. The technique utilizes dilute bupivacaine 0.125–0.25% infused via catheters placed within the neurovascular sheath. Brachial plexus block for shoulder surgery is best accomplished via the interscalene approach, whereas supraclavicular or axillary block is employed for forearm and hand procedures.

NEW IDEAS IN PAIN MANAGEMENT

Preemptive Analgesia

In the late 1980s, Wall proposed the concept of preemptive preoperative analgesia, suggesting that analgesic intervention is most effective when performed in advance of the pain stimulus rather than in reaction to it. Preincisonal administration of opioids and NSAIDs alone or in combination with local anesthetic blockade provides measurable reductions in postsurgical pain and acute disability. Preemptive administration may also provide longer term convalescent–rehabilitative benefits and minimize the severity of persistent pain syndromes.

Multimodal Analgesia

Complete abolition of postsurgical pain (pain prevention) is difficult to achieve with a single drug or analgesic technique. In order to avoid dose-dependent adverse effects and potential toxicity associated with reliance on one agent or technique, "balanced" or multimodal analgesic regimens have been advocated. The combination of NSAIDS that block pain at the peripheral receptor neural conduction blockade and spinal modulation of pain with small amounts of opioids and/or clonidine can significantly reduce pain scores, adverse effects, and parenteral opioid requirements.

PAIN CONTROL AND POSTSURGICAL OUTCOME

Patients who benefit most from spinal/epidural opioid analgesia include debilitated individuals and others recovering from surgical procedures associated with severe pain and high parenteral opioid dose requirements. Optimally administered epidural analgesia can suppress the release of catecholamines, maintain hemodynamic stability, reduce myocardial oxygen requirements, improve respiratory function, and facilitate physical therapy. Such therapy has also been shown to reduce mortality, hospital stay, and overall costs. Yeager and colleagues noted that debilitated patients treated with epidural morphine benefited from significant reductions in cardiac and respiratory failure and the incidence of major infections when compared with individuals administered iv opioids. Similar results were reported by Christopherson and coworkers in patients recovering from major vascular surgery.

CONCLUSION

Poorly controlled acute pain following surgery and trauma incites several pathophysiological responses that can increase morbidity. By appreciating the severity and character of the pain stimulus, optimal control may be provided at each phase of the recovery process. Analgesic regimens including opioid infusions, iv and epidural patient-controlled analgesia, and continuous regional blockade not only provide effective pain relief and high patient satisfaction but also lead to improved functionality, decreased recovery time, and shortened hospitalization.

—*Raymond S. Sinatra*

See also–**Analgesics, Non-Opioid and Other; Coma, Postoperative; Opioids and Their Receptors; Phantom Limb and Stump Pain**

Further Reading

Allen, H. W., Liu, S. S., Ware, P. D., et al. (1998). Peripheral nerve block improves analgesia after total knee replacement surgery. *Anesth. Analg.* 87, 93–97.

Bach, S., Noreng, M. F., and Tjellden, N. U. (1988). Phantom limb pain in amputees during the first 12 months following limb amputation after preoperative lumbar epidural blockade. *Pain* 33, 297–301.

Beattie, W. S., Buckley, D. N., and Forrest, J. B. (1993). Epidural morphine reduces the risk of postoperative myocardial ischemia in patients with cardiac risk factors. *Can. J. Anaesth.* 40, 523–541.

Bonica, J. J. (1990). Definitions and taxonomy of pain. In *Management of Pain* (J. J. Bonica, Ed.), pp. 18–27. Lea & Febiger, Philadelphia.

Breslow, M. J. (1990). Neuroendocrine responses to surgery. In *Perioperative Management* (M. J. Breslow, C. F. Miller, and M. C. Rogers, Eds.), pp. 331–344. Mosby-Year Book, St. Louis.

Chaplan, S. R., Duncan, S. R., Brodsky, J. B., et al. (1992). Morphine and hydromorphone epidural analgesia: A prospective, randomized comparison. *Anesthesiology* 77, 1090–1094.

Christopherson, R., Beattie, C., Meinert, C. L., et al. (1993). Perioperative morbidity in patients randomized to epidural or general anesthesia for lower extremity vascular surgery. *Anesthesiology* 79, 1–12.

Cousins, M. J. (1989). Acute pain and the injury response: Immediate and prolonged effects. *Reg. Anesth.* 16, 162–176.

Cousins, M. J., and Mather, L. E. (1984). Intrathecal and epidural administration of opioids. *Anesthesiology* 61, 276.

Ferrante, F. M., Orav, E. J., Rocco, A. G., et al. (1988). A statistical model for pain in patient controlled analgesia and conventional intramuscular opioid regimens. *Anesth. Analg.* 67, 457–461.

Ginsberg, B., Sinatra, R. S., Crews, J., et al. (1998). Conversion from IV patient controlled analgesia morphine to oral controlled-release oxycodone tablets for postoperative pain management. *Anesth. Analg.* 86, 271S.

Hord, A. H., and Kelly, P. M. (1992). University-based acute pain treatment service. In *Acute Pain: Mechanisms and Management* (R. S. Sinatra, A. H. Hord, B. Ginsberg, and L. M. Preble, Eds.), pp. 532–538. Mosby-Year Book, St. Louis.

Kehlet, H., and Dahl, J. B. (1993). The value of "multimodal" or "balanced analgesia" in postoperative pain treatment. *Anesth. Analg.* 77, 1048–1056.

Loper, K. A., Ready, L. B., Downey, M., et al. (1990). Epidural and intravenous fentanyl infusions are clinically equivalent after knee surgery. *Anesth. Analg.* 70, 72–75.

McQuay, H. J., Carrol, D., and Moore, R. A. (1988). Postoperative orthopaedic pain—The effect of opiate premedication and local anesthetic blocks. *Pain* 33, 291–295.

Parker, A. J., Sinatra, R. S., and Glass, P. S. A. (1992). Patient-controlled analgesia systems. In *Acute Pain: Mechanisms and Management* (R. S. Sinatra, A. H. Hord, B. Ginsberg, and L. M. Preble, Eds.), pp. 205–224. Mosby-Year Book, St. Louis.

Parker, R. K., and White, P. F. (1992). Epidural patient-controlled analgesia: An alternative to intravenous patient-controlled analgesia for pain relief after cesarean delivery. *Anesth. Analg.* 75, 245–251.

Preble, L., and Sinatra, R. S. (1992). Patient characteristics influencing postoperative pain management. In *Acute Pain Mechanisms and Management* (R. S. Sinatra, A. H. Hord, B. Ginsberg, and L. M. Preble, Eds.), pp. 140–150. Mosby-Year Book, St. Louis.

Reuben, S. S., and Connelly, N. R. (2000). Postoperative analgesic effects of Celecoxib or Rofecoxib after spinal fusion surgery. *Anesth. Analg.* 91, 1221–1225.

Rueben, S. S., Connelly, N. R., Lurie, S., et al. (1998). Dose response of ketorolac as an adjunct to patient-controlled analgesia morphine in patients after spinal fusion. *Anesth. Analg.* 87, 98–102.

Sinatra, R., Chung, K. S., Silverman, D. G., et al. (1989). An evaluation of morphine and oxymorphone administered via patient controlled analgesia or patient controlled analgesia plus basal infusion. *Anesthesiology* 71, 20–25.

Stevens, D. S., and Dunn, W. T. (1992). Acute pain management for the trauma patient. In *Acute Pain: Mechanisms and Management* (R. S. Sinatra, A. H. Hord, B. Ginsberg, and L. M. Preble, Eds.), pp. 412–421. Mosby-Year Book, St. Louis.

Wall, P. D. (1988). The prevention of postoperative pain [Editorial]. *Pain* 33, 289–290.

Woolf, C. J., and Chong, M. S. (1993). Preemptive analgesia-treating postoperative pain by preventing the establishment of central sensitization. *Anesth. Analg.* 77, 362–379.

Yeager, M. P., Glass, D. G., and Neff, R. K. (1987). Epidural anesthesia and analgesia in high-risk surgical patients. *Anesthesiology* 66, 729–736.

Pain, Referred

Encyclopedia of the Neurological Sciences
Copyright 2003, Elsevier Science (USA). All rights reserved.

THE CONCEPT OF PAIN REFERRAL has been well-known since the time of Henry Head; it indicates pain perceived in an area other than that in which the noxious stimulation takes place—that is, pain localized not at the site of origin but in an area that may be adjacent to or at a distance from such a site. Pain can be referred from both internal organs (referred pain from viscera) and deep somatic structures such as muscles and joints (referred pain from somatic structures) to areas of the body wall that are usually included in the same dermatome or myotome as the structure of origin of the painful input. Pain is normally never referred from the skin; in fact, cutaneous pain is characteristically very well localized and circumscribed at the site of injury.

Whether originating from a viscus or a deep somatic structure, referred pain is very often accompanied by a condition of secondary hyperalgesia (increased sensitivity to pain and decreased pain threshold) and by trophic changes involving to a various extent the three tissues of the body wall (skin, subcutaneous tissue, and muscle).

Referred pain is extremely frequent in the clinical setting, given the large number of potentially pain-producing conditions that can occur in viscera and deep somatic tissues. Despite its prominence, its correct diagnosis in the patient has posed numerous problems. This is partly due to the relatively scarce knowledge, with respect to other forms of pain, about the mechanisms of referred pain. In recent years, however, referred pain and referred sensory–trophic changes have been the subject of renewed research interest in both human and animal studies, and significant advancement has thus been made in the field.

In addition to clinical studies in patients affected with various pathologies of internal organs and deep somatic structures, human research has involved investigations in which experimental noxious stimuli have been applied to either a viscus or a deep somatic structure and in which the appearance, location, and extension of the referred area could be evaluated in relation to the modalities of application of the primary stimulus. Of notable importance is the characterization of the sensory and trophic changes of the tissues in the referred zone via quantitative techniques. Such techniques include pain threshold measurement to various stimuli (mechanical, thermal, electrical, or chemical) or measurement of tissue thickness with ultrasound. Animal studies using models of clinically relevant forms of referred pain/hyperalgesia have further contributed to a better understanding of the pathophysiology of referred phenomena, especially in experiments involving electrophysiological evaluations at the spinal cord level.

This entry provides a concise outline of recent advances in the field of referred pain by analyzing separately referred pain from viscera and referred pain from somatic structures.

REFERRED PAIN FROM VISCERA

Referred pain from viscera is the most paradigmatic form of the phenomenon because the process of "referral" is practically the rule in visceral nociception. In fact, visceral pain begins with a transitory phase of direct pain, which is a vague and poorly defined sensation, always located along the midline and accompanied by marked neurovegetative signs and emotional reactions (true visceral pain). Following this, diseases of viscera refer pain to areas of the body wall usually within the dermatomal or myotomal field of the specific organ (referred pain from viscera). In these areas of the body wall, a condition of secondary hyperalgesia most often arises that may involve all three somatic tissues—skin, subcutis, and muscle—but is primarily localized at the muscle level. Two types of referred pain from viscera are thus classically distinguished: referred pain without hyperalgesia and referred pain with hyperalgesia. The second, by far the more frequent, can be extinguished or diminished through infiltration with local anesthetic of the painful area, whereas this same procedure lacks any effect in the case of referred pain without hyperalgesia.

A typical example of the described processes is provided by myocardial infarction. In the early phases, true visceral pain is perceived in the lowest sternal or epigastric areas and sometimes also in the interscapular region. The symptom has only vague localization, an oppressive and constrictive quality, and is generally accompanied by pallor, sweating, nausea, and vomiting, with associated strong alarm reactions (such as a feeling of impending death). After 10 min to several hours, however, the pain reaches the structures of the body wall. It becomes sharper in quality, tends to be located in the thoracic region, either anteriorly or posteriorly, and very often extends to the upper limbs, usually the left one (referred pain). Hyperalgesia, mostly at the muscle level, often accompanies the symptom so that additional stimuli exerted on the area of referral increase the pain. Hyperalgesia mostly involves the pectoralis major and muscles of the interscapular region and forearm. In a low percentage of cases, pain is also referred to the skin, within dermatomes C8–T1 on the ulnar side of the arm and forearm, and hyperalgesia is found at the same level.

The phenomenon of hyperalgesia in the areas of referred pain from viscera has been extensively studied in recent years. These studies have permitted the establishment of a precise relationship between the presence of the primary pain-generating focus in the viscus and the occurrence and extent of the referred hyperalgesia. The conclusion is that referred hyperalgesia is an early phenomenon (i.e., it appears relatively soon after the first painful visceral episodes), it mainly involves the muscle tissues, and it tends to be accentuated by the repetition of the painful visceral attacks. Most important, hyperalgesia is long lasting; in fact, it persists for a long time after the spontaneous pain has ceased. Moreover, it can be detected even after the primary focus in the viscus has been eliminated. It has been shown that residual hyperalgesia is present at the muscle level in the lumbar region of patients who suffered from renal/ureteral colics in the past but had eliminated the stone through the urine, either spontaneously or after fragmentation obtained through lithotripsy.

Together with the hyperalgesia, a number of trophic changes have been documented in the areas of referred pain from viscera, ranging from alterations of skin reactivity to increased thickness and consistency of the subcutaneous tissue and reduced thickness of the muscle.

Several theories have been put forward to account for the phenomenon of referred pain from viscera. An initial, simple model for interpreting referred pain without hyperalgesia was based on the idea of viscerosomatic convergence occurring in primary afferent fibers, with the same nerves having branches that innervate both viscera and somatic structures. The number of such fibers, however, is so limited that it is extremely unlikely that they play a major role in the mechanisms of referred pain.

In contrast, convergence of both visceral and somatic afferent inputs in the central nervous system is widely documented. This convergence–projection theory thus provides a convincing explanation for the phenomenon of referred pain without hyperalgesia.

Interpreting referred pain with hyperalgesia is more complex, and the simple convergence–projection mechanism is inadequate to account for the sensory and trophic changes that occur in the area of referral. A convergence–facilitation theory has been put forward, according to which the visceral input would produce an "irritable focus" in the relevant spinal cord segment (sensitization of viscerosomatic convergent neurons, which would become hyperactive and hyperexcitable), causing facilitation of messages normally arising in somatic structures. This hypothesis has received experimental support. For example, signs of central sensitization have been documented in electrophysiological studies using animal models of referred muscle hyperalgesia from viscera, such as the model of artificial ureteral calculosis in rats. In this model, the oblique muscle ipsilateral to the ureter implanted with a stone becomes hypersensitive.

The persistence of hyperalgesia in the clinical setting beyond the presence of the original visceral focus has been interpreted by some as an indicator of how central neuronal changes (plastic changes), once established, may persist, becoming relatively independent of the primary triggering event. However, results of recent studies on ureter motility in rats with artificial ureteral calculosis (abnormal hypermotility persisting long after stone elimination) suggest that a number of "clinically inapparent" peripheral visceral changes are likely to outlive the presence of the primary focus and thus maintain the state of central hyperexcitability via persistence of the peripheral drive.

The intervention of further mechanisms in the genesis of referred pain with hyperalgesia from viscera should not be ruled out, especially because trophic changes are present in addition to the hyperalgesia in the referred zone. According to the reflex arc theory, the afferent barrage from the internal organ would activate several viscerocutaneous and visceromuscular reflexes in the peripheral area of referral, resulting in sensitization of nociceptors and trophic changes locally. The afferent branch of the reflex arc would thus be sensory afferent fibers from the viscera, whereas the efferent branch would differ for superficial and deep somatic tissues (sympathetic efferents for the former and somatic efferents for the latter). This hypothesis is being actively investigated in current animal models, such as that of experimental uterine inflammation in rats in which referred muscle hyperalgesia has been documented in conjunction with trophic tissue changes in the referred area.

REFERRED PAIN FROM SOMATIC STRUCTURES

There are several examples of referred pain from somatic structures (e.g., from muscles or from joints). Myofascial pain syndromes (MPSs) are typical of referred pain from muscles. MPSs are characterized by pain and dysfunction due to the presence, in muscles or their fascia, of the so-called trigger points (TrPs). A TrP is a site of hyperirritability included in a taut, palpable band of muscle fibers. When stimulated, it gives rise to pain not only locally but also at a distance. The area of referred pain is characteristic for each muscle and is the site not only of spontaneous pain but also of sensory changes. These consist of hyperalgesia, which is a function of the degree of hyperirritability of the TrP (i.e., the more irritable the TrP, the greater the degree and extension of hyperalgesia). The dependence of these changes on the presence of TrPs is indicated by their regression after the TrPs are extinguished through local infiltration.

A typical example of referred muscle pain from a joint regards the painful symptomatology in patients affected with osteoarthritis of the knee. The pain from this condition is deep, fairly well localized, and of varying intensity, sometimes making walking difficult. It spreads upward to the lower part of the thigh and downward as far as the middle of the calf. It begins when walking, increases as walking continues, and decreases at rest. The skin appears pale and hypothermic to touch in an area covering the anterior surface of the knee. The underlying subcutis is tender and thickened. The skeletal muscles connected to the joint are tender and tense. Pain thresholds of all three tissues of the body wall in the painful area are decreased (hyperalgesia). Both sensory and trophic changes are reversible when the intraarticular focus is extinguished, testifying to their referred nature.

From the aforementioned clinical examples (MPSs and osteoarthritis), it can be deduced that referred pain from deep somatic structures is almost exclusively of the type referred with hyperalgesia, although the extent of the hyperalgesic involvement of the tissues of the body wall can vary.

Similar to what has been described for visceral nociception, referred pain from deep somatic structures (whether from a muscle or a joint) has been attributed primarily to phenomena of central sensitization triggered by the primary algogenic focus. To account for the phenomenon of referral, however, central hyperexcitability should involve neurons receiving convergent input from the site of injury and the referred zone, whereas it is known that in dorsal horn neurons there is little convergence from deep tissues. Thus, referred pain from somatic structures is not easily explained on the basis of the convergence–facilitation theory in its original form. In this respect, Mense suggested an interesting theory to account for referred pain from one muscle to another, as is the case for MPSs. According to the author, convergent connections from deep tissues to dorsal horn neurons would not be present from the beginning but are opened by nociceptive input from skeletal muscle, and referral to myotomes outside the lesion is due to the spread of central sensitization to adjacent spinal segments. Regarding visceral nociception, central mechanisms alone are not adequate to account for all phenomena observed in the area of referred pain, especially the trophic changes. Thus, in line with the hypothesis put forward for internal organs, it has been suggested that the afferent barrage from the deep focus (whether in the muscle or the joint) triggers the activation of reflex arcs toward the periphery (area of referral) via both

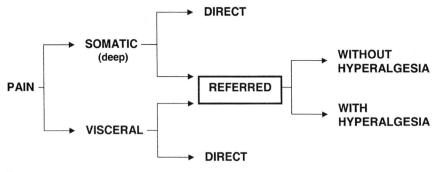

Figure 1
Classification of referred pain.

somatic (towards the muscle) and sympathetic (toward subcutis and skin) efferent fibers.

CONCLUSION

Referred pain is a notable component of the pain complaints of patients and a crucial diagnostic issue in the clinical setting. Knowledge about its existence, modalities of presentation, and possible mechanisms of generation is essential to interpret the symptomatology. This knowledge, in fact, prevents the mistake of focusing only on the painful area and leads one to consider other distant structures (deep somatic or visceral) as possible sources of the noxious impulses (Fig. 1). A comprehensive diagnostic orientation is thus permitted, with the identification of a range of structures potentially responsible for the pain observed. Specific examinations can subsequently be planned, targeting the various structures suspected to be involved; their outcome normally allows one to identify precisely the site of origin of the noxious stimuli. A final diagnosis can then be made, which is an indispensable step toward the most appropriate therapeutic approach.

—*Leonardo Vecchiet and Maria Adele Giamberardino*

See also–Pain, Assessment of; Pain, Basic Neurobiology of; Pain, Overview; Pain, Visceral; Phantom Limb and Stump Pain

Further Reading

Arendt-Nielsen, L. (1997). Induction and assessment of experimental pain from human skin, muscle and viscera. *Prog. Pain Res. Manage.* **8**, 393–425.
Bonica, J. J. (Ed.) (1990). *The Management of Pain*. Lea & Febiger, Philadelphia.
Cervero, F., and Laird, J. M. (1999). Visceral pain. *Lancet* **19**, 2145–2148.
Giamberardino, M. A. (2000). Visceral hyperalgesia. *Prog. Pain Res. Manage.* **16**, 523–550.
Mense, S. (1994). Referral of muscle pain. *Am. Pain Soc. J.* **3**, 1–9.
Procacci, P., and Maresca, M. (1999). Referred pain from somatic and visceral structures. *Curr. Rev. Pain* **3**, 96–99.
Simons, D. G., Travell, J. G., and Simons, L. S. (1999). *Travell & Simons' Myofascial Pain and Dysfunction. The Trigger Point Manual, Vol. 1: Upper Half of Body*, 2nd ed. William & Wilkins, Baltimore.
Vecchiet, L., Albe-fessard, D., Lindblom, U., *et al.* (Eds.) (1993). *New Trends in Referred Pain and Hyperalgesia, Pain Research and Clinical Management, Vol. 7.* Elsevier Science, Amsterdam.
Vecchiet, L., Vecchiet, J., and Giamberardino, M. A. (1999). Referred muscle pain: Clinical and pathophysiological aspects. *Curr. Rev. Pain* **3**, 489–498.
Wesselmann, U., and Lai, J. (1997). Mechanisms of referred visceral pain: Uterine inflammation in the adult virgin rat results in meurogenic plasma extravasation in the skin. *Pain* **73**, 309–317.

Pain, Visceral

Encyclopedia of the Neurological Sciences
Copyright 2003, Elsevier Science (USA). All rights reserved.

PAIN is the symptom that most frequently compels patients to seek medical attention and is often an adjunct to many neurological disorders. However, most practitioners regard the symptom of pain as a component of the underlying disease and therefore not a prime subject of neurological interest. The only exception is neuropathic pain, which statistically amounts to a very small proportion of all forms of pain. As a rule, pain is viewed by medical practitioners of all specialties as part of the causal disorder or as a post-traumatic or postoperative event.

Pain of internal origin, or visceral pain, is also a subject of lesser neurological interest. However, visceral pain is the most frequent manifestation of disorders of internal organs and, as a functional sign of neural activity, it is a common neurological symptom. If pain is the most frequent neurological symptom of disease, visceral pain is arguably the most common form of pain.

FEATURES OF VISCERAL PAIN

There are five basic clinical characteristics of visceral pain that make this form of pain unique. Visceral pain is not evoked from all viscera, may not be linked to visceral injury, is referred to other locations, is diffuse and poorly localized, and is accompanied by motor and autonomic reflexes (Table 1).

Table 1   SENSORY CHARACTERISTICS OF VISCERAL PAIN AND THEIR RELATED MECHANISMS

Psychophysics	Neurobiology
Not evoked from all viscera	Not all viscera are innervated by sensory receptors
Not linked to injury	Functional properties of visceral sensory afferents
Referred to body wall	Viscerosomatic convergence in central pain pathways
Diffuse and poorly localized	Few sensory visceral afferents; extensive divergence in the CNS
Intense motor and autonomic reactions	Mainly a warning system, with a substantial capacity for amplification

The referral of visceral pain to other locations, the diffuse nature of visceral pain, and the strong reflexes it evokes are due to the central organization of visceral nociceptive mechanisms. Particularly important are the lack of a separate visceral sensory pathway and the low proportion of visceral afferent fibers compared to those of somatic origin.

The clinical observation that visceral pain cannot be evoked from all viscera and the lack of a direct relationship between visceral injury and pain generated the idea that some viscera lacked an afferent innervation. However, it is now clear that all internal organs are innervated and that these features of visceral pain are due to the functional properties of the sensory receptors that innervate different visceral organs. Many viscera are innervated by receptors whose activation does not evoke conscious perception and they are not sensory receptors in the strict sense. These are receptors concerned with the homeostatic regulation of the internal environment and mainly activated by chemical and mechanical signals that do not reach consciousness (e.g., the level of blood pressure or the pH of the stomach).

VISCERAL NOCICEPTORS

Three distinct classes of nociceptive sensory receptor innervate internal organs:

• *High-threshold receptors:* These are sensory receptors with a high threshold to natural stimuli (mainly mechanical) and an encoding function contained entirely within the noxious range of stimulation. High-threshold receptors have been identified in the heart, veins, lungs and airways, esophagus, biliary system, small intestine, colon, ureter, urinary bladder, and uterus. Their functional properties indicate that these sensory receptors will be activated by intensities of stimulation perceived as painful. In addition, these receptors can be sensitized by prolonged and intense stimuli so that their threshold decreases and their excitability increases in the presence of tissue injury and inflammation.

• *Intensity-encoding receptors:* A number of reports have described sensory receptors in internal organs with a low threshold to natural stimuli (mainly mechanical) and an encoding function that spans innocuous and noxious intensities of stimulation. These receptors have been described mainly in the gastrointestinal tract and the urinary bladder. It is thought that these receptors constitute a category of sensory receptors that encode the stimulus intensity

in the magnitude of their discharges (intensity encoding) and may be responsible for those visceral sensations that start as nonpainful but that evolve toward pain as the stimulus intensity or duration increase (e.g., fullness and urge to void).

• *"Silent" nociceptors:* It has been found that a component of the afferent innervation of internal organs consists of mechanically insensitive afferent fibers that become mechanosensitive after inflammation of the peripheral organ (silent nociceptors). Like the high-threshold population, they can be sensitized by prolonged and intense stimuli. Because of their relative lack of excitability in the normal state, it has been suggested that these afferents are mainly concerned with chemical stimuli such as those resulting from ischemia, tissue injury, or inflammation. This type of sensory receptor can contribute to the signaling of chronic visceral pain, to long-term alterations of spinal reflexes, and to abnormal autonomic regulation of internal organs.

All three kinds of sensory receptors contribute to the peripheral encoding of noxious events in viscera. Brief, acute visceral pain, such as acute colic pain or the pain produced by an intense contraction of a hollow organ, could be triggered by the activation of high-threshold and intensity-encoding afferents. More prolonged forms of visceral stimulation, including those leading to hypoxia and inflammation of the tissue, result in the sensitization of high-threshold receptors and the activation of previously unresponsive silent nociceptors. In the sensitized state, nociceptors are able to respond to innocuous stimuli of the type normally occurring in internal organs. As a consequence, the central nervous system (CNS) receives an increased afferent barrage from peripheral nociceptors that is initially related to the acute injury but that, for the duration of the inflammatory process, is also dependent on the physiological activity of the internal organ until the process of peripheral sensitization is complete. This in turn triggers central mechanisms that enhance and sustain the peripheral input. Visceral pain is thus enhanced by a central mechanism brought into action by a peripheral barrage.

CENTRAL PROCESSING OF VISCERAL PAIN

Spinal Neurons

Spinal neurons are the first point of processing and integration of visceral pain-related information within the CNS. Visceral afferent fibers with cell bodies in the dorsal root ganglia convey visceral information to the spinal cord. Visceral afferents terminate in the outermost layer of the spinal gray matter (lamina I), the neck of the dorsal horn (lamina V), and around the central canal (lamina X). In contrast, afferents from the skin terminate in the upper layers of the gray matter (fine afferents in laminae I and II, with a few in lamina V; large myelinated afferents in laminae III–IV) (Fig. 1).

The major feature of spinal processing of visceral information is the convergence of visceral and

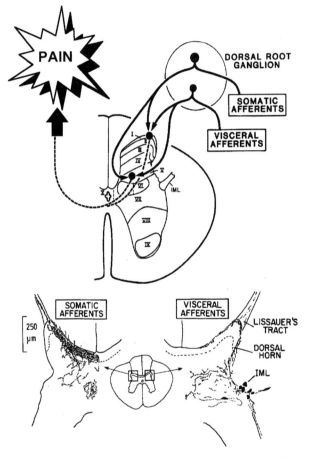

Figure 1
(Top) Schematic diagram showing viscerosomatic convergence of primary afferent fibers onto neurons of lamina I and lamina V of the spinal dorsal horn. The output of these neurons contributes to the perception of visceral pain. (Bottom) Patterns of termination of somatic (left) and visceral (right) primary afferent fibers in the spinal cord. Note their different patterns of termination and the absence of visceral afferent projections to the substantia gelatinosa, whose ventral border is indicated by the dotted line [modified from Cervero, F., and Foreman, R. D. (1990). In *Central Regulation of Autonomic Functions*, pp. 104–125. Oxford Univ. Press, Oxford].

somatic afferents onto the same population of spinal neurons. There is no evidence for a population of spinal neurons receiving purely visceral information that would provide a "private pathway" for the signaling of visceral sensation. The viscerosomatic afferent convergence in the spinal cord underlies the referral of visceral pain to somatic tissue in the same segments. Electrophysiological recordings from single neurons in the spinal cord of animals indicate that neurons excited by stimulation of a particular viscus are also activated by stimulation of somatic tissues in the appropriate dermatomes. For example, neurons with an excitatory input from the ureter are also activated by stimulation of the flanks of the animal.

The area of somatic tissue whose stimulation affects the activity of the neurons, known as the somatic receptive field of the neuron, is larger in spinal neurons with both visceral and somatic input (viscerosomatic neurons) than in neighboring neurons with a purely somatic input. Many viscerosomatic neurons, even those excited by one side of a bilateral viscus such as the ureter, have bilateral somatic receptive fields. These observations explain the diffuse, poorly localized nature of visceral pain sensations.

Visceral sensation depends on a relatively small population of afferent fibers compared to the numbers innervating somatic targets. Even in the midthoracic segments, in which visceral innervation is at its greatest and somatic innervation density is low, there are approximately 10-fold more somatic than visceral afferent fibers. Visceral afferent fibers nonetheless branch extensively within the spinal cord and excite many spinal neurons. This diffuse termination pattern within the spinal cord further contributes to the poor localization of visceral pain sensations. The extensive branching also serves to amplify the visceral nociceptive input at the level of the spinal cord and may contribute to the strong autonomic and skeletal muscle reflex responses evoked by visceral noxious stimulation.

Some spinal neuronal populations receive excitatory inputs from more than one viscus. This visceroviscrally convergence likely explains the similarities of the sensations evoked by stimulation of certain viscera. For example, afferents from the esophagus and the heart converge onto a population of thoracic spinal neurons. This convergence may underlie the phenomenon of noncardiac chest pain, in which patients present with symptoms typical of angina but upon exploration have normal heart function. In some cases, such patients have been shown to suffer from esophageal reflux.

The characteristics of visceral stimuli that excite spinal neurons reflect the response properties of visceral afferents and, in turn, underlie the characteristics of sensation from the organ in question. For example, neurons excited by distension of the colon show a range of thresholds from very low to above the normal pain threshold. Almost all encode in the noxious range, with the exception of a very small number of neurons that have low thresholds. The afferent innervation of the colon includes a large population of intensity encoding afferents and a smaller proportion of fibers that have high thresholds. Both nonpainful and painful sensations can be experienced from distension of the colon. In contrast, stimulation of organs such as the ureter or gallbladder exclusively evokes the sensation of pain. Spinal neurons excited by distension of the ureter or gallbladder recorded in animals have relatively high thresholds, similar to the thresholds of pain sensation in man, and the afferents innervating these organs include a large proportion of high-threshold fibers.

Transmitters Involved in Visceral Pain

There are two distinct biochemical classes of fine-caliber unmyelinated primary afferents—those that contain peptide neurotransmitters, such as substance P and calcitonin gene-related peptide, and those that do not. There is also a range of other receptors that are expressed by one group and not the other, and the two groups seem to have different trophic requirements to maintain their normal phenotypes. Furthermore, there are anatomical differences in the termination patterns of the two classes in the gray matter of the spinal cord. The peptide-containing afferents terminate in the outermost layers of the posterior horn, lamina I, outer lamina II, and lamina V, whereas the nonpeptide groups terminate in inner lamina II.

Somatic fine afferent fibers include both biochemical classes, and the functional role of the two classes in somatic pain is unclear. However, almost all visceral afferent fibers contain peptides, and they do not express the carbohydrate membrane markers that are characteristic of the nonpeptide class. Furthermore, the distinctive termination pattern in laminae I and V of the spinal cord of visceral afferent fibers corresponds to their biochemical identification as peptide-containing afferents. The biochemical identification of visceral afferents as part of the peptide-containing class suggests that peptides are particularly important in the transmission of information from viscera.

Pathways

Several pathways originating in the spinal gray matter and terminating in the brain have been identified as carrying information related to visceral pain. Of these, the spinothalamic tract is thought to be the most important for sensory-discriminative functions (i.e., the localization and quality of pain sensation). Recent evidence suggests that the postsynaptic dorsal column pathway, generally considered most important for cutaneous tactile discrimination, may also have an important role in the transmission of signals related to visceral nociceptive processing. Other pathways that carry axons of viscerosomatic spinal neurons, such as the spinohypothalamic or spinoparabrachialamygdaloid pathways, are obvious candidates for carrying signals related to the affective components of the sensation of visceral pain. Spinal viscerosomatic neurons also project rostrally in the spinosolitary and spinoreticular tracts.

Higher Processing of Visceral Pain

Information on the processing of visceral pain in higher centers has come from animal experiments and, in recent years, from studies in man—from both imaging studies and microstimulation during intracranial surgery in conscious patients. Imaging experiments in normal subjects and visceral pain patients have revealed the activation of the hypothalamus and periaqueductal gray, the thalamus, and various cortical regions in response to visceral stimuli. Comparisons of nonpainful somatic and visceral stimuli suggest that visceral sensations have a greater representation in the limbic cortex, as might be expected. Painful visceral stimuli produce activation of the anterior cingulate cortex and insular cortex, in addition to regions of the prefrontal cortex. Studies in animals have demonstrated a viscerotopic representation of the viscera in the thalamus and cortex.

Microstimulation of the thalamus in patients can evoke visceral pain experiences such as angina or labor pain, sometimes many years after the original episode. These observations suggest the existence of long-term neural mechanisms capable of storing the results of a previous pain experience. The pain memories evoked in these studies are almost all of visceral pain experiences, presumably because they are frequent in the general population and relatively intense.

VISCERAL HYPERSENSITIVITY

Sensitization and Hyperalgesia

In psychophysical terms, hyperalgesia is best understood as the consequences of the leftward shift that occurs, following a peripheral injury, in the curve that relates stimulus intensity to pain sensation (Fig. 2). This shift causes the lower portion of the pain curve to fall in the innocuous stimulus intensity range (allodynia), whereas the top portion shows an increased pain sensation to noxious stimuli (hyperalgesia).

The areas of hypersensitivity produced by an injury to the skin include a zone that incorporates the injury site and a much larger area of undamaged skin around the site of injury. These regions are known as areas of primary and secondary hyperalgesia, respectively. This nomenclature is still used today, even though the word hyperalgesia, strictly speaking, should be reserved to describe only one of the components of hypersensitivity states, namely the increased pain sensitivity to noxious stimuli.

An injury to visceral tissue also produces areas equivalent to primary and secondary hyperalgesia seen after cutaneous lesions. The primary hyperalge-

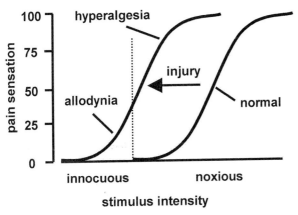

Figure 2
Diagram illustrating the changes in pain sensation induced by injury. The normal relationship between stimulus intensity and the magnitude of pain sensation is represented by the curve on the right. Pain sensation is only evoked by stimulus intensities in the noxious range (the dotted line indicates the pain threshold). Injury provokes a leftward shift in the curve relating stimulus intensity to pain sensation. Under these conditions, innocuous stimuli evoke pain (allodynia) and noxious stimuli are amplified (hyperalgesia).

sia zone, as for the skin, is the damaged area. The secondary hyperalgesia area (i.e., undamaged tissue showing hypersensitivity as a result of a nearby lesion) similarly includes adjacent undamaged regions of the same viscus. However, visceral damage may also result in hypersensitivity in other, undamaged viscera. This is known as viscerovisceral hyperalgesia. Furthermore, visceral lesions may also give rise to hyperalgesia in the area to which the visceral pain is referred—on the body wall. This is known as referred hyperalgesia.

Within the area of primary hyperalgesia, low-intensity stimuli evoke pain. Tissue injury induces a process of nociceptor sensitization whereby the excitability of the nociceptors is increased and their thresholds are lowered. Primary hyperalgesia can thus be explained in terms of nociceptor sensitization. For example, primary hyperalgesia can be demonstrated in patients and animals after visceral inflammation or injury by distension of the gut with an intraluminal balloon. However, the viscera are normally inaccessible to external stimuli; thus, is primary visceral hyperalgesia really of any relevance?

Visceral nociceptors in principle innervate motile, secretory tissue. Thus, sensitization of these nociceptors to chemical or mechanical stimuli may result in their activation by the normal physiological activity of the viscus. Furthermore, this effect may be potentiated by increases in motility or secretion induced by the lesion, either directly or by activation of reflex arcs. Thus, sensitization of visceral nociceptors will lead to visceral pain by a dual mechanism—as a result of any spontaneous activity induced and also by lowering their threshold such that they are excited by normal physiological activity of the viscus.

The situation with secondary hyperalgesia (referred or viscerovisceral hyperalgesia) is quite different since secondary hyperalgesia is mediated by changes in central processing of the sensory input. These central alterations are produced and maintained by the afferent barrage in peripheral nociceptors evoked by the originating injury.

Referred Hyperalgesia

Hyperalgesia of the somatic area to which visceral pain is referred, or referred hyperalgesia, is a common clinical observation. It is particularly obvious in conditions in which visceral pain occurs intermittently (e.g., dysmenorrhea or ureteric colic) since the referred hyperalgesia often continues during the pain-free periods. Patients generally report experiencing tenderness in the referral zone. Referred hyperalgesia has been quantified using electrical and natural stimulation in patients with a variety of different visceral pain states and has also been measured in animal models of visceral pain. Referred hyperalgesia is more pronounced in subcutaneous tissues than in the skin and is directly related to the duration and intensity of visceral pain episodes. The referral zone may also present trophic changes in visceral pain patients. For example, increases in the thickness of the subcutis and a reduction in muscle volume have been quantified ipsilateral to painful ureteric colics.

Referred hyperalgesia can be explained by an extension of the viscerosomatic convergence that underlies referred pain. A continuous low-level activity in nociceptors innervating an area of visceral damage may not produce sufficient spinal activation to evoke pain. However, if the somatic area of referral is stimulated, the somatic input summates with the ongoing visceral activity and the threshold to evoke pain sensations is reached more quickly. Referred hyperalgesia is correlated with the intensity and duration of visceral pain, suggesting that this reflects the level of activity in visceral nociceptors. However, noxious inputs can also change the way in which subsequent inputs are processed, usually resulting in an enhanced response. Thus, visceral hyperalgesia also reflects these "memory traces" or changes in spinal processing.

Viscerovisceral Hyperalgesia

Painful events in one viscus may affect the responses to noxious stimuli of another viscus with partially overlapping innervation. For example, fertile women with repeated ureteric colics have been shown to be more likely to suffer a colic attack at a specific moment in their monthly cycle. The effect of the monthly cycle on the timing of colics was especially pronounced in women with dysmenorrhea.

There is evidence for single visceral afferent fibers that innervate more than one viscus and a good deal of evidence for viscerovisceral convergence onto neurons of the spinal cord. These findings could provide the anatomical substrate for viscerovisceral hyperalgesia. The underlying spinal mechanism is probably similar to that of referred hyperalgesia. However, in addition to the pain sensation per se, another factor in viscerovisceral hyperalgesia may be the activation of reflex pathways by disease in one viscus that initiate or exacerbate problems in another organ. Since reflexes are segmentally organized, the

greatest effects are likely to occur in viscera innervated by the same or adjacent spinal segments.

—*Fernando Cervero and Jennifer M. A. Laird*

See also–Pain, Assessment of; Pain, Basic Neurobiology of; Pain, Referred; Sensation

Further Reading

Cervero, F. (1994). Sensory innervation of the viscera: Peripheral basis of visceral pain. *Physiol. Rev.* **74**, 95–138.

Cervero, F. (1995). Mechanisms of visceral pain: Past and present. *Prog. Pain Res. Manage.* **5**, 25–40.

Cervero, F. (1996). Visceral nociceptors. In *Neurobiology of Nociceptors* (C. Belmonte and F. Cervero, Eds.), pp. 220–240. Oxford Univ. Press, Oxford.

Cervero, F., and Jänig, W. (1992). Visceral nociceptors: A new world order? *Trends Neurosci.* **15**, 374–378.

Cervero, F., and Laird, J. M. A. (1999). Visceral pain. *Lancet* **353**, 2145–2148.

Foreman, R. D. (1999). Mechanisms of cardiac pain. *Annu. Rev. Physiol.* **61**, 143–167.

Gebhart, G. F. (2000). Pathobiology of visceral pain: Molecular mechanisms and therapeutic implications—IV. Visceral afferent contributions to the pathobiology of visceral pain. *Am. J. Physiol. Gastrointest. Liver Physiol.* **278**, G834–G838.

Giamberardino, M. A. (2000). Visceral hyperalgesia. In *Proceedings of the 9th World Congress on Pain* (M. Devor, M. Rowbotham, and Z. Wiesenfeld-Hallin, Eds.), pp. 523–550. IASP Press, Seattle, WA.

Mayer, E. A., and Gebhart, G. F. (1994). Basic and clinical aspects of visceral hyperalgesia. *Gastroenterology* **107**, 271–293.

Sengupta, J. N., and Gebhart, G. F. (1994). Gastrointestinal afferent fibers and sensation. In *Physiology of the Gastrointestinal Tract* (L. R. Johnson, Ed.), pp. 483–519. Raven Press, New York.

Pallidotomy

Encyclopedia of the Neurological Sciences
Copyright 2003, Elsevier Science (USA). All rights reserved.

PALLIDOTOMY, or more specifically posteroventral pallidotomy, is the surgical lesioning of the posteroventral globus pallidus for the treatment of medically refractory symptoms of Parkinson's disease.

INDICATIONS

Parkinson's disease is a progressive neurodegenerative disorder that results from the loss of nigrostriatal dopaminergic neurons and leads to progressive tremor, rigidity, bradykinesia (slowness in initiating movement), and cognitive symptoms. Anticholinergic medications and dopamine agonists relieve symptoms of Parkinson's disease and are standard initial treatments; levodopa therapy is not a standard initial treatment and the prolonged use of levodopa results in dyskinesias (involuntary movements) and, in some instances, major management problems later. Patients often develop disabling fluctuations in motor function between an "on" state (when levodopa effects are maximal) and an "off" state (when therapeutic effects are minimal). Patients with severely refractory parkinsonian symptoms, severe motor fluctuations, and disabling dyskinesias that prevent dose escalation of levodopa are candidates for pallidotomy. Contraindications to surgery include marked cerebral atrophy, major depression or psychiatric disorder, advanced dementia, or a serious concurrent medical illness; a major contraindication to surgery is a diagnosis of atypical parkinsonism.

PHYSIOLOGICAL RATIONALE FOR PALLIDOTOMY

The neurophysiology of the basal ganglia has been studied in detail in animal models, but much remains unknown. The basal ganglia receive input from motor areas of the cerebral cortex, process this input along with input from other brain regions, and provide feedback to the motor areas via the thalamus. This basal ganglia–thalamocortical motor circuit is thought to regulate and refine movement, and disturbances in this circuit are the basis of all movement disorders including Parkinson's disease. Parkinson's disease results from the loss of dopamine-secreting neurons that project from the substantia nigra pars compacta to the striatum. Through a complex series of neurophysiological alterations, this neuronal loss leads to excessive activity of the globus pallidus interna. The globus pallidus interna then excessively inhibits thalamocortical and brainstem pathways, causing the characteristic bradykinesia, tremors, and gait abnormalities of Parkinson's disease. This (highly oversimplified) scheme explains why lesions of the globus pallidus interna reverse parkinsonian symptoms.

HISTORY AND SURGICAL TECHNIQUE

The initial surgical treatment for patients with Parkinson's disease involved open craniotomies with open lesioning of the caudate nucleus and later of the globus pallidus. Briefly in the 1950s, a surgical procedure was performed to ligate the anterior choroidal artery causing an infarction of the medial globus pallidus. The procedure was beneficial for some parkinsonian symptoms but ultimately was abandoned because it caused several side effects. Contemporary surgery for Parkinson's disease incorporates stereotactic methods that usually involve only a small frontal burr hole. Contemporary pallidotomies usually incorporate image guidance with microelectrode recordings.

Patients are fitted with a stereotactic headframe and then undergo magnetic resonance imaging (MRI) or computed tomography to allow registration points to be calculated relative to the target in the globus pallidus. Most neurosurgeons now use the target, first described by Lars Leksell in Sweden in the 1950s, that lies in the posteroventral globus pallidus just lateral and dorsal to the optic tract. After the target has been determined, the stereotactic arc is set to the appropriate trajectory and the patient undergoes placement of a frontal burr hole under local anesthesia. Typically, the microelectrode recording follows, and differences in firing patterns and electrical impedance are used to confirm the target physiologically. Some surgeons forego this physiological monitoring and rely only on MRI guidance, but this approach is controversial. Once the target has been confirmed, a thermal lesion is made. The patient usually leaves the hospital within 1 or 2 days.

COMPLICATIONS

Surgical complications include rare instances of intracranial hemorrhage and seizures. Occasional damage to the optic tract with resultant visual symptoms has been reported. The two most recent prospective studies demonstrated no permanent complications or operative mortality.

RESULTS

In initial reports from pallidotomies performed in the 1950s and 1960s, success rates ranged from 50 to 85%, but follow-up was short in these series. The use of pallidotomy as a treatment for Parkinson's patients diminished in the 1960s and 1970s due to the introduction and widespread use of levodopa. The procedure regained popularity in the past two decades as the long-term effects of levodopa became more apparent.

Two contemporary prospective series examining pallidotomy reported marked or moderate improvement in parkinsonian symptoms in 82% of patients

3 months after surgery and an 18% reduction in scores on a Parkinson's disease rating scale 4 years after surgery. The most significant results involved dyskinesias contralateral to the lesion side. More modest effects were noted for contralateral "off" state motor scores. No effect was noted for ipsilateral motor scores or dyskinesias. Neither study demonstrated any change in usage of parkinsonian medications as a result of the procedure. However, this outcome is not surprising. Some patients undergo the procedure to eliminate drug-induced dyskinesias and may actually be able to tolerate higher doses of levodopa after surgery. Some, but not all, studies have also found that rigidity and gait function improve as a result of pallidotomy. Studies of cognitive and language function have failed to demonstrate any significant benefit as a result of pallidotomy. Patients with asymmetric motor symptoms tend to have better outcomes from unilateral pallidotomy. Patients' initial response in the first few weeks after surgery is the best predictor of long-term success. Limited experience with bilateral pallidotomies in Parkinson's disease suggests an unacceptable risk of speech and cognitive deficits.

Overall, pallidotomy appears to significantly improve tremor, rigidity, bradykinesia, and the drug-induced dyskinesias of patients with severe Parkinson's disease. It is ideal for patients with predominantly unilateral symptoms, especially dyskinesias. However, the procedure does not alter the underlying neurodegeneration responsible for the disease. The progression of symptoms is delayed but not eliminated. It also has no demonstrable effect on cognitive function and the progressive dementia associated with Parkinson's disease. Consequently, patients being referred for the procedure must be informed of the goals and limitations of this surgical treatment.

ALTERNATIVES TO PALLIDOTOMY

An important advance in the surgical treatment of movement disorders has been the development of implantable stimulators. These stimulators can be placed stereotactically into the various nuclei of the basal ganglia, where they act as lesions that can be modified by adjusting the intensity of the stimulus. The results of chronic stimulation of the globus pallidus compare favorably with the results of pallidotomy. Compared to pallidotomy, the advantages of chronic stimulation include the ability to control the size of the "lesion," the greater safety associated with bilateral procedures, and the

potential reversibility of any side effects. The disadvantages of implanted stimulators include the possibility of an infection that would require the stimulator to be removed and the need to monitor and adjust the device, which can be time-consuming and expensive. In some series, chronic stimulation of the subthalamic nucleus has been more effective for the treatment of the off symptoms of Parkinson's disease, including bradykinesia and rigidity, than pallidotomy or stimulation of the globus pallidus. A prospective study comparing chronic stimulation of the globus pallidus with stimulation of a subthalamic nucleus is under way.

Patients who predominately suffer from tremor but not from other symptoms of Parkinson's disease may benefit from thalamotomy or chronic stimulation of the thalamic nucleus.

PALLIDOTOMY FOR DYSTONIA AND HEMIBALLISM

A unilateral pallidotomy can also significantly reduce dystonic movement disorders and the associated disability. The involuntary movements of the limbs observed in hemiballism can also be abolished successfully by a pallidotomy. The improvements in symptomatology tend to persist except in patients with predominantly axial dystonia, who show better results after bilateral pallidotomies. A decrease in speech or speech difficulties after this procedure, which sometimes follows bilateral pallidotomies for Parkinson's disease, has not been reported consistently. Thalamotomy has also been described as a potential treatment for dystonia. Overall, patient series on lesioning the basal ganglia structures for the treatment of this condition are lacking, and accurate and reliable conclusions cannot be drawn.

—Sam P. Javedan, Iman Feiz-Erfan, Patrick P. Han,
and Andrew G. Shetter

See also—Basal Ganglia; Corpus Striatum; Deep Brain Stimulation; Dyskinesias; Dystonia; Globus Pallidus; Parkinsonism; Parkinson's Disease

Further Reading

Burchiel, K. J., Anderson, V. C., Favre, J., *et al.* (1999). Comparison of pallidal and subthalamic nucleus deep brain stimulation for advanced Parkinson's disease: Results of a randomized, blinded pilot study. *Neurosurgery* 45, 1375–1384.

Fine, J., Duff, J., Chen, R., *et al.* (2000). Long-term follow-up of unilateral pallidotomy in advanced Parkinson's disease. *N. Engl. J. Med.* 342, 1708–1714.

Josefson, D. (2000). Pallidotomy relieves some symptoms of Parkinson's disease. *Br. Med. J.* **320,** 1622.

Lai, E. C., Jankovic, J., Krauss, J. K., *et al.* (2000). Long-term efficacy of posteroventral pallidotomy in the treatment of Parkinson's disease. *Neurology* **55,** 1218–1222.

Laitinen, L. V., Bergenheim, A. T., and Hariz, M. I. (1992). Leksell's posteroventral pallidotomy in the treatment of Parkinson's disease. *J. Neurosurg.* **76,** 53–61.

Obeso, J. A., Rodriguez-Oroz, M. C., Rodriguez, M., *et al.* (2000). Pathophysiology of the basal ganglia in Parkinson's disease. *Trends Neurosci.* **23,** S8–S19.

Ondo, W. G., Desaloms, J. M., Jankovic, J., *et al.* (1998). Pallidotomy for generalized dystonia. *Movement Disord.* **13,** 693–698.

Rettig, G. M., York, M. K., Lai, E. C., *et al.* (2000). Neuropsychological outcome after unilateral pallidotomy for the treatment of Parkinson's disease. *J. Neurol. Neurosurg. Psychiatry* **69,** 326–336.

Vitek, J. L., Chockkan, V., Zhang, J.-Y., *et al.* (1999). Neuronal activity in the basal ganglia in patients with generalized dystonia and hemiballismus. *Ann. Neurol.* **46,** 22–35.

Panic Disorder

Encyclopedia of the Neurological Sciences

PANIC DISORDER is a clinical syndrome characterized by recurrent spontaneous episodes of intense fear and discomfort known as "panic attacks." During a panic attack, the individual experiences a sense of overwhelming fear and anxiety accompanied by somatic and cognitive symptoms, such as palpitations, trembling, shortness of breath, sweating, chest pain, and often a fear of dying, having a life-threatening medical condition, or of experiencing a "mental breakdown." The symptoms associated with panic attacks can occur in a variety of psychiatric and medical conditions. It is when the attacks are recurrent and unexplained by medical factors or other psychiatric conditions that a diagnosis of panic disorder is made. Some patients with panic disorder develop such an intense fear of experiencing another panic attack that they begin to avoid situations in which escape might be difficult, such as riding in elevators or crowds, or in which they would be in a public place where others might observe them experiencing the panic attack. This condition is called agoraphobia, and it can significantly interfere with an individual's ability to function in work and social situations outside the home. Panic disorder is thus subdivided into two major subgroupings: with agoraphobia and without agoraphobia.

EPIDEMIOLOGY

Although there have been descriptions in the literature of syndromes resembling what is now designated panic disorder since the mid-1800s, it was not formally codified in the American Psychiatric Association *Diagnostic and Statistical Manual* until 1980. Epidemiological studies report lifetime prevalence rates of 1.5–5% for panic disorder and 3–5.6% for panic attacks. Women are two to three times more likely to be diagnosed with panic disorder, but some researchers believe that there may be a bias toward under-reporting in men. Rates vary little between racial groups. Panic disorder typically develops in young adulthood, although both panic disorder and agoraphobia can develop at any age. Studies on agoraphobia have yielded wider ranges in estimates of prevalence, from as low as 0.6% to as high as 6%.

ETIOLOGY

A number of studies have shown abnormalities in the autonomic nervous systems of persons with panic disorder. Those with panic disorder are significantly more likely to experience a panic attack when given certain "panic-inducing" substances, such as intravenous lactate, than are controls. Genetic studies show a consistent and distinct genetic component. Functional brain imaging and positron emission tomography research has demonstrated dysregulation of cerebral blood flow in panic disorder patients. At one time, it was thought that mitral valve prolapse was correlated with panic disorder, but subsequent large-scale studies have shown that this is not the case.

Psychoanalytical theories postulate that panic attacks are the result of a failure of defense mechanisms against unconscious impulses. Behavior theory views the syndrome through a process of modeling parental behavior or through classic conditioning, pairing a sensation of anxiety with a specific situation. However, this does not explain the occurrence of the initial panic attack.

Other research has suggested that stressful psychological events may produce neurophysiological changes that render the individual more susceptible to panic attacks. Studies have shown that separation from mother early in life is significantly correlated with the development of panic disorder later. Additional support for the interaction of psychology and physiology is provided by a study of cognitive behavior therapy for panic disorder. Patients with a history of intravenous lactate-triggered panic attacks who then had a successful clinical response to cognitive behavior therapy no longer developed panic symptoms when subsequently infused with lactate.

CLINICAL FEATURES

The first panic attack typically occurs in young adulthood. Although there is no identifiable immediate precipitant, often the attacks follow a recent period of emotional or physical stress. The symptoms begin suddenly and escalate in intensity over a period of a few minutes. The attack may last from approximately 20 min to several hours. Most patients immediately experience a sense of escalating panic and are bewildered as to why they should be feeling so frightened but are unable to suppress the symptoms. Patients often describe a desperate fear of impending disaster, serious medical illness or death, or of "going crazy." Associated somatic symptoms include palpitations, hyperventilation and shortness of breath, sweating, trembling, extreme restlessness, tightness or pain in the chest, dizziness, and numbness or tingling in the face or extremities. The attack usually tapers off gradually or may sometimes end abruptly. Many patients rush to emergency rooms with the belief that they are having a heart attack. Between attacks, patients may develop a degree of anticipatory anxiety due to fear of having another panic attack.

Those patients who develop agoraphobia begin to avoid situations that they associate with precipitating the panic attack or from which it would be difficult to escape or obtain help. Sometimes, they insist on being accompanied by a friend or relative when leaving the house; others become so severely incapacitated that they find it difficult to leave home at all, even accompanied.

Symptoms of depression are frequently present in panic disorder, often sufficient to merit a comorbid diagnosis of major depressive disorder. Phobias, obsessive–compulsive disorder, and substance abuse also occur more frequently in individuals with panic disorder than in the general population.

DIFFERENTIAL DIAGNOSIS

The symptoms of a panic attack may closely resemble those of acute angina or myocardial infarction. Patients with new-onset symptoms char-

acteristic of panic attacks should have a thorough medical evaluation. A urine drug screen is an important and often overlooked component of the evaluation because ingestion of stimulants, such as cocaine or amphetamines, or withdrawal from sedatives, such as alcohol, benzodiazepines, or barbiturates, can mimic panic attack symptoms. If there are atypical symptoms, such as neurological abnormalities, loss of bladder control, or loss of consciousness, further diagnostic studies are warranted to rule out an underlying medical/neurological condition.

If the medical evaluation is negative for an illness that could explain the symptoms, a thorough psychiatric assessment is indicated. Psychiatric illnesses that occasionally resemble panic disorder must be considered in the differential. These include phobias, obsessive–compulsive disorder, malingering, factitious disorder, substance abuse, hypochondriasis, depressive disorders, and even schizophrenia. A careful history is essential in making the diagnosis. A key diagnostic distinction is that panic attacks associated with specific settings or situations are characteristic of specific or social phobia or obsessive–compulsive disorder, whereas in panic disorder the attacks are unexpected and do not have a situational focus.

Untreated, panic disorder tends to be a chronic condition, but the course is highly variable. If the patient has frequent attacks, the likelihood of comorbid depression, substance abuse, and psychosocial consequences secondary to the illness (e.g., relationship, work, or school problems) increases. Patients with good premorbid functioning and a brief duration of symptoms, or those with very infrequent attacks, tend to have a better prognosis.

TREATMENT

Pharmacotherapy and cognitive behavior therapy have consistently been shown to be the most effective treatments for panic disorder, and the combination of the two works better than either one alone. Most patients respond very well to treatment, with response rates of 80% reported in the literature.

The first-line treatment of choice is a selective serotonin reuptake inhibitor (SSRI). All SSRIs are effective and the clinician can make a decision based on side effect profiles and tolerability. Panic disorder patients are often especially susceptible to the activating effects of SSRIs, and it is generally advisable to start at low doses and titrate upward gradually. Studies show good response at the same doses used to treat major depression, but it may be possible to achieve good results with lower doses in some patients.

Benzodiazepines are also effective and have a more rapid onset of action in the treatment of panic disorder. Alprazolam has been the most widely used benzodiazepine, but controlled studies have shown that lorazepam and clonazepam are equally effective. Some clinicians use benzodiazepines concurrently while starting the patient on a SSRI in order to achieve rapid control of symptoms and then gradually withdraw the benzodiazepine once the SSRI takes effect. Benzodiazepines have the potential for abuse/dependence and cognitive/psychomotor impairment as well as a well-documented discontinuation syndrome. This has been reported to be especially problematic with alprazolam. For these reasons, benzodiazepines are considered second-line treatment after the SSRIs. Tricyclic and monoamine oxidase inhibitor (MOI) antidepressants are also effective, but because of their far less favorable side effect profile and danger of overdose (and drug/food interactions in the case of MAOIs), they have been overwhelmingly supplanted by the SSRIs.

If several SSRI trials at adequate doses fail, a benzodiazepine may be considered. Tricyclics, MAOIs, and combination therapy with agents of different classes may be considered in treatment-refractory patients. There have been case reports of effectiveness with anticonvulsants. Once the patient demonstrates remission of symptoms, the medication should be continued for 8–12 months and then gradually tapered off. If symptoms recur, the medication should be immediately reinstituted and it is likely that lifelong treatment will be necessary.

Cognitive behavior therapy has been shown to be an effective treatment for panic disorder. Several studies have shown that patients who have a good response to cognitive behavior therapy have long-lasting remission of symptoms. Other research has demonstrated the highest response rates with combinations of cognitive behavior therapy with pharmacotherapy.

Panic disorder is a common psychiatric condition that can lead to significant morbidity and disruption of an individual's life. Advances in diagnosis and treatment have had a major impact in improving outcomes for afflicted persons.

—*Douglas Vanderburg*

See also–Antianxiety Pharmacology; Anxiety Disorders, Overview; Cognitive Behavioral Psychotherapy; Obsessive–Compulsive Disorder; Paranoia; Parasomnias; Phobias; Substance Abuse

Further Reading

American Psychiatric Association (1994). *Diagnostic and Statistical Manual of Mental Disorders*, 4th ed. American Psychiatric Association, Washington, DC.
Coplan, J. D., and Lydiard, R. B. (1998). Brain circuits in panic disorder. *Biol. Psychiatry* **44**, 1264–1276.
den Boer, J. A., and Slaap, B. R. (1998). Review of current treatment in panic disorder. *Int. Clin. Psychopharmacol.* **13**, S25–S30.
Hochman, N. K. S. (1997, September 7). Many more seek help for panic disorder. *The New York Times on the Web*.
Kaplan, H. I., and Sadock, B. J. (1998). *Synopsis of Psychiatry: Behavioral Sciences/Clinical Psychiatry*, 8th ed. Williams & Wilkins, Baltimore.

Paralysis

Encyclopedia of the Neurological Sciences
Copyright 2003, Elsevier Science (USA). All rights reserved.

THE WORD PARALYSIS derives from the Greek *paralyein* (to loosen, disable). In neurology, it is generally used to mean complete loss of motor power. When the loss is partial, the word paresis is used instead. The word palsy also implies loss of power, but it does not define the severity of the loss. Paralysis is most often focal. When it affects one of the cranial nerves, it is named after the cranial nerve affected (e.g., facial paralysis). Paralysis that affects all four extremities is called quadriplegia or tetraplegia. When it affects the limbs of one side of the body or, more often, the lower face and limbs of one side of the body, it is called hemiplegia. The presence of hemiplegia suggests involvement of the corticospinal tract. Finally, when both legs are paralyzed, the term used is paraplegia. Paraplegia often results from lesions of the spinal cord. With corticospinal tract lesions, the paralysis is accompanied by spasticity; therefore, it is often called spastic paralysis. Paralysis can result from damage of the peripheral nerves, neuromuscular junction, or muscle. In these cases, there is no spasticity.

Paralysis can also be used in other contexts. Sleep paralysis is the loss of the ability to move that patients with narcolepsy experience for brief periods of time during wakefulness, typically when awaking from sleep. Poliomyelitis was known as infantile paralysis in the 19th and early 20th centuries. In 1817, paralysis agitans was the name used by Sir James Parkinson for the disease that today bears his name. Periodic paralysis is the transient loss of motor power in the entire body while the patient remains awake. It is due to any of a number of congenital disorders of electrolyte channels in the muscle membrane.

—*José C. Masdeu*

See also—Paraparesis and Paraplegia; Paresis; Quadriplegia; Sleep Paralysis; Tick Paralysis

Further Reading

Brazis, P. W., Masdeu, J. C., and Biller, J. (Eds.) (2001). *Localization in Clinical Neurology*, 4th ed. Lippincott Williams & Wilkins, Philadelphia.

Davies, N. P., and Hanna, M. G. (2001). The skeletal muscle channelopathies: Basic science, clinical genetics and treatment. *Curr. Opin. Neurol.* **14**, 539–551.

Krahn, L. E., Black, J. L., and Silber, M. H. (2001). Narcolepsy: New understanding of irresistible sleep. *Mayo Clin. Proc.* **76**, 185–194.

Paraneoplastic Syndromes, Central

Encyclopedia of the Neurological Sciences
Copyright 2003, Elsevier Science (USA). All rights reserved.

PARANEOPLASTIC neurological diseases are clinical syndromes that develop in a cancer patient but cannot be attributed to metastatic disease or any nonmetastatic complication, such as treatment toxicities, infections, or nutritional disturbances. Paraneoplastic syndromes can affect every level of the neuraxis from the cortex to the neuromuscular junction and even the muscle. Patients often present first to neurologists because the neurological dysfunction in most instances precedes identification of the malignancy. Specific paraneoplastic syndromes may even suggest the particular underlying cancer or where to look (e.g., cerebellar degeneration is frequently associated with gynecological malignancies in women). Often, the cancer is small and potentially curable if detected immediately, so recognition of the paraneoplastic syndromes affords the neurologist the opportunity for early identification and treatment of a potentially aggressive cancer. Occasionally, this ameliorates the neurological dysfunction as well.

Diagnosis of the paraneoplastic neurological diseases is based in part on the detection of cancer, exclusion of other causes of neurological impairment by neuroimaging, cerebrospinal fluid (CSF) analysis and electroencephalogram (EEG), and the detection of specific autoantibodies. Autoantibodies are not identified in every patient with paraneoplastic neurological disease, but they are seen in the majority, especially those with the more common syndromes such as encephalomyelitis and cerebellar degeneration. These autoantibodies are important diagnostically and prognostically since it appears that in some syndromes the underlying cancer has a better prognosis in patients with detectable autoantibodies. Furthermore, these autoantibodies are believed to be critical in the pathogenesis of the neurological dysfunction, although a direct link has not been established. The major syndromes are discussed individually in the following sections.

PARANEOPLASTIC LIMBIC ENCEPHALITIS

This disorder is characterized by the subacute development of depression, irritability, seizures, and short-term memory loss. Symptoms usually precede the diagnosis of the tumor. The tumor most frequently involved is small-cell lung cancer (SCLC). The magnetic resonance imaging (MRI) findings of paraneoplastic limbic encephalitis include uni- or bilateral mesial temporal lobe abnormalities that are best seen on T2-weighted images. On T1 sequences the temporal–limbic regions may be hypointense and atrophic and sometimes enhance with contrast. Some patients develop hyperthermia, hyperphagia, hypersomnia, catalepsy, and MRI abnormalities indicating hypothalamic involvement. In two-thirds of patients, analysis of the CSF shows mild pleocytosis, an increased protein concentration, intrathecal synthesis of IgG, and oligoclonal bands. The EEG is useful in assessing whether changes in level of consciousness or behavior are related to temporal lobe seizures.

Pathological findings include perivascular and interstitial inflammatory infiltrates, neuronal loss, and microglial proliferation that predominate in the limbic system (hippocampus, amygdala, hypothalamus, and insular and cingulate cortex) (Fig. 1).

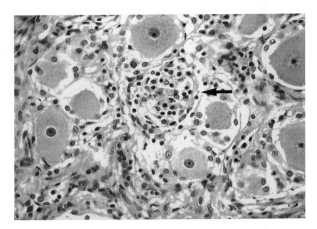

Figure 1
Neuronal degeneration and infiltrates of T cells (arrow) in the dorsal root ganglia of a patient with paraneoplastic sensory neuronopathy.

Anti-neuronal antibodies associated with limbic encephalitis include anti-Hu, anti-Ma2, and anti-CV2 antibodies and anti-PCA2. However, limbic encephalopathy may be paraneoplastic in origin, even when anti-neuronal autoantibodies are not detected. In a study of 50 patients with paraneoplastic limbic encephalitis, tumors unassociated with antibodies included cancer of the breast, colon, and ovary, Hodgkin's lymphoma, plasma cell dyscrasia, chronic myeloid leukemia, teratoma, and thymoma. Paraneoplastic limbic encephalitis may improve with treatment of the tumor.

PARANEOPLASTIC CEREBELLAR DEGENERATION

Presenting symptoms of this disorder usually include dizziness, nausea, blurry or double vision (sometimes with oscillopsia), and gait instability. Subsequently, patients develop variable degrees of truncal and limb ataxia, dysarthria, and dysphagia. These symptoms are similar for most types of paraneoplastic cerebellar degeneration, irrespective of the type of cancer or autoantibody detected, but the course of the disease may be different depending on the associated immune response. In general, neurological symptoms usually precede the tumor diagnosis.

MRI of the brain is usually normal in the early stages of the disease and may show global cerebellar atrophy months after symptom development. The CSF often shows pleocytosis, an increased protein concentration, intrathecal synthesis of IgG, and oligoclonal bands.

The pathological hallmark of paraneoplastic cerebellar degeneration is a diffuse loss of Purkinje cells accompanied by thinning of the molecular and granular layers and degeneration of the dentate and olivary nuclei and long tracts of the spinal cord. These findings can be associated with mild or prominent lymphocytic infiltrates (encephalomyelitis), or inflammation may be absent.

Anti-neuronal antibodies associated with paraneoplastic cerebellar dysfunction include anti-Yo, anti-Ri, anti-Tr, anti-Hu, anti-Ma, anti-CV2, anti-GluR1α, and anti-PCA2. Several-primary cancers are associated with cerebellar degeneration; certain cancer types are linked to particular antibodies (Table 1). Symptoms of paraneoplastic cerebellar dysfunction may occur in the absence of anti-neuronal antibodies, in which case the tumors most frequently involved are non-Hodgkin's lymphoma and lung cancer (non-SCLC and SCLC).

Treatment should be directed to the tumor. Although clear improvement of the neurological dysfunction is rare, a complete tumor response may result in stabilization of neurological symptoms.

PARANEOPLASTIC ENCEPHALOMYELITIS

The term paraneoplastic encephalomyelitis (PEM) describes patients with cancer who develop multifocal neurological deficits and signs of inflammation involving two or more areas of the nervous system, including brain, cerebellum, brainstem, and spinal cord. This gives rise to a mixture of symptoms, including limbic encephalitis, cerebellar degeneration, brainstem encephalitis, myelitis, and autonomic dysfunction.

Symptoms of paraneoplastic brainstem encephalitis include oscillopsia, diplopia, dysarthria, dysphagia, gaze abnormalities (both internuclear or supranuclear), subacute hearing loss, and facial numbness. The spinal cord symptoms of patients with PEM usually result from an inflammatory degeneration of the lower motor neurons (myelitis). Autonomic dysfunction produces gastrointestinal paresis and pseudoobstruction, orthostatic hypotension, cardiac dysrhythmias, erectile insufficiency, sweating abnormalities, and abnormal pupillary responses.

PEM usually precedes the tumor diagnosis. In patients with prominent limbic dysfunction, the MRI of the brain may show medial temporal lobe abnormalities; otherwise, the MRI is usually normal. Since 75% of PEM patients have SCLC, the antibody

Table 1   ANTIBODY-ASSOCIATED PARANEOPLASTIC SYNDROMES OF THE CENTRAL NERVOUS SYSTEM

Antibody	Paraneoplastic syndrome	Tumor[a]
Anti-Hu	Encephalomyelitis	*SCLC*, neuroblastoma sarcoma, prostate
	Sensory neuronopathy	
	Autonomic dysfunction	
Anti-Yo	Cerebellar degeneration	*Ovary, breast*
Anti-Ri	Ataxia, opsoclonus	Breast, gynecological, lung
Anti-Tr	Cerebellar degeneration	*Hodgkin's lymphoma*
Anti-CV2 (anti-CRMP-5)[23]	Encephalomyelitis	SCLC, thymoma, gynecological
	Cerebellar degeneration	
	Sensorimotor neuronopathy	
Anti-Ma1 and -2	Limbic encephalitis	*Germ cell tumors*, lung, breast, colon, salivary gland
	Brainstem encephalitis	
	Cerebellar degeneration	
Anti-PCA2	Limbic encephalitis	SCLC
	Brainstem encephalitis	
	Cerebellar degeneration	
Anti-amphiphysin	Stiff-man syndrome	*Breast*, SCLC
	Encephalomyelitis	

[a]Tumors in *italics* are the most frequently encountered in association with the corresponding antibody. SCLC; small-cell lung cancer.

most frequently detected in serum and CSF is anti-Hu. Other antibodies include anti-CV2 and anti-amphiphysin (commonly associated with stiff-person syndrome). The paraneoplastic disorder associated with antibodies to Ma proteins affects only the limbic, hypothalamic, brainstem, and cerebellar structures, and it may respond to treatment of the tumor. PEM rarely responds to treatment of the tumor or immunotherapy.

PARANEOPLASTIC OPSOCLONUS–MYOCLONUS

Approximately 50% of children with paraneoplastic opsoclonus–myoclonus (POM) have neuroblastoma, and approximately 2% of children with this tumor develop opsoclonus. POM usually affects children younger than 4 years of age (median age, 18 months) and is often associated with hypotonia, ataxia, and irritability. In half of the patients with POM, the opsoclonus precedes the diagnosis of neuroblastoma. Symptoms usually fluctuate and may have a prolonged course. POM frequently responds to treatment of the tumor, steroids, and IVIg, but relapses are common, often as a result of intercurrent infections. Approximately 65% of patients are left with deficits, including psychomotor retardation and behavioral abnormalities. Patients with POM have a

better tumor prognosis than patients without paraneoplastic symptoms.

In adults, POM develops in association with truncal ataxia resulting in gait difficulty and frequent falls. In more than half of patients, POM precedes the diagnosis of the tumor, usually an SCLC. Patients with breast cancer may harbor anti-Ri antibodies. There have been clinical responses to immune suppressants, depletion of serum IgG using protein A columns, clonazepam, and thiamine, and treatment of the tumor. Interpretation of these results is confounded by the possibility of spontaneous improvement.

PARANEOPLASTIC STIFF-PERSON SYNDROME

This disorder is characterized by muscle stiffness and rigidity that predominate in the paraspinal and abdominal muscles resulting in abnormal postures and exaggeration of the normal lumbar lordosis. In addition, patients have muscle spasms precipitated by voluntary movement, emotional upset, and auditory and somesthetic stimuli. Electrophysiological studies show continuous motor unit activity in at least one axial muscle. A focal variety of the disorder, or stiff-limb syndrome, has been described.

Stiff-person syndrome can occur as a paraneoplastic manifestation of cancer or, more frequently, in the absence of cancer. When it develops as a paraneo-plastic disorder, the patient's sera and CSF usually contain antibodies to amphiphysin I. In patients without cancer the major autoantigen is glutamic acid decarboxylase, and 70% of these patients develop diabetes.

Neurological symptoms may develop before or after tumor diagnosis; the common cancers include breast and colon cancer and Hodgkin's disease. Symptomatic improvement can be obtained with diazepam, clonazepam, or baclofen, but more definitive improvement is often obtained with treatment of the tumor and steroids.

—*Josep Dalmau*

See also–Neurooncology, Overview; Paraneoplastic Syndromes, Immunology; Stiff-Person Syndrome

Further Reading

Anderson, N. E., Budde-Steffen, C., Rosenblum, M. K., *et al.* (1988). Opsoclonus, myoclonus, ataxia, and encephalopathy in adults with cancer: A distinct paraneoplastic syndrome. *Medicine (Baltimore)* 67, 100–109.

Cher, L. M., Hochberg, F. H., Teruya, J., *et al.* (1995). Therapy for paraneoplastic neurologic syndromes in six patients with protein A column immunoadsorption. *Cancer* 75, 1678–1683.

Dalmau, J., Graus, F., Rosenblum, M. K., *et al.* (1992). Anti-Hu-associated paraneoplastic encephalomyelitis/sensory neuronopathy. A clinical study of 71 patients. *Medicine* 71, 59–72.

Dalmau, J., Gultekin, S. H., Voltz, R., *et al.* (1999). Ma1, a novel neuron- and testis-specific protein, is recognized by the serum of patients with paraneoplastic neurological disorders. *Brain* 122, 27–39.

Folli, F., Solimena, M., Cofiell, R., *et al.* (1993). Autoantibodies to a 128-kd synaptic protein in three women with the stiff-man syndrome and breast cancer. *N. Engl. J. Med.* 328, 546–551.

Gultekin, S. H., Rosenfeld, M. R., Voltz, R., *et al.* (2000). Paraneoplastic limbic encephalitis: Neurological symptoms, immunological findings and tumour association in 50 patients. *Brain* 123, 1481–1494.

Honnorat, J., Antoine, J. C., Derrington, E., *et al.* (1996). Antibodies to a subpopulation of glial cells and a 66 kDa developmental protein in patients with paraneoplastic neurological syndromes. *J. Neurol. Neurosurg. Psychiatry* 61, 270–278.

Keime-Guibert, F., Graus, F., Broet, P., *et al.* (1999). Clinical outcome of patients with anti-Hu-associated encephalomyelitis after treatment of the tumor. *Neurology* 53, 1719–1723.

Koh, P. S., Raffensperger, J. G., Berry, S., *et al.* (1994). Long-term outcome in children with opsoclonus–myoclonus and ataxia and coincident neuroblastoma. *J. Pediatr.* 125, 712–716.

Russo, C., Cohn, S. L., Petruzzi, M. J., *et al.* (1997). Long-term neurologic outcome in children with opsoclonus–myoclonus

associated with neuroblastoma: A report from the Pediatric Oncology Group. *Med. Pediatr. Oncol.* 28, 284–288.

Solimena, M., Folli, F., Aparisi, R., *et al.* (1990). Autoantibodies to GABA-ergic neurons and pancreatic beta cells in stiff-man syndrome. *N. Engl. J. Med.* 322, 1555–1560.

Voltz, R., Gultekin, S. H., Rosenfeld, M. R., *et al.* (1999). A serologic marker of paraneoplastic limbic and brain-stem encephalitis in patients with testicular cancer. *N. Engl. J. Med.* 340, 1788–1795.

Yu, Z., Kryzer, T. J., Griesmann, G. E., *et al.* (2001). CRMP-5 neuronal autoantibody: Marker of lung cancer and thymoma-related autoimmunity. *Ann. Neurol.* 49, 146–154.

Paraneoplastic Syndromes, Immunology

Encyclopedia of the Neurological Sciences
Copyright 2003, Elsevier Science (USA). All rights reserved.

PARANEOPLASTIC neurological disorders (PNDs) are disorders of nervous system function that cannot be ascribed to invasion of the nervous system by neoplastic cells or by any other mechanisms related to the presence of a cancer, including coagulopathy, infection, metabolic and nutritional deficits, and toxic effects of cancer therapy. In recent years, the detection of immune responses to proteins with expression that is highly restricted to the nervous system and tumors (onconeuronal antigens) has led to the concept that most PNDs are immune mediated. According to the immunological mechanisms involved, PNDs can be classified into three categories (Table 1). The first category includes those disorders directly mediated by antibodies. The second category includes disorders that are likely mediated by cytotoxic T cells, although antibodies to onconeuronal antigens are also present. The third category comprises a group of disorders in which the neoplastic cells synthesize immunoglobulins that may affect the peripheral nerves. For most disorders in the first two categories, it is believed that the expression of neuronal proteins by the tumor is a crucial step in the process of breaking immune tolerance for these proteins and eventually leading to the PNDs. In the third group, immunoglobulins synthesized by the neoplastic cells may be the cause of the neurological dysfunction due to antibody activity against peripheral nerve antigens, nonspecific deposition of immunoglobulin fragments (amyloid) in peripheral nerves, or through unknown mechanisms.

Table 1 CLASSIFICATION OF PNDS ACCORDING TO IMMUNOLOGICAL FINDINGS[a]

Group no.	Immunological findings	Antibody	Tumor	Neurological disorder
1	Mediated by antibodies	Anti-P/Q-type VGCC	SCLC	Lambert–Eaton myasthenic syndrome
	Removal of antibodies results in neurological improvement	Anti-acetylcholine receptor	Thymoma	Myasthenia gravis
	Passive transfer of antibodies causes the disease in animals	Anti-VGKC	Thymoma, SCLC	Neuromyotonia
2	Likely mediated by cytotoxic T cells	Anti-Hu (or ANNA1)	SCLC	Encephalomyelitis; sensory neuronopathy
	Antibodies are present but a pathogenic role has not been proven	Anti-Yo (or PCA-1)	Ovary, breast	Cerebellar degeneration
	Removal of antibodies does not result in neurological improvement	Anti-Ri (or ANNA2)	Breast, SCLC, bladder	Opsoclonus, ataxia, myoclonus
	No animal model	Anti-amphiphysin	Breast, SCLC	Stiff-man syndrome, encephalomyelitis
		Anti-CV2	Thymoma, SCLC	Encephalomyelitis, sensory neuronopathy
		Anti-Ma	Several	Brainstem encephalitis/cerebellar degeneration
		Anti-Ma2 (also called Ta)	Testis	Limbic/brainstem encephalitis
		Anti-Tr	Hodgkin's lymphoma	Cerebellar degeneration
		Anti-PCA-2	SCLC	Several
3	Direct synthesis of IgM by tumor cells	Anti-MAG	Waldenström's macroglobulinemia	Peripheral neuropathy
	Removal of antibodies may result in some neurological improvement	Anti-gangliosides	B cell lymphoma	Peripheral neuropathy

[a] Abbreviations used: VGCC, voltage-gated calcium channel; VGKC, voltage-gated potassium channel; SCLC, small-cell lung cancer; MAG, myelin-associated glycoprotein.

ANTIBODY-MEDIATED DISORDERS

Immune-mediated mechanisms have been demonstrated for the Lambert–Eaton myasthenic syndrome (LEMS), myasthenia gravis, and neuromyotonia. These three disorders share several features: They affect the peripheral nervous system and spare the neuronal body, they are directly mediated by antibodies to antigens (ion channels or receptors) located on the cell surface, removal of serum antibodies (plasma exchange) usually results in neurological improvement, and the disorders have been modeled in animals by passive transfer of patients' sera or IgG.

Patients with LEMS develop antibodies against the P/Q-type voltage-gated calcium channel located in the presynaptic neuromuscular junction. These anti-bodies block the entry of calcium necessary for the quantal release of acetylcholine, resulting in neuromuscular weakness. An antibody-mediated mechanism has also been demonstrated in myasthenia gravis, which in 10% of patients is a paraneoplastic manifestation of a thymic epithelial tumor (thymoma or thymic carcinoma). These patients, as well as most myasthenic patients without thymic tumors, develop antibodies against the acetylcholine receptor of the postsynaptic neuromuscular junction, resulting in muscle weakness and fatigability. Patients with paraneoplastic myasthenia gravis are more likely to harbor anti-titin antibodies than are patients with myasthenia of nonparaneoplastic origin (thymic hyperplasia).

Thymoma is also the tumor most frequently associated with paraneoplastic neuromyotonia.

Patients with this disorder develop antibodies against voltage-gated potassium channels. Patients with neuromyotonia frequently develop an associated peripheral sensorimotor neuropathy and hyperhidrosis.

ANTIBODY-ASSOCIATED DISORDERS THAT ARE LIKELY MEDIATED BY CYTOTOXIC T CELL MECHANISMS

Compared with the disorders in group 1, the PNDs of group 2 share other features: They affect the central nervous system (CNS); the location of the target antigens is intracellular, either predominantly cytoplasmic (CDR, Tr, Ulip, and amphiphysin) or nuclear (Hu proteins and Nova); plasma exchange does not usually improve the neurological symptoms; and passive transfer of patients' sera or IgG, or animal immunization with the onconeuronal antigens, has not modeled the disease.

To date, there is no evidence that the antibodies associated with the PNDs of group 2 are pathogenic. However, a recent report of two patients with a remote history of Hodgkin's disease and cerebellar dysfunction associated with antibodies to mGluR1α demonstrated that intrathecal injection of these antibodies reproduced the disease in animals.

For most PNDs of group 2, there is increasing evidence that cytotoxic T cell-mediated mechanisms play a major pathogenic role. The antigens targeted by these T cells are probably the same as those identified by the accompanying anti-neuronal antibodies, which serve as surrogate markers of the immunological disorder causing the PNDs. The pathogenic role of cytotoxic T cell responses and the mechanisms involved in antigen recognition in the tumor and nervous system have been explored in several studies.

First, autopsies of patients with PNDs of the CNS show intense inflammatory infiltrates of $CD4^+$ and $CD8^+$ T cells, which predominate in the symptomatic areas of the nervous system. Some of these T cell infiltrates are in close contact with neurons, suggesting neuronophagia. Extensive T cell infiltrates have been demonstrated in the nervous system of patients with anti-Hu (also known as ANNA1), anti-Ri (also known as ANNA2), anti-Ma, and anti-Ma2 (also known as anti-Ta) antibodies. Less intense infiltrates of mononuclear cells have also been encountered in the brainstem and deep cerebellar nuclei of patients with anti-Yo (also known as PCA-1) antibodies. The early presence of pleocytosis and

activated Th1 cells in the cerebrospinal fluid of patients with anti-Yo-associated symptoms also suggests that T cell-mediated mechanisms play a pathogenic role.

Second, in patients with the anti-Hu syndrome, specific T cell-mediated immunity has been shown by analysis of peripheral blood lymphocytes. *In vitro* exposure of peripheral blood mononuclear cells from patients with and without the anti-Hu syndrome to the HuD antigen resulted in a significant increase in memory helper T cells in anti-Hu seropositive patients only. The finding of a significant increase in the γ-interferon/interleukin 4 ratio in the anti-Hu seropositive group suggested that the HuD protein is an antigenic target for autoreactive $CD4^+$ T cells of the Th1 subtype, which are capable of directing cell-mediated injury. A pathogenic role of the T cell arm of the immune response was also suggested by the demonstration that the peripheral blood lymphocytes of patients with the anti-Hu syndrome were cytotoxic for autologous fibroblasts manipulated to express HuD and class I major histocompatibility complex (MHC). Furthermore, analysis of T cell receptor usage in the inflammatory infiltrates of the CNS and tumors of patients with immunity to Hu proteins showed overrepresentation of several Vβ families with *in situ* clonal expansion, suggesting that the T cells were specifically targeting neuronal and tumor antigens.

Third, how tumors break immune tolerance for onconeuronal proteins is unknown. Studies suggest that dendritic cells located in tumor-draining lymph nodes play a crucial role in the process of antigen presentation by engulfing tumor cells, processing and presenting the antigen to the immunological system, and thus priming T cell responses. This mechanism has been demonstrated in patients with immunity to CDR2 (a Yo antigen), and a similar mechanism is likely involved in patients with immunity to Hu proteins, accounting for the almost constant and often exclusive detection of small-cell lung cancer in the pulmonary draining lymph nodes of the mediastinum.

Finally, the mechanisms involved in antigen recognition and neuronal damage in the CNS also remain speculative. The conventional view that neurons are immunoprivileged by their location behind the blood–brain barrier and lack of immune recognition molecules has recently been challenged. Activated lymphocytes are able to cross the blood–brain barrier, and recent studies indicate that under certain biological conditions some neurons express high levels of class I MHC. Interestingly, there is a predilection for this to occur in neurons of the limbic region, Purkinje cells, and brainstem, which are common targets of most PNDs.

ANTIBODIES PRODUCED BY TUMORS

The third group of PNDs associated with immunological activity against the nervous system includes the sensory motor neuropathies associated with plasma cell malignancies (i.e., myeloma and Waldenström's macroglobulinemia), leukemias, or lymphomas. In some of these disorders, such as Waldenström's macroglobulinemia, the monoclonal gammopathy may have antibody activity against known peripheral nervous system antigens, including myelin-associated glycoprotein and gangliosides. In other disorders, such as myeloma and Castleman's disease, the specific target antigens are unknown.

Symptoms of lower and upper motor neuron dysfunction, sometimes identical to those of amyotrophic lateral sclerosis, have been identified more frequently than expected in patients with lymphoma. Some of these patients have paraproteinemia and increased cerebrospinal fluid protein and oligoclonal bands, suggesting an immune-mediated pathogenesis; however, no specific B cell or T cell mechanisms have been identified.

—Josep Dalmau

See also–Lambert–Eaton Myasthenic Syndrome; Myasthenia Gravis; Neuroimmunology, Overview; Neurooncology, Overview; Paraneoplastic Syndromes, Central; Stiff-Person Syndrome

Further Reading

Albert, M. L., Austin, L. M., and Darnell, R. B. (2000). Detection and treatment of activated T cells in the cerebrospinal fluid of patients with paraneoplastic cerebellar degeneration. *Ann. Neurol.* 47, 9–17.

Benyahia, B., Liblau, R., Merle-Béral, H., *et al.* (1999). Cell-mediated auto-immunity in paraneoplastic neurologic syndromes with anti-Hu antibodies. *Ann. Neurol.* 45, 162–167.

Corriveau, R. A., Huh, G. S., and Shatz, C. J. (1998). Regulation of class I MHC gene expression in the developing and mature CNS by neural activity. *Neuron* 21, 505–520.

Dalmau, J., and Posner, J. B. (1997). Paraneoplastic syndromes affecting the nervous system. *Semin. Oncol.* 24, 318–328.

Dalmau, J., Graus, F., Rosenblum, M. K., *et al.* (1992). Anti-Hu-associated paraneoplastic encephalomyelitis/sensory neuronopathy. A clinical study of 71 patients. *Medicine* 71, 59–72.

Dimopoulos, M. A., Panayiotidis, P., Moulopoulos, L. A., *et al.* (2000). Waldenstrom's macroglobulinemia: Clinical features, complications, and management. *J. Clin. Oncol.* 18, 214–226.

Drachman, D. B., Angus, C. W., Adams, R. N., *et al.* (1978). Myasthenic antibodies cross-link acetylcholine receptors to accelerate degradation. *N. Engl. J. Med.* 298, 1116–1122.

Ropper, A. H., and Gorson, K. C. (1998). Neuropathies associated with paraproteinemia. *N. Engl. J. Med.* 338, 1601–1607.

Sillevis, S. P., Kinoshita, A., De Leeuw, B., *et al.* (2000). Paraneoplastic cerebellar ataxia due to autoantibodies against a glutamate receptor. *N. Engl. J. Med.* 342, 21–27.

Tanaka, K., Tanaka, M., Inuzuka, T., *et al.* (1999). Cytotoxic T lymphocyte-mediated cell death in paraneoplastic sensory neuronopathy with anti-Hu antibody. *J. Neurol. Sci.* 163, 159–162.

Tanaka, M., Tanaka, K., Shinozawa, K., *et al.* (1998). Cytotoxic T cells react with recombinant Yo protein from a patient with paraneoplastic cerebellar degeneration and anti-Yo antibody. *J. Neurol. Sci.* 161, 88–90.

Voltz, R. D., Albrich, W. C., Nagele, A., *et al.* (1997). Paraneoplastic myasthenia gravis: Detection of anti-MGT30 (titin) antibodies predicts thymic epithelial tumor. *Neurology* 49, 1454–1457.

Voltz, R., Dalmau, J., Posner, J. B., *et al.* (1998). T-cell receptor analysis in anti-Hu associated paraneoplastic encephalomyelitis. *Neurology* 51, 1146–1150.

Younger, D. S., Rowland, L. P., Latov, N., *et al.* (1990). Motor neuron disease and amyotrophic lateral sclerosis: Relation of high CSF protein content to paraproteinemia and clinical syndromes. *Neurology* 40, 595–599.

Paranoia

Encyclopedia of the Neurological Sciences
Copyright 2003, Elsevier Science (USA). All rights reserved.

PARANOIA is a mental phenomenon whereby individuals have a tendency to attribute adverse events to external factors and ascribe threatening intent to the motives of others. In misunderstanding the intentions of others, they blame others for personal difficulties. The severity of paranoia ranges from situation specific, transient mistrust or suspicion on one end of the clinical continuum to chronic delusional beliefs on the other end.

Those with paranoid personality disorder display qualities that endure over time and across situations. They are often suspicious, arrogant, mistrusting, blaming, and unforgiving. Their interpersonal relations are hindered by these characteristics as well as their heightened need for self-sufficiency and control over others.

When stressed, these individuals may develop brief psychotic episodes with prominent delusions. Ongoing psychotic states begin to resemble a delusional disorder or paranoid schizophrenia.

Paranoid or persecutory delusions are found in a variety of disorders. They are one of the most common forms of delusional beliefs. Individuals believe they are monitored, spied on, threatened, controlled, or manipulated. Such beliefs may be present in combination with grandiose, jealous, or other types of delusions. These beliefs may increase the risk of suicidal or assaultive behavior. Deluded individuals may pursue litigation to redress imagined wrongs. They may periodically flee a setting to try to protect themselves.

From a neural circuitry perspective, paranoid or persecutory beliefs may derive from dysregulation of pattern generators that infer causation and assume hostile intent in the face of confusing or upsetting experiences. Aside from the neurobiological basis for paranoid delusions, these thinking disturbances are associated with a broad range of conditions. Substance use, medical and central nervous system disorders, schizophrenia, and mood disorders may generate paranoid delusions.

Treatment involves identifying and managing the underlying disorder. The clinician may reduce the patient's suspicions and sense of vulnerability through respectful and compassionate attention to stated fears, clarification of catalysts of paranoia, and joint exploration and challenge of the evidence supporting the beliefs. The treating clinician may also help the patient to develop a hierarchy of appropriate responses to increased paranoia, review the interpersonal impact from open expression of paranoid delusions, and arrange sufficient physical security.

Antipsychotic medication is most effective in treating acute, poorly organized, and affectively charged delusions. Treatment is often only partially effective with long-standing paranoid delusions. Medication side effects may be perceived and interpreted within the persecutory frame of reference, increasing patient resistance to taking medication. In the case of full-blown or partially symptomatic mood disorders with persecutory delusions, clinicians include antidepressant and/or mood-stabilizer medications in the treatment regimen.

—*Herbert N. Ochitill*

See also–Antidepression Pharmacology; Antipsychotic Pharmacology; Delusions; Mood Disorders, Treatment; Mood Stabilizer Pharmacology; Panic Disorder; Personality Types and Disorders; Phobias

Further Reading
Bentall, R., and Kinderman, P. (1998). Psychological processes and delusional beliefs: Implications for the treatment of paranoid states. In *Outcome and Innovation in Psychological Treatment of Schizophrenia* (T. Wykes and N. Tarrier, Eds.), pp. 119–144. Wiley, Chichester, UK.
Blaney, P. (1999). Paranoid conditions. In *Oxford Textbook of Psychopathology* (T. Millon and P. Blaney, Eds.), pp. 339–361. Oxford Univ. Press, New York.
Fried, Y., and Agassi, J. (1976). *Paranoia: A Study in Diagnosis.* Reidel, Boston.
Kinderman, P., and Bentall, R. (1998). The clinical implications of a psychological model of paranoia. In *Behavior and Cognitive Therapy Today* (E. Sanavio, Ed.), pp. 131–162. Elsevier, Oxford.
Kreitler, S., and Kreitler, H. (1997). The paranoid person: Cognitive motivations and personality traits. *Eur. J. Pers.* **11**, 101–132.
Post, F. (1966). *Persistent Persecutory States of the Elderly.* Pergamon, New York.
Swanson, D., Bohnert, P., and Smith, J. (1970). *The Paranoid.* Little, Brown, Boston.

Paraparesis and Paraplegia

Encyclopedia of the Neurological Sciences
Copyright 2003, Elsevier Science (USA). All rights reserved.

PARAPARESIS is weakness affecting both lower extremities, and paraplegia is paralysis of the lower extremities. Motor control of the legs involves a two-part neuronal system—the upper motor neuron and lower motor neuron pathways. Paraparesis due to lesions of the upper motor neuron is characterized by weakness (affecting flexors more than extensors), spasticity, hyperactivity of the tendon reflexes of the knee and ankle, and the presence of an extensor toe reflex (Babinski sign). The lower motor neuron syndrome, which occurs as a result of injury in the lumbosacral segments or the spinal cord, the corresponding spinal roots, or the peripheral nerves, causes bilateral leg weakness, flaccidity, and loss of tendon reflexes.

Injuries to the upper motor neuron system causing paraparesis can occur at different levels, from the brain down to the spinal cord. In the brain, the lesion seldom affects the cortex in the leg areas of the precentral gyrus, which is located on the medial side of the hemisphere in the paracentral lobule. Because the leg areas from each hemisphere face each other in the interhemisphere fissure, a lesion in this area such as a parasagital meningioma can affect both legs at the same time. Also rare is the paraparesis produced by bilateral lesions in the leg area of the corona radiata or internal capsule. Lesions of the suprathalamic white matter or those of the ventrolateral nucleus of the thalamus may give rise to a marked disequilibrium, with inability to stand but without any apparent limb weakness. This is not strictly paraparesis but may be confused with it in the clinical situation because ambulation is affected and these patients lack signs of vestibular or cerebellar dysfunction.

Most cases of paraparesis from upper motor neuron lesions are due to spinal cord disease. Motor and sensory findings depend on the level of the lesion. Slowly progressive compressive lesions of the cervical cord, as with cervical spondylosis, can cause progressive gait impairment, with brisk reflexes in the legs, Babinski signs, and proprioceptive impairment in the lower extremities. A thoracic spinal cord lesion may cause paraparesis, normal reflexes in the arms, and a thoracic sensory level (loss of sensory sensation below this level), whereas a lumbar spinal cord lesion may cause paraparesis, loss of reflexes in the legs, and sphincter disturbances, with a flaccid bladder and a patulous anal sphincter. The cutaneous sensory level of extramedullary lesions can occur several or many levels lower than the actual lesion. Cervical lesions may present with a thoracic level.

Paraparesis may also result from bilateral involvement of the peripheral nerves or muscles of the legs. As a rule, when the lower motor neuron syndrome affects the peripheral nerves, motor loss tends to involve the distal muscles of the legs more than the proximal ones, whereas the opposite is true of most muscle disorders causing paraparesis. In both instances, sphincter functions are usually spared.

For clinical purposes it is helpful to separate acute (rapid-onset) paraparesis from the chronic (long-standing) ones. The most frequent cause of acute paraparesis is spinal cord trauma. Other causes include demyelinating disease, cord compression by spine metastases, spinal cord stroke, hemorrhage, infections, and acute polyneuritis (Guillain–Barré syndrome). Chronic paraparesis can be classified as those occurring in infancy or those beginning in adult life. Infantile paraparesis can be caused by cerebral palsy, congenital malformation of the spinal cord, or

birth injury. Familial neurodegenerative diseases tend to appear later during childhood and adolescence and are slowly progressive. In adult life, multiple sclerosis, vitamin deficiency, tumors, cervical spondylosis, and infections such as syphilis, fungal, tuberculosis, and other rare spinal cord disturbances such as syringomyelia are relatively common causes of paraparesis.

—*Esther Cubo and Jose Masdeu*

See also–Paralysis; Paresis; Quadriplegia (see also specific disorders)

Further Reading

Adams, R. D., Victor, M., and Ropper, A. H. (1997). *Principles of Neurology*, 6th ed. McGraw-Hill, New York.

Paraplegia
see **Paraparesis and Paraplegia**

Parasites and Neurological Disease, Overview

Encyclopedia of the Neurological Sciences
Copyright 2003, Elsevier Science (USA). All rights reserved.

Whenever an animal is too small and too imperfectly armed to overcome and destroy another living being upon which its instincts direct it to seek nourishment, it must be contented with robbing it, by feasting upon its blood, juices, and solid parts.
—Leuckart (Parasiten and parasitismus, in *Vierordt's Archive*, 1852)

IT IS more than 100 years since Nobel Laureate Sir Ronald Ross, having with others identified the Anopheline vector of malaria, confidently predicted that the disease would be eradicated by draining or otherwise neutralizing stagnant water in the vicinity of human habitation. Sadly, World Health Organization data suggest that more than 40% of the world's population still lives in malarial endemic zones, and there are between 0.5 and 2.5 million fatal cases each year, predominantly in African children. Two thousand cases are imported each year into the United Kingdom and 1000 cases are found in the United States. Despite the clarion advice to travelers, fatal cerebral malaria still occurs in these countries.

Human infection with protozoa and helminths is a major global problem. Recent estimates suggest that

200 million people have schistosomiasis, more than 100 million are infected with lymphatic filiariasis, cysticercosis is present in 1–4% of the population in endemic areas, more than 60 million are at risk of African trypanosomiasis, and similar numbers are at risk of onchocerciasis. For every success story, such as the worldwide eradication of guinea worm or the large-scale clearance of river blindness by invermectin treatment of whole populations, there is the depressing resurgence of other diseases, such as sleeping sickness in war-torn and poverty-stricken central and east Africa.

Transmitted by insect vector, in impure water sources and via the feco-oral route, zoonotic infections are commonly associated with poor hygiene, inadequate living conditions, malnourishment, and deficient health care facilities. These factors are often found combined in poor developing countries in tropical regions where resources are not available for prevention and treatment, and where health education may be nonexistent. Wars and corrupt administration may further compound the problem, whereas in a well-organized local or global campaign, great achievements can be made, such as the successful obliteration of smallpox or near eradication of poliomyelitis worldwide. The spread of parasitic disease is assisted by the modern massive movement of individuals, families, and whole groups in and out of endemic regions. The baleful geographical association of HIV immunosuppression with endemic parasitosis is a potential additional factor in the dissemination of these diseases, such as the case in which toxoplasmosis seizes the opportunity to infect the brain of an AIDS sufferer.

CLASSIFICATION

The only animals which occur as parasites in or upon the human body belong to the classes of insecta and worms, and perhaps also to the infusoria.
—F. Küchenmeister (On Animal and Vegetable Parasites of the Human Body. New Sydenham Society, London, 1887)

Pathogenic human protozoa are found in the phyla Sarcodina, Ciliospora, Mastigophora, and Saporozoa. The helminths that cause disease in man are classified into nematodes (roundworms), trematodes (flatworms), and cestodes (segmented worms). Many protozoal and helminth parasites infest the nervous system and cause neurological disease. These are summarized in Table 1, and some of the more important ones are briefly described in this entry.

PROTOZOA

American trypanosomiasis (Chagas' disease; *Trypanosoma cruzi*) and African trypanosomiasis (sleeping sickness; *T. brucei rhodesiense* and *gambiense*) are clinically distinct conditions, but the organisms share biological characteristics. Chagas' disease develops after an infected assassin bug bites its human prey, inoculating the trypanosome into its new host. Natural reservoirs of infection are found in domestic and wild animals. Hematogenous spread follows, but in many cases the infection is trivial. However, in some cases, especially where immunity is defective, a serious and sometimes fatal illness may follow. The characteristic features of Chagas' disease occur due to involvement of the heart causing cardiomyopathy and the gut giving megaesophagus and megacolon. When the nervous system is affected, patients exhibit cognitive impairment and other signs of encephalopathy, strokes due to embolization from the diseased heart, and also peripheral neuropathy. The trypanosome can be identified in the blood or cerebrospinal fluid or by means of serological tests. Treatment with nifurtimox or benznidazole in the acute phase may be helpful, but the chronic neurological features are often resistant. Although prevalent in South America, this disease is also seen in migrants to North America.

The tsetse fly is the vector of African trypanosomiasis, of which infection reservoirs are present in cattle and other animals. Following inoculation and hematogenous spread, the parasite may lay dormant for months or years before the chronic encephalopathy of sleeping sickness develops. Lassitude, somnolence, and initially subtle psychiatric disturbance are followed by a progressive dementia as well as impairment of coordination, movement, and gait, leading eventually to a bedbound stupor and death. Doctors in the endemic areas of sub-Saharan Africa recognize the characteristic features of this encephalopathy, differentiating it from other conditions. Suramin and pentamidine can be used in early infections, but these drugs do not cross the blood–brain barrier; therefore, for later cases, the toxic arsenical melarsoprol is used, sometimes with a good response. For a disease to which 60 million people are exposed, more effective and safer therapies are desperately needed.

Cerebral malaria is recognized when a severe infection with *Plasmodium falciparum* leads to a state of unrousable coma. This is common in Africa and Southeast Asia, where it is a major killer of

Table 1 PARASITES CAUSING NEUROLOGICAL DISEASE[a]

Group	Organism	Neurological features	Main geographic regions
Protozoa	*Plasmodium falciparum*	Cerebral malaria	Throughout the tropics and subtropics
	Trypanosoma cruzi	Peripheral neuropathy, myositis, and stroke	Central and South America
	Trypanosoma brucei (gambiense and *rhodesiense)*	Sleeping sickness	Equatorial, west and east Africa
	Entamoeba histolytica	Meningoencephalitis, cerebral abscess	Throughout the tropics and subtropics
	Free-living amoebae *(Naegleria fowleri* and *Acanthamoeba)*	Meningitis, granulomatous meningoencephalitis	Worldwide (rare)
	Toxoplasma gondii	Encephalitis, cerebral abscess	Worldwide
	Sarcocystis	Muscle pain and swelling	Worldwide (rare)
	Microsporidiosa	Encephalitis	Japan (case report)
Helminths Nematodes	*Angiostronglyus cantonensis*	Eosinophilic meningoencephalitis	Widespread in tropics, especially Southeast Asia, Pacific Islands
	Gnathostoma spinigerum	Eosinophilic meningoencephalitis	Widespread in tropics, especially Thailand and Japan
	Trichinella spiralis	Muscle pain, meningoencephalitis	Temperate and tropical areas
	Stronglyoides stercoralis	Meningitis, encephalopathy	Patchy in tropics and subtropics
	Toxocara canis	Eosinophilic meningitis, myelitis, encephalitis	Worldwide
	Loa loa	Meningoencephalitis	Central and west Africa
	Dracunculus medinensis	Spinal cord compression	Africa and Asia
	Onchocerca volvulus	Optic atrophy, epilepsy	Mainly west Africa; also South America and Middle East
Trematodes	*Wuchereria bancrofti*	Filariae in CNS	India, widely in tropics and subtropics
	Dipetalonema perstans	Meningoencephalitis	Tropical Africa and America
	Micronema deletrix	Meningoencephalitis	North America (case reports)
Cestodes	*Schistosoma mansoni*	Spinal cord (especially in *S. mansoni* and *hematobium*) and cerebral lesions (especially in *S. japonicum*)	Africa, Brazil, Arabia
	Schistosoma japonicum		China, Indonesia, Philippines
	Schistosoma hematobium		Africa, Arabia, Southwest Asia
	Paragonimus	Epilepsy, cerebral mass lesion, encephalopathy, cord compression	Widespread in tropics, especially the Far East
	Echinococcus granulosus and *multilocularis*	Cerebral or spinal hydatid cysts	Worldwide
	Taenia solium	Fits, cerebral cysts, rarely spinal	Widespread, especially Latin America and India Southeast Asia, east Africa and North America
	Spirometra	Cerebral and spinal sparaganosis (mass lesions)	Temperate and tropical areas (rare)
	Taenia (multiceps)	Similar to *T. solium*	Northern temperate areas and worldwide
	Diphyllobothrium latum	B_{12} deficiency	

[a] Reproduced with permission from Blair, P., and Harris, J. (Eds.) (1999), *Medical Neurotoxicology*, p. 128. E. Arnold, London.

children. Less serious infections with *P. malariae*, *P. vivax*, and *P. ovale* do not cause this complication. Following inoculation of the sporozoite by the female mosquito, the parasite develops in the host liver into a schizont that then spills back into the blood, infecting erythrocytes as the merozoite. This undergoes a cycle through ring forms, trophozoite, and multinucleated schizonts, which rupture to release merozoites capable of infecting fresh erythrocytes to perpetuate the cycle. When some merozoites develop into gametocytes, these can be taken up by another mosquito to complete the sexual cycle and produce another generation of sporozoites.

The clinical hallmark of cerebral malaria is the onset of coma in a febrile patient, and this may develop with frightening rapidity in children. Generalized convulsions occur in 50% of adults and even more commonly in children. Even with successful treatment there may be neurological sequelae in at least 10% of children, including mental deterioration or epilepsy. The mortality of cerebral malaria is as high as 25%.

The pathogenesis of the condition is not fully understood, but it is associated with metabolic and vascular phenomena triggered by the stasis of parasitized erythrocytes in the cerebral circulation. Mechanical effects, activation of abnormal clotting processes, and release of cytokines may all be important. The diagnosis is confirmed by the identification of heavy parasitemia during the examination of thick and thin blood smears or with newer dipstick techniques. Urgent treatment with antimalarial drugs is essential, and most patients are treated with intravenous quinine because of the high prevalence of chloroquine-resistant strains. Recent evaluation of the ancient Chinese remedy extracted from the plant *Artemisia annua* shows that artemisin derivatives are at least as potent as quinine. In addition to chemotherapy, other supportive measures may be necessary to deal with the complications of anemia, renal failure, shock, and hypoglycemia.

Toxoplasmosis has become an increasingly important protozoal parasite, causing neurological disease in the modern AIDS era in which 5–20% of cases have cerebral toxoplasmosis. This ubiquitous obligate intracellular sporozoan can infect congenitally to cause cerebral calcification, mental retardation, ocular abnormality, or hydrocephalus, and it may lead to intrauterine death, although infection is often silent. Acquired toxoplasmosis develops after ingestion of tainted meat or by feco-oral spread from infected pets. The primary infection may be silent or give an acute febrile illness, but after a latent period the immune-incompetent patient is at risk from a subacute encephalitis or cerebral mass lesions. There is a high index of suspicion in people with HIV; the condition can be readily confirmed by computed tomography (CT) or magnetic resonance imaging (MRI), and treatment with a pyrimethamine–sulfadiazine combination or alternative such as clindamycin is usually successful.

Other protozoan causes of neurological diseases are rare.

HELMINTHS

Neurocysticercosis is the most common worm infestation causing central nervous system disease. Man is the definitive host, harboring the mature *Taenia solium* cestode worm in the gut, from which proglottide segments containing ova are regularly excreted. The pig is the usual intermediate host and reservoir for human taeniasis; hence, the life cycle only continues where man and pig are in close proximity. When eggs are ingested by the feco-oral route as a result of poor hygiene, man also becomes an intermediate host. The eggs migrate from the gut to other tissues, including the brain, and transform into the larval cysticercus stage. Thus, consumption of infected pork leads to intestinal infestation with an adult worm, but non-pork eaters may be infected with eggs transmitted by an unclean food handler and develop neurocysticercosis. This explains cases in Muslims and the recent outbreak in an orthodox Jewish community in New York.

Cysticercosis is common in rural populations in Latin America, Asia, and Africa, and cases are seen in large Western cities that accommodate migrants from these areas. It is often asymptomatic and has been found in up to 3.6% of autopsies conducted in Mexico. Cerebral cysts commonly cause seizures, and it is thought that worldwide, cysticercosis is the most prolific cause of epilepsy. Less commonly, parenchymal cysts present as mass lesions or with increased intracranial pressure. Meningeal cysts may obstruct cerebrospinal fluid circulation and cause hydrocephalus, as also occurs with intraventricular cysts. Strokes are seen in parenchymal or meningeal disease. Spinal cord cysts are much rarer. The appearance of the cysts on a CT or MRI brain scan can be characteristic, showing the scolex surrounded by the cyst wall, both of which eventually calcify. Other tests for cysticercosis, including serological investigation, are often less helpful.

Cysticidal drugs are effective in neurocysticercosis, although treatment is futile in cases in which the cysts are shown to already be dead and calcified. The common problem in India and South America of a solitary calcified cerebral cyst presenting with focal or generalized epileptic seizures is best treated by anticonvulsants and sequential observation. Where antihelminthic drugs are indicated, albendazole is usually the first choice, with praziquantel as an alternative. Steroids are sometimes necessary to prevent a potentially dangerous immune-mediated encephalopathic reaction as the cerebral larvae are killed.

Cysticercosis could be eradicated in endemic zones if human and animal living environments were separated, food handlers practiced thorough personal hygiene, and pigs were effectively inspected before meat entered the food market.

Schistosomiasis causes human disease throughout Africa (*Schistosoma mansoni* and *S. hematobium*), in Southeast Asia, China, and Japan (*S. japonicum*), and it is also found in South America and the Caribbean. Man is the host for the adult worm, which resides in the bladder or bowel and excretes eggs that develop into larvae and find their way to freshwater snails, in which further transition into free-swimming cercariae takes place, followed by penetration of submerged skin to reinfect a human host. The disease is common in endemic regions, affecting the local population and also visitors, as many people have discovered after swimming in Lake Malawi and other infected African lakes.

Cerebral or spinal schistosomiasis is relatively rare but should be suspected in an endemic area when patients present with an acute or chronic encephalopathy (cerebral) or with a painful paraparesis (spinal). Identification of the correct diagnosis is understandably difficult because sophisticated or even simple investigations are unlikely to be available to help differentiate cerebral schistosomiasis from brain tumor, cerebral complication of HIV or sleeping sickness, or spinal schistosomiasis from HTLV-1 infection or malignant cord compression. However, if the diagnosis is considered likely, then there is usually a good response to praziquantel treatment augmented by steroids.

Eosinophilic meningoencephalitis is seen in Southeast Asia, Japan, Korea, Taiwan, and China, as well as in Papua New Guinea and the Pacific Islands. Infections by the rat lungworm *Angiostrongylus cantonensis*, *Gnathostoma spinigerum*, or *Paragonimus* sp. may be suspected in the appropriate endemic region. Ingestion of raw snails, raw shellfish, and unwashed vegetables is unwise in these areas.

The characteristic clinical features are subacute or chronic meningitis or meningoencephalitis in which blood and cerebrospinal fluid examination reveals plentiful eosinophils. Antihelminthic drugs (praziquantel) and, in some cases, surgery may be successful in removing the worm, but in other cases the disease follows its course and can be fatal.

Hydatid disease is caused by two species of the cestode worm Echinococcus (*Echinococcus granulosus* and *E. multilocularis*) where there is close proximity to infected domestic animals (dog, cat, sheep, and cattle). Usually, the liver or the lungs are affected, but cysts can grow in the brain and rarely invade the spinal extradural space and compress the spinal cord. Albendazole is effective in extracerebral disease, but surgical treatment is necessary in cerebral hydatid disease, in which the cyst has to be aspirated or delivered whole without spilling its contents and disseminating infective daughter cysts (protoscolices). Recurrence rates are high in this condition, occurring in at least 25% of cases.

Other rare helminth infestations of the nervous system are beyond the scope of this entry but are discussed in the references listed under Further Reading.

CONCLUSION

Parasitic neurological disorders should be considered in residents in endemic regions, in patients returning from travel to these areas, and in people who are immunosuppressed due to medication or concurrent disease. Some conditions, such as a solitary cerebral cyst in neurocysticercosis, are benign, but others, if untreated, will follow a progressive and sometimes fatal course. In most cases, correct identification of the clinical entity will lead to successful treatment. Careful precautions by travelers to avoid infection and good hygiene practice in endemic regions should prevent most cases.

—Peter K. Newman

***See also*—Tropical Neurology (see also specific entries in the Parasitic Infections section)**

Further Reading

Cetron, M. S., Chitsulo, L., Sullivan, J. J., *et al.* (1996). Schistosomiasis in Lake Malawi. *Lancet* 348, 1274–1278.

Cook, G. C. (Ed.) (1996). *Manson's Tropical Disease*, 20th ed. Saunders, London.

Kirchhoff, L. V. (1993). American trypanosomiasis (Chagas' disease): A tropical disease now in the United States. *N. Engl. J. Med.* **329**, 639–644.

Liu, L. X., and Weller, P. F. (1996). Drug therapy. Antiparasitic drugs. *N. Engl. J. Med.* **334**, 1178–1184.

Newton, C. R., Tran, T. H., and White, N. (2000). Cerebral malaria. *J. Neurol. Neurosurg. Psychiatry* **69**, 433–441.

Porter, S. B., and Sande, M. A. (1992). Toxoplasmosis of the central nervous system in the acquired immune deficiency syndrome. *N. Engl. J. Med.* **327**, 1643–1648.

Schantz, P. J. M., Moore, A. C., Munoz, J. L., *et al.* (1992). Neurocysticercosis in an orthodox Jewish community in New York City. *N. Engl. J. Med.* **327**, 692–695.

Shakir, R. A., Newman, P. K., and Poser, C. M. (1996). *Tropical Neurology.* Saunders, London.

Strickland, G. T. (Ed.) (1991). *Hunter's Tropical Medicine*, 7th ed. Saunders, Philadelphia.

Parasomnias

Encyclopedia of the Neurological Sciences

PARASOMNIAS are defined as experiential or unpleasant or undesirable behavioral phenomena that occur predominately or exclusively during the sleep period. These were initially thought to represent a unitary phenomenon, often attributed to psychiatric disease. Recent clinical and polygraphic analysis has revealed that they are, in fact, the result of a large number of completely different conditions, most of which are diagnosable and treatable. Most are not the manifestation of psychiatric disorders and are far more prevalent than previously suspected. There are many parasomnias, and they may be conveniently categorized as primary (disorders of the sleep states per se) and secondary (disorders of other organ systems that manifest themselves during sleep). The primary sleep parasomnias can be classified according to the sleep state of origin: rapid eye movement (REM) sleep, non-rapid eye movement (N-REM) sleep, or miscellaneous (those not respecting sleep state). The secondary sleep parasomnias can be further classified by the organ system involved. Only the most common will be discussed in this entry.

PATHOPHYSIOLOGY

Integral to the understanding of the parasomnias is the concept of state-dependent reorganization of the central nervous system (CNS). Decades ago, it was believed that sleep was a unitary phenomenon and simply represented the passive absence of wakefulness, a period of relative brain inactivity. It is now known that sleep is actually an active, bimodal process (REM and N-REM), indicating that humans, as most mammals, spend their lives in three completely different states of being: wakefulness, REM sleep, and N-REM sleep. Each of these states has its unique neuroanatomical, neurophysiological, neurochemical, and neuropharmacological correlates.

Parasomnias are clinical phenomena that appear as the brain becomes reorganized across states; therefore, they are particularly apt to occur during the transition periods from one state to another. There is compelling evidence that there is extensive reorganization of CNS activity during sleep. Almost all portions of the nervous system are active across all three states of being, but they are active in a different mode. The concept of state dissociation in animals and humans has been extensively reviewed. Such waking-dissociated states likely play a role in many human parasomnias.

COMMON PARASOMNIAS

Primary Sleep Phenomena

REM Phenomena—Normal: Conventional dreams are normal events that occur during sleep. Dreaming may occur in all stages of sleep and may even occur during relaxed wakefulness.

Dream anxiety attacks (nightmares) are simply frightening dreams, frequently associated with moderate autonomic activity (tachycardia, tachypnea, and diaphoresis) and arousal. There is usually immediate return of complete alertness, with recollection of the dream events that resulted in arousal. The immediate postarousal alertness and the vivid memory of the dream content differentiate nightmares from disorders of arousal.

Sleep paralysis and hypnagogic (occurring at sleep onset) or hypnopompic (occurring upon awakening) hallucinations are experienced by many normal individuals, particularly in the setting of sleep deprivation.

REM Phenomena—Abnormal: REM sleep behavior disorder (RBD) is discussed elsewhere in this encyclopedia.

N-REM Sleep Phenomena—Normal: There are a number of normal N-REM phenomena that may result in clinical symptoms or complaints, often resulting in medical consultation.

First, the oft-stated dichotomy between REM and N-REM and dreaming and not-dreaming is not always the case. Prominent vivid dream-like mentation may occur at sleep onset, during light N-REM sleep, and even during relaxed wakefulness.

Second, sleep starts (hypnic jerks) are experienced by many normal individuals during the transition between wake and sleep. The most common is the motor sleep start, which is a sudden jerk of all or part of the body, occasionally awakening the victim or bed partner. However, variations on this theme are less well-known and may result in unnecessary neurological consultation. These include the visual (flashes of light and fragmentary visual hallucinations), auditory (loud bangs and snapping noises; also termed the exploding head syndrome), or somesthetic (pain, floating, or something flowing through the body) sleep start. These sensory phenomena may occur without the body jerk.

N-REM Phenomena—Abnormal: Disorders of arousal are the most impressive and most frequent of the N-REM sleep phenomena. The disorders of arousal are prevalent (and perfectly normal) in childhood and are far more common in adults (4–10%) than generally acknowledged. These share common features: They tend to arise from any stage of N-REM sleep, most commonly from the deepest stages (slow-wave sleep), and therefore usually occur in the first third of the sleep cycle (and rarely during naps); and they are common in childhood, usually decreasing in frequency with increasing age. There is often a family history of disorders of arousal. Disorders of arousal occur on a broad spectrum ranging from confusional arousals to somnambulism (sleep walking) and sleep terrors (also termed pavor nocturnus). Some take the form of "specialized" behaviors, such as sleep-related eating and sleep-related sexual activity, without conscious awareness.

Confusional arousals are often seen in children and are characterized by movements in bed, occasionally thrashing about, or inconsolable crying. "Sleep drunkenness" is probably a variation on this theme.

Sleepwalking may be either calm or agitated, with varying degrees of complexity and duration. It is characterized by complex, automatic behaviors, such as aimlessly wandering about, nonsensically carrying objects from one place to another, rearranging furniture, inappropriately eating, urinating in closets, going outdoors, and, very rarely, driving an automobile. The eyes are usually wide open and have a glassy stare, and there may be some mumbling.

However, communication with a sleepwalker is usually poor or impossible. The episodes usually occur 15–120 min after sleep onset but can occur throughout the entire sleep period in adults. The duration of each episode can vary widely. Frenzied or aggressive behavior, the wielding of weapons (knives or guns), or the calm suspension of judgment (e.g., going out a bedroom window or wandering far outdoors) can result in inadvertent injury or death to self or others.

Sleep terrors are the most dramatic form of disorder of arousal. They are frequently initiated by a loud, blood-curdling scream associated with extreme panic, followed by prominent motor activity such as hitting the wall, running around or out of the bedroom or even out of the house, resulting in bodily injury or property damage. A universal feature is inconsolability. Although the victim appears to be awake, they usually misperceive the environment, and attempts at consolation are fruitless and may serve only to prolong and intensify the confusional state. Some degree of perception may be evident—for example, running for and opening a door or window. Complete amnesia for the activity is typical but may be incomplete. Although usually benign, these behaviors may be violent, resulting in considerable injury to the victim or others or damage to the environment, occasionally with forensic implications.

Disorders of arousal may be triggered by febrile illness, alcohol, prior sleep deprivation, physical activity, and emotional stress. Medication-induced cases have been reported with sedative/hypnotics, neuroleptics, minor tranquilizers, stimulants, and antihistamines, often in combination with each other.

Persistence of these behaviors beyond childhood or their development in adulthood is often taken as an indication of significant psychopathology. Numerous studies have dispelled this myth, indicating that significant psychopathology is usually not present in adults with disorders of arousal. These arousals may not be the culmination of ongoing psychologically significant mentation because sleepwalking can be induced in normal children by standing them up during slow-wave sleep and sleep terrors can be precipitously triggered in susceptible individuals by sounding a buzzer during slow-wave sleep.

Treatment is often not necessary. Reassurance of their typically benign nature, lack of psychological significance, and the tendency to diminish over time is often sufficient. The tricyclic antidepressants and benzodiazepines may be effective, and they should be administered if the behaviors are dangerous to person or property or extremely disruptive to family members. Nonpharmacological treatment such as hypnosis is recommended for long-term management. The avoidance of precipitants such as drugs, alcohol, and sleep deprivation is also important.

Miscellaneous Primary Sleep Parasomnias

There are a number of poorly understood primary sleep phenomena that appear not to respect sleep stages. Bruxism (tooth grinding) and enuresis are often classified as parasomnias, but are beyond the scope of this entry. Importantly, there is little, if any, evidence that these disorders are the manifestation or consequence of underlying psychiatric or psychological conditions.

Rhythmic movement disorder (RMD) (formerly termed jactatio capitis nocturna) refers to a group of behaviors characterized by stereotyped movements (rhythmic oscillation of the head or limbs, head banging or body rocking during sleep) seen most frequently in childhood and rarely in adults. It may be familial in some cases. RMD may arise from all stages of sleep, including REM sleep, and may occur in the transition from wake to sleep.

Posttraumatic stress disorder (PTSD) is often associated with subjective sleep complaints, including nightmares and sleep terror-like experiences. Recent detailed objective studies of sleep in PTSD sufferers have generally been strikingly unremarkable, suggesting a discrepancy between subjective sleep perception and objective sleep evaluation in those individuals.

Somniloquy (sleep talking) is very common in the general population, may have a genetic component, may occur in either REM or N-REM sleep, and is of no apparent clinical or psychological significance.

Secondary Sleep Phenomena

The secondary phenomena are those parasomnias representing either abnormal or excessive autonomic or physiological events arising from specific organ systems and occurring preferentially during the sleep period. These can be approached by the organ system involved.

Central Nervous System Parasomnias

Nocturnal Seizures: Most nocturnal seizures present little diagnostic difficulty; however, it must be remembered that any behavior or experience, regardless of the clinical feature, that is recurrent,

stereotyped, and inappropriate may be the manifestation of a seizure. Exclusively nocturnal seizures with extremely bizarre behaviors are not uncommon, but they are routinely misdiagnosed. Seizures emanating from the frontal lobe are a common culprit: Their tendency for bizarre behaviors, exclusively nocturnal timing, and clustering in time all predispose to a psychiatric misdiagnosis. Interictal (and often ictal) electroencephalograms may be unrevealing. Treatment with anticonvulsant medication is often effective.

"Vascular" Headaches: The headache symptoms of cluster headache, chronic paroxysmal hemicrania, and possibly migraines in some cases tend to be REM sleep related, explaining the common report of sleep-related headaches in these conditions.

Cardiopulmonary Parasomnias

In some individuals, cardiac arrhythmias, angina pectoris, and asthma may be sleep-period related, but no generalizations are possible.

Gastrointestinal Parasomnias

Numerous gastrointestinal events may result in paroxysmal arousals during sleep, often mimicking disorders of other organ systems. These include gastroesophageal reflux and sleep-related diffuse esophageal spasm.

Miscellaneous Secondary Parasomnias

Nocturnal Panic Attacks: Sleep-related panic attacks may occur in many (one-third to one-half) patients with diurnal panic, may precede the appearance of diurnal panic, or may be exclusively nocturnal in nature. The striking similarity of the symptoms of dream anxiety attacks, sleep terrors, nocturnal seizures, sleep apnea, and nighttime panic indicates that caution should be used in diagnosis.

Psychogenic Dissociative States: Complex, potentially injurious behavior, occasionally confined to the sleep period, may be the manifestation of a psychogenic dissociative state. Unlike the other parasomnias that arise precipitously from sleep, the psychogenic dissociative disorders arise from a period of wakefulness during the sleep period. A history of childhood physical and/or sexual abuse is virtually always present (but may be difficult to elicit).

Nocturnal Muscle Cramps: The complaint of muscle cramping, frequently nocturnal, is extremely common but poorly understood. The true incidence

Table 1 CLASSIFICATION OF THE COMMON PARASOMNIAS

Primary sleep phenomena
  REM phenomena
    Normal
      Dreams and dream anxiety attacks (nightmares)
      Sleep paralysis, hypnagogic and hypnopompic
        hallucinations
    Abnormal
      REM sleep behavior disorder
  N-REM phenomena
    Normal
      Hypnagogic imagery
      Sleep starts (hypnic jerks)
    Abnormal—disorders of arousal
      Confusional arousals
      Sleepwalking
      Sleep terrors
    Miscellaneous
      Bruxism
      Enuresis
      Rhythmic movement disorder
      Posttraumatic stress disorder
      Somniloquy
Secondary sleep phenomena
  Central nervous system
    Seizures
    Headaches
  Cardiopulmonary
    Cardiac arrhythmias
    Nocturnal angina pectoris
    Nocturnal asthma
  Gastrointestinal
    Gastroesophageal reflux
    Diffuse esophageal spasm
  Miscellaneous
    Nocturnal panic attacks
    Psychogenic dissociative states
    Nocturnal muscle cramps

and etiology are unknown, and there has been no systematic study of nocturnal muscle cramps.

Table 1 outlines the common parasomnias.

CLINICAL AND LABORATORY EVALUATION

Isolated, often bizarre, sleep-related events may be experienced by perfectly normal people, and most do not warrant further extensive or expensive evaluation. The initial approach to the complaint of unusual sleep-related behavior is to determine whether further evaluation is necessary. The patient should be queried regarding the exact nature of the events. Because many of these episodes may be associated with partial or complete amnesia, additional descriptive information from a bed partner or other observer may prove invaluable. Home video-

tapes of the clinical event may be quite helpful. In general, indications for formal evaluation of parasomnias include behaviors that (i) are potentially violent or injurious; (ii) are extremely disruptive to other household members; (iii) result in the complaint of excessive daytime sleepiness; or (iv) are associated with medical, psychiatric, or neurological symptoms or findings.

Evaluation by experienced sleep medicine professionals usually leads to a specific diagnosis, with effective therapeutic recommendations.

CONCLUSION

The three states of mammalian being—wakefulness, REM sleep, and N-REM sleep—are not mutually exclusive and may occur simultaneously, oscillate rapidly, or appear in dissociated or incomplete form to produce primary sleep parasomnias. Dysfunction of a wide variety of organ systems may present during the sleeping state, resulting in the secondary sleep parasomnias. Contrary to popular opinion, the majority of these often bizarre and frightening experiences are not the manifestation of underlying psychological or psychiatric conditions. Formal study in an experienced sleep disorders center will usually reveal a diagnosable and treatable condition. Various parasomnias may result in injurious or violent behavior.

—*Mark W. Mahowald and Carlos H. Schenck*

***See also**–Dreaming; Nightmares; NREM (Non Rapid Eye Movement) Sleep; Panic Disorder; REM (Rapid Eye Movement) Sleep; Sleep Disorders; Sleep, Overview; Wakefulness*

Further Reading

Hurwitz, T. D., Mahowald, M. W., Kuskowski, M., *et al.* (1998). Polysomnographic sleep is not clinically impaired in Vietnam combat veterans with chronic posttraumatic stress disorder. *Biol. Psychiatry* **44**, 1066–1073.

Lavigne, G. J., and Manzini, C. (2000). Sleep bruxism and concomitant oro-motor activity. In *Principles and Practice of Sleep Medicine* (M. H. Kryger, T. Roth, and W. C. Dement, Eds.). Saunders, Philadelphia.

Mahowald, M. W., and Ettinger, M. G. (1990). Things that go bump in the night—The parasomnias revisited. *J. Clin. Neurophysiol.* **7**, 119–143.

Mahowald, M. W., and Schenck, C. H. (1996). NREM parasomnias. *Neurol. Clin.* **14**, 675–696.

Mahowald, M. W., and Schenck, C. H. (1997). Sleep disorders. In *Epilepsy: A Comprehensive Textbook* (J. Engel, Jr., and T. A. Pedley, Eds.), pp. 2705–2715. Lippincott-Raven, Philadelphia.

Mahowald, M. W., and Schenck, C. H. (2000). Parasomnias: Sleepwalking and the law. *Sleep Med. Rev.* **4**, 321–339.

Mahowald, M. W., and Schenck, C. H. (2001). Evolving concepts of human state dissociation. *Arch. Ital. Biol.* **139**, 269–300.

Mahowald, M. W., Bundlie, S. R., Hurwitz, T. D., *et al.* (1990). Sleep violence–forensic science implications: Polygraphic and video documentation. *J. Forensic Sci.* **35**, 413–432.

Nielsen, T. A. (1999). Mentation during sleep: The NREM/REM distinction. In *Handbook of Behavioral State Control. Cellular and Molecular Mechanisms* (R. Lydic and H. A. Baghdoyan, Eds.), pp. 101–128. CRC Press, Boca Raton, FL.

Nielsen, T. A., and Zadra, A. (2000). Dreaming disturbances. In *Principles and Practice of Sleep Medicine* (M. H. Kryger, T. Roth, and W. C. Dement, Eds.). Saunders, Philadelphia.

Schenck, C. H., Milner, D., Hurwitz, T. D., *et al.* (1989). Dissociative disorders presenting as somnambulism: Polysomnographic, video and clinical documentation (8 cases). *Dissociation* **2**, 194–204.

Parasympathetic System, Overview

Encyclopedia of the Neurological Sciences
Copyright 2003, Elsevier Science (USA). All rights reserved.

THE PARASYMPATHETIC NERVOUS SYSTEM is critical for pupil constriction in response to light, lacrimal and salivary secretion, beat-to-beat control of the heart rate, coordinated gastrointestinal motility and secretion, evacuation of the bladder and rectum, and reflex penile erection. Like the sympathetic system, the parasympathetic system is a two-neuron outflow. It is referred to as craniosacral system because its preganglionic neurons are located either in brainstem nuclei or at the sacral spinal cord segments S2–S4. The parasympathetic ganglia are located just outside or even within the wall of the target organ. Both the preganglionic neurons and the neurons of the parasympathetic ganglia utilize acetylcholine as their primary neurotransmitter. Preganglionic inputs excite the parasympathetic ganglion cells via cholinergic nicotinic receptors. Neurotransmission in parasympathetic ganglia is regulated by presynaptic autoreceptors in preganglionic nerve terminals. Acetylcholine acts via different subtypes of muscarinic receptors in the target organs. The M1 receptors stimulate gastric acid and bronchial secretions, the M2 receptors are responsible for cardiac inhibition, and the M3 receptors stimulate smooth muscle and secretomotor activity. Many parasympathetic cholinergic neurons also release vasoactive intestinal polypeptide (VIP) and other neuropeptides as well as nitric oxide (NO).

The cranial parasympathetic neurons are located in the general visceral efferent column of the midbrain, pons, and medulla. Their preganglionic axons are components of cranial nerves III, VII, IX, and X. Parasympathetic axons innervating the eye originate in the Edinger–Westphal nucleus and are carried via the oculomotor nerve (cranial nerve III) through the cavernous sinus and superior orbital fissure to reach the orbit, where they synapse on the ciliary ganglion, located against the surface of the optic nerve. The ciliary ganglion axons form the short ciliary nerves that innervate the sphincter of the iris to elicit constriction of the pupil and the smooth muscle of the ciliary body to elicit accommodation of the lens. The preganglionic neurons of the superior salivatory nucleus, located in the pons, project via the intermediate portion of the facial nerve (cranial nerve VII), and their axons pass by way of the greater petrosal nerve to reach the pterygopalatine ganglion or the chorda tympani to reach the submandibular ganglion. Neurons of the pterygopalatine ganglion stimulate secretion of the lacrimal gland and glands of the mucous membrane of the nose and palate, and they elicit vasodilation of blood vessels of the face. The submandibular ganglion stimulates secretion of the submandibular and sublingual salivary glands. The preganglionic neurons of the inferior salivatory nucleus project via the glossopharyngeal nerve (cranial nerve IX) by way of the minor petrosal nerve to synapse in the otic ganglion, which stimulates secretion of the parotid gland. The cholinergic muscarinic secretomotor effect of the parasympathetic system is potentiated by the potent vasodilator effect of VIP.

The vagus nerve (cranial nerve X) provides the most widespread brainstem parasympathetic output. Vagal motoneurons located in the compact region of the nucleus ambiguus innervate the esophagus, and those in the ventrolateral portion of the nucleus provide the major preganglionic output to the heart. The largest source of vagal preganglionic fibers is the dorsal nucleus of the vagus nerve (DVN), which innervates essentially all thoracic and abdominal viscera except the distal colon and rectum. The DVN together with the nucleus of the solitary tract and the area postrema form an anatomofunctional unit referred to as the dorsal vagal complex. The DVN has a viscerotopic and columnar organization; this functional topography allows selective effects of afferent and descending influences on specific vagal-mediated functions. Its main effects are cardioinhibitory, visceromotor, and secretomotor. Most of the postganglionic neurons in the vagal pathways are located in ganglia that form plexuses located close to the target tissues. The major effect of the vagus in the heart is to reduce heart rate by reducing the firing discharge frequency of the sinoatrial node via muscarinic M2 receptors coupled to G protein-activated inward rectifying K^+ channels. Spontaneous and baroreflex-induced firing of central cardiovagal neurons is inhibited during inspiration and is maximal during early expiration. This is the basis of the respiratory sinus arrhythmia. Heart rate variability is inversely correlated with age in resting normal subjects. The vagus also reduces atrioventricular conduction and increases the ventricular refractory period. Vagal stimulation also reduces contractility of the atria and to a much lesser extent the ventricles. The vagal control of the airways is mediated via microganglia associated with the pulmonary plexus. The postganglionic neurons are of two types. Most neurons are cholinergic and stimulate bronchial constriction via M3 muscarinic receptors. Some neurons mediate relaxation of the tracheobronchial smooth muscles, which may be mediated by VIP or NO. Vagal inputs to the alimentary tract influence primarily the esophagus and stomach. The vagus provides both excitatory and inhibitory inputs to its final effectors. The vagus input is tonically active and mediated via postganglionic cholinergic neurons activating muscarinic receptors. The alternative pathways may involve postganglionic neurons that release VIP or other substances or cholinergic muscarinic activation of the release of local hormones. The esophageal branches are located above and below the pulmonary branches and form the esophageal plexus. The vagus may elicit contraction of the lower esophageal sphincter, via activation of postganglionic cholinergic neurons, or relaxation, perhaps via VIP-containing neurons. The vagus causes relaxation of smooth muscle in the proximal stomach (receptive relaxation) that may be mediated by VIP. At other times, the vagus stimulates motility in the distal stomach and thus gastric emptying, which is mediated by intrinsic cholinergic neurons. The vagus stimulates hydrochloric acid secretion via activation of postganglionic cholinergic neurons that directly excite parietal cells or via intrinsic neurons that release gastrin-releasing peptide and stimulate the release of gastrin from gastric mucosal G cells. In addition, the vagus may inhibit gastrin secretion via a postganglionic cholinergic stimulation of D cells that release somatostatin. In the gut, vagal efferents modulate a variety of local reflexes mediated by neurons of the enteric nervous system (ENS). The ENS contains approximately 100 million neurons that receive inputs from approximately 30,000 vagal efferents. The ENS consists of sensory neurons, interneurons, and motor neurons that form integrative local circuits and reflexes involved in the control of peristalsis and secretion. These reflexes are modulated both by vagal cholinergic inputs from the dorsal vagal nucleus and by sympathetic noradrenergic inputs from the prevertebral ganglia. The ENS consists of two major ganglionated plexuses, the myenteric plexus (of Auerbach), located between the longitudinal and circular muscle layers and extending from the pharyngoesophageal junction to the internal anal sphincter, and the submucosal plexus (of Meissner), which is confined to the small and large intestines. The hepatic branches of the vagus reach the gallbladder and stimulate contractility through intrinsic cholinergic neurons via muscarinic receptors, VIP-containing neurons, or an excitatory effect on secretion of cholecystokinin from the duodenum. Vagal preganglionic branches to the celiac and superior mesenteric plexuses reach small ganglia in the pancreas. At least some of these neurons are cholinergic and some contain VIP. The vagus stimulates a resting secretion of bicarbonate, but its main effect is to increase enzyme secretion via cholinergic muscarinic mechanisms. Branches of the right vagus innervate the pancreatic islets. Vagal inputs increase secretion of somatostatin and pancreatic polypeptide, which in turn inhibit enzyme and bicarbonate secretion.

The sacral parasympathetic nucleus (SPN), located at the S2–S4 segments of the spinal cord, contains preganglionic neurons that project pelvic splanchnic nerves to ganglion cells in the pelvic plexus and in the ganglia located in the walls of the bladder, rectum, and sexual organs. The sacral parasympathetic outflow is critical for evacuation of the bladder and rectum and reflex vasodilatation of the erectile tissue in sexual organs of men and women. Transmission in the bladder ganglia is mediated by nicotinic cholinergic receptors and can be modulated by muscarinic, adrenergic, and peptidergic receptors. For example, lumbar sympathetic noradrenergic inputs presynaptically modulate transmission in the bladder parasympathetic ganglia. The excitatory effect of the parasympathetic system on the bladder detrusor is mediated both by acetylcholine, via M2- and M3-type receptors, and by ATP, via P2X purinergic receptors. Modulatory prejunctional receptors, including M1 excitatory and M4 inhibitory auto-receptors, regulate the release of acetylcholine in the bladder. Parasympathetic fibers also release NO, which relaxes the urethral smooth muscle. The central reflex control of the pelvic organs involves coordinated activity between the sacral parasympathetic outflow and the lumbar sympathetic and sacral somatomotor outflow. The lumbar sympathetic output originates in the T11–L2 segments, relays either in the lumbar paravertebral or in the inferior mesenteric ganglia, and via the hypogastric and pelvic nerves produces relaxation of the bladder or rectum and contraction of the smooth muscle of the internal sphincters, thus promoting urinary and fecal retention. The sympathetic system promotes emission of sperm and contributes to psychogenic erection. The sacral somatomotor output arises from alpha motoneurons in the Onuf nucleus at segments S2 and S3; via the pudendal nerves, it produces activation of the striated muscle of the external urinary and anal sphincters, pelvic floor, and bulbo- and ischiocavernous muscles. During the storage and expulsion phases of the bladder and rectum, there is a reciprocal activation of the SPN and the Onuf nucleus. Normal micturition depends on a suprasp-inal pathway integrated at the level of the pons and is critical for the coordinated activation of sacral parasympathetic and inhibition of sacral sphincter motoneurons. The rostral dorsolateral pons contains a medial (M) region that corresponds to the classic pontine micturition center, stimulates sacral parasympathetic neurons, and inhibits a more laterally located region in the pons (L region) that innervates the motor neurons of the Onuf nucleus. The preganglionic neurons of the SPN provide an excitatory input to parasympathetic ganglion cells of the pelvic plexus that via the cavernous nerves elicit vasodilatation of penile arteries and relaxation of venous sinusoids in the erectile tissue, resulting in increase in blood flow, expansion of the sinusoidal spaces, and penile erection. The primary neurochem-ical transmitter involved is NO via accumulation of cyclic GMP (cGMP), a potent vasodilator. An increase in the level of cGMP by inhibiting the activity of the cGMP phosphodiesterase 5 isoenzyme is the mechanism by which sildenafil (Viagra) improves male erectile dysfunction. VIP coexists with acetylcholine in postganglionic fibers innervat-ing the penis and may contribute to erection. The parasympathetic input to the distal colon and rectum passes through the pelvic nerve, pelvic plexus, colonic ganglia, and colonic fiber bundles to the large intestine. Sacral parasympathetic inputs provide phasic excitation to the rectal smooth muscle and inhibition of the circular smooth muscle of the internal anal sphincter during defecation. Pregan-glionic fibers in the pelvic nerve synapse with neurons in the peripheral ganglia on the serosal surface of the distal colon and rectum; synaptic inputs are excitatory and mediated by cholinergic nicotinic receptors. Some preganglionic neurons also contain enkephalin, which may produce inhibition of synaptic transmission at the level of the ganglia. Sacral preganglionic fibers synapse with both choli-nergic and nonadrenergic, noncholinergic (NANC) neurons of the myenteric plexus. Cholinergic neurons excite longitudinal smooth muscle, whereas NANC neurons inhibit the internal anal sphincter, perhaps via release of VIP or NO.

—*Eduardo E. Benarroch*

See also–Autonomic Nervous System, Overview; Central Nervous System Infections, Overview; Motor System, Overview; Sensory System, Overview; Sympathetic System, Overview; Vagus Nerve (Cranial Nerve X); Vertebrate Nervous System, Development of

Further Reading

de Groat, W. C. (1999). Neural control of the urinary bladder and sexual organs. In *Autonomic Failure. A Textbook of Clinical Disorders of the Autonomic Nervous System* (C. J. Mathias and R. Bannister, Eds.), 4th ed., pp. 151–165. Oxford Univ. Press, Oxford.

Eckberg, D. L., Nerhed, C., and Wallin, B. G. (1985). Respiratory modulation of muscle sympathetic and vagal cardiac outflow in man. *J. Physiol. (London)* **365**, 181–196.

Gibbins, I. (1990). Peripheral autonomic nervous system. In *The Human Nervous System* (G. Paxinos, Ed.), pp. 93–124. Academic Press, New York.

Shields, R. W. (1993). Functional anatomy of the autonomic nervous system. *J. Clin. Neurophysiol.* **10**, 2–13.

Spyer, K. M., Brooks, P. A., and Izzo, P. N. (1994). Vagal preganglionic neurons supplying the heart. In *Vagal Control of the Heart: Experimental Basis and Clinical Implications* (M. N. Levy and P. J. Schwartz, Eds.), pp. 45–64. Futura, New York.

Paresis

Encyclopedia of the Neurological Sciences
Copyright 2003, Elsevier Science (USA). All rights reserved.

PARESIS is a clinical sign consisting of a loss of power of any muscle group. Very mild weakness or paresis may not be identified by formal manual muscle

Table 1 TERMS USED TO DESIGNATE PARESIS ACCORDING TO THE PART OF THE BODY AFFECTED AND THE MOST LIKELY LOCALIZATION OF THE RESPONSIBLE LESION

Extent of involvement	Term used	Lesion location
A single limb	Monoparesis	Peripheral nerve
		Motor cortex
The limbs on one side of the body	Hemiparesis	Corticospinal tract in the brainstem or cerebrum
The lower extremities	Paraparesis	Spinal cord
		Peripheral nerves
All four limbs	Quadriparesis or tetraparesis	Cervical spinal cord
		Peripheral nerves
		Muscle
Face	Facial paresis	Corticobulbar tract
		Facial nerve

Table 2 THE MEDICAL RESEARCH COUNCIL RATING OF MUSCLE STRENGTH[a]

Degree of weakness	Scale
No contraction	0
Flicker or trace of contraction	1
Active movement with gravity eliminated	2
Active movement against gravity	3
Active movement against gravity and resistance	4
Normal strength	5

[a] From Medical Research Council (1976). Aids to the examination of the peripheral nervous system, Memorandum No. 45. Crown, London.

testing of isometric strength, but it may lead to movements that are abnormally slow or clumsy. A complete loss of motor power is called plegia or paralysis. In the older literature, paresis was often referred to specifically as paretic neurosyphilis.

"General paresis" and "general paralysis" may still carry that connotation. The term paresis derives from the Greek παρεσισ or *pa/resiv*, which means neglecting or disregarding.

Often, the term paresis is modified by a prefix indicating the location of the weakness, as shown in Table 1. When referring to a limb that has paresis, the adjective used is "paretic," as in "the patient had a paretic left hand."

To grade paresis, the classification of the Medical Research Council is commonly used (Table 2). This system of classification is based on isometric strength and therefore fails to recognize the mildest forms of paresis with normal isometric strength but abnormal motility. As the diagnosis in neurology becomes more accurate, it is precisely the milder degrees of paresis that become important in clinical practice. The cause of the paresis should be identified and treated before it can cause frank weakness. Tests that can detect mild paresis include the pronator sign for the upper extremity and heel walking for the lower extremity. The pronator sign is elicited by asking the patient to hold the arms outstretched in front of them, with the palms up, while keeping their eyes closed. A positive sign is elicited when the hand tends to pronate and, often, the elbow tends to become slightly flexed. Heel walking will facilitate the recognition of mild paresis in the leg by enhancing the difference between the two feet, with the weak one showing foot dorsiflexion weakness that may not be appreciated in regular gait or by isometric manual testing.

Lesions of the motor or sensory systems can cause paresis, although typically the lesion is in the motor pathways, most often in the corticobulbar–corticospinal tract, peripheral nerves (including the cranial nerves), or muscle. The etiology of the lesion can be inferred from the tempo of the development of the paresis. Some of the more common etiologies are listed in Table 3 according to the type of onset and site of involvement.

Table 3 COMMON ETIOLOGIES CAUSING PARESIS

Onset of the paresis	Corticobulbar–corticospinal	Cranial nerve or peripheral nerve	Muscle
Acute (minutes to few hours)	Stroke, ischemic or hemorrhagic	Diabetes	Periodic paralysis
	Trauma	Other vasculitis	
		Trauma	
Subacute (hours to days)	Demyelinating disease	Demyelinating neuropathies	Toxic myopathies
	Infection	Toxic neuropathies	
Chronic (weeks to months)	Neoplasms	Genetic disorders	Other genetic disorders
	Motor neuron disease	Repeated microtrauma	

Lesions in the proprioceptive pathways of the upper extremities can also cause clumsiness of movements of the affected limb, which can mimic the paresis caused by lesions of the corticospinal tract. In these cases, the distal part of the extremity is often unsteady when the patient is asked to close his or her eyes and extend the affected limb (piano-playing movements of the fingers), and the finger-to-nose test performed with eyes closed is inaccurate.

—*Joseph C. Masdeu*

***See also**–Paralysis; Paraparesis and Paraplegia; Quadriplegia (see also specific disorders)*

Further Reading

Brazis, P. W., Masdeu, J. C., and Biller, J. (Eds.) (2001). *Localization in Clinical Neurology*, 4th ed. Lippincott Williams & Wilkins, Philadelphia.

Brochier, T., Boudreau, M. J., Pare, M., *et al.* (1999). The effects of muscimol inactivation of small regions of motor and somatosensory cortex on independent finger movements and force control in the precision grip. *Exp. Brain Res.* **128**, 31–40.

Ghika, J., Ghika-Schmid, F., and Bogousslasvky, J. (1998). Parietal motor syndrome: A clinical description in 32 patients in the acute phase of pure parietal strokes studied prospectively. *Clin. Neurol. Neurosurg.* **100**, 271–282.

Haerer, A. F. (1992). *DeJong's the Neurological Examination*, 5th ed. Lippincott, Philadelphia.

Parietal Lobe

Encyclopedia of the Neurological Sciences

THE PARIETAL lobe's location and connections place it strategically between other areas of cerebral cortex dedicated to the initial processing of different modalities of sensory experience. Accordingly, this part of the brain contains neuronal assemblies that integrate multiple streams of sensory data into cohesive structures to direct attention and determine the relationship of parts of the body to each other (e.g., body schema), the orientation of our bodies to other objects in extrapersonal space, and the orientation of different objects in extrapersonal space to each other. This entry reviews the pertinent anatomy of the parietal lobes and summarizes the cardinal behavioral manifestations associated with brain injuries that involve this region of the central nervous system.

ANATOMY

The parietal lobe extends posteriorly from the central sulcus nearly to the occipital pole (Fig. 1). The Sylvian fissure forms the parietal lobe's inferior boundary, a border that becomes increasingly obscure in the zone shared by the parietal, temporal, and occipital lobes. The parietal region can be further classified into major divisions. On the outer surface of the hemisphere, these include the postcentral gyrus, the supramarginal gyrus, the angular gyrus, and the superior parietal lobule. The interparietal sulcus separates the superior parietal lobule from the supramarginal and angular gyri. On the hemisphere's inner surface, the paracentral lobule straddles the central sulcus, as does a region termed the precuneus. A posterior portion of the cingulate gyrus, known as the retrosplenial cortex, abuts the mesial portion of the parietal lobe, although it is anatomically designated as part of the limbic system.

The postcentral gyrus receives afferent projections from the ventral tier of thalamic nuclei. These fibers, conveying somatosensory information from the contralateral side of the body, terminate in a somatotopic arrangement on the posterior bank of the central sulcus. Somatosensory information from this area projects to association cortex in the superior parietal lobe. A substantial portion of the parietal cortex, including the supramarginal and angular gyri, consists of heteromodal cortex, wherein neurons receive convergent inputs from other regions of cortex dedicated to the processing of individual sensory modalities. These data include visual system projections from the so-called dorsal visuofugal pathway, in which a combination of elementary retinotopic and visuomotor information results in computation of extrapersonal events in terms of

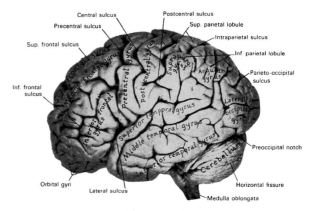

Figure 1
Lateral view of the human brain (left hemisphere).

head- and body-centered frames of reference. Other sensory modalities converging on heteromodal parts of the parietal cortex include vestibular inputs that contribute to computation of body position and motion in three-dimensional space. In addition, all parts of the parietal cortex receive extensive projections from parts of the intralaminar thalamic nuclear groups, a structure that acts as a gate to refine the nature of input passing via the ventral thalamus to the cortex. Information from heteromodal parietal cortex projects via reciprocal corticocortical tracts to premotor frontal cortex and cingulate gyrus. The parietal lobe also projects reciprocally to the intralaminar thalamus and to other extrapyramidal motor systems such as the caudate nucleus.

CLINICAL DEFICITS ASSOCIATED WITH PARIETAL LOBE INJURY

The complexity of the anatomical relationships between the parietal lobe and other parts of the brain guarantees that damage to this region will cause a vast spectrum of disorders at the highest levels of information processing. For example, the parietal lobes are part of a distributed neural network that is important for directed attention. However, the clinical consequences of parietal lobe injury may also involve a number of elemental functions. These problems, which can be detected on routine physical examination, follow directly from the anatomical arrangement of lower level sensory structures mentioned previously.

Receptors for different types of tactile stimuli (e.g., light touch, vibration, and temperature) project somatotopically via the ventrolateral thalamus to neurons in the postcentral gyrus, which constitute the primary somatosensory region. The somatotopic organization of sensory projections in this area approximates that found in the adjacent primary motor cortex of the precentral gyrus. Disruption of this most anterior aspect of the parietal cortex results in disorders of somatic sensation, with affected patients reporting a distortion of the quality of exteroceptive and proprioceptive sensations rather than profound hypalgesia or anesthesia that can result from interruption of more caudal components of the somatosensory system. Parietal lesions typically raise the sensory threshold of the contralateral distal extremities more than the proximal extremities, trunk, or face.

Two-point discrimination refers to the threshold distance between two cutaneous stimuli at which individuals misperceive the separate stimuli as one. Using a device such as a pair of calipers, the examiner initially probes performance in a body part with two points relatively far apart, varying unpredictably between single and double stimuli. The examiner progressively adjusts the caliper points into closer proximity, noting the distance at which the patient fails to accurately distinguish between single and double stimuli. Homologous body parts should demonstrate nearly identical two-point discrimination. The specific distance normally varies widely (e.g., approximately 2 mm on a fingertip and more than 20 mm on the dorsum of the hand). Parietal injuries increase the distance required to make accurate two-point discriminations on body parts contralateral to the brain lesion. Hence, findings on one side of the body must always be compared with those of homologous body parts on the opposite side of the body.

Parietal lobe injury may cause disruption of functions that direct attention and integrate more basic sensations across time and space. A striking example of such a disorder is the neglect syndrome, which is discussed later. Discriminatory tactile sensibility depends on sensory inputs conducted in the heavily myelinated fibers that mediate transduction of tactile, vibratory, and proprioceptive stimuli. In the context of preserved elementary sensory function, deficits in these "cortical" sensory discriminations distinguish parietal lobe injury from damage involving more peripheral portions of the neuronal pathway from body surface to brain. Note, however, that disruption of some integrative sensory capacities will also occur when more basic stimulus perception is disrupted.

Visual projections from the lateral geniculate nucleus pass through the parietal region on their way to the upper bank of the calcarine (primary visual) cortex in the occipital lobe. Information from the contralateral visual field maintains a retinotopic arrangement throughout this course, thereby conveying information about the lower half of the visual world. Corresponding input from upper visual space is transmitted via inferior geniculocalcarine projections that traverse the hemisphere through the temporal lobe. Thus, the elemental visual deficits associated with parietal brain injuries include either inferior quadrantanopsia or incomplete hemianopsia. The parietal lobes are also important for higher level processing underlying visuospatial functions and direction of attention to external space.

Another function of parietal cortex entails guiding volitional movements within extrapersonal space. Thus, certain ocular and motor findings may also signify the presence of parietal cortex injury. Rapid shifts of gaze known as saccades occur after a delay and fall short of their target after posterior parietal damage, although detection of this abnormality may require specialized apparatus. In addition, parietal injury impedes normal rhythmic eye movements induced by pursuing moving visual targets across space (optokinetic nystagmus). Lesions involving the area of angular and supramarginal gyri inhibit or abolish this response when the target moves toward the affected hemisphere. When patients with parietal injury attempt to maintain the contralateral limbs in a stationary position, writhing movements similar to choreoathetosis may be elicited, presumably as a consequence of disturbed proprioceptive function. Ataxic contralateral limb movements, similar in quality to those observed with cerebellar dysfunction, may also accompany unilateral parietal damage, presumably a result of interrupted corticopontine projections from the parietal cortex to the cerebellum. Lesions of parietal and other regions in the hemisphere may result in hypometric (i.e., smaller) movements toward contralateral (i.e., opposite) space when guided by proprioception rather than vision.

The higher level functions of the parietal lobes are different for the left and right sides of the brain in individuals with typical cerebral lateralization. Regardless of handedness, most humans have the majority of language functions lateralized to the left brain, resulting in its designation as the dominant cerebral hemisphere. It is estimated that more than 95% of right-handed individuals exhibit left hemisphere dominance for language, whereas the corresponding figure for left-handed individuals is approximately 70%. In distinction, the right brain is frequently referred to as the nondominant brain with respect to language functions, even though it is actually dominant for certain functions as described later.

BEHAVIORAL CONSEQUENCES OF PARIETAL INJURY: DOMINANT HEMISPHERE

Aphasia

Patients with injuries to the parietal cortex typically can demonstrate language deficits (aphasia) characterized by retained fluency. Aphasia from parietal injury generally is classified into one of three categories: Wernicke's aphasia, transcortical sensory aphasia, and conduction aphasia.

Patients with Wernicke's aphasia produce speech effortlessly with normal pace and melody, but their speech conveys little or no meaning. Less severe cases commit errors that bear discernible relationships to normal words, known as paraphasic errors. In addition, they show impairment when attempting to repeat phrases spoken by the examiner. Lastly, these individuals characteristically fail to comprehend the examiner's speech, even for elementary commands. In general, a patient's comprehension of written language parallels their deficiency in comprehension of spoken language. Wernicke's aphasia occurs most commonly after lesions of the posterior superior temporal gyrus (Wernicke's area, which is a cortical region important in decoding speech sound), but the adjacent inferior parietal lobe is frequently involved.

Patients with transcortical sensory aphasia also produce fluent speech devoid of content and fail to comprehend the speech of others. In contrast to Wernicke's aphasia, however, these individuals retain the ability to repeat phrases out of proportion to their comprehension. For example, they may repeat complex phrases from which they can derive no meaning. Intact repetition implies that they can decode strings of language sound but that the results of such processes fail to activate the parts of the brain that store information linked to words (the semantic system). Accordingly, responsible lesions usually involve more posterior and superior parietal cortex outside the perisylvian language zones.

Patients with conduction aphasia retain relatively intact auditory comprehension and often produce meaningful expressions that can be understood by others. Paraphasic errors may also contaminate their speech. Paraphasic errors may include successive approximations that frequently bring them closer to the intended word with each attempt (e.g. "fesk … fisk … fist"). The most characteristic deficit in conduction aphasia consists of extreme difficulty repeating phrases or even single words. The lesion responsible for conduction aphasia can involve the left inferior parietal cortex and underlying white matter, functionally disconnecting otherwise intact areas that decode speech sound in the auditory association areas of the posterior–superior temporal lobe from areas that program speech movements in the frontal cortex.

Dyslexia

A comprehensive review of acquired reading disorders secondary to brain injury exceeds the scope of this entry. However, no discussion of the behavioral consequences of parietal lobe injury would be complete without at least mention of dyslexia.

More than a century ago, Dejerine distinguished between two major forms of reading impairment based on whether disturbed reading was associated with trouble writing. The first form, called alexia with agraphia, resulted from an injury to the left parietal lobe, leading him to speculate that the region of the angular gyrus contained a store of "word images" required for both reading and writing. The second form, termed alexia without agraphia, was associated with right homonymous visual field loss. Although the responsible lesions were outside the parietal region in the left occipital lobe and the corpus callosum, Dejerine asserted that the tandem injuries prohibited visual input from accessing the critical site in the left angular gyrus and other critical left perisylvian language regions. Since word images could be invoked in other tasks, such as writing, dyslexia developed in relative isolation.

Detailed analysis of the reading patterns in other types of acquired dyslexia resulted in elaboration of information processing models that parse the complex process of reading into more elementary operations. Although not strictly informed by anatomic–function relationships that are the focus of this entry, these models retain some heuristic value with respect to the distinctive ways in which the system fails after brain injury. A diagram of the operations and their organization is presented in Fig. 2. The first step entails elementary visual processing (i.e., extracting primitive features and shapes), invoking functions common to all forms of visual perception. At this point, information flow diverges depending on characteristics of both the reader and the character string to be read. Assuming a reader is literate, information from elementary visual analysis may activate a stored entry from the lexicon, a memory bank of previously learned words. From the lexicon, information can further activate entries in the semantic system, where it links with previously learned associations regarding the specific features and concepts represented by the word. By now, printed material reaches a level at which it corresponds to mental images or thoughts; this sequence of operations is termed the lexical route (Fig. 2, A). Another path of information flow,

designated the sublexical reading system, presumably accounts for the capacity of most individuals to pronounce words they never previously encountered. When confronted by a novel nonword character string (e.g., FLIG), an appropriate pronunciation can be derived through an operation that involves a direct translation of letters to their corresponding sounds (Fig. 2, B).

What happens if an individual forgets the appearance of words he or she had previously learned? If the person retained knowledge about letter–sound correspondences, he or she could still rely on the sublexical route to pronounce character strings. However, the individual would compensate much more readily for strings whose pronunciation corresponds to standard spelling-to-sound "rules" (i.e., regular words such as "hand"), and nonword character strings would pose no particular problem. In contrast, the individual would fail to accurately pronounce words that break these rules (e.g., irregular words such as "yacht" would sound like "hatched"). This pattern of reading dysfunction is termed surface dyslexia.

What happens if a person loses sublexical processes, forgetting how to derive pronunciation from letter–sound correspondence rules? Such an individual would rely exclusively on an intact lexical route

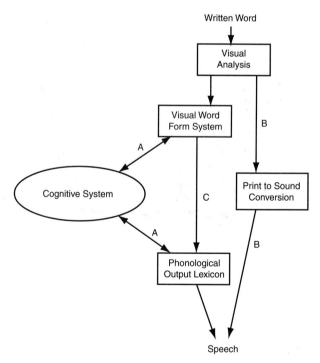

Figure 2
Schematic model of cognitive operations involved in reading.

and read previously learned words relatively well. However, the person would fail to accurately pronounce novel, meaningless nonwords. As one might predict, patients do not often seek evaluation for an inability to read nonword letter strings. In fact, this type of dyslexia, termed phonological dyslexia, was predicted from the information processing model and detected only after direct assessment of brain-injured individuals.

Apraxia

Clinicians apply the term apraxia to many different situations. The form of apraxia most often associated with parietal lobe injury, ideomotor apraxia, entails a disorder of learned, skilled movements executed primarily by the upper extremity. For all types of apraxia, the operational definition specifies that disordered movements cannot be accounted for by weakness, proprioceptive defect, abnormal tone, poor cooperation, or general intellectual deterioration. The types of apraxia that implicate damage in the dominant parietal region are described here. Other deficits, termed constructional apraxia and dressing apraxia, are mentioned later in the entry. Still other varieties of apraxia, such as buccofacial or gait, generally result from injuries outside the parietal lobe and are not further considered in this entry.

Ideomotor Apraxia: Patients with ideomotor apraxia demonstrate improper temporal and spatial organization of movements. Proper execution of skilled movements requires the brain to organize and implement a deceptively complex series of motor commands. Cognitive neuropsychological models of praxis posit that the nervous system stores information about previously learned sequences of movement. Such "programs" allow an individual to execute learned movements automatically rather than inefficiently recreating them part by part. This knowledge is presumably stored as an abstract representation containing general spatial and temporal information (e.g., hammering → striking flat surface of tool onto object to propel object in direction perpendicular to surface). For movement production to occur, however, this general code must be translated into a specific pattern of innervation taking into account the context of the movement (e.g. driving tent stakes into ground with sledge hammer versus tapping a pin into the hinge on spectacle frames). If one accepts these premises, then two primary defects could impair production of

skilled movement: defective "motor memory" storage or normal motor memory but improper translation into an "innervatory pattern" or motor program.

Defects at either level would hinder a patient's ability to perform a limb gesture to the examiner's command. However, by testing recognition of movements made by others, different patterns of deficit are observable. For example, patients with disrupted motor memory would fail gesture to command and also fail to recognize the nature of a pantomimed action performed by the examiner. Individuals behave in this manner after injury to the dominant inferior parietal structures, especially the supramarginal and angular gyri. In contrast, other patients who fail to produce learned, skilled movements retain the capacity to discriminate between proper and improper gestures made by others. In this situation, movement representations in the parietal region presumably remain intact and the defect arises at the level of implementation, a deficit associated more with damage to motor systems in the prefrontal cerebral cortex.

Conceptual Apraxia: Patients with conceptual apraxia can perform individual gestures well but select improper tools/gestures for a given context. The processing failure may occur on at least three levels: loss of knowledge of the type of action associated with certain tools (e.g., hammers strike), inability to associate tools with the recipients of their actions (e.g., hammers strike nails), and impairment of knowledge about the mechanical advantage afforded by given tools (e.g., hammers strike nails better than do wrenches).

Patients with conceptual apraxia produce well-executed actions but in inappropriate circumstances, leading to peculiar and disabling behavior. An example of such content errors is tool substitution (e.g., the patient selects and uses the toothbrush when attempting to shave). Detailed study of this type of patient has revealed that patients retain the ability to name the tools they misuse, arguing against improper selection on the basis of recognition failure (agnosia). In contrast, they fail to name or point to tools when their function was described, indicating a restricted knowledge deficit limited only to the use of tools and the relationship between tools and the objects on which they act. Disruption of tool–object knowledge can result in less bizarre but equally ineffective behavior. For example, a patient may show that they need to rotate a screw to drive it but select a pair of pliers to carry out the rotation.

Patients with conceptual apraxia often harbor diffuse or bilateral posterior cerebral involvement.

Gerstmann Syndrome

This term refers to a constellation of findings that accompany damage to the left parietal cortex, typically involving the angular gyrus or subjacent white matter tracts. Characteristic features include problems naming or designating the different fingers on both hands (finger agnosia), confusion between left and right, defective writing (dysgraphia), and defective calculating (dyscalculia). Authorities debate whether this constellation of findings represents a common, unifying cognitive disturbance or whether these findings present a serendipitous aggregation of "neighborhood signs." In fact, it is very unusual to see this constellation of deficits in isolation without other deficits associated with parietal lobe lesions. Nevertheless, the syndrome does highlight several deficits that may occur with damage to the left parietal lobe.

According to some authorities, most patients with Gerstmann syndrome show preservation of route-finding ability, indicating that right–left disorientation reflects a lexical deficit rather than a sign of spatial disorientation. Indeed, disambiguating aphasic limitations from a disturbance of egocentric organization requires tests that do not require verbal response. For example, one task requires the patient to touch a lateralized location on their body that corresponds to the same point on the examiner's body that is indicated by the examiner.

Finger recognition, a skill accomplished at different ages during normal development, actually comprises multiple basic spatial and linguistic operations. Elementary abilities mastered before the first grade entail nonverbal tasks such as having patients point to fingers that the examiner touches or points to on themselves. More complex skills require patient recognition based on isolated tactile stimulation. For example, out of the patient's view, an examiner touches a digit on one of the patient's hands and then asks the patient to indicate which digit on the other hand corresponds to the one touched. Even more challenging tasks require patients to localize the touched finger on a schematic representation of the hands or require the mediation of language, such as naming the individual fingers or indicating specific fingers named by the examiner. As summarized by Benton and Sivan, the deficit termed finger agnosia by Gerstmann can reflect any of these deficits that impair finger recognition.

Because the capacity to calculate entails the operation of multiple, simultaneous cognitive operations, calculation difficulty can take several forms. At one level, manipulation of numerical quantities presumes some degree of attentional capacity and linguistic competence, such as when the examiner asks a patient to subtract one digit from another "in their head." Performance of the same task presented in written form entails proper visual processing of symbols as well as their spatial relationship to each other. At another level, conducting basic arithmetical operations presented graphically (e.g. "carrying") requires mastery of specific rules, similar to syntactical structure required by spoken and written language. Disruption in one or more of these functions results in acalculia.

In general, dysgraphia can be classified into forms in which the defect relates to motor dysfunction and forms in which the defect reflects language dysfunction. In the former case, termed apractic dysgraphia, patients retain the capacity to spell words and can produce words through arrangement of letters or the use of keyboards. Although they can often copy letters or letter strings, their productions are slow and deliberate, revealing unusual features, such as producing the letter "X" by joining four small lines at the center rather than simply crossing two larger lines. In contrast, patients with aphasic agraphia often fail to spell words and produce legible individual letters arranged in unintelligible strings.

BEHAVIORAL CONSEQUENCES OF PARIETAL INJURY: NONDOMINANT HEMISPHERE

Neglect Syndrome

Although the term neglect subserves many connotations in clinical practice, the neglect syndrome refers specifically to a complex behavioral disorder in which affected patients with brain damage fail to report, respond, or orient to meaningful or novel stimuli and this failure cannot be explained by elemental deficits in sensory or motor functions (e.g., anesthesia or paralysis). The disorder primarily involves stimuli from the side contralateral to an injured hemisphere. Although the neglect syndrome can develop after injury to many different sites of the central nervous system in either hemisphere, it is most common and severe with large acute right brain lesions. When smaller focal lesions occur, neglect is most common and severe with damage to the right parietal region. Note that behavior similar to neglect might also occur when, for example, patients fail to acknowledge or act on stimuli based on hemisensory or hemimotor defects induced by brain lesions. However, neglect refers more specifically to a failure that cannot be explained by such elemental deficits.

The neglect syndrome encompasses many forms, not all of which can be identified within an individual patient. For the purposes of this entry, only the most basic and practical means of assessment and interpretation are considered.

Extrapersonal (Hemispatial) Neglect: Patients who neglect extrapersonal space, termed hemispatial neglect, fail to respond or orient to stimuli in their immediate environment contralateral to the brain lesion (e.g., left hemibody and hemispace for a right brain lesion). This type of behavior may be first observed informally during interviews or conversations with the patient wherein individuals with neglect may often manifest deviation of their head and eyes in the direction of the injured hemisphere (i.e., away from the neglected side). Examiners who address such patients from their neglected side might observe them turn away and orient responses toward their "good side," even if no one is present in this part of space. Note that contraversive movement of the head and eyes is not synonymous with neglect; other problems can produce this phenomenon and not all patients with hemispatial neglect display head/eye deviation.

Immediately after brain injury, patients with neglect may actually fail to detect contralesional sensory stimuli presented in isolation, a finding that may suggest deafferentation rather than neglect. Later in the recovery period, patients may detect simple sensory stimuli but mislocalize them (i.e., allesthesia), claiming that a sight, sound, or touch on the contralesional side of space actually occurred at the analogous place on the ipsilesional side, a phenomenon known as allochiria. Likewise, other patients may fail to detect contralesional stimuli only under specific conditions. Specifically, some individuals fail to respond to a contralesional stimulus only when presented simultaneously with an ipsilesional stimulus, a phenomenon known as extinction.

When neglect is not evident on informal assessment during the history and physical examination,

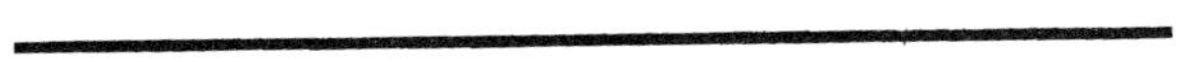

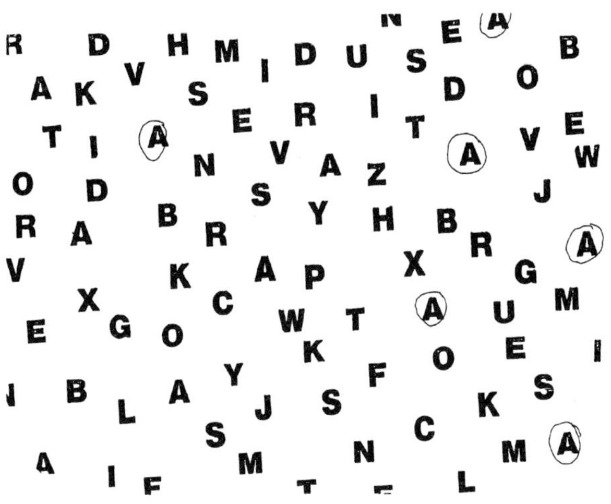

Figure 4
Target cancellation in patient with left hemispatial neglect; targets are omitted primarily from the (patient-centered) left side of the array.

clinicians can elicit neglect behavior using several easy bedside tests. Such tasks include line bisection, in which the subject attempts to divide a line into two equal segments; patients with neglect tend to displace their mark toward the side of their brain injury (Fig. 3). Using longer lines and performing the task in the contralesional hemispace can improve detection of bisection errors. In the target cancellation task, in which patients locate target objects from an array, patients with neglect often fail to mark items from the contralesional side of the array (Fig. 4). Using greater numbers of targets and distributing them among multiple nontarget foils can increase the likelihood of omissions. Additional information can be obtained through qualitative analysis of cancellation performance: Individuals with neglect initiate their search on the right side of an array, a distinctly uncommon behavior in otherwise normal people. Finally, hemispatial neglect can be identified by asking the patient to draw simple figures, either through copying the examiner's test stimulus or producing a drawing to verbal prompt. Patients may fail to draw the figure's contralesional components because they fail to register that part of the stimulus or fail to move their pencil to that side of the page (Fig. 5). In contrast, patients who spontaneously omit details from one side of the target object may harbor deficiency at the level of a mental representation or memory of the object. Defects in spatial representation can also be elicited by asking the patient to describe the layout of commonly known public places or their home from a

Figure 3
Line bisection in patient with left hemispatial neglect; the bisection mark falls to the right of the true midpoint.

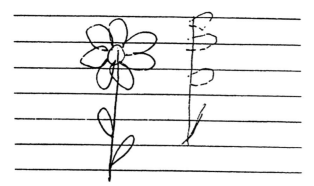

Figure 5
Figure copy of patient with left hemispatial neglect; elements on the object's left side are omitted.

specific vantage point (i.e., "Describe the floor plan of your house looking in from the front door"). Patients with representational neglect will not include structures or items located on the contralesional side of their mental image.

Personal Neglect—Asomatognosia: When neglect affects personal space, patients fail to recognize their own body parts on the side opposite the brain lesion. Such patients may deny ownership of their own hand opposite to the brain lesion, often misattribute the paretic limb to others, and may voice distress at the uncomfortable proximity of the "alien" limb to their own body. They often fail to groom or dress the neglected parts, shaving half of the face, washing half of the body, combing half of their hair, and brushing half of their teeth. This remarkable behavior is most common after acute large lesions of the right brain, which usually involve the right temporoparietal region.

Anosognosia: This term refers to a clinical condition in which patients deny or fail to recognize their own neurological deficits. As originally described, anosognosia referred specifically to denial of hemiparesis. However, over the years, anosognosia has been described in association with a wide variety of disorders, including visual field loss, aphasia, and amnesia. Anosognosia for hemiparesis most frequently occurs after large acute right brain lesions but can be seen with smaller lesions of the right parietal area. It almost always coexists with other aspects of neglect behavior.

Denial of deficit may result from reduced deficit awareness, although individuals may display either denial or lack of insight separately. Some patients adamantly reject assertions that they are weak but act disabled, whereas others freely acknowledge

hemiparesis but betray lack of insight when they unsuccessfully attempt to walk or perform bimanual tasks. Patients with anosognosia may concede impairment but underestimate its severity or appear unmoved by its consequences, a phenomenon termed anosodiaphoria. In addition to disturbed awareness of bodily function, patients with anosognosia may exhibit "productive" manifestations. For example, when asked to use the weak extremity, they move their intact appendage and then claim with conviction that they followed the examiner's instructions. Other patients report peculiar and complex delusions regarding the affected body parts. Sometimes, patients will reduplicate limbs, claiming to possess two arms on the paretic side, a type of delusion termed somatoparaphrenia. Similar examples include individuals who personify a paralyzed extremity, asserting that their weak arm is in fact that of one of their relatives.

Visuospatial and Constructional Dysfunction

The ability to properly perceive visuospatial relations is obviously impaired in patients with neglect. However, even patients without neglect will frequently exhibit deficits in visuospatial perceptual abilities following lesions of the parietal lobe, especially the right parietal lobe. In fact, tasks involving visuospatial perception and reconstruction (e.g., copying a figure) are among the most sensitive to right parietal dysfunction. It should be noted that the deficit is not specific to the parietal lobe.

The capacity to recreate a visually presented stimulus, either through drawing or assembling pieces like a puzzle, presupposes other more elementary functions. For example, an individual must possess requisite visual acuity as well as the basic motor skills. However, an individual who fails to negotiate the construction process even with intact basic sensorimotor functions shows defective constructional ability. Many clinicians designate such a finding as constructional apraxia. Although some constructional capacities call on learned skilled movements (e.g., holding and manipulating a pencil), reproducing the spatial orientation of different parts into a cohesive unit does not share many characteristics of apraxia as defined by Liepmann.

Several well-established measures can be employed to assess visuoconstructive capacity. In common screening tasks, the patient is asked to copy a simple figure such as a cross, interlocking pentagons, or a "transparent" cube. Performance on these tests is typically graded on a binary pass/fail basis. Another commonly employed task is clock drawing, for which simple scoring rules can permit semiquantitative judgment of performance; this task requires the patient to draw a clock with the hands placed at a given time. Drawing figures with more detail permits both quantitative and qualitative analysis of constructional ability (Fig. 6). Other techniques that avoid the necessity of holding and manipulating a pen or pencil include assembly of blocks to match a model.

Although injuries to either parietal lobe can disrupt constructional ability, such a disorder most frequently follows injury to the nondominant hemisphere. In this case, impaired productions can also reflect concomitant left hemispatial neglect. Patients with right hemisphere injury also dwell to a fault on the details of the target stimulus without conveying the overall outline or Gestalt of the object (Fig. 7). In contrast, defective constructional ability after left brain damage typically features omissions or distortions of internal details while preserving the model's general contour. Constructional disorders observed after left hemisphere injury may occur in association with either aphasia or elements of the Gerstmann syndrome. Lesions to the frontal lobes may impair constructional abilities by interfering with planning and sequencing. Furthermore, patients with diffuse cerebral disease (e.g., degenerative dementias) often exhibit impairment on constructional tasks. Thus, although the parietal lobes are critical to constructional abilities, constructional dysfunction is not specific to parietal lobe injury.

Astereognosis

Stereognosis refers to the capacity to perceive the nature of an object through its tactile properties, allowing individuals to identify objects by touch. Loss of this ability is called astereognosis. In contrast, the term tactile agnosia is typically reserved for the

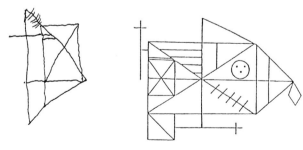

Figure 6
Gross constructional disturbance on copy of a complex figure (patient copy on left; model on right).

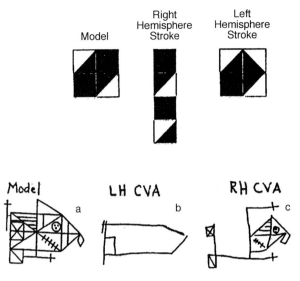

Figure 7
Lateralized forms of constructional deficit. Patients with right hemisphere injury can get correct internal relationships and features while losing the global configuration, whereas patients with left hemisphere injury maintain the overall organization but omit specific details.

inability to identify objects through touch despite the ability to recognize the same objects via other sensory modalities (e.g., vision) and despite relatively intact access to the objects' tactile features (i.e., size and shape). Failing object identification, some preserved stereognostic function might allow for discrimination of basic physical features such as stimulus size or texture. Less affected patients might also be able to distinguish simple shapes, such as the contour of a circle. Both astereognosis and tactile agnosia are most often associated with injury to inferior aspects of the right parietal lobe. Tests of stereognostic sensibility usually involve the manual exploration of a stimulus. Tactile exploration of an object requires relatively intact fine motor function, a requirement proportionally more critical for complex objects.

Agraphesthesia

Graphesthesia entails the ability to recognize symbols such as letters through their tactile properties, and loss of this function is called agraphesthesia. Language disorders might impair recognition of characters, although such problems should influence performance across multiple sensory modalities. Parietal lobe damage may disrupt graphesthetic discrimination more predominantly in the hand contralateral to brain injury. The term agraphesthesia is usually limited to the situation in which the deficit cannot be explained by a language disorder or the loss of elemental sensory perception. When agraphesthesia is not due to dysphasia or lower level sensory deficits, it is most commonly associated with lesions of the right parietal lobe.

Dressing Apraxia

Although taken for granted as a skill mastered in early childhood, the capacity to place clothes on one's body likely entails complicated manipulation of multiple spatial relationships. Because the act of dressing calls on such a diverse set of cognitive operations, some authorities take issue with using the term apraxia in this particular behavioral disorder. However, the employment of such clinical terms over many years creates a certain momentum that, in the absence of a concise alternative, nearly guarantees their perpetuation. For present purposes, the term dressing apraxia refers to a patient's inability to properly position clothing over the appropriate body parts as well as problems with fastening the clothing to the body. Although dressing apraxia may result from unilateral right parietal injury, it most commonly develops in the setting of multiple brain lesions (e.g., bilateral parietal injury or multiple infarcts) or diffuse cerebral degeneration (e.g., Alzheimer's disease).

Sometimes, the deficit may involve only the contralesional half of the body, in which case it almost certainly represents a manifestation of the neglect syndrome, such as denial of the limbs opposite the lesion. Other patients show more global defects in the capacity to properly orient the parts of a garment to itself, becoming baffled by one sleeve being turned inside out. This behavior could, in principle, result from simultanagnosia, whereby the patient cannot simultaneously attend to and compare different parts of the garment to each other. Dressing apraxia can also result from the failure to make correspondences between the parts of a garment and a person's own body parts. These patients will, for example, tie the sleeves of their shirt around their waist like a belt, arranging the remainder of the garment in the manner of an apron or kilt. Such behavior may accompany a rare, more pervasive disturbance of body knowledge termed autotopagnosia. Less conspicuous deficits might include individuals who improperly line up a row of buttons with their corresponding holes. Problems with dressing may reflect defective sequencing and organization of otherwise correctly executed actions. In this case, patients confronted with multiple items of clothing make errors such as putting their underwear on over their trousers, thereby resembling a limited form of conceptual or ideational apraxia.

Aprosodia

Prosody refers to the ability to understand and express emotional meaning through variable intonations of speech. Although the left brain is dominant for the propositional components of language (e.g., comprehending the meaning of words), the right brain is dominant for prosody. Lesions of the right parietal lobe may result in aprosodia, in which the patient is unable to understand the emotional tone of the speaker's voice (e.g., anger and sadness) even though they understand the meaning of the words per se. In contrast, more anterior lesions in the right brain typically impair the expression of emotional tone.

BEHAVIORAL CONSEQUENCES OF BILATERAL PARIETAL INJURY

Balint's syndrome

Balint's syndrome refers to a conspicuous disorder of spatial analysis characterized by three cardinal features: optic ataxia, ocular apraxia, and simultanagnosia. According to Damasio et al., the syndrome's essence involves disturbed ability to perceive the visual field as a whole despite relative preservation of adequate visual acuity. This perceptual disorder develops in association with impairments of limb movements toward visually guided targets and eye movements toward new visual stimuli. As a consequence, other complex behaviors that depend on effective distribution of visual attention (e.g., reading) can also be disrupted. The triad's individual behavioral constituents can be observed in isolation, and thus the term Balint's syndrome should be reserved for cases demonstrating all three components.

Optic ataxia refers to the inability to reach toward or point to a location under visual guidance. Although Balint's original patient made reaching errors primarily with the right hand, most cases demonstrate ataxic movements with either hand. Clinically, patients or their family describe "near miss" incidents in which, for example, the affected individual gropes for objects at the dinner table. Upon examination, a patient asked to touch the examiner's finger may initially contact the examiner proximally and then extend their tactile search down the extremity until the fingers are located. In contrast, the patient's ability to manually locate parts of their own body under proprioceptive guidance remains intact. Such individuals may also be able to accurately reach with one hand for an object held by the other hand.

Patients with ocular apraxia show difficulty shifting their direction of gaze with quick eye movements called saccades. The failure to refixate on new targets can occur even when patients receive verbal warning about the impending stimulus. If the individual can redirect their gaze, the movement is often inadequate to bring the target stimulus into fixation range.

Bilateral parietal injury can result in defective detection of visual stimuli from one or both inferior quadrants. However, the visual fields in patients with Balint's syndrome may be normal by standard perimetric testing. Assessment of visual acuity can be challenging due to problems with fixation on the stimuli of standard visual acuity charts. Even when patients demonstrate that they can detect motion in the visual periphery, they perceive objects sufficiently to identify them only within the very narrow field of fixation. Such patients cannot effectively maintain "focus" on objects in their visual environment; when presented with a visual stimulus, they may fail to report any experience unless their fixation stumbles inadvertently onto the object. Just as swiftly, a momentarily perceived object can disappear from view as fixation moves just as randomly to another location. These individuals show the disconcerting tendency to look in the general direction of the examiner when conversing rather than making direct eye contact. As a consequence, patients with severe visual disorientation "act blind," leading earlier clinicians to term the deficit psychic blindness.

Similar perceptual dysfunction may account for simultanagnosia, a term referring to a patient's inability to apprehend the "meaning" of a complex visual scene as a whole even though component parts can be recognized individually. A person with Balint's syndrome may report only a small fraction of the depicted activities. Even when the patient can produce an accurate list of multiple elements in a visual scene, they may not be able to report the relationships of these parts to each other or to the scene as a whole. Practical bedside tests consist of presenting patients with a random array of several dots on a page or two simple figures occupying the same part of a page (e.g., a cross within a circle). Patients with Balint's syndrome will typically be unable to count the number of dots and may respond that they see only one of the simple figures.

—*J. C. Adair and K. J. Meador*

See also–Alexia; Angular Gyrus Syndrome; Anosognosia; Aphasia; Apraxia; Balint's Syndrome; Brain Anatomy; Cerebral Cortex: Architecture and Connections; Motion and Spatial Perception; Neglect Disorders; Reading and Acquired Dyslexia

Further Reading

Benton, A., and Sivan, A. B. (1993). Disturbances of body schema. In *Clinical Neuropsychology* (K. M. Heilman and E. Valenstein, Eds.), 2nd ed., pp. 123–140. Oxford Univ. Press, New York.

Bisiach, E., and Luzzatti, C. (1978). Unilateral neglect of representational space. *Cortex* **14**, 129–133.

Coslett, H. B. (2000). Acquired dyslexia. *Semin. Neurol.* **20**, 419–426.

Coslett, H. B., and Saffran, E. (1991). Simultanagnosia. To see but not two see. *Brain* **114**, 1523–1545.

Damasio, A. R. (1992). Aphasia. *N. Engl. J. Med.* **326**, 531–539.

Damasio, A. R., Tranel, D., and Rizzo, M. (2000). Disorders of complex visual processing. In *Principles of Behavioral and Cognitive Neurology* (M. M. Mesulam, Ed.), 2nd ed., pp. 332–372. Oxford Univ. Press, New York.

Feinberg, T. E., Haber, L. D., and Leeds, N. E. (1990). Verbal asomatognosia. *Neurology* **40**, 1391–1394.

Haerer, A. F. (1992). *De Jong's The Neurological Examination*, 5th ed. Lippincott, Philadelphia.

Heilman, K. M., and Gonzaez-Rothi, L. J. (1993). Apraxia. In *Clinical Neuropsychology* (K. M. Heilman and E. Valenstein, Eds.), 2nd ed., pp. 141–163. Oxford Univ. Press, New York.

Heilman, K. M., Watson, R. T., and Valenstein, E. V. (1993). Neglect and related disorders. In *Clinical Neuropsychology* (K. M. Heilman and E. Valenstein, Eds.), 2nd ed., pp. 279–336. Oxford Univ. Press, New York.

Heilman, K. M., Barrett, A., and Adair, J. (1998). Possible mechanisms of anosognosia: A defect in self-awareness. *Philos. Trans. R. Soc. London Ser. B* **353**, 1903–1909.

Mayer, E., Martory, D., Pegna, A. J., *et al.* (1999). A pure case of Gerstmann syndrome with a subangular lesion. *Brain* **122**, 1107–1120.

Mesulam, M. M. (1994). The multiplicity of neglect phenomenon. *Neuropsychol. Rehab.* **4**, 173–176.

Roeltgen, D. P. (1993). Agraphia. In *Clinical Neuropsychology* (K. M. Heilman and E. Valenstein, Eds.), 2nd ed., pp. 63–90. Oxford Univ. Press, New York.

Seltzer, B., and Pandya, D. N. (1980). Converging visual and somatic sensory cortical input to the intraparietal sulcus of the rhesus monkey. *Brain Res.* **192**, 339–351.

Srinivas, K., and Ogas, J. (1999). Disorders of somesthetic recognition: A theoretical review. *Neurocase* **5**, 83–93.

Swanda, R. M., Haaland, K. Y., and La Rue, A. (2000). Clinical neuropsychology. In *Comprehensive Textbook of Psychiatry* (H. I. Kaplan and B. J. Sadock, Eds.), 7th ed., pp. 689–702. Williams & Wilkins, New York.

Weintraub, S. (2000). Mental state assessment of young and elderly adults in behavioral neurology. In *Principles of Behavioral and Cognitive Neurology* (M. M. Mesulam, Ed.), 2nd ed., pp. 332–372. Oxford Univ. Press, New York.

Parkinson, James

Encyclopedia of the Neurological Sciences
Copyright 2003, Elsevier Science (USA). All rights reserved.

PARKINSON'S DISEASE affects that part of the brain (basal ganglia) which governs movement. Sufferers therefore show limb weakness, slowness of movements, and shaking, particularly of the hands.

James Parkinson (1755–1824) was born in London and worked as a general practitioner, as did his father and grandfather before him. He was baptized, married, and buried at St. Leonard's Church, Hoxton.

No portrait of Parkinson exists, but his friend, Dr. Mantell, described him as "rather below middle stature, with an energetic intellect, and pleasing expression of countenance, and of mild and courteous manners; readily imparting information, either on his favourite science, or on professional subjects."

Apprenticed to his father, he studied for 6 months at the London Hospital Medical College in 1776. In the following year, he was awarded the Honorary Silver Medal of the Royal Humane Society for resuscitating a Hoxton man who had hanged himself.

In 1784 and 1785, he attended a course of lectures by John Hunter, the "father of British surgery," and was able, because of his knowledge of shorthand, to take down a verbatim account that is still preserved in the Royal College of Surgeons of England. In 1787, he was elected a fellow of the Medical Society of London (founded 1773) and communicated his first paper on the injurious effects of lightning that struck two men in Shoreditch (neighboring Hoxton).

He was a radical in politics, supporting parliamentary reform and women's suffrage. He wrote several political pamphlets under the pseudonym of "Old Hubert" and, as a result, was prosecuted for publishing seditious libel several times and had to give evidence before the Privy Council in the "popgun" plot to assassinate King George III.

He was a leading paleontologist as well as medical attendant to a private madhouse. He published many medical tracts for laymen, but it was his *Essay on the Shaking Palsy*, published in 1817, that makes him a household name today. He and other contemporaries knew nothing of the underlying pathology. At the time, they were unaware of rigidity, the increase of resistance to passive movement, but his clinical description of six cases could hardly be bettered:

> So slight and nearly imperceptible are the first inroads of this malady, and so extremely slow is its progress, that it rarely happens, that the patient can form any recollection of the precise periods of its commencement. The first symptoms perceived are, a slight sense of weakness, with a proneness to trembling in some particular part; sometimes in the head, but most commonly in one of the hands and arms. These symptoms gradually increase in the part first affected; and at an uncertain period, but seldom in less than 12 months or more, the morbid influence is felt in some other part. Thus assuming that one of the hands and arms to be first attacked, the other, at this period becomes similarly affected. After a few more months the patient is found to be less strict than usual in preserving an upright posture; this being most observable whilst walking, but sometimes whilst sitting or standing. Sometime after the appearance of this symptom, and during its slow increase, one of the legs is discovered slightly to tremble, and is also found to suffer fatigue sooner than the leg on the other side. And in a few months this limb becomes agitated by similar tremblings, and suffers a similar loss of power.

After publication of his essay in 1817, Parkinson continued to practice as a general practitioner in Hoxton until his death seven years later. Cooke, whose *Treatise on the Nervous System* was published in 1821, took note of the *Essay*, stating "Mr. Parkinson's *paralysis agitans* or shaking palsy ... appears to me to be highly deserving of our attention." It was not until 1861 that the condition was called maladie de Parkinson (Parkinson's disease) by Charcot (qv).

On December 19, 1824, Parkinson had a sudden onset of right hemiplegia and aphasia and died two days later presumably from a stroke.

—*F. Clifford Rose*

See also–Charcot, Jean-Martin; Parkinsonism; Parkinson's Disease; Parkinson's Disease, Epidemiology (see Index entry Biography for complete list of biographical entries)

Further Reading

Morris, A. D. (1981). In *James Parkinson: His Life and Times* (F. C. Rose, Ed.). Birkhauser, Boston.
Rose, F. C. (1999). James Parkinson (1755–1824). In *A Short History of Neurology: The British Contribution 1660–1910* (F. C. Rose, Ed.), pp. 108–116. Butterworth-Heinemann, London.

Parkinsonism

Encyclopedia of the Neurological Sciences
Copyright 2003, Elsevier Science (USA). All rights reserved.

PARKINSONISM is a descriptive term that refers to the presence of tremor (usually at rest), bradykinesia or slowness of movements without weakness, rigidity or increased muscle tone, and poor balance. The prototype of parkinsonism is Parkinson's disease (PD). Because parkinsonism relates to underactivity of the neurotransmitter system involving dopamine, in the pathway traveling from the substantia nigra to the striatum, drugs that block striatal dopamine receptor can induce the same features and provoke drug-induced parkinsonism. In addition to PD, several other primary neurodegenerative conditions have parkinsonism as one of the major clinical features. However, because they all have additional features not typical of PD and have a poorer response to antiparkinsonian therapy, they share an overall worse prognosis. They are often grouped together with the conglomerate term parkinsonism-plus syndromes. Within this grouping, each condition has distinctive characteristics that are important to recognize and distinguish from one another and from PD.

DRUG-INDUCED PARKINSONISM

The drugs called neuroleptics are the most commonly used agents associated with drug-induced parkinsonism. Neuroleptics are usually used to treat psychosis but sometimes are used as tranquilizers in other situations. Neuroleptic-induced parkinsonism is the result of basal ganglia dopaminergic underactivity due to dopaminergic receptor blockade. Clinically, the parkinsonism cannot be distinguished from PD. Parkinsonism symptoms resolve a few weeks to 6 months after stopping the neuroleptic or with the use of antiparkinsonian drugs. Proposed risk factors for development of neuroleptic-induced parkinsonism are female gender, older age, and the use of high-potency agents. Metoclopramide is an agent used widely in the treatment of gastric complaints and it also blocks dopaminergic receptors and induces parkinsonism. In addition to neuroleptics, several drugs have been related to parkinsonism, such as calcium channel blockers, methyl-phenyl-tetrahydropyridine, and anticancer drugs including fluorouracil, cyclophosphamide, cytosine arabinoside, and methotrexate.

Drug-induced parkinsonism treatment consists of discontinuing or reducing the dose of the offending agent. In psychotic agents, low doses of neuroleptics or one of several novel neuroleptics that lack prominent striatal dopamine receptor blockade, such as clozapine or quetiapine, can be used.

NEURODEGENERATIVE DISORDERS

Multiple-System Atrophy

Multiple-system atrophy (MSA) is a group of closely related disorders that include degeneration in the extrapyramidal, pyramidal, autonomic, and cerebellar systems. The MSA group includes striatonigral degeneration, Shy–Drager syndrome, and olivopontocerebellar atrophy. Neuronal degeneration is much more widespread than in PD, and Lewy bodies are absent. Pathogenic mechanisms for MSA are unknown.

The population prevalence, which refers to the total number of people with the disease in a population at a given time, is unknown; however, in a review of autopsied cases of parkinsonism, reported frequencies ranged from 3.6 to 22%, with a mean of 8.2% (68/833 cases) and a median onset age of 53 years (range, 33–76 years). Based on autopsy-proven cases of MSA, average survival is expected to be less than a decade.

The hallmark features of MSA are parkinsonism that is poorly responsive to dopaminergic therapy and varying degrees of autonomic, cerebellar, and pyramidal dysfunction. Early onset of frequent falling, lack of resting tremor, myoclonic jerks, and significant speech disturbances are characteristic and distinctive from PD. Shy–Drager syndrome is characterized by parkinsonism and prominent autonomic dysfunction, including orthostatic hypotension associated with lightheadedness, impotence, urinary incontinence, and sweating abnormalities. Severe speech disturbances, sleep apnea (severe breathing difficulties during sleep), and psychiatric changes may also occur. Olivopontocerebellar atrophy is characterized by prominent cerebellar abnormalities, and the parkinsonian symptoms may be early or late manifestations. Speech difficulties, swallowing impairment, dementia, and visual disturbances may also occur. Olivopontocerebellar atrophy may be inherited in some families. Familial cases usually begin at a younger age, progress more slowly, and exhibit less autonomic failure than nonhereditary cases. Striatonigral degeneration is characterized by a symmetric bradykinetic-rigid disorder with early falling, speech, and swallowing disturbances. Pyramidal dysfunction including hyper-reflexia is usually prominent. Age of onset is comparable to that of PD, but progression of disability is much more rapid.

There are several neurological conditions that may mimic MSA and can be particularly difficult to distinguish, especially in the first 5 years of clinical illness. These include PD, with prominent postural instability and gait disturbance, PSP (a neurological condition characterized by slowness, eye movement disturbances, and gait problems with loss of balance), and other parkinsonisms including cerebrovascular disease with multiple strokes. The diagnosis of MSA is made by clinical evaluation, but in some cases additional tests may support the diagnosis. Magnetic resonance imaging (MRI) and computed tomography scans of the brain may be useful to rule out strokes or other causes of parkinsonism. In MSA, striatonigral degeneration variant, MRI scan may demonstrate marked basal ganglia abnormalities that suggest iron deposition. In the olivopontocerebellar atrophy variant, prominent cerebellar and brainstem atrophy is usually seen on MRI. Other tests less routinely used include external urethral and rectal sphincter neurophysiological studies that are usually abnormal in almost all patients with MSA. Resting, supine, and standing chemical products such as norepinephrine levels are of questionable value, but supine and standing norepinephrine levels have been found to be slightly elevated in MSA, whereas in other neurological conditions, such as pure autonomic failure, they are usually decreased. Genetic tests are sometimes requested to rule out spinocerebellar ataxias that may mimic MSA.

There is no known effective treatment for this disorder. Dopaminergic therapy including levodopa may provide some, usually short-term, benefit for rigidity, bradykinesia, and postural instability. Patients with MSA usually require larger dosages of levodopa than do patients with PD, but side effects such as increased orthostatic hypotension and facial dystonia often limit the usefulness of levodopa. Patients rarely derive any meaningful benefit from other dopaminergic drugs, including dopaminergic agonists, anticholinergics, amantadine, or other antiparkinsonian drugs. When the patient becomes symptomatic because of significant orthostatic hypotension, this can be treated with salt and fluids. Supplementary measures include wearing elastic stockings to increase central venous volume, and elevating the head of the bed six inches may also be attempted but often proves uncomfortable. Fludrocortisone, an adrenal hormone, often improves orthostatic symptoms by increasing vascular volume, and many patients benefit from constriction of the caliber of the vessels with pro-amatine. Urinary urgency or incontinence may respond to anticholinergic agents such as oxybutinin, desmopressin, or propantheline at bedtime. Impotence may respond to yohimbine, papaverine, sildenafil, or penile implant. Constipation can be treated with cisapride, stool softeners, and bulk-forming agents.

Corticobasal Ganglionic Degeneration

Corticobasal ganglionic degeneration (CBGD) is a progressive, adult-onset bradykinetic-rigid syndrome characterized by the presence of both parkinsonism and cognitive dysfunction. Neither familial predisposition nor environmental factors increase subject risk. Clinically, patients usually develop symptoms after age 60, and neurological signs of CBGD include marked asymmetric limb rigidity, bradykinesia, postural and action tremor, and marked dystonia. Cognitive features include limb apraxia and parietal lobe dysfunction with severe cortical sensory loss. In most instances, the condition starts as an apparent case of PD, but the cortical sensory loss, dystonia, and apraxia quickly become noticeable. Because PSP and MSA can be presented with these signs, they must always be considered in the differential diagnosis.

On pathology, the disease is characterized by asymmetrical atrophy of the frontal and parietal lobes and substantia nigra. The parkinsonism can be treated with modest success in some cases by introducing levodopa or dopaminergic agonists, but the marked disability from the limb apraxia is progressive, untreatable, and markedly disabling. Botulinum toxin can relieve elements of the dystonia. The condition usually progresses steadily, with death occurring within 10 years of diagnosis.

Parkinsonism–Dementia Amyotrophic Lateral Sclerosis Complex

Parkinsonism–dementia amyotrophic lateral sclerosis complex (PDALS) is a distinctive condition that occurs on the island of Guam and is locally known as Lytico–Bodig. It has been the focus of significant research because of the possibility of genetic and environmental causes. A study of more than 2000 affected and nonaffected individuals on Guam showed that the incidence of this disorder peaked in the 1950s and has gradually declined since that time. Early studies focusing on possible environmental dietary toxins were encouraging, but recent work has failed to identify a consistent agent, and the onetime hypothesis that native flour contains a causative neurotoxin is no longer considered tenable. Pathologically, PDALS shows cell loss in the substantia nigra and several histological disturbances in the substantia nigra, anterior horn cells, and pyramidal tracts.

Clinical findings in PDALS range from motor neuron disease in younger patients to parkinsonism with severe dementia in the older population. The ALS form is predominantly seen in the Chamorros, whereas the parkinsonism–dementia presentation may be seen in both Chamorro and Filipino residents. ALS on Guam does not clinically differ from the motor neuron disease seen throughout the world and is characterized by severe motor weakness. Conditions that may mimic PDPALS include Alzheimer's disease, diffuse Lewy body disease, postencephalitic parkinsonism, PD, other atypical parkinsonism syndromes as well as ALS and the various forms of motor neuron disease. Regardless of the form of clinical presentation, the disorder is relentlessly progressive, with death usually occurring within 10 years of diagnosis. Only the benzothiazole riluzole has been shown to provide some benefit in ALS patients, although it has not been extensively studied in the ALS Guam variety. The role of this drug in the parkinsonian features is unclear.

Hemiatrophy/Hemiparkinsonism

Hemiatrophy/hemiparkinsonism (HA/HP) is an uncommon disorder that involves the onset of parkinsonism on one side of the body in association with decreased size of a side of the face, arm, or leg in varying combinations (hemiatrophy). First described by Klawans, the patient presents with parkinsonism just in one side of the body, and the hemiatrophy is completely unnoticed by the patient. Therefore, a hemiparkinsonian patient, comparative examination of the size of the hands and feet may be needed to diagnose the condition. When compared to PD, the parkinsonism of HA/HP usually begins at a younger age and generally remains on the hemiatrophic side for several years before sometimes progressing to a bilateral condition, and it responds poorly to dopaminergic therapy. The etiology is unknown, but early birth injury, from hypoxia or trauma has been posited as a possibility, and there may be some relationship between this syndrome and a distinct form of dystonia termed dopa-responsive dystonia. Hemiatrophy of the contralateral cortex may be seen on MRI in some patients.

Arteriosclerotic Parkinsonism

Arteriosclerotic or vascular parkinsonism is usually characterized by bradykinesia and rigidity without tremor, and there may be other neurological evidence of stroke. Patients with multiple strokes may experience a stepwise progression of symptoms with sudden worsenings. An MRI should confirm the presence of cerebrovascular disease. Multi-infarct parkinsonism rarely shows a positive response to dopaminergic drugs. The main objective in vascular parkinsonism is the prevention of stroke with adequate therapy and the control of risk factors for cerebrovascular disease.

Normal Pressure Hydrocephalus

Normal pressure hydrocephalus (abnormal accumulation of the cerebrospinal fluid in the brain) is an acquired condition leading to mental changes in mentation, gait disturbances, and urinary incontinence. Patients develop overt bradykinesia without tremor. The diagnosis is made by a combination of clinical and imaging findings. Some, but not all, patients will respond to shunting.

MISCELLANEOUS

Infections, including viruses such as HIV and tuberculosis, can cause parkinsonism. Postencephalitic parkinsonism has been considered the most important infectious cause of parkinsonism. Encephalitis lethargic or von Economo disease occurred as an epidemic from 1919 to 1926. It commonly affected young adults in their 20s and 30s, but also involved a substantial number of children. Early symptoms included fever, mental changes, and several neurological deficits. Mortality rates were high. Those who survived were left with various neurological deficits, including parkinsonism, and eye movement abnormalities. Pathological changes were seen in the substantia nigra, subthalamus nucleus, and hypothalamus.

Trauma can also cause parkinsonism. Boxers who endure repeated trauma to the head may develop a syndrome of dementia, parkinsonism, and pyramidal and cerebellar signs. *Dementia pugilistic* refers to the cognitive changes boxers experience years after the trauma occurred. Multiple concussions may cause diffuse brain injury and may initiate dopamine neuronal degeneration.

—*Esther Cubo and Christopher G. Goetz*

See also–Amyotrophic Lateral Sclerosis (ALS); Boxing, Neurology of; Hemiatrophy; Hydrocephalus; Movement Disorders, Overview; Motor System, Overview; Multisystem Atrophy (MSA); Pallidotomy; Parkinson, James; Parkinson's Disease, Epidemiology; Progressive Supranuclear Palsy (PSP); Shy–Drager Syndrome

Further Reading

Hughes, A. J., Colosimo, C., Kleedorfer, B., *et al.* (1992). The dopaminergic response in multiple system atrophy. *J. Neurol. Neurosurg. Psychiatry* **55**, 1009–1013.

Jankovic, J., McDermott, M., Carter, J., *et al.* (1991). Variable expression of Parkinson's disease: A baseline analysis of the DATATOP cohort. *Neurology* **41**, 1529–1534.

Klawans, H. L. (1981). Hemiparkinsonism as a late complication of hemiatrophy: A new syndrome. *Neurology* **31**, 625–628.

Polinsky, R. J. (1993). Shy–Drager syndrome. In *Parkinson's Disease and Movement Disorders* (J. Jankovic and E. Tolosa, Eds.), pp. 191–204. Williams & Wilkins, Baltimore.

Quinn, N. (1994). Multiple system atrophy. In *Movement Disorders* (C. D. Marsden and S. Fahn, Eds.), pp. 263–281. Butterworth, Oxford.

Rinne, J. O., Lee, M. S., Thompson, P. D., *et al.* (1994). Corticobasal degeneration: A clinical study of 36 cases. *Brain* **117**, 1183–1196.

Stacy, M. (1996). Parkinsonism–dementia-amyotrophic lateral sclerosis complex of Guam. In *Neurobase* (J. Jankovic, Ed.). Arbor, San Diego.

Wenning, G. K., Ben Shlomo, Y., Magalhaes, M., *et al.* (1994). Clinical features and natural history of multiple system atrophy: An analysis of 100 cases. *Brain* **117**, 835–845.

Parkinson's Disease

Encyclopedia of the Neurological Sciences

JAMES PARKINSON, a London physician, first described Parkinson's disease in 1817. Its distinctive features of tremor, rigidity, and gait difficulties were appreciated in this early monograph. More than 50 years later, in his teaching at the Salpêtrière Hospital, Jean-Martin Charcot was more thorough in describing the varied features of the illness and distinguished the hallmark of bradykinesia. In the 1960s, the biochemical and pharmacological discoveries that the neurochemical dopamine was depleted in Parkinson's disease and that levodopa, as the precursor to this neurotransmitter, could improve Parkinson's disease signs were described in landmark studies. Although public awareness of Parkinson's disease has been heightened by recognition of the disease in certain actors, political leaders, and public figures, probably the most notorious historical figure afflicted with Parkinson's disease was Adolph Hitler.

After essential tremor, Parkinson's disease is the most common movement disorder and affects approximately 500,000 people in the United States. It is most frequently seen after the age of 50, and approximately 1% of this age group has the disorder. There is a modest (1.5:1) male predominance.

Several studies have suggested that Caucasians are affected more often than African Americans, but this issue is unsettled.

Parkinsonism is a general term that refers to the presence of signs typical of Parkinson's disease: resting tremor (a rhythmic, sinusoidal movement that resolves with movement but is often present with sustained postures), bradykinesia or slowness of movement, rigidity (inflexibility or stiffness), and loss of postural reflexes with unsteadiness (Fig. 1). Several diseases can be associated with these signs and are termed parkinsonian syndromes as a group; Parkinson's disease is the prototype. Signs that additionally help the clinician to distinguish Parkinson's disease clinically from other parkinsonian disorders are asymmetry of parkinsonian signs, marked rest tremor, and a clinically significant response to levodopa. In addition, after several years of levodopa therapy, patients with Parkinson's disease tend to develop irregular medication responses, termed wearing off or motor fluctuations. Patients with other parkinsonian syndromes tend not to develop irregular medication responses. There are few or no balance problems during the first months and years of the disease. Other common signs of Parkinson's disease include shuffling gait, stooped posture, difficulty with fine coordinated movements, soft speech (hypophonia), decreased facial expression (hypomimia), and micrographia (small handwriting).

Moderate and advanced Parkinson's disease patients develop increasing gait and balance difficulties, bradykinesia, and tremor. In the very late stages of the illness, tremor sometimes decreases. The major problems that patients usually experience after 5 years of treatment for Parkinson's disease are motor fluctuations (unpredictable motor response to levodopa in patients with chronic Parkinson's disease) and behavioral or cognitive changes. The emergence of long-term complications probably occurs as a result of the combination of disease progression and levodopa side effects. There are several forms of motor fluctuations. Most commonly, a predictable decline in motor performance occurs near the end of each medication dose. Patients change gradually from an "on" period (the time during which a patient with Parkinson's disease is benefiting from therapy) to an "off" period (the time during which a patient with Parkinson's disease is not benefiting from pharmacotherapy) 30 min to 1 hr before the next medication dose is due. Often, patients experience involuntary movements, termed dyskinesias, as a peak dose complication (when the concentration of

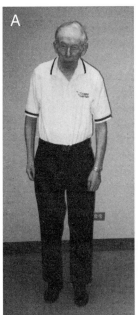 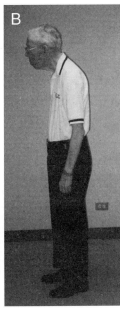 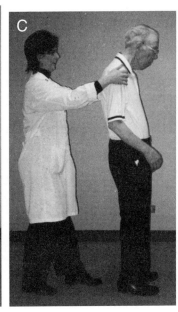 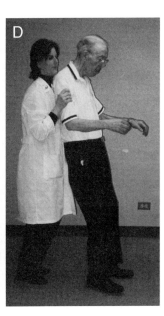

Figure 1
Patient with Parkinson's disease. (A) Front view showing expressionless face and slightly flexed arms. (B) Side view showing stooped posture. (C and D) Compromised postural reflexes whereby when the examiner pulls on the patient's shoulders to test for balance and stability, the patient tilts backwards and falls against the examiner because his feet do not move quickly to compensate.

levodopa is highest in the blood), and sometimes similar movements occur at the end of the dose. Rarely, sudden and severe cataclysms of motor fluctuation occur, with ambulatory patients becoming immobilized over seconds ("freezing").

Among the behavioral and cognitive troubles experienced by Parkinson's disease patients, depression occurs in approximately one-third of patients, especially in patients who have bradykinesia and rigidity as their predominant symptoms. Dementia occurs in approximately one-third of patients, and hallucinations and psychotic behavior occur in approximately one-fourth of chronically treated patients. Dementia is more likely to develop in patients whose parkinsonism did not include tremor in the early phases of clinical disease. The loss of intellectual function almost always involves memory impairment and may be associated with personality changes, impaired judgment, and difficulty with abstract thinking. Olfactory disturbances in odor identification, recognition, and detection thresholds occur in Parkinson's disease and resemble patterns seen in Alzheimer's disease patients.

As many as 70–80% of Parkinson's disease patients experience some degree of autonomic nervous system impairment in later stages of the disease, including decreased salivation, impotence,

orthostatic hypotension, urinary urgency or incontinence, constipation, swallowing difficulties, and sweating abnormalities. Sleep disruption is another common complaint of Parkinson's disease patients, with inability to get a full night of restful sleep. Patients describe both an inability to fall asleep and numerous nighttime awakenings.

The diagnosis of Parkinson's disease is made by evaluation of the patient's history, neurological examination, and response to dopamine replacement therapy. There are no blood tests that make the diagnosis, and brain computed tomography and magnetic resonance imaging (MRI) are typically unremarkable. The definitive diagnosis of Parkinson's disease is made by autopsy. The typical histopathological features found in the brain of Parkinson's disease patients include degeneration of cells in the pigmented brainstem region called the substantia nigra and other deep brain structures, including locus ceruleus, thalamus, cerebral cortex, and autonomic nervous system, and also the determination of abnormal inclusions in these affected neurons, called Lewy bodies. Chemical abnormalities occur in the dopaminergic system as well as the cathecholaminergic and serotonergic systems. After approximately 60–80% of the dopamine-producing neurons of the substantia nigra are lost, the extrapyramidal system can no longer promote movement, and the symptoms of Parkinson's disease appear.

In order to describe the severity of Parkinson's disease, the Hoehn and Yahr scale is used, which describes five stages of Parkinson's disease: stage 1, with unilateral features of Parkinson's disease, including the major features of tremor, rigidity, or bradykinesia; stage 2, with bilateral features as mentioned previously; stage 3, with worsening bilateral features of Parkinson's disease, along with balance difficulties, but patients are still able to function independently; stage 4, patients have severe gait difficulties and are unable to live alone independently; and stage 5, patients need wheelchair assistance or are unable to get out of bed.

The cause of Parkinson's disease is unknown; current research efforts focus on hereditary factors, including several genetic defects, and on environmental toxins that could damage substantia nigra cells selectively. Between 6 and 41% of Parkinson's disease patients have a relative who is also affected with Parkinson's disease. A follow-up study from the World War II Veteran Twins Registry demonstrated overall similarity in concordance for monozygotic (identicals) and dizygotic (no identicals) twins. The study concluded that genetic influences were not important to the etiology of typical Parkinson's disease with onset after age 50, but among the few pairs of early onset Parkinson's disease, genetic influences appeared stronger. Two genes have been identified with familial Parkinson's disease—the α-synuclein gene located in the long arm of chromosome 4 and the parkin gene located in the long arm of chromosome 6. In addition, the tau gene has been shown to be the disease gene for familial frontotemporal dementia and parkinsonism. Many other families with frequent Parkinson's disease have been studied. In these families certain chromosome loci have been mapped: One is in the short arm of chromosome 2, and the two other forms are in the different loci of the short arm of chromosome 4. In familial Parkinson's disease, the age of onset is usually younger than that of nonfamilial Parkinson's disease.

There is also interest in whether exposure to a toxin or multiple toxins might cause Parkinson's disease. Several associations between environmental exposures and Parkinson's disease have been identified, including rural living, well water intake, vegetable farming, exposure to wood pulp, and exposure to pesticides. Some of these associations

are controversial and no single environmental toxin has been identified that might be causative for most patients with Parkinson's disease. Nonetheless, interest in environmental toxins was greatly bolstered by the discovery that MPTP, a heroin derivative, caused a Parkinson's disease-like illness in young adults who injected themselves with this contaminant.

The biological basis of complications that occur in the context of advanced Parkinson's disease after patients have been treated with medication for several years is not well understood. Whereas many aspects of motor fluctuations relate to peripheral delivery problems such as gastrointestinal absorption of medication, changes also occur in the dopaminergic striatal system itself.

Since the cause of Parkinson's disease is unknown, prevention measures and risk factor identification have been elusive. Prevention of rapid disease progression has been clinically studied with antioxidant and vitamin E therapies. The results of these large population studies suggest that antioxidant therapy in the form of the monoamine oxidase B inhibitor selegiline, but not vitamin E, slows the clinical progression of early Parkinson's disease disability. Among demographic factors, young age of onset is associated with a slower clinical progression. Protective factors against the risk of developing Parkinson's disease include cigarette smoking and possibly estrogen in women.

Essential tremor is the movement disease most frequently confused with Parkinson's disease, and some investigators have found a link between Parkinson's disease and essential tremor. There are several variants of Parkinson's disease, termed parkinsonism-plus syndromes. Although patients with the parkinsonism-plus syndromes are generally less responsive to levodopa than Parkinson's disease patients, they may show brisk improvement in the early years. Because clinical features can overlap with Parkinson's disease, MRI scans of the brain have been suggested to help in differentiating the parkinsonism-plus disorders from Parkinson's disease. In the differential diagnosis of early Parkinson's disease, a few additional conditions have been highlighted in recent years.

The current evaluation for a parkinsonian patient is not extensive. Medication history will establish likely drug-induced disease, and if the parkinsonism occurs in the context of other neurological signs, extrapyramidal or otherwise, more extensive metabolic and scanning evaluations may be of higher yield. Computed tomography scans, electroencephalography (brain waves), and MRI scans of the brain are typically normal in patients with Parkinson's disease. In young patients, more extensive biochemical tests, including evaluations for Wilson's disease, should be undertaken. Single photon emission computed tomography and positron emission tomography scans are of little clinical practical use, and their use is largely experimental.

Parkinson's disease is known to be a slowly progressive disorder. Although an average rate of progression can be defined, it is not possible to accurately predict prognosis for an individual patient. After the discovery of specific therapy for Parkinson's disease, mortality figures changed. Prior to the availability of levodopa, the mortality rate for Parkinson's disease patients was almost three times that of the general population. Later reports argued that life expectancy in Parkinson's disease was normal; however, recent studies suggest that mortality may still be increased in Parkinson's disease patients relative to the general population. Added dementia is the highest risk factor for shortened life.

Treatment of Parkinson's disease focuses on two distinct concepts—arresting the progressive natural history of the disorder and developing new and effective symptomatic therapies. Neuroprotective therapies are those that slow neuronal degeneration, thereby delaying disease progression. No neuroprotective therapy has been identified. Selegiline (a monoamine oxidase B inhibitor) has been associated with a slower progression of clinical Parkinson's disease impairment, similarly to another monoamine oxidase B inhibitor, lazabemide. Likewise, based on evidence that levodopa may have trophic effects, early treatment with levodopa is currently being tested for neuroprotective efficacy and safety.

Symptomatic therapies are those that improve signs and symptoms without affecting the underlying disease state. Degeneration of the substantia nigra in Parkinson's disease causes a striatal dopamine deficiency. Administration of levodopa, the chemical precursor of dopamine, increases dopamine concentration in the striatum, especially when its peripheral breakdown is inhibited by carbidopa. Levodopa therapy is currently the gold standard of symptomatic therapy for Parkinson's disease. The most common side effect of levodopa is nausea. If a patient has difficulty initiating levodopa due to nausea, the patient may take it with meals or with additional carbidopa. Other potential side effects of levodopa include orthostatic hypotension, confusion, hallucinations, psychosis, and hypersexuality. Cognitive side effects typically occur later in the disease in patients who have developed underlying dementia. Confusion may improve with a decrease in levodopa dose. Hallucinations and hypersexuality can be treated with clozapine or quetiapine, which are atypical neuroleptics with minimal parkinsonian side effects. Levodopa therapy is generally initiated when signs of decreasing independence develop. A long-acting form of levodopa, Sinemet-CR, is a newer formulation of levodopa with slow-release properties. Theoretically, a more continuous dopaminergic stimulation could provide improved efficacy and fewer motor fluctuations. Alternatively, motor fluctuations have been managed by frequent (hourly) ingestion of levodopa in liquid form. A chemical variant of levodopa termed levodopa ethyl ester has been used as a rapidly acting "rescue" therapy in patients with severe motor fluctuations (with frequent and severe episodes of freezing or immobility). Other mild medications that can often be used for early symptoms include anticholinergics for young tremorous patients and amantadine for mild bradykinesia, rigidity, and gait disturbance.

Dopamine agonists, drugs that stimulate striatal dopaminergic receptors and mimic dopamine effects, are used as adjuncts to levodopa and as a monotherapy at the beginning of the disease. In moderate and advanced disease, patients with motor fluctuations on levodopa may benefit from the addition of a dopamine agonist to smooth motor fluctuations and improve symptoms control. Dopamine agonists include bromocriptine, pergolide, ropirinole, and pramipexole. Side effects of agonists when used alone, and especially when used in conjunction with levodopa, include hypotension, dyskinesia, and hallucinations. Recently, catechol-O-methyl transferase inhibitor agents that enhance delivery of levodopa to the brain have also been studied in patients concurrently on levodopa. Entacapone, which acts primarily extracerebrally, and tolcapone, which acts both extracerebrally and intracerebrally, increase central availability of levodopa. Both drugs have been associated with antiparkinsonian efficacy, fewer motor fluctuations, and reduced daily levodopa dosing requirements. Because of hepatotoxicity concerns, tolcapone treatment must include regular hepatic enzyme monitoring. Two nondopaminergic therapies have recently been advocated in select patients with Parkinson's disease—estrogen for women and vitamin D for elderly patients—but extensive studies on these agents have not been conducted.

Neurosurgical treatments have emerged as new experimental possibilities for advanced Parkinson's disease. The three basic types of surgery for Parkinson's disease are implantation, lesioning, and stimulation. Implantation involves the delivery of tissue or other material into a target site. It is thought that implanted cells can replace lost neurons to restore in this case dopaminergic function. Adrenal medullary cells that can produce dopamine were found to provide some benefit in animal studies, but in humans the patients who were transplanted experienced only modest and transient improvement in the context of significant surgical complications. This procedure has been abandoned. Fetal brainstem tissue has been transplanted to the striatum with positive results, including clinical improvement, PET scans demonstrating enhanced dopaminergic activity, and excellent graft survival in autopsy examinations. Genetically engineered cells that produce levodopa or dopamine are in preclinical development. Trophic factors or chemicals that alter the environment or growth of neurons are also investigative but offer potential application for primary neurodegenerative disorders such as Parkinson's disease.

Lesioning involves the destruction of a target site to modify overall brain function. The target is usually identified by electrophysiological techniques. Thalamotomy (lesion of the ventral intermediate nucleus of the thalamus) has been shown to be effective in reducing tremor and, to a less extent, rigidity. Bradykinesia and postural instability are not improved. Unilateral pallidotomy has been extensively employed and has been shown to be very effective in alleviating dyskinesia and to improve motor function during the off state. Both contralateral and ipsilateral tremor showed significant improvement, and other parkinsonian motor disability measures also improved. Side effects of pallidotomy and thalamotomy include intracerebral hemorrhages, weakness, seizures, speech and swallowing difficulties, behavioral changes, and weight gain.

Deep brain stimulation involves the implantation of an electrode with an exposed tip into a target site. The electrode is then connected to a wire run beneath the skin to a stimulator placed in the chest wall. Stimulation is a reversible form of lesions since the stimulation is high frequency and modifies the function of the target site. The principal advantage of stimulation is that it provides a degree of control, and if a side effect occurs due to electrical stimulation, the stimulation can be reduced and the side effects will resolve. High-frequency stimulation of thalamic nuclei, globus pallidus, or subthalamic nucleus is supposed to interrupt presumed overactive basal ganglia circuits, but the mechanism of action is not known. Patients with severe functional disability due to medically refractory tremor are the best candidates for chronic thalamic stimulation. This procedure does not improve other parkinsonian features, such as rigidity and incoordination. Subthalamic stimulation has been shown to be superior to pallidal stimulation with regard to parkinsonian features, especially bradykinesia. In addition, pallidal stimulation has been associated with cognitive decline in some patients, especially in older subjects on high preoperative doses of levodopa.

In addition to pharmacological and surgical concerns, rehabilitation with physical therapy programs, including therapeutic exercises, gait training, and psychosocial support, improves mobility and quality of life. A major concern among families and patients is driving safety and the need for an objective and clear safety evaluation procedures. Supportive care and continued guidance are perceived by patients to be important, and nurse specialists may provide other community services and support in addition to those available in medical centers.

—*Esther Cubo and Christopher G. Goetz*

***See also*—Basal Ganglia; Corpus Striatum; Deep Brain Stimulation; Degenerative Disorders; Movement Disorders, Overview; Motor System, Overview; Pallidotomy; Parkinson, James; Parkinsonism; Parkinson's Disease, Epidemiology; Progressive Supranuclear Palsy (PSP)**

Further Reading

Bajaj, N. P., Shaw, C., Warner, T., *et al.* (1998). The genetics of Parkinson's disease and parkinsonian syndromes. *J. Neurol.* **245**, 625–633.

Gorell, J. M., Johnson, C. C., Rybicki, B. A., *et al.* (1998). The risk of Parkinson's disease with exposure to pesticides, farming, well water, and rural living. *Neurology* **50**, 1346–1350.

Koller, W. C., and Tolosa, E. (1998). Current and emerging drug therapies in the management of Parkinson's disease. *Neurology* **50**, S1.

Limousin, P., Greene, J., Pollak, P., *et al.* (1997). Changes in cerebral activity pattern due to subthalamic nucleus or internal pallidum stimulation in Parkinson's disease. *Ann. Neurol.* **42**, 283–291.

Mizuno, Y., Hattori, N., and Mori, H. (1999). Genetics of Parkinson's disease. *Biomed. Pharmacother.* **53**, 109–116.

Olanow, C. W., Kordower, J. H., and Freeman, T. B. (1996). Fetal nigral transplantation for the treatment of Parkinson's disease. *Trends Neurosci.* **19**, 102–108.

Poewe, W. H., and Wenning, G. K. (1998). The natural history of Parkinson's disease. *Ann. Neurol.* **44**, S1–S9.

Shannon, K. M., Penn, R. D., Kroin, J. S., *et al.* (1998). Stereotactic pallidotomy for the treatment of Parkinson's disease. *Neurology* **50**, 434–438.

Soto-Otero, R., Mendez-Alvarez, E., Riguera-Vega, R., *et al.* (1998). Studies on the interaction between 1,2,3,4-tetrahydro-beta-carboline and cigarette smoke: A potential mechanism of neuroprotection for Parkinson's disease. *Brain Res.* **802**, 155–162.

Parkinson's Disease, Epidemiology

Encyclopedia of the Neurological Sciences
Copyright 2003, Elsevier Science (USA). All rights reserved.

PARKINSON'S DISEASE is a neurodegenerative disorder of mid- to late life characterized clinically by resting tremor, bradykinesia, cogwheel rigidity, and postural reflex impairment. Pathologically, Parkinson's disease is distinguished by specific areas of nerve cell loss, most notably pigmented aminergic brainstem neurons, and by the presence of characteristic α-synuclein positive intracytoplasmic inclusion bodies (Lewy bodies). Specific genetic or environmental causes of parkinsonism resembling Parkinson's disease have been described, but these account for only a small proportion of disease. The cause or causes of most cases remain unknown.

Epidemiology is the study of the distribution and dynamics of diseases in human populations and of the factors that affect these characteristics. Knowledge of these patterns can be important for public health planning. In addition, investigation of the pattern of disease in populations may provide clues to the determinants of disease. Since the etiology of Parkinson's disease is unknown, epidemiological studies can be a powerful tool in the investigation of this disease. The epidemiological investigation of Parkinson's disease presents specific challenges, however. Since there is no antemortem diagnostic test for Parkinson's disease, diagnosis can vary with the skill of the examiner as well as the diagnostic criteria applied. Diagnostic criteria have varied over time. As a result, direct comparisons of epidemiological studies is difficult. For example, persons with atypical parkinsonism, essential tremor, or secondary parkinsonism may have been included in some studies.

DISEASE FREQUENCY

James Parkinson described the first cases of Parkinson's disease in 1817, but community-based incidence and prevalence studies of Parkinson's disease were not performed until the 1950s. In these studies, Parkinson's disease was found to be one of the most common neurodegenerative disorders of the elderly.

Incidence

The frequency of a disease can most accurately be measured by estimating incidence, which is the number of new cases of a disorder identified in a defined population during a specific time interval. Incidence is particularly important for a slowly progressive disorder such as Parkinson's disease because it is relatively unaffected by factors affecting disease survival. There are few studies of Parkinson's disease and almost all have been conducted in North America or Europe. Estimated annual incidence ranges from 4.5 to 19 new cases per 100,000 persons, although direct comparison of these estimates is not appropriate because the age and gender of the underlying populations may differ. When comparisons are made after adjustment to a standard population, variability is reduced. For North America, Western Europe, and Japan, the incidence of Parkinson's disease is similar. In all countries reported, Parkinson's disease occurs only rarely before age 50. Incidence increases with increasing age so that incidence in the ninth decade of life is typically 20 or more times greater than that in the sixth decade of life. Men are typically affected more frequently than women.

Prevalence

Prevalence is the total number of existing cases of disease in a population at a specific time. Prevalence is determined not only by the incidence of disease but also by factors determining survival after diagnosis. In the case of Parkinson's disease, prevalence is typically much greater than incidence because persons with Parkinson's disease typically live many years. Reported estimates of prevalence show tremendous variability internationally. Although differences in the age distribution in the populations studied, as well as differences in the methods used to identify cases, can account for some of this variation, it is possible that there are real differences in disease prevalence worldwide. For North America or Europe, overall crude prevalence is typically estimated to be between 100 and 200/100,000 population, although Parkinson's disease prevalence greater than 400/100,000 has been reported. For Asia or Africa, however, reported Parkinson's disease prevalence may be as much as 10 times lower. Parkinson's disease prevalence is typically greater in men and increases with increasing age. For persons in the eighth and ninth decades of life, estimated Parkinson's disease prevalence of 1000–2000/100,000 is not unusual in North America or Europe. As the percentage of older persons in the United States and Europe increases in the next decades, the number of persons with Parkinson's disease in these countries, and the consequent societal tolls, is expected to increase dramatically.

Mortality

Mortality is the least reliable measure of Parkinson's disease frequency because Parkinson's disease is rarely a direct cause of death. Consequently, reporting of Parkinson's disease on death certificates is inconsistent. Several studies have shown that in approximately 50% of known Parkinson's disease cases, Parkinson's disease is not listed as a primary or contributing cause on the death certificate. Therefore, it is particularly problematic to use death certificates to estimate geographic distribution of disease since recording on death certificates can vary with local practices. One consistent observation is a trend in recent years of lower death rates from Parkinson's disease in the sixth and seventh decades but higher rates in the eighth and ninth decades of life. This pattern likely represents improved survival due to advances in therapy, beginning with the introduction of levodopa in the 1970s.

Temporal Variation

A number of studies have attempted to examine changes in the frequency of Parkinson's disease over time, searching for patterns that could provide important etiological clues. For example, a steady increase or decrease in incidence over decades might be explained by corresponding changes in exposure to causative or protective factors. Alternatively, periodic fluctuations in incidence might suggest a sporadically present causative agent. Unfortunately, comparison of Parkinson's disease frequency at more than one point in time has been possible for only a few populations. In these, the period of observation has typically been only one or two decades, perhaps not long enough to allow observation of any but the most dramatic temporal trends. Also, because Parkinson's disease is relatively rare, and the populations studied have often been small, precision has sometimes been poor.

No study has reported a decrease in Parkinson's disease frequency in recent times. Whether the frequency of Parkinson's disease has been stable during the past few decades or has increased more recently remains less certain. Modest to moderate increases in Parkinson's disease incidence have been reported for populations in Minnesota, Finland, Australia, England, and Taiwan. Others have reported no change in frequency in Hawaii and Japan. Whether these apparent increases in Parkinson's disease reflect changes in risk factors in these populations or simply increased disease recognition is unknown.

Geographic Variation

Many studies suggest that the frequency of Parkinson's disease varies from country to country. When all published studies are considered, Parkinson's disease incidence and prevalence are most often reported to be greatest in North America and Western Europe. Parkinson's disease incidence and prevalence are lower in east Asia and Africa, even when comparable methods are used to ascertain cases (such as door-to-door surveys). However, these contrasts are most obvious in studies performed in the 1980s and 1990s. The most recent estimates of incidence and prevalence are similar to those reported for Western countries. These apparent geographic variations may be due to differences in study methods. Alternatively, there may be real differences in Parkinson's disease frequency internationally. Because there is a temporal trend to higher rates in recent years, it is not likely that this pattern is due solely to genetic differences in the populations studied. Instead, this pattern suggests that environmental differences in the populations studied could account for the differences in Parkinson's disease frequency observed in prior decades.

RISK FACTORS

Risk Factors Suggested by Demographic Patterns

The patterns of Parkinson's disease in populations may provide clues to the cause(s) of the disease. The most universally observed demographic characteristics of Parkinson's disease are the associations of Parkinson's disease with increasing age and male gender. Whether or not whites are at greater risk of Parkinson's disease remains controversial.

Age: Increasing age is the only unequivocal risk factor for Parkinson's disease. Parkinson's disease incidence increases with increasing age throughout the life span. This is true in all community-based studies, regardless of the absolute prevalence of disease in the population. Parkinson's disease occurs rarely before the age of 50, but rates increase steadily thereafter. The reasons for this relationship are not known. Possible explanations for the near-exponential correlation between increasing age and Parkinson's disease prevalence include age-related neuronal vulnerability or an accumulation of toxins due to exposure over a period of time. In some populations, Parkinson's disease appears to decline after the eighth or ninth decade. This apparent decline among the most elderly is probably not a reflection of the true underlying frequency of disease but instead due to difficulties ascertaining Parkinson's disease in this age group.

Because of the strength and consistency of this risk factor, comparisons of disease frequency among populations must be adjusted for their differing age distributions. Similarly, evaluation of any putative risk factor requires concomitant adjustment for the distribution of that risk factor with respect to age.

Gender: Men are more commonly affected with Parkinson's disease than women in almost all populations studied. Male preponderance of Parkinson's disease is most remarkable after the sixth decade. Thereafter, on average, of every five persons with Parkinson's disease, three are men and two are women. The reason for this pattern is unknown. Evidence suggests different determinants for earlier and later onset Parkinson's disease, however. If earlier onset disease includes a greater proportion of inherited forms of parkinsonism, distribution in men and women might be expected to be equal. If environmental determinants are important in later onset Parkinson's disease, differences in exposures between men and women might explain the difference in disease frequency. Alternatively, biological differences, such as those related to sex hormones, might explain the pattern observed.

Race: The prevalence of Parkinson's disease appears to be highest for whites in Europe and North America. Until recently, Parkinson's disease was found less frequently in Japanese and Chinese and even less often in blacks in Africa. Comparisons of Parkinson's disease prevalence in African and U.S. blacks found higher rates in the United States. Recent reports from Japan and China have also found Parkinson's disease to be as frequent as in white populations. These observations argue against the proposal that whites are at greater risk of Parkinson's disease. Rather, greater Parkinson's disease frequency seems to be determined by geography and time. Such patterns may in part reflect differences in awareness and diagnosis of Parkinson's disease. However, differences in environmental risk factors could also explain these patterns.

Environmental Risk Factors

The idea that environmental exposure might cause Parkinson's disease was triggered by the observation of a cluster of parkinsonism in narcotics addicts. The causative agent was identified as 1-methyl-4-phenyl-1,2,4,6-tetrahydropyridine (MPTP). When injected intravenously, MPTP caused irreversible parkinsonism remarkable for its clinical similarities to Parkinson's disease. Although toxicants had long been known to cause parkinsonism, MPTP-induced parkinsonism was the first to cause a syndrome of levodopa-responsive parkinsonism without other symptoms or signs, compellingly similar to "idiopathic" Parkinson's disease. In postmortem studies of animals and a few humans, the distribution of nerve cell injury within the brain also paralleled that seen in Parkinson's disease, although whether Lewy bodies occur was uncertain. This observation sparked a search for environmental factors that might be causally related to idiopathic Parkinson's disease either by increasing or by decreasing the risk of disease. In this sense, "environmental" refers to all exposures not intrinsic to the organism. Among these are exposures due to occupation, place of residence, lifestyle, diet, and infectious agents.

Cigarette Smoking: The most frequently observed association between an exposure and Parkinson's disease is the inverse association between cigarette smoking and Parkinson's disease risk. This pattern has been seen in nearly every population in which it has been investigated, independent of race, nationality, or time. In the most compelling studies, smoking histories were collected well in advance of the diagnosis of Parkinson's disease, obviating any bias that may have been caused by selective recall or smoking-associated illnesses. The "dose" of smoking also appears to be important; that is, smoking more cigarettes makes one less likely to develop Parkinson's disease.

However, despite the strength of this association, the underlying biological rationale is not established. In the few laboratory studies done to date, nicotine, a key component of cigarette smoke, appears to protect against experimental parkinsonism. However, cigarette smoke contains hundreds of compounds, and most have not been investigated. Additional work in this area is a priority. Although smoking cigarettes has unequivocal health hazards, the identification of the underlying Parkinson's disease-causing agent could lead to the development of a safe preventive agent.

Coffee/Caffeine: A recent but equally strong observation is that coffee and caffeine consumption is associated with a decreased risk of Parkinson's disease. Consumption of coffee or caffeine-containing beverages in midlife lowers the risk of developing Parkinson's disease. In one study, coffee has also been shown to be inversely associated with pathological changes thought to represent presymptomatic Parkinson's disease ("incidental" Lewy bodies). As with cigarette smoking, coffee drinking has been proposed by some to simply represent a preparkinsonian personality profile. Most, however, believe that pharmacological properties of caffeine more likely explain this association. For example, some laboratory studies suggest that caffeine may have neuroprotective effects on dopaminergic neurons.

Industrialization-Associated Exposures: Parkinson's disease appears to be less common in countries with lower levels of industrialization, providing indirect support for the idea that industrial chemical exposure might cause Parkinson's disease. Several studies using indirect measures of Parkinson's disease suggested associations between Parkinson's disease and specific industries, including steel mining and manufacturing, farming, and wood pulp and paper manufacturing. Very similar results were found in a Michigan study using county-specific Parkinson's disease mortality rates. Parkinson's disease mortality was reported more often in counties with chemical, iron, copper, paper, and pulp industries. In case–control studies, persons with Parkinson's disease (cases) are compared to otherwise similar persons without Parkinson's disease (controls). Numerous case–control studies, primarily investigating populations in North America or Europe, have implicated specific broad categories of industry, including farming, chemical manufacturing, and the steel industry. The determination of specific chemicals related to Parkinson's disease is the next challenge.

Pesticides: The association of Parkinson's disease with farming was the most consistent finding among studies performed early after the description of MPTP-induced parkinsonism. Interest in a possible association between chemicals used in farming, such as pesticides, and Parkinson's disease ensued. The structural and mechanistic resemblances of some common agricultural chemicals to the toxin MPTP are particularly intriguing. For example, the herbicide paraquat is a structural analog of MPTP. The pesticide rotenone and MPTP both inhibit mitochondrial complex I. In mice, rotenone or paraquat can produce biochemical and behavioral changes thought to be the equivalent of those of human parkinsonism, including selective reduction in striatal dopamine. When paraquat is combined with the fungicide maneb, even greater damage results. *In vitro*, rotenone, dieldrin, and paraquat cause aggregation of the protein α-synuclein. Aggregation of α-synuclein is thought to be an important determinant of Lewy body formation *in vivo*.

These observations in the laboratory have parallels in human populations, although the associations are less clear. In many case–control studies, Parkinson's disease risk is increased in association with farming or pesticide exposure. In a few studies, specific classes of agents have been identified, including alkylated phosphates, organochlorines, and thiocarbamates, but these findings have not been consistent across studies. In a few populations, specific agents have been identified, including paraquat, rotenone, and dieldrin. In a combined analysis of the published results of 19 case–control studies, the risk of Parkinson's disease was 90% greater in persons reporting pesticide exposure than in those with no exposure.

Although reproducibility of the associations over many different studies lends strength to these observations, a cause–effect relationship cannot be assumed. Biological plausibility is provided by the laboratory investigations. Nonetheless, the significance of these associations should be weighed cautiously, pending further investigations in human populations and experimental settings.

Metal Exposure: Although less consistently observed than the association with pesticides, metal exposure has also been proposed to increase the risk of Parkinson's disease. Occupational manganese exposure has long been known to produce parkinsonism, but manganese-induced parkinsonism is recognized to be a distinct disorder from Parkinson's disease. Specific associations between metals and Parkinson's disease have rarely been carefully investigated. Preliminary evidence suggests that occupational exposures to combinations of lead and copper, iron and copper, and lead and iron can increase the risk of Parkinson's disease. In postmortem studies, elevated iron levels have been observed in the substantia nigra of Parkinson's disease patients. In laboratory investigations, metal exposure can cause increased aggregation of α-synuclein and predispose to oxidative nerve cell death under certain conditions, lending biological plausibility to the proposed role for these compounds in the pathogenesis of Parkinson's disease.

Infection: The observation that parkinsonism was a common delayed sequela of encephalitis lethargica, a disorder that was pandemic in the 1910s and 1920s, prompted the postulate that all cases of parkinsonism were the result of exposure to that infectious agent. The corollary prediction, that Parkinson's disease would ultimately disappear as survivors of that epoch died, has proven incorrect. Today, few cases of parkinsonism are postencephalitic, but the incidence of Parkinson's disease is unchanged or even increased.

Many have sought to identify an infectious agent in Parkinson's disease, but definitive evidence of such an association has not been obtained. One study suggested a periodic pattern of Parkinson's disease incidence consistent with *in utero* exposure to influenza virus, but this observation was not confirmed. Early childhood measles was inversely associated with Parkinson's disease in one population, but this observation was not replicated. Others have used biological measures, such as serum or spinal fluid antibody titers, to investigate an association between Parkinson's disease and infectious agents. Occasional associations have been observed, but none has been consistent across populations.

The most intriguing of the infectious hypotheses of Parkinson's disease is the proposal that *Nocardia asteroides*, a common soil pathogen, may cause Parkinson's disease. In mice and primates, infection with *N. asteroides* causes a slowly progressive degeneration of nigral dopaminergic neurons accompanied by a levodopa-responsive movement disorder. There are no clinical signs of an acute infectious process following exposure. In humans, the evidence is less straightforward. Increased antibody titers to the common soil pathogen *N. asteroides* have been found in Parkinson's disease patients compared to controls, but not consistently. This may reflect difficulties in making such a determination in

humans because *N. asteroides* is ubiquitous, and the significance of serum antibodies is uncertain. Moreover, only certain strains of *N. asteroides* cause the movement disorder in animals, and there is no assay available to determine whether humans have been exposed to these specific strains. Nonetheless, *N. asteroides* exposure is agriculture–related, and it is an alternate exposure for the farming-associated patterns observed in case–control studies.

Diet: It has been proposed that oxidative mechanisms, such as oxidative stress and free radical formation by toxic compounds, play an important role in the pathogenesis of Parkinson's disease. This observation has resulted in the complimentary hypotheses that diets rich in antioxidants may prevent Parkinson's disease and those causing increased oxidative stress may cause Parkinson's disease. To date, epidemiological findings lend support to the latter but not the former hypothesis. Parkinson's disease risk is increased in persons with midlife diets high in calories and animal fat. Lipids are a major source of oxygen radicals through peroxidation, and when consumed in high concentrations they can have toxic effects on tissue function in different regions including the brain. In accordance, diets rich in vitamins with antioxidant activity, such as carotenoids, vitamin C, and vitamin E, have been proposed to protect against oxidative damage. However, dietary studies have not found such a protective association for Parkinson's disease.

Head Trauma: Parkinsonism is recognized to occur in pugilists following repeated head injuries, although this form of parkinsonism is clinically and pathologically distinct from Parkinson's disease. Retrospective case–control studies have often reported an association between head trauma and Parkinson's disease. However, this association has been viewed skeptically because subjects with a chronic illness typically seek explanations for their disease in prior experiences, and those with central nervous system injuries might be particularly thoughtful about an association between head injuries and parkinsonism. Recently, one study confirmed an association of head trauma with increased risk of Parkinson's disease by examining a medical database, thus removing any effect of selective recall. As with all single observations, replication in additional populations is desirable.

Emotional Stress: Stress has been cited as a possible cause of Parkinson's disease. Laboratory studies suggest that stress-produced changes in central dopamine systems could theoretically increase dopamine turnover and result in an increased risk of oxidative nerve cell death, thus contributing to the development of parkinsonism. Similarly, persons with Parkinson's disease experience transient worsening of their symptoms during stressful periods. Three reports have linked the extreme emotional and physical hardship of concentration camp imprisonment with the subsequent development of Parkinson's disease, whereas one study did not find such an association. Whether these observations reflect an accelerated nigral injury as a result of a stress-related increase in dopamine turnover with resultant increased oxidative injury, nutritional deficiencies of dietary protective agents, or other factors cannot be determined. Evaluation of the relationship of less severe emotional or physical stress and the development of Parkinson's disease poses a methodological challenge.

GENETIC FORMS OF PARKINSONISM

Genes Causing Parkinsonism

Several specific genes causing parkinsonism have been identified. First identified was the gene encoding α-synuclein, responsible for a rare, dominantly inherited disorder limited to fewer than 100 individuals worldwide. More common is the recessively inherited disorder caused by mutations in the *Parkin* gene, accounting for most cases of parkinsonism beginning before age 30. However, parkinsonism with onset before age 50 accounts for less than 10% of all disease worldwide, so this genetic form is also not a common cause of parkinsonism. An unusual form of parkinsonism and dementia has been linked to chromosome 17, but these cases also seem to be rare. Other families with apparently inherited parkinsonism have been identified, but a causative gene has not. Similarly, two recent reports of genomewide screens in familial parkinsonism obtained conflicting results. Apart from replicating the association of *Parkin* mutations and early onset parkinsonism, none of the chromosomal associations found in one study were reproduced in the other. One study did find an association of several single nucleotide polymorphisms in the gene encoding tau on chromosome 17 and familial parkinsonism. Careful cognitive testing was not performed at ascertainment, which is problematic since tau abnormalities are implicated in Alzheimer's disease and

in several forms of atypical parkinsonism with cognitive impairment, including the chromosome-linked familial parkinsonism previously mentioned, progressive supranuclear palsy, and cortical basal ganglionic degeneration. Whether these findings pertain to Parkinson's disease or to one of the forms of atypical parkinsonism requires further investigation.

In general, the genetic forms of parkinsonism described to date are characterized by younger age at onset and some atypical clinical features in at least some family members. Investigation of the biological function of the genes identified can provide important clues to the causes of all forms of Parkinson's disease. Determination of the relationship of any of these forms of familial parkinsonism to most cases of Parkinson's disease, in which there is not a family history, will require additional studies.

Familial Aggregation Studies

Investigating whether there are genetic determinants of later onset Parkinson's disease has many challenges. Case–control studies have suggested a genetic component to Parkinson's disease by the finding that cases more frequently report affected family members than do controls. However, it is important to remember when considering familial patterns that in addition to genes, families also share behaviors and environments. Furthermore, because Parkinson's disease begins in later life, most studies have had to obtain information from Parkinson's disease patients regarding whether the disease was present in deceased relatives. Because Parkinson's disease patients are probably more prone to investigate whether other relatives have had Parkinson's disease than are persons without Parkinson's disease, an overestimation of disease in cases and an underestimation in controls can result. Moreover, whether or not Parkinson's disease patients who have affected family members carry mutations associated with known genetic causes of parkinsonism has not been determined in case–control studies. Despite these cautions, case–control studies have consistently found Parkinson's disease risk to be greater in those with a relative with the disease (first or second degree)—from 2 to 14 times greater, depending on study methods. In population-based studies that have attempted to take into account family makeup (number and ages of family members) and more stringent diagnostic criteria (history of a physician diagnosis rather than report of symptoms resembling Parkinson's disease), lower risks have been observed.

Evidence for a genetic component to parkinsonism was reported in a study of the population of Iceland, for which genealogical information is known over many generations. The Icelandic parkinsonian population differs from other populations, however, because Parkinson's disease is more common in the younger age groups and less frequent as the population ages. Perhaps genetic forms of parkinsonism in which younger age at onset is common account for a larger proportion of parkinsonism in Iceland.

Twin Studies

Twin studies can provide information concerning the relative contribution of genetic and environmental factors to disease through comparisons of disease concordance in monozygotic and dizygotic twins. Monozygotic twins have identical nuclear DNA (although mitochondrial DNA can differ). Dizygotic twins share genes as frequently as do other siblings—on average, approximately 50%. If concordance in monozygotic twins is greater than that in dizygotic twins, a genetic cause of disease is indicated, whereas similar rates suggest shared environment. Twin studies support a strong genetic component for early onset parkinsonism, consistent with the observation that disease onset is early in families with identified genetic mutations. Environmental causes have been suggested for typical later onset Parkinson's disease (beginning after age 50). Later onset disease has been observed with equal frequency in monozygotic and dizygotic twins in cross-sectional studies (in which twin pairs have been evaluated only once). These studies may have missed concordant pairs if there was a long interval between onset in the first and second twin. Two small studies have evaluated twins at two points in time. One study found no difference in concordance after 8 years of follow-up. In this study, no pairs were lost to follow-up. A second study found newly concordant monozygotic pairs but no newly concordant dizygotic pairs after follow-up of 2.5–8 years, suggesting a genetic contribution to later onset Parkinson's disease. However, only a few of the original twins were included. Population-based studies with more pairs are needed to determine which of these findings best represents typical Parkinson's disease.

Gene–Environment Interaction

Recent interest has focused on the interaction of genes and environmental exposures in causing Parkinson's disease. Evidence supports such an interaction as a cause of Parkinson's disease. A person with a genetic susceptibility factor would manifest disease only if a specific exposure were encountered. Such interactions have been observed in other diseases. In Parkinson's disease, an interaction between cigarette smoking and one variant of the gene encoding the dopamine-metabolizing enzyme monoamine oxidase B has been described. Others have sought interactions between genes encoding enzymes metabolizing xenobiotics, but results have been inconsistent.

CONCLUSION

Parkinson's disease will become increasingly important in the following decades as the number of persons older than age 50 (and thus at risk for Parkinson's disease) increases in many countries. Understanding the distribution of the disease will be critical for planning adequate health services. More important, identifying the determinants of Parkinson's disease may lead to improved strategies for treating the disease. Even more important is the goal of preventing Parkinson's disease. Achieving this goal will most likely not be simple. Work to date suggests that Parkinson's disease is a complex disorder. Determining the interactions of genes and exposures that result in Parkinson's disease is a major challenge. Continued identification of genetic forms of parkinsonism will no doubt assist in this goal. Collaboration between epidemiologists and researchers attempting to identify disease mechanisms is necessary so that early identification and, ultimately, prevention of Parkinson's disease may become possible.

—*Robert D. Field and Caroline M. Tanner*

See also–Brain Injury, Traumatic: Epidemiological Issues; Degenerative Disorders; Epilepsy, Epidemiology; Movement Disorders, Overview; Motor System, Overview; Neuroepidemiology, Overview; Parkinson, James; Parkinsonism; Parkinson's Disease

Further Reading

Bower, J. H., Maraganore, D. M., McDonnell, S. K., *et al.* (1999). Incidence and distribution of parkinsonism in Olmsted County, Minnesota, 1976–1990. *Neurology* **52**, 1214–1220.
Gorell, J. M., Rybicki, B. A., Cole Johnson, C., *et al.* (1999). Occupational metal exposures and the risk of Parkinson's disease. *Neuroepidemiology* **18**, 303–308.

Grandinetti, A., Morens, D. M., Reed, D., *et al.* (1994). Prospective study of cigarette smoking and the risk of developing idiopathic Parkinson's disease. *Am. J. Epidemiol.* **139**, 1129–1138.

Kuopio, A. M., Marttila, R. J., Helenius, H., *et al.* (1999). Changing epidemiology of Parkinson's disease in southwestern Finland. *Neurology* **52**, 302–308.

Langston, J. W., Ballard, P. A., Tetrud, J. W., *et al.* (1983). Chronic parkinsonism in humans due to a product of meperidine analog synthesis. *Science* **219**, 979–980.

Logroscino, G., Marder, K., Cote, L. J., *et al.* (1996). Dietary lipids and antioxidants in Parkinson's disease: A population-based, case–control study. *Ann. Neurol.* **39**, 89–94.

Marder, K., Tang, M., Mejia, H., *et al.* (1996). Risk of Parkinson's disease among first-degree relatives: A community-based study. *Neurology* **47**, 155–160.

Mayeux, R., Marder, K., Cote, L. J., *et al.* (1995). The frequency of idiopathic Parkinson's disease by age, ethnic group, and sex in northern Manhattan, 1988–1993. *Am. J. Epidemiol.* **142**, 820–827.

Ross, G. W., Abbott, R. D., Petrovitch, H., *et al.* (2000). Association of coffee and caffeine intake with the risk of Parkinson disease. *J. Am. Med. Assoc.* **283**, 2674–2679.

Schoenberg, B. S., Osuntokun, B. O., Adeuja, A. O. G., *et al.* (1988). Comparison of the prevalence of Parkinson's disease in the rural United States and in rural Nigeria: Door-to-door community studies. *Neurology* **38**, 645–646.

Tanner, C. M., Ottman, R., Goldman, S. M., *et al.* (1999). Parkinson disease in twins: An etiologic study. *J. Am. Med. Assoc.* **281**, 341–346.

Paroxysmal Movement Disorders

Encyclopedia of the Neurological Sciences
Copyright 2003, Elsevier Science (USA). All rights reserved.

PAROXYSMAL movement disorders are characterized by a sudden onset of intermittent (paroxysmal) dyskinesias including choreoathetosis, dystonia, or both. The condition can be hereditary or secondary to a variety of neurological disorders. The familial paroxysmal dyskinesias are subdivided into action induced (kinesigenic) and non-action induced (non-kinesigenic), depending on whether or not they are induced by sudden voluntary movements. A variety of sensory phenomena (warning sensations) may herald an attack, such as feelings of "pins and needles" or "tugging" in the involved body parts, that last from several seconds up to 5 min. In the familial kinesigenic paroxysmal choreoathetosis, the movements are brief, usually lasting seconds to less than 3 min. These occur many times daily, some-times up to 100 times per day. Nonkinesigenic paroxysmal dyskinesias may also be hereditary, and the movements in these forms tend to be more dystonic than choreic in nature. The dyskinesia is usually more prolonged (2 min to 4 hr) and less frequent (3–5 per day). In both types, attacks can sometimes be precipitated by alcohol, coffee, fatigue, stress, or excitement. Nocturnal paroxysmal dyskinesias are similar to daytime dyskinesias, and the contortions are isolated to sleep or to awakening in the morning. They can be either prolonged or brief. The majority of patients with nocturnal episodes do not usually have daytime attacks.

Pathophysiologically, these conditions offer an interface between movement disorders and seizures since they are short duration and episodic involuntary movements of sudden onset without loss of consciousness. Frontal lobe or basal ganglia disturbances, multiple sclerosis, thyroid disturbances, stroke, and hypocalcemia are sometimes associated with paroxysmal dyskinesias. In order to complete the evaluation of a patient with paroxysmal dyskinesias, the patient should have a magnetic resonance imaging or computed tomography scan of the brain, electroencephalogram (EEG) (brain waves) while awake and sleep deprived, and metabolic screen. Special elective examinations including an EEG with double-density electrodes are used to detect very tiny seizures. Kinesigenic dyskinesias respond well to anticonvulsant medications, such as phenytoin, carbamazepine, or phenobarbital. In contrast, non-kinesigenic dyskinesias respond poorly to most medical therapy, although some patients improve with clonazepam. The treatment of paroxysmal dyskinesias due to metabolic or structural disturbances of the brain is closely tied to the underlying disease.

—*Esther Cubo and Christopher G. Goetz*

See also–Choreoathetosis; Dyskinesias; Dystonia; Movement Disorders, Overview

Further Reading

Bakdash, T., and Goetz, C. G. (1999). Familial and primary sporadic paroxysmal dyskinesias. In *Movement Diosrders in Neurology and Neuropsychiatry* (A. B. Joseph and R. R. Young, Eds.), pp. 502–508. Blackwell, Oxford.

Jankovic, J., and Stacy, M. (1998). Movement disorders. In *Textbook of Clinical Neurology* (C. G. Goetz and E. J. Pappert, Eds.), pp. 655–679. Saunders, Philadelphia.

PCP (Phencyclidine Hydrochloride)

Encyclopedia of the Neurological Sciences
Copyright 2003, Elsevier Science (USA). All rights reserved.

PHENCYCLIDINE [1-(1-phenylcyclohexyl)-piperidine hydrochloride] is an arylcyclohexylamine derivative (Fig. 1) that is colloquially referred to as PCP, angel dust, or elephant tranquilizer. The initial development and marketing of phencyclidine (under the trade names Sernyl or Sernylan) was related to its anesthetic and analgesic actions in both humans and animals. Both PCP and its congener ketamine can produce decreases in pain perception and loss of consciousness. Both drugs exhibit additional psychoactive effects even at subanesthetic doses; PCP intoxication is associated with delirium, agitated or violent behavior, impairments of psychomotor functions, catatonia, and psychosis/hallucinosis. Neurological signs of PCP intoxication include nystagmus, ataxia, and tremor. These effects can also be observed in individuals emerging from PCP-induced anesthesia.

PCP-induced psychosis is of heuristic interest because the spectrum of psychopathology produced by the drug uniquely bears strong similarity to schizophrenia. For this reason, it has been argued that PCP acts on substrates in the brain that are implicated in the pathophysiology of psychotic disorders. Scientists have therefore used PCP and related drugs to model the schizophrenic process in humans and, increasingly, in animals.

In the late 1950s, PCP became a recreationally abused drug (angel dust) in the United States and Europe. PCP is frequently consumed orally or intranasally or it is smoked (sometimes in combination with marijuana). Increasing abuse of PCP ultimately led to its classification as a Schedule II controlled substance. Incidence rates for phencyclidine abuse have traditionally been comparatively low (currently $<0.5\%$); however, the profound side effects associated with chronic PCP consumption (including psychosis and impairments of learning and memory) make PCP abuse a significant medical concern. PCP abuse is also a significant concern to law enforcement because persons intoxicated with PCP frequently exhibit aggravated and violent behavior coupled with resistance to physical pain.

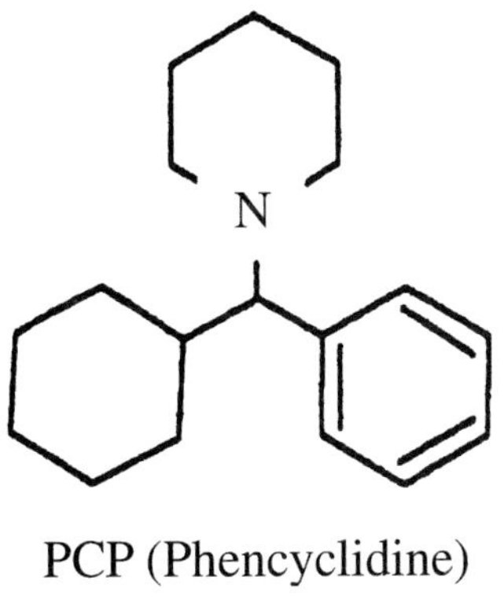

PHARMACOLOGY

PCP acts at a number of receptors in the central and peripheral nervous systems to produce its psychoactive effects. Principally, PCP acts to block the *N*-methyl-D-aspartate (NMDA)-sensitive glutamate receptor. The NMDA receptor is a pentameric structure (consisting of five subunits); when assembled, the subunits form an ionophore that fluxes sodium, potassium, and calcium ions when activated by glutamate binding. The receptor is also activated by coagonists (e.g., glycine and spermine) that act through allosteric regulatory sites.

PCP binds to a site within the ion channel and produces a blockade of receptor function; the antagonism is noncompetitive in nature because PCP inhibits receptor function without directly interfering with the binding of the agonist (glutamate). Importantly, PCP can only gain access to its binding site when the receptor channel is otherwise activated and "open"; therefore, the blockade is referred to as use dependent.

In addition to NMDA receptor antagonism, PCP binds to two other families of proteins with high affinity. First, PCP can affect sigma receptors. Initially, it was thought that these sites were receptors for endogenous opiates; however, this appears not be the case. Although the nature of PCP's interactions with the sigma receptor is unclear, there is limited evidence that the sigma receptor may be involved in schizophrenia and, hence, in the psychotomimetic actions of PCP.

PCP also binds to a set of brain proteins called dopamine transporters. These proteins function to remove the neurotransmitter dopamine from intracellular space, and PCP inhibits this transport. Hence, PCP indirectly acts to promote dopaminergic neurotransmission. This finding is thought to be relevant to the psychiatric effects of PCP because

PCP (Phencyclidine)

Figure 1
PCP (phencyclidine).

most drugs of abuse stimulate dopaminergic function, and heightened dopamine release has been implicated in the pathophysiology of schizophrenia.

Despite these additional pharmacological actions of PCP, blockade of the NMDA receptor is likely the most important mechanism by which PCP supports addictive behavior and produces psychosis. The involvement of NMDA receptor blockade in its psychoactive effects is supported by the fact that another noncompetitive NMDA receptor antagonist, ketamine, also produces psychosis and is an abused drug. Taken together, it seems likely that NMDA receptor blockade, either alone or in combination with the sigma/dopamine transporter actions of PCP, is primarily implicated in the psychiatric and neurological effects of PCP.

NEUROTOXICITY

PCP and related noncompetitive NMDA receptor antagonists produce neurotoxicity in animal models. Although not confirmed in humans, PCP has been observed to damage cells within certain regions of the cerebral cortex and basal ganglia of rats, sometimes irreversibly. Despite the lack of direct evidence for cell damage produced by PCP in humans, chronic intake of the drug by recreational abusers is associated with metabolic changes in many of the same cerebral cortical regions that are implicated in the rat studies. Therefore, PCP can produce long-lasting changes in brain function, particularly after chronic usage of the drug.

The neurotoxic effects of PCP are paradoxical in that PCP and related NMDA antagonists, including dizocilpine (MK801) and amantadine, are antiischemic. Despite this clinical indication for NMDA antagonists, the psychosis-provoking effects of the drugs, as well as the indications of neurotoxicity in animals, have limited the development of noncompetitive NMDA antagonists for the treatment of ischemic damage.

CLINICAL IMPLICATIONS

PCP abuse is a persistent problem with significant associated clinical consequences. Both alkylating agents and anti-PCP antibodies have been developed to reduce the acute effects of PCP intoxication; however, their usage in humans is not yet permitted. Alkalinization of urine is recommended to promote excretion; PCP-induced agitation and organic symptoms may also be managed with benzodiazepines. Moreover, evidence suggests that PCP-induced

psychosis can be managed with neuroleptic drugs, particularly atypical antipsychotics. However, very little is known about the management of the persistent side effects of chronic PCP abuse.

—*J. David Jentsch*

See also–Amphetamine Toxicity; Antipsychotic Pharmacology; Cocaine; Dopamine; Marijuana; Schizophrenia, Biology; Schizophrenia, Treatment; Substance Abuse

Further Reading
Javitt, D. C., and Zukin, S. R. (1991). Recent advances in the phencyclidine model of schizophrenia. *Am. J. Psychiatry* **148**, 1301–1308.
Jentsch, J. D., and Roth, R. H. (1999). The neuropsychopharmacology of phencyclidine: From NMDA receptor hypofunction to the dopamine hypothesis of schizophrenia. *Neuropsychopharmacology* **20**, 201–225.

Pediatric Brain Tumors
see Childhood Brain Tumors

Peduncular Hallucinosis

Encyclopedia of the Neurological Sciences
Copyright 2003, Elsevier Science (USA). All rights reserved.

PEDUNCULAR HALLUCINOSIS (Lhermitte's syndrome) consists of vivid hallucinations (usually visual but occasionally auditory, tactile, or visual with these components) that are similar to hypnagogic hallucinations. They usually consist of variable sequential scenes, often coming on in the evening with eye closure, and are associated with insight that the phenomena are not real. They differ from the hallucinations of schizophrenia in that they do not have symbolic significance and are not incorporated into delusional thinking.

Associated lesions are most commonly vascular and are located in the rostral brainstem, usually with involvement of the reticular formation. The thalamus (pulvinar and medial thalamic nuclei) has been coinvolved in some cases. In one case, the pars reticulata of the substantia nigra was selectively affected.

It has been proposed that a neurotransmitter imbalance, involving a relative increase in the ratio of serotonin (acting on 5-HT$_2$ and 5-HT$_3$ receptors) to acetylcholine activity, may be responsible for the syndrome. The association of visual hallucinations with drowsiness has led to the suggestion that there is a disturbance in the control of rapid eye movement sleep mechanisms that are under the control of serotonergic and cholinergic systems in the brainstem. The thalamic gating mechanism for processing incoming sensory information may be enhanced, and the activity of the cerebral cortical visual system, especially that of visual association areas, could be "disinhibited."

Peduncular hallucinations are individually brief and often do not recur for many days, although there are exceptions. They usually do not require therapy for symptomatic relief. Drugs that are often effective against visual hallucinations of various causes and that have anti-5-HT$_2$ activity, including clozapine (for psychoses) and methysergide (for migraine), might also be considered.

—*G. Bryan Young*

See also—Acetylcholine; Hallucinations, Visual and Auditory; Lhermitte's Symptom; Serotonin

Further Reading

Geller, T. J., and Bellur, S. N. (1987). Peduncular hallucinosis: Magnetic resonance imaging confirmation of mesencephalic infarction during life. *Ann. Neurol.* **21**, 602–604.

Lhermitte, J., Levy, G., and Trelles, J. (1932). L'hallucinose pédonculaire (étude anatomique d'un cas). *Rev. Neurol.* **1**, 382–388.

Manford, M., and Andermann, F. (1998). Complex visual hallucinations: Clinical and neurobiological aspects. *Brain* **121**, 1819–1840.

Penfield, Wilder

Encyclopedia of the Neurological Sciences
Copyright 2003, Elsevier Science (USA). All rights reserved.

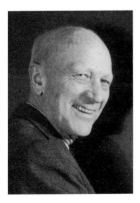

WILDER PENFIELD (1891–1976), a skillful neurosurgeon, brought to the operating room his insight from physiology, microscopic anatomy, and neurology. At the forefront of his achievements was the foundation in 1934 of the Montreal Neurological Institute (MNI). Here, he directed scientific and surgical teams toward teaching, research, and treatment related to disorders of the brain and nerves. The institute became recognized as a leading world center for the study and surgery of epilepsy. Penfield will be remembered by many for his personal warmth, his insistence on excellence as a teacher, his inspiration as a leader, and his physical stamina, whether at surgery or sports. His influence touched people in many walks of life, extending outside the special field of neurology and far beyond Canada.

EDUCATION

Wilder Penfield was born in Spokane, Washington. He graduated from Princeton University in 1913, and in 1915 he attended Oxford on a Rhodes Scholarship. Two great teachers there deeply influenced the direction of his career. From Sir William Osler, then Regius Professor of Medicine, he derived intellectual inspiration and the sympathetic approach to patients. In the physiological laboratory of the methodical genius Sir Charles Sherrington, he learned to observe, document, and summarize experimental findings; he became aware of the "undiscovered country of the brain in which the mystery of the mind of man might someday be explained."

He completed his medical degree in 1918 at Johns Hopkins Medical School. He then studied for a year in Oxford with Sherrington and at the National Hospital for the Paralyzed and Epileptic, Queen Square, London. Here, he came under the tutelage of Sir Gordon Holmes in neurology, Dr. Godwin Greenfield in neuropathology, and Sir Percy Sargent in neurosurgery.

NEW YORK PERIOD

From 1921 to 1928, Penfield was a surgical associate with Allen Whipple at Columbia University and with Charles Elsberg at the Neurological Institute of New York. To observe neurosurgical techniques, he visited Dandy, Frazier, and Cushing, adopting many details of Cushing's "surgical ritual." Two important "brain dustings," as Osler called these overseas study trips, gave substantial input to Penfield's future career. In 1924, as the first English-speaking investigator to work with Ramón y Cajal and Río-Hortega in Madrid, he learned the metallic methods for demonstrating the glia. Back in New York, he and his new energetic partner, Dr. William Cone, applied these techniques to original studies on brain tumors and glial scars. In 1928, he went abroad again to the clinic of Professor Otfrid Foerster in Breslau, Germany. Here, he learned how precise brain mapping, by electrical stimulation in a patient during surgery under local anesthesia, allowed exact and safe excision of cortical scars as a means of treating focal epilepsy. This surgical approach became the focus of his life's work.

MONTREAL AND THE MNI

In September 1928, Penfield came with Cone to the Royal Victoria Hospital and McGill University in Montreal. Their success at McGill led in September 1934 to the opening of the MNI, made possible by a $1 million grant for research from the Rockefeller Foundation and matched by generous Montreal donors and annual pledges from the city and province to cover hospital costs. Combining a hospital for nervous diseases and advanced research resources in the same building, the institute quickly gained an international reputation. It became a model for similar units elsewhere, most notably the prestigious National Institute of Neurological Diseases in Bethesda, Maryland, established in 1951. Graduates of the MNI in various disciplines returned to many lands, not least of all to the United States, where they were sought after to fill some of the most distinguished professorial positions. The first neurosurgeons to form training programs in such far-flung countries as Norway, China, India, and Hungary were all former fellows of the "Neuro," as it came to be known.

PENFIELD'S CONTRIBUTIONS

Derived from accurate observations of the responses to cortical stimulation and electrical recording from the human brain during surgery, Penfield's numerous publications on cerebral localization with a succession of neurosurgical associates became classics. Continuing contributions appeared on motor and sensory function popularized by recurrent cartoons of the homunculi, which represented the body's image on the cortex. In the early 1950s, he and his team defined the pathogenesis of temporal lobe seizures coming from the mesial temporal structures; based on this, they described the operation for tailored temporal lobe excision that became known

as the Montreal procedure. This provided successful seizure-free cure in more than 75% of well-selected patients; it became widely adopted as one of the most satisfactory and cost-effective therapies in the field of neurosurgery. These studies also identified the role of the amygdala and hippocampus in memory function. Penfield postulated what he termed a centrencephalic integrating system to explain diffuse bilateral seizure activity and the mechanism of consciousness.

SECOND CAREER

In 1960, Penfield closed his surgical practice to take up what he called his second career. He wrote two historical novels and an excellent biography of Dr. Alan Gregg, medical director of the Rockefeller Foundation who had been a key figure in the negotiations of the MNI. At the urging of Governor General of Canada and Madame Vanier, he took on the first presidency of the Vanier Institute of the Family and devoted his time to lecturing and promoting the financial basis of this organization. He summarized his research findings on human brain function in his book *The Mystery of the Mind*. This gave him an opportunity to debate his courageous and provocative views in the controversial brain–mind arena. A few weeks before he died on April 5, 1976, he turned over the final draft of his autobiography that recounted his life up to the time of the foundation in 1934 of the MNI. He was well satisfied with the beginning of an expansion to the institute that would be named the Penfield Pavilion.

HONORS AND AWARDS

Penfield received the highest award of his own country, Companion of the Order of Canada, and of Great Britain, the Order of Merit (which had been bestowed earlier upon Sherrington, Adrian, and Dale, his teachers and friends). He was recognized by the US Medal of Freedom with Silver Palm and by the Cross of Chevalier of the Legion d'honneur of France. Elected to learned and medical societies of many countries, he was often referred to as Canada's most distinguished citizen.

Penfield wrote,

If it seems to neurologists today that the present understanding of the brain and mind of man is hardly more than the beginning of science, it may be reassuring to recall that our task is the ultimate one. The problem of neurology is to understand man himself.

—*William Feindel*

Further Reading

Eccles, J., and Feindel, W. (1978). Wilder Graves Penfield 1891–1976. *Biogr. Mem. Fellows R. Soc.* **24,** 473–513.

Feindel, W. (1977). Wilder Penfield (1891–1976): The man and his work. *Neurosurgery* **1,** 93–100.

Feindel, W. (Ed.) (1977). Wilder Penfield: His legacy to neurology. *Can. Med. Assoc. J.* **116,** 1–16.

Feindel, W. (1982). The contributions of Wilder Penfield to the functional anatomy of the human brain. *Hum. Neurobiol.* **1,** 231–234.

Feindel, W. (1996). Neurosurgery at the Montreal Neurological Institute and McGill University Hospitals. *Neurosurgery* **39,** 830–839.

Lewis, J. (1981). *Something Hidden. A Biography of Wilder Penfield.* Doubleday, Garden City, NY.

Penfield, W. (1936). The significance of the Montreal Neurological Institute. *Neurological Biographies and Addresses; Foundation Volume Published for the Staff, to Commemorate the Opening of the Montreal Neurological Institute of McGill University [on September, 27, 1934],* pp. 37–54. Oxford Univ. Press, London.

Penfield, W. (1975). *The Mystery of the Mind.* Princeton Univ. Press, Princeton, NJ.

Penfield, W. (1977). *No Man Alone. A Neurosurgeon's Life.* Little, Brown, Boston.

Penfield, W., and Erickson, T. C. (1941). *Epilepsy and Cerebral Localization; A Study of the Mechanism, Treatment and Prevention of Epileptic Seizures.* Thomas, Springfield, IL.

Penfield, W., and Jasper, H. (1954). *Epilepsy and the Functional Anatomy of the Human Brain.* Little, Brown, Boston.

Penfield, W., and Rasmussen, T. (1950). *The Cerebral Cortex of Man. A Clinical Study of Localization of Function.* Macmillan, New York.

Preul, M. C., and Feindel, W. (1991). Origins of Wilder Penfield's surgical technique. *J. Neurosurg.* **75,** 812–820.

Peptides
see Neuropeptides

Perception and Perceptual Disorders

Encyclopedia of the Neurological Sciences
Copyright 2003, Elsevier Science (USA). All rights reserved.

PERCEPTION involves conscious awareness of a sensation along with some interpretation of its meaning or significance. There are a number of linked processes, including sensation, attention to the sensation, processing the information, along with links to memory and other systems.

Higher levels of visual processing achieve conscious perception. The lowest level of perception appears to be the appreciation of "qualia" or certain discrete properties, such as wavelength of light (color) or luminance intensity. There is at least an awareness of this, even though it is a crude or fundamental perception, requiring integrity of the visual pathway up to and including the primary visual cortex, also called V1 or area 17. At this level, however, there is no object vision, which involves the ability to segment the image into background and foreground and to fuse the impressions into shapes and objects.

The next level of conscious vision is object recognition, a complex process involving the primary visual cortex, visual association areas, and reciprocal connections with memory stores. It is likely that meaning and significance are given to parallel and serially processed sensory information by feedback and feedforward connections involving multiple hierarchical levels.

Libet *et al.* reported that thalamic stimulation must usually last more than 500 msec to achieve conscious detection, even though subjects can indicate that they were stimulated in a forced choice paradigm. There was an intermediate state of partial awareness with some stimuli that lasted less than 500 msec; the transition from detection without awareness to detection with awareness is not an abrupt change. This somewhat variable temporal threshold may have some value with respect to attending to stimuli that last longer and are more important for behavioral decision making. Longer duration stimuli are processed to greater degrees. The awareness of time is dependent on the growth and decay of perceptions and stored abstractions in memory. Since 500 msec or longer is required for perception, the awareness of the present is likely an averaged series of very recent events from the immediate past. Some disorders of perception are discussed next.

The effects of occipital lesions further our understanding of the relative roles of these regions in visual perception. For example, cortical color blindness can result from lesions of a discrete part of area 19; a lesion in area 19 may also lead to reduced perception of movement (akinetopsia). Thus, area 19 is intimately involved in the appreciation of color and movement. Where color and movement are "perceived," however, is more difficult to answer.

Lesions that destroy or isolate the primary visual cortex, but spare extrageniculostriate and the extrastriate cortical areas, allow some reactions to "unseen" visual stimuli. This is referred to as blindsight. Such individuals can make accurate projections into a visual field for which there is no sensation of vision but deny conscious awareness of the existence of the object in extrapersonal space. Experimentally, responses in the hemianopic field interfere with simultaneous stimuli applied to the intact field; in forced choice paradigms, the responses are better than chance. Thus, there is an effect on conscious activity even though the stimuli do not achieve conscious perception. It is proposed that this phenomenon occurs because visual information relayed to the superior colliculus (by-passing the optic radiations) is transmitted to extrastriate cerebral cortex. Awareness without detection also occurs with central somatosensory thalamic stimulation in humans.

In neglect syndromes there is loss of conscious awareness of primary sensory stimuli in the presence of intact sensory pathways. These are most common in parietal or frontal lesions. Unilateral neglect with nondominant parietal lesions can extend from the person to extrapersonal space. The person may fail to wash the left side of the body, to comb the hair or shave on the left side, and may wear a glove only on the right hand. There may be decreased associated movements of the left limbs for simple tasks, even though there is no paresis. This disordered body image may relate to an interruption of sensory processing that moves from primary sensations to hierarchical processing in the parietal and frontal lobes. The highest level of modeling of self and extrapersonal space is reflected in goals and behavior. Presumably, neglect relates to disrupted processing at an intermediate level.

Individuals with lesions in certain cortical areas may have selective associative agnosias. Agnosias are failures of perception despite preservation of at least some sensation. A good example is prosopagnosia, the failure to recognize faces with which the patient is familiar. These cases usually have lesions that involve inferior temporal regions bilaterally. Even though the patient knows the image is a face and can discriminate it from the background, they are unable to recognize the individual. There is still debate as to the level of dysfunction—that is, does the problem lie with (i) basic sensations and early processing (e.g., perception of simple forms), (ii) synthesizing sensations to produce a "gestalt" or concept, or (iii) linking sensations to stored memories? For example, larger lesions affecting multiple prestriate regions bilaterally may cause a visual agnosia such as simultagnosia, in which the patient cannot synthesize the information into a general shape (e.g., a hamburger) but may perceive lines and/or parts of the object. Patients who cannot segment images to differentiate the foreground from the background or fuse impressions into shapes have apperceptive visual agnosia, usually due to lesions involving the extrastriate cortex bordering on but sparing V1 and V2. Formulating background from foreground, or grouping parts of images, and higher ordering visual processes rest on the integrity of qualia as serial processing. There is a dissociation, however, from some primary visual defects (i.e., some qualia may be missing).

—*G. Bryan Young*

See also–**Agnosia; Awareness; Consciousness; Memory, Overview; Motion and Spatial Perception; Neglect Disorders; Perceptual-Motor Integration; Sensation; Sensory Testing, Quantitative; Vision, Color and Form**

Further Reading

Moskovitch, M. (1979). Information processing and the cerebral hemispheres. In *Handbook of Behavioral Neurobiology, Vol. 2: Neuropsychology* (M. S. Gazzinga, Ed.), pp. 379–446. Plenum, New York.

Perceptual-Motor Integration

Encyclopedia of the Neurological Sciences

THIS PHASE of processing involves the use that is made of the visual information, or perceptual-motor integration. Examples include verbally describing what is seen, reading aloud, or hitting a ball with a bat. This relies on the integrity of pathways and structures that link vision, memory, and motor systems.

Stimulus processing refers to various learning paradigms that can function independently of each other (e.g., different memory systems for different sensory inputs). Patients with right parietal lesions characteristically show reduced awareness of visual stimuli presented to the left visual hemifield, especially if a competing stimulus is simultaneously presented in the right hemifield. In one tachistoscopic study in which stimuli were flashed separately or simultaneously onto both hemifields, patients often neglected the left field stimulus when they verbally reported their experience. However, when they manually registered their observations (by pressing buttons), they reported the left field stimuli significantly less than with verbal reporting. There may be different pathways or mechanisms for sensorimotor integration.

Neglect also shows a spatial continuum rather than abrupt transitions. Patients with right cerebral lesions tend to bisect a horizontal line at a point to the right of center. If a mirror is used so that movements appear to be in the opposite direction, the error rate decreases, especially in patients with right frontal lesions. Probably both perceptual and premotor processing are involved in performing this task. A further distinction between the perceptual and premotor components of a task was shown by a test in which the images were reversed by a mirror so the lines on the left of midline were projected to the left cerebrum. When subjects were asked to cross out lines, some crossed out lines projected to the left hemisphere, but they had to perform the act in the left side of hemispace. These individuals had parietal perceptual problems, whereas those who could not operate in left hemispace and crossed out lines on the opposite side had premotor deficits. Such directional hypokinesia is a feature of lesions affecting the frontal lobe or basal ganglia.

—G. Bryan Young

See also–Learning, Motor; Motion and Spatial Perception; Motor System, Overview; Neglect Disorders; Perception and Perceptual Disorders; Sensation

Further Reading

Ewert, J. P. (1997). Neural correlates of key stimulus and releasing mechanism: A case study and two concepts. *Trends Neurosci.* 20, 332–339.

Periodic Limb Movements in Sleep (PLMS)

Encyclopedia of the Neurological Sciences
Copyright 2003, Elsevier Science (USA). All rights reserved.

PERIODIC LIMB MOVEMENTS IN SLEEP (PLMS) are repetitive, nearly periodic movements frequently found when limb activity is monitored during sleep. PLMS are common in younger adults, may be found in the majority of seniors, and are seen frequently in a wide variety of sleep, neurological, and medical disorders. The closest association is with restless legs syndrome (RLS), but important associations include uremia and neurological disorders with dopamine abnormalities. Diagnosis generally requires a sleep study to enumerate PLMS, establish whether they are associated with respiratory abnormalities, and to confirm that movements during the night are PLMS rather than a variety of other abnormal sleep-associated movements. The pathophysiology of PLMS is unclear but appears to focus on the dopamine system and to include oscillators located within the spinal cord. The clinical significance of the associated disorder, periodic limb movement disorder (PLMD), is controversial, but selected patients may have sleep disruption and sleep complaints based on PLMS. Sometimes, treatment of associated or causative conditions can alleviate the impact of PLMS. Patients with otherwise unexplained PLMD can be treated with a variety of medication approaches focusing on dopaminergic agents and benzodiazepines given at low doses and titrated to therapeutic efficacy. Successful treatment should involve abolition of sleep complaints with or without suppression of most PLMS.

HISTORY

Disturbing movements during sleep have been known to occur perhaps as long as history. More than 300 years ago, Willis described a case that is now assumed to be one of RLS in which he mentioned a "flying about" of the limbs due to an excitatory phenomenon. However, until recently, most of these abnormal movements remained vague and undefined. The study of PLMS began half a century ago with Symonds, who coined the term nocturnal myoclonus. He described a series of cases that, from a modern perspective, appear to have included a variety of both epileptic and nonepileptic phenomena, including PLMS. Clarification of the syndrome awaited the development of methodologies for observing and recording sleep, in particular, the polysomnographic sleep study or polysomnogram (PSG). PSGs record a variety of physiological phenomena, such as the electroencephalogram (EEG), electrooculogram, respiratory flow and effort, electrocardiogram, and muscle activity through electromyograms (EMGs). Based on the variation in these phenomena, sleep and its stages can be determined. Using such a study, Lugaresi and colleagues, particularly Coccagna, discovered that a patient with familial restless legs suffered through much of the night with repetitive leg movements that recurred in approximately 30-sec intervals. They were subsequently able to show that most patients with RLS have these movements.

Approximately a decade later, Weitzmann and his group, including Guilleminault and later Coleman, explored these movements further and found that they were present in a wide variety of patients as well as in those otherwise without a sleep abnormality. To emphasize the most significant aspect of these movements, they called them periodic movements in sleep. Subsequently, the term was modified until today the most generally accepted term is periodic limb movements in sleep. Since it is now recognized that very similar movements can occur when awake, the general term is periodic limb movements (PLMs) (Table 1). The disorder presumptively caused by PLMS has been termed periodic limb movement disorder.

CLINICAL FEATURES OF PLMS

Description and Phenomenology of PLMS

Most remarkable about PLMS are their periodicity and repetitiveness. Although the range of intermovement intervals is quite broad, most movements repeat with a period of approximately 20–30 sec. Rarely do movements repeat at intervals less than 10 or more than 50 sec. In a given series of movements, this period is fairly regular, with a variability much smaller than the possible range of periods. This is more true of the movements in the sleep state than in the wake state (Fig. 1). Studies have shown that in the waking state, movements have a shorter period and are less regular. Movements during quiet, non-rapid eye movement (NREM) sleep decrease in intensity and increase in duration as sleep deepens from transitional to regular to slow-wave sleep (stages 1–4). The movements are less common and less intense in REM sleep, but it is unclear whether there is a further increase in duration. The movements also occur in series, typically of tens or even hundreds of movements that last from a few minutes to 1 hr or more. These characteristics have been incorporated into the definition of PLMS by the American Academy of Sleep Medicine (AASM). As part of the formal definition, the movements must

Table 1   **ABBREVIATIONS**

PLM—Periodic limb movement(s): One or more of a series of movements (minimum, four in series) that occur at intervals of approximately 5–90 sec. They have a typical form (Fig. 1), minimum amplitude (one-fourth maximum as measured in the tibialis anterior muscle), and are most pronounced in legs but may involve arms or include other muscle groups.

PLMS—Periodic limb movement(s) in sleep: PLM occurring during a sleep stage (NREM or REM). Formerly called nocturnal myoclonus. Waking movements have been called dyskinesias while awake or PLMW (PLM wake state). Only PLMS, not PLMW, are typically reported in a sleep study.

PLMD—Periodic limb movement disorder: Condition of disturbed sleep with symptoms attributable to sleep disruption by PLMS. Implies exclusions of other sources of sleep complaint (insomnia and excessive daytime somnolence).

PLMI—Periodic limb movement index: Generally calculated as the number of PLMS per hour of sleep but can be extended to the wake state.

PLMA—Arousal(s) associated with PLMS: Arousal has been defined by the AASM as a 3-sec or longer period of changed EEG activity involving high-amplitude slow waves, higher frequency waves (alpha), or both that interrupts an established sleep stage.

PLMAI—PLMA index: The number of arousals associated with PLMS per hour of sleep.

RLS—Restless legs syndrome: A condition with clinical definition based on history of an urge to move, usually associated with unpleasant leg or limb sensations; motor restlessness evident in increased movement inappropriate to context; aggravation by inactivity and relief by activity; and a circadian pattern with worsening of symptoms late in the wake period (usually evening or night).

have a duration between 5 and 90 sec and occur in a series of four or more movements (Table 2).

The individual PLMS typically are flexion movements of the legs with extension of the great toe, dorsiflexion of the ankle, and flexion of the knee and hip. As a result, they have been likened both to the Babinski reflex and to a flexion withdrawal reflex. However, although this form is most typical, there are actually a wide variety of forms. PLMS vary in intensity from subtle, almost imperceptible foot movements to large-scale, rapid contractions of both legs that can cause whole-body movement and lead to arousal or awakening of a sleeping person. Although the legs are most often involved, the arms can be involved, either by themselves or, more commonly, in conjunction with leg movements. Within a series of movements, PLMS tend to be fairly stereotypic with a similar intensity and distribution that changes only slowly. One or both sides of the body may be involved at a given moment,

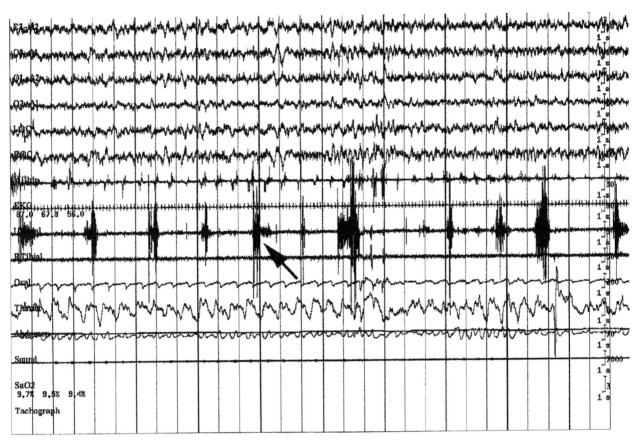

Figure 1

Series of periodic limb movements in a sleeping patient. These occur almost exclusively in the left leg. The burst at the arrow shows several initial high-amplitude brief components. The middle burst in the record is prolonged, consistent with an arousal leading to prolonged movement. After this burst, there is an altered EEG rhythm and EMG activity spreading to the chin and right leg, as well as altered respiratory rhythm. (Chin EMG has respiratory artifacts through tracing.) Note the approximate but not exact periodicity. Traces 1–4, EEG from vertex (traces 1 and 2) and occiput (traces 3 and 4) referenced to the opposite ear; traces 5 and 6, left and right electrooculograms; trace 7, chin EMG; trace 8, electrocardiogram; traces 9 and 10, left and right tibialis anterior EMGs; trace 11, oral air flow; traces 12 and 13, thoracic and abdominal respiratory effort; bottom trace, sound recording. The trace superimposed on abdominal effort is a displaced oximeter tracing indicating oxygen saturation. The entire record is 160 sec long; thick vertical lines indicate 16-sec divisions.

but most persons with PLMS will show bilateral involvement. The side on which movements occur can shift on different nights or even within a given night or within a given series of movements. Posture can also influence the form of movements, perhaps because of sensory input modulating the excitability of different generators. A characteristic set of movements will begin with low-amplitude movements that gradually increase in intensity until an arousal or gross body movement occurs, at which point the series may resume, terminate, or shift in form. Most PLMS have a moderate speed, similar to that of voluntary movements. However, movements may begin abruptly with one to several jerks of almost myoclonic speed, evident as brief EMG pulses in the PSG. These are more common and sustained in

movements that occur while awake. For the majority of movements, however, it is clear that these movements are not really myoclonic and so the original terminology was somewhat misleading.

For operational purposes, the AASM states that movements, as represented in the associated anterior tibialis muscle EMG, must have a duration of 0.5–5 sec and exceed 25% of the EMG amplitude of a maximal voluntary foot dorsiflexion. It has recently been suggested that when these movements occur in the waking state, their associated EMG may last as long as 10 sec. Such movements are commonly seen only in RLS patients who are temporarily immobile. The long duration probably reflects a voluntary response to the initial involuntary movement and can resemble a dystonic fixation at the end point of the

Table 2 OPERATIONAL DEFINITIONS OF PLMS AND PLMD[a]

Operational definition of PLMS
  Movements repeat at intervals of 5–90 sec
  During a regular sleep stage
  In a series of four or more movements each meeting other
    criteria
  Lasting between 0.5 and 5 sec as recorded
Diagnostic criteria: PLMD (780.52–4)
  A. The patient has a complaint of insomnia or excessive
     sleepiness. The patient occasionally will be asymptomatic,
     and the movements are noticed by an observer.
  B. Repetitive, highly stereotyped limb muscle movements are
     present; in the leg, these movements are characterized by
     extension of the big toe in combination with partial flexion of
     the ankle, knee, and sometimes hip.
  C. Polysomnographic monitoring demonstrates repetitive
     episodes of muscle contraction (0.5–5 sec in duration)
     separated by an interval of typically 20–40 sec.
     Arousal or awakenings may be associated with the
     movements.
  D. The patient has no evidence of a medical or mental disorder
     that can account for the primary complaint.
  E. Other sleep disorders (e.g., obstructive sleep apnea syndrome)
     may be present but do not account for the movements.

Minimal criteria: A + B

Categorization of PLMD
  Severity
    Mild: Associated with an PLMI of 5–24 per hour and results
     in mild insomnia or mild sleepiness
    Moderate: Associated with a PLMI of 25–49 per hour and
     results in moderate insomnia or sleepiness
    Severe: Associated with a PLMI >50 per hour or a PLMI
     >25 per hour and results in severe insomnia or sleepiness
  Duration
    Acute: 1 month or less
    Subacute: Longer than 1 month but less than 6 months
    Chronic: 6 months or longer

[a] Diagnostic criteria and categorizations from Diagnostic Classification Steering Committee of the American Sleep Disorders Association (1997).

original movement. I have observed patients who maintained a flexed posture, seemingly as a means of inhibiting PLMS while awake (PLMW, originally called dyskinesias while awake).

Diagnosis of PLMS and PLMD

PLMS can only be enumerated from a sleep record. Based on the AASM criteria (Table 2), they can generally be readily recognized and counted on the PSG if recording is made from one or both anterior tibialis muscles (Fig. 1). It is generally agreed, however, that movements that occur in association with periodic respiratory phenomena, especially apneas, are not considered PLMS. In the case of more subtle respiratory phenomena, such as the upper airway resistance syndrome (UARS), special recordings may need to be made in order to exclude such an association. Until recently, such recordings were not made; in the future, reassessment of our understanding of the prevalence and significance of PLMS may be necessary. In general, PLMS also require a determination that the patient is asleep, as determined from the PSG. Waking movements, PLMSW, are not counted in a sleep study. However, as a general rule, when PLMSW are also assessed, as in RLS, the same rules for scoring apply. It has become clear that many, if not most, patients with PLMS are likely to also have PLMSW, if only during brief waking episodes in the course of a night's sleep. In reporting PLMS, it is the usual case to also calculate a PLMS index (PLMI), which is the number of PLMS per hour of recorded sleep.

Recently, it has become possible to enumerate PLMS using activity recording. Using miniaturized devices that rely on accelerometry to determine movement, special routines can extract periodic activity from the background and count PLMS fairly accurately. Such devices permit low-cost, sustained recordings and can be useful for monitoring PLMS for research purposes, therapeutic trials, or clinical monitoring. However, without additional instrumentation, they cannot establish sleep–wake state exactly (although approximations can be made), determine if arousals occur, or eliminate PLMS associated with respiratory events.

Important aspects of PLMS are their ability to disturb sleep and to cause awakenings or, more often, arousals that temporarily disrupt the sleep state. Although the exact role of arousals in impairing sleep quality remains unclear, it is generally believed that arousals do have an adverse impact on sleep quality. Arousals have been defined by the AASM to require a minimum of a 3-sec interruption of the EEG appearance characteristic of sleep, either by the development of an alpha rhythm, associated with the wake state, or by evidence of a cortical response, a vertex wave, or both, as in a K complex when they occur within the EEG frequency shift. Arousals associated with PLMS are often separately counted and an arousal index (PLMAI) calculated (arousals associated with PLMS per hour of sleep).

The sleep disorder associated with PLMS, PLMD, has also been defined by the AASM. The diagnosis of PLMD has three components. First, the patient must have a sleep complaint. This may be either one of insomnia (difficulty initiating or maintaining sleep) or one of excessive daytime somnolence. Second, a sleep study must confirm the presence of PLMS. It is generally agreed that to be significant, there must be at least five PLMS per hour of sleep. Finally, the sleep complaint must not be reasonably explained by some other condition, such as nocturnal respiratory disturbance or the use of sleep-impairing medications.

The AASM also grades PLMD according to duration (acute, subacute, and chronic) and severity, with higher grades of severity requiring a greater complaint and a larger PLMI or PLMAI.

Differential Diagnosis of PLMS

The differential diagnosis of PLMS is quite broad, including a spectrum of parasomnias, nocturnal respiratory disturbances, movement disorders, and ictal phenomena. The patient may not be able to provide much information about the condition, except for the sleep-related complaint and awareness of disturbed, restless sleep. Bed partners may provide more accurate information about the nature and timing of abnormal movements and should always be interviewed, if feasible.

In addition, PLMS may commonly occur in many other sleep disorders so that the clinical picture may be compound or mixed. Common conditions with large numbers of PLMS include RLS, narcolepsy, REM sleep behavior disorder (RBD), and many cases of respiratory disturbance in sleep. Teasing out these various disorders may require a sleep study with more elaborate leads (to exclude seizures) and with video recording to establish more exactly the phenomenology of the movements. To exclude UARS, special pressure recording such as esophageal manometry may be required.

From the history, the presence of vivid dreams and arousals may suggest RBD, whereas snoring or gasping during sleep may indicate a respiratory disorder. Classic signs of narcolepsy include daytime sleep attacks and cataplexy as well as hallucinatory experiences at onset and end of the sleep state.

On the standard sleep study (Fig. 1), PLMS are indicated by the presence of a regularly recurring motor activity with standard features that can be readily recognized. More difficult is the discrimination of movements associated with a cyclical respiratory deficiency such as UARS, although typical apneas or hypopneas associated with recurrent, periodic arousals and movements can be readily noted on the standard PSG.

Almost all other sleep-related movements lack the repetitive, periodic character of PLMS and can thus be discriminated by their recurrence. Videos can support this finding by showing more elaborate, behaviorally suggestive if automaton-like movements more typical of parasomnias or seizures. Sleep state can assist since PLMS typically occur more often in the lighter stages of NREM sleep, whereas some parasomnias may arise from deeper NREM sleep and RBD is associated with REM sleep.

Epidemiology and Genetics

Because the detection of PLMS requires objective monitoring, such as PSG, there have been relatively few broad, population-based studies of PLMS. However, more studies, generally using ambulatory instruments to record PLMS, have been carried out in the elderly. The studies have shown a relatively low percentage of PLMS in those younger than age 50 (<10%) but a rapid increase in prevalence in those older than age 50, and the majority of those older than age 65 have a PLMI of more than 5. Studies of symptoms that might be related to PLMS have found that as many as 10% of the North American population complains of symptoms related to PLMS.

In general, PLMS have not been systematically studied in other conditions. Large-scale studies conducted by Coleman and colleagues did show that approximately 10% of those with a wide variety of sleep disorders have a significant number (>5/hr) of PLMS. PLMS, like RLS, are increased in renal failure and carry a poor prognosis. They have also been reported to occur in heart failure, COPD, genitourinary disorders, and rheumatic conditions.

PLMS have also been reported in a wide variety of degenerative and neuromuscular and other neurological disorders, but most studies have been performed on small series and have not controlled for patient age. Montplaisir proposed that PLMS may occur in a wide spectrum of disorders that have deficiencies or abnormalities of the dopamine system, including Parkinson's disease (PD), Lewy body disease, RBD, and narcolepsy. Increased PLMS have been found in children with attention deficit hyperactivity disorder, another disorder with presumptive dopamine abnormalities. In contrast, in one condition with presumed dopamine excess, schizophrenia, it has been reported that patients have fewer PLMS than age-matched controls. Disorders with spinal cord pathology, including multiple sclerosis, spinal neoplasms, syringomyelia, and spinal cord transection, have also been associated with a frequent occurrence of PLMS, often in younger individuals.

The genetics of PLMS have not been extensively studied. Insofar as PLMS coexist with RLS, a variety of surveys and family studies have shown that there is a strong family aggregation of RLS. However, 15 years of investigations on the genetic basis of RLS have yet to yield any linkage or genetic basis for that condition. In at least one family, a person with PLMD was an obligate carrier for the genetic disorder underlying RLS.

PATHOPHYSIOLOGY AND LESIONS

Like that of RLS, the pathophysiology of PLMS is largely unknown. Given the very high percentage of elderly with at least some PLMS, it is possible that the generators for these movements are a normal component of the central nervous system, perhaps a variety of "primitive" reflexes suppressed during most of life and reemergent in older individuals. This would explain the presence of PLMS in association with a wide variety of nervous system disorders.

Because PLMS, like RLS, respond particularly well to dopaminergic medications, this clinical result supports the idea that there is some dopamine deficiency in PLMD. Indeed, in recent studies using dopamine agonists to treat RLS, the suppression of PLMS has been more impressive than the alleviation of other aspects of RLS. Some of the imaging studies done for RLS have included patients with only PLMS, and results have shown decreased binding to dopamine receptors in the striatum. PLMS in RLS have been shown by functional magnetic resonance imaging to involve activation of the red nucleus as well as regions near the pontine reticular formation. However, it is not clear to what extent these abnormalities are of pathogenetic significance and the brainstem loci require further specification.

Attempts to establish nervous system hyperexcitability in PLMS have produced mixed results. There has been no clear finding of generally increased reflexes, but there is support from magnetic stimulation studies that there are deficiencies in inhibitory mechanisms that govern motor neuron excitability. Motor pathways and motor control appear to be largely intact. Bara-Jimenez and colleagues showed that the spinal flexion reflex was increased in patients with PLMS and did not show the expected degree of suppression during NREM sleep. These reflexes are also known to be modulated by dopaminergic input;

thus, this result also supports the idea of a dopamine abnormality associated with PLMS.

The presence of PLMS in patients with clinically complete spinal cord transections suggests that much of the machinery for PLMS, if not their overall neural control, lies within the spinal cord. One study suggested that patterns of progression of excitation in different muscles at different cord levels indicates that a likely transmission is via the propriospinal pathways. However, this finding has not been replicated, and contrary evidence has been presented. Evidence from patients with different periods of activation in different limbs also suggests that each limb has enough machinery to generate its own idiosyncratic rhythm. This is similar to the presence of locomotor or other motor oscillators that are present somewhat distinctly for each limb, although the usual situation is coordinated and synchronized activation.

CLINICAL SIGNIFICANCE

In recent years, there has been a growing controversy about the clinical significance of PLMS. In patients with hypersomnolence and PLMS but no other sleep abnormality, treatment of PLMS in one series did not improve daytime sleepiness. In the elderly with PLMS, it has been very difficult in large series to associate increased numbers of PLMS with any sleep complaint. The concern that many patients with possible PLMD have subtle or pronounced respiratory abnormalities has also led some to question the validity of PLMD as a significant clinical syndrome. However, there are contrary cases in which PLMS provide the only explanation for a sleep complaint, and treatment to suppress PLMS leads to improvement. As a result of this persistent, if poorly documented, clinical impression, it seems that PLMD should be entertained and treated in those cases in which no other problem can be ascertained.

TREATMENT

The general approach to the PLMD patient has been examined by the AASM, which has set forth standards for treatment of RLS and PLMD (Table 3). These include the need to make an adequate diagnosis, to be aware of complicating or associated conditions, and to follow patients with clinical management.

Lifestyle and nutritional approaches to PLMS have not been thoroughly studied. Although RLS may respond to iron or magnesium supplementation, this

Table 3   STANDARDS FOR MANAGEMENT OF PLMD[a]

Pharmacological treatment of PLMD should be limited to patients who meet specific diagnostic criteria (**standard**).[b]

The physician who treats patients with PLMD should be aware of the existence of idiopathic and secondary forms and should be knowledgeable about risk factors and comorbid conditions for these disorders (**standard**).

Individuals with PLMD who are being treated with medication should be followed by a physician at appropriate intervals and monitored for adverse side effects, augmentation, and tolerance (**standard**).

The following medication recommendation was endorsed as a **guideline:**
  Treatment of RLS or PLMD using L-Dopa with a decarboxylase inhibitor

The following medication recommendation was endorsed as an **option:**
  Treatment of PLMD (and possibly RLS) with clonazepam

[a] Modified from Chesson *et al.* (1999).

[b] A **standard** is a generally accepted strategy that reflects near certainty about the clinical procedure and that is based on large-scale randomized, controlled studies. A **guideline** is a moderately certain procedure based on more restricted randomized, controlled studies or a large set of nonrandomized compartive studies. An **option** is an uncertain strategy based on conflicting evidence or opinion.

is less clear for PLMD. An approach to increase blood flow to the legs, based on the clinical impression that PLMD patients may have an increased incidence of cold feet or vascular insufficiency in the legs, has not been clearly successful. Behavioral approaches may alleviate the sleep complaints of PLMD patients but have not been shown to actually decrease PLMS. This finding is consistent with the observation that placebo responders in RLS studies may report substantial subjective improvement but little or no decrease in PLMS.

Medications that may be useful in PLMD include most of those successful for RLS. Dopaminergic medications, in particular, work very well for PLMS. Other medications of some use are benzodiazepines, other sedatives, opioids, and anticonvulsants.

PLMD patients may respond to low-dose carbidopa/levodopa combinations, either regular or sustained release, using a total levodopa dose of 200 mg per night or less. Keeping doses low may avoid the iatrogenic complications of rebound (late night or morning wearing off) or augmentation (aggravation of the underlying disorder when therapeutic blood levels are low before evening doses). Higher doses of levodopa may, in fact, provoke RLS in patients who previously had PLMD alone. As a substitute, any one of the dopamine agonists may be helpful at very low

doses, much below the typical range for PD. Exact doses have not been determined, but these should be lower than those typically used for RLS (up to 20 mg bromocriptine, 1 mg pergolide, 1.5 mg pramipexole, or 6 mg ropinirole per day). Treatment with dopaminergic agents, as other treatments for PLMD, should start with the lowest possible dose and then gradually increase (i.e., begin with 50 or 100 mg of levodopa, 2.5 mg bromocriptine, 0.05 mg pergolide, 0.125 mg pramipexole, or 0.25 mg ropinirole per day). Ideally, a pill taken 1 or 2 hr before bedtime should be adequate for the entire night. Typical dopaminergic problems (gastrointestinal upset, skin rashes, headache, sleepiness, insomnia, nasal congestion, and orthostatic hypotension) can be alleviated with low doses and cautious titration. The psychotic and dyskinetic complications for treatment of PD are rarely seen with RLS; similarly, those without PD or associated major dopaminergic disorders should not be so affected during treatment of PLMD.

Benzodiazepines were among the first medications used to treat PLMD. Clonazepam at doses of 0.5–2.0 mg per night is usually well tolerated but may accumulate and cause problems for the elderly because of its long half-life. It is generally feasible to substitute benzodiazepines with a shorter half-life (temazepam, lorazepam, and triazolam). Doses should be kept low. The newer, nonbenzodiazepine sedatives (zopiclone, zolpidem, and zaleplon) have not been studied for PLMD, but could also be considered. There are clinical reports of effectiveness for RLS. In general, benzodiazepines (and other sedatives) do not suppress PLMS to the same degree as dopaminergic medications, but they appear to have greater benefit in consolidating sleep and reducing the impact of the movements. Major problems with benzodiazepines are sedation and possible confusion in susceptible individuals.

Other medications that have been used for PLMD include opioids and anticonvulsants (carbamazepine, valproate, and gabapentin). Experience with these is more limited, and they are not as specific as dopaminergic agents in suppressing PLMS. In one trial with baclofen, the amplitude and impact of PLMS were reduced, but the numbers of the movements actually increased. In some cases, combination therapy may be needed, such as low doses of levodopa combined with a low-dose dopamine agonist or a dopaminergic agent combined with a benzodiazepine, opioid, or anticonvulsant.

The key to successful treatment is management aimed at obtaining a successful therapeutic result, with alleviation of the sleep complaint more important than simple reduction of the PLMS. This should be based on a clear analysis of the PLMD and possible associated conditions. Treatment should be cautious, with titration to clinical success and, in almost all cases, restriction to relatively low doses of the selected agents.

—*Wayne A. Hening*

See also–Polysomnography, Clinical; Restless Legs Syndrome (RLS); Sleep, Effects of Aging and; Sleep Disorders

Further Reading

Atlas Task Force of the American Sleep Disorders Association (1993). Recording and scoring leg movements. *Sleep* 16, 748–759.

Bara-Jimenez, W., Aksu, M., Graham, B., *et al.* (2000). Periodic limb movements in sleep: State-dependent excitability of the spinal flexor reflex. *Neurology* 54, 1609–1616.

Chabli, A., Michaud, M., and Montplaisir, J. (2000). Periodic arm movements in patients with the restless legs syndrome. *Eur. Neurol.* 44, 133–138.

Chesson, A. I., Jr., Anderson, W. M., Littner, M., *et al.* (1999). Practice parameters for the treatment of restless legs syndrome and periodic limb movement disorder. An American Academy of Sleep Medicine Report. Standards of Practice Committee of the American Academy of Sleep Medicine. *Sleep* 22, 961–968.

Coleman, R. M. (1982). Periodic movements in sleep (nocturnal myoclonus) and restless legs syndrome. In *Sleeping and Waking Disorders: Indications and Techniques* (C. Guilleminault, Ed.), pp. 265–295. Addison-Wesley, Menlo Park, CA.

Diagnostic Classification Steering Committee of the American Sleep Disorders Association (M. J. Thorpy, Chairperson) (1997). *The International Classification of Sleep Disorders: Diagnostic and Coding Manual.* American Sleep Disorders Association, Rochester, MN.

Hening, W., Allen, R., Early, C., *et al.* (1999). The treatment of restless legs syndrome and periodic limb movement disorder. An American Academy of Sleep Medicine Review. *Sleep* 22, 970–999.

Hening, W. Walters, A., and Chokroverty, S. (1999). Motor functions and dysfunctions of sleep. In *Sleep Disorders Medicine* (S. Chokroverty, Ed.), pp. 441–507. Butterworth-Heinemann, Boston.

Lugaresi, E., Cirignotta, F., Coccagna, G., *et al.* (1986). Nocturnal myoclonus and restless legs syndrome. *Adv. Neurol.* 43, 295–307.

Montplaisir, J., Michaud, M., Denesli, R., *et al.* (2000). Periodic leg movements are not more prevalent in insomnia or hypersomnia but are specifically associated with sleep disorders involving a dopaminergic impairment. *Sleep Med.* 1, 163–167.

Picchietti, D. L., Underwood, D. J., Farris, W. A., *et al.* (1999). Further studies on periodic limb movement disorder and restless legs syndrome in children with attention-deficit hyperactivity disorder. *Move. Disord.* 14, 1000–1007.

Symonds, C. P. (1953). Nocturnal myoclonus. *J. Neurol. Neurosurg. Psychiatry* 16, 166–171.

Peripheral Nervous System, Immunology of

Encyclopedia of the Neurological Sciences
Copyright 2003, Elsevier Science (USA). All rights reserved.

THE PERIPHERAL NERVOUS SYSTEM (PNS) has traditionally been considered as "immunologically privileged." This view has undergone revision within recent years, and currently differences from other organs appear to be more quantitative than qualitative. The PNS is separated from the external environment by the blood–nerve barrier, which restricts access of immune cells and soluble mediators to a certain degree. However, this restriction is not complete, either anatomically (it is absent or relatively deficient at the roots, in the ganglia, and in the motor terminals) or functionally. Immune surveillance, as found in most organs, is present in the PNS as well: Activated T lymphocytes can cross the blood–nerve barrier irrespective of their antigen specificity, and antigen-presenting cells can be detected in peripheral nerve tissue.

Four cell types armed with immunocompetent properties and found in normal PNS play distinct roles in immune-mediated neuropathies: macrophages, lymphocytes, mast cells, and Schwann cells.

IMMUNOCOMPETENT CELLULAR COMPONENTS OF THE PNS

Macrophages

Macrophages constitute 2–10% of total cells in peripheral nerves. Their predominant perivascular distribution makes them uniquely suited to act as antigen presenting cells in the PNS. Indeed, they express constitutively the major histocompatibility complex (MHC) class II molecules, which are required for antigen presentation. Under inflammatory conditions these molecules are upregulated. Macrophages are involved in myelin destruction, immune regulation, and removal of myelin debris.

T Lymphocytes

In normal nerves, T lymphocytes can only rarely be identified, although they normally traffic into and through the endoneurium of the PNS. The local activation of T cells requires antigen presentation in the context of MHC class II antigens, which can be found on a restricted number of cells in the peripheral nerve. In immune-mediated disorders the number of T cells within the PNS increases dramatically by invasion and clonal expansion, indicating the important role of this cell type in the local immune response.

Mast Cells

There is an extensive mast cell population within the PNS; however, their physiological role remains largely unexplained. Through degranulation endoneurial mast cells contribute to the genesis of immune-mediated demyelination by releasing vasoactive amines and arachidonic acid-derived metabolites that augment vascular permeability and disturb nerve conduction.

Schwann Cells

Besides forming the myelin sheath, Schwann cells express MHC class II antigens, which enables these cells to act as antigen presenters. Moreover, it has been shown that they also exhibit MHC class I antigens, which mark these cells as targets for T cell-mediated cellular cytotoxicity. Schwann cells are endowed with an enzyme, the so-called inducible nitric oxide synthase, producing nitric oxide, which is a toxic and immunosuppressive mediator. This raises the possibility that Schwann cells act as antigen presenters as well as immunoregulators within the PNS.

PERIPHERAL NERVE ANTIGENS

Immune-mediated disorders within the PNS are generally regarded to be antigen-mediated; however, the putative (auto-)antigens still need to be defined. Several protein, lipid, and glycoconjugate antigens have been considered to exhibit immunological relevant antigenetic properties.

Protein Antigens

The myelin sheath is composed of three major proteins: P0, P1, and P2, all of which represent more than 70% of the total protein content. P0 accounts for more than 50% of total membrane protein in human PNS myelin, where it is exclusively found. It is physiologically involved in starting and stabilizing the compaction of the extracellular apposition of the myelin membrane in the PNS. P1 represents approximately 2–16% of all myelin proteins, and P2 can be found in large amounts in the PNS and also, to a lesser extent, in the central nervous system. Its

primary localization is in the paranodal loops and in Schmidt–Lantermann incisures.

Lipid and Glycoconjugate Antigens

Lipids make up approximately 75% of the total nerve dry weight. Major myelin lipids are cholesterol, galactosylceramide (galactocerbroside), and galactosylceramide-3-O-sulfate (sulfatide), whereas gangliosides and complex neutral glycolipids occur in smaller amounts. Carbohydrate structures are shared extensively with glycolipids and glycoproteins. Functionally, gangliosides have been implicated in controlling cell interactions, receptor function, and growth. They can be localized in the membranes of many cells and are concentrated in neuronal membranes and processes but also occur in low concentrations in glia and myelin. Antibodies to a large variety of these lipids and glycoconjugates have been reported to be associated with inflammatory demyelinating diseases of the peripheral nerve.

Most of our current knowledge about the relevance of these antigens and the mechanisms involved in the pathogenesis of immune-mediated demyelination was obtained in the animal model experimental autoimmune neuritis (EAN).

EXPERIMENTAL AUTOIMMUNE NEURITIS

EAN is an acute inflammatory demyelinating polyradiculoneuropathy that can be induced in rats, mice, rabbits, and monkeys by active immunization with whole peripheral nerve homogenate, myelin, myelin proteins P0 and P2, or peptides thereof. It can also be produced by adoptive transfer of P2, P2 peptide-specific, P0, and P0 peptide-specific T cell lines, reflecting the essential role of myelin-reactive T lymphocytes in the initiation of the disease.

EAN mirrors many of the immunological, electrophysiological, and morphological aspects of the human Guillain–Barré syndrome and has therefore been widely used as a model to study its pathogenesis.

Pathology of EAN

The pathological hallmark of EAN is the infiltration of the PNS by lymphocytes and macrophages, which results in multifocal demyelination of axons predominantly around venules. Macrophages actively strip off myelin lamellae from axons, induce vesicular disruption of the myelin sheath, and phagocytose both intact and damaged myelin.

Cellular Immune Response

Crucial to the pathogenesis of inflammatory demyelination is the early invasion of the PNS by leukocytes. Circulating autoreactive T cells need to be activated in the periphery in order to cross the blood–nerve barrier and to incite a local immunoinflammatory response. The process of lymphocyte migration from the blood into the PNS, called trafficking or homing, depends on a complex interaction of adhesion molecules, chemokines, and proteases. Breakdown of the blood–nerve barrier is one of the earliest morphologically demonstrable events in lesion development in EAN. Blood-borne T lymphocytes, having reached the PNS, are locally reactivated when they engage with macrophages presenting the antigen in the context of MHC class II molecules. T cells expand clonally and release cytokines to orchestrate the subsequent immune response. Interferon-γ and tumor necrosis factor-α appear to be particularly important cytokines. Both have multiple proinflammatory effects and mediate myelin damage through activation of macrophages to enhance phagocytosis and the release of noxious molecules, such as reactive oxygen and nitrogen oxide metabolites, complement, and proteases.

Various mechanisms appear to be involved in terminating the immune response within the PNS. From the animal model, it was learned that down-regulatory cytokines, such as transforming growth factor-β, interleukin (IL)-4, and IL-10, are critically involved in abolishing the local immune response in the peripheral nerve tissue. Another mechanism may be the induction of apoptosis (i.e., programmed cell death) of activated T lymphocytes accumulating in the PNS.

Humoral Immune Response

A role for antibodies has clearly been documented in chronic rabbit EAN induced by immunization with the galactosylceramide Gal C. Moreover, antibodies to Gal C have been shown to demyelinate axons upon intranerval transfer.

Antibodies can conceivably induce myelin damage by three mechanisms: (i) Upon binding to the Fc receptor of macrophages, they can direct these cells to the putative (auto-)antigenic structures and induce a so-called antibody-dependent cellular cytotoxicity; (ii) by opsonizing (i.e., coating) target structures, they can promote their internalization by macrophages; and (iii) upon binding to the antigenic epitopes, they can activate the classic complement

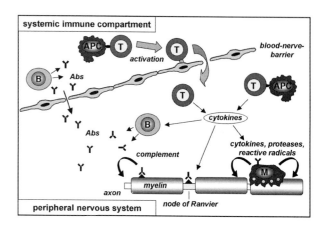

Figure 1
Autoreactive T cells (T) in the systemic circulation, on activation and guided by adhesion molecules and chemokines, can migrate into the peripheral nervous system. Proteases are utilized to penetrate the blood–nerve barrier. Such T cells, when recognizing their specific antigen on an antigen presenting cell (APC) in the peripheral nervous system, are reactivated, proliferate, and secrete cytokines. These can in turn activate macrophages (M) to elaborate noxious inflammatory molecules. Cytokines can also impede impulse propagation. Autoreactive B cells (B) and antibodies (Abs) can pass through the damaged blood–nerve barrier and through activation of the complement system damage myelin. Antibodies can also bind to macrophages and stimulate them to antibody-dependent cytotoxicity.

pathway with subsequent formation of the terminal complement complex (C5b-9). An important role of complement in the pathogenesis of inflammatory demyelination was identified by the observation that blocking the complement system partly suppressed EAN. Current knowledge suggests that complement may be important in recruiting macrophages into the endoneurium, in opsonizing myelin for phagocytosis, in amplifying ongoing inflammatory reactions, and in disintegrating the myelin sheath. In addition to mediating structural damage, antibodies may impair nerve impulse propagation and neuromuscular transmission when binding at or close to the node of Ranvier or the motor terminals (Fig. 1).

The local immune response within the peripheral nerve tissue incorporates cell-mediated and humorally mediated immune mechanisms. Experimental evidence suggests that myelin-reactive T cells and antibodies can synergize to produce myelin destruction. Thus, the local immune setting in inflammatory disorders of the PNS is apparently based on a synergistic interaction of T and B cell responses.

—Bernd C. Kieseier and Hans-Peter Hartung

See also–Neuroimmunology, Overview;
Neuropathies, Overview

Further Reading

Hartung, H.-P., Gold, R., and Jung, S. (1998). Local immune responses in the peripheral nervous system. In *Clinical Neuroimmunology* (J. Antel, G. Birnbaum, and H.-P. Hartung, Eds.), pp. 40–54. Blackwell, Malden, MA.

Ho, T. W., McKhann, G. M., and Griffin, J. W. (1998). Human autoimmune neuropathies. *Annu. Rev. Neurosci.* **21,** 187–226.

Kiefer, R., Kieseier, R. C., Stoll, G., *et al.* (2001). The role of macrophages in immune-mediated damage to the peripheral nervous system. *Prog. Neurobiol.* **64,** 109–127.

Linington, C., and Brostoff, S. W. (1993). Peripheral nerve antigens. In *Peripheral Neuropathy* (P. J. Dyck, P. K. Thomas, J. W. Griffin, P. A. Low, and J. F. Podesto, Eds.), 3rd ed., Vol. 1, pp. 404–417. Saunders, Philadelphia.

Peroneal Nerve

Encyclopedia of the Neurological Sciences

THE COMMON peroneal nerve (CPN), also called the lateral popliteal nerve, and the tibial nerve, also named the medial popliteal nerve, share a common sheath to form the sciatic nerve but never exchange fascicles. In the upper thigh, the CPN innervates the short head of biceps femoris, whereas the tibial nerve innervates the rest of the hamstring muscles. In the upper popliteal fossa, the CPN separates from the tibial nerve and gives off the lateral cutaneous nerve of the calf that innervates the upper third of the lateral leg (Fig. 1). Then, the CPN winds around the fibular neck and divides into its terminal branches, the deep and superficial peroneal nerves.

The deep peroneal nerve (DPN), also called the anterior tibial nerve, innervates the tibialis anterior, extensor hallucis, peroneus tertius, and extensor digitorum longus. Slightly proximal to the ankle joint, the DPN passes under the extensor retinaculum to innervate the extensor digitorum brevis (EDB) and the skin of the web space between the first and second toes (Fig. 2).

The superficial peroneal nerve (SPN) gives motor branches to the peroneus longus and brevis. Then, it pierces the crural fascia approximately 10 cm proximal to the lateral malleolus to become subcutaneous and innervates the skin of the lower two-thirds of the lateral leg and the dorsum of the foot, except for the first web space (Fig. 1).

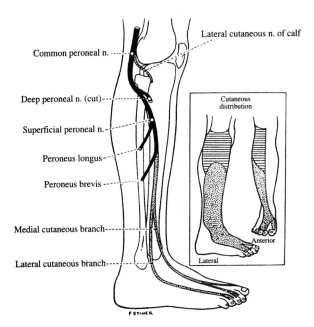

Figure 1
The common and superficial peroneal nerves with their terminal branches and cutaneous innervation [reproduced with permission from Haymaker, W., and Woodhall, B. (1953). *Peripheral Nerve Injuries. Principles of Diagnosis.* Saunders, Philadelphia].

The accessory deep peroneal nerve is a common anomaly occurring in 18–28% of the population. It arises as a motor branch of superficial peroneal nerve, usually a continuation of the muscular branch that innervates the peroneus brevis muscle, and passes behind the lateral malleolus to innervate the lateral EDB muscle.

Peroneal mononeuropathy is the most common compressive neuropathy in the lower extremity. All age groups are equally affected but the disorder is more common in males. Peroneal nerve lesions are usually unilateral. Bilateral lesions constitute approximately 10% of all cases. Lesions of the CPN at the fibular neck are most common, with DPN lesions comprising a small percentage. Selective proximal (high) CPN lesions are rare since most injuries in the upper thigh affect the entire sciatic nerve.

PERONEAL MONONEUROPATHY AT THE FIBULAR NECK

Clinical Presentation

Peroneal mononeuropathy at the fibular neck is a frequent cause of acute foot drop. However, the onset may be subacute, developing gradually over

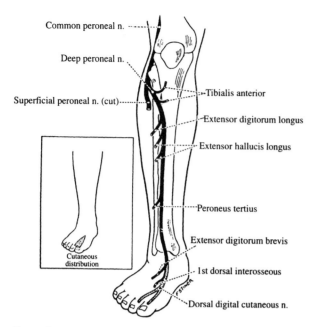

Figure 2
The deep peroneal nerve and its terminal branches and cutaneous innervation [reproduced with permission from Haymaker, W., and Woodhall, B. (1953). *Peripheral Nerve Injuries. Principles of Diagnosis.* Saunders, Philadelphia].

days or weeks, or occasionally cannot be determined. Subjective numbness, mostly on the dorsum of foot, often extending into the lower lateral leg, is common. Pain, usually mild, is rare. A steppage gait may be evident with significant foot drop. Neurological examination reveals weakness of ankle and toe dorsiflexion (extension). There is also weakness of ankle eversion, whereas ankle inversion, toe flexion, and plantar flexion are spared since muscles controlling these functions are innervated by the tibial nerve. Deep tendon reflexes are normal. Hypesthesia or hyperesthesia is common, limited to the lower two-thirds of the lateral leg and dorsum of foot. Tinel's sign may be elicited by percussing the peroneal nerve around the fibular neck. In selective DPN lesions, ankle eversion is normal and there is no sensory loss (except possibly in the first web space).

Etiology

Peroneal mononeuropathies around the fibular neck are usually caused by nerve compression or by knee trauma (Table 1). In compressive lesions, the CPN is often trapped between an external object and the fibular neck. Typically, the DPN is more severely affected than the SPN, and occasionally only the DPN is compressed. This phenomenon is related to the

Table 1   CAUSES OF PERONEAL NERVE LESIONS AT THE FIBULAR NECK[a]

Compression
  During anesthesia
  Weight loss
  Habitual leg crossing[b]
  Prolonged hospitalization[b]
  Prolonged bed rest[b]
  Anorexia nervosa[b]
  Coma
  Diabetes mellitus
  Peripheral polyneuropathy
  Prolonged squatting
    Yoga
    Crop harvesting "strawberry pickers"
    Childbirth
  Iatrogenic
    Above or below knee cast
    Ankle–foot orthosis (brace)
    Pneumatic compression device
    Antithrombotic stocking
    Bandage
    Strap
    Lithotomy position with stirrups
  Intrauterine (with breech presentation)
Trauma
  Blunt
    Fibular fracture
    Ligamental knee joint rupture
    Knee dislocation
    Tibiofibular joint dislocation
      Ankle sprain
  Open
    Laceration
    Gunshot wound
    Animal bite
  Iatrogenic
    Conventional knee surgery
    Knee joint replacement
    Arthroscopic knee surgery
Mass lesion
  Extrinsic
    Osteochondroma
    Baker's cyst
    Ganglion cyst
    Hematoma
    Pseudoaneurysm
  Intrinsic
    Schwannoma
    Neurofibroma
    Neurogenic sarcoma
Infection
  Leprosy

[a] Adapted with revision from Katirji, B. (2002). Compressive and entrapment mononeuropathies of the lower extremity. In *Neuromuscular Disorders in Clinical Practice* (B. Katirji, H. J. Kaminski, D. C. Preston, R. L. Ruff, and B. E. Shapiro, Eds.). Butterworth-Heinemann, Boston.
[b] Usually with weight loss.

topographical arrangement of the CPN around the fibular neck, where the exiting fascicles, forming the SPN, are placed laterally, whereas the DPN is located medially in direct contact with the fibular bone.

Electrodiagnostic Evaluation

Electrodiagnostic (EDX) studies in patients with foot drop and suspected peroneal nerve lesion are extremely useful, with the following objectives:

1. Confirm that the foot drop is due to a lesion of the CPN or DPN, and exclude other causes of foot drop, such as L5 radiculopathy and sciatic mononeuropathy.
2. Localize the site of the peroneal nerve lesion (CPN at fibular neck or upper thigh or DPN).
3. Define the lesion's primary pathophysiological mechanism (demyelinating versus axonal versus mixed).
4. Predict the prognosis and expected course of recovery.
5. Assess the presence and extent of reinnervation (in axonal loss lesions).

The EDX findings in peroneal mononeuropathies may reveal a demyelinative conduction block, axonal loss, or mixed patterns (Table 2). The axonal lesions may be further localized to the upper thigh or between the fibular and upper thigh based on denervation of the short head of the biceps femoris. Selective deep peroneal mononeuropathies are much less common and often axonal.

Based on low-amplitude distal peroneal compound muscle action potentials, significant axonal loss is present in approximately 80% of cases of peroneal mononeuropathies, which accounts for the poor outcome in patients with such lesions. This occurs independent of its mode of onset (i.e., in acute, subacute, or undetermined onset lesions) and equally applies to all compressive peroneal lesions. In particular, patients developing peroneal nerve injury during anesthesia have similar findings and prognosis, despite the common belief that acute perioperative compressive peroneal lesions are due to neurapraxia (i.e., segmental demyelination) and recovery should be rapid.

Differential Diagnosis

Unilateral peroneal mononeuropathy should be differentiated from L5 radiculopathy, sciatic nerve lesion, or lumbosacral plexopathy. In general, radicular pain and positive straight leg test (Lasègue test) are common in L5 radiculopathy and may be present in sciatic nerve lesions, but they are not seen in common peroneal mononeuropathy at the fibular neck. Weakness of ankle inversion, toe flexion, or plantar flexion or absent/depressed ankle jerk are inconsistent with peroneal nerve lesion. Establishing the diagnosis of peroneal mononeuropathy may be based on clinical grounds but often requires EDX confirmation.

Management and Prognosis

Peroneal nerve injury may result in significant disability mostly due to foot drop, which may not recover completely or in a timely manner, particularly when axonal loss is severe. Ankle foot orthosis to improve gait and prevent ankle contractures and sprains is indicated when the foot drop is profound, axonal, or expected to have a protracted course. Active foot exercises and passive range of movements are useful. Patients with significant weight loss should be warned about leg crossing and should wear protective knee pads, properly placed over the fibular head and neck, to prevent recurrent external compression.

Patients with axon-loss peroneal nerve lesions around the fibular neck should be observed for 4–6 months to allow for improvement by spontaneous reinnervation. Severe lesions often require sequential EDX examination to search for early evidence of reinnervation and follow its progression.

Surgical intervention on the peroneal nerve is indicated with nerve laceration or a mass lesion, and it is often appropriate with progressive peroneal mononeuropathies and in severe axonal lesions with no clinical or electromyographic (EMG) evidence for reinnervation 4–6 months after injury.

EDX studies are essential in the planning of management and prognostication of peroneal nerve lesions. Apart from nerve lacerations or gunshot injuries, which result in axonal injury, clinical assessment often cannot predict the prognosis in these patients. Even patients with acute perioperative compressive nerve lesions at the fibular neck have a higher likelihood of harboring axon loss, which carries relatively poor prognosis. EDX evaluation distinguishes lesions with a predominant segmental demyelination from those with extensive axonal loss. Compressive peroneal neuropathies at the fibular neck due to demyelinative conduction block often have good prognosis with spontaneous recovery in 2 or 3 months as long as further compression is

Table 2 ELECTROPHYSIOLOGICAL PATTERNS OF PERONEAL MONONEUROPATHIES[a]

Pattern	Site of lesion	Frequency (%)	Superficial peroneal SNAP	Distal peroneal CMAPs[b]	Conduction block at fibular head	Focal slowing across the fibular head	Needle EMG of peroneus longus	Needle EMG of biceps femoris (short head)	Prognosis for recovery
Conduction block	Fibular head	20–30	Normal	Normal	Present	Rare	Abnormal	Normal	Excellent
Axonal loss	Mid-thigh and fibular head[c]	45–50	Usually absent	Low amplitude or absent	Absent	Absent	Abnormal	Normal	Protracted
	Deep peroneal	5	Normal	Low amplitude or absent	Absent	Absent	Normal	Normal	Fair
	Proximal[d]	<5	Usually absent	Low amplitude or absent	Absent	Absent	Abnormal	Abnormal	Very poor
Mixed	Fibular head	25–30	Low amplitude or absent	Low amplitude	Present	Rare	Abnormal	Normal	Biphasic

[a] Reproduced with permission from Katirji (1999). Abbreviations used: SNAP, sensory nerve action potential; CMAP, compound muscle action potential; EMG, electromyography.
[b] Recording tibialis anterior and extensor digitorum brevis.
[c] Usually around the fibular neck.
[d] High-proximal to the gluteal fold.

prevented. However, the prognosis of axon-loss peroneal lesions is less promising.

COMMON PERONEAL MONONEUROPATHY IN THE UPPER THIGH (SCIATIC MONONEUROPATHY AFFECTING THE PERONEAL NERVE SELECTIVELY)

Clinical Presentation

Selective CPN lesions in the upper thigh are rare and present with foot drop with neurological findings similar to those of lesions at the fibular neck. The only possible clinical sign is that the numbness in the lateral leg may extend into the knee by following the distribution of the lateral cutaneous nerve of the calf (Fig. 1). Although the short head of biceps femoris is weak with high CPN lesions, this muscle cannot be evaluated satisfactorily in isolation on manual muscle testing since its function is often overshadowed by the more powerful hamstring muscles (semitendinosus, semimembranosus, and long head of biceps femoris), all innervated by the tibial nerve. Also, it cannot be palpated during such testing because of its location deep to the long head of the biceps femoris.

Etiology

Partial lesions of the sciatic nerve in the upper thigh usually affect the lateral division (peroneal nerve) more than the adjacent medial division (tibial nerve). On rare occasions, the common peroneal nerve is the only nerve injured, leaving the tibial nerve completely intact. The greater vulnerability of the peroneal division of the sciatic nerve to physical injury is due to the following:

1. *The difference in the fascicular pattern of the perineurium among these two nerves in the upper thigh:* The peroneal nerve has fewer and larger fascicles with limited supportive tissue, whereas the tibial nerve is composed of many cushioning fascicles, well placed between the elastic epineurial tissue. This renders the peroneal division of the sciatic nerve more susceptible to external pressure.

2. *The anatomical course of the common peroneal and tibial nerves:* The peroneal nerve is taut and secured at the sciatic notch and fibular neck, whereas the tibial nerve is loosely fixed posteriorly. Hence, traction of the sciatic nerve in the upper thigh (such as during total hip replacement) will result in earlier and more extensive damage to the peroneal nerve than the tibial nerve.

Causes of high CPN lesions are similar to those of sciatic nerve lesions in general, including total hip replacement, hip fracture/dislocation, femur fracture, gluteal injection, gluteal compartment syndrome, gunshot or knife wounds, and acute compression during coma, drug overdose, intensive care unit, or prolonged sitting.

Differential Diagnosis

A proximal (high) CPN lesion often presents a diagnostic challenge since it imitates CPN at the fibular neck. When the tibial component of the sciatic nerve is also involved, there is often sensory loss in the sole, depressed or absent ankle jerk, and weakness of plantar flexion and depressed/absent ankle jerk. EDX study reveals additional nonperoneal nerve findings, such as asymmetrically low (or sometimes absent) sural sensory nerve action potential (SNAP) amplitude, borderline or low tibial compound muscle action potential (CMAP) amplitude, asymmetrically abnormal H-reflex, or minimal neurogenic changes in tibial-innervated muscles (such as gastrocnemius, tibialis posterior, or flexor digitorum longus). However, when the sciatic nerve lesion is selective to the CPN, the nerve conduction studies (NCSs) are identical to an axon-loss common peroneal mononeuropathy at the fibular neck. However, needle EMG of the short head of biceps femoris reveals signs of denervation only in proximal (high) common peroneal mononeuropathies and is normal in distal lesions such as at the fibular neck. In contrast to manual muscle testing, this muscle is easily accessible during needle EMG examination.

DEEP PERONEAL MONONEUROPATHY AT THE ANKLE (ANTERIOR TARSAL TUNNEL SYNDROME)

Etiology

Lesions of the distal segment of the DPN, which occur on the dorsum of the ankle beneath the extensor retinaculum, are sometimes referred to as the anterior tarsal tunnel syndrome. Causes of the anterior tarsal tunnel syndrome include direct trauma to the dorsum of the ankle; chronic pressure from shoe rims or straps; fractures, dislocations, or sprains of the ankle; ganglion cyst; and osteophyte. Other causes include unusual positioning of the foot, such as with marked foot plantar flexion accompanied by dorsiflexion of the toes (e.g., wearing high-heeled shoes), or extreme inversion of the foot (e.g., with spasticity or dystonia).

Clinical Presentation

The syndrome is slightly more common in women, probably related to the use of high-healed shoes. It may be unilateral or bilateral. Anterior tarsal tunnel syndrome is often asymptomatic, detected incidentally during EDX testing of the lower limb for other symptoms such as lumbosacral radiculopathy. This has raised many questions regarding the true existence of this entity.

In the few symptomatic cases, there is often numbness and paresthesias limited to the web space between the first and second toes. Ankle and foot pain, worse at night, is common, whereas foot weakness is not part of the syndrome. On examination, there is diminished sensation in the web space between the first and second toes (i.e., in the region innervated by the terminal portion of the deep peroneal nerve) and wasting of the EDB muscle. Weakness of the EDB is difficult to assess due to the more powerful toe dorsiflexors, the extensor hallucis, and extensor digitorum longus. Occasionally, a Tinel's sign over the deep peroneal nerve at the ankle may be elicited.

Electrodiagnostic Evaluation

EDX findings in the anterior tarsal tunnel syndrome are limited to low CMAP amplitude and prolongation of peroneal motor distal latency recording EDB, with a normal proximal conduction velocity, and chronic neurogenic motor unit action potential changes, usually with fibrillation potentials, in the EDB muscle. All other peroneal NCSs and needle EMG of common peroneal and L5 or S1 innervated muscles are normal. The findings may be unilateral or bilateral.

In asymptomatic patients, it may difficult to separate the previously mentioned findings from the common occurrence of denervation of the EDB, with or without slowing of peroneal motor distal latency. It is advised to reserve the diagnosis of anterior tarsal tunnel syndrome to patients with typical manifestations and EDX findings.

Treatment

Avoiding high heels or tight shoes and correcting ankle malposition (e.g., by bracing) are often helpful. Occasionally, surgical exploration may be necessary to remove a ganglion cyst or an osteophyte or to simply divide the extensor retinaculum.

SUPERFICIAL PERONEAL MONONEUROPATHY

Clinical Manifestations

It is extremely rare for peroneal nerve lesions at the fibular neck to affect only the SPN without greater damage to the DPN. Lesions to the SPN, which are uncommon, are purely sensory since they occur in the distal leg or ankle (i.e., distal to the takeoff of the motor branches to the peroneus longus and brevis muscles). Hence, they manifest with sensory loss in the lower lateral third of the leg and dorsum of the foot, excluding the first web space, with sparing of ankle eversion (a function of the peroneus longus and brevis muscles). Pain in the distal anterolateral leg is common. Both numbness and pain may be worse with walking or running. Tenderness, swelling, or both may be evident over the fascial defect in the distal leg. Occasionally, Tinel's sign may be induced there. The typical EDX finding is a low-amplitude or absent superficial peroneal SNAP.

Etiology

Most superficial peroneal mononeuropathies are purely sensory since the site of entrapment is at the fascial defect, 10 cm above the lateral malleolus, where the nerve become subcutaneous. Most reported cases are in athletes, and common precipitating events include long marches, tight boots, or direct blunt trauma. Rarely, tumors such as lipoma or herniation of muscle through the fascial defect may entrap the superficial peroneal nerve. Near the ankle, superficial peroneal nerve injuries may be iatrogenic, such as during ankle arthroscopy or needle insertion.

Treatment

Conservative treatment of patients with external compression may be accomplished by changing precipitating factors such as footwear. Patients with persistent symptoms may require exploration and nerve decompression near the fascial defect.

—*Bashar Katirji*

See also—Foot Drop; Sciatic Nerve; Tibial Nerve

Further Reading

Blair, J. M., and Botte, M. J. (1994). Surgical anatomy of the superficial peroneal nerve in the ankle and foot. *Clin. Orthop.* 305, 229–238.

Jones, H. R., Felice, Z. K. J., and Gross, P. T. (1993). Pediatric peroneal mononeuropathy: A clinical and electromyographic study. *Muscle Nerve* 16, 1167–1173.

Katirji, B. (1999). Peroneal neuropathy. *Neurol. Clin.* **17**, 567–591.

Katirji, M. B., and Wilbourn, A. J. (1988). Common peroneal mononeuropathy: A clinical and electrophysiologic study of 116 lesions. *Neurology* **38**, 1723–1728.

Katirji, M. B., and Wilbourn, A. J. (1994). High sciatic lesions mimicking peroneal neuropathy at the fibular head. *J. Neurol. Sci.* **121**, 172–175.

Katirji, B. (2002). Electrodiagnostic approach to the patient with suspected mononeuropathy of the lower extremity. *Neurol. Clin.* **20**, 479–501.

Kernohan, J., Levack, B., and Wilson, J. N. (1985). Entrapment of the superficial peroneal nerve. Three case reports. *J. Bone Jt. Surg. (Br)* **67**, 60–61.

Kim, D. H., and Kline, D. G. (1996). Management and results of peroneal nerve lesions. *Neurosurgery* **39**, 312–319.

Mont, M. A., Dellon, A. L., Chen, F., *et al.* (1996). The operative treatment of peroneal nerve palsy. *J. Bone Jt. Surg.* **78**, 863–869.

Sourkes, M., and Stewart, J. D. (1991). Common peroneal neuropathy: A study of selective motor and sensory involvement. *Neurology* **41**, 1029–1033.

Sunderland, S. (1978). *Nerve and Nerve Injuries*, 2nd ed. Churchill Livingstone, Edinburgh, UK.

Wilbourn, A. J. (1986). Common peroneal mononeuropathy at the fibular head. *Muscle Nerve* **9**, 825–836.

Yuen, E. C., Olney, R. K., and So, Y. T. (1994). Sciatic neuropathy: Clinical and prognostic features in 73 patients. *Neurology* **44**, 1669–1674.

Peroxisomes

Encyclopedia of the Neurological Sciences
Copyright 2003, Elsevier Science (USA). All rights reserved.

THE PEROXISOME is a subcellular organelle that is present in all human cells other than the mature erythrocyte. The organelle was described first by de Duve and associates and derives its name from its role in the production and degradation of hydrogen peroxide. It has since been shown that it is the site of 60 or more biochemical reactions. These include the degradation of hydrogen peroxide by catalase; the synthesis of ether lipids and bile acids and of certain polyunsaturated fatty acids such as docosahexanoic acid (DHA); many of the enzymatic reactions involved in the biosynthesis of cholesterol; and the beta oxidation of fatty acids, including very long chain and branched-chain fatty acids, D-amino acid oxidases, and alanine-glyoxalate transaminase. Peroxisomes are particularly abundant in the liver and kidney. In these tissues they appear under the electron microscope as round or oval organelles bounded by one membrane, with an average diameter of approximately 0.5 µm. In other organs, such as the brain and cultured skin fibroblasts, they are much less abundant and smaller, with diameters of approximately 0.1–0.25 µm.

Peroxisome matrix proteins are synthesized on cytoplasmic polyribosomes and imported posttranslationally. Two sequences that target proteins to the matrix of the organelle have been identified. Most matrix proteins contain peroxisome targeting sequence (PTS) 1, which is a carboxy-terminal tripeptide with a consensus sequence of -SKL or a conservative variant. PTS2 contains the sequence -R/KLX5Q/HL- located 2–12 residues from the amino terminus of the protein. The targeting of peroxisomal membrane proteins is less well understood, but sequences required for the import of membrane proteins have been identified. Proteins that contain these targeting sequences interact with a variety of import factors that are now referred to as peroxins in accordance with a recently developed nomenclature. The peroxin category encompasses all proteins involved in peroxisome biogenesis, inclusive of peroxisomal matrix protein import, membrane biogenesis, peroxisome proliferation, and peroxisome proliferation and peroxisome inheritance. The peroxins are numbered by the date of published characteristics and currently number 23. The recognition and definition of peroxins was aided by the study of human disease states in which one of these genes is defective. These disorders are referred to as disorders of peroxisome biogenesis.

HUMAN PEROXISOMAL DISORDERS

At least 25 genetically determined human peroxisomal disorders have been described and are classified into two major categories (Table 1). The first category is disorders of peroxisome biogenesis (PBDs). In these disorders, the organelle fails to be formed normally and this causes defects in multiple peroxisomal proteins. In the second category, the defects involve single peroxisomal enzymes. The molecular defects that underlie nearly all these disorders have been defined during the past 5 years. These new developments have facilitated diagnosis, greatly increased the effectiveness of genetic counseling and disease prevention, and provided new therapeutic leads. The Kennedy Krieger Institute conducted a testing program for peroxisomal disorders. Table 2 shows the number of patient in these various disease categories that have been identified through this program.

Table 1 GENETICALLY DETERMINED PEROXISOMAL DISORDERS

Assembly deficiencies or disorders of peroxisome biogenesis	Single peroxisomal enzyme deficiencies
Zellweger syndrome	X-linked adrenoleukodystrophy
Neonatal adrenoleukodystrophy	Acyl-coenzyme A oxidase deficiency
Infantile Refsum disease	Bifunctional enzyme deficiency
Rhizomelic chondrodysplasia punctata	Peroxisomal thiolase deficiency
	DHAP alkyl transferase deficiency
	Alkyl DHAP synthase deficiency
	Glutaric aciduria type III
	Classic Refsum disease
	Hyperoxaluria type I
	Acatalasemia

DISORDERS OF PEROXISOME BIOGENESIS

PBDs are associated with four different clinical syndromes: the Zellweger syndrome (ZS), neonatal adrenoleukodystrophy (NALD), infantile Refsum disease (IRD), and rhizomelic chondrodysplasia punctata. These disorders were named before their relationship to the peroxisome was recognized. Table 3 lists their principal clinical features. The classification and understanding of these disorders have been enhanced greatly by the technique of complementation analysis. The underlying principle

Table 2 PEROXISOMAL DISORDERS DIAGNOSED AT THE KENNEDY KRIEGER INSTITUTE, 1981–SEPTEMBER 2000

Peroxisomal biogenesis disorders (PBDs)		816
Zellweger syndrome	369	
Neonatal adrenoleukodystrophy	206	
Rhizomelic chondrodysplasia punctata	101	
Infantile Refsum disease	48	
Other PBDs or PBDs suspect	92	
Defects that involve single peroxisomal enzymes		4916
X-linked adrenoleukodystrophy, males	3109	
X-linked adrenoleukodystrophy, heterozygotes	1700	
Bifunctional enzyme defect	72	
Other single enzyme defects	35	
Total		5732

of this technique is that cultured skin fibroblasts from two different patients, both deficient in a peroxisomal process, are induced to fuse. The resulting multinucleated cells are examined for their ability to carry out this metabolic process. Restoration of activity can occur only if each cell line provides the gene product defective in the other, and cell lines that complement each other in this way therefore represent distinct genotypes. The PBDs have been subdivided into 13 complementation groups. Complementation analyses were conducted concurrently in Europe, the United States, and Japan, and group designations were assigned to each. Exchange of cell lines has permitted correlation between the groups established in each of these centers (Table 4). The molecular defects have been defined in 10 of these groups and are listed in Table 4. Each of these defects involves one of the peroxins.

These complementation studies and molecular analyses have had a profound effect on the classification of the PBDs. The ZS, NALD, and IRD phenotypes can be associated with 11 different complementation groups and with nine different molecular defects. This finding, combined with the analysis of the clinical features of these disorders, indicates that they represent a clinical continuum, with ZS the most severe, IRD the least severe, and NALD intermediate. In contrast, among the PBDs, rhizomelic chondrodysplasia punctata is associated only with a defect of *PEX7*, the receptor of PTS2.

GENETIC DEFECTS THAT INVOLVE A SINGLE PEROXISOMAL ENZYME

As shown in Table 2, X-linked adrenoleukodystrophy (X-ALD) is by far the most common peroxisomal disorder, and it is discussed in more detail later. Brief comments are presented here about the other disorders in this category. The clinical manifestations associated with defects of the peroxisomal bifunctional enzyme, peroxisomal acyl-CoA oxidase, and peroxisomal thiolase mimic those with the PBD ZS–NALD–IRD continuum (Table 3). The clinical manifestations of defects of dihydroxyacetone phosphate (DHAP) alkyl transferase or alkyl DHAP synthase, enzymes that are required for the synthesis of the ether lipid plasmalogen, mimic those of rhizomelic chondrodysplasia punctata. The gene that is deficient in Refsum disease was identified in 1997, more than 50 years after the

Table 3 MAJOR CLINICAL FEATURES OF DISORDERS OF PEROXISOME ASSEMBLY AND THEIR OCCURRENCE IN VARIOUS PEROXISOMAL DISORDERS[a]

Feature	ZS	NALD	IRD	Oxidase deficiency	Bifunctional enzyme deficiency	Thiolase deficiency	RCDP	DHAP synthase deficiency	DHAP alkyl transferase deficiency
Average age at death or last follow-up (years)	0.76	2.2	6.4	4.0	0.75	0.9	1.0	0.5	?
Facial dysmorphism	2+	+	+	0	73%	+	2+	2+	2+
Cataract	80%	45%	7%	0	0	0	72%	+	+
Retinopathy	71%	82%	100%	2+	+	0	0	0	0
Impaired hearing	100%	100%	93%	2+	?	?	71%	33%	100%
Psychomotor delay	4+	3–4+	3+	2+	4+	4+	4+	4+	?
Hypotonia	99%	82%	52%	+	4+	+	±	±	?
Neonatal seizures	80%	82%	20%	50%	93%	+	±	?	?
Large liver	100%	79%	83%	0	+	+	0	?	
Renal cysts	93%	0	0	0	0	+	0	0	0
Rhizomelia	3%	0	0	0	0	0	93%	+	+
Chondrodysplasia punctata	69%	0	0	0	0	0	100%	+	+
Neuronal migration defect	67%	20%	±	?	88%	+	±	?	?
Coronal vertebral cleft	0	0	0	0	0	0	+	+	+
Demyelination	22%	50%	0	60%	75%	±	0	0	0

[a] Percentages indicate the percentage of patients in whom the abnormality is present; 0, abnormality is absent; ± to 4+, degree to which an abnormality is present. Abbreviations used: ZS, Zellweger syndrome; NALD, neonatal adrenoleukodystrophy; IRD, infantile Refsum disease; RCDP, rhizomelic chondrodysplasia punctata; DHAP, dihydroxyacetone phosphate.

Table 4   GENOTYPE–PHENOTYPE CORRELATIONS IN DISORDERS OF PEROXISOME BIOGENESIS[a]

Pex defect	Complementation group			No. of patients, KKI	Phenotypes
	U.S.	Japan	Netherlands		
1	1	E	2	99	ZS, NALD, IRD
2	10	F	5	2	ZS
5	2		4	2	ZS, NALD
6	4	C	3	16	ZS, NALD
7	11		1	43	RCDP
10	7	B		5	ZS, NALD
12	3			5	ZS, NALD
13		H		2	ZS, NALD
16	9	D		1	ZS
19		J			ZS
Unidentified	8	A		7	ZS, NALD, IRD
Unidentified		G			ZS

[a] Abbreviations used: ZS, Zellweger syndrome; NALD, neonatal adrenoleukodystrophy; IRD, infantile Refsum disease; KKI, Kennedy Krieger Institute.

Table 5   PHENOTYPES IN MALES AND IN FEMALE X-ALD CARRIERS

Phenotype	Description	Estimated relative frequency
Males		
Childhood cerebral	Onset at 3–10 years of age; progressive behavioral, cognitive, and neurological deficit, often leading to total disability within 3 years; inflammatory brain demyelination	31–35%
Adolescent	Like childhood cerebral; onset age 11–21 years; somewhat slower progression	4–7%
Adrenomyeloneuropathy (AMN)	Onset 28 ± 9 years, progressive over decades; involves spinal cord mainly, distal axonopathy; inflammatory response mild or absent; approximately 40% have or develop cerebral involvement with varying degrees of inflammatory response and more rapid progression	40–46%
Adult cerebral	Dementia, behavioural disturbances; sometimes focal deficits, without preceding AMN; white matter inflammatory response present; progression parallels that of childhood cerebral form	2–5%
Olivopontocerebelllar	Mainly cerebellar and brain stem involvement in adolescence or adulthood	1–2%
Addison only	Primary adrenal insufficiency without apparent neurological involvement; onset common before 7.5 years; most eventually develop AMN	Varies with age: up to 50% in childhood
Asymptomatic	Biochemical and gene abnormality without demonstrable adrenal or neurological deficit; detailed studies often show adrenal hypofunction or subtle signs of AMN	Diminishes with age: common, <4 years; very rare, >40 years
Female X-ALD carriers		
Asymptomatic	No evidence of adrenal or neurological involvement	Diminishes with age: most women, <30 years; neurologically uninvolved
Mild myelopathy	Increased deep tendon reflexes and distal sensory changes in lower extremities with absent or mild disability	Increases with age; approximately 50% >40 years
Moderate to severe myeloneuropathy	Symptoms and pathology resemble AMN, but milder and later onset	Increases with age; approximately 15% >40 years
Cerebral involvement	Rarely seen in childhood and slightly more common in middle age and later	Approximately 2%
Clinically evident adrenal insufficiency	Rare at any age	Approximately 1%

disease was defined as a clinical entity. Primary hyperoxaluria type 1 is associated with a defect of alanine:glyoxalate aminotransferase, which in man is localized to the peroxisome. This condition can be treated successfully with liver and kidney transplantation.

X-LINKED ADRENOLEUKODYSTROPHY

X-ALD affects mainly the nervous system, adrenal cortex, and the testis. It has been reported in all ethnic groups and its prevalence in males is estimated to be between 1:20,000 and 1:50,000. It shows a wide range of phenotypic expression (Table 5) that often cooccurs within the same family. The childhood cerebral form is the most severe phenotype, and it is associated with an inflammatory demyelinating process in the cerebral hemispheres. Its manifestations contrast with those of adrenomyeloneuropathy (AMN), which is the most common phenotype and presents as a slowly progressive paraparesis in young or middle-aged adults. AMN affects mainly the long tracts in the spinal cord. Its pathological basis is a noninflammatory distal axonopathy.

The principal biochemical abnormality is the accumulation of saturated very long-chain fatty acids (VLCFAs) in tissues and body fluids due to the impaired capacity to degrade these substances—a reaction that normally takes place in the peroxisome. It was surprising when it was shown that the gene that is defective in X-ALD does not code for one of the enzymes known to be involved in VLCFA oxidation. It codes for a peroxisomal membrane protein referred to as ALDP, which is a member of the ATP binding cassette transporter protein family that also includes the cystic fibrosis protein. More than 200 mutations in ALDP have been identified. The mechanisms through which the ALDP defect leads to VLCFA accumulation and the pathogenesis of X-ALD have not been clarified. Bone marrow transplantation can be of long-term benefit to boys and adolescents who show early evidence of the cerebral inflammatory response, but it carries a high risk and patients must be selected with care. Dietary therapy with a 4:1 mixture of glyceryl trioleate and glyceryl trierucate, referred to as Lorenzo's oil, can normalize the levels of VLCFA in plasma, but its clinical effectiveness is limited. Therapeutic approaches are being tested in a mouse model of X-ALD and provide the hope that effective therapies can be developed.

—*Hugo W. Moser*

See also–Leukodystrophy

Further Reading

Braverman, N., Steel, G., Obie, C., *et al.* (1997). Human PEX7 encodes the peroxisomal PTS2 receptor and is responsible for rhizomelic chondrodysplasia punctata. *Nat. Genet.* **15**, 369–376.

Danpure, C. J., Jennings, P. R., Leiper, J. M., *et al.* (1996). Targeting of alanine: Glyoxylate aminotransferase in normal individuals and its mistargeting in patients with primary hyperoxaluria type 1. *Ann. N. Y. Acad. Sci.* **804**, 477–490.

De Duve, C., and Baudhuin, P. (1966). Peroxisomes (microbodies and related particles). *Physiol. Rev.* **46**, 323–357.

Distel, B., Erdmann, R., Gould, S. J., *et al.* (1996). A unified nomenclature for peroxisome biogenesis factors. *J. Cell Biol.* **135**, 1–3.

Ghaedi, K., Honsho, M., Shimozawa, N., *et al.* (2000). PEX3 is the causal gene responsible for peroxisome membrane assembly-defective Zellweger syndrome of complementation group G. *Am. J. Hum. Genet.* **67**, 976–981.

Gould, S. J., Raymond, G. V., and Valle, D. (2000). The peroxisome biogenesis disorders. In *The Metabolic and Molecular Bases of Inherited Disease* (C. R. Scriver, A. L. Beaudet, W. S. Sly, D. Valle, and B. Vogelstein, Eds.), 8th ed. McGraw-Hill, New York.

Jansen, G. A., Ofman, R., Ferdinandusse, S., *et al.* (1997). Refsum disease is caused by mutations in the phytanoyl-CoA hydroxylase gene. *Nat. Genet.* **17**, 190–193.

Kemp, S., Wei, H. M., Lu, J. F., *et al.* (1998). Gene redundancy and pharmacological gene therapy: Implications for X-linked adrenoleukodystrophy. *Nat. Med.* **4**, 1261–1268.

Lazarow, P. B., and Fujiki, Y. (1985). Biogenesis of peroxisomes. *Annu. Rev. Cell Biol.* **1**, 489–530.

Lazo, O., Contreras, M., Hashmi, M., *et al.* (1988). Peroxisomal lignoceroyl-CoA ligase deficiency in childhood adrenoleukodystrophy and adrenomyeloneuropathy. *Proc. Natl. Acad. Sci. USA* **85**, 7647–7651.

Matsumoto, N., Tamura, S., Moser, A., *et al.* (2001). The peroxin pex6p is impaired in peroxisomal biogenesis disorders in complementation group 6. *J. Hum. Genet.* **46**, 273–277.

Moser, H. W. (1997). Adrenoleukodystrophy: Phenotype, genetics, pathogenesis and therapy. *Brain* **120**, 1485–1508.

Moser, H. W. (1999). Genotype–phenotype correlations in disorders of peroxisome biogenesis. *Mol. Genet. Metab.* **68**, 316–327.

Moser, H. W., Loes, D. J., Melhem, E. R., *et al.* (2000). X-linked adrenoleukodystrophy: Overview and prognosis as a function of age and brain magnetic resonance imaging abnormality. A study involving 372 patients. *Neuropediatrics* **31**, 227–239.

Mosser, J., Douar, A. M., Sarde, C. O., *et al.* (1993). Putative X-linked adrenoleukodystrophy gene shares unexpected homology with ABC transporters. *Nature* **361**, 726–730.

Muntau, A. C., Mayerhofer, P. U., Paton, B. C., *et al.* (2000). Defective peroxisome membrane synthesis due to mutations in human PEX3 causes Zellweger syndrome, complementation group G. *Am. J. Hum. Genet.* **67**, 967–975.

Powers, J. M., DeCiero, D. P., Ito, M., *et al.* (2000). Adrenomyeloneuropathy: A neuropathologic review featuring its noninflammatory myelopathy. *J. Neuropathol. Exp. Neurol.* **59**, 89–102.

Smith, K. D., Kemp, S., Braiterman, L. T., *et al.* (1999). X-linked adrenoleukodystrophy: Genes, mutations, and phenotypes. *Neurochem. Res.* **24,** 521–535.

Subramani, S. (1998). Components involved in peroxisome import, biogenesis, proliferation, turnover, and movement. *Physiol. Rev.* **78,** 171–188.

van den Bosch, H., Schutgens, R. B., Wanders, R. J., *et al.* (1992). Biochemistry of peroxisomes. *Annu. Rev. Biochem.* **61,** 157–197.

van Geel, B. M., Assies, J., Haverkort, E. B., *et al.* (1999). Progression of abnormalities in adrenomyeloneuropathy and neurologically asymptomatic X-linked adrenoleukodystrophy despite treatment with "Lorenzo's oil". *J. Neurol. Neurosurg. Psychiatry* **67,** 290–299.

van Grunsven, E. G., van Berkel, E., Ijlst, L., *et al.* (1998). Peroxisomal D-hydroxyacyl-CoA dehydrogenase deficiency: Resolution of the enzyme defect and its molecular basis in bifunctional protein deficiency. *Proc. Natl. Acad. Sci. USA* **95,** 2128–2133.

Persistent Vegetative State (PVS)

Encyclopedia of the Neurological Sciences
Copyright 2003, Elsevier Science (USA). All rights reserved.

PATIENTS with the persistent vegetative state (PVS) have the capacity for wakefulness but not awareness. Although the patient has wake and sleep cycles and can be roused from sleep, there is no interaction with stimuli. The patient cannot respond other than reflexively and cannot carry out any motor act that requires planning or cognitive function. There is no evidence of cognition or awareness of self or the environment. Reactions to stimuli are simple, automatic, stereotypical, and predictable rather than goal directed. Hypothalamic functions and cranial nerve and spinal reflexes are usually, but not necessarily completely, preserved.

In PVS, the arousal system is functioning, but the cognitive component of consciousness is lacking. Because we cannot know what an unresponsive person is thinking, our clinical conclusions must be inferred. Supportive evidence for "wakefulness without awareness" includes the following: Behavior occurs in stereotypic responses that are thought to arise at subcortical regions in a reflexive or almost reflexive fashion; positron emission tomography (PET) studies show a marked reduction in cerebral metabolism compared to normals and patients with locked-in syndrome; and all available pathological material indicates that PVS is associated with lesions that would have made conscious awareness highly improbable.

When Jennett and Plum coined the term persistent vegetative state, "persistent" meant that the state was consistently sustained over the period of observation. The term was not meant to imply permanency. To prognosticate that the vegetative state is permanent requires time and observation. "Vegetative" refers to the preservation of vegetative or simple homeostatic processes that are regulated by subcortical centers, without requiring cognitive capacity. Ancillary tests are very helpful when appropriately applied.

EPIDEMIOLOGY

The estimated prevalence of PVS in the United States is 10,000–25,000 for adults and 4000–10,000 for children.

ETIOLOGIES OF PVS

There are three classifications of etiologies. First, acute brain insults are acute brain disorders that lead to a vegetative state following a period of coma lasting days to weeks. During the comatose period there may be compromise of ventilatory drive, autonomic functions, etc., but these basic functions recover along with reappearance of arousal and wake–sleep behavior. The succeeding vegetative state may become permanent or the patient may have various degrees of cognitive recovery. The most common acute causes of the vegetative state in both children and adults are head trauma and hypoxic–ischemic encephalopathy. Certain encephalitides (e.g., St. Louis, Eastern and Western equine, and Japanese B) may also produce a coma followed by a vegetative state, related to diffuse cerebral cortical damage.

Second, subacute and chronic disorders include various degenerative, metabolic, and infectious conditions: This category includes those conditions that cause progressive or cumulative brain damage, progressing through cognitive and multifocal deficits to dementia and loss of all cognitive function, but with preservation of basic arousal and wake–sleep cycles. From an epidemiological perspective, the most common condition is Alzheimer's disease. Other relentlessly progressive disorders such as Creutzfeldt–Jakob disease, subacute sclerosing panencephalitis, and metabolic storage diseases of infancy, such as Tay–Sachs disease, can produce terminal PVS.

Finally, developmental malformations are conditions that develop during embryogenesis in which the cerebral structures (in which cognition would take place) never develop into functioning anatomical structures. Thus, these patients do not have the potential for cognition, based on our knowledge of the nervous system. Even before cognitive function would develop in the normal neonate, it should be possible to identify those extreme cases of brain maldevelopment who could never achieve self- and environmental awareness.

ANATOMICAL BASIS OF PVS

There are three basic topographical patterns of neuropathology in patients who have died of PVS that was persistent to death.

Predominantly Neocortical

The most common finding in PVS patients who suffered severe anoxic–ischemic insult is diffuse laminar cortical necrosis. This involves the larger cell layers, especially 3, 5, and 6, but the necrosis can involve all layers. In addition, there is almost invariable involvement of the hippocampus (especially the CA1 and CA4–6 regions) and variable involvement of subcortical gray matter structures and the cerebellar Purkinje cells. A markedly suppressed or "flat" electroencephalograph (EEG) is commonly found.

Predominantly Thalamic

An alternative pattern was recently proposed following a very careful study of the brain of Karen Ann Quinlan, who suffered a cardiopulmonary arrest at age 21. She survived for nearly a decade in a persistent vegetative state, in which she showed wake and sleep cycles, spontaneous eye opening, as well as eye opening to auditory stimuli. She had simple withdrawal-type responses to stimuli—more than spinal reflex movements but not goal-directed, purposeful movements.

At postmortem, the thalamus was severely affected, especially in the paramedian and lateral regions of the central and posterior portions. It is of special interest that the "nonspecific" and reticular thalamic nuclei were severely ravaged, given their proposed function in arousal. The forniceal system and mammillary bodies were badly damaged. Her cerebral cortex was especially affected in the parasagittal watershed zones posteriorly and in the occipital lobes. However, other cortical regions were

relatively spared. Thus, her PVS appears to have been largely due to diencephalic disease.

The postmortem study gives reasonable evidence that (i) the thalamus plays an important role in cognitive function, and that (ii) extrathalamic mechanisms may cause alerting and "activation" of the cerebral cortex, as an alternative pathway to the traditional ascending reticular activating system (ARAS).

Diffuse Axonal Injury and Subcortical White Matter Damage

Diffuse axonal injury results from acute trauma, in which shearing decelerating–accelerating and rotational forces tear white matter axons. This effectively isolates the cortex from subcortical structures. There may be associated brainstem injury, but this is not an essential or consistent feature.

Leukoencephalopathies following anoxic insults or carbon monoxide poisoning (often appearing a week or two after apparent recovery), necrotizing hemorrhagic leukoencephalopathy, or necrotizing leukoencephalopathies from methotrexate radiation damage could produce PVS.

CLINICAL FEATURES

The following criteria for the diagnosis of PVS have been established by the Multi-Task Force on PVS:

1. No evidence of awareness of self or environment and an inability to interact with others
2. No evidence of sustained, reproducible, purposeful, or voluntary behavioral responses to visual, auditory, tactile, or noxious stimuli
3. No evidence of language comprehension or expression
4. Intermittent wakefulness manifested by the presence of wake–sleep cycles
5. Sufficiently preserved hypothalamic and brainstem autonomic functions to permit survival with medical and nursing care
6. Bladder and bowel incontinence
7. Variably preserved cranial nerve reflexes (pupillary, oculocephalic, corneal, vestibuloocular, and gag) and spinal reflexes

The patient in PVS is not immobile, but moves the eyes, limbs, and trunk in meaningless ways. There is no goal-directed behavior and the patient does not visually track or show a behavioral, emotional, or avoidance response to the image projected on the retina. Primitive orienting reflexes, such as turning the head and eyes toward the source of a sound or tactile stimulus, may be present. As a corollary, when patients do visually track or show more than reflexive or instinctive behavior on testing and retesting, they are no longer in PVS.

Recovery form PVS occurs in some patients. Usually, the first feature is the return of visual tracking, followed by primitive behaviors, the obeying of commands, and then spontaneous purposeful activity. Speech, cognitive function, and motor abilities have fully or nearly fully recovered in a small number of patients. Significant improvement is very unlikely in a child or adult who has been in a PVS for more than 12 months. Some very exceptional cases have occurred in which recovery of reactivity occurs after more than 1 year in PVS. Laboratory assessment of cerebral function should allow more reliable predictors than clinical features alone. Better guidelines are needed.

DIFFERENTIAL DIAGNOSIS

The main conditions to be differentiated are those of reduced responsiveness. It should be noted that decreased responsiveness does not necessarily imply decreased consciousness or cognitive function. Patients may have psychogenic unresponsiveness (e.g., from malingering, psychosis, or conversion reaction) or may be locked-in [either from the classic basis pontis lesion or from peripheral de-efferentation (e.g., severe Guillain–Barré syndrome, myopathy, or neuromuscular transmission defect)].

MANAGEMENT

Management decisions are dependent on the accurate diagnosis of PVS and determination of prognosis. The value of adherence to valid guidelines in arriving at a diagnosis in PVS was emphasized in a recent survey in London's Royal Hospital for Neurodisability. Seventeen of 40 patients deemed to be in PVS were, in fact, aware. A similar American study showed inaccurate diagnosis in 18 of 49 (37%) patients thought to be in PVS.

With developmental abnormalities (e.g., hydranencephaly) and chronic progressive degenerative and subacute and chronic infectious disorders (discussed previously), there is no hope of meaningful recovery when PVS is reached. Establishing

the prognosis in the acute brain disorder category is the most difficult because the outcome is often not as clear in the early phase of the illness. Consulting the literature for guidance is problematic because (i) most studies are retrospective and therefore biased; (ii) in some studies, outcome measures in some patients are often not clearly defined (e.g., "poor outcome" refers to PVS as well as patients with various degrees of disability who are not vegetative); and (iii) the effect of perceived prognosis on quality of care (i.e., the care is less vigorous in patients who are perceived to have a poor outcome).

ESTABLISHING THE PROGNOSIS CLINICALLY

With trauma in either adults or children, recovery of consciousness after 6 months is unusual but does occasionally occur. In contrast, recovery of consciousness after nontraumatic PVS is uncommon (15% of adults and 13% of children) and rare after 3 months in both adults and children. This led the American Academy of Neurology to issue the following diagnostic standards for a permanent vegetative state:

1. PVS can be judged to be permanent after traumatic injury in adults and children. Special attention to signs of awareness should be devoted to children during the first year after traumatic injury.
2. PVS can be judged to be permanent for nontraumatic injury in adults and children after 3 months.
3. The chance for recovery after these periods is exceedingly low, and recovery is almost always to a severe disability.

A ROLE FOR INVESTIGATIVE/ CONFIRMATORY TESTS

EEG

EEGs have shown varied results because they are heavily dependent on the anatomical site of maximum damage. Since the EEG records only cerebral cortical synaptic activity, it is most helpful in cases in which the cortex is primarily affected. Thus, in severe anoxic–ischemic insult, the EEG shows suppression of various degrees. Complete suppression in such cases is associated with a PVS if the patient survives several weeks or more.

With white matter and thalamic lesions, EEG rhythms are better preserved. These show various degrees of slowing and reactivity as well as differences between wakefulness and sleep.

Evoked Potential Studies

Somatosensory evoked potentials are useful in the early assessment probability of death or PVS following all three anatomical types of insult. They are most reliable in the coma after anoxic–ischemic insult, where bilateral absence of N_{20} after median nerve stimulation (in the presence of intact earlier potentials such as N_{14}) is reliably predictive that PVS is permanent. They are also of considerable value in the post-trauma patient.

Neuroimaging

Standard neuroimaging is of value in PVS. Patients with PVS are more likely to have abnormal computed tomography or magnetic resonance imaging scans than those who recover. Predictive guidelines for PVS based on degrees of structural change have not been developed, but cases of large bihemispheric near total destruction, as in cases of hydranencephaly or complete bilateral middle cerebral artery territory infarctions, would be predictive of PVS.

Functional Imaging

The tests that have potential value in prognosis include PET and blood flow studies. PET studies of regional cerebral oxygen and glucose metabolism show widespread reduced metabolism in the cerebral cortex by at least 40% of normal or patients with locked-in syndrome. It is not certain whether this consistently reflects irreversible damage (e.g., could recovering multiple "penumbra" in cases of multiple infarcts show improvement?) or what extent this represents the metabolism of neuronal versus nonneuronal cells.

Cerebral blood flow (CBF) studies show variable patterns shortly after coma-producing insult. However, after PVS is established, there is a reduction in CBF. Hexamethylpropylamine oxime single photon emission tomography indicated similar results in at least one preliminary study.

—*G. Bryan Young*

See also–Akinetic Mutism; Awareness; Coma; Coma Scales; Consciousness; Diffuse Axonal Injury (DAI); Evoked Potentials (EPs); Sleep–Wake Cycle; Wakefulness

Further Reading

Kinney, H. C., and Samuels, M. A. (1994). Neuropathology of the persistent vegetative state. A review. *J. Neuropathol. Exp. Neurol.* **53**, 548–558.
Multi-Society Task Force on PVS (1994). Medical aspects of the persistent vegetative state. *N. Engl. J. Med.* **330**, 1499–1908.

Personality Types and Disorders

Encyclopedia of the Neurological Sciences
Copyright 2003, Elsevier Science (USA). All rights reserved.

THE CONCEPT of personality has a long history in psychological science; conceptualizations of personality and personality types date back at least to the ancient Greeks. One well-known example is the theory of humors (e.g., phlegm and bile) that posited an excess of the offending bodily substance as the explanation for the stable individual differences in emotional functioning, thinking style, interpersonal relationships, and other behavior patterns that characterize human functioning. Other classification systems, such as Jung's or William Sheldon's somatotypes (body types), have also been proposed, but none has been supported by empirical research.

A related conceptualization of personality type was offered by the Harvard psychologist Gordon Allport in 1937, who advocated understanding stable differences between individuals in terms of "cardinal traits." This is a salient characteristic that clearly describes "who" the person is. Examples of cardinal traits are the altruism of Mother Theresa and the sophistication of Jacqueline Kennedy Onassis. This approach is consistent with lay understanding, but it, too, has little scientific empirical support.

These typological or quasi-typological conceptualizations notwithstanding, current knowledge about normal personality functioning has simply not produced an agreed upon classification or personality typology, despite major advances in the study of personality. What is now agreed upon is that personality is a useful and predictive organizing concept for human functioning. The study of personality traits is valuable and has validity, and it is what comprises most of current personality research.

In this regard, personality can be defined as the enduring, relatively stable inner cognitive and emotional experience and outer behavioral and interpersonal activities that differentiate one person from another and are characteristic of the person across time and across situations or contexts. These features characterize both normal personality functioning and personality pathology.

NORMAL PERSONALITY

In the area of so-called "normal" personality functioning, there is wide agreement that there are five underlying constructs or dimensions that comprehensively cover the descriptive lexicon of personality traits. This set of dimensions captures the majority of the variability across people in temperament and behavior and is currently the dominant conceptualization in normal personality. These traits are openness, conscientiousness, extraversion, agreeableness, and neuroticism. The name of each dimension is a fairly accurate description of the nature of the hypothesized underlying construct.

PSYCHOPATHOLOGY

In the arena of psychopathology, there is considerably less agreement about whether an individual's disordered functioning in personality is best understood as very high or very low standing on a few or several of the panoply of traits that have different relative salience for each person or whether there is a more coherent organization that includes true types, categories, or taxa. The research evidence that is available does not particularly support the typological conjecture. Nonetheless, the current practice in the assessment and diagnosis of dysfunction in personality is a typological or categorical approach that gives rise to the terminology of personality disorders. In this respect, the personality disorders represent a disjunction with normal personality because the disorders are by definition categorical in nature.

The diagnostic nomenclature of both the World Health Organization [*International Statistical Classification of Diseases and Related Health Problems (ICD)*] and the American Psychiatric Association [*Diagnostic and Statistical Manual of Mental Disorders (DSM)*] include disorders of adult personality as categories of mental disorders. Personality disorder is defined in the *DSM-IV* as

an enduring pattern of inner experience and behavior that deviates markedly from the expectations of the individual's culture, is pervasive and inflexible, has an onset in adolescence or early adulthood, is stable over time, and leads to distress or impairment.

The *ICD-10* defines personality disorders as

deeply ingrained and enduring behavior patterns, manifesting as inflexible responses to a broad range of personal and social situations. They represent extreme or significant deviations from the way in which the average individual in a given culture perceives, thinks, feels, and, particularly, relates to others. Such behavior patterns tend to be stable and to encompass multiple domains of behavior and psychological functioning. They are frequently, but not always, associated with various degree's of subjective distress and problems of social performance.

Thus, the key features of a personality disorder are its pervasiveness across a wide array of areas of functioning, its stability over time, its onset relatively early in development, and its resultant compromise of functioning in social and occupational domains. There is considerable debate in the field about the etiology of personality disorders in terms of nature and/or nurture and their relationship to other psychiatric disorders (e.g., the relationship of schizoid and schizotypal personality disorder to schizophrenia). No consensus has emerged, although there are active programs of research into genetic factors as well as environmental and childhood experiences.

PREVALENCE

The personality disorders are much less well studied than other disorders, and therefore data about their prevalence are considerably less available than for the major psychiatric syndromes, such as major depression and schizophrenia. In a recent community sample study from Norway, the estimated prevalence of meeting criteria for at least one personality disorder was approximately 13%, with the rates in men and women not meaningfully different. Such disorders were most prevalent among those with a high school education and those who were single. The latter finding is not surprising because personality disorders exact a toll on interpersonal relationships.

In the *DSM-IV*, personality disorders are grouped on Axis II, reserved only for personality disorders, as opposed to the disorders on Axis I. There are 10 personality disorders grouped into three clusters, with a final diagnostic category, Not Otherwise Specified, for situations in which the specific criteria for any of the others are not met. Those with disorders in cluster A often seem odd or eccentric. Cluster A includes paranoid, schizoid, and schizotypal personality disorders. Those with disorders in the B cluster often appear dramatic, emotional, or erratic. Cluster B includes antisocial, borderline, histrionic, and narcissistic personality disorders. Those with disorders in cluster C often appear anxious or fearful. Cluster C includes avoidant, dependent, and obsessive–compulsive personality disorders (Table 1).

The *ICD-10* includes the same categories as the *DSM-IV* with mainly minor changes. Schizotypal disorder is listed with schizophrenia and is not part of the personality disorders. Antisocial personality disorder is termed dissocial personality disorder, borderline personality disorder is termed emotionally unstable personality disorder, obsessive–compulsive personality disorder is termed anankastic personality disorder, and narcissistic personality disorder is one among several under the category of other specific personality disorders: eccentric, haltlose type, immature, narcissistic, passive–aggressive, and psychoneurotic. There is little empirical evidence to choose between these somewhat arbitrary specific personality disorders.

For medical disorders for which the etiology is not known or is only suspected, specific signs and symptoms take on more diagnostic significance since it is not known whether a particular feature is definitory or just an accessory. Similarly, in the personality disorders, there has been a relatively complete abandonment of the connection between etiology and the definition of any particular personality disorder. Indeed, specifically in the *DSM-IV* nomenclature, the diagnostic criteria are purely

Table 1 DIAGNOSTIC CRITERIA: MAIN CHARACTERISTICS OF *DSM-IV* PERSONALITY DISORDERS

Disorder	Characteristics
Paranoid	Distrust and suspicion; interpretation of others' motives as malevolent
Schizoid	Detachment from others; restricted range of emotional expression
Schizotypal	Marked distress in close relationships; thinking or perceptual distortions; behavioral eccentricities
Antisocial	Disregard for and violation of the rights of others
Borderline	Instability in relationships; unstable self-image; impulsivity in actions; emotional dyscontrol
Histrionic	Attention seeking in an emotionally excessive manner
Narcissistic	Grandiosity; exploitation; need to be admired
Avoidant	Overly sensitive to criticism; feels inadequate; socially inhibited
Dependent	Excessive need to be cared for; submissive and clinging
Obsessive–compulsive	Preoccupied with control, perfection, and order

polythetic, meaning that there is no characteristic that everyone with a particular personality disorder must have. Instead, the diagnostic criteria require the presence of only several (exactly how many is specified for each disorder) of a larger subset of characteristics. Also, unlike for major depression, for example, for which everyone with this disorder must either have depressed mood or loss of interest in previously pleasurable activities, it is possible for two people with the same personality disorder diagnosis to overlap on only one characteristic and have three or four that are not shared in common.

These diagnostic decision rules provide for the possibility of considerable phenotypic diversity in those sharing a personality disorder diagnosis, although to the degree that individuals meet most or all of the criteria, this heterogeneity will be reduced. Currently, research on these issues is underdeveloped.

COMORBIDITY WITH OTHER PSYCHIATRIC DISORDERS

There is substantial comorbidity of the personality disorders with other Axis I psychiatric disorders, especially the mood and anxiety disorders. In one study, among those with a diagnosis of depressive disorder, personality disorder prevalence was as follows: avoidant, 31.6%; borderline, 30.8%; and obsessive–compulsive, 30.8%. Among those with bipolar disorder, the comparable data were as follows: obsessive–compulsive, 32.4%; borderline, 29.6%; and avoidant, 19.7%.

It is not uncommon for individuals who meet diagnostic criteria for one personality disorder (e.g., borderline) to also meet criteria for one or more other personality disorders (e.g., narcissistic and histrionic). This situation is a direct result of the decisions made in forming the nomenclature and is one of the arguments that some have advanced for considering personality psychopathology in terms of dimensions rather than categories.

TREATMENT CONSIDERATIONS

Evidence-based treatments for the personality disorders lag behind evidence-based treatments for other psychiatric disorders, such as depression or schizophrenia. Since the severity of disability and distress can vary widely both within and across personality disorder categories, treatment decisions will often be based on the key issues that the patient presents (e.g., suicidality or emptiness) as well as whether diagnostic criteria for an Axis I disorder are met. Such considerations will govern whether or not psychotropic medications (e.g., antidepressants or low-dose neuroleptics) are part of the treatment.

There are various forms of psychological therapies for personality disorders, including the more classic forms of psychoanalytic psychotherapy, couples or family therapy, group psychotherapy, and some forms of behavioral or cognitive behavioral therapy. Treatment of the personality disorders should be conceptualized more along the lines of treatment or management of a chronic disorder and less along the lines of remission or cure, which are more appropriate for Axis I disorders.

—*Daniel S. Weiss*

See also—Anxiety Disorders, Overview; Borderline Personality Disorder; Diagnostic and Statistical Manual of Mental Disorders (DSM-IV); Mood Disorders, Biology; Mood Disorders, Treatment; Obsessive–Compulsive Disorder; Paranoia

Further Reading

American Psychiatric Association (1994). *Diagnostic and Statistical Manual of Mental Disorders*, 4th ed. American Psychiatric Association, Washington, DC.

Cloninger, C. R. (2000). A practical way to diagnosis personality disorder: A proposal. *J. Pers. Disord.* 14, 99–108.

New, A. S., Gelernter, J., Goodman, M., *et al.* (2001). Suicide, impulsive aggression, and HTR1B genotype. *Biol. Psychiatry* 50, 62–65.

Rossi, A., Marinangeli, M. G., Butti, G., *et al.* (2001). Personality disorders in bipolar and depressive disorders. *J. Affect. Disord.* 65, 3–8.

Torgersen, S., Kringlen, E., and Cramer, V. (2001). The prevalence of personality disorders in a community sample. *Arch. Gen. Psychiatry* 58, 590–596.

Widiger, T. A., and Sanderson, C. J. (1997). Personality disorders. In *Psychiatry* (A. Tasman, J. Kay, and J. A. Lieberman, Eds.), pp. 1291–1317. Saunders, Philadelphia.

World Health Organization (1994). *ICD-10: International Statistical Classification of Diseases and Related Health Problems.* World Health Organization, Geneva.

Zanarini, M. C., Frankenburg, F. R., Reich, D. B., *et al.* (2000). Biparental failure in the childhood experiences of borderline patients. *J. Pers. Disord.* 14, 264–273.

Phakomatoses

see **Neurofibromatosis; Tuberous Sclerosis Complex; Von Hippel–Lindau Disease**

Phantom Limb and Stump Pain

Encyclopedia of the Neurological Sciences

MANY PATIENTS awake from the anesthetic after an amputation feeling certain that the operation has not been performed. They feel the lost limb so vividly that only when they reach out to touch it or peer under the bed sheets to see it do they realize it has been cut off. The startling realization does nothing to subdue the reality of the limb they experience. More than 125 years ago, Mitchell provided the first detailed description of this phenomenon and coined the term phantom limb to describe the persisting sensory awareness of a limb after amputation. The term so accurately captures the nature and subjective experience of the phenomenon that it has been used ever since.

STUMP PAIN

Pain in the amputation stump or residual limb is frequently confused with phantom limb pain, especially in amputations that have been performed below the elbow or knee. Stump pain is a normal consequence of amputation and subsides in the majority of patients by approximately 1 week after the operation. Stump pain that persists after the initial phase of healing usually is accompanied by peripheral pathology (e.g., circulatory problems, infection, bone spurs, and formation of neuromas), but it can also occur in the presence of a perfectly healed stump, in which case the problem may arise from activity in supraspinal structures. There is an approximately 20% frequency of stump pain 2 years after amputation.

PHANTOM LIMB PAIN

For many amputees, a distressing problem is phantom limb pain. Painful phantom experiences vary along a number of dimensions, including intensity, quality, location, frequency, and duration. Many amputees report a painful intensification (dysesthesias) of the common nonpainful paresthesias that occur after amputation. Some sufferers describe bouts of paroxysmal shooting pain that travels up and down the limb. Others report the phantom to be in a cramped or otherwise unnatural posture that gives rise to excruciating pain. Many amputees describe the pain in the phantom limb as indistinguishable from the pain they experienced in the limb before amputation. In still others, the phantom may be immobile or paralyzed so that attempts to move it generate pain. Finally, the phantom is often the seat of an intense burning pain, as if the hand or foot were held too close to an open flame. Frequently, amputees suffer from several types of pain. Phantom limb pain appears to be equally prevalent among men and women and is not related to side, level, age, or cause of amputation.

Surveys based on several thousand amputees reveal that 78–85% of patients continue to experience significant amounts of phantom limb pain more than 25 years after amputation. Results of prospective studies of the frequency of phantom limb pain are consistent with these estimates. Between 50 and 71% of amputees report phantom limb pain 2 years after amputation. There is a reduction in the frequency and duration of attacks over time. Equally striking is the low success rate of treatment for phantom limb pain: In the long term, only 7% of patients are helped by the more than 50 types of therapy used to treat phantom limb pain.

The different qualities of phantom limb pain, its high prevalence, and low treatment success rate highlight the complexity of the problem. This complexity is reflected in the suggestion that phantom limb pain is not a unitary syndrome with a single underlying casual mechanism. Rather, it is likely that there are multiple types of phantom limb pain, with each type subserved by one or more separate mechanisms. The development and severity of this disorder are determined by the interaction of multiple factors that vary both within and across individuals. These include past experience with pain and the immediate physiological, motivational, and psychological states of the individual.

PSYCHOGENIC EXPLANATIONS OF PHANTOM LIMB PAIN

Psychogenic explanations of phantom limb pain have been advanced as evidence of the amputee's difficulty in adapting to the mutilated state. Denial (of the loss or the associated affect) and repression are the most common defense mechanisms proposed to explain the presence of a painful phantom as well as various alterations in the form of the phantom limb. In addition to the role of specific defense mechanisms in the psychogenesis of phantom limb pain, it has been postulated that phantom limb pain may be psycho-

logically determined by characterological disturbances. Although often elegantly formulated, psychodynamic and other psychological explanations are not consistent with the physiological and psychological data. The foregoing does not imply that denial of the loss, affect, illness, or future implications plays no part in the overall adaptation to amputation. Patients may demonstrate their denial of the importance of these realities in a variety of ways, but these do not include having phantom limb pain. The presence of a phantom limb, whether painful or painless, is not a symptom of a psychological disorder.

PAIN MEMORIES IN PHANTOM LIMBS

A striking property of phantom limb pain is the presence of a pain that existed in a limb prior to its amputation. This class of phantom limb pain is characterized by the persistence or recurrence of a previous pain, has the same qualities of sensation, and is experienced in the same region of the limb as the preamputation pain. Case studies of amputees have revealed pain "memories" of painful diabetic foot ulcers, bedsores, gangrene, corns, blisters, ingrown toenails, cuts and deep tissue injuries, and damage to joints and bony structures. Also, the phantom limb may assume the same painful posture as that of the real limb prior to amputation, especially if the arm or leg had been immobilized for a prolonged period.

The proportion of amputees who report similar pain before and after amputation may be as high as 79%, although according to prospective studies, the frequency is approximately 10% 1 year after amputation. Pain also persists in patients with deafferentation that does not involve amputation. In these conditions, the involved body part is still present but it is devoid of sensibility due to an interruption in the supply of sensory (afferent) information. Brachial plexus avulsions, in which the sensory nerve roots supplying the arm and hand are torn from the spinal cord, often produce pain that is felt in the deafferented and anesthetic region. Similarly, patients with spinal cord injuries may complain of pain referred to body parts below the level of the transection.

Pain also persists or recurs after surgical removal or deafferentation of body structures other than the limbs, such as breasts, teeth, and internal and special sense organs. Ulcer pain has been reported to persist after subtotal gastrectomy with removal of the ulcer.

Patients have reported labor pain and menstrual cramps after total hysterectomy, rectal pain and hemorrhoids after removal of the rectum and anus, the burning pain of cystitis after complete removal of the bladder, and the pain of a severely ulcerated cornea after enucleation of an eye.

Taken together, these case reports and studies of amputees indicate that pain memories are not merely images or cognitive recollections; they are direct experiences of pain that resemble an earlier pain in location and quality. They are perceptually complex experiences that may even involve information from multiple sensory modalities, including visual, olfactory, tactile, and motor components that accompanied the original experience. The precise details of the experiences of pain involve localization, discrimination, affect, and evaluation (i.e., all the dimensions of perceptual experience), and these properties are a function of integrated brain activity. It is likely that the outputs of sensitized spinal cells activate the neural structures in the brain that subserve memories of earlier events.

SYMPATHETIC NERVOUS SYSTEM CONTRIBUTIONS TO PHANTOM LIMB PAIN

Another class of phantom limb pain may derive from involvement of the sympathetic nervous system, although its role in triggering or maintaining pathological pain has been a source of considerable confusion and debate. Sympathetic nervous system involvement in pain has been attributed to a cycle of sympathetic-efferent, somatic-afferent activity in which neural and/or vascular mechanisms participate. Pain is hypothesized to arise from sympathetically triggered ephaptic transmission, sympathetic activation of nociceptors, or low-threshold mechanoreceptors that terminate on sensitized spinal cord cells or from injury-induced alteration in the pattern of postganglionic cutaneous vasoconstrictor neurons that lose their normal thermoregulatory function leading to trophic changes and ischemia.

One mechanism that accounts for the dysesthetic component of the phantom limb pain is a cycle of sympathetic-efferent, somatic-afferent activity. Changes in the intensity of phantom limb paresthesias reflect the joint activity of cholinergic (sudomotor) and noradrenergic (vasomotor) postganglionic sympathetic fibers on primary afferents located in the stump and stump neuromas. Release of acetylcholine and norepinephrine from postganglionic sympathetic fibers produces transient vasoconstriction and heigh-

tened skin conductance responses. Also, neurotransmitter release onto apposing peripheral fibers trapped in stump neuromas increases primary afferent discharge. This information is transmitted rostrally, where it gives rise to referred phantom sensations upon reaching central structures subserving the amputated parts of the limb. The moment-to-moment fluctuations in the intensity of phantom limb pain reported by many amputees may, in part, reflect a cycle of sympathetic-efferent, somatic-afferent activity. Increases in the intensity of phantom limb paresthesias would follow bursts of sympathetic activity and decreases would correspond to periods of relative sympathetic inactivity. If central sensitization has also developed through prior injury, trauma during amputation, inflammation, or ectopia, or if the sympathetic sensory coupling involves nociceptors, the sensation may be one of dysesthesia.

PSYCHOLOGICAL AND EMOTIONAL PROCESSES INFLUENCE PHANTOM LIMB PAIN

Traditionally, the idea that emotional and psychological processes can cause pain has been tied to the notion of psychopathology. However, it is becoming increasingly clear that in certain circumstances pain may be triggered by these processes in psychologically healthy individuals as well. The aggravation or alleviation of pain referred to phantom body parts may be mediated in part by psychological processes that alter anxiety levels. Attacks of phantom limb pain are triggered by emotional distress as many as 7 years after amputation. A combination of progressive relaxation training and electromyography biofeedback of stump and forehead muscles results in significant reductions of phantom limb pain and anxiety that are sustained for up to 3 years.

The model schematically represented in Fig. 1 outlines a mechanism through which cognitive and affective processes associated with higher cortical and limbic centers may alter phantom limb sensations and pain. The reciprocal connections between cortical, limbic, and lateral hypothalamic structures are well documented. The lateral hypothalamus is involved in the control and integration of neural activity associated with affectively charged behavior and has direct projections to the lateral horn of the spinal cord. The intensity of phantom limb pain may thus be modulated by higher brain centers involved in cognitive and affective processes via a multisynaptic network of descending inputs that impinge

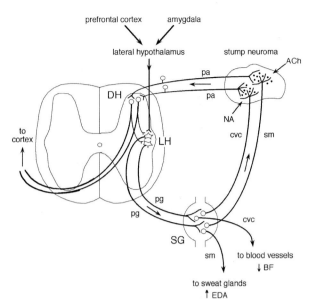

Figure 1

Schematic diagram illustrating a mechanism of sympathetically generated phantom limb paresthesias. Spontaneous sympathetic activity or excitatory inputs descending from cortex (e.g., due to the perception of a salient event, loud noise, thought, and feeling) increase the discharge rate of preganglionic (pg) sympathetic neurons with cell bodies in the lateral horn (LH) of the spinal cord and terminals in the sympathetic ganglion (SG). These neurons excite postganglionic noradrenergic (NA) cutaneous vasoconstrictor (cvc) and cholinergic (ACh) sudomotor (sm) fibers that impinge on effector organs (vascular smooth muscle and sweat glands) in the stump and on sprouts from large-diameter primary afferent (pa) fibers that have been trapped in a neuroma. The release of ACh and NA on effector organs results in increased electrodermal activity (EDA) and decreased blood flow (BF) to the stump. Release of these chemicals in the neuroma activates primary afferents that project to spinal cord dorsal horn (DH) cells subserving the amputated parts of the limb. These neurons, in turn, feed back to the preganglionic sympathetic neurons and project rostrally where the impulses contribute to the perception of phantom limb paresthesias. If DH cells have been sensitized due to injury, or nociceptive primary afferents are activated, then the perception may be one of dysesthesias (adapted with permission from Fields, 1987).

on preganglionic sympathetic neurons, producing diffuse peripheral autonomic discharge and activation of primary afferent fibers located in stump neuromas.

EFFORTS TO PREVENT PHANTOM LIMB PAIN

Traditional methods of postoperative analgesia do not provide adequate control of pain, in part because they focus on treating the patient only after the pain is well entrenched. Patients are ordinarily transported to the recovery room in considerable pain,

where they receive high doses of morphine in an attempt to bring the pain under control. The idea behind preemptive analgesia is to administer analgesics or local anesthetics before the start of surgery with the aim of reducing postoperative pain intensity and postoperative analgesic requirements. The idea is not simply that preemptive analgesia reduces pain during the procedure, although that in itself is a worthwhile goal. The hypothesis is that the transmission of noxious afferent input from the periphery (e.g., brought about by preamputation pain, incision and subsequent noxious intraoperative events, and postoperative noxious inputs from the amputation stump) to the spinal cord induces a prolonged state of central neural sensitization or hyperexcitability that amplifies subsequent input from the wound and leads to increased postoperative pain. By interrupting the transmission of noxious perioperative inputs to the spinal cord, a preemptive approach is hypothesized to prevent the establishment of central sensitization and to result in reduced pain and analgesic requirements after the analgesic effects of the (preemptive) agents have worn off.

Recent studies of patients undergoing lower limb amputation show that epidural anesthesia started before and continuing for the duration of surgery or for several days after amputation confers the most protection from long-term pain. The exception to this is a randomized, controlled trial evaluating the long-term effects on phantom limb and stump pain of continuous epidural morphine and bupivacaine administered 18 hr before, during, and for approximately 1 week after lower limb amputation. Discovering the relative contributions to long-term pain of factors such as preexisting pain, noxious perioperative events, and postoperative pain will enable us to design multiagent, preemptive treatments aimed specifically at minimizing the detrimental effects of these factors.

CONCLUSIONS

Phantom limb pain is not a unitary phenomenon but a frequently changing perceptual experience dependent on the current sensory input, emotional state, and past experience of the individual amputee. Phantom limb pains range from simple, diffuse sensations of dysesthesias to perceptually complex experiences of pains and lesions that originally were felt in the limb prior to amputation. Although phantom pains and other sensations are frequently triggered by the perception of salient events, thoughts, and feelings, there is no evidence that the painful or painless phantom limb is a symptom of a psychological disorder. The sympathetic nervous system may provide an important link between higher brain centers involved in cognitive and affective processes and phantom limb sensations through its peripheral actions on primary afferents located in stump neuromas.

—Joel Katz

See also–Mitchell, Silas Weir; Pain, Cancer and; Pain, Postoperative; Pain, Referred

Acknowledgments

This work was supported by an Investigator Award from the Canadian Institutes of Health Research (CIHR) and CIHR Grants MCT-38144 and MOP-37845.

Further Reading

Fields, H. L. (1987). *Pain*. McGraw-Hill, New York.
Jensen, T. S., and Nikolajsen, L. (1999). Phantom pain and other phenomena after amputation. In *Textbook of Pain* (P. D. Wall and R. Melzack, Eds.), 4th ed., pp. 799–814. Churchill Livingstone, Edinburgh, UK.
Katz, J. (1997). Phantom limb pain. *Lancet* **350**, 1338–1339.
Katz, J., and Gagliese, L. (1999). Phantom limb pain: A continuing puzzle. In *Psychosocial Factors in Pain: Critical Perspectives* (R. J. Gatchel and D. C. Turk, Eds.), pp. 284–300. Guilford, New York.
Katz, J., and Melzack, R. (1990). Pain "memories" in phantom limbs: Review and clinical observations. *Pain* **43**, 319–336.
Nikolajsen, L., Ilkjaer, S., Krøner, K., *et al.* (1997). Randomised trial of epidural bupivacaine and morphine in prevention of stump and phantom pain in lower-limb amputation. *Lancet* **350**, 1353–1357.
Sherman, R. A. (1989). Stump and phantom limb pain. *Neurol. Clin.* **7**, 249–264.

Phenylketonuria (PKU)

A DEFICIENCY in the activity of phenylalanine hydroxylase (PAH), a hepatic enzyme that converts phenylalanine to tyrosine, causes phenylketonuria (PKU). In patients with PKU, the biochemical block results in the accumulation of phenylalanine, which is converted to phenylketones that are excreted in the urine. PKU is treated by selective restriction of phenylalanine intake (and tyrosine supplementation) while providing enough additional protein and nutrients to support normal growth. Mandatory population newborn screening for PKU, in combination with postnatal presymptomatic therapy, was begun more than 40 years ago. The presymptomatic institution of specific dietary therapy prevents mental retardation. On the other hand, therapeutic success has been tempered by the unfortunate occurrence of congenital anomalies, secondary to the teratogenic effects of phenylalanine, in children born to mothers with PKU who are in poor dietary control.

Elevated blood phenylalanine levels may infrequently be caused by inherited disorders of the biosynthesis of tetrahydrobiopterin, a cofactor in the PAH reaction. The biopterin disorders are also briefly discussed in this entry.

CLINICAL FEATURES

Mental retardation (IQs often 50 or lower) is the most significant clinical finding in untreated or poorly treated PKU. Patients with PKU appear normal at birth and appear to have normal early development, even if untreated. Metabolic encephalopathy does not occur in PKU, but neurological manifestations of the disease appear insidiously and include changes in muscle tone, reduced rate of growth of head circumference, and failure of acquisition of milestones. Patients may present with lighter pigmentation than other family members (reduced melanin synthesis) and have a musty odor (phenylacetic acid). Eczema and decreased bone mineral density may occur. Patients exposed to chronically elevated phenylalanine levels ultimately develop microcephaly, seizures, athetosis, and spasticity, and they may be misdiagnosed as having cerebral palsy. Autistic behavior(s) and hyperactivity are common. Magnetic resonance imaging (MRI) of the brain may show dysmyelination, a finding that is potentially reversible with the initiation of dietary therapy. In the past, most untreated PKU patients were institutionalized.

As a rule, treated PKU patients have normal IQs; however, careful psychological testing has shown degrees of impairment in abstract reasoning and problem solving, even in well-treated individuals. Emotional disorders, as well as hyperactive behavior, are more frequently encountered in patients with PKU than in the general population.

Patients with PKU are classified into clinical subtypes on the basis of blood phenylalanine levels and phenylalanine tolerance. A blood phenylalanine level higher than the normal range (31–110 µM) is referred to as hyperphenylalaninemia. Patients are classified as having non-PKU hyperphenylalaninemia if their blood phenylalanine levels without dietary therapy are 360–600 µM, whereas classic PKU is characterized by untreated phenylalanine levels of >1200 µM. A range of reduced PAH specific activity correlates broadly with the severity of the phenotype. When it has been measured, residual liver PAH specific activity is relatively high in milder hyperphenylalaninemic patients, whereas enzyme activity is low, and often zero, in the more severe classic PKU. Classification of PKU into subtypes based on blood phenylalanine levels is arbitrary; some patients, referred to as having mild, variant, or atypical PKU, fall between the two extreme biochemical phenotypes.

BASIC DEFECT

PKU is an autosomal recessive disorder with a population prevalence of approximately 1/10,000 in Caucasians of northern European ancestry. The gene for PAH on chromosome 12q24.1 has been cloned, and more than 400 different mutations have been reported. Most patients are compound heterozygotes, carrying a different mutant allele on each chromosome. Prevalences of specific mutant alleles differ from population to population.

The precise etiology of the mental retardation in untreated PKU is not understood. Since cerebral protein synthesis is inhibited by excessive phenylalanine, it is possible that defective brain myelination may be related to decreased biosynthesis of myelin proteins. Central nervous system effects may be ascribed to more global amino acid imbalances. Elevated phenylalanine may affect the central nervous system concentrations of neutral amino acids by competitive inhibition of a shared amino acid transporter. Brain tyrosine deficiency, with resultant perturbations in brain neurochemistry, may also contribute to pathogenesis.

PKU and non-PKU hyperphenylalaninemia are single gene, autosomal recessive disorders caused by mutations in the PAH gene. However, the final biochemical phenotype (blood phenylalanine level and phenylalanine tolerance) and clinical phenotype (neurodevelopmental status) are not only dependent on the severity of the mutation(s) but also influenced by patient compliance and by the effects of modifying genetic factors. Such modifier genes may encode proteins mediating interindividual rates of protein synthesis (and phenylalanine utilization), synthesis and degradation of the PAH enzyme protein, hepatic uptake of circulating phenylalanine, metabolism of the tetrahydrobiopterin cofactor, and the rate of phenylalanine transported across the blood–brain barrier. PKU is an example of how a simple Mendelian disorder actually constitutes a complex multifactorial trait. Since patients, including sibling patients, with identical mutations can show divergent neurodevelopmental progress, mutation identification may not predict the severity of the disease with certainty in a given patient.

DIAGNOSIS

The Guthrie bacterial inhibition assay was a technical breakthrough, allowing newborn screening of large populations. Fluorometric assays or tandem-mass spectrometry (MS/MS) are methodologies currently being utilized in screening and monitoring. False positives may be seen in neonates with liver disease or in infants on parenteral alimentation. Confirmation of the diagnosis is made by analysis of blood phenylalanine concentration by high-performance liquid chromatography, fluorescent methods, or MS/MS. The phenylpyruvic acid present in urine causes the appearance of a deep green color when ferric chloride is added. This ferric chloride test is sometimes performed as part of a metabolic screen for the evaluation of patients suspected of having an inborn error of metabolism, but it should not be used to confirm a diagnosis of PKU. All patients with confirmed hyperphenylalaninemia must have further screening for tetrahydrobiopterin defects. Finally, PKU may be suspected in a child or adult, or it can reasonably be included in the differential diagnosis of a given patient of any age, presenting with neurodevelopmental delay of unknown etiology. In such settings, diagnostic testing for PKU must be done, even if there is a history or a record of a normal newborn screen.

TREATMENT

A diet low in phenylalanine is the basis of PKU therapy. If a neonate has an initial positive screen and a confirmation of an elevated blood phenylalanine level (more than 600 µM) is obtained, dietary restriction of phenylalanine is begun. If the low-phenylalanine diet is initiated in the neonatal period (between 7 and 14 days) and maintained throughout life, the underlying biochemical toxicity is ameliorated and mental retardation is prevented. The goal of dietary therapy is the maintenance of blood phenylalanine concentrations between 120 and 360 μM. (Normal phenylalanine levels are usually lower than 120 μM.) Significant restriction of dietary phenylalanine is required for treatment (intake limited to 200–500 mg of phenylalanine/day), but the exact level of daily phenylalanine intake will vary from patient to patient and will also vary with age in a given individual patient. Although severe mutations, in general, require a greater limitation of phenylalanine intake in order to maintain acceptable blood phenylalanine levels, individual variations of phenylalanine tolerance may occur, even in patients with identical genotypes. Therefore, the diet must be adjusted with care for each patient. The regimen must be initiated and overseen by experts in PKU at a specialized center, and referral of the patient to such a specialized center is mandatory.

In earlier therapeutic protocols, treatment was only continued through the first few years of life, theoretically corresponding to the age at which brain myelination is complete. As developmental data accumulated, it became evident that treatment throughout childhood and adolescence was the best course to preserve intelligence. In recent studies, it has been shown that brain abnormalities as demonstrated on MRI, and electrophysiological testing abnormalities referable to the central nervous system, are observed in adults who are on unrestricted phenylalanine intake. Accordingly, it is reasonable to continue treatment into adulthood, and most centers recommend treatment for life.

Patients who are diagnosed in the neonatal period and who adhere to the phenylalanine-restricted diet have normal overall intelligence. However, learning problems can occur in well-treated patients and include problems in spelling, reading, and mathematical skills. Patients may also be more prone to depression, anxiety, phobic tendencies, and isolation from their peers. Such potentially adverse and unpredictable manifestations should be brought to the attention of parents and carefully explained with care and support during the ongoing and long-term management process.

Somatic gene therapy experiments using retroviral vectors or DNA/protein complexes carrying a PAH transgene have targeted PAH-deficient hepatocytes and T lymphocytes from patients and mouse models *in vitro* with some success. However, theoretical restraints limit the use of these delivery systems *in vivo*. Adenoviral vectors have corrected the PAH deficiency in mouse models following direct intraportal injection, but the effect is short-lived. Newer vector systems are being explored, but gene therapy for PKU is still in an early phase.

A novel therapeutic approach employs the enzyme phenylalanine lyase (PAL). PAL converts phenylalalnine to *trans*-cinnamic acid, a harmless compound, and has been shown to reduce hyperphenylalaninemia in a PKU mouse model. Enteral PAL therapy has the theoretical potential to substantially increase dietary phenylalanine tolerance, but it has not been studied in humans.

Finally, a number of recent reports have documented the lowering of serum phenylalanine concentrations in response to oral administration of the naturally occurring cofactor tetrahydrobiopterin (BH_4). These patients have mutations in the PAH gene and not in one of the genes encoding enzymes involved in BH_4 biosynthetic. It has been suggested that the PAH mutations in such patients affect the structure of domains that are involved in the binding of BH_4 to the PAH enzyme. If these observations and hypotheses are borne out, it may be possible to define by mutation analysis a subset of patients who would predictably benefit from cofactor supplementation.

MATERNAL PKU SYNDROME

Elevated maternal blood phenylalanine levels can cross the placenta and cause fetal birth defects, including microcephaly, dysmorphic features, and congenital heart defects. More than 90% of children born to women with untreated classic PKU have mental retardation, with microcephaly being present in 70% of cases, intrauterine growth retardation in 40%, and congenital heart disease in 12%. The risk to the fetus is greatest with increasing maternal blood phenylalanine levels. The maternal PKU syndrome is especially tragic given that these children are typically heterozygous for the mutant PAH gene and would not be affected with PKU. For optimal physical and cognitive fetal outcomes, it is strongly recommend that dietary control be achieved before conception and that mothers with PKU be monitored carefully by an experienced center throughout pregnancy. Blood phenylalanine levels should be maintained between 120 and 360 μM.

BIOPTERIN DISORDERS

Neonatal hyperphenylalaninemia may rarely be the result of autosomal recessive defects in the synthesis or recycling of BH_4, an essential cofactor in the PAH reaction. Up to 1 or 2% of patients with hyperphenylalaninemia have a defect in one of the four enzymes responsible for maintaining BH_4 levels. Guanosine triphosphate cyclohydrolase I (GTPCH) and 6-pyruvoyl-tetrahydrobiopterin synthase (PTPS) are essential enzymes for BH_4 biosynthesis, whereas pterin-4α-carbinolamine dehydratase (PCD) and dihydropteridine reductase (DHPR) are responsible for BH_4 recycling. (An autosomal dominant form of GTPCH deficiency (dopa-responsive dystonia, Segawa disease, hereditary progressive dystonia) presents with dystonia but is not associated with elevated phenylalanine levels.) Because the tyrosine and tryptophan hydroxylases also require BH_4 for proper functioning, these disorders also result in deficiencies of the neurotransmitters L-dopa and 5-hydroxytryptophan (5-HTP). The hyperphenylalaninemia, in association with neurotransmitter deficits, causes the neurological manifestations associated with the defects in BH_4 synthesis and recycling.

All children with persistent hyperphenylalaninemia must be screened for biopterin disorders by measuring the levels of pterin metabolites (neopterin and biopterin). Patients with GTPCH deficiency have decreased urinary excretion of both neopterin and biopterin. In PTS deficiency, neopterin is increased and biopterin decreased, resulting in a greatly elevated neopterin:biopterin ratio. The neopterin:biopterin ratio in PCD deficiency is also increased but not to the same extent as in PTS deficiency. In PCD deficiency, the characteristic feature is the presence of primapterin (7-biopterin) in the urine. In DHPR deficiency the percentage of biopterin is elevated ($>80\%$ in most cases), and the measurement of DHPR activity in neonatal dried blood spots is employed for diagnosis. Urine pterin analysis and DHPR activity screening should be performed early in the management of a new patient with persistent hyperphenylalaninemia or these disorders may be missed.

Untreated patients typically develop neurological manifestations by 4 months, although symptoms can appear in the neonatal period. Clinical manifestations include progressive neurological deterioration, microcephaly, movement disorders, seizures, tone disturbances, oculogyric spasms, swallowing difficulties, hypersalivation, hyperthermia, and eczema. Transient forms of both PTPS and PCD deficiencies exist. Importantly, such symptoms can appear even if the blood phenylalanine level is maintained in the therapeutic range for classic PAH-deficiency PKU.

The goals of therapy are to decrease the level of phenylalanine to an acceptable range (120–360 μM) by dietary restriction and to correct the neurotransmitter deficiencies with exogenous supplementation. Accordingly, patients are given BH_4 supplementation, and L-dopa and 5-HTP are administered, in doses that are determined for each patient. Adjunctive agents (e.g., carbidopa and L-deprenyl), which reduce the catabolism of L-dopa and 5-HTP, may be added to the therapeutic protocol in order to enable the use of lower doses of these compounds. Measuring levels of cerebrospinal fluid neurotransmitter metabolites (homovanillic acid and 5-hydroxyindolacetic acid) is useful in monitoring the efficacy of treatment.

Side effects of therapy include choreoathetosis and dystonia, which are also features of the underlying disorders. Tachycardia, diarrhea, and anorexia are associated with 5-HTP administration. Low cerebrospinal fluid folate concentration is typically present in DHPR deficiency and is treated by folinic acid supplementation. Neurological function may improve with therapy, but the overall prognosis for these disorders is largely unknown. There are mild forms of DHPR, PTPS, and PCD deficiencies, and some forms of PTPS and PCD deficiencies may be transient.

—*Seymour Packman*

See also–Mental Retardation

Further Reading

Blau, N., Thöny, B., Cotton, R. G. H., *et al.* (2001). Disorders of tetrahydrobiopterin and related biogenic amines. In *The Metabolic and Molecular Bases of Inherited Disease* (C. R. Scriver, A. L. Beaudet, W. S. Sly, and D. Valle, Eds.), 8th ed., pp. 1725–1778. McGraw-Hill, New York.

Centerwall, S., and Centerwall, W. (2000). The discovery of phenylketonuria: The story of a young couple, two retarded children, and a scientist. *Pediatrics* **105**, 89–103.

Enns, G. M., Martinez, D. R., Kuzmin, A. I., *et al.* (1999). Molecular correlations in phenylketonuria: Mutation patterns and corresponding biochemical and clinical phenotypes in a heterogeneous California population. *Pediatr. Res.* **46**, 594–602.

Kayaalp, E., Treacy, E., Waters, P., *et al.* (1997). Human phenylalanine hydroxylase mutations and hyperphenylalaninemia phenotypes: A meta-analysis of genotype–phenotype correlations. *Am. J. Hum. Genet.* **61**, 1309–1317.

Scriver, C. R., and Kaufman, S. (2001). Hyperphenylalaninemia: Phenylalanine hydroxylase deficiency. In *The Metabolic and Molecular Bases of Inherited Disease* (C. R. Scriver, A. L. Beaudet, W. S. Sly, and D. Valle D, Eds.), 8th ed., pp. 1667–1724. McGraw-Hill, New York.

Phobias

Encyclopedia of the Neurological Sciences
Copyright 2003, Elsevier Science (USA). All rights reserved.

PHOBIAS are very common psychiatric disorders in the anxiety spectrum and are sometimes confused with fear. An example of the difference is that fear of flying can interfere with enjoyment of travel, but a true airplane phobia causes an inability to travel by airplane. Similarly, social phobia, also called social anxiety disorder, is more than just shyness. The functional impairment associated with social phobia is so severe that it leads to dropping out of school or the complete inability to apply for a job.

SPECIFIC PHOBIA

Specific phobias affect between 5 and 10% of the population. The object of the phobia can be animate or inanimate objects or specific situations. The essence of specific phobia is that whenever people come into contact with the intensely feared object or situation, or even suspect that they might, they must either flee from it or tolerate it with severe anxiety. Such ongoing monitoring or vigilance, and the concurrent avoidance, cause phobias to be extremely disabling. Everyday life can be a minefield of potential horrors. Fear, on the other hand, is not associated with such an intense reaction. A feared object can be confronted without a high degree of functional impairment.

The most common phobia is of illness or injury, such as blood phobia, whereas the most frequent intense fear is of snakes. There are wide gender differences among the specific phobias, with fear of storms, for example, occurring almost entirely among women and agoraphobia occurring approximately equally between men and women. Age of onset varies widely among the phobias. Most phobias typically begin in early childhood; for example, blood phobia usually starts at approximately age 7 years. The age of onset for agoraphobia and claustrophobia ranges from the late teens to the early twenties.

Agoraphobia and claustrophobia are linked in other ways. In agoraphobia, there is severe anxiety about being in places or situations from which escape would be difficult or extremely embarrassing or in which help would not be available in the event that the person has a panic attack or symptoms. In claustrophobia there is severe fear of closed spaces, with similar intense worry about lack of help or escape.

Panic disorder, agoraphobia, and claustrophobia all have similar ages of onset, with frequent comorbidity.

SOCIAL PHOBIA

Social phobia has become more widely recognized, in large part due to advertising of medication remedies. Social phobia affects approximately 3% of the population. Those with social phobia tend to think that their extreme shyness is "part of their personality" and do not typically seek psychiatric treatment. More than half of those with social phobia develop major depression, and many present for treatment at that point.

The central diagnostic feature of social phobia is severe fear of acting in such a way to cause embarrassment or humiliation in a wide array of normal social situations. Panic attacks can occur in anticipation of these situations. Avoidance of these situations becomes disabling since they can include attending classes, speaking to people in any level of authority, going to a restaurant, or using public phones and restrooms. In its most severe form, social phobia can generalize to all social situations, causing a complete inability to leave home.

There is debate over whether avoidant personality disorder and social phobia are essentially the same since both share many characteristics. Personality disorders, by definition, must begin in adolescence or early adulthood and represent a pattern of illness that affects patients in most aspects of their lives. Avoidant personality disorder may be more of a trait-like condition and social phobia a more treatable state.

TREATMENT

Most treatments for phobia, whether specific or social, involve behavioral therapy. The most common therapy employed is desensitization, in which the patient is exposed to the feared stimulus. Progressive desensitization involves gradual exposure and can also be "covert," where the patient imagines exposure to the stimulus. The most extreme form, flooding, involves suddenly placing the patient in the most feared situation.

Pharmacotherapy is also useful. Beta-blockers such as propranolol can reduce the physical manifestations of anxiety, such as sweating and tremulousness. Medications that increase brain serotonin, such as the MAO inhibitors and serotonin reuptake inhibitors, have proven effective for the treatment of social phobia. In general, benzodiazepines such as diazepam are recommended only for the occasional treatment of phobic anxiety not only because they are potentially addicting but also because they are so effective that they can impair the progress of behavioral therapy. Ironically, patients need to experience an uncomfortable degree of anxiety in order to appreciate that their reaction to a feared stimulus has been reduced.

CONCLUSION

Specific phobia and social phobia share a common characteristic: profoundly disturbing anxiety reactions when patients are presented with objects or situations of which they have developed an intense, disabling fear. Fortunately, through proven therapeutic methods, patients can learn to master their fears in ways that can be as satisfying as their old fears were demoralizing.

—*Mark H. Townsend*

***See also*–Antianxiety Pharmacology; Anxiety Disorders, Overview; Freudian Psychology; Hysteria; Obsessive–Compulsive Disorder; Panic Disorder; Paranoia; Personality Types and Disorders**

Further Reading

Agras, W. S., and Jacob, R. G. (1981). Phobia: Nature and measurement. In *Phobia: Psychological and Pharmological Treatment* (M. Mavissakalian and D. H. Barlow, Eds.). Guilford, New York.

Barlow, D. H. (1988). Simple phobia. In *Anxiety and Its Disorders: The Nature and Treatment of Anxiety and Panic* (D. H. Barlow, Ed.). Guilford, New York.

Cox, B. J., and Taylor, S. (1999). Anxiety disorders: Panic and phobias. In *Oxford Textbook of Psychophatology: Oxford Texbooks in Clinical Psychology* (T. Million and P. H. Blaney, Eds.), Vol. 4. Oxford Univ. Press, New York.

Emmelkamp, P. M. G., and Van Oppen, P. (2001). Anxiety disorders. In *Advanced Abnormal Psychology* (M. Hersen and V. B. Van Hasselt, Eds.). Kluwer/Plenum, New York.

Rettew, D. C. (2000). Avoidant personality disorder, generalized social phobia, and shyness: Putting the personality back into personality disorders. *Harvard Rev. Psychiatry* **6**, 283–297.

Phonology

Encyclopedia of the Neurological Sciences
Copyright 2003, Elsevier Science (USA). All rights reserved.

LANGUAGE is a complex and intricate system within the brain and relies on other systems to complete the process of communication, such as the motor speech system. Speech production is an important part of language and communication processes. A study of the spoken language system is called phonology. The sounds placed together or the systematic organization of selected speech sounds to form vocalized words in individual languages is part of phonology.

Three distinct phonological processes have an affect on sound production. One is the set of sounds used in a language. An example is the tonal production of words in Chinese. The tone of similar-sounding words gives each word its different meaning. Another process is the arrangement of sounds to produce distinct and understandable words. The third process that affects sound production is that of sound addition and deletion.

Within the phonological processes there are physical elements. The "articulatory" organs, which are attributed to sound production, comprise the tongue, lips, palate, and teeth. These articulatory organs are controlled by the pyramidal tract, the nervous system pathway that controls voluntary muscle movements. The physical elements are further broken down into two categories for which these processes are responsible. The resonance and articulation of sounds involve the hard palate and teeth. For example, a missing tooth can cause a person to have trouble with pronunciation because they lack the sharpness in sound production with the /s/ and /z/. The soft palate, lips, and tongue are responsible for phonetic components such as the pronouncing of vowels, consonant, and the consonant–vowel syllables. Each vowel is produced based on the positioning of the tongue and the shape of the lips. Consonants are produced with the help of the levator veli palatani muscle, which controls the soft palate, and the narrowing of the vocal tract. These organs are important to the phonological process of speech. Also, the size of the articulatory organs plays a role in one's ability to make precise speech articulation.

DISORDERS

A type of disorder that interferes with phonological processes is called dysarthria. It is a motor problem but more specifically a neurological disorder of speech (articulation) caused by damage to the motor cortex (located in the frontal lobe) or the cranial nerves. Not only can dysarthria be caused by lesions to the upper motor neurons but also any weakness or malfunctioning to any structures related to speech production can be caused by a series of lesions that occur at different levels in the nervous system: to the upper motor neurons bilaterally at any level, from the cortex to the nuclei of the cranial nerves; to the extrapyramidal system; to the cerebellum; and to the lower motor neurons. Dysarthria is defined as any disturbance of articulation or speech, but a more refined definition is needed to distinguish it from other speech disorder such as speech apraxia. In a more narrow definition, dysarthria is a motor speech disturbance of phonation, articulation, and resonance due to the abnormal neuromusculature actions that change the speed, strength, range, timing, or accuracy of the speech output. The symptoms of dysarthria are slurred speech or paralysis of the speech musculature.

There are many types of dysarthria, depending on the affected structure. One subtype of dysarthria is paralytic dysarthria, categorized by paralysis of the lower motor neurons of the cranial nerves. An example is paralysis of the hypoglossal nerve that controls the articulatory movements resulting in the impairment of movements of the tongue. The inability to move the tongue results in loss of controlled speech. There are other types of disorders of the tongue that prevent precise phonological output, such as Beckwith–Wiedeman syndrome, which also causes difficulty in producing precise articulation or speech. A feature associated with Beckwith–Wiedeman syndrome is macroglossia (enlargement of the tongue). This enlargement prevents the patient from placing their tongue within the oral space either when resting or when speaking, thus preventing the tongue from functioning properly during speech. Macroglossia can be resolved through surgical reduction and with the help of a speech pathologist.

A lesion of the upper motor neuron in the motor cortex or in the fiber tracts that originate from the motor cortex causes another type of dysarthria called spastic dysarthria. This type of dysarthria is characterized by inaccurate speech production of consonants, monopitch, and reduced stress speech. A weak voice in spastic dysarthric is due to excessive muscle tone.

A cerebellar lesion produces a type of dysarthria called ataxic dysarthria. The symptoms of ataxic dysarthria are the incoordination of speech due to reduced muscle tone, thus causing slowness, and inaccuracy in timing, range, force, and direction of speech actions. Therefore, it is unlike spastic dysarthria, in which there is weak speech production, but there is more uncoordinated speech in ataxic dysarthria.

A lesion in the basal ganglia causes hypokinetic dysarthria. This subtype of dysarthria is caused by rigidity and/or reduced range of movements. One of the prominent symptoms of hypokinetic dysarthria is the "inappropriate silences" caused by trouble initiating movements. In addition to the symptoms mentioned previously, dysphonia (involuntary contractions of the laryngeal muscles) can also be associated with dysarthria. An early sign of hypokinetic dysarthria is breathiness and reduction in loudness. In particular, there are three forms of dysphonia—adductor, abductor, and mixed—that have either a neurogenic (a neurological lesion) or psychogenic (psychological stress) cause. The adductor type is a more common spasmodic dysphonia and is differentiated by a strained, tight, and strangled voice. The abductor type generates a breathy voice, which can be found in some hypokinetic dysarthria. The mixed type of dysphonia produces intermittent strained and breathy qualities.

CONCLUSION

The study of phonology provides a better understanding of the correlation between the motor cortex, cranial nerves, and the articulatory organs. The motor cortex is the control center for speech production, and if there is an insult to this area then controlled speech production will be difficult to retain. This also holds for the cranial nerves, which provide the connection from the motor cortex to the articulatory organs. If speech disorder is the result of a damaged articulatory system, then controlled speech production may be restored to a certain degree.

Tests have been developed to help diagnose probable speech disorder and locate problematic areas of speech production. Neurologists use these tests to diagnose speech disorders such as dysarthria in patients with dementia. Phonology is one of the more concrete areas of language and language problems.

—La Phengrasamy and Bruce Miller

See also–Apraxia; Communication, Nonhuman; Language and Discourse; Language Disorders, Overview; Language, Overview; Memory, Semantic; Reading and Acquired Dyslexia; Speech Disorders, Overview

Further Reading

Bentin, S. (1989). Electrophysiological studies of visual word perception, lexical organization, and semantic processing: A tutorial review. *Lang. Speech* **32**, 205–220.

Bernthal, J. E., and Bankson, N. W. (1988). *Articulation and Phonological Disorders*. Prentice-Hall, Englewood Cliffs, NJ.

Bosman, A. M., van Leerdam, M., and de Gelder, B. (2000). The/ O/in OVER is different from the/O/in OTTER: Phonological effects in children with and without dyslexia. *Dev. Psychol.* **36**, 817–825.

Duffy, J. R. (1995). *Motor Speech Disorders: Substrates, Differential Diagnosis, and Management*. Mosby, St. Louis.

Fiez, J. A. (1997). Phonology, semantics, and the role of the left inferior prefrontal cortex. *Hum. Brain Mapping* **5**, 79–83.

Fiez, J. A., and Raichle, M. E. (1997). Linguistic processing. *Int. Rev. Neurobiol.* **41**, 233–254.

Grunwell, P. (1987). *Clinical Phonology*. Williams & Wilkins, Baltimore.

Honjo, I. (1999). *Language Viewed from the Brain*. Karger, New York.

Jenkins, L. (2000). *Biolinguistics*. Cambridge Univ. Press, New York.

Moller, K. T. (1994). Dental-occlusal and other conditions and speech. In *Child Phonology: Characteristics, Assessment, and Intervention with Special Populations* (J. E. Bernthal and N. W. Bankson, Eds.), pp. 3–28. Thieme, New York.

Muma, J. R. (1978). *Language Handbook*. Prentice-Hall, Englewood Cliffs, NJ.

Phosphofructokinase Deficiency
see Glycogen Storage Diseases

Phrenic Nerve

Encyclopedia of the Neurological Sciences
Copyright 2003, Elsevier Science (USA). All rights reserved.

THE WORD PHRENIC derives from the Greek word *phren*, meaning diaphragm or mind. Although phrenic had been used in the 19th century to mean "of or relating to the mind," this usage is now considered obsolete. This latter meaning is still preserved, however, in words such as phrenology (the theory of character and mental faculties based on the study of the shape and protuberances of the skull) and schizophrenia.

Each phrenic nerve provides motor innervation for its half of the diaphragm. The diaphragm is the principal inspiratory muscle and performs the main work of breathing.

ANATOMY AND FUNCTION

The phrenic nerve is derived from the motor neurons (in the anterior spinal cord segments) and corresponding nerve roots of C3–C5. As part of the cervical plexus (C1–C4), it leaves the roots proximally in the neck (before the C5 root joins the upper trunk of the brachial plexus). It travels medially and then descends vertically over the anterior surface of the scalenus anterior muscle, posterolateral to the internal jugular vein. It continues into the superior mediastinum of the chest between the subclavian artery and vein, and it passes down the middle of the anterior mediastinum within the pericardial sac, anterior to the pleural cavity. Finally, it reaches the diaphragm and supplies it. The phrenic nerve also contains some sensory fibers from the mediastinal and diaphragmatic pleura, pericardium, diaphragmatic peritoneum, and serosa of the liver, gall bladder, and pancreas.

The diaphragm (formed by the left and right hemidiaphragm) separates the thoracic cavity from the abdominal cavity. Voluntary contraction of the diaphragm causes it to draw down, resulting in a vacuum in the thoracic cavity. This causes inspiration and inflation of the lungs with air. Other respiratory muscles of inspiration include the external intercostals, scalenes, sternocleidomastoid, and trapezius.

CAUSES OF PHRENIC NERVE DYSFUNCTION

Neck

Various injuries to the cervical motor neurons, roots, and actual phrenic nerve can occur within the narrow confines of the neck. Traumatic wounds and traction injuries can occur during motor vehicle accidents. Congenital brachial plexus (Erb's) palsy of newborns can be associated with phrenic nerve palsy, especially when the nerve is primarily supplied by the C5 root. Variable trauma, where phrenic nerve damage is usually temporary and asymptomatic, can occur during hospital procedures. These entities include central venous catheterization of the internal jugular or subclavian vein, prolonged infusion with an indwelling central venous catheter (e.g., Hickman line), and regional anesthetic block of the adjacent brachial plexus. Metastatic cancer can infiltrate the phrenic nerve in the neck; this can also involve the sympathetic chain (causing ipsilateral Horner's syndrome) and the recurrent laryngeal nerve (causing ipsilateral vocal cord paralysis).

Chest

Phrenic nerve dysfunction is well documented as a complication of open-heart surgery (e.g., coronary bypass and valve replacement). The cause is probably a combination of nerve hypothermia due to topical cooling with iced slush of the pericardial sac, nerve stretch by sternal retractors, and prolonged pericardial stretch. Injury to the phrenic nerve may be increased when the internal mammary artery is harvested for use in coronary artery bypass. This artery is closely associated with the phrenic nerve as the latter enters the chest, and the harvesting procedure can result in direct nerve contusion or electrocoagulation injury. Phrenic nerve palsy is considered a relatively minor cause of the frequent postoperative pulmonary complications that occur with cardiac surgery; approximately 10% or less of open-heart surgical cases have apparent phrenic nerve dysfunction. It may involve only the left phrenic nerve (closer to the pericardium), and it completely resolves in almost all cases. Other causes of phrenic nerve injury usually accompany chest disease or its treatment. These entities include mediastinal tumors (bronchial carcinoma, lymphoma, and thymoma) and masses (substernal thyroid and aortic aneurysm), tuberculosis (with mediastinal fibrosis), sarcoidosis (with granulomas and lymphadenopathy), chest surgery (pericardiectomy, removal of mediastinal masses, repair of tracheoesophageal fistula, and intercostal drainage), and chest radiation for tumor.

Neuromuscular Diseases

Motor neuron diseases can cause bilateral phrenic nerve dysfunction by destruction of the C3–C5 anterior horn cells. The most devastating and rapid of these diseases is amyotrophic lateral sclerosis (ALS; Lou Gehrig's disease), in which severe phrenic nerve degeneration, and hence respiratory failure, is the usual cause of death. Less common motor neuron diseases that can affect the phrenic nerve include progressive muscular atrophy, infantile and juvenile spinal muscular atrophy, and Kennedy's disease (spinal–bulbar muscular atrophy). Certain infections can also damage anterior horn cells. Poliomyelitis, although uncommon today, was a major source of prolonged respiratory failure in the first half of the 20th century. Herpes zoster with cervical motor neuron or root involvement is usually unilateral and asymptomatic.

Neuropathies frequently affect the phrenic nerves. The most common entity with serious disruption of phrenic nerve function is Guillain–Barré syndrome, an acute inflammatory polyneuropathy that can be either demyelinating in type or the less common but more devastating axonal loss type. Other demyelinating neuropathies (chronic inflammatory demyelinating polyneuropathy, multifocal motor neuropathy with conduction block, and Charcot–Marie–Tooth disease) are rare causes of associated phrenic nerve damage. Axonal neuropathies, which constitute most of the common metabolic and toxic entities, occasionally involve the phrenic nerve; these include neuropathies due to diabetes mellitus and sarcoid. Recently, a polyneuropathy has been recognized that is limited to chronically sick patients in the intensive care unit—this is the so-called critical care neuropathy, which can damage the phrenic nerve and cause prolonged ventilator dependence. Brachial plexus neuropathy (neuralgic amyotrophy or Parsonage–Turner syndrome), although usually causing unilateral arm weakness, rarely can involve the unilateral phrenic nerve. Finally, an entity called idiopathic phrenic neuropathy can occur, but it is probably a variant of brachial plexus neuropathy.

EVALUATION OF PHRENIC NEUROPATHY

Symptoms depend on whether phrenic nerve dysfunction is unilateral or bilateral. Unilateral paralysis is often asymptomatic but may cause dyspnea on exertion or with underlying pulmonary disease. Bilateral paralysis causes dyspnea (worse in the supine position) and, later, symptoms of hypercarbia (morning headaches, insomnia, and excessive daytime somnolence). This may be followed by hypoxia and respiratory failure, with prolonged ventilator dependence. Phrenic nerve dysfunction can be the cause of unexplained failure to wean a patient from the ventilator.

The following signs suggest phrenic nerve involvement (either unilateral or bilateral): decreased or absent diaphragmatic excursions, dullness to lower chest percussion, and use of accessory muscles of respiration with "paradoxical" abdominal breathing (i.e., inward movement of the abdominal wall during inspiration). Occasionally, severe chronic unilateral phrenic nerve damage (usually seen in the pediatric population) can result in acquired diaphragmatic eventration, in which the paralyzed hemidiaphragm elevates into the chest cavity, bringing with it intraabdominal viscera. The physician must consider nonpulmonary symptoms and signs associated with the various causes of phrenic nerve dysfunction (e.g., various neuromuscular diseases and C3–C4 nerve root injury).

Tests and Procedures

The chest x-ray, usually with fluoroscopy, is evaluated for raised hemidiaphragm and lack of movement. Atelectasis and infiltrates in the lung may occur but are not specific for phrenic nerve palsy. Chest fluoroscopy (accompanied by the sniff test) may show reduced excursion or paradoxical motion of the hemidiaphragm. Real-time sonography of each hemidiaphragm has been used to serially follow diaphragm excursion. Routine pulmonary function tests will show a restrictive pattern, whereas maximum inspiratory (and transdiaphragmatic) pressures are reduced. Pulse oximetry and arterial blood gases show hypoxemia and respiratory acidosis.

Nerve conduction study (NCS) of the phrenic nerve is often used in cases of respiratory failure to evaluate for slowing or blocking of impulse conduction and to measure the size of the diaphragmatic response. The most common NCS technique is to stimulate the phrenic nerve percutaneously in the posterior cervical triangle of the neck and to record over the area of the diaphragm (with surface electrodes on the anterior axillary line near the costal margin and on the sternum). Needle electromyography (EMG) of the diaphragm via the anterior chest wall may show diaphragmatic denervation or decreased motor unit recruitment. Repetitive nerve stimulation of the phrenic nerve is performed to check for neuromuscular junction defect (e.g., myasthenia gravis). When neuromuscular disease is suspected as the cause of phrenic nerve dysfunction, a complete NCS/EMG/repetitive stimulation study (including limb, bulbar, and chest muscles) should be performed by an experienced electromyographer. Newer and less commonly used tests include transcortical or cervical magnetic stimulation (recording diaphragmatic muscle action potential or transdiaphragmatic pressure) and somatosensory evoked potentials of the phrenic nerve; both have been used to evaluate impaired central respiratory drive.

Differential Diagnosis

Dyspnea due to diaphragmatic weakness can be caused by primary muscle disease rather than dysfunction of the phrenic nerve that innervates that muscle; such myopathies include the muscular dystrophies, some congenital myopathies, and polymyositis. Following open-heart surgery, atelectasis and pneumonia of the left lower lobe are common but usually not due to phrenic nerve palsy. Entities to consider are lung trauma from surgical retraction (especially of the left lung), eventration of the diaphragm, infradiaphragmatic disease, chest pain with decreased ability to cough, and sedation.

TREATMENT OF PHRENIC NEUROPATHY

Most patients with unilateral paralysis do not require treatment and recover in several months; those with bilateral disease have a longer course. Regrowth and reinnervation of the phrenic nerve depend on the nature and severity of the lesion (i.e., the extent of nerve fiber disruption) and the location of the lesion. When the nerve is stretched (but not totally disrupted) in the neck, recovery of diaphragmatic function usually takes approximately 6 months. Lesions in the chest take less time to recover. Demyelinating nerve lesions can improve more quickly, often within days or a few weeks. NCS/EMG can be helpful in predicting prognosis of phrenic nerve palsy. Prognosis for recovery of phrenic nerve dysfunction in neuromuscular diseases is mainly dependent on the natural history and the proper treatment of the underlying disease.

Several surgical modifications have been described that attempt to avoid phrenic nerve injuries during open-heart surgery. Hypothermic nerve injury may be avoided by using cardiac insulation pads to isolate the phrenic nerve from the cooled pericardial sac. Many surgeons avoid harvesting the internal mammary artery; if this artery is harvested for coronary bypass, the phrenic nerve must be carefully identified during arterial dissection.

Phrenic nerve pacing is a specialized treatment of diaphragmatic paralysis due to a traumatic spinal cord lesion above the C3 cord level. Typically, the patient is apneic (with ventilator dependence) and quadriplegic. If pacing is to be successful, the entire phrenic nerve must be intact and viable, including the corresponding anterior horn cells of the spinal cord. Bilateral phrenic nerve stimulation is accomplished with the use of an external radiofrequency transmitter/antenna assembly that transmits electrical pulses to two small radio receivers implanted in the subcutaneous chest wall. Each receiver transmits the pulses to wire electrodes directly in contact with the phrenic nerves in the neck. The two sides of the diaphragm are stimulated alternately in a repetitive fashion, which results in rhythmic contractions (i.e., pacing) of the diaphragm and resultant electrophrenic respiration. Phrenic nerve pacing, when performed in the correct setting, can improve strength and endurance of the diaphragm. It can provide full-time or part-time electrophrenic respiration in patients previously ventilator dependent.

Recently, research has been undertaken on the use of a nerve transfer from one of the intercostal nerves to the phrenic nerve to treat patients with either a severely damaged phrenic nerve or a spinal cord injury with damage to anterior horn cells at the C3–C5 levels. In successful grafts, performed approximately 5 cm above the diaphragm, nerve regeneration occurs in approximately 9 months. The fused phrenic nerve can then stimulate the diaphragm (diaphragmatic reanimation), often with the help of an implanted phrenic nerve pacemaker. Diaphragmatic eventration due to phrenic nerve palsy can be treated by surgical plication of the redundant tissue of the paralyzed diaphragm. In cases of extensive brachial plexus injury, reconstruction has been aided by the transfer of the unilateral phrenic nerve to either the musculocutaneous nerve or the suprascapular nerve.

—Jerry M. Belsh

See also—Amyotrophic Lateral Sclerosis (ALS); Brachial Plexopathies; Nerve Conduction Studies; Nerve Roots; Thoracic Nerve, Long

Further Reading

Bolton, C. F. (1993). AAEM Minimomograph #40: Clinical neurophysiology of the respiratory system. *Muscle Nerve* 16, 809–818.

Krieger, L. M., and Krieger, A. (2000). The intercostal to phrenic nerve transfer: An effective means of reanimating the diaphragm in patients with high cervical spine injury. *Plast. Reconstr. Surg.* 105, 1255–1261.

Markand, O. M., Moorthy, S. S., Mahomed, Y., et al. (1985). Postoperative phrenic nerve palsy in patients with open-heart surgery. *Ann. Thorac. Surg.* 39, 68–73.

Stewart, J. D. (2000). *Focal Peripheral Neuropathies*, 3rd ed., pp. 85–88. Lippincott Williams & Wilkins, Philadelphia.

Physiological Brain Imaging

Encyclopedia of the Neurological Sciences
Copyright 2003, Elsevier Science (USA). All rights reserved.

PHYSIOLOGICAL brain imaging is the branch of neuroimaging that is concerned with measuring biological processes in the brain and their alteration in disease states. A similar term, functional brain imaging, is often used interchangeably. Alternatively, the term functional brain imaging is used synonymously with brain mapping. Physiological brain imaging is distinguished from structural brain imaging. Structural brain imaging provides information about the macroscopically visible structure of the brain and blood vessels as a substitute for direct visualization at surgery or autopsy. Angiography, X-ray computed tomography (CT), proton magnetic resonance imaging (MRI), and ultrasound all use the regional signal characteristics of the tissue to produce structural images. Because of the close correspondence of these images to visible changes in diseased tissue, structural brain imaging techniques are the cornerstone of clinical diagnostic neuroradiology. For structural brain imaging, the physical or chemical explanation for a relationship between the image and the visible structure is less important than the empirical demonstration that a reliable relationship exists.

Physiological brain imaging also utilizes images to obtain information. However, in this case, an understanding of the physical or chemical basis for the tissue signal that produces the image is essential since the goal is to use this signal to measure a physiological or biological process. This relationship between signal and biology can take many forms. Molecules labeled with radioactive atoms have been utilized extensively for many years to investigate physiology and pathology. These radioactive molecules are administered in such small quantities that they do not affect the physiological process under study (radiotracers), but the radioactivity is sufficient that it can be measured by an external detection system, such as positron emission tomography (PET) or single photon emission computed tomography (SPECT). For physiological imaging based on radiotracers, a mathematical model that quantitatively relates tissue concentration of radioactivity to the physiological variable under study is required. This model must take into account a variety of factors, including delivery of the radiotracer to the tissue, distribution and metabolism of the radiotracer within the tissue, egress of radiotracer and radioactive metabolites from the tissue, recirculation of radiotracer and radioactive metabolites, and the amount of radiotracer and radioactive metabolites remaining in the blood. Furthermore, the model must be practically applicable given the constraints imposed by PET and SPECT designs and the amount of radioactivity that can be safely administered to human subjects. Finally, the validity of the underlying assumptions and possible sources of error for each model when applied to the study of both normal physiology and disease states must be clearly understood. Ideally, such techniques should be validated by pairwise comparison to a gold standard under the conditions for which they will be used. Similar considerations apply to the use of nonradioactive agents used to assess cerebral hemodynamics with X-ray CT and proton MRI. An additional factor is that these agents are not administered in tracer quantities and experiments must be performed to determine that the agents do not disturb the biological process under study.

In the field of physiological imaging, measurement of cerebral blood flow (CBF) has received the greatest amount of attention. Techniques to measure whole brain CBF in humans were first developed in the late 1940s by Kety and Schmidt. Techniques for regional CBF measurements based on intracarotid arterial injection of radiotracers were developed by Ingvar and Lassen several decades later. These techniques have been largely superseded by PET and SPECT radiotracer methods. PET provides quantitatively accurate measurements of regional CBF in ml blood per 100 g brain per min. SPECT suffers from some limitations in its ability to accurately quantitate regional radioactivity *in vivo* and in the availability of suitable radiotracers for accurate CBF measurements. An X-ray CT method for measuring CBF using inhaled xenon gas in high doses provides reliable regional CBF data. Both X-ray CT and proton MRI methods for measuring CBF using intravascular contrast agents have been described. Most of these have been based on incorrect tracer kinetic models and do not produce accurate measurements. Recently, methodologically correct techniques have been introduced. Although conceptually straightforward, these have proven difficult to implement. Carotid and transcranial Doppler ultrasonography measure the frequency shift induced in an ultrasound pulse by red blood cells to determine the velocity of the blood flowing through a vessel. This Doppler shift is dependent on the angle between the ultrasound beam and the blood vessel, so it is best at demonstrating changes in velocity and not absolute values. The relationship between Doppler velocity and CBF is complex. It is dependent not only on the angle of insonation but also on the vessel diameter and the volume of tissue perfused by that vessel. Measurements of regional cerebral blood volume

using agents that remain intravascular can provide information about dilation and constriction of cerebral vessels. Both PET and SPECT radiotracers and proton MRI intravascular contrast agents are useful for this purpose.

Measurements of cerebral metabolism have proven to be more difficult than measurements of CBF. Kety and Schmidt combined arterial–jugular venous differences of oxygen and glucose with whole brain CBF measurements to yield measurements of whole brain oxygen and glucose consumption. Currently, measurements of regional cerebral oxygen and glucose metabolism are a unique capability of PET. SPECT lacks suitable radiotracers for this purpose. Proton MRI can produce a signal that is related to the amount of deoxy-hemoglobin [blood oxygen level dependent (BOLD)]. This signal provides information about the relative balance between CBF and cerebral oxygen consumption but has not proved to be useful for quantitative measurements of cerebral oxygen metabolism. Magnetic resonance spectroscopy (MRS) can provide quantitative measurements of different tissue constituents such as glucose and lactate.

Both PET and SPECT can be used with highly specific radiolabeled neuroreceptor ligands to study the neuropharmacology of disease *in vivo*. The most common applications of this approach has been the study of alterations in dopamine and serotonin receptors; however, within the constraints of practical consideration of chemical synthesis, the possibilities are almost limitless. Imaging of specific radioligands can be used for other purposes as well, such as assessment of cortical neuronal density with the central benzodiazepine receptor ligand ^{11}C-flumazenil.

Modern physiological brain imaging techniques have proven to be invaluable research tools for investigating human physiology and pathophysiology. Regional CBF increases when regional neuronal activity increases. Methods for measuring regional CBF have therefore made it possible to map the regional activation of brain structures during cognitive tasks and provide insight into higher brain function. The discovery that CBF increased in excess of cerebral oxygen metabolism during physiological brain activation provides the basis for the increasingly widespread use of the BOLD proton MRI signal for this purpose (Fig. 1).

Physiological imaging of human diseases has provided a means to study pathophysiology *in vivo*. The combination of hemodynamic and metabolic

882 PHYSIOLOGICAL BRAIN IMAGING

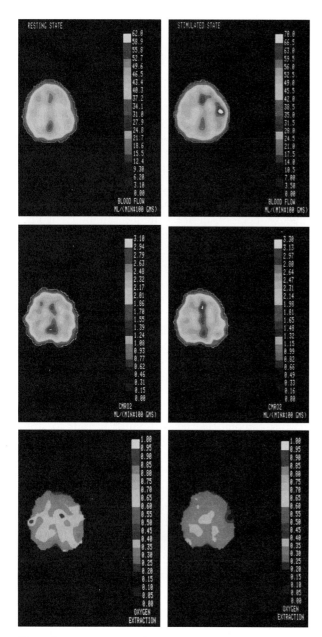

Figure 1
The effect of physiological brain stimulation on regional cerebral blood flow (CBF) and oxygen metabolism. All images are from the same subject. The left-hand column shows images of cerebral blood flow, cerebral oxygen metabolism ($CMRO_2$), and oxygen extraction fraction (OEF) obtained with the eyes closed. OEF is the fraction of the oxygen delivered to the brain (CBF × arterial oxygen content) that is metabolized. OEF is normally uniform throughout the resting brain, reflecting the close coupling of CBF and $CMRO_2$. The corresponding images in the right-hand column were obtained during vibrotactile stimulation of the left fingers. During stimulation, there is increased CBF in the contralateral sensori-motor cortex (upper right) but no increase in $CMRO_2$ (middle right). OEF is decreased (lower right), reflecting the fact the CBF has increased more than $CMRO_2$. This decrease in OEF results in increased oxygen content of venous blood which can be detected by BOLD MRI [reproduced with permission from Fox, P. T., and Raichle, M. E. (1986). *Proc. Natl. Acad. Sci. USA* 83, 1140–1144]. (See color plate section.)

measurements has proven especially valuable for understanding the changes that take place during physiological brain activation and during cerebral ischemia. Measurements of receptor ligands have proven especially useful in neurological and psychiatric diseases in which structural changes are minor or nonexistent. These are only a few of the examples of the importance of physiological brain imaging in modern neuroscience research.

The value of physiological brain imaging in the clinical care of patients with neurological disease has proven to be more elusive. Many of these techniques provide new information, the value of which will take time to demonstrate by properly designed and conducted studies. Others provide information, such as CBF measurements which would seem to be valuable in diagnosis and treatment of conditions such as ischemic stroke, yet has never been shown to reduce medical costs or improve patient outcome. Until such data are obtained, the role of physiological brain imaging in clinical care will remain undefined.

—*William J. Powers*

***See also*–Angiography; Cerebral Blood Flow, Measurement of; Computerized Axial Tomography (CAT); Magnetic Resonance Imaging (MRI); Neuroimaging, Overview; Positron Emission Tomography (PET); Single-Photon Emission Computed Tomography (SPECT); Ultrasound, Carotid; Ultrasound, Transcranial Doppler**

Further Reading

Calamante, F., Thomas, D. L., Pell, G. S., *et al.* (1999). Measuring cerebral blood flow using magnetic resonance techniques. *J. Cereb. Blood Flow Metab.* 19, 701–735.
Iacoboni, M., Baron, J.-C., Frackowiak, R. S. J., *et al.* (1999). Emission tomography contributions to clinical neurology. *Clin. Neurophys.* 110, 2–23.
Lee, C. C., Jack, C. R., Jr., and Riederer, S. J. (1996). Use of functional magnetic resonance imaging. *Neurosurg. Clin. North Am.* 7, 665–683.
Mullan, B. P., O'Connor, M. K., and Hung, J. C. (1996). Single photon emission computed tomography brain imaging. *Neurosurg. Clin. North Am.* 7, 617–651.
von Schulthess, G. K. (Ed.) (2000). *Clinical Positron Emission Tomography (PET).* Lippincott Williams & Wilkins, Philadelphia.
Wagner, H. N., Jr., Szabo, Z., and Buchanan, J. W. (1995). *Principles of Nuclear Medicine.* Saunders, Philadelphia.
Watson, J. D. G. (1997). Images of the working brain: Understanding human brain function with positron emission tomography. *J. Neurosci. Methods* 74, 245–256.